GUIDE TO AMBULATORY SUPPLEMENTS

Ambulatory Supplements are provided for five [guidelines]. The Supplements outline additional considerations for perioperative ambulatory surgery centers or physician office-based surgery centers.

The *Amb* symbol in the text of a guideline indicates that there is additional information in an Ambulatory Supplement at the end of the document.

TRANSMISSIBLE INFECTIONS

Recommendation XI

Documentation should reflect activities related to infection prevention. *Amb*

Documentation is a professional medicolegal standard.¹⁶⁷ Documentation related to infection prevention is applicable at the systems level and the patient care level. At [...] basis for [...] mance, [...] exposure [...] mentation [...] clear co[...] between [...]

XI.a. E[...]

XI.b. A[...]

XI.b.1. [...]

- an explanation of how the incident occurred.

Some health care employers may be exempt from maintaining a sharps injury log. The requirement to establish and maintain a sharps injury log applies to any employer who is required to maintain a log of occupational injuries and illnesses under [...]

PATIENT AN[D WORKER SAFETY]

AMBULATORY SUPPLEMENT: TRANSMISSIBLE INFECTIONS

Recommendation III

Droplet precautions should be used throughout the perioperative environment (ie, preoperative, intraoperative, postoperative) when providing care to patients who are known or suspected to be infected with microorganisms that can be transmitted by large droplets.^A1

Amb The facility should screen individuals for infectious agents (eg, influenza, pertussis) transmitted by droplets.^A1 Identification of infected individuals before their admission to the ambulatory surgery center (ASC) may prevent infection transmission.^A1

Recommendation IV

Airborne precautions should be used when providing care to patients who are known or suspected to be infected with microorganisms that can be transmitted by the airborne route.

IV.h. Elective surgery should be postponed for patients who have suspected or confirmed [tuberculosis] TB until the patient is determined to be noninfectious. If surgery cannot be postponed, perioperative personnel should follow airborne precautions and consult with an infection preventionist.

Amb Personnel in an ASC that provides care to patients with confirmed or suspected TB should follow recommendation IV.

Amb Unless the facility has the capability of establishing a negative pressure room, patients with suspected or confirmed cases of TB should be transferred to or re-scheduled at a facility with a negative pressure room. A negative pressure airborne infection isolation room and a respiratory protection program are needed for airborne infection isolation. Airborne infection isolation is needed for any patient with suspected or confirmed active pulmonary TB.^A1-A3

Recommendation X

Perioperative personnel should receive initial and ongoing education and competency validation of their understanding of the principles of infection prevention and the performance of standard, contact, droplet, and airborne precautions for prevention of transmissible infections and [multidrug-resistant organisms] MDROs.

Amb An ASC that is certified by the Ce[nters for Medicare] care & Medicaid Services (CMS) m[ust designate a] staff member trained in infection prev[ention to lead] the facility's infection prevention progr[am.]

> **Interpretive Guidelines: §416.51(b)[(1)]**
> *The ASC must designate in writin[g a quali-]fied licensed health care professio[nal to] lead the facility's infection control program. The ASC must determine that the individual has had training in the principles and methods of infection control.*
>
> Interpretative Guidelines: §416.51(b)(1). In: Centers for Medicare & Medicaid Services. *State Operations Manual Appendix A—Survey Protocol, Regulations and Interpretive Guidelines for Hospitals.* Rev. 89; 2013.

Amb Ambulatory surgery center personnel, including
- medical personnel,
- nursing personnel,
- personnel responsible for on-site sterilization/high-level disinfection processes, and
- environmental services personn[el]

should receive infection prevention ed[ucation.]

Amb Infection prevention educati[on should be] conducted
- upon hire,
- annually, and
- periodically as needed.^A5

Recommendation XI

Documentation should reflect activities related to infection prevention.

Amb A CMS-certified facility's infection prevention program must document the process of consideration, selection, and implementation of a nationally recognized infection control guideline,^A4 such as the AORN *Perioperative Standards and [Recommended] Practices.*^A6

Amb Supporting documentation for th[e facility's] infection tracking and surveill[ance activities] should be maintained.^A5

Amb Infection prevention education rec[ords should be] maintained for all personnel.^A7

Recommendation XII

Policies and procedures for the prevention and control of transmissible infections and MDROs should be developed, reviewed periodically, revised as necessary, and readily available within the practice setting.

452 | 2015 Guidelines for Perioperative Practice
First published: January 2014. Copyright © 2015 AORN, Inc. All rights reserved.

Where applicable, the Ambulatory Supplements include text from the Centers for Medicare & Medicaid Services State Operations Manual. *This text appears within purple brackets.*

Relevant text from the guideline is repeated in the Supplement for easy reference and to give context to the ambulatory considerations.

The Amb *symbol in the Supplement indicates information specific to ambulatory settings.*

Copyright © 2015 AORN, Inc.

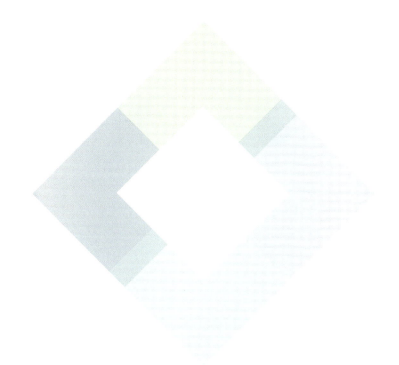

GUIDELINES
FOR PERIOPERATIVE PRACTICE
2015 EDITION

Association of periOperative Registered Nurses

Clinical Editor
Ramona Conner, MSN, RN, CNOR

Contributing Authors
Byron Burlingame, MS, BSN, RN, CNOR
Bonnie Denholm, MS, BSN, RN, CNOR
Terri Link, MPH, BSN, CNOR, CIC
Mary J. Ogg, MSN, RN, CNOR
Lisa Spruce, DNP, RN, ACNS, ACNP, ANP, CNOR
Cynthia Spry, MA, MS, RN, CNOR, CBSPDT
Sharon A. Van Wicklin, MSN, RN, CNOR, CRNFA, CPSN, PLNC
Amber Wood, MSN, RN, CNOR, CIC, CPN

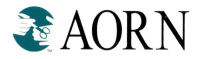

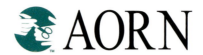

2170 South Parker Road
Suite 400
Denver, CO 80231-5711
(800) 755-2676
(303) 755-6300

Guidelines for Perioperative Practice, 2015 Edition
Copyright © 2015 AORN, Inc

Director of Publishing: Richard L. Wohl, MFA, MBA
Managing Editor: Liz Cowperthwaite
Associate Editor: Zac Wiggy
Graphic Design Manager: Colleen Ladny
Graphic Designer: Kurt Jones
Cover Design: Jacob Blocker
Marketing Manager: Holly Tripp

NOTICE
No responsibility is assumed by AORN, Inc, for any injury and/or damage to persons or property as a matter of products liability, negligence, or otherwise, or from any use or operation of any standards, guidelines, methods, products, instructions, or ideas contained in the material herein. Because of rapid advances in the health care sciences, independent verification of diagnoses, medication dosages, and individualized care and treatment should be made. The material contained herein is not intended to be a substitute for the exercise of professional medical or nursing judgment.

The content in this publication is provided on an "as is" basis. TO THE FULLEST EXTENT PERMITTED BY LAW, AORN, INC, DISCLAIMS ALL WARRANTIES, EITHER EXPRESS OR IMPLIED, STATUTORY OR OTHERWISE, INCLUDING BUT NOT LIMITED TO THE IMPLIED WARRANTIES OF MERCHANTABILITY, NON-INFRINGEMENT OF THIRD PARTIES' RIGHTS, AND FITNESS FOR A PARTICULAR PURPOSE.

No part of this book may be used, reproduced, or transmitted in any manner whatsoever without written permission from the publisher, except in the case of brief quotations embodied in critical articles and reviews. All requests to reprint, reproduce, or license any portion of the content must be submitted in writing. Send requests via e-mail to permissions@aorn.org or by mail to AORN Publications Department, 2170 South Parker Road, Suite 400, Denver, CO 80231-5711.

ISBN 978-1-888460-87-2   Printed in the United States of America

TABLE OF CONTENTS

Introduction to the 2015 Edition 1

   AORN Mission, Vision, and Values 8

Section I: Guidelines for Perioperative Practice

Aseptic Practice

Environmental Cleaning 9

Hand Hygiene 31

Patient Skin Antisepsis* 43

Sterile Technique 67

Surgical Attire* 97

Equipment and Product Safety

Electrosurgery 121

Laser Safety 139

Pneumatic Tourniquet 153

Product Selection 179

Patient and Worker Safety

Autologous Tissue Management* 187

Environment of Care, Part 1 239

   Amb Ambulatory Supplement 264

Environment of Care, Part 2* 265

Medication Safety 291

   Amb Ambulatory Supplement 330

Reducing Radiological Exposure 335

   Amb Ambulatory Supplement 345

Retained Surgical Items 347

   Amb Ambulatory Supplement 364

Sharps Safety 365

Specimen Management* 389

Transmissible Infections 419

   Amb Ambulatory Supplement 452

---

* *Documents appearing in print for the first time in 2015 and new/revised items published electronically in 2014.*

Amb *Indicates that an Ambulatory Supplement is available for the preceding topic.*

TABLE OF CONTENTS

Patient Care

Complementary Care Interventions* 455

Deep Vein Thrombosis 469

Hypothermia 479

Information Management 491

Local Anesthesia* 513

Minimally Invasive Surgery 525

Moderate Sedation/Analgesia 553

Positioning the Patient 563

Transfer of Patient Care Information 583

Sterilization and Disinfection

Flexible Endoscopes 589

High-Level Disinfection 601

Instrument Cleaning* 615

Packaging Systems 651

Sterilization 665

Section II: Standards of Perioperative Nursing 693

Exhibit A: Historical Perspectives 709

Exhibit B: Perioperative Explications 711

Section III: Additional Resources

Guidance Statement: Safe Patient Handling and Movement in the Perioperative Setting 733

Listing of AORN Position Statements 753

AACD Glossary of Procedural Times 755

Quality and Performance Improvement Standards 761

Index 771

* *Documents appearing in print for the first time in 2015 and new/revised items published electronically in 2014.*

INTRODUCTION TO THE AORN *GUIDELINES FOR PERIOPERATIVE PRACTICE*

AORN began publishing recommended practices in March 1975. A compilation was printed in March 1978 in *AORN Standards of Practice.* Beginning in 1981, compilations were published annually under various names, most recently *Perioperative Standards and Recommended Practices* (2008-2014).

Effective with this edition, AORN has changed the title of the compilation to *Guidelines for Perioperative Practice.* This new title better describes the documents comprising this publication. The Institute of Medicine defines clinical practice guidelines as "systematically developed statements to assist practitioner and patient decisions about appropriate health care for specific clinical circumstances."[1(p38)] AORN's documents meet this definition of a guideline. The AORN guidelines are evidence-based; the individual references are appraised and scored, and the recommendations are rated according to strength and quality of the evidence supporting the recommendation using the recently developed AORN Evidence Rating Model. This approach enables AORN to meet the submission criteria for acceptance by the National Guideline Clearinghouse. The decision to change the title was primarily driven by the acceptance of AORN's most recently updated evidence-based recommended practices documents to the National Guideline Clearinghouse as nationally recognized guidelines for perioperative practice.

AORN is committed to promoting excellence in perioperative nursing practice, advancing the profession, and supporting the professional perioperative registered nurse (RN). AORN promotes safe care for patients undergoing operative and other invasive procedures by providing practice support to the perioperative RN and other perioperative personnel. Perioperative RNs function in a variety of roles that include circulator, scrub person, first assistant, advanced practice nurse, manager, administrator, educator, informatics nurse specialist, and researcher. The descriptive and comprehensive documents in this publication reflect the perioperative RN's scope of professional responsibility and provide essential information for the delivery of safe perioperative patient care and a safe work environment.

New in this Edition

All previously titled "Recommended Practices" documents have been retitled as "Guidelines." There are eight new evidence-rated guidelines on the following topics:

- Autologous Tissue Management
- Complementary Care Interventions
- Cleaning and Care of Surgical Instruments
- Care of the Patient Receiving Local Anesthesia
- Preoperative Patient Skin Antisepsis
- A Safe Environment of Care, Part 2
- Specimen Management
- Surgical Attire

Section I: Guidelines for Perioperative Practice

The AORN guidelines are based on a comprehensive review of the research and non-research evidence. Each guideline consists of practice recommendations based on the highest level of evidence available. The guidelines are authored by perioperative nursing specialists in the AORN Nursing Department and selected members of the AORN Guidelines Advisory Board in collaboration with liaisons from the American Association of Nurse Anesthetists, the American College of Surgeons, the American Society of Anesthesiologists, the Association for Professionals in Infection Control and Epidemiology, the International Association of Healthcare Central Service Materiel Management, and the Society for Healthcare Epidemiology of America. These guidelines represent the Association's official position on questions regarding perioperative practice, and they have been approved by the AORN Guidelines Advisory Board.

The guidelines describe perioperative practices that promote patient and health care worker safety. They are intended to be achievable and represent what is believed to be an optimal level of patient care and perioperative practice within operative and invasive procedure settings. These settings include hospital operating rooms, ambulatory surgery centers, physicians' offices, cardiac catheterization laboratories, endoscopy suites, radiology departments, and all other areas where operative and other invasive procedures may be performed.

As used within the context of the guidelines, the word "should" indicates that a certain course of action is recommended. "Must" is used only to describe requirements mandated by government regulation. The use of "may" indicates that a course of action is permissible within the limits of the recommendation, and "can" indicates possibility and capability.

The printed book is a snapshot in time: all updated content approved by the Guidelines Advisory Board as of October of the year preceding publication appears in the annual print edition and on CD. An all-digital workflow launched in 2007 has enabled AORN to publish new and revised guidelines electronically throughout the year as the guidelines are

INTRODUCTION TO THE 2015 EDITION

updated and to make them available via electronic subscription (e-Subscription), mobile application, or individual chapter purchase.

Implementation in Practice

Individual commitment, professional conscience, and the setting in which perioperative nursing is practiced should guide the RN in implementing these guidelines. Implementation of the guidelines in perioperative settings requires close examination of existing policies and procedures. This review may indicate that new or revised policies and procedures are needed. Although the guidelines are considered to represent the optimal level of practice, variations in practice settings and clinical situations may limit the degree to which each guideline can be implemented.

Development, Review, and Revision Process

The guidelines are living documents that are developed, reviewed, and revised on an ongoing basis in an effort to provide current recommendations based on the highest level and quality of evidence available. Differences in format and content organization may occur as the guidelines continue to evolve over time; differences in design and layout also may occur.

Each guideline is reviewed and revised as appropriate at periodic intervals. Although only a portion of the documents may be updated for publication in any given year, all 32 guidelines are under continual scrutiny by the AORN Guidelines Advisory Board. The titles of previously released recommended practices documents have been changed to "Guideline"; however, the name "Recommended Practices" will continue to appear within the text and references of some of the documents until these documents are fully reviewed and revised.

Evidence Review

AORN is dedicated to providing guidelines for perioperative practice that are an indispensable and credible resource for perioperative RNs and other members of the perioperative team. Using the highest level of evidence available to support national recommendations about clinical practice has become an expectation of perioperative health care professionals. Evidence-based practice is an essential element for improving patient care by promoting decisions based on evidence rather than on tradition. A list of references has always been provided with each document; however, beginning with the 2013 edition, individual references have been rigorously assessed for their individual level of strength and quality, and a rating has been applied to the collective body of evidence supporting each recommendation.

In 2010, the AORN Board of Directors formed the Evidence Rating Task Force to evaluate evidence rating

Table 1. Research Appraisal Scores

Strength levels

I: Randomized controlled trial or experimental study

II: Quasi-experimental (no manipulation of independent variable, may have random assignment or control)

III: Non-experimental (no manipulation of independent variable; includes descriptive, comparative, and correlational studies; uses secondary data)

III: Qualitative (exploratory [eg, interviews, focus groups] starting point for studies where little research exists, small sample sizes, results used to design empirical studies)

Quality levels

Studies

A (High): Consistent, generalizable results; sufficient sample size for the study design; adequate control; definitive conclusions; consistent recommendations based on comprehensive literature review that includes thorough reference to scientific evidence

B (Good): Reasonably consistent results, sufficient sample size for the study design, some control, fairly definitive conclusions, reasonably consistent recommendations based on fairly comprehensive literature review that includes some reference to scientific evidence

C (Low): Little evidence with inconsistent results, insufficient sample size for the study design, conclusions cannot be drawn

Summaries

A (High): Well-defined, reproducible search strategies; consistent results with sufficient numbers of well-defined studies; evaluation of strength and quality of included studies; definitive conclusions

B (Good): Reasonably thorough and appropriate search, reasonably consistent results with sufficient numbers of well-defined studies, evaluation of strengths and limitations of included studies, fairly definitive conclusions

C (Low): Undefined, poorly defined, or limited search strategies; insufficient evidence with inconsistent results; conclusions cannot be drawn

REFERENCE
Dearholt S, Dang D. Johns Hopkins Nursing Evidence-Based Practice: Model and Guidelines. 2nd ed. Indianapolis, IN: Sigma Theta Tau International; 2012.

TABLE 2. NON-RESEARCH APPRAISAL SCORES

Strength levels

IV: Clinical practice guidelines, consensus or position statement

V: Literature review, expert opinion, case report, community standard, clinician experience, consumer experience, organizational experience: quality improvement, organizational experience: financial

Quality levels

Clinical practice guidelines, consensus or position statement

A (High): Application of standardized evidence appraisal for well-defined, reproducible search strategies; criteria-based evaluation of overall scientific strength and quality of included studies with definitive conclusions; national expertise is clearly evident

B (Good): Reasonably thorough and appropriate search strategies, reasonably consistent results, sufficient numbers of well-designed studies, evaluation of strengths and limitations of included studies with fairly definitive conclusions, national expertise is clearly evident

C (Low): Undefined, poorly defined, or limited search strategies; no evaluation of strengths and limitations of included studies; insufficient evidence with inconsistent results; conclusions cannot be drawn

REFERENCE
Dearholt S, Dang D. Johns Hopkins Nursing Evidence-Based Practice: Model and Guidelines. *2nd ed. Indianapolis, IN: Sigma Theta Tau International; 2012.*

---

methodologies and recommend a method that could be used to direct the review of evidence and evaluate the overall strength of the evidence used in creating a recommended practices document. The task force members included Victoria M. Steelman, PhD, RN (chair); Kathleen Gaberson, PhD, RN; Paula Graling, DNP, RN; Cecil King, MS, RN, CNS; and Theresa Pape, PhD, RN. Based on the recommendations of the task force, the document development and review process was redesigned using a systems approach for evidence review that incorporates evidence-rated recommendations into the guidelines.

Following the recommendation of the Evidence Rating Task Force, the Oncology Nursing Society Putting Evidence Into Practice (ONS PEP®) schema was used to rate the collective evidence supporting each recommendation for the newly revised recommended practices documents published in the 2013 edition. Based on the experience of the authors who used the ONS PEP model and on input from readers, the Recommended Practices Advisory Board approved the development and implementation of the AORN Evidence Rating Model, a model better suited to the content of the recommended practices documents. The AORN model is used to rate the collective evidence of each recommendation within the newly revised evidence-rated guideline. Previously published evidence-rated recommended practices documents were revised in 2014 to reflect the AORN evidence ratings. All evidence-rated guidelines in this edition have been rated according to the AORN Evidence Rating Model.

Each guideline focuses on a specific question or topic. The evidence review begins with a systematic literature search conducted using the MEDLINE®, CINAHL®, and Scopus® databases and the Cochrane Database of Systematic Reviews for meta-analyses, randomized and nonrandomized trials and studies, systematic and nonsystematic reviews, and opinion documents and letters to identify articles related to the topic. The search is conducted by a medical librarian employed by AORN. As relevant research and other evidence is located, it is independently evaluated and critically appraised according to the strength and quality of the evidence (Tables 1 and 2) using the AORN Evidence Appraisal Tools (Research and Non-Research). These tools were adapted with permission from the *Johns Hopkins Evidence-Based Practice: Model and Guidelines*[2] for use in the AORN Authoring System™. The reviewers participate in conference calls to discuss their individual appraisal scores and to establish consensus. Each article or study is assigned an appraisal score as agreed upon by the reviewers. The appraisal scores of individual references are noted in brackets after each citation in the references section of the guideline as applicable.

Evidence Rating

After the evidence is individually appraised, the collective evidence supporting each intervention within a specific recommendation is rated using the AORN Evidence Rating Model. The model includes a crosswalk comparison of the appraisal score and the recommendation rating (Table 3). Factors considered when applying the evidence-rating model to the collective body of evidence are the quality of research, the quantity of similar studies on a given topic, and the consistency of results supporting a recommendation. The recommendations in each guideline are given one of the following ratings:
- 1: Strong Evidence
- 1: Regulatory Requirement
- 2: Moderate Evidence
- 3: Limited Evidence
- 4: Benefits Balanced with Harms
- 5: No Evidence

The evidence ratings are noted in brackets after each recommended intervention and activity statement within the guideline.

INTRODUCTION TO THE 2015 EDITION

TABLE 3. AORN CROSSWALK: APPRAISAL SCORE TO EVIDENCE RATING

Appraisal score		AORN Evidence Rating Model	
Research	Non-research	Evidence rating	Evidence requirements
IA	IVA Regulatory	1: Strong Evidence 1: Regulatory Requirement	Interventions or activities for which effectiveness has been demonstrated by strong evidence from rigorously designed studies, meta-analyses, or systematic reviews; rigorously developed clinical practice guidelines; or regulatory requirements • Evidence from a meta-analysis or systematic review of research studies that incorporated evidence appraisal and synthesis of the evidence in the analysis • Supportive evidence from a single, well-conducted, randomized controlled trial • Guidelines developed by a panel of experts that derive from an explicit literature search methodology and include evidence appraisal and synthesis of the evidence
IB IIA, IIB IIIA, IIIB	IVB VA, VB	2: Moderate Evidence	Interventions or activities for which the evidence is less well established than for those listed under "1: Strong Evidence" • Supportive evidence from a well-conducted research study • Guidelines developed by a panel of experts that are primarily based on the evidence but not supported by evidence appraisal and synthesis of the evidence • Non-research evidence with consistent results and fairly definitive conclusions
IC IIC IIIC	IVC VC	3: Limited Evidence	Interventions or activities for which there currently is insufficient evidence or evidence of inadequate quality • Supportive evidence from a poorly conducted research study • Evidence from non-experimental studies with high potential for bias • Guidelines developed largely by consensus or expert opinion • Non-research evidence with insufficient evidence or inconsistent results • Conflicting evidence, but where the preponderance of the evidence supports the recommendation
		4: Benefits Balanced with Harms	Selected interventions or activities for which the AORN Guidelines Advisory Board is of the opinion that the desirable effects of following this recommendation outweigh the harms
		5: No Evidence	Interventions or activities for which no supportive evidence was found during the literature search completed for the recommendation • Consensus opinion

Copyright © 2015 AORN, Inc.

Document Structure

Each evidence-rated guideline is composed of eight elements.

1. Introduction: a general introductory statement.
2. Purpose: a description of the intent and scope of the document.
3. Evidence Review: a description of the systematic literature search and review of the evidence and the processes used to evaluate and rate the evidence.
4. Recommendation: a broad recommendation for optimal practice. The recommendation statements are in bold font and identified by a Roman numeral (eg, I). Each recommendation statement is followed by a rationale.
5. Intervention: a specific recommendation for treatment or action. Interventions are identified by an alphabetic character after the recommendation Roman numeral (eg, I.a.). The intervention statement is followed by a rationale detailing the evidence that supports the recommendation. The level of each intervention is rated using the AORN Evidence Rating Model. The evidence rating is noted in brackets after the intervention statement (eg, *[1: Strong Evidence]*).
6. Activity: a statement that describes the actions necessary to implement the intervention. Activities are noted by a number following the recommendation Roman numeral and the intervention alphabetic character (eg, I.a.1). The level of each activity may be rated using the AORN Evidence Rating Model. If so, the evidence rating is noted in brackets after the activity statement (eg, *[1: Strong Evidence]*).
7. Glossary: a list of defined terms used in the text of the document with which the reader may be unfamiliar.
8. References: a list of all references used within the document and the assigned appraisal scores. The appraisal score is noted in brackets after each citation (eg, *[IA], [IVA]*).

INTRODUCTION TO THE 2015 EDITION

Ambulatory Supplements

Each document was reviewed and vetted for applicability to ambulatory surgery centers, and supplemental information has been provided related to recommendations that may have additional considerations for these perioperative practice settings. The Ambulatory Supplements are intended to be used as additional information for the perioperative RN practicing in a free-standing ambulatory surgery center or a physician office-based surgery center.

The *Amb* symbol in the text of a guideline indicates that there is additional information in the Ambulatory Supplement following the document. Relevant text from the guideline is repeated in the Supplement for easy reference and to give context to the ambulatory considerations. New text is denoted with the *Amb* symbol in the Supplement. Where applicable, the Ambulatory Supplements include text from the Centers for Medicare & Medicaid Services *State Operation Manual Appendix L—Guidance for Surveyors: Ambulatory Surgical Centers*.

The Ambulatory Supplement is intended to be an adjunct to the guideline upon which it is based and is not intended to be a replacement for that document. Perioperative personnel who are developing and updating organizational policies and procedures should review and cite the full guideline.

AORN Guidelines and the PNDS

The Perioperative Nursing Data Set (PNDS) is the standardized nursing language developed by AORN and recognized by the American Nurses Association to describe the nursing care, from preadmission to discharge, of patients undergoing operative or other invasive procedures. As a controlled vocabulary, the PNDS organizes the unique knowledge of perioperative nursing for computerization and easy accessibility. The PNDS enables nursing care to be documented in a standardized manner and allows the collection of reliable and valid comparable clinical data to evaluate the effectiveness of nurse-sensitive interventions and the relationship between these interventions and patient outcomes.

This standardized language consists of a collection of unique concepts that reflect the nursing process as described in the *Guidelines for Perioperative Practice*. The perioperative patient and his or her family members are at the core of the Perioperative Patient Focused Model, the conceptual framework for the PNDS. The model depicts perioperative nursing in four domains and illustrates the relationship among the patient, his or her family members, and the care provided by the professional perioperative RN. Within the PNDS, the Safety, Physiological Responses, and Behavioral Responses domains contain nursing diagnoses, interventions, and outcomes representing patient care concerns. The Health System domain focuses on the structural elements that describe the environment in which care is provided. Each uniquely identified concept in the PNDS is clearly defined, common to all procedures, relates to the delivery of care, and is appropriate for use in any surgical setting.

The *Guidelines for Perioperative Practice* is the foundation of clinical knowledge from which the PNDS is derived. An initial attempt to map the PNDS outcomes and interventions to the recommended practices was reflected in recommended practices documents published from 2004 to 2009, and PNDS codes appeared in parentheses after the purpose and intervention statements. The guidelines do not display the PNDS codes. AORN continues to develop and refine the PNDS language.

The AORN guidelines and the *Perioperative Nursing Data Set*, 3rd edition, concepts are mapped to the clinical content within the AORN Syntegrity® perioperative documentation solution for the electronic health record. The AORN Syntegrity solution provides standardized content for electronic perioperative nursing documentation. The *Perioperative Nursing Data Set*, 3rd edition, is distributed only through an AORN Syntegrity license. To learn more about the AORN Syntegrity solution and implementation of the PNDS with the electronic health record, contact the AORN Syntegrity team via e-mail at syntegrity@aorn.org or visit http://www.aorn.org/syntegrity.

Section II: Standards of Perioperative Nursing

The AORN Standards of Perioperative Nursing define the scope, responsibilities, and dimensions of professional perioperative nursing practice. This document guides individual practitioners in performing safe and effective care and reflects the value-based behaviors and priorities of the profession.

The standards serve as the foundation for AORN's guidelines, competency statements, and the PNDS. They are consistent with *Nursing: Scope and Standards of Practice*,[3] *Nursing's Social Policy Statement*, 2nd edition,[4] and *Nursing Administration: Scope and Standards of Practice*, 3rd edition,[5] published by the American Nurses Association. The Standards of Perioperative Nursing focus on the process of providing nursing care and performing professional role activities; they also provide a mechanism to delineate the responsibilities of the RN engaged in practice in the perioperative setting.

Section III: Additional Resources

Additional resources feature the AORN Guidance Statement: Safe Patient Handling and Movement in the Perioperative Setting, which provides suggested strategies to assist practitioners in developing organization-specific processes related to clinical and administrative issues. Additional resources include a listing of AORN Position Statements, the AACD Glossary of Times Used for Scheduling and Monitoring of Diagnostic and Therapeutic Procedures, and Quality and Performance Improvement Standards for Perioperative Nursing.

INTRODUCTION TO THE 2015 EDITION

Editor's note: ONS PEP is a registered trademark of the Oncology Nursing Society, Pittsburgh, PA. MEDLINE is a registered trademark of the US National Library of Medicine's Medical Literature Analysis and Retrieval System, Bethesda, MD. CINAHL, Cumulative Index to Nursing and Allied Health Literature, is a registered trademark of EBSCO Industries, Birmingham, AL. Scopus is a registered trademark of Elsevier B.V., Amsterdam, The Netherlands. AORN Authoring System is a trademark of AORN, Inc, Denver, CO. Syntegrity is a registered trademark of AORN, Inc, Denver, CO.

References

1. Dearholt S, Dang D. *Johns Hopkins Nursing Evidence-Based Practice Model and Guidelines.* 2nd ed. Indianapolis, IN: Sigma Theta Tau International; 2012.
2. Institute of Medicine. Field MJ, Lohr KN, eds. *Clinical Practice Guidelines: Directions for a New Program.* Washington, DC: National Academy Press; 1990:38.
3. *Nursing: Scope and Standards of Practice.* Washington, DC: American Nurses Association; 2004.
4. *Nursing's Social Policy Statement.* 2nd ed. Washington, DC: American Nurses Association; 2003.
5. *Nursing Administration: Scope and Standards of Practice.* 3rd ed. Washington, DC: American Nurses Association; 2009.

AORN Staff Support

Ramona Conner, MSN, RN, CNOR
Manager, Standards and Guidelines

Linda Groah, MSN, RN, CNOR, NEA-BC, FAAN
Executive Director/CEO

Lisa Spruce, DNP, RN, ACNS, ACNP, ANP, CNOR
Director of Evidence-based Perioperative Practice

Janet Knox
Executive Project Coordinator

Perioperative Nursing Specialists
Byron Burlingame, MS, RN, CNOR
Bonnie Denholm, MS, BSN, RN, CNOR
Mary J. Ogg, MSN, RN, CNOR
Sharon A. Van Wicklin, MSN, RN, CNOR, CRNFA, CPSN, PLNC
Amber Wood, MSN, RN, CNOR, CIC, CPN

Director, Ambulatory Surgery Division
Jan Davidson, MSN, RN, CNOR, CASC

Product Manager, Guideline Implementation Tools
Terri Link, MPH, BSN, CNOR, CIC

AORN Research and Information Center
Sara Katsh, MA, AHIP, Manager
Melissa Kovac, MA, MLIS, AHIP, Research Librarian
Ronda Gunnett, Librarian

AORN Publications Department
Liz Cowperthwaite, Senior Managing Editor
Zac Wiggy, Associate Editor
Bonnie Kibbe, Administrative Assistant

INTRODUCTION TO THE 2015 EDITION

AORN gratefully acknowledges the work of the 2013–2014 Recommended Practices Advisory Board and 2014–2015 Guidelines Advisory Board

Members

Rodney W. Hicks, PhD, ARNP, RN, FAANP, FAAN
Professor
Western University of Health Science
Pomona, California
(Chair 2014-2015, Member 2013-2014)

Antonia B. Hughes, MA, BSN, RN, CNOR
Perioperative Education Specialist
Baltimore Washington Medical Center
Glen Burnie, Maryland
(Chair 2013-2014)

George D. Allen, PhD, CIC, CNOR
Director Infection Control
Downstate Medical Center
Clinical Assistant Professor
SUNY College of Health Related Professions
Brooklyn, New York
(Member 2013-2014)

Patricia A. Graybill-D'Ercole, MSN, RN, CNOR, CHL, CRCST
Clinical Specialist
Integra Life Sciences Instrument Division
York, Pennsylvania
(Member 2013-2015)

Deborah S. Hickman, MS, RN, CNOR, CRNFA
Director of Surgical Services
Renue Plastic Surgery
Brunswick, Georgia
(Member 2013-2015)

Paula J. Morton, MS, RN, CNOR
Director Perioperative Services
Advocate Sherman Health Care
Elgin, Illinois
(Member 2013-2014)

Deborah F. Mulloy, PhD, RN, CNOR
Associate Chief Nurse
Quality & Center for Nursing Excellence
Brigham and Women's Hospital
Boston, Massachusetts
(Member 2013-2015)

Barbara L. Nalley, MSN, CRNP, CNOR
Manager
Jackson Surgical Assistants
Crofton, Maryland
(Member 2014-2015)

Advisory Board Liaisons

Leslie Ann Jeter, RN, CRNA, MSNA
American Association of Nurse Anesthetists
(2013-2015)

Amy L. Halverson, MD
American College of Surgeons
(2013-2015)

Armin Schubert, MD, MBA
American Society of Anesthesiologists
(2013-2015)

Marcia R. Patrick, MSN, RN, CIC
Association for Professionals in Infection Control and Epidemiology
(2013-2014)

Heather Hohenberger, BSN, RN, CIC, CNOR
Association for Professionals in Infection Control and Epidemiology
(2014-2015)

Paula Berrett, BS, CRCST
International Association of Healthcare Central Service Materiel Management
(2013-2014)

Michelle R. Dempsey-Evans, MSN, RN, CNOR, CRCST
International Association of Healthcare Central Service Materiel Management
(2014-2015)

Angela Hewlett, MD, MS
Society for Healthcare Epidemiology of America
(2014-2015)

AORN Board Liaison

Donna A. Ford, MSN, RN-BC, CNOR, CRCST
Nursing Education Specialist
Assistant Professor of Nursing
Mayo Clinic College of Medicine
Rochester, Minnesota
(Board Liaison 2014-2015, Member 2013-2014)

Judith L. Goldberg, MSN, RN, CNOR, CRCST
Nurse Manager
Pequot Surgery Center
Lawrence Memorial Hospital
Groton, Connecticut
(2013-2014)

INTRODUCTION TO THE 2015 EDITION

AORN and Perioperative Nursing

AORN is a nonprofit membership association that represents the professional interests of more than 160,000 perioperative nurses by providing nursing education, standards, and clinical practice resources to enable optimal outcomes for patients undergoing operative and other invasive procedures. AORN's 40,000 registered nurse members manage, teach, and practice perioperative nursing, are enrolled in nursing education, or are engaged in perioperative research.

AORN Mission, Vision, and Values

Mission
AORN's mission is to promote safety and optimal outcomes for patients undergoing operative and other invasive procedures by providing practice support and professional development opportunities to perioperative nurses. AORN will collaborate with professional and regulatory organizations, industry leaders, and other health care partners who support the mission.

Vision
AORN will be the indispensable resource for evidence-based practice and education that establishes the standards of excellence in the delivery of perioperative nursing care.

Values
AORN's core values reflect what is important to the association:
- Communication—open, honest, respectful
- Innovation—creative, risk taking, leading edge
- Quality—reliable, timely, accountable
- Collaboration—teamwork, inclusion, diversity

GUIDELINES
FOR PERIOPERATIVE PRACTICE

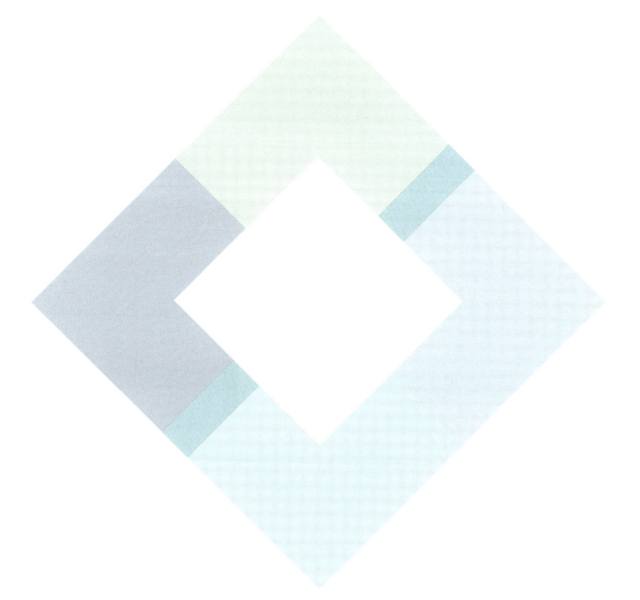

SECTION I

ASEPTIC PRACTICE

GUIDELINE FOR ENVIRONMENTAL CLEANING

The Guideline for Environmental Cleaning was approved by the AORN Recommended Practices Advisory Board. It was presented as proposed recommendations for comments by members and others. The guideline is effective November 15, 2013. The recommendations in the guideline are intended to be achievable and represent what is believed to be an optimal level of practice. Policies and procedures will reflect variations in practice settings and/or clinical situations that determine the degree to which the guideline can be implemented. AORN recognizes the many diverse settings in which perioperative nurses practice; therefore, this guideline is adaptable to all areas where operative and other invasive procedures may be performed.

Purpose

Historically, perioperative registered nurses (RNs) have played a critical role in providing a clean environment for patients undergoing operative or other invasive procedures. In recent years, researchers have developed an increasing awareness of the role of the environment in the development of health care-associated infections and transmission of multidrug-resistant organisms (MDROs).[1-4]

The literature describes a high risk of pathogen transmission in the perioperative setting due to multiple contacts among patients, perioperative team members, and environmental surfaces.[1] Thus, thorough cleaning and disinfection of perioperative areas is essential to preventing the spread of potentially pathogenic microorganisms.[1] Because surfaces that health care providers touch frequently may present a high risk for pathogen transmission to patients,[2] routine cleaning of high-touch objects is an effective approach to limiting transmission of pathogens[5] when implemented as part of a comprehensive environmental cleaning and disinfection program.

Researchers have shown that cleaning practices in the operating room (OR) have not been adequately thorough or consistent with the policies of the health care organization.[1,6,7] Jefferson et al observed a mean cleaning rate of 25% for objects monitored in the OR setting in six acute care hospitals.[7] These findings demonstrate that some ORs may not be as clean as previously thought,[1] although the literature has not defined the concept of cleanliness. All perioperative team members have a responsibility to provide a clean environment for patients. Perioperative and environmental services leaders can cultivate an environment where perioperative and environmental services personnel work collaboratively to accomplish adequately thorough cleanliness in a culture of safety and mutual support.

This document provides guidance for environmental cleaning and disinfection in the perioperative practice setting and are based on the highest quality evidence available. The quality of the research investigating environmental cleaning has not yet achieved a level of rigor to thoroughly define and evaluate best practices for environmental cleaning in health care, including the perioperative setting.[3] According to Carling, published studies have not separated cleaning thoroughness from the cleaning chemicals being evaluated, and there is a need for outcome studies to determine the impact of environmental cleaning on the transmission of disease.[3]

Donskey found that although much of the evidence for environmental disinfection as a control strategy for reducing health care-associated infections is suboptimal, the practice of environmental cleaning is supported by several high-quality investigations.[8] Conscientious application of these recommendations should result in a clean environment for perioperative patients and minimize the exposure risk of health care personnel and patients to potentially infectious microorganisms. Any patient could be infected with bloodborne or other pathogens, so all surgical procedures should be considered potentially infectious. This document provides specific guidance for cleaning procedures; selection of appropriate cleaning chemicals, materials, tools, and equipment; ongoing education and competency verification; policies and procedures; and quality assurance and performance improvement processes.

Although these recommendations include references to cleaning a wide variety of surfaces, the focus of this document is specific to the environmental cleaning of perioperative areas. These recommendations may be applicable to sterile processing areas. Laundering of textiles is outside the scope of these recommendations. Environmental cleaning includes considerations for a safe environment of care, prevention of transmissible infections, and hand hygiene. These topics are addressed in other AORN guidelines, and although they are mentioned briefly where applicable (eg, standard precautions), broader discussions are outside the scope of this document.[9-11]

Evidence Review

A medical librarian conducted systematic searches of the databases MEDLINE, CINAHL, and the Cochrane Database of Systematic Reviews for meta-analyses, systematic reviews, randomized controlled and nonrandomized trials and studies, opinion documents, case reports, letters, reviews, and guidelines. Scopus was also consulted, although not searched systematically.

ENVIRONMENTAL CLEANING

Search terms included *operating room, operating theater, operating suite, surgical suite, recovery room, post-anesthesia, post-anaesthesia, perioperative nursing, ambulatory care facilities, surgicenters, ambulatory surgery, outpatient surgery, healthcare facilities, terminal cleaning, terminal disinfecting, terminal decontamination, cleaning schedule, cleaning program, cleaning regimen, prior patient, prior room occupant, previous patient, cleaning standard, cleaning policies, cleaning guideline, cleaning protocol, routine cleaning, hospital housekeeping, housekeeping department, environmental services, cross infection, infection control, decontamination, room decontamination, disinfection, disinfectants, adenosine triphosphate, detergents, solvents, phenols, disinfectants, hydrogen peroxide, ultraviolet rays, fluorescent light, quaternary ammonium disinfectant, sodium hypochlorite, ozone, silver, copper, gram-negative bacteria, gram-positive bacteria, viruses, Staphylococcus aureus, methicillin resistance, vancomycin, multi-drug resistant organism, clostridium, chickenpox, measles, varicella, rubeola, tuberculosis, prion diseases, prions, Creutzfeldt-Jakob, disease reservoir, dust, surgical wound infection, blood, body fluids, tissues, blood spill, semen, cerebrospinal fluid, synovial fluid, vaginal secretions, pericardial fluid, peritoneal fluid, saliva, amniotic fluid, air microbiology, air pollution, bacterial load, microbial colony count, environmental microbiology, environmental cleaning, green cleaning, mop, mopping, bucket, wringer, brush, buffers, floor machine, sweepers, microfiber, microfibre, paper towel, cloths, wiping, vacuum, environmental surface, contact surface, fomites, floors and floor coverings, interior design and furnishings, mites, lice, fleas, cockroaches, vermin, flies, ants, insects, pest control, textiles, bedding and linens, beds and mattresses, curtains, laundry, laundry service, cellular phone, cellphones, cell phones, telephones, wireless communications, mobile devices, iPad, tablets, laptops, computer systems, computers, keyboards, mouse, tables, beds, operating tables, mattress, stretcher, examination tables, patient transfer board, trolleys, carts, scrub sink, durable medical equipment, disposable equipment, equipment reuse, storage areas, hospitals, eye wash, operating room waste, clinical waste, medical waste, medical waste disposal, biohazardous waste, hazardous materials, formaldehyde, formalin, methyl methacrylate, storage, disposal, transport, handling, safety management, occupational health, occupational-related injuries, occupational exposure, contact precautions, standard precautions, droplet precautions, universal precautions, eye protective devices, masks, respiratory protective devices, protective clothing, gloves, goggles, gowns, environmental monitoring, luminescent measurements, checklists, visual inspection, fluorescent light, audit, tacky mat, sticky mat, hospital design and construction, demolition, construction materials, aspergillus, aspergillosis, central service department, sterile processing, sterile supply, central supply, central processing, task performance and analysis, job performance, competency-based education, continuing education,* and *human factors.*

The search was originally limited to literature published in English between 2008 and 2013. The lead author and the medical librarian identified relevant guidelines from government agencies and standards-setting bodies, and the lead author requested additional articles that either did not fit the original search criteria or were discovered during the evidence appraisal process. The medical librarian also established continuing alerts on the environmental cleaning topics and provided relevant results to the lead author.

Articles identified by the search were provided to the project team for evaluation. The team consisted of the lead author, three members of the Recommended Practices Advisory Board, and two doctorally prepared evidence appraisers. The lead author divided the search results into topics and assigned members of the team to review and critically appraise each article using the Johns Hopkins Evidence-Based Practice Model and the Research or Non-Research Evidence Appraisal Tools as appropriate. The literature was independently evaluated and appraised according to the strength and quality of the evidence. Each article was then assigned an appraisal score. The appraisal score is noted in brackets after each reference, as applicable.

The collective evidence supporting each intervention within a specific recommendation was summarized and used to rate the strength of the evidence using the AORN Evidence Rating Model. Factors considered in review of the collective evidence were the quality of research, quantity of similar studies on a given topic, and consistency of results supporting a recommendation. The evidence rating is noted in brackets after each intervention.

Editor's note: *MEDLINE is a registered trademark of the US National Library of Medicine's Medical Literature Analysis and Retrieval System, Bethesda, MD. CINAHL, Cumulative Index to Nursing and Allied Health Literature, is a registered trademark of EBSCO Industries, Birmingham, AL. Scopus is a registered trademark of Elsevier B.V., Amsterdam, Netherlands.*

Recommendation I

A multidisciplinary team should establish cleaning procedures and frequencies in the perioperative practice setting.

Involvement of a multidisciplinary team (eg, perioperative nursing, sterile processing, environmental services, infection prevention) allows input from personnel who perform environmental cleaning in perioperative areas and from personnel with expertise beyond clinical end-users (eg, infection prevention personnel). As part of a bundled approach to implementing best practices for environmental cleaning, Havill recommended developing cleaning procedures as part of a multidisciplinary team.[12]

Operational guidelines for frequency of cleaning in the perioperative setting were identified as a gap in the literature based on the evidence review.

ENVIRONMENTAL CLEANING

I.a. A multidisciplinary team should select cleaning chemicals for use in the perioperative setting. *[2: Moderate Evidence]*

A standardized product selection process assists in the selection of functional and reliable products that are safe, cost-effective, and environmentally friendly and promote quality care, as well as decreases duplication or rapid obsolescence.[13]

I.a.1. A multidisciplinary team should evaluate the following factors during selection of a cleaning detergent or disinfectant chemical:
- Environmental Protection Agency (EPA) registration and rating as hospital grade[14,15]; *[1: Strong Evidence]*
- targeted microorganisms[14]; *[1: Strong Evidence]*
- dwell times (ie, contact times)[14]; *[1: Strong Evidence]*
- chemical manufacturers' instructions for use[14,15]; *[1: Strong Evidence]*
- compatibility with surfaces, cleaning materials, and equipment[15]; *[3: Limited Evidence]*
- patient population (eg, neonatal)[14,15]; *[1: Strong Evidence]*
- cost[15]; *[3: Limited Evidence]*
- safety[15-17]; *[2: Moderate Evidence]* and
- effect on the environment.[15] *[3: Limited Evidence]*

I.a.2. High-level disinfectants or liquid chemical sterilants should not be used to clean and disinfect environmental surfaces or noncritical devices.[14] *[1: Strong Evidence]*

These chemicals are not intended for use on environmental surfaces and are not labeled for use as low-level disinfectants.[14]

I.a.3. Alcohol should not be used to disinfect large environmental surfaces.[14] *[1: Strong Evidence]*

Alcohol is not an EPA-registered disinfectant. Alcohol is an antiseptic and not a detergent. Alcohol does not remove soil or debris.

I.a.4. An EPA-registered disinfectant in the concentration indicated in the manufacturer's instructions for nurseries and neonatal patient care areas should be used when the perioperative patient population includes neonates and infants.[14,15] *[1: Strong Evidence]*

Hyperbilirubinemia in newborns has been linked to poor ventilation and cleaning of incubators and other nursery surfaces with inadequately diluted phenolic solutions.[14]

I.b. A multidisciplinary team should select cleaning materials, tools, and equipment for use in the perioperative practice setting.[13,15] *[2: Moderate Evidence]*

A standardized product selection process assists in the selection of functional and reliable products that are safe, cost-effective, and environmentally friendly and promote quality care, as well as decreases duplication or rapid obsolescence.[13,15]

I.b.1. A multidisciplinary team should evaluate the following factors during selection of cleaning materials, tools, and equipment:
- manufacturers' instructions for use on surfaces to be cleaned[15];
- manufacturers' instructions for use for cleaning materials and equipment[15];
- compatibility with detergents and disinfectants[15];
- effect on environmental conditions in the OR (eg, temperature, humidity);
- cost[15];
- personnel ergonomics and safety[15]; and
- effect on the environment.[15]

I.b.2. Reusable or single-use disposable cleaning materials (eg, mop heads, cloths) may be used.[14]

I.b.3. Mops that dispense cleaning solutions may be used.

Using mops that dispense cleaning solutions may decrease the risk of contaminating multi-use containers of cleaning solution and reduce the risk of chemical splashes.

I.b.4. Microfiber or low-linting cotton cleaning materials (eg, mop heads, cloths) may be used.[15,18,19]

In a comparative study, Rutala et al reported that microfiber mopping systems were more effective than cotton string mops at microbial removal, 95% and 68% respectively, and that microbial removal with microfiber was equally effective with and without use of a disinfectant.[18] Diab-Elschahawi et al found in another comparative study that although microfiber cloths were best for decontamination, cotton was most effective after multiple launderings.[19] However, the laundering methods used to process the microfiber cloths in this study were at a higher temperature than that recommended by the Centers for Disease Control and Prevention (CDC), which may have altered their effectiveness.

Additional research is needed to determine the most effective material for cleaning and disinfecting environmental surfaces in perioperative areas.

I.c. A multidisciplinary team should establish cleaning frequencies for high-touch objects and surfaces.[2,14,20,21] *[1: Strong Evidence]*

In a literature review, Dancer found that contamination of environmental surfaces that are touched frequently provides an opportunity for

ENVIRONMENTAL CLEANING

hands to acquire pathogens, which could be transmitted to patients.[2,20] Stiefel et al demonstrated in an observational study that touching environmental surfaces in the inpatient room of a patient colonized with methicillin-resistant *Staphylococcus aureus* (MRSA) was just as likely to contaminate the gloved hands of health care personnel as was touching the patient's skin.[21] The results of this study showed that environmental surfaces may be a reservoir for pathogens that can contaminate the hands of health care personnel.[21]

I.d. A multidisciplinary team and the infection prevention committee should determine when enhanced environmental cleaning procedures should be implemented to prevent the spread of infections or outbreaks.[22-26] (See Recommendation VII.) *[1: Strong Evidence]*

I.e. A multidisciplinary team should designate personnel responsible for cleaning perioperative areas and equipment.[15,20] *[2: Moderate Evidence]*

Designating cleaning responsibilities is an important component of defining cleaning procedures. In a literature review, researchers identified the importance of assigning cleaning responsibilities to reduce the number of items that personnel forget to clean.[20]

I.f. A multidisciplinary team should develop cleaning and disinfection procedures for construction, renovation, repair, demolition, or disaster remediation.[14] (See Recommendation VII.) *[1: Strong Evidence]*

Development of cleaning procedures during construction is a critical component of an infection control risk assessment that should be completed before the start of any construction project.[14]

I.g. A multidisciplinary team should develop cleaning and disinfection procedures for managing environmental contamination (eg, condensation, air contamination).[14] (See Recommendation VII.) *[1: Strong Evidence]*

Defining cleaning procedures before contamination occurs will guide personnel in selecting appropriate actions to decrease the risk of transmitting pathogens in the event of environmental contamination.[14]

Recommendation II

The patient should be provided with a clean, safe environment.

In a literature review by Ibrahimi et al, the authors stated that the amount of bacteria present in the operative site is one of the most important factors associated with surgical site infection (SSI) development, although the minimum number of bacteria that causes an infection varies depending on the qualities of the organism, the host, and the procedure being performed. The authors also found that fomites near the surgical field may harbor bacteria. These fomites may serve as a reservoir for wound contamination and SSI development through either fomite-to-skin contact with the patient or personnel contact with fomites and subsequent skin-to-skin contact with the patient.[27]

In another literature review, Dancer found that unless a pathogen is removed from fomite surfaces by some cleaning process, the microorganism may persist in the environment for weeks, depending on the qualities of the organism, and may contaminate the hands of perioperative personnel or be deposited on or near a patient if the organism is uplifted by air currents.[20]

II.a. The perioperative RN should assess the perioperative environment frequently for cleanliness and take action to implement cleaning and disinfection procedures. *[2: Moderate Evidence]*

Environmental cleaning and disinfection is a team effort involving perioperative personnel and environmental services personnel. The responsibility for verifying a clean surgical environment before the start of an operative or invasive procedure rests with perioperative nurses.[28]

II.a.1. The perioperative RN should visually inspect the OR for cleanliness before case carts, supplies, and equipment are brought into the room.

II.b. All horizontal surfaces in the OR (eg, furniture, surgical lights, booms, equipment) should be damp dusted before the first scheduled surgical or other invasive procedure of the day.[14,20,29] *[1: Strong Evidence]*

Dust is known to contain human skin and hair, fabric fibers, pollens, mold, fungi, insect parts, glove powder, and paper fibers, among other components.[10,14] Airborne particles range from 0.001 micrometers to several hundred micrometers. In settings with dry conditions, gram-positive cocci (eg, coagulase negative *Staphylococcus* species) found in dust may persist; in settings with surfaces that are moist and soiled, the growth of gram-negative bacilli may persist.[14]

II.b.1. Damp dusting of the OR should be completed before case carts, supplies, and equipment are brought into the room.

II.b.2. A clean, low-linting cloth moistened with an EPA-registered hospital-grade disinfectant should be used to damp dust.[15]

The purpose of damp dusting is to remove dust, not to perform surface disinfection, which is completed after each procedure and at terminal cleaning. Therefore, achieving disinfectant dwell times for surface disinfection is not necessary when using disinfectants for damp dusting purposes.

II.b.3. Damp dusting should be performed methodically, from top to bottom.[15]

ENVIRONMENTAL CLEANING

II.c. Environmental protection agency-registered hospital-grade disinfectants should be used to disinfect surfaces in the perioperative practice setting. *[1: Strong Evidence]*

The CDC recommends that EPA-registered disinfectants be used in health care settings.[14,30]

II.c.1. Environmental surfaces should be cleaned with a detergent prior to disinfection, according to the manufacturer's instructions for use, in either a one-step (ie, combined detergent and disinfectant product) or two-step (ie, two separate detergent and disinfectant products) process.[15]

The presence of visible soil, dirt, and organic material inhibits the process of disinfection by preventing the disinfectant from interacting with the surface.[15]

II.c.2. Safety data sheets must be available and reviewed for each cleaning chemical used in the perioperative setting.[10]

II.c.3. Cleaning chemicals must be prepared, handled, stored, and disposed of according to manufacturers' instructions for use and local, state, and federal regulations.[10,14,30]

Microbial contamination of disinfectants has been reported with improper dilution of the disinfectant.[30]

II.c.4. If the cleaning chemical is removed from the original container, the secondary container should be labeled with the chemical name, concentration, and expiration date.

II.c.5. Disinfectants should be applied and reapplied as needed, per manufacturers' instructions, for the dwell time required to kill the targeted microorganism (eg, *Clostridium difficile*).[30]

II.c.6. Spray and misting methods (eg, a spray bottle) should not be used to apply cleaning chemicals in the perioperative practice setting.[14]

Cleaning chemicals that are sprayed produce more aerosols than solutions that are poured or ready to use.[14] If the cleaning solution is contaminated, the spray mechanism may provide a route for airborne transmission of disease.[14] Aerosols generated may contaminate the surgical wound, sterile supplies, or the sterile field, or may cause respiratory symptoms (acute or chronic) in personnel and patients.

II.d. Floors should be mopped with damp or wet mops. Dry methods of environmental cleaning (ie, dusting, sweeping) should not be used in semi-restricted and restricted areas.[14,31] *[1: Strong Evidence]*

In an observational study, Andersen et al found that wet and moist mopping was most effective in reducing organic soil on floors.[31] Although all methods of mopping in the study increased bacterial counts in the air just after mopping, wet methods of mopping produced fewer aerosols than dry methods.[31]

II.e. Floors in the perioperative practice setting should be considered contaminated at all times.[1,31] *[2: Moderate Evidence]*

Munoz-Price et al found that the OR floor was a potential reservoir for microorganisms due to inadvertent contamination of items during routine patient care.[1] When patient care items (eg, intravenous tubing, safety straps) inadvertently touched the floor, the items were potentially contaminated by the floor and could transmit pathogens to the patient if they were not disinfected before contact with the patient.[1] Andersen et al investigated the reduction of bacterial contamination of the floor using various cleaning methods, and found that even with the best results, the floor was contaminated with more than 25 colony-forming units and the air was contaminated after use of each method.[31] Even in the best scenario, the floor is essentially contaminated as soon as it is cleaned due to air contaminants settling on the floor after mopping and new contaminants being introduced by air currents or traffic.

II.e.1. Items that contact the floor for any amount of time should be considered contaminated. Noncritical items (eg, safety straps, positioning devices) should be disinfected after contact with the floor per manufacturers' instructions before patient use.[14,30]

II.e.2. Reusable cleaning materials should be changed after each use.[14] Disposable cleaning materials should be discarded after each use.

Using a dirty mop or cloth on a clean area or to clean for multiple patients may increase the possibility of cross-contamination.

I.e.3. Used cleaning materials (eg, mop heads, cloths) should not be returned to the cleaning solution container.[14,15]

Used cleaning materials are considered contaminated and returning them to the cleaning solution container contaminates the solution.[15]

II.e.4. Tacky mats should not be used to decrease floor contamination in the OR.[14]

Tacky mats have not been shown to reduce the number of organisms on shoes or equipment wheels, nor do they reduce the risk of SSI.[14]

II.f. A protective barrier covering should be used to protect noncritical equipment surfaces if the surface cannot withstand disinfection or is difficult to clean (eg, computer keyboards, foot pedals).[14] *[1: Strong Evidence]*

ENVIRONMENTAL CLEANING

Protecting surfaces that cannot withstand disinfection, in accordance with the equipment manufacturer's instructions for cleaning, provides a mechanism to prevent surfaces from becoming a reservoir for microorganisms. Equipment that is difficult to clean may harbor pathogens in crevices that are not amenable to disinfection. Using a barrier covering may prevent contamination of these areas and other areas that are difficult to reach.[14]

II.f.1. Noncritical items in the perioperative setting that cannot be covered and cannot withstand disinfection (eg, monitor screens, telephones, other electronic devices) should be cleaned in accordance with the equipment manufacturers' cleaning recommendations.[14]

Computers and other sensitive electronic devices are likely to become contaminated and may be difficult to clean. Sensitive computer components, such as monitors, may be damaged by cleaning disinfectants.

II.f.2. If a protective barrier covering is used, the cover should be removed or cleaned and disinfected per the manufacturer's instructions after each patient use.

II.g. Equipment should be cleaned and disinfected before being brought into the semi-restricted area. *[5: No Evidence]*

Equipment may harbor dust and microorganisms that can contaminate the OR environment.

II.h. Mattresses and padded positioning device surfaces (eg, OR beds, arm boards, patient transport carts) should be moisture-resistant and intact.[14] *[1: Strong Evidence]*

Absorbent or nonintact surfaces may become reservoirs for microorganisms and may harbor pathogens.

II.h.1. Damaged or worn coverings should be replaced.[14]

II.h.2. Penetration of the mattress cover by needles and other sharp items should be avoided.[14]

II.i. Cleaning equipment should be disassembled according to manufacturers' instructions for use, cleaned, disinfected with an EPA-registered disinfectant, and dried before storage and reuse.[14] *[1: Strong Evidence]*

Cleaning the equipment prevents the growth of microorganisms during storage and prevents subsequent contamination of the perioperative area.[14]

II.j. Measures should be taken to prevent vermin infestation of the perioperative environment.[14] These measures should include removing food sources or environmental factors that attract pests and keeping windows and doors closed. *[1: Strong Evidence]*

Vermin may cause disease and microorganism transmission by serving as a vector.[14,32-38] Insects in health care settings have been shown to carry more pathogens than insects in residential settings. Pathogens isolated from insects in health care settings also have been shown to have antibiotic resistance.[14]

II.j.1. If preventive measures fail, a credentialed pest control specialist should be contracted to eliminate the cause of the infestation.

II.j.2. After an infestation is resolved, the area should be terminally cleaned. (See Recommendation V.)

Recommendation III

A clean environment should be reestablished after the patient is transferred from the area.[14,15,39,40]

Reestablishing a clean environment after the patient leaves the area decreases the risk of cross-contamination and disease transmission. Environmental cleaning has been associated with a decreased risk of the patient acquiring MRSA or vancomycin-resistant enterococci (VRE) when the previous room occupant was infected or colonized with one of these MDROs.[23] In an observational study, Morgan et al demonstrated that contamination of health care workers' clothing, gloves, and gowns with MDROs was mainly attributed to contact with contaminated environmental surfaces.[25]

III.a. Reusable noncritical, nonporous surfaces such as mattress covers, pneumatic tourniquet cuffs, blood pressure cuffs, and other patient equipment should be cleaned and disinfected according to manufacturers' instructions after each patient use.[14] *[1: Strong Evidence]*

The CDC recommends low-level disinfection of noncritical patient care items.[14]

III.a.1. Single-use items should be discarded after each patient use.

III.b. Cleaning of high-touch objects after each patient use should include cleaning of any soiled surface of the item and any frequently touched areas of the item (eg, control panel, switches, knobs, work area, handles).[14] *[1: Strong Evidence]*

Contamination of environmental surfaces that are touched frequently provides a risk for hands to acquire pathogens, which could be transmitted to patients.[2,20]

III.c. Operating and procedure rooms must be cleaned after each patient.[14,39,40] (Figure 1) *[1: Regulatory Requirement]*

III.c.1. Environmental cleaning, including trash and contaminated laundry removal, should not begin until the patient has left the area.

III.c.2. Trash and used linen should be removed from the room.[15] (See Recommendation VI.)

ENVIRONMENTAL CLEANING

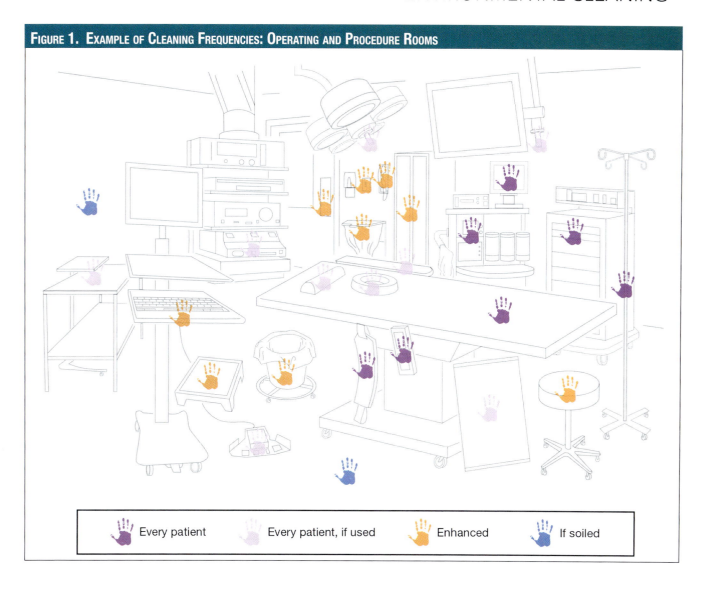

FIGURE 1. EXAMPLE OF CLEANING FREQUENCIES: OPERATING AND PROCEDURE ROOMS

Every patient | Every patient, if used | Enhanced | If soiled

III.c.3. Items that are used during patient care should be cleaned and disinfected after each patient use, including
- anesthesia carts and equipment (eg, IV poles, IV pumps)[1,15];
- anesthesia machines[1,7,41];
- patient monitors[42];
- OR beds[1,14,15]; and
- reusable table straps.[5,15]

III.c.4. Items that are used during a surgical or invasive procedure should be cleaned and disinfected, including
- OR bed attachments (eg, arm boards, stirrups, head rests)[1,15];
- positioning devices (eg, viscoelastic polymer rolls, vacuum pack positioning devices);
- patient transfer devices (eg, roll boards)[43];
- overhead procedure lights[1,5,7,15];
- tables and Mayo stands[1,15]; and
- mobile and fixed equipment (eg, suction regulators, medical gas regulators, imaging viewers, viewing monitors, radiology equipment, electrosurgical units, microscopes, robots, lasers).[7,15]

III.c.5. The floors and walls of operating and procedure rooms should be cleaned and disinfected after each surgical or invasive procedure if soiled or potentially soiled (eg, by splash, splatter, or spray).[1,14,15,18,31]

III.d. Preoperative and postoperative patient care areas must be cleaned after each patient has left the area.[14,15,39,40] (Figure 2) *[1: Regulatory Requirement]*

III.d.1. Items that are used during patient care should be cleaned and disinfected after every patient use, including
- patient monitors,[42]
- patient beds,[2,42,44-48]
- over-bed tables,[2,6,42,45-52]
- television remote controls,[45-48,52] and
- call lights.[2,6,44,49,50]

III.d.2. Mobile and fixed equipment (eg, suction regulators, medical gas regulators, imaging

ENVIRONMENTAL CLEANING

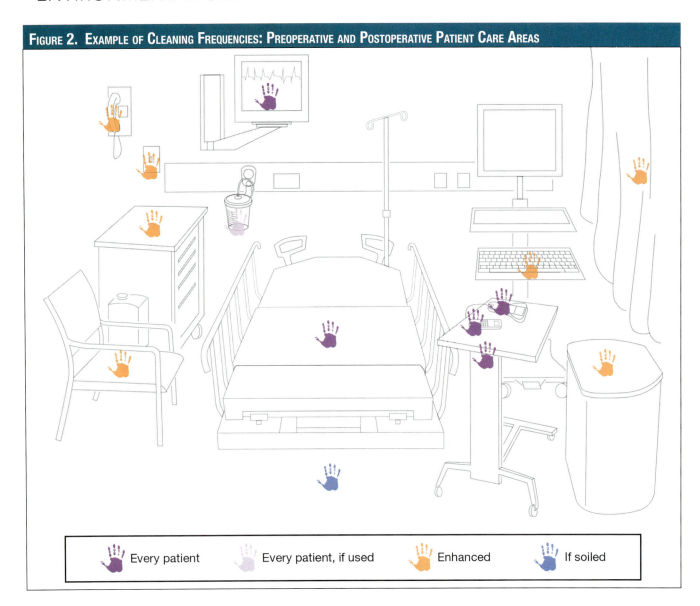

FIGURE 2. EXAMPLE OF CLEANING FREQUENCIES: PREOPERATIVE AND POSTOPERATIVE PATIENT CARE AREAS

Every patient | Every patient, if used | Enhanced | If soiled

viewers, radiology equipment, warming equipment) that is used during patient care should be cleaned and disinfected after each patient use.[7,15]

III.d.3. Preoperative and postoperative patient care area floors and walls should be cleaned after each patient has left the area, if soiled or potentially soiled (eg, by splash, splatter, or spray) during patient care.[1,14,15,18,31,42]

III.e. Patient transport vehicles including the straps, handles, side rails, and attachments should be cleaned and disinfected after each patient use.[14] *[1: Strong Evidence]*

The CDC recommends that noncritical surfaces be cleaned and disinfected after each use.[14,30]

III.e.1. Single-use straps should be discarded after one use according to the manufacturer's instructions.

Recommendation IV

Perioperative areas should be terminally cleaned.

Terminal cleaning and disinfection of the perioperative environment decreases the number of pathogens and the amount of dust and debris.[29] The CDC recommends that floors in the OR be wet vacuumed or mopped after the last procedure of the day or night.[14,29] The Centers for Medicare & Medicaid Services (CMS) states that surveyors should inspect inpatient and outpatient operative rooms and suites at participating hospitals and ambulatory surgery centers to observe that "appropriate terminal cleaning [is] applied," although the procedures and frequencies of appropriate terminal cleaning are not defined.[53,54]

IV.a. Terminal cleaning and disinfection of perioperative areas, including sterile processing areas, should be performed daily when the areas are being used.[14,29,55] *[1: Strong Evidence]*

ENVIRONMENTAL CLEANING

The Association for the Advancement of Medical Instrumentation recommends that floors and horizontal work surfaces in sterile processing areas be cleaned daily.[55] However, neither the CMS nor the CDC provides guidance for the time frame required for terminal cleaning frequencies in perioperative areas. The literature search did not reveal any studies related to the optimal frequency of terminal cleaning.

IV.a.1. For terminal cleaning in semi-restricted and restricted areas (eg, operating or procedure rooms, sterile processing areas, corridors, storage areas), a multidisciplinary team should determine the frequency and extent of cleaning required when areas are not occupied (eg, unused rooms, weekends).
- If the area is closed with no personnel present, the team may determine that terminal cleaning is unnecessary.
- If perioperative team members are present in the area briefly, the team may determine that the area may only need damp dusting on horizontal surfaces.
- If perioperative team members are present in the area for an extended period or are performing patient care activities, the team may determine that thorough terminal cleaning of the area is necessary.

The presence of personnel generates dust from shedding skin squames, which can harbor bacteria.[14,20,56] However, further evidence is needed to determine ideal terminal cleaning frequencies and the extent of cleaning required in perioperative areas.

IV.b. All floors in the perioperative and sterile processing areas should be disinfected.[14,15] *[1: Strong Evidence]*

Floor cleaning procedures and frequencies were identified as a gap in the literature during the evidence review, although guidance is provided by the CDC Healthcare Infection Control Practices Advisory Committee and the Association for the Healthcare Environment.[14,15] Additional research is needed in perioperative areas to define the role of the floor in disease transmission and recommendations for cleaning procedures and frequencies.

IV.b.1. Floors may be terminally cleaned with either a wet vacuum or a single-use mop and a disinfectant.[14,15] The floor should be wet with the disinfectant for the dwell time indicated on the manufacturer's instructions for use.[15]

IV.b.2. Cleaning should progress from the cleanest to dirtiest areas of the floor.

IV.b.3. Floor surfaces at the perimeter of the room should be disinfected before floor surfaces in the center of the room.

The center of the room, where the majority of patient care occurs, is most likely to be have higher levels of contamination.

IV.b.4. The entire floor surface should be disinfected, including areas under the OR bed and mobile equipment.

IV.c. Terminal cleaning of operating and procedure rooms should include cleaning and disinfecting of all exposed surfaces, including wheels and casters, of all items, including
- anesthesia carts and equipment (eg, IV poles, IV pumps)[1,15];
- anesthesia machines[1,7,41];
- patient monitors[42];
- OR beds[1,14,15];
- reusable table straps[5,15];
- OR bed attachments (eg, arm boards, stirrups, head rests)[1,15];
- positioning devices (eg, viscoelastic polymer rolls, vacuum pack positioning devices);
- patient transfer devices (eg, roll boards)[43];
- overhead procedure lights[1,5,7,15];
- tables and Mayo stands[1,15];
- mobile and fixed equipment (eg, suction regulators, medical gas regulators, imaging viewers, viewing monitors, radiology equipment, electrosurgical units, microscopes, robots, lasers)[7,15];
- storage cabinets, supply carts, and furniture[7,15];
- light switches[5,7,15];
- door handles and push plates[5,7,15,57];
- telephones and mobile communication devices[5,15,58];
- computer accessories (eg, keyboard, mouse, touch screen)[1,51,59];
- chairs, stools, and step stools[15]; and
- trash and linen receptacles.[7,14,15,29] *[1: Strong Evidence]*

IV.d. Terminal cleaning of preoperative and postoperative patient care areas should include cleaning and disinfecting all exposed surfaces, including wheels and casters, of all items, including
- patient monitors[42];
- patient beds[2,42,44-48];
- over-bed table[2,6,42,45-52];
- television remote controls[45-48,52];
- call lights[2,6,44,49,50];
- mobile and fixed equipment (eg, suction regulators, medical gas regulators, imaging viewers, radiology equipment, warming equipment)[7,15];
- storage cabinets, supply carts, and furniture[7,15];
- light switches[5,7,15];
- door handles and push plates[5,7,15,57];
- telephones and mobile communication devices[5,15,58];
- computer accessories (eg, keyboard, mouse, touch screen)[1,51,59];
- chairs and stools[15]; and
- trash and linen receptacles.[14,15,60,61] *[1: Strong Evidence]*

ENVIRONMENTAL CLEANING

IV.e. Sterile processing areas should be terminally cleaned.[55] *[3: Limited Evidence]*

Sterile processing personnel conduct critical processes, such as decontaminating, assembling, and sterilizing surgical instrumentation, in support of operating and invasive procedure rooms. As such, the recommendations for terminal cleaning apply in sterile processing areas as in areas where surgical and other invasive procedures are performed. Furthermore, sterile processing areas where decontamination occurs have some of the highest risks for environmental contamination of all perioperative areas. Environmental cleaning in sterile processing areas is critical for reducing the risk of disease transmission from reservoirs of bloodborne pathogens and microorganisms in the decontamination environment.

IV.e.1. During cleaning of sterile processing areas, the clean work areas, such as the packaging area and sterile storage area, should be cleaned before the dirty work areas, such as the decontamination area, to reduce the possibility of contaminating the clean areas.[55]

IV.e.2. All horizontal surfaces (eg, sterilizers, countertops, furniture, shelving) should be damp dusted daily with an EPA-registered disinfectant and a clean, low-linting cloth.[55]

IV.e.3. All work surfaces and high-touch objects should be cleaned with an EPA-registered disinfectant and a clean, low-linting cloth.[55]

IV.e.4. Trash should be removed from receptacles in sterile processing areas when they are full, but at least daily.[55]

IV.e.5. Terminal cleaning should not commence when personnel are actively decontaminating instruments.

IV.f. A multidisciplinary team may choose to evaluate emerging technologies for room decontamination (eg, ozone, peroxide vapor,[62-67] ultraviolet light,[42,48,68-70] saturated steam[71]) as adjuncts to terminal cleaning procedures.[20] (See Recommendation I.) *[2: Moderate Evidence]*

Barbut et al demonstrated in a randomized controlled trial that a hydrogen peroxide mist system was significantly more effective than 0.5% sodium hypochlorite solution at eradicating *C difficile* spores in patient rooms at two French hospitals.[62] Bartels et al used a dry-mist hydrogen peroxide and silver ion vapor to decrease environmental contamination in intensive care unit (ICU) settings as an adjunct to terminal cleaning procedures, but did not find sustained lowering of contamination in ICUs with a MRSA epidemic.[63] Boyce et al found that a hydrogen peroxide vapor effectively eradicated *C difficile* spores from contaminated surfaces in patient rooms.[64] Chan et al used hydrogen peroxide vapor to effectively decontaminate ward rooms in an Australian hospital.[65] Manian et al reported that hydrogen peroxide vapor, in addition to a round of cleaning and disinfection, effectively reduced the number of persistently contaminated room sites in hospital rooms contaminated with MRSA.[66] Passaretti et al found a reduction of patient acquisition of MDROs when a hydrogen peroxide vapor system was used as part of room cleaning procedures.[67]

In a prospective cohort study by Anderson et al, the researchers found a significant decrease in environmental contamination of VRE, *C difficile*, and *Acinetobacter* spp in patient rooms after exposure to an automated ultraviolet (UV)-C emitter.[68] Boyce et al found that use of a mobile UV-C light in conjunction with routine terminal cleaning procedures significantly reduced colony counts and *C difficile* spores on five high-touch surfaces in patient rooms.[48] Nerandzic et al reported that a novel automated UV-C emitting device significantly reduced hospital surface contamination of *C difficile*, MRSA, and VRE.[69] Rutala et al determined that a UV-C emitting device effectively eliminated vegetative bacteria from contaminated surfaces within approximately 15 minutes and eliminated *C difficile* spores within 50 minutes.[42] Umezawa et al reported that a portable pulsed UV device was practical for daily disinfection of housekeeping surfaces and decreased the labor burden.[70]

Sexton et al showed that a portable steam vapor system effectively reduced microbial contamination of high-touch objects in patient rooms.[71]

Use of emerging technologies may enhance environmental cleanliness, although additional clinical studies are needed to determine their applicability in the perioperative setting.[72]

Recommendation V

All areas and equipment that are not terminally cleaned should be cleaned according to an established schedule.

A clean environment will reduce the number of microorganisms present.

V.a. A multidisciplinary team should establish a cleaning schedule for perioperative areas and equipment that should be cleaned on a regular (eg, weekly, monthly) basis.[14,15] (See Recommendation I.) *[1: Strong Evidence]*

Areas and equipment that are not cleaned according to a schedule may be missed during routine cleaning procedures and become environmental reservoirs for dust, debris, and microorganisms.

V.a.1. Areas and items that should be cleaned on a schedule include
- clean and soiled storage areas;
- sterile storage areas;

- shelving and storage bins;
- corridors, including stairwells and elevators;
- walls and ceilings;
- privacy curtains;
- pneumatic tubes and carriers;
- sterilizers and loading carts;
- sterilizer service access rooms;
- unrestricted areas (eg, lounges, waiting rooms, offices); and
- environmental services closets.

V.b. Ventilation ducts, including air vents and grilles, should be cleaned and have their filters changed on a routine basis according to manufacturers' instructions for use.[14] *[1: Strong Evidence]*

Clean ventilation ducts and filters support optimal performance of the ventilation system.

V.c. Linen chutes in the perioperative environment should be cleaned and disinfected on a routine basis.[14] *[1: Strong Evidence]*

Linen chutes become contaminated by dirt and debris with use.

V.d. All refrigerators and ice machines in perioperative patient care areas should be cleaned and disinfected on a routine basis according to manufacturers' instructions for use.[14] *[1: Strong Evidence]*

Refrigerators and ice machines become contaminated with use.

V.e. Sinks and wash basins, including eye wash stations, should be cleaned and disinfected on a routine basis.[14] *[1: Strong Evidence]*

V.e.1. Aerators on faucets should be cleaned and disinfected.

Recommendation VI

All personnel should take precautionary measures to limit transmission of microorganisms when performing environmental cleaning and handling waste materials.

The Occupational Safety and Health Administration (OSHA) regulates the implementation of the bloodborne pathogens standard to protect health care workers from exposure to bloodborne pathogens.[73] Because of the increased risk for exposure to bloodborne pathogens during cleaning procedures in the perioperative practice setting, personnel must comply with the bloodborne pathogens standard to protect themselves, their colleagues, and patients from exposure to blood, body fluids, and other potentially infectious materials.

VI.a. Health care personnel who are cleaning must follow standard precautions to prevent contact with blood, body fluids, or other potentially infectious materials.[11,73] *[1: Regulatory Requirement]*

All body fluids except sweat (eg, semen, vaginal secretions, cerebrospinal fluid, synovial fluid, pleural fluid, pericardial fluid, peritoneal fluid, amniotic fluid, saliva) are potentially infectious.[73]

VI.a.1. Health care personnel handling contaminated items or cleaning contaminated surfaces must wear personal protective equipment (PPE) to reduce the risk of exposure to blood, body fluids, and other potentially infectious materials.[14,73]

VI.a.2. Personnel must wear gloves when it is reasonably anticipated that they may have contact with blood, body fluids, or other potentially infectious materials while handling or touching contaminated items or surfaces.[73]

VI.a.3. Personnel must wear masks, eye protection, and face shields whenever contact with splashes, spray, splatter, or droplets of blood, body fluids, or other potentially infectious materials is anticipated.[73]

VI.a.4. If cleaning procedures are expected to generate infectious aerosols, personnel should wear proper respiratory protection (ie, an N95 respirator, a powered air-purifying respirator).[14]

VI.a.5. Hand hygiene should be performed when PPE is removed and as soon as possible after hands are soiled.[9]

VI.b. Cleaning and disinfection activities should be performed in a methodical pattern that limits the transmission of microorganisms.[15,74] *[3: Limited Evidence]*

Cleaning an area in a methodical pattern establishes a routine for cleaning so that items are not missed during the cleaning process.[15] The method for cleaning may limit the transmission of microorganisms to reduce the risk of cross contamination of environmental surfaces.[74]

In an observational study, Bergen et al evaluated the spread of bacteria on surfaces when cleaning with microfiber cloths in a 16-side method and found that although bacterial counts (*Enterococcus faecalis, Bacillus cereus*) were decreased after cleaning, the bacteria from contaminated surfaces were spread to clean surfaces.[74] Additional research is needed to determine optimal cleaning methods for the perioperative setting and to evaluate the risk for microbial transmission across environmental surfaces during cleaning and disinfection activities.

VI.b.1. Cleaning should progress from clean to dirty areas.[15,74]

VI.b.2. Cleaning should progress from top to bottom areas.[15]

During cleaning of top areas, dust, debris, and contaminated cleaning solutions may contaminate bottom areas. If bottom areas are cleaned first, these areas could

ENVIRONMENTAL CLEANING

potentially be recontaminated with debris from the top areas.[15]

VI.b.3. Clockwise or counter-clockwise cleaning may be performed when used in conjunction with clean-to-dirty and top-to-bottom methods.[15]

VI.c. When visible soiling by blood, body fluids, or other potentially infectious materials appears on surfaces or equipment, the area must be cleaned and disinfected as soon as possible.[14,73] The responsibility for verifying disinfection of a contaminated surface rests with the perioperative team member who is aware of the contamination. *[1: Regulatory Requirement]*

Soil on environmental surfaces increases the risk of cross-contamination and is more difficult to remove the longer it remains on the surface.

VI.c.1. If perioperative team members are performing critical patient care activities when the contamination occurs, the contaminated surface should be cleaned as soon as a perioperative team member is available.

VI.c.2. Spills that contain blood, body fluids, or other potentially infectious materials must be removed with an absorbent material as soon as possible, and then the area must be cleaned and disinfected.[14,73] *[1: Regulatory Requirement]*

VI.c.3. If the spill involves a large amount of blood, a 1:10 dilution of sodium hypochlorite solution (5,000 ppm to 6,150 ppm available chlorine), preferably an EPA-registered product, should be applied to the spill before cleaning when feasible.[14]

VI.d. Items that are contaminated with blood or tissue and that would release blood, body fluids, or other potentially infectious materials in a liquid or semi-liquid state if compressed, and items that are caked with dried blood, body fluids, or other potentially infectious materials must be placed in closable, leak-proof containers or bags that are color coded, labeled, or tagged for easy identification as biohazardous waste.[73] *[1: Regulatory Requirement]*

Leak-proof containers prevent exposure of personnel to blood, body fluids, and other potentially infectious materials and prevent contamination of the environment. Color coding and/or labeling alert personnel and others to the presence of items potentially contaminated with infectious microorganisms, prevent exposure of personnel to infectious waste, and prevent contamination of the environment.[73]

VI.d.1. Single-use items that do not release blood, body fluids, or other potentially infectious materials in a liquid or semi-liquid state if compressed and that are not caked with dried blood, body fluids, or other potentially infectious materials are considered noninfectious and should be placed in a separate receptacle designated for noninfectious waste.[73]

VI.d.2. Waste generated during care of patients on isolation precautions should be managed with the same methods as waste in other patient care areas.[14,75]

VI.e. Contaminated sharps (eg, needles, blades, sharp disposable instruments) must be discarded immediately in a closeable, puncture-resistant container that is leakproof on its sides and bottom and is labeled or color coded.[14,73] *[1: Regulatory Requirement]*

VI.e.1. Sharps containers should be replaced routinely and not overfilled.[73]

VI.e.2. Broken glassware must not be handled with unprotected hands.[73]

VI.f. Contaminated liquid waste must be disposed of according to state and federal regulations (eg, by adding a solidifying powder to the liquid, using a medical liquid waste disposal system, pouring the liquid down a sanitary sewer).[14] *[1: Regulatory Requirement]*

VI.g. Laundry contaminated with blood, body fluids, or other potentially infectious materials must be handled as little as possible.[14,73] *[1: Regulatory Requirement]*

Handling contaminated laundry with a minimum of agitation avoids contamination of air, surfaces, and personnel.[14]

VI.g.1. Contaminated laundry must be placed in labeled or color coded containers or bags at the location where it was used.[14,73]

VI.g.2. Contaminated laundry that is wet and may soak or leak through the container or bag must be placed and transported in containers or bags that prevent soak-through or leakage of fluids to the exterior.[14,73]

VI.h. Regulated waste must be stored in a ventilated area that is inaccessible to pests until transported for treatment and disposal according to state and federal regulations.[14] *[1: Regulatory Requirement]*

VI.i. Containers or bags containing regulated medical waste must be transported in closed, impervious containers, according to state and federal regulations.[14] *[1: Regulatory Requirement]*

Recommendation VII

Procedures for environmental cleaning and disinfection should be established for circumstances that may require special cleaning procedures (ie, multidrug-resistant organisms, *C difficile*, prion diseases, construction, environmental contamination).

Some situations require a deviation from routine cleaning procedures. Having cleaning procedures in place

ENVIRONMENTAL CLEANING

for special cleaning situations guides personnel in cleaning the perioperative environment in an efficient and consistent manner in accordance with the health care organization's policies and procedures.

VII.a. Enhanced environmental cleaning procedures, which are intended to decrease environmental contaminates on high-touch surfaces, should be implemented for cleaning following the care of patients who are infected or colonized with MDROs, including
- MRSA,
- VRE,
- Vancomycin-intermediate *Enterococcus* spp,
- Vancomycin-resistant *Staphylococcus aureus*,
- Vancomycin-intermediate *Staphylococcus aureus*,
- Carbapenem-resistant enterobacteriacae,
- Multidrug-resistant *Acinetobacter* spp,
- Extended spectrum beta-lactamase-producing organisms, and
- *Klebsiella pneumoniae* carbapenemase-producing organisms.[22-26,75] (See Recommendation I.) [1: Strong Evidence]

Decreasing environmental contaminates on high-touch surfaces may decrease the risk of MDRO transmission. In a randomized controlled trial, Hess et al evaluated enhanced cleaning procedures in the ICU setting and found that intense cleaning of patient rooms contaminated with identified MRSA or multi-drug-resistant *Acinetobacter baumanii* did not significantly decrease contamination of health care workers' gowns and gloves.[26] However, an observational study by Morgan et al found that environmental contamination was the main determinant of transmission of MDROs to health care workers' clothing, gloves, and gowns.[25]

In a quasi-experimental study, Datta et al found that enhanced cleaning may reduce MRSA and VRE contamination and decrease the risk of transmission from the room's previous occupant.[23]

VII.a.1. All high-touch objects, in addition to objects cleaned as part of routine cleaning, should be cleaned and disinfected as part of enhanced environmental cleaning procedures after the patient leaves the room or area (ie, bay), including
- storage cabinets, supply carts, and furniture[7,15];
- light switches[5,7,15];
- door handles and push plates[5,7,15,57];
- telephones and mobile communication devices[5,15,58];
- computer accessories (eg, keyboard, mouse, touch screen)[1,51,59];
- chairs, stools, and step stools[15];
- trash and linen receptacles[15]; and
- privacy curtains in the perioperative patient care areas.[60,61]

VII.a.2. In addition to standard precautions, perioperative personnel should wear gowns and gloves when performing enhanced environmental cleaning procedures.[11,14]

VII.b. An EPA-registered disinfectant that is effective against *C difficile* spores should be used during cleaning following the care of patients diagnosed with or suspected of infection with *C difficile*.[11,14,30] [1: Strong Evidence]

C difficile presents unique challenges for environmental cleaning. In its spore form, *C difficile* can survive for prolonged periods of time, up to five months, on environmental surfaces. *C difficile* spores also are resistant to several cleaning chemicals (eg, alcohols, phenols, quaternary ammonium compounds).[51] Selection of a cleaning chemical that is effective against *C difficile* spores and removal of the spores from environmental surfaces are crucial when disinfecting a surface contaminated with *C difficile*. Thorough cleaning of environmental surfaces using a chemical that effectively kills *C difficile* spores remains a foundational requirement for preventing the transmission of *C difficile* infection and colonization.[2,51,62,64,76-79]

VII.c. Room access should be restricted following the care of patients diagnosed with or suspected of infection with an airborne transmissible disease (eg, tuberculosis) and following aerosolization activities (eg, intubation, extubation, cough-generating activities) of a droplet transmissible disease (eg, influenza) until adequate time has passed for air exchanges per hour to clean 99% of airborne particles from the air (eg, 15 air exchanges per hour for 28 minutes to remove 99.9% of airborne contaminants).[11,14,80] [1: Strong Evidence]

Patients and personnel entering a room that has transmissible disease particles in the air are at risk for contracting the disease.[11]

VII.c.1. Personnel entering the room before a complete air exchange occurs must wear respiratory protection (eg, an N95 respirator).[11]

VII.c.2. After the air has exchanged by 99%, personnel may proceed with environmental cleaning without respiratory protection.

VII.d. Special cleaning procedures should be used if environmental contamination with high-risk tissue (ie, brain, spinal cord, eye tissue) from a patient who is diagnosed with or suspected of having Creutzfeldt-Jakob disease (CJD) occurs. If the environment is not contaminated with high-risk tissue, routine cleaning procedures should be used.[14,30,81] [1: Strong Evidence]

Currently, no EPA-registered disinfectants claim to inactivate prions on environmental surfaces.[81] When the environment is contaminated

ENVIRONMENTAL CLEANING

with tissue that is high risk for containing prions, the causative infectious agent in CJD, extraordinary cleaning procedures are necessary in accordance with recommendations from the CDC and the Society for Healthcare Epidemiology of America.[14,30,81]

VII.d.1. Before the operative or invasive procedure begins, personnel should cover work surfaces with a disposable, impervious material that can be removed and decontaminated after the procedure if contaminated with high risk tissue.[14,81]

Covering environmental surfaces minimizes contamination of the environment.

VII.d.2. If not contaminated with high-risk tissue, linens may be laundered in accordance with routine laundering processes when the patient is suspected of having CJD.[81]

VII.d.3. Noncritical environmental surfaces contaminated with high-risk tissues should be cleaned with a detergent and then decontaminated with a solution of either sodium hypochlorite (1:5 to 1:10 dilution with 10,000 ppm to 20,000 ppm available chlorine) or sodium hydroxide (1N NaOH), depending on surface compatibility.[14,81]

No transmissions of prion diseases from environmental surfaces have been reported; however, it remains prudent to eliminate highly infectious material from OR surfaces that will be contacted during subsequent surgeries.[14,30,81]

VII.d.4. Cleaning and disinfection of surfaces contaminated with high-risk tissues should be performed in the following order:
1. Remove the gross tissue from the surface.
2. Clean the area with a detergent solution.[81]
3. Apply the disinfectant solution for a contact time of 30 minutes to one hour.[14]
4. Use an absorbent material to soak up the solution.
5. Discard the cleaning material in an appropriate waste container.
6. Rinse the treated surface thoroughly with water.

VII.d.5. Standard cleaning procedures should be used to disinfect surfaces that are not contaminated with high-risk tissue.[81]

VII.d.6. Regulated medical waste generated during patient care, including waste contaminated by high-risk tissue that is decontaminated, should be managed in accordance with standard waste management procedures per local, state, and federal regulations.[14]

No epidemiological evidence has linked CJD transmission to waste disposal practices.[14]

VII.e. Cleaning and disinfection procedures should be implemented for construction, renovation, repair, demolition, and disaster remediation.[14] *[1: Strong Evidence]*

According to the CDC, cleaning and disinfection measures during internal and external construction projects reduce contamination of environmental air and surfaces with dust and potential pathogens, such as *Aspergillus* and *Bacillus*, and are key elements of an infection prevention program.[14] Several reports have linked environmental air and surface contamination from construction projects to outbreaks of infection in the health care setting.[82-85]

VII.e.1. Cleaning and disinfection of environmental surfaces should be performed to remove dust and debris caused by construction, renovation, remediation, repair, or demolition.[14,85] If dust is contaminating areas outside of the construction barriers, the barriers should be assessed to determine their effectiveness and reestablished.

While investigating an outbreak of deep bacterial eye infections, Gibb et al reported that fine dust from a construction project was found on horizontal surfaces in the OR. After the ORs were cleaned of dust and reopened, no additional eye infections were reported during the surveillance period.[85]

VII.e.2. Terminal cleaning should be performed before equipment and supplies are placed in the area where the construction, renovation, repair, demolition, or disaster remediation has been completed.[14] (See Recommendation IV.)

VII.e.3. A cleaning and disinfection process should be implemented when environmental contamination occurs.[14]

VII.e.4. If flooding or a water-related emergency occurs, including sewage intrusion, terminal cleaning of the affected areas should be performed after the water is removed; the area is inspected for water damage according to local, state, and federal regulations; and remediation for identified water damage is completed.[14] (See Recommendation IV.)
- When hard surfaces remain in good repair, these areas should be allowed to dry for 72 hours prior to cleaning.[14]
- If items cannot be thoroughly cleaned and dried within 72 hours, the surface should be replaced with new materials after the facility engineer determines that the underlying structure is dry.[14]

VII.e.5. When condensation is observed on surfaces in the semi-restricted and restricted areas, terminal cleaning of the affected areas should be performed. (See Recommendation IV.) *[5: No Evidence]*

VII.e.6. When contamination of the air occurs, terminal cleaning of the affected areas, including ventilation ducts, air vent, and grilles, should be performed and air filters should be changed after the source of the contamination is identified and contained.[82] *[2: Moderate Evidence]*

Recommendation VIII

Perioperative and environmental services personnel should receive initial and ongoing education and competency verification on their understanding of the principles and the performance of the processes for environmental cleaning in perioperative areas.[86]

Health care organizations are responsible for providing initial and ongoing education and evaluating the competency of perioperative and environmental services personnel on the principles of and the performance of environmental cleaning.

Initial and ongoing education of perioperative and environmental services personnel on the principles of and the performance of environmental cleaning facilitates the development of knowledge, skills, and attitudes that affect safe patient care. Ongoing development of knowledge and skills and documentation of personnel participation is a regulatory and accreditation requirement for both hospitals and ambulatory settings.[53,54,87-90]

Periodic education programs provide the opportunity to reinforce the principles and processes of environmental cleaning and to introduce relevant new equipment or practices.

Competency assessment measures individual performance, provides a mechanism for documentation, and verifies that perioperative personnel have an understanding of facility policies and potential environmental hazards to patients and personnel. Every nurse is personally accountable for maintaining competency.[28,91]

There are no universally accepted or mandated ways to perform or verify competency, and strategies to accomplish this differ among states. The goal of competency verification is to reassure the public that nurses have the knowledge, skills, and judgment to provide safe and effective care.[92]

VIII.a. Perioperative and environmental services personnel must receive education and complete competency verification activities that address specialized knowledge and skills related to the principles and processes of environmental cleaning.[39,40] *[1: Regulatory Requirement]*

Hota et al found that surface contamination with VRE was related to a failure to clean rather than failure of a product or cleaning procedure; cleaning thoroughness and site contamination improved significantly after implementation of an education program for housekeeping personnel.[93]

In a literature review, Dancer found that cleaning processes were often no more than a "perfunctory introduction to the cleaning process" and that a lack of understanding of the basic microbiologic principles underlying cleaning processes can allow potential reservoirs of pathogens in the environment to go unrecognized.[20] Dancer further described the consequences of limited training in environmental cleaning, such as improper maintenance of cleaning equipment, inappropriate use of cleaning chemicals, and exposure of the patient to contaminated surfaces.[20]

VIII.a.1. Education and competency verification should include topics related to the principles and processes of environmental cleaning, including
- basic principles of microbiology[20];
- explanation of signs and labels and/or color coding required for contaminated items;
- an explanation of the modes of transmission of bloodborne pathogens and an explanation of the employer's exposure control plan[73];
- an explanation of the use and limitation of methods for reducing the exposure (eg, engineering controls, work practices, PPE)[73];
- information on the hepatitis B vaccine, its efficacy and safety, the method of administration, and the benefits of vaccination[73];
- location and use of eye wash stations[10];
- information on the types, proper selection, proper use, location, removal, handling, decontamination, and disposal of PPE[11,73];
- location of safety data sheets[10];
- hazardous and medical waste disposal[10];
- handling of hazardous chemicals[10];
- review of the organization's policies and procedures;
- selection of cleaning chemicals, materials, and equipment based on the intended use; and
- access to manufacturers' instructions for cleaning and disinfection.[14]

VIII.a.2. Educational materials should be appropriate in content, vocabulary level, literacy, and language for the target personnel.[73]

VIII.a.3. Continuing education should be provided when new equipment or processes are introduced.

VIII.b. Personnel who are occupationally exposed to blood, body fluids, or other potentially infectious materials must receive training before assignments to tasks where occupational exposure may occur, at least annually, and when changes to procedures or tasks effect occupational exposure.[73] *[1: Regulatory Requirement]*

ENVIRONMENTAL CLEANING

Employers are required by OSHA to provide training on the bloodborne pathogens standard during working hours at no cost to employees.[73]

VIII.c. Perioperative and environmental services personnel should receive education that addresses human factors related to the principles and processes of environmental cleaning.[94,95] *[2: Moderate Evidence]*

Human factors include the interpersonal and social aspects of the perioperative environment (eg, coordination of activities, teamwork, collaboration, communication). Effectively implementing the principles and processes of environmental cleaning requires that perioperative and environmental services personnel demonstrate not only procedural knowledge and technical proficiency but also the ability to anticipate needs, coordinate multiple activities, work collaboratively with other team members, and communicate effectively.

Matlow et al conducted focus groups and administered questionnaires to evaluate ICU environmental service workers' attitudes and beliefs and intent about their jobs and found that the environmental services workers' attitudes and beliefs may affect intent and effectiveness of their cleaning practices.[95]

Recommendation IX

Policies and procedures for environmental cleaning processes and practices should be developed, reviewed periodically, revised as necessary, and readily available in the practice setting.

Policies and procedures assist in the development of patient and workplace safety, quality assessment, and performance improvement activities. Policies and procedures establish authority, responsibility, and accountability within the facility. Policies and procedures also serve as operational guidelines that are used to minimize patient and health care worker risks, standardize practice, and direct perioperative personnel.

IX.a. Policies and procedures for the implementation of environmental cleaning must be developed. *[1: Regulatory Requirement]*

Policies and procedures that guide and support patient care, treatment, and services are regulatory and accreditation requirements for both hospitals and ambulatory settings.[39,40,89,96-98]

IX.a.1. Policies and procedures regarding the principles and processes of environmental cleaning should include
- standard cleaning and disinfection procedures[14,30];
- frequency of cleaning and disinfection[99];
- identification of responsible personnel[20,100,101];
- cleaning chemicals, materials, and equipment approved for use[14,30];
- preparation, handling, storage, and disposal of cleaning chemicals;
- required PPE[11,14,30,73];
- enhanced cleaning procedures; and
- special cleaning and disinfection procedures for MDROs, *C difficile*, prion diseases, construction, and environmental contamination.[11,14,30]

IX.b. Policies and procedures designed to minimize or eliminate exposure of health care personnel to blood, body fluids, and other potentially infectious materials must be developed and implemented.[73] *[1: Regulatory Requirement]*

A written bloodborne pathogens exposure plan consistent with federal, state, and local rules and regulations that is readily available in the practice setting promotes safety.[73]

IX.c. Policies and procedures must include processes for initial education, training, ongoing competency verification, and annual review for issues related to environmental cleaning. *[1: Regulatory Requirement]*

Policies and procedures assist in the development of activities that support patient safety, quality assessment, and the establishment of guidelines for continuous performance improvement.[39,40,89,96-98]

Recommendation X

Perioperative personnel should participate in a variety of quality assurance and performance improvement activities that are consistent with the health care organization's plan to improve understanding of and compliance with the principles and processes of environmental cleaning.

Quality assurance and performance improvement programs assist in evaluating worker safety and formulating plans for corrective actions. These programs provide data that may be used to determine whether an individual organization is within benchmark goals and, if not, identify areas that may require corrective actions. These programs also may provide ongoing feedback regarding whether problems are improving, stabilizing, or worsening.

X.a. Process monitoring must be a part of every perioperative setting as part of an overall environmental cleaning program.[39,40,89,96-98] Process monitoring should include
- compliance with regulatory standards[39,40];
- a review of products and manufacturers' instructions for use[14];
- cleaning procedures;
- monitoring cleaning and disinfection practices; and
- reporting and investigation of adverse events (eg, outbreaks, product issues, corrective actions, evaluation). *[1: Regulatory Requirement]*

X.b. Performance improvement should focus on thoroughness of cleaning.[1] *[2: Moderate Evidence]*

In a prospective study conducted at a large teaching hospital affiliated with the University of Miami, Munoz et al used UV markers and cultures of environmental surfaces to evaluate cleaning thoroughness in the OR. The researchers found that improvement in thoroughness of cleaning practices in the OR significantly decreased surface contamination with organisms that are potentially pathogenic.[1]

X.c. Cleaning practices should be measured with qualitative measures[6,7,46,49,50,102] (eg, visual observation of cleaning process, visual inspection of cleanliness, fluorescent marking) and quantitative measures[5,45,100,101,103-105] (eg, culture, adenosine triphosphate [ATP] monitoring).[106-108] Multiple measures should be used as part of a comprehensive assessment of environmental cleaning practices.[6,46,103] *[2: Moderate Evidence]*

Carling and Bartley reported that environmental monitoring programs allow health care organizations to provide measurable, objective data to support proof of a clean environment.[106] The CDC tool kit *Options for Evaluating Environmental Cleaning* describes a multidisciplinary approach to implementing a comprehensive environmental monitoring program that is specific to the level of monitoring desired by the health care organization.[108]

Malik et al found in an observational study that visual inspection of cleanliness was less effective than use of an audit tool for inspecting cleanliness.[102] Jefferson et al used a novel fluorescent technique and found improved thoroughness of daily terminal cleaning in the OR.[7] Boyce et al determined that fluorescent marking is useful for determining the frequency of high-touch surface cleaning during terminal cleaning.[46] Carling et al evaluated environmental hygiene in 27 ICUs and found that an objective fluorescent targeting method and feedback to environmental services personnel led to significant improvements in room cleaning.[49] In 23 acute care hospitals, Carling et al found that use of a novel fluorescent targeting method provided significant opportunity to improve cleaning of high-touch objects in the patient's immediate environment.[50]

Aiken determined in a laboratory study that although there is no ideal method for detecting bacteria on hospital surfaces, the viable count culture technique was the most suitable for detecting *Staphylococcus aureus*.[104] Vande Leest et al used ATP and culture methods to evaluate the effectiveness of cleaning five high-touch locations in ORs at an ambulatory surgery center. These researchers determined that their cleaning practices were effective, and they gained insight into the practical applications of cleaning procedures in the perioperative setting.[5] Boyce et al reported that use of an ATP assay showed suboptimal cleaning practices and improved cleaning of high-touch objects when implemented with an education and feedback program.[45] Sherlock et al found in an observational study that ATP may be useful to assess cleaning efficacy because ATP trends can identify surfaces that need additional cleaning or need to be cleaned more frequently.[105] Dumigan et al used an ATP monitoring system to quantitatively measure cleanliness after delegating cleaning responsibilities and found that the program improved cleanliness across the nursing service.[100] Havill et al also used an ATP monitoring system in combination with aerobic cultures to assess cleaning practices among nurses; the results suggested that periodic education of nurses and monitoring of cleaning practices was warranted.[101]

In a study of 36 acute care hospitals, Carling et al found that cleaning can be significantly improved with a combined approach of a highly objective targeting method, repeat performance feedback to environmental services personnel, and administrative interventions.[6] Al-Hamad and Maxwell reported that combined methods for assessing hospital cleanliness may be useful.[103] Boyce et al found that although fluorescent marking was useful for determining cleaning frequency, this method was not as reliable for detecting surface contamination levels as were quantitative measures.[46]

Data generated by measurement of cleaning practices provides complementary information that can be used to drive process improvement activities, encourage compliance with established cleaning protocols, educate personnel, and verify personnel competency.

X.c.1. Immediate feedback of assessment findings should be provided to perioperative and environmental services personnel when possible.[45,49]

Boyce et al reported in a prospective intervention study conducted at a university-affiliated community teaching hospital that use of an ATP assay showed suboptimal cleaning practices and implementation of an education and feedback program improved cleanliness of high-touch objects in patient rooms. The researchers found that the instant results of the ATP assay were useful in improving cleaning practice.[45]

Carling et al found that repeated performance feedback to environmental services personnel as part of an objective fluorescent targeting method led to significant improvements in ICU room cleaning.[49]

X.d. Completion of terminal and scheduled cleaning procedures should be documented on a checklist or log sheet.[109] *[2: Moderate Evidence]*

ENVIRONMENTAL CLEANING

Checklists that outline the health care organization's cleaning procedures guide cleaning personnel in performing terminal and scheduled cleaning procedures so that items are not missed due to human factors. A checklist or log sheet also facilitates communication between perioperative team members and environmental services personnel that the environment is safe and clean for patients.

Glossary

Clean: The absence of visible dust, soil, debris, blood, or other potentially infectious material.

Disinfection: A process that kills most forms of microorganisms on inanimate surfaces. Disinfection destroys pathogenic organisms (excluding bacterial spores) or their toxins or vectors by direct exposure to chemical or physical means.

Dwell time: The amount of time required for contact of a chemical agent with a surface.

Enhanced environmental cleaning: Environmental cleaning practices implemented to prevent the spread of infections or outbreaks; enhanced cleaning practices promote consistent and standardized cleaning procedures that extend beyond routine cleaning.

Fomite: An inanimate object which, when contaminated with a viable pathogen (eg, bacterium, virus), can transfer the pathogen to a host.

High touch: Frequently touched object or surface.

Low-level disinfection: A process by which most bacteria, some viruses, and some fungi are killed.

Noncritical item: An item or instrument that comes in contact with intact skin, but not with mucous membranes, sterile tissue, or the vascular system.

Noninfectious waste: Materials with no inherent hazards or infectious potential (eg, packaging materials, paper).

Personal protective equipment (PPE): Specialized equipment or clothing for eyes, face, head, body, and extremities; protective clothing; respiratory devices; and protective shields and barriers designed to protect the worker from injury or exposure to a patient's blood, tissue, or body fluids. Used by health care workers and others whenever necessary to protect themselves from the hazards of processes or environments, chemical hazards, or mechanical irritants encountered in a manner capable of causing injury or impairment in the function of any part of the body through absorption, inhalation, or physical contact.

Regulated medical waste: Liquid or semi-liquid blood or other potentially infectious materials, contaminated items that would release blood or other potentially infectious materials in a liquid or semi-liquid state if compressed, items that are caked with dried blood or other potentially infectious materials and are capable of releasing these materials during handling, contaminated sharps, and pathological and microbiological wastes containing blood or other potentially infectious materials.

Standard precautions: The primary strategy for successful infection control and reduction of worker exposure. Precautions used for care of all patients regardless of their diagnosis or presumed infectious status.

Terminal cleaning: Thorough environmental cleaning that is performed at the end of each day when the area is being used.

References

1. Munoz-Price LS, Birnbach DJ, Lubarsky DA, et al. Decreasing operating room environmental pathogen contamination through improved cleaning practice. *Infect Control Hosp Epidemiol.* 2012;33(9):897-904. [IIIA]

2. Dancer SJ. The role of environmental cleaning in the control of hospital-acquired infection. *J Hosp Infect.* 2009;73(4):378-385. [VB]

3. Carling PC, Huang SS. Improving healthcare environmental cleaning and disinfection: current and evolving issues. *Infect Control Hosp Epidemiol.* 2013;34(5):507-513. [VA]

4. Otter JA, Yezli S, French GL. The role played by contaminated surfaces in the transmission of nosocomial pathogens. *Infect Control Hosp Epidemiol.* 2011;32(7):687-699. [VA]

5. Vande Leest L, Kawczynski R, Esser Lipp F, Barrientos R. Identifying potential areas of infectivity on high-touch locations in the OR. *AORN J.* 2012;96(5):507-512. [IIIC]

6. Carling PC, Parry MM, Rupp ME, et al. Improving cleaning of the environment surrounding patients in 36 acute care hospitals. *Infect Control Hosp Epidemiol.* 2008;29(11):1035-1041. [IIIA]

7. Jefferson J, Whelan R, Dick B, Carling P. A novel technique for identifying opportunities to improve environmental hygiene in the operating room. *AORN J.* 2011;93(3):358-364. [IIIB]

8. Donskey CJ. Does improving surface cleaning and disinfection reduce health care-associated infections? *Am J Infect Control.* 2013;41(5 Suppl):S12-S19. [VB]

9. Guideline for hand hygiene. In: *Guidelines for Perioperative Practice.* Denver, CO: AORN, Inc; 2015:31-42. [IVB]

10. Guideline for a safe environment of care, part 1. In: *Guidelines for Perioperative Practice.* Denver, CO: AORN, Inc; 2015:239-263. [IVA]

11. Guideline for prevention of transmissible infections. In: *Guidelines for Perioperative Practice.* Denver, CO: AORN, Inc; 2015:419-451. [IVA]

12. Havill NL. Best practices in disinfection of noncritical surfaces in the health care setting: creating a bundle for success. *Am J Infect Control.* 2013;41(5 Suppl):S26-S30. [VB]

13. Guideline for product selection. In: *Guidelines for Perioperative Practice.* Denver, CO: AORN, Inc; 2015:179-186. [IVB]

14. Sehulster L, Chinn RY; CDC, HICPAC. Guidelines for environmental infection control in health-care facilities. Recommendations of CDC and the Healthcare Infection Control Practices Advisory Committee (HICPAC). *MMWR Recomm Rep.* 2003;52(RR-10):1-42. [IVA]

15. *Practice Guidance for Healthcare Environmental Cleaning.* 2nd ed. Chicago, IL: Association for the Healthcare Environment; 2012. [IVC]

16. Arif AA, Delclos GL. Association between cleaning-related chemicals and work-related asthma and asthma symptoms among healthcare professionals. *Occup Environ Med.* 2012;69(1):35-40. [IIIB]

17. Bello A, Quinn MM, Perry MJ, Milton DK. Characterization of occupational exposures to cleaning products

used for common cleaning tasks—a pilot study of hospital cleaners. *Environ Health*. 2009;8:11. [IIIB]

18. Rutala WA, Gergen MF, Weber DJ. Microbiologic evaluation of microfiber mops for surface disinfection. *Am J Infect Control*. 2007;35(9):569-573. [IIIB]

19. Diab-Elschahawi M, Assadian O, Blacky A, et al. Evaluation of the decontamination efficacy of new and reprocessed microfiber cleaning cloth compared with other commonly used cleaning cloths in the hospital. *Am J Infect Control*. 2010;38(4):289-292. [IIIB]

20. Dancer SJ. Hospital cleaning in the 21st century. *Eur J Clin Microbiol Infect Dis*. 2011;30(12):1473-1481. [VA]

21. Stiefel U, Cadnum JL, Eckstein BC, Guerrero DM, Tima MA, Donskey CJ. Contamination of hands with methicillin-resistant *Staphylococcus aureus* after contact with environmental surfaces and after contact with the skin of colonized patients. *Infect Control Hosp Epidemiol*. 2011;32(2):185-187. [IIIC]

22. Siegel JD, Rhinehart E, Jackson M, Chiarello L; Healthcare Infection Control Practices Advisory Committee. *Management of Multidrug-Resistant Organisms in Healthcare Settings*. Atlanta, GA: Centers for Disease Control and Prevention; 2006. [IVA]

23. Datta R, Platt R, Yokoe DS, Huang SS. Environmental cleaning intervention and risk of acquiring multidrug-resistant organisms from prior room occupants. *Arch Intern Med*. 2011;171(6):491-494. [IIB]

24. Landman D, Babu E, Shah N, et al. Transmission of carbapenem-resistant pathogens in New York City hospitals: progress and frustration. *J Antimicrob Chemother*. 2012;67(6):1427-1431. [IIIA]

25. Morgan DJ, Rogawski E, Thom KA, et al. Transfer of multidrug-resistant bacteria to healthcare workers' gloves and gowns after patient contact increases with environmental contamination. *Crit Care Med*. 2012;40(4):1045-1051. [IIIA]

26. Hess AS, Shardell M, Johnson JK, et al. A randomized controlled trial of enhanced cleaning to reduce contamination of healthcare worker gowns and gloves with multidrug-resistant bacteria. *Infect Control Hosp Epidemiol*. 2013;34(5):487-493. [IA]

27. Ibrahimi OA, Sharon V, Eisen DB. Surgical-site infections and routes of bacterial transfer: which ones are most plausible? *Dermatol Surg*. 2011;37(12):1709-1720. [VB]

28. Standards of perioperative nursing. In: *Perioperative Standards and Recommended Practices*. Denver, CO: AORN, Inc; 2012:3-20. [IVB]

29. Mangram AJ, Horan TC, Pearson ML, Silver LC, Jarvis WR. Guideline for prevention of surgical site infection, 1999. Centers for Disease Control and Prevention (CDC) Hospital Infection Control Practices Advisory Committee. *Am J Infect Control*. 1999;27(2):97-132. [IVA]

30. Rutala WA, Weber DJ; Healthcare Infection Control Practices Advisory Committee. *Guideline for Disinfection and Sterilization in Healthcare Facilities*, 2008. Atlanta, GA: Centers for Disease Control and Prevention; 2008. [IVA]

31. Andersen BM, Rasch M, Kvist J, et al. Floor cleaning: effect on bacteria and organic materials in hospital rooms. *J Hosp Infect*. 2009;71(1):57-65. [IIIB]

32. Cotton MF, Wasserman E, Pieper CH, et al. Invasive disease due to extended spectrum beta-lactamase-producing *Klebsiella pneumoniae* in a neonatal unit: the possible role of cockroaches. *J Hosp Infect*. 2000;44(1):13-17. [IIIB]

33. Faulde M, Spiesberger M. Role of the moth fly *Clogmia albipunctata* (Diptera: Psychodinae) as a mechanical vector of bacterial pathogens in German hospitals. *J Hosp Infect*. 2013;83(1):51-60. [IIIB]

34. Fotedar R, Nayar E, Samantray JC, et al. Cockroaches as vectors of pathogenic bacteria. *J Commun Dis*. 1989;21(4):318-322. [IIIA]

35. Lemos AA, Lemos JA, Prado MA, et al. Cockroaches as carriers of fungi of medical importance. *Mycoses*. 2006;49(1):23-25. [IIIC]

36. Munoz-Price LS, Safdar N, Beier JC, Doggett SL. Bed bugs in healthcare settings. *Infect Control Hosp Epidemiol*. 2012;33(11):1137-1142. [VB]

37. Pai HH, Chen WC, Peng CF. Cockroaches as potential vectors of nosocomial infections. *Infect Control Hosp Epidemiol*. 2004;25(11):979-984. [IIIC]

38. Saitou K, Furuhata K, Kawakami Y, Fukuyama M. Biofilm formation abilities and disinfectant-resistance of Pseudomonas aeruginosa isolated from cockroaches captured in hospitals. *Biocontrol Sci*. 2009;14(2):65-68. [IIIB]

39. *42 CFR 416: Ambulatory Surgical Services*. 2011. US Government Printing Office. http://www.gpo.gov/fdsys/granule/CFR-2011-title42-vol3/CFR-2011-title42-vol3-part416/content-detail.html. Accessed September 30, 2013.

40. *42 CFR 482: Conditions of Participation for Hospitals*. US Government Printing Office. http://www.gpo.gov/fdsys/granule/CFR-2011-title42-vol5/CFR-2011-title42-vol5-part482/content-detail.html. Accessed September 30, 2013.

41. Loftus RW, Brown JR, Koff MD, et al. Multiple reservoirs contribute to intraoperative bacterial transmission. *Anesth Analg*. 2012;114(6):1236-1248. [IIA]

42. Rutala WA, Gergen MF, Weber DJ. Room decontamination with UV radiation. *Infect Control Hosp Epidemiol*. 2010;31(10):1025-1029. [IIIB]

43. van 't Veen A, van der Zee A, Nelson J, Speelberg B, Kluytmans JA, Buiting AG. Outbreak of infection with a multiresistant *Klebsiella pneumoniae* strain associated with contaminated roll boards in operating rooms. *J Clin Microbiol*. 2005;43(10):4961-4967. [VB]

44. Blue J, O'Neill C, Speziale P, Revill J, Ramage L, Ballantyne L. Use of a fluorescent chemical as a quality indicator for a hospital cleaning program. *Can J Infect Control*. 2008;23(4):216-219. [IIIC]

45. Boyce JM, Havill NL, Dumigan DG, Golebiewski M, Balogun O, Rizvani R. Monitoring the effectiveness of hospital cleaning practices by use of an adenosine triphosphate bioluminescence assay. *Infect Control Hosp Epidemiol*. 2009;30(7):678-684. [IIB]

46. Boyce JM, Havill NL, Havill HL, Mangione E, Dumigan DG, Moore BA. Comparison of fluorescent marker systems with 2 quantitative methods of assessing terminal cleaning practices. *Infect Control Hosp Epidemiol*. 2011;32(12):1187-1193. [IIIA]

47. Boyce JM, Havill NL, Lipka A, Havill H, Rizvani R. Variations in hospital daily cleaning practices. *Infect Control Hosp Epidemiol*. 2010;31(1):99-101. [IIIC]

48. Boyce JM, Havill NL, Moore BA. Terminal decontamination of patient rooms using an automated mobile UV light unit. *Infect Control Hosp Epidemiol*. 2011;32(8):737-742. [IIIB]

49. Carling PC, Parry MF, Bruno-Murtha LA, Dick B. Improving environmental hygiene in 27 intensive care units to decrease multidrug-resistant bacterial transmission. *Crit Care Med*. 2010;38(4):1054-1059. [IIA]

50. Carling PC, Parry MF, Von Beheren SM; Healthcare Environmental Hygiene Study Group. Identifying opportunities to enhance environmental cleaning in 23 acute care hospitals. *Infect Control Hosp Epidemiol*. 2008;29(1):1-7. [IIIB]

51. Weber DJ, Rutala WA, Miller MB, Huslage K, Sickbert-Bennett E. Role of hospital surfaces in the

transmission of emerging health care-associated pathogens: norovirus, *Clostridium difficile*, and Acinetobacter species. *Am J Infect Control*. 2010;38(5 Suppl 1):S25-S33. [VA]

52. Friedman ND, Walton AL, Boyd S, et al. The effectiveness of a single-stage versus traditional three-staged protocol of hospital disinfection at eradicating vancomycin-resistant Enterococci from frequently touched surfaces. *Am J Infect Control*. 2013;41(3):227-231. [IIIB]

53. Centers for Medicare & Medicaid Services. *State Operations Manual Appendix A: Survey Protocol, Regulations and Interpretive Guidelines for Hospitals*. Rev 78; 2011.

54. Centers for Medicare & Medicaid Services. *State Operations Manual Appendix L: Guidance for Surveyors: Ambulatory Surgical Centers*. Rev 76; 2011.

55. *ANSI/AAMI ST79:2010 & A1:2010, & A2:2011, & A3:2012: Comprehensive Guide to Steam Sterilization and Sterility Assurance in Health Care Facilities*. Arlington, VA: Association for the Advancement of Medical Instrumentation; 2012. [IVC]

56. Carlesso AM, Artuso GL, Caumo K, Rott MB. Potentially pathogenic acanthamoeba isolated from a hospital in Brazil. *Curr Microbiol*. 2010;60(3):185-190. [IIIB]

57. Wojgani H, Kehsa C, Cloutman-Green E, Gray C, Gant V, Klein N. Hospital door handle design and their contamination with bacteria: a real life observational study. Are we pulling against closed doors? *PLoS ONE*. 2012;7(10):e40171. [IIIC]

58. Brady RR, Verran J, Damani NN, Gibb AP. Review of mobile communication devices as potential reservoirs of nosocomial pathogens. *J Hosp Infect*. 2009;71(4):295-300. [VA]

59. Wilson AP, Ostro P, Magnussen M, Cooper B; Keyboard Study Group. Laboratory and in-use assessment of methicillin-resistant *Staphylococcus aureus* contamination of ergonomic computer keyboards for ward use. *Am J Infect Control*. 2008;36(10):e19-e25. [IIIB]

60. Trillis F 3rd, Eckstein EC, Budavich R, Pultz MJ, Donskey CJ. Contamination of hospital curtains with healthcare-associated pathogens. *Infect Control Hosp Epidemiol*. 2008;29(11):1074-1076. [IIIC]

61. Ohl M, Schweizer M, Graham M, Heilmann K, Boyken L, Diekema D. Hospital privacy curtains are frequently and rapidly contaminated with potentially pathogenic bacteria. *Am J Infect Control*. 2012;40(10):904-906. [IIIB]

62. Barbut F, Menuet D, Verachten M, Girou E. Comparison of the efficacy of a hydrogen peroxide dry-mist disinfection system and sodium hypochlorite solution for eradication of *Clostridium difficile* spores. *Infect Control Hosp Epidemiol*. 2009;30(6):507-514. [IB]

63. Bartels MD, Kristoffersen K, Slotsbjerg T, Rohde SM, Lundgren B, Westh H. Environmental methicillin-resistant *Staphylococcus aureus* (MRSA) disinfection using dry-mist-generated hydrogen peroxide. *J Hosp Infect*. 2008;70(1):35-41. [IIIB]

64. Boyce JM, Havill NL, Otter JA, et al. Impact of hydrogen peroxide vapor room decontamination on *Clostridium difficile* environmental contamination and transmission in a healthcare setting. *Infect Control Hosp Epidemiol*. 2008;29(8):723-729. [IIIB]

65. Chan HT, White P, Sheorey H, Cocks J, Waters MJ. Evaluation of the biological efficacy of hydrogen peroxide vapour decontamination in wards of an Australian hospital. *J Hosp Infect*. 2011;79(2):125-128. [IIB]

66. Manian FA, Griesenauer S, Senkel D, et al. Isolation of *Acinetobacter baumannii* complex and methicillin-resistant *Staphylococcus aureus* from hospital rooms following terminal cleaning and disinfection: can we do better? *Infect Control Hosp Epidemiol*. 2011;32(7):667-672. [IIIB]

67. Passaretti CL, Otter JA, Reich NG, et al. An evaluation of environmental decontamination with hydrogen peroxide vapor for reducing the risk of patient acquisition of multidrug-resistant organisms. *Clin Infect Dis*. 2013;56(1):27-35. [IIA]

68. Anderson DJ, Gergen MF, Smathers E, et al. Decontamination of targeted pathogens from patient rooms using an automated ultraviolet-C-emitting device. *Infect Control Hosp Epidemiol*. 2013;34(5):466-471. [IIIB]

69. Nerandzic MM, Cadnum JL, Pultz MJ, Donskey CJ. Evaluation of an automated ultraviolet radiation device for decontamination of *Clostridium difficile* and other healthcare-associated pathogens in hospital rooms. *BMC Infect Dis*. 2010;10:197. [IIB]

70. Umezawa K, Asai S, Inokuchi S, Miyachi H. A comparative study of the bactericidal activity and daily disinfection housekeeping surfaces by a new portable pulsed UV radiation device. *Curr Microbiol*. 2012;64(6):581-587. [IIA]

71. Sexton JD, Tanner BD, Maxwell SL, Gerba CP. Reduction in the microbial load on high-touch surfaces in hospital rooms by treatment with a portable saturated steam vapor disinfection system. *Am J Infect Control*. 2011;39(8):655-662. [IIIB]

72. Otter JA, Yezli S, Perl TM, Barbut F, French GL. The role of "no-touch" automated room disinfection systems in infection prevention and control. *J Hosp Infect*. 2013;83(1):1-13. [VB]

73. *29 CFR 1910.1030. Occupational Exposure. Bloodborne Pathogens*. 2012. Occupational Safety & Health Administration. https://www.osha.gov/pls/oshaweb/owadisp.show_document?p_table=standards&p_id=10051. Accessed September 30, 2013.

74. Bergen LK, Meyer M, Hog M, Rubenhagen B, Andersen LP. Spread of bacteria on surfaces when cleaning with microfibre cloths. *J Hosp Infect*. 2009;71(2):132-137. [IIIB]

75. Siegel JD, Rhinehart E, Jackson M, Chiarello L; Health Care Infection Control Practices Advisory Committee. 2007 Guideline for isolation precautions: preventing transmission of infectious agents in health care settings. *Am J Infect Control*. 2007;35(10 Suppl 2):S65-S164. [IVA]

76. Abbett SK, Yokoe DS, Lipsitz SR, et al. Proposed checklist of hospital interventions to decrease the incidence of healthcare-associated *Clostridium difficile* infection. *Infect Control Hosp Epidemiol*. 2009;30(11):1062-1069. [IIB]

77. Carter Y, Barry D. Tackling *C difficile* with environmental cleaning. *Nurs Times*. 2011;107(36):22-25. [IIIB]

78. Doan L, Forrest H, Fakis A, Craig J, Claxton L, Khare M. Clinical and cost effectiveness of eight disinfection methods for terminal disinfection of hospital isolation rooms contaminated with *Clostridium difficile* 027. *J Hosp Infect*. 2012;82(2):114-121. [IA]

79. Dubberke E. Strategies for prevention of *Clostridium difficile* infection. *J Hosp Med*. 2012;7(Suppl 3): S14-S17. [IVA]

80. Jensen PA, Lambert LA, Iademarco MF, Ridzon R; CDC. Guidelines for preventing the transmission of *Mycobacterium tuberculosis* in health-care settings, 2005. *MMWR Recomm Rep*. 2005;54(RR-17):1-141. [IVA]

81. Rutala WA, Weber DJ, Society for Healthcare Epidemiology of America. Guideline for disinfection and sterilization of prion-contaminated medical instruments. *Infect Control Hosp Epidemiol*. 2010;31(2):107-117. [IVA]

82. Balm MN, Jureen R, Teo C, et al. Hot and steamy: outbreak of *Bacillus cereus* in Singapore associated with

construction work and laundry practices. *J Hosp Infect.* 2012;81(4):224-230. [VA]

83. Campbell JR, Hulten K, Baker CJ. Cluster of Bacillus species bacteremia cases in neonates during a hospital construction project. *Infect Control Hosp Epidemiol.* 2011;32(10):1035-1038. [VA]

84. Fournel I, Sautour M, Lafon I, et al. Airborne Aspergillus contamination during hospital construction works: efficacy of protective measures. *Am J Infect Control.* 2010;38(3):189-194. [IIIB]

85. Gibb AP, Fleck BW, Kempton-Smith L. A cluster of deep bacterial infections following eye surgery associated with construction dust. *J Hosp Infect.* 2006;63(2):197-200. [VB]

86. Kak N, Burkhalter B, Cooper M-A. *Measuring the Competence of Healthcare Providers.* Operations Research Issue Paper 2(1). Bethesda, MD: Quality Assurance Project for the US Agency for International Development; 2001. http://www.hciproject.org/sites/default/files/Measuring%20the%20Competence%20of%20HC%20Providers_QAP_2001.pdf. Accessed September 30, 2013. [VA]

87. HR.01.05.03: Staff participate in ongoing education and training. In: *Comprehensive Accreditation Manual: CAMH for Hospitals.* Oakbrook Terrace, IL: Joint Commission Accreditation; 2012.

88. Quality management and improvement. In: *2012 Accreditation Handbook for Ambulatory Health Care.* Skokie, IL: Accreditation Association for Ambulatory Health Care; 2012:34-39.

89. Personnel: personnel records. In: *Procedural Standards and Checklist for Accreditation of Ambulatory Surgery Facilities.* Version 3 ed. Gurnee, IL: American Association for Accreditation of Ambulatory Surgery Facilities; 2011:77-79.

90. Quality assessment /quality improvement: quality improvement. In: *Procedural Standards and Checklist for Accreditation of Ambulatory Surgery Facilities.* Version 3 ed. Gurnee, IL: American Association for Accreditation of Ambulatory Surgery Facilities; 2011:67.

91. Sportsman S. Competency education and validation in the United States: what should nurses know? *Nurs Forum.* 2010;45(3):140-149. [VA]

92. Jordan C, Thomas MB, Evans ML, Green A. Public policy on competency: how will nursing address this complex issue? *J Contin Educ Nurs.* 2008;39(2):86-91. [VA]

93. Hota B, Blom DW, Lyle EA, Weinstein RA, Hayden MK. Interventional evaluation of environmental contamination by vancomycin-resistant enterococci: failure of personnel, product, or procedure? *J Hosp Infect.* 2009;71(2):123-131. [IIIA]

94. Gillespie BM, Hamlin L. A synthesis of the literature on "competence" as it applies to perioperative nursing. *AORN J.* 2009;90(2):245-258. [VA]

95. Matlow AG, Wray R, Richardson SE. Attitudes and beliefs, not just knowledge, influence the effectiveness of environmental cleaning by environmental service workers. *Am J Infect Control.* 2012;40(3):260-262. [IIIC]

96. Governance. In: *2012 Accreditation Handbook for Ambulatory Health Care.* Skokie, IL: Accreditation Association for Ambulatory Health Care; 2012:20-27.

97. LD.04.01.07: The hospital has policies and procedures that guide and support patient care, treatment, and services. In: *Hospital Accreditation Standards 2012.* 2012 ed. Oakbrook Terrace, IL: Joint Commission Resources; 2012.

98. LD.04.01.07: The organization has policies and procedures that guide and support patient care, treatment, or services. In: *Standards for Ambulatory Care 2012: Standards, Elements of Performance Scoring Accreditation Polices.* Oakbrook Terrace, IL: The Joint Commission; 2012.

99. Rutala WA, Weber DJ. Sterilization, high-level disinfection, and environmental cleaning. *Infect Dis Clin North Am.* 2011;25(1):45-76. [VA]

100. Dumigan DG, Boyce JM, Havill NL, Golebiewski M, Balogun O, Rizvani R. Who is really caring for your environment of care? Developing standardized cleaning procedures and effective monitoring techniques. *Am J Infect Control.* 2010;38(5):387-392. [VB]

101. Havill NL, Havill HL, Mangione E, Dumigan DG, Boyce JM. Cleanliness of portable medical equipment disinfected by nursing staff. *Am J Infect Control.* 2011;39(7):602-604. [IIIB]

102. Malik RE, Cooper RA, Griffith CJ. Use of audit tools to evaluate the efficacy of cleaning systems in hospitals. *Am J Infect Control.* 2003;31(3):181-187. [IIIC]

103. Al-Hamad A, Maxwell S. How clean is clean? Proposed methods for hospital cleaning assessment. *J Hosp Infect.* 2008;70(4):328-334. [IIIC]

104. Aiken ZA, Wilson M, Pratten J. Evaluation of ATP bioluminescence assays for potential use in a hospital setting. *Infect Control Hosp Epidemiol.* 2011;32(5):507-509. [IIIB]

105. Sherlock O, O'Connell N, Creamer E, Humphreys H. Is it really clean? An evaluation of the efficacy of four methods for determining hospital cleanliness. *J Hosp Infect.* 2009;72(2):140-146. [IIIA]

106. Carling PC, Bartley JM. Evaluating hygienic cleaning in health care settings: what you do not know can harm your patients. *Am J Infect Control.* 2010;38(5 Suppl 1):S41-S50. [IIB]

107. Carling P. Methods for assessing the adequacy of practice and improving room disinfection. *Am J Infect Control.* 2013;41:S20-25. [VA]

108. Guh A, Carling P; Environmental Evaluation Workgroup. CDC toolkit: options for evaluating environmental cleaning. 2010. Centers for Disease Control and Prevention. http://www.cdc.gov/HAI/toolkits/Evaluating-Environmental-Cleaning.html. Accessed September 30, 2012. [VC]

109. Gawande Atul. *The Checklist Manifesto: How to Get Things Right.* New York, NY: Metropolitan Books; 2010. [VA]

Acknowledgements

Lead Author
Amber Wood, MSN, RN, CNOR, CIC, CPN
Perioperative Nursing Specialist
AORN Nursing Department
Denver, Colorado

Contributing Author
Ramona Conner, MSN, RN, CNOR
Manager Standards and Guidelines
AORN Nursing Department
Denver, Colorado

The authors and AORN thank Philip Carling, MD, Department of Clinical Medicine, Boston University School of Medicine, Department of Infectious Diseases, Carney Hospital, Boston, Massachusetts; George Allen, PhD, MS, RN, CNOR, CIC, Director Infection Control, Downstate Medical Center and

ENVIRONMENTAL CLEANING

Clinical Assistant Professor, SUNY College of Health Related Professions, Brooklyn, New York; Marcia R. Patrick, MSN, RN, CIC, Association for Professionals in Infection Control and Epidemiology liaison to the AORN Recommended Practices Advisory Board and Independent Consultant, Tacoma, Washington; Deborah F. Mulloy, PhD, RN, CNOR, Associate Chief Nurse, Quality & Center for Nursing Excellence, Brigham and Women's Hospital, Boston, Massachusetts; Lisa Spruce, DNP, RN, ACNS, ACNP, ANP, CNOR, Director of Evidence-based Perioperative Practice, AORN, Inc, Denver, Colorado; Elayne Kornblatt Phillips, PhD-BSN, MPH, RN, International Healthcare Worker Safety Center, University of Virginia, Charlottesville; and Janice A. Neil, PhD, RN, Associate Professor and Chair, Department of Undergraduate Nursing Science, College of Nursing, East Carolina University, Greenville, North Carolina, for their assistance in developing this guideline.

PUBLICATION HISTORY

Originally published June 1975, *AORN Journal* as "Recommended practices for sanitation in the surgical practice setting."

Format revised March 1978; March 1982; July 1982. Revised April 1984; November 1988; December 1992.

Revised June 1996; published October 1996, *AORN Journal*. Reformatted July 2000.

Revised; published December 2002, *AORN Journal*.

Revised 2007; published in *Perioperative Standards and Recommended Practices*, 2008 edition.

Minor editing revisions made to omit PNDS codes; reformatted September 2012 for publication in *Perioperative Standards and Recommended Practices*, 2013 edition.

Revised September 2013 for online publication in *Perioperative Standards and Recommended Practices*.

Minor editing revisions made in November 2014 for publication in *Guidelines for Perioperative Practice*, 2015 edition.

GUIDELINE FOR HAND HYGIENE

The Guideline for Hand Hygiene was developed by the AORN Recommended Practices Committee and was approved by the AORN Board of Directors. It was presented as proposed recommendations for comments by members and others. The guideline is effective July 1, 2009. The recommendations in this guideline are intended to be achievable and represent what is believed to be an optimal level of practice. Policies and procedures will reflect variations in practice settings and/or clinical situations that determine the degree to which the guideline can be implemented. AORN recognizes the various settings in which perioperative nurses practice; therefore, this guideline is adaptable to various practice settings. These practice settings include traditional operating rooms (ORs), ambulatory surgery centers, physicians' offices, cardiac catheterization laboratories, endoscopy suites, radiology departments, and all other areas where operative and other invasive procedures may be performed.

Purpose

This document provides guidance for hand hygiene for surgical and other invasive procedures. Microorganism transfer from the hands of health care workers to patients is an important factor in health care-associated infections and has been recognized since the observations of Ignaz Semmelweis and others more than 100 years ago. Skin is a major potential source of microbial contamination in the surgical environment. Hand hygiene has been recognized as a primary method of decreasing health care-associated infections.[1] Prevention of health care-associated infections is a priority of all health care personnel. Health care-associated infections can result in untoward outcomes such as escalating cost of care, increased morbidity and mortality, longer length of stay, as well as the pain and suffering a patient may experience.[2] Hand hygiene, hand washing, and surgical hand scrubs are the most effective way to prevent and control infections and represent the least expensive means of achieving both.

The normal skin flora on the hands include transient and resident microorganisms. The transient flora are microorganisms that colonize the superficial layers of the skin. These microorganisms are acquired by health care personnel while caring for patients and from coming into contact with contaminated surfaces where patients reside. Transient bacteria are easier to remove during hand washing. Resident flora are bacteria seated in the deeper layers of skin and are more difficult to remove. The transient and resident bacteria usually maintain a constant level on individuals' hands.[3,4]

The term "hand hygiene" is used to describe all measures related to hand condition and decontamination. Decontamination of hands can be done by one or more methods:

- **hand washing** using
  - soap and water,
  - antiseptic and water, or
  - antiseptic hand rub if visible soil is not present, or
- **surgical hand scrub** using
  - water-aided brushless surgical antiseptics,
  - waterless brushless surgical antiseptics, or
  - traditional surgical hand scrub using a sponge.[3,4]

Recommendation I

All health care personnel should follow established hand hygiene practices for maintaining healthy skin and fingernail condition and regarding the wearing of jewelry in the perioperative setting.

A direct route of transmission of microorganisms occurs when person-to-person contact results in transmission of microorganisms from a person who is infectious or colonized to a susceptible host. An indirect route of transmission of microorganisms occurs when inanimate objects such as a contaminated surface, instrument, or health care personnel's hands transfer microorganisms to a susceptible host.[5,6] An example of an outbreak involved a cardiac surgeon's infected fingernail. When cultured, it grew *Pseudomonas aeruginosa*. Two patients treated by the surgeon developed a surgical site infection with the same strain of *P aeruginosa*.[7]

I.a. Health care personnel should keep natural fingernails no more than one-quarter inch (0.64 cm) long.[3,8,9]

The subungual area of fingernails has the largest number of microorganisms on the hands. Pathogens most frequently isolated from the subungual area are coagulase-negative staphylococci, gram-negative rods (including *Pseudomonas* spp), corynebacteria, and yeasts.[10,11]

Long fingernails pose a risk of developing tears in gloves and also the possibility of injuring a patient during positioning and caring for the patient. There is also the concern that hand washing, hand rub, and surgical hand scrubbing may not be performed as well due to the health care personnel protecting their fingernails.[12,13] Short fingernails collect less debris, and debris is more easily removed when fingernails are short. Short fingernails have a decreased risk of being colonized with *P aeruginosa* compared to health care personnel with long or artificial fingernails. Long

HAND HYGIENE

fingernails make washing and drying of hands difficult and may result in hand colonization.[9]

I.b. Chipped fingernail polish should be removed prior to entry into the restricted area of the perioperative environment.

Fingernail polish that is chipped may harbor pathogens in large numbers.[4,8,13] It has been shown that fingernail polish becomes chipped by the fourth day of wear.[13] Chipped fingernail polish should be removed to prevent possible contamination of the environment or the patient.[4,8] Glove tears occasionally occur during a surgical procedure; chipped fingernail polish could be deposited on the sterile field or in the wound.

I.c. Artificial fingernails should not be worn by health care personnel in the perioperative environment.

Any fingernail enhancement or resin bonding product is considered artificial. Fingernail extensions or tips, gels and acrylic overlays, resin wraps, or acrylic fingernails constitute types of artificial fingernails.[14] Over time, gel or acrylic fingernails can become chipped and lift from the nail plate if moisture gets under the overlay. Adding artificial fingernails to an area of fingernails that is colonized may increase the microorganisms on the native fingernails.[12] The greater the length of time artificial fingernails are worn, the greater the number of microorganisms isolated.[12] Health care personnel who wear artificial fingernails may also limit hand hygiene and surgical hand scrub practices as a result of a need to protect their manicure.[12,15] Patients at risk of infection may be at increased risk of exposure to pathogens that have been known to be colonized on artificial fingernails of health care personnel.[12,15] Studies have shown the correlation of microorganisms from health care personnel's hands to patients that result in surgical site infections. One such study showed three patients who developed a surgical site infection with *Candida albicans*; the strains isolated were identical. It was found that the surgical technician who scrubbed on all three cases had long artificial fingernails at the time of the patients' surgeries. A throat culture of the surgical technician later grew *C albicans*.[3,16]

I.d. Rings should not be worn by health care personnel in the perioperative setting.

Studies have shown that wearing rings may result in colonization of the hands with pathogens such as gram-negative and gram-positive pathogens.[2-4,17] With an increasing number of rings worn, the pathogens recovered may also increase in number.[4] In one study, isolates recovered from swabbing the area adjacent to the ring included coagulase-negative staphylococci, other skin flora, gram-negative cocci, *Pseudomonas* spp and *Staphylococcus aureus*.[18] There is a strong link between wearing rings and contamination of hands by health care personnel; removing rings will decrease the potential for pathogens remaining on hands before and after hand hygiene.[19]

I.e. Watches and bracelets should be removed prior to washing hands.[2,3,20]

One study found that persons wearing watches or bracelets wash the wrist area less. Removing watches and bracelets allows for thorough hand hygiene.[2,20]

I.f. Health care organization-approved hand lotions should be readily available and used frequently to maintain good hand skin condition following surgical hand hygiene.

Skin irritation and dermatitis from frequent hand washing can increase the risk of infection for both the health care worker and the patient.[21] Failure to follow practices that maintain intact skin may create breaks in intact epithelium, which compromises the barrier properties of the skin and presents the opportunity for microbial transmission into the tissues.[22]

I.f.1. Lotions selected for use in the perioperative setting should be evaluated and approved by an interdisciplinary group that has the designated authority to evaluate and select hand lotions.

I.f.2. Hand lotions used in the perioperative setting should
- be compatible with antiseptics and barrier products in use,
- list water as the first ingredient on the label,[23]
- contain no anionic-based materials or chemicals, and
- contain no petroleum or other ingredients with a demonstrated detrimental effect on the barrier properties of gloves in use.

Many lotions found in over-the-counter products contain an anionic-based ingredient that interferes with the residual effect of chlorhexidine gluconate and chloroxylenol. Chlorhexidine gluconate and chloroxylenol are in many hand antiseptic products used in health care organizations for their antiseptic properties.[3,23]

Petroleum may affect the barrier properties of latex gloves that may be worn by health care personnel.[24] A study on latex glove compatibility has shown petroleum to have adverse effects on the integrity of latex gloves.[25] Some gloves have been demonstrated to be compatible with some lotions.

I.g. Health care personnel with cuts, abrasions, weeping dermatitis, or fresh tattoos on exposed skin should not provide direct patient care. Health care personnel should not have patient contact until these conditions are healed and they have been cleared by an infection preventionist, employee health nurse, occupational health nurse, or other health care personnel with specialized knowledge in making a determination regarding the safety of the employee returning to work in the perioperative setting.[22,24]

Health care personnel with breaks in their skin integrity may be at risk for acquiring or transmitting infection to patients.

Recommendation II

A standardized procedure for hand washing should be followed.

The purpose of hand washing is to
- remove soil, organic material, and transient microorganisms from fingernails, hands, and forearms;
- decrease the resident microorganism count to a minimum; and
- inhibit the rapid rebound of microorganisms.[3]

Application technique, length of exposure to the product, and correct concentration of the product impact the effectiveness of hand washing.[26] Inconsistent compliance with recommended procedures may result in the transmission of pathogens to patients.

II.a. A hand wash should be performed
- upon arrival at the health care facility,
- before and after every patient contact,
- before putting gloves on and after removing gloves or other personal protective equipment,
- any time there is a possibility that there has been contact with blood or other potentially infectious materials or surfaces,
- before and after eating,
- before and after using the restroom,
- before leaving the health care facility, and
- when hands are visibly soiled.[3,27]

Hand washing remains one of the most important measures in maintaining patient and health care personnel safety. Following these hand washing practices will prevent transmission of infection and reduce health care-associated infections for the patient and health care personnel.[27]

Contamination of hands may occur
- as a result of holes or tears in gloves that are not visible;
- when gloves are removed; and
- when continuing to wear gloves following the care of a patient, which may lead to transmission of microorganisms from patient to patient.

Wearing gloves will not replace hand hygiene.[28] One study found a 15% rate of colonization from methicillin-resistant *Staphylococcus aureus* (MRSA)-positive patients to health care personnel's hands after removal of gloves. Another study found a 17% rate of colonization from MRSA-colonized patients to gloves of health care personnel.[29,30]

II.a.1. Hands should be washed with soap and water for at least 15 seconds.

Hand washing for 15 seconds has been shown to reduce soil, spores, and microorganism counts on the hands.[3,27,31-33]

II.a.2. Hand washing with soap and water should be performed in the following order:
(1) Remove jewelry from hands and forearms.
(2) Adjust water to a comfortable temperature.
(3) Wet hands thoroughly with water.
(4) Follow the manufacturer's directions for application of soap.
(5) Rub hands covering all surfaces including the backs of hands, fingertips, inner webs, and palms.
(6) Wash for at least 15 seconds.
(7) Rinse well to remove all soap.
(8) Dry hands thoroughly with an absorbent, non-abrasive, disposable towel.[27]
(9) Use a disposable towel to turn the water off and open the door if hands-free controls are not available.[3]

Drying hands thoroughly assists in removing soil, stratum corneum, and microorganisms that have been loosened during the process of hand washing.

Touching faucet handles provides an opportunity for cross-contamination.[34] Moisture remaining on the hands can create a transfer of microorganisms remaining on the hands to surfaces in the environment.[34]

II.b. Hand washing stations should be placed in convenient locations according to local and state building codes.

Hand washing stations located close to patient care areas, medication preparation areas, and food storage and dispensing areas encourage health care personnel to wash their hands. Convenient hand washing stations result in a higher frequency of hand washing.[35]

II.b.1. Water temperature at the faucet should be controlled between 105° F and 120° F (40° C and 49° C).[35]

Dermatitis can be prevented by using tap water that is adjusted to a comfortable temperature.

II.b.2. Hand washing stations in new or remodeled facilities should have hands-free water and soap dispensing controls.[35]

Hands-free water and soap dispensing controls reduce the risk of cross-contamination.[34]

II.b.3. Paper towel dispensers should be designed to prevent recontamination when removing towels. The towel dispenser should dispense cleanly without the need to touch the towel dispenser.[36]

Paper towel dispenser design is important, as the process of drying hands is the final step in hand washing; ease of use is important in preventing recontamination of

HAND HYGIENE

hands.[36] Towels that jam when the towel dispenser does not work properly can result in hands becoming contaminated by touching the dispenser.[36]

II.c. Hand washing may be performed using an alcohol-based antiseptic hand rub when soil is not present on hands.[3] The hand rub manufacturer's written directions for the amount of product and technique for application should be followed.[27]

Alcohol-based hand rubs are easy to use, fast acting, and provide activity against most bacteria, most viruses, and fungi.[37]

II.c.1. Care should be taken in the placement of alcohol-based hand antiseptic product dispensers in areas where surgical and other invasive procedures are performed and where oxygen and ignition sources are present.[38] Dispensers should be installed following the 2004 National Fire Protection Association (NFPA) Life Safety Code as well as state and local regulations. Alcohol-based hand hygiene product dispensers should
- be at least four feet apart;
- only hold 1.2 L in rooms, corridors, and areas open to corridors; and
- not be placed over an electrical outlet or switch.[27,39]

Hand antiseptic product dispensers containing flammable antiseptics may be a fire hazard. Following the NFPA Life Safety Code will decrease the risk of fire.[27,39]

II.c.2. Hand rubs should be performed in the following manner:
(1) Follow the manufacturer's written directions for use of product.
(2) Use the recommended amount of hand rub product.
(3) Rub hands, covering all surfaces, including the backs of hands, fingertips, inner webs, and palms.
(4) Rub hands until they are dry.

A sufficient amount of product is required to ensure antimicrobial effect.

Recommendation III

A surgical hand scrub should be performed by health care personnel before donning sterile gloves for surgical or other invasive procedures. Use of either an antimicrobial surgical scrub agent intended for surgical hand antisepsis or an alcohol-based antiseptic surgical hand rub with documented persistent and cumulative activity that has met US Food and Drug Administration (FDA) regulatory requirements for surgical hand antisepsis is acceptable.

The objective of a surgical hand scrub is the reduction of transient and resident flora, which also may reduce health care-associated infections.[3,26] Although the skin can never be rendered sterile, it can be made surgically clean by reducing the number of microorganisms. A surgical hand scrub will decrease transient and resident microorganisms on the hands and maintain the bacterial level below baseline.[40] The mechanical action associated with hand scrubbing removes debris and microorganisms. This can be accomplished by rubbing the skin with or without a sponge to produce friction. With the addition of a health care organization-approved antiseptic soap, which acts as a surfactant, transient and some resident microorganisms can be lifted and flushed away under running water. Surgical hand antisepsis/hand scrubs are effective only if all surfaces are exposed to the mechanical cleaning and chemical antisepsis processes.

III.a. A multiuser scrub sink should be located near the entrance to the OR. A multiuser scrub sink may serve two ORs to provide ready access to the adjacent ORs.[35]

III.b. A standardized surgical hand scrub using an alcohol-based surgical hand rub product with demonstrated persistence and cumulative activity should be performed according to the manufacturer's written directions for use. An alcohol and chlorhexidine product that is fast drying and has residual effect is preferred.[3]

III.b.1. A standardized surgical hand scrub procedure using an alcohol-based surgical hand rub product should include, but may not be limited to, the following:
(1) Remove jewelry including rings, watches, and bracelets.
(2) Don a surgical mask. If others are at the scrub sink, a surgical mask should be worn in the presence of hand scrub activity.
(3) If visibly soiled, prewash hands and forearms with plain soap and water or antimicrobial agent.
(4) Clean the subungual areas of both hands under running water using a disposable nail cleaner.
(5) Rinse hands and forearms under running water.
(6) Dry hands and forearms thoroughly with a disposable paper towel.
(7) Dispense the manufacturer-recommended amount of the surgical hand rub product.
(8) Apply the product to the hands and forearms according to the manufacturer's written instructions.
(9) Repeat the product application process as directed.
(10) Rub hands thoroughly until completely dry.[2,27]
(11) In the OR or other invasive procedure room, don a sterile surgical gown and gloves.

III.c. A traditional, standardized, surgical hand scrub procedure should include, but may not be limited to, the following:

HAND HYGIENE

(1) Remove jewelry including rings, watches, and bracelets.
(2) Don a surgical mask. If others are at the scrub sink, a surgical mask should be worn in the presence of hand scrub activity.
(3) Wash hands and forearms if visibly soiled with soap and running water immediately before beginning the surgical scrub.
(4) Clean the subungual areas of both hands under running water using a disposable nail cleaner.
(5) Rinse hands and forearms under running water.
(6) Dispense the approved antimicrobial scrub agent according to the manufacturer's written directions.
(7) Apply the antimicrobial agent to wet hands and forearms using a soft, nonabrasive sponge.
(8) A three- or five-minute scrub should be timed to allow adequate product contact with skin, according to the manufacturer's written directions.
(9) Visualize each finger, hand, and arm as having four sides. Wash all four sides effectively, keeping the hand elevated. Repeat this process for opposite fingers, hand, and arm.
(10) For water conservation, turn water off when it is not directly in use, if possible.
(11) Avoid splashing surgical attire.
(12) Discard sponges, if used, in appropriate containers.
(13) Hands and arms should be rinsed under running water in one direction from fingertips to elbows as often as needed.
(14) Hold hands higher than elbows and away from surgical attire.
(15) In the OR, dry hands and arms with a sterile towel before donning a sterile surgical gown and gloves.[4]

The use of a brush for surgical hand scrubs is not necessary for adequate reduction of bacterial counts. Scrubbing with a brush is associated with an increase in skin cell shedding. The skin on hands can become damaged with the use of brushes, resulting in an increase in bacterial load. Use of a sponge or soft brush rather than a hard bristle brush will reduce damage to the epidermis.[2,41] A study of the duration of surgical hand scrubs using ranges of three to five minutes showed that three-minute surgical hand scrubs are as effective as five-minute surgical hand scrubs.[42] Appropriate disposal of sponges, if used, prevents cross-contamination of the surgical scrub sink area.

Hands and forearms should be held higher than the elbows and away from surgical attire to prevent contamination and allow water to run from the clean to the less clean area down the arm. A sterile gown cannot be put on over wet or damp surgical attire without resultant potential contamination of the gown by strike-through moisture.

Recommendation IV

Surgical hand hygiene products should be selected following an analysis of product effectiveness, application requirements, and user acceptance.

Acceptability of products is a key factor in health care personnel compliance with good hand hygiene practices.[21]

IV.a. Surgical hand hygiene products and hand lotions should be approved by the organization's infection prevention and control committee or designated authority with specialized knowledge in hand products.

The organization's infection prevention and control committee is made up of a multi-disciplinary team that includes the infection preventionist, epidemiologist, administrative staff, perioperative member, pharmacist, as well as other department representatives. This allows for a collaborative discussion on what products would be appropriate.[3] A health care facility that does not have an infection control committee should utilize guidance from health care personnel with specialized knowledge in infection prevention and control.

IV.a.1. Written criteria should be used to evaluate surgical hand hygiene products and their application. Criteria should include, but is not limited to,
- safety,
- purpose and use,
- ease of use,
- skin comfort and reaction,
- fragrance,
- consistency,
- color,
- compatibility with other products,
- patient and health care personnel outcomes,
- efficacy,
- regulatory control, and
- cost.[21,43,44]

IV.a.2. Health care personnel's selection of products should be made with the guidance of an infection preventionist or other health care personnel with specialized knowledge in infection prevention and control.

IV.a.3. End-user evaluations should be completed to determine acceptability prior to final selection of products.

Some of the key concerns that can influence health care personnel regarding hand hygiene products include fragrance, consistency, and color.[44]

HAND HYGIENE

IV.a.4. Following the end-user evaluation of the products tested, written evaluations should be completed by the health care personnel and collected and reviewed by authorized personnel.[45,46]

Written questionnaires or evaluations give valuable validation of product acceptability. Written evaluations should be completed to verify acceptability.

IV.b. Surgical hand hygiene products should be selected and used according to manufacturers' written instructions.[45]

IV.b.1. Antimicrobial surgical hand hygiene products should
- significantly reduce microorganisms on intact skin,
- contain emollients and humectants to prevent skin irritation,[21]
- be broad spectrum,
- be fast acting, and
- have a persistent and cumulative effect[45] (Table 1).

Recommendation V

Health care personnel should receive education, training, and competency validation on surgical hand hygiene products and procedures.

Competency assessment verifies that health care personnel have an understanding of the application and purpose for surgical hand hygiene in infection prevention and control. This knowledge is essential in reducing the risk of health care-associated infections. Health care personnel also understand the potential risk of their becoming colonized or infected by microorganisms from the patient and are better able to protect themselves and the patient.

V.a. Health care personnel should receive education and guidance on hand hygiene products and their application.

Health care personnel should be knowledgeable about surgical hand hygiene products and their application. This includes the indications, contraindications, and special precautions used when handling flammable antiseptic products.[38,47]

V.a.1. Health care personnel should receive education and guidance on the identification and reporting of symptoms of irritant contact dermatitis and allergic contact dermatitis.

Skin irritation conditions may be difficult to differentiate. Skin health is related to its lipid barrier, and the lipid barrier can be compromised by lipid-emulsifying detergents and lipid-dissolving alcohols.[48,49] Education to prevent skin irritation has proven to be effective. Research has shown that by providing educational theory, didactics, and evaluation of surgical hand hygiene practices, improvement in surgical hand hygiene compliance may be achieved.[50]

V.a.2. Health care personnel should participate in surgical hand hygiene product evaluation.

Participation in product evaluations assures health care personnel that they have input into choice of products. A higher level of compliance may be achieved in this manner.

V.b. Health care personnel should demonstrate proficiency in surgical hand hygiene practices and the use of surgical hand hygiene products periodically and when new products are introduced. Periodic performance monitoring also should take place.

Proficiency in surgical hand hygiene practices allows health care personnel to prevent the transmission of pathogens.

V.c. Fire safety education and training should be provided to all health care personnel working in the perioperative area where alcohol and alcohol-based hand hygiene products are used. Fire safety education should include periodic fire drills.

Alcohol and alcohol/combination hand products pose a fire safety concern.

V.c.1. All members of the perioperative surgical team should participate in fire drills.[38]

Fire drills assist the surgical team in promoting a culture of fire safety.[3,38] Participation in fire drills promotes and maintains a fire-safe environment.[38]

Recommendation VI

Policies and procedures for surgical hand hygiene should be written, reviewed annually, and readily available within the practice setting.

Policies and procedures serve as a source of information for preventing health care-associated infections by delineating products to be used as well as the correct technique. Policies and procedures establish authority, responsibility, and accountability and serve as operational guidelines. Policies and procedures establish guidelines for performance improvement activities to be used when monitoring and evaluating surgical hand hygiene in the perioperative setting.

VI.a. Policies regarding hand hygiene should be developed in collaboration with the surgical team as well as the infection preventionist and employee health nurse.

A collaborative approach to policy development and the provision of access to policies for all health care personnel will result in a better team approach to appropriate hand hygiene. The health care organization's infection prevention and control committee should be made up of a multidisciplinary team that may include the infection preventionist, epidemiologist, perioperative registered nurse, pharmacist, administrative staff, as well as nursing and other department representatives. This allows informed discussion on what products would be appropriate.[4] Smaller facilities with no infection prevention and control committee may utilize individuals with specialized knowledge in infection prevention and control.[21]

VI.a.1. Hand hygiene policies should include, but are not limited to,
- standardized procedures for surgical hand scrub,
- removal of jewelry for hand rubs and surgical hand antisepsis,
- health care personnel education in the use of hand scrub products,
- health care organization-approved hand antiseptic products,
- identification and reporting of irritant and allergic contact dermatitis,
- maintenance and location of material safety data sheets (MSDS),
- precautions when flammable antiseptics are used,
- proper storage of flammable hand antiseptic agents,
- reporting of adverse events, and
- performance monitoring.

VI.b. Policies and procedures should be introduced and reviewed in the initial orientation, when new products are introduced, and with ongoing education for health care personnel.

Access to policies and procedures allows health care personnel to have ongoing information. Review of policies and procedures assists health care professionals in the development of knowledge.

Recommendation VII

A quality management program should be in place to evaluate surgical hand hygiene procedures and to identify and respond to opportunities for improvement.

Quality control programs that enhance personal performance and monitor surgical hand hygiene practices are established to promote patient and health care personnel safety. It is the responsibility of professional perioperative registered nurses to ensure safe, high-quality nursing care to patients undergoing operative and invasive procedures.[43]

VII.a. Adverse events (eg, fire, bacterial contamination of multiuse containers) related to the use of hand products should be reported to the health care organization's quality review program.

Open communication is important in determining why adverse events occur. The use of a root cause analysis will facilitate the identification of the cause of the event and assist in determining steps to be taken to prevent future adverse events.

VII.b. Symptoms of irritant or allergic contact dermatitis should be identified and treated as soon as health care personnel report a concern.

Skin dryness, irritation, itching, cracking, and bleeding may be diagnosed as irritant contact dermatitis.[21] These symptoms should be identified and treated quickly to prevent further damage to health care personnel's hands. Allergic contact dermatitis results from an allergic reaction to ingredients in antiseptic products. Allergic contact dermatitis may be mild, localized, or severe, resulting in respiratory distress or possible anaphylaxis.[21] These symptoms should be determined quickly to prevent continued damage to health care personnel's hands and to mitigate anaphylaxis reactions. A change in hand hygiene product can prevent further allergic reactions.

VII.b.1. Cuts, abrasions, weeping dermatitis, or fresh tattoos should be documented in the employee's health record by the infection preventionist, employee health nurse, occupational health nurse, or other health care personnel with specialized knowledge in making a determination regarding the employee's returning to work in the perioperative setting.

VII.c. Barriers that may exist for surgical hand hygiene should be recognized and addressed.

Health care personnel hand washing practice studies note inadequate hand washing compliance.[51] However, another study notes that failure of health care personnel to wash their hands is not due to intentional negligence.[52] Removing barriers to hand hygiene will help health care personnel improve adherence to these procedures. Some of the identified barriers are hand hygiene products causing irritation, sinks not conveniently located, lack of supplies, understaffing, and patient needs that take priority.[53]

VII.c.1. A study of usage patterns of surgical hand hygiene products should be done on an ongoing basis.

VII.c.2. Antiseptic products for surgical hand hygiene that minimize skin irritation should be used.

Health care personnel compliance with the recommended use of antiseptic products is improved when the product does not irritate the skin.

VII.c.3. Staffing levels of health care personnel should be evaluated as a barrier to hand washing.

Staffing levels that are inadequate may result in cross-contamination when health care personnel have an increased workload. A decrease in hand washing may result. Having the right level of health care personnel

HAND HYGIENE

TABLE 1. ACTIVITY AND CONSIDERATIONS FOR HAND HYGIENE AGENTS

Antiseptic agent	Mechanism of action	Gram + bacteria	Gram − bacteria	Viruses	Rapidity of action
Soap and water	Cleansing activity is due to detergent property of soap and water as a solvent[1,2]	Minimal[1]	Minimal[1]		Limited
Alcohol	Denatures proteins[1]	Excellent[1]	Excellent[1]	Good[1]	Excellent. Optimal concentration 60% to 80%[2]
Chlorhexidine	Disrupts cell membrane[1]	Excellent[1]	Good[1]	Good against enveloped viruses, less active against non-enveloped viruses[1]	Slower than alcohol[1]
Chlorhexidine gluconate with alcohol	Disrupts cell membrane and denatures proteins[1,3]	Excellent[1]	Excellent[1]	Good	Excellent
Chloroxylenol	Inactivates bacterial enzymes and disrupts cell walls[1]	Excellent[1]	Fair[1]	Fair[1]	Intermediate[4]. Not as rapidly active as chlorhexidine or iodophors[1]
Iodine and iodophors	Disrupts cell membrane[1]	Excellent[1]	Excellent[1]	Good[1]	Intermediate[1]
Quaternary ammonium compounds	Believed to work by absorbing the cytoplasmic membrane, which creates leakage of the molecular weight cytoplasmic components[2]	Fair[1,2]	Good[1,2]	Fair[1]	Slow[1]
Triclosan	Affects the cytoplasmic membrane and syntheses of RNA, fatty acids, and proteins when it enters bacterial cells[1]	Good[1]	Fair	Fair	Slow

REFERENCES
1. Centers for Disease Control and Prevention. Guideline for hand hygiene in health-care settings. MMWR. October 25, 2002;51(RR-16):1-44.
2. WHO Guidelines on Hand Hygiene in Health Care (Advanced Draft). Geneva, Switzerland: World Health Organization; 2006. http://www.who.int/patient safety/information_centre/ghhad_download_link/en/. Accessed October 19, 2009.
3. Boyce JM, Kelliher S, Vallande N. Skin irritation and dryness associated with two hand-hygiene regimens: soap-and-water hand washing versus hand antisepsis with an alcoholic hand gel. Infect Control Hosp Epidemiol. 2000;21(7):442-448.
4. Larson E. Guideline for use of topical antimicrobial agents. Am J Infect Control. 1988;16(6);253-266.
5. Sicherer SH. Risk of severe allergic reactions from the use of potassium iodide for radiation emergencies. J Allergy Clin Immunol. 2004;114(6);1395-1397.
6. Rotter ML. Hand washing and hand disinfection. In: Mayhall CG, ed. Hospital Epidemiology and Infection Control. 3rd ed. Philadelphia, PA: Lippincott Williams & Wilkins; 2004:1727-1746.

available enables personnel to be compliant with hand hygiene.[54]

VII.d. Hand hygiene practices should be measured to determine compliance.

Following hand hygiene policies and procedures is an important step in infection prevention and control in protecting health care personnel and patients. Measurement involves adhering to and following the manufacturer's written product directions. Studies have been conducted but may need to be expanded.[54]

VII.d.1. Measures to evaluate surgical hand hygiene practices may include, but are not limited to,
- direct observation (considered the most effective measurement);
- measuring the amount of product used;
- monitoring by using technology plus scanning;
- electronically monitoring entrance and exits into rooms with the use of video surveillance[55];
- electronically monitoring hand washing and surgical hand scrub dispensers[55]; and
- automated hand washing stations that read ID badges and record both the length of time the process takes and where the hand washing is performed.

Observational surveillance of surgical hand hygiene practices provides direct information on compliance by health care personnel.[3] Direct observation also can determine the areas

HAND HYGIENE

TABLE 1 CONTINUED. ACTIVITY AND CONSIDERATIONS FOR HAND HYGIENE AGENTS

Antiseptic agent	Persistent/ residual activity	Contraindications	Cautions	Soil removal
Soap and water	None[1]		May result in an increase of bacterial counts,[1,2] can result in skin dryness and irritation with frequent use[3]	Yes
Alcohol	None[1]		Flammable, does not penetrate organic material, very poor activity against bacterial spores[1]	No
Chlorhexidine	Excellent[1]	Keep out of eyes and inner ears[1]	Known sensitivity to any of the ingredients; activity can be affected by natural soaps, different inorganic anions, non-ionic surfactants and hand lotions that contain anionic emulsifying agents[3]; very poor activity against bacterial spores[1]	Yes
Chlorhexidine gluconate with alcohol	Excellent[1]	Keep out of eyes and inner ears[1]	Known sensitivity to any of the ingredients, very poor activity against bacterial spores, flammable[1]	Limited
Chloroxylenol	Good[1]		Safe up to 5% concentration[4]	Yes
Iodine and iodophors	Intermediate[1]	Sensitivity to povidone iodine	Products prone to contamination by gram negative bacteria, shellfish allergy is not a contraindication[5]	No
Quaternary ammonium compounds	None	Incompatible with anionic detergents[1,4]	Products prone to contamination by gram negative bacteria,[1] antimicrobial activity reduced by organic material[1]	No
Triclosan	Good[1]		Antimicrobial activity reduced by organic material,[6] minimally effective against gram-negative bacteria, product prone to contamination by gram-negative bacteria[6]	Yes

of strengths and weaknesses in hand hygiene practices and allows for improvement in the process.[1]

A disadvantage of this method is that direct observation of hand hygiene can be labor-intensive and expensive. In addition, one study showed there was little clinical improvement because the direct observer viewed only 0.4% of the hand washing and hand scrubbing that was done.[56] The Hawthorne effect may result in health care personnel improving how they do hand hygiene while being observed.[56] Over time, however, health care personnel forget why the observer is there. The observation process, if kept simple, can monitor one type of hand hygiene at a time (eg, surgical hand scrub).[4]

Measuring the amount of hand hygiene product used requires less time and fewer productive hours to monitor but may not take into account patient-case mix.[4] Studies have shown that this method may not be as effective as direct observation and may not change hand hygiene practices.[4] Therefore, this may not be a reliable method of monitoring hand hygiene or hand antisepsis.

Electronic monitoring can be an efficient and effective method of tracking hand hygiene compliance.[55] The advantages of video surveillance are that the camera is less obvious and may prevent the Hawthorne effect. Review of the recordings can be labor-intensive,[55] however, and electronic monitoring measures may not capture all of the possible times that hand hygiene should be performed.

Automated hand washing stations that read badges and record the length of time the process takes and where hand washing is performed is a technology utilized in the food industry to measure hand hygiene practice compliance. This technology provides the ability to record and produce reports that can be evaluated for hand hygiene compliance. This method is beginning to be adopted in the health care arena. It is more expensive than other methods but may become another useful tool for monitoring hand hygiene practices within health care organizations.[57]

VII.e. The health care organization's financial plan should include sufficient funds for hand hygiene products, performance monitoring, and feedback, as well as periodic training on surgical hand hygiene and the use of surgical hand hygiene products.[4]

Health care personnel involvement in product selection and acceptance of the product can result in better hand hygiene and savings.[4] Motivating health care personnel to change and practice good hand hygiene will have no value if there are no resources to make these changes.[58]

Glossary

Alcohol-based hand rub: An alcohol-containing preparation designed for application to the hands for reducing the number of viable microorganisms on the hands.

Artificial nails: Substances or devices applied or added to the natural nails to augment or enhance the wearer's own nails. They include, but are not limited to, bonding, tips, wrapping, and tapes.

Cumulative effect: A progressive decrease over time, usually measured in days, in the number of microorganisms present after repeated applications of a product.

Hand hygiene: a generic term that applies to all measures related to hand condition and decontamination.

Persistence: Prolonged or extended antimicrobial activity, usually measured in hours, which prevents or inhibits the regrowth of microorganisms after application of the product.

Subungual: Under the nail (eg, fingernail).

Surgical hand antiseptic agent: A product that is a broad-spectrum, fast-acting, and nonirritating preparation containing an antimicrobial ingredient designed to significantly reduce the number of microorganisms on intact skin. Surgical hand antiseptic agents demonstrate both persistent and cumulative activity.

References

1. Haas JP, Larson EL. Measurement of compliance with hand hygiene. *J Hosp Infect*. 2007;66(1):6-14.
2. Graves PB, Twomey CL. Surgical hand antisepsis: an evidence-based review. *Perioperative Nursing Clinics*. 2006;1(3):235-246.
3. Centers for Disease Control and Prevention. Guideline for hand hygiene in health-care settings. *MMWR*. October 25, 2002;51(RR-16):1-44.
4. *WHO Guidelines on Hand Hygiene in Health Care* (Advanced Draft). Geneva, Switzerland: World Health Organization; 2006. http://www.who.int/patientsafety/information_centre/ghhad_download_link/en/. Accessed October 19, 2009.
5. Friedman C, Petersen KH. *Infection Control in Ambulatory Care*. Boston, MA: Jones and Bartlett Publishers; 2004.
6. Siegel JD, Rhinehart E, Jackson M, Chiarello L; the Healthcare Infection Control Practices Advisory Committee. *Guideline for Isolation Precautions: Preventing Transmission of Infectious Agents in Healthcare Settings 2007*. Atlanta, GA: Centers for Disease Control and Prevention; 2007. http://www.cdc.gov/ncidod/dhqp/gl_isolation.html. Accessed October 19, 2009.
7. Mermel LA, McKay M, Dempsey J, Parenteau S. Pseudomonas surgical-site infections linked to a healthcare worker with onychomycosis. *Infect Control Hosp Epidemiol*. 2003;24(10):749-752.
8. Wynd CA, Samstag DE, Lapp AM. Bacterial carriage on the fingernails of OR nurses. *AORN J*. 1994;60(5):796-805.
9. Moolenaar RL, Crutcher JM, San Joaquin VH, et al. A prolonged outbreak of *Pseudomonas aeruginosa* in a neonatal intensive care unit: did staff fingernails play a role in disease transmission? *Infect Control Hosp Epidemiol*. 2000;21(2):80-85.
10. McGinley KJ, Larson EL, Leyden JJ. Composition and density of microflora in the subungual space of the hand. *J Clin Microbiol*. 1988;26(5):950-953.
11. Hedderwick SA, McNeil SA, Lyons MJ, Kauffman CA. Pathogenic organisms associated with artificial fingernails worn by healthcare workers. *Infect Control Hosp Epidemiol*. 2000;21(8):505-509.
12. Toles A. Artificial nails: are they putting patients at risk? A review of the research. *J Pediatr Oncol Nurs*. 2002;19(5):164-171.
13. Baumgardner CA, Maragos CS, Walz J, Larson E. Effects of nail polish on microbial growth of fingernails. Dispelling sacred cows. *AORN J*. 1993;58(1):84-88.
14. Porteous J. Artificial nails . . . very real risks. *Can Oper Room Nurs J*. 2002;20(3):16-17.
15. McNeil SA, Foster CL, Hedderwick SA, Kauffman CA. Effect of hand cleansing with antimicrobial soap or alcohol-based gel on microbial colonization of artificial fingernails worn by health care workers. *Clin Infect Dis*. 2001;32(3):367-372.
16. Parry MF, Grant B, Yukna M, et al. *Candida osteomyelitis* and diskitis after spinal surgery: an outbreak that implicates artificial nail use. *Clin Infect Dis*. 2001;32(3):352-357.
17. Salisbury DM, Hutfilz P, Treen LM, Bollin GE, Gautam S. The effect of rings on microbial load of health care workers' hands. *Am J Infect Control*. 1997;25(1):24-27.
18. Kelsall NK, Griggs RK, Bowker KE, Bannister GC. Should finger rings be removed prior to scrubbing for theatre? *J Hosp Infect*. 2006;62(4):450-452.
19. Trick WE, Vernon MO, Hayes RA, et al. Impact of ring wearing on hand contamination and comparison of hand hygiene agents in a hospital. *Clin Infect Dis*. 2003;36(11):1383-1390.
20. Field EA, McGowan P, Pearce PK, Martin MV. Rings and watches: should they be removed prior to operative dental procedures? *J Dent*. 1996;24(1-2):65-69.
21. Larson E, Girard R, Pessoa-Silva CL, Boyce J, Donaldson L, Pittet D. Skin reactions related to hand hygiene and selection of hand hygiene products. *Am J Infect Control*. 2006;34(10):627-635.
22. Molinari JA, Harte JA, eds. *APIC Text of Infection Control and Epidemiology*. Dental services. Washington, DC: Association for Professionals in Infection Control and Epidemiology; 2005: 51-1–51-22.

23. Marino C, Cohen M. Washington State hospital survey 2000: gloves, handwashing agents, and moisturizers. *Am J Infect Control.* 2001;29(6):422-424.

24. CPL 02-02-069–CPL 2-2.69: Enforcement procedures for the occupational exposure to bloodborne pathogens. Occupational Safety & Health Administration. http://www.osha.gov/pls/oshaweb/owadisp.show_document?p_table=DIRECTIVES&p_id=2570. Accessed October 19, 2009.

25. Jones RD, Jampani H, Mulberry G, Rizer RL. Moisturizing alcohol hand gels for surgical hand preparation. *AORN J.* 2000;71(3):584-587.

26. Widmer AE, Dangel M. Alcohol-based handrub: evaluation of technique and microbiological efficacy with international infection control professionals. *Infect Control Hosp Epidemiol.* 2004;25(3):207-209.

27. Hand hygiene. In: Underwood MA, ed. *APIC Text of Infection Control and Epidemiology.* Washington, DC: Association for Professionals in Infection Control and Epidemiology; 2005:19-1–19-7.

28. Kim PW, Roghmann MC, Perencevich EN, Harris AD. Rates of hand disinfection associated with glove use, patient isolation, and changes between exposure to various body sites. *Am J Infect Control.* 2003;31(2):97-103.

29. Grundmann H, Hori S, Winter B, Tami A, Austin DJ. Risk factors for the transmission of methicillin-resistant *Staphylococcus aureus* in an adult intensive care unit: fitting a model to the data. *J Infect Dis.* 2002;185(4):481-488.

30. McBryde ES, Bradley LC, Whitby M, McElwain DL. An investigation of contact transmission of methicillin-resistant *Staphylococcus aureus. J Hosp Infect.* 2004; 58(2):104-108.

31. Hubner NO, Kampf G, Kamp P, Kohlmann T, Kramer A. Does a preceding hand wash and drying time after surgical hand disinfection influence the efficacy of a propanol-based hand rub? *BMC Microbiol.* 2006;6:57.

32. Hubner NO, Kampf G, Loffler H, Kramer A. Effect of a 1 min hand wash on the bactericidal efficacy of consecutive surgical hand disinfection with standard alcohols and on skin hydration. *Int J Hyg Environ Health.* 2006;209(3):285-291.

33. Mangram AJ, Horan TC, Pearson ML, Silver LC, Jarvis WR. Guideline for prevention of surgical site infection, 1999. Hospital Infection Control Practices Advisory Committee. *Infect Control Hosp Epidemiol.* 1999; 20(4):250-278.

34. Griffith CJ, Malik R, Cooper RA, Looker N, Michaels B. Environmental surface cleanliness and the potential for contamination during handwashing. *Am J Infect Control.* 2003;31(2):93-96.

35. AIA Academy of Architecture for Health, Facilities Guidelines Institute. *Guidelines for Design and Construction of Health Care Facilities.* Washington, DC: American Institute of Architects; 2006.

36. Harrison WA, Griffith CJ, Ayers T, Michaels B. Bacterial transfer and cross-contamination potential associated with paper-towel dispensing. *Am J Infect Control.* 2003;31(7):387-391.

37. Hugonnet S, Pittet D. Hand hygiene-beliefs or science? *Clin Microbiol Infect.* 2000;6(7):350-356.

38. AORN guidance statement: Fire prevention in the operating room. In: *Perioperative Standards and Recommended Practices.* Denver, CO: AORN, Inc; 2009:195-203.

39. *NFPA 99 Standard for Health Care Facilities.* Quincy, MA: National Fire Protection Association; 2005.

40. Rotter ML, Kampf G, Suchomel M, Kundi M. Long-term effect of a 1.5 minute surgical hand rub with a propanol-based product on the resident hand flora. *J Hosp Infect.* 2007;66(1):84-85.

41. Gupta C, Czubatyj AM, Briski LE, Malani AK. Comparison of two alcohol-based surgical scrub solutions with an iodine-based scrub brush for presurgical antiseptic effectiveness in a community hospital. *J Hosp Infect.* 2007;65(1):65-71.

42. Hingst V, Juditzki I, Heeg P, Sonntag HG. Evaluation of the efficacy of surgical hand disinfection following a reduced application time of 3 instead of 5 min. *J Hosp Infect.* 1992;20(2):79-86.

43. Recommended practices for product selection in perioperative practice settings. In: *Perioperative Standards and Recommended Practices.* Denver, CO: AORN, Inc; 2009:387-390.

44. Larson E, Leyden JJ, McGinley KJ, Grove GL, Talbot GH. Physiologic and microbiologic changes in skin related to frequent handwashing. *J Infect Control.* 1986;7(2):59-63.

45. Department of Health and Human Services. Tentative final monograph for healthcare antiseptic drug products: proposed rules. *Fed Regist.* 1994;59(116):31402-31452.

46. Ojajarvi J. The importance of soap selection for routine hand hygiene in hospital. *J Hyg (Lond).* 1981;86(3):275-283.

47. Recommended practices for a safe environment of care. In: *Perioperative Standards and Recommended Practices.* Denver, CO: AORN, Inc; 2009:415-437.

48. Kownatzki E. Hand hygiene and skin health. *J Hosp Infect.* 2003;55(4):239-245.

49. Boyce JM, Kelliher S, Vallande N. Skin irritation and dryness associated with two hand-hygiene regimens: soap-and-water hand washing versus hand antisepsis with an alcoholic hand gel. *Infect Control Hosp Epidemiol.* 2000;21(7):442-448.

50. Schwanitz HJ, Riehl U, Schlesinger T, Bock M, Skudlik C, Wulfhorst B. Skin care management: educational aspects. *Int Arch Occup Environ Health.* 2003;76(5):374-381.

51. Pittet D. Improving compliance with hand hygiene in hospitals. *Infect Control Hosp Epidemiol.* 2000;21(6):381-386.

52. Voss A, Widmer AF. No time for handwashing!? Handwashing versus alcoholic rub: can we afford 100% compliance? *Infect Control Hosp Epidemiol.* 1997; 18(3):205-208.

53. Pittet D. Compliance with hand disinfection and its impact on hospital-acquired infections. *J Hosp Infect.* 2001;48(Suppl A):S40-S46.

54. Kampf G. The first hand scrub: why it does not make much sense. *J Hosp Infect.* 2007;65(1):83-84.

55. Venkatesh AK, Lankford MG, Rooney DM, Blachford T, Watts CM, Noskin GA. Use of electronic alerts to enhance hand hygiene compliance and decrease transmission of vancomycin-resistant *Enterococcus* in a hematology unit. *Am J Infect Control.* 2008;36(3):199-205.

56. van de Mortel T, Murgo M. An examination of covert observation and solution audit as tools to measure the success of hand hygiene interventions. *Am J Infect Control.* 2006;34(3):95-99.

57. Paulson DS. *Independent Laboratory Studies Summary. Automated Handwashing Stations.* Bozeman, MT: BioScience Laboratories, Inc; 2008.

58. Bandura A. Health promotion by social cognitive means. *Health Education & Behavior.* 2004;31(2):143-164.

HAND HYGIENE

Acknowledgments

LEAD AUTHORS

Joan Blanchard, RN, BSN, MSS, CNOR, CIC
Perioperative Nursing Specialist
AORN Center for Nursing Practice
Denver, Colorado

Renae Battié, RN, MN, CNOR
Regional Director Perioperative Services
Franciscan Health System
Tacoma, Washington

CONTRIBUTING AUTHORS

Nancy Bjerke, RN, MPH, CIC
Consultant
Association for Professionals in Infection Control and Epidemiology, Inc (APIC)
San Antonio, Texas

Elizabeth Bolyard, RN, MPH
Technical Information Specialist
Centers for Disease Control and Prevention
Atlanta, Georgia

Peter Graves, RN, BSN, CNOR
Consultant
Molnlycke Health Care US
Corinth, Texas

Ardene L. Nichols, RN, MSN, CNS, CNOR
Consultant
Association for Professionals in Infection Control and Epidemiology, Inc (APIC)
Conroe, Texas

PUBLICATION HISTORY

Originally published May 1976, *AORN Journal*, as "Recommended practices for surgical hand scrubs."

Revised March 1978, July 1982, May 1984, October 1990. Published as proposed recommended practices August 1994.

Revised November 1998; published April 1999, *AORN Journal*. Reformatted July 2000.

Revised November 2003; published in *Standards, Recommended Practices, and Guidelines,* 2004 edition. Reprinted February 2004, *AORN Journal*.

Revised March 2009 for online publication in *Perioperative Standards and Recommended Practices*. Revised July 2009 for online publication in *Perioperative Standards and Recommended Practices*.

Minor editing revisions made in October 2009 for publication in *Perioperative Standards and Recommended Practices,* 2010 edition.

Reformatted September 2012 for publication in *Perioperative Standards and Recommended Practices*, 2013 edition.

Minor editing revisions made in November 2014 for publication in *Guidelines for Perioperative Practice,* 2015 edition.

GUIDELINE FOR PREOPERATIVE PATIENT SKIN ANTISEPSIS

The Guideline for Preoperative Patient Skin Antisepsis has been approved by the AORN Guidelines Advisory Board. It was presented as a proposed guideline for comments by members and others. The guideline is effective August 15, 2014. The recommendations in the guideline are intended to be achievable and represent what is believed to be an optimal level of practice. Policies and procedures will reflect variations in practice settings and/or clinical situations that determine the degree to which the guideline can be implemented. AORN recognizes the many diverse settings in which perioperative nurses practice; therefore, this guideline is adaptable to all areas where operative and other invasive procedures may be performed.

Purpose

This document provides guidance for preoperative patient skin preparation, including preoperative patient bathing; preoperative hair removal; selection of skin antiseptics; application of antiseptics; and safe handling, storage, and disposal of antiseptics.

The goal of preoperative patient skin antisepsis is to reduce the risk of the patient developing a surgical site infection (SSI) by removing soil and transient microorganisms at the surgical site.[1] Reducing the amount of bacteria on the skin near the surgical incision lowers the risk of contaminating the surgical incision site.[1] As part of preparing the skin for antisepsis, preoperative bathing and hair management at the surgical site contribute to a reduction of microorganisms on the skin.[2-4] Effective skin antiseptics rapidly and persistently remove transient microorganisms and reduce resident microorganisms to subpathogenic levels with minimal skin and tissue irritation.[1]

Perioperative registered nurses (RNs) play a critical role in developing protocols for preoperative bathing, selecting and applying preoperative patient skin antiseptics, and facilitating appropriate hair removal when necessary. The guideline provides the perioperative RN and other perioperative team members with evidence-based practice guidance for preoperative patient skin antisepsis to promote patient safety and reduce the risk of SSI.

The following topics are outside the scope of this document: patient skin antisepsis after incision; antiseptic irrigation; preoperative patient skin antisepsis with no incision; patient skin antisepsis for postoperative wound care, including suture removal; preoperative patient bathing not intended for surgical preparation; preoperative patient bathing for decolonization of *Staphylococcus aureus*; mechanical and oral antimicrobial bowel preparation; adhesive incise drapes; microbial sealants; and antimicrobial prophylaxis to reduce the microbial load on skin.

Evidence Review

A medical librarian conducted a systematic literature search of the databases MEDLINE®, CINAHL®, and the Cochrane Database of Systematic Reviews for meta-analyses, systematic reviews, randomized controlled and nonrandomized trials and studies, case reports, letters, reviews, and guidelines. Search terms included *surgical skin preparation, skin preparation, skin prep, skin antisepsis, skin antiseptic, sterile preparation, disinfectants, local anti-infective agents, antiseptic solution, preoperative care, perioperative nursing, preoperative, surgical procedures, surgical wound infection, skin, skin care, paint, scrub, antiseptic shower, antiseptic cloth, chlorhexidine wipe, preoperative shower, preoperative wash, preoperative bathing, bathing and baths, hair removal, shaving, depilation, depilatory, nonshaved, razor, clipping, clipper, povidone-iodine, chlorhexidine, iodine, iodophors, iodine compounds, 2-propanol, alcohols, baby shampoo, isopropyl alcohol, alcohol-based, parachoroxylenol, chloroxylenol, PCMX, DuraPrep, pHisoHex, Prevantics, Hibiclens, Techni-Care, ChloraPrep, Betadine, Betasept, PVP-I Prep, ExCel AP, Castile, iodophor, cyanoacrylates, tissue adhesives, chemical burns, skin diseases, dermatitis, skin sensitivity, surgical fires, fires, flammability, flammable, penis, vagina, mucous membrane, stoma, fingernails, nail polish, artificial nails, jewelry, body piercing, body jewelry,* and *subdermal implant*.

The initial search, conducted on December 5, 2013, was limited to literature published in English between January 2006 and December 2013; however, the time restriction was not considered in subsequent searches. At the time of the search, the librarian also established weekly alerts on the topics included in the search and until February 2014, presented relevant alert results to the lead author.

Before the systematic search, the medical librarian had provided the lead author with a list of the citations from the 2008 revision of the AORN Recommended Practices for Preoperative Patient Skin Antisepsis for consideration for the 2014 revision. During the development of the guideline, the lead author requested additional articles that either did not fit the original search criteria or were discovered during the evidence appraisal process. Finally, the lead author and medical librarian identified relevant guidelines

PATIENT SKIN ANTISEPSIS

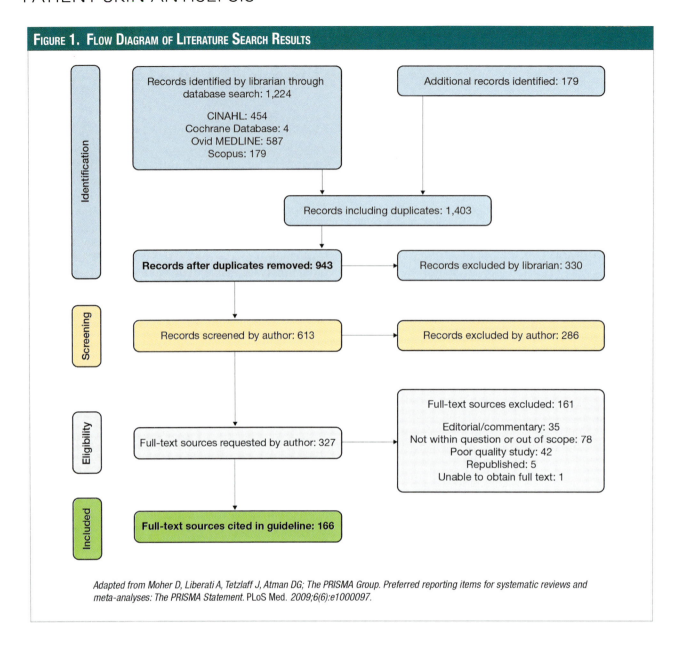

Figure 1. Flow Diagram of Literature Search Results

Adapted from Moher D, Liberati A, Tetzlaff J, Atman DG; The PRISMA Group. Preferred reporting items for systematic reviews and meta-analyses: The PRISMA Statement. *PLoS Med.* 2009;6(6):e1000097.

from government agencies and standards-setting bodies.

Excluded were non-peer–reviewed publications, studies that evaluated skin antisepsis as part of a bundle to prevent SSI, and low-quality evidence when higher-quality evidence was available.

Articles identified in the search were provided to the project team for evaluation. The team consisted of the lead author and three evidence appraisers. The lead author divided the search results into topics and assigned members of the team to review and critically appraise each article using the AORN Research or Non-Research Evidence Appraisal Tools as appropriate. The literature was independently evaluated and appraised according to the strength and quality of the evidence. Each article was then assigned an appraisal score. The appraisal score is noted in brackets after each reference, as applicable.

The collective evidence supporting each intervention within a specific recommendation was summarized, and the AORN Evidence-Rating Model was used to rate the strength of the evidence. Factors considered in the review of the collective evidence were the quality of evidence, the quantity of similar evidence on a given topic, and the consistency of evidence supporting a recommendation. The evidence rating is noted in brackets after each intervention.

Note: The evidence summary table is available at http://www.aorn.org/evidencetables/.

Editor's note: *MEDLINE is a registered trademark of the US National Library of Medicine's Medical Literature Analysis and Retrieval System, Bethesda, MD. CINAHL, Cumulative Index to Nursing and Allied Health Literature, is a registered trademark of EBSCO*

Industries, Birmingham, AL. DuraPrep is a registered trademark of 3M, St Paul, MN. pHisoHex is a registered trademark of Aspen Pharmacare Australia Pty Ltd, New South Wales, Australia. Prevantics is a registered trademark of Professional Disposables International, Inc, Parsippany, NJ. Hibiclens is a registered trademark of Mölnlycke Health Care AB, Gothenburg, Sweden. Techni-Care is a registered trademark of Care-Tech Laboratories, Inc, St Louis, MO. ChloraPrep is a registered trademark of CareFusion, San Diego, CA. Betadine and Betasept are registered trademarks of The Purdue Frederick Company, South Norwalk, CT. ExCel AP is a registered trademark of Aplicare, Meriden, CT.

Recommendation I

Patients should bathe or shower before surgery with either soap or an antiseptic.

The collective evidence supports that preoperative patient bathing may reduce the microbial flora on the patient's skin before surgery.

The limitations of the evidence are that research has not confirmed the effect of preoperative bathing on SSI development. Additional research is needed to define optimal preoperative bathing procedures, including whether antiseptics are more effective than soaps (eg, plain, antimicrobial), whether bathing the whole body or only the surgical site is more effective, the optimal timing of bathing before surgery, and the optimal number of baths or showers before surgery.

The benefits of preoperative patient bathing outweigh the harms. Benefits include reduction of transient and resident microorganisms on the skin that may lower the risk of the patient developing an SSI.[2] The harms of preoperative patient bathing with an antiseptic may include skin irritation, allergic reaction, or unnecessary treatment with antiseptics.[2]

I.a. The patient should be instructed to bathe or shower before surgery with either soap or a skin antiseptic on at least the night before or the day of surgery.[2,4-14] *[1: Strong Evidence]*

Preoperative patient bathing before surgery may reduce microbial skin contamination. Additional research is needed to determine the optimal soap or antiseptic product, interval between bathing and surgery, and number of baths or showers.

In 1973, findings of a nonexperimental study of 23,649 surgical wounds suggested that preoperative bathing was effective by showing a 2.3% infection rate for patients who did not bathe, 2.1% for patients who bathed with soap, and 1.3% for patients who bathed with an antiseptic before surgery.[5] No similar study has since been published that compares bathing with antiseptics or soaps to not bathing.

Three clinical practice guidelines make recommendations for preoperative bathing. National Institute for Health and Care Excellence (NICE) guidelines advise that the patient should shower or bathe with soap the day of or the day before surgery.[4] The NICE guidelines state that the evidence on the use of antiseptics is inconclusive.[4] The Society for Healthcare Epidemiology of America (SHEA) guidelines note gaps in evidence related to preoperative bathing, such as the effect of bathing on SSI development and the effectiveness of chlorhexidine gluconate (CHG).[6] Guidelines from the National Association of Orthopaedic Nurses (NAON) support the nursing practice of providing the patient with instructions for preoperative bathing protocols and advise providing written instructions.[7]

In a Cochrane systematic review of seven randomized controlled trials (RCTs), Webster and Osborne[2] concluded that there is not a soap or antiseptic product that is clearly the best to use for preoperative bathing for reducing the incidence of SSI. One of the RCTs included in the Cochrane review was a classic European study by Rotter et al[8] that compared a whole-body, two-bath protocol of CHG (n = 1,413) with placebo (n = 1,400) in 2,813 patients. This study found that preoperative bathing had no effect on SSI rates.[8] Another RCT in this Cochrane review, conducted by Veiga et al[9] in Brazil, compared 150 patients undergoing clean plastic surgery: one group took 4% CHG showers two hours before surgery (n = 50), one group showered with a placebo (n = 50), and one group received no instructions for showering (n = 50). The researchers found that the CHG showers effectively reduced skin contamination with coagulase-negative *Staphylococcus* but found no differences in postoperative infection rates.[9]

Randomized controlled trials with conflicting results were examined in the evidence review. A trial by Veiga et al[10] examined preoperative showers with 10% povidone-iodine two hours before surgery (n = 57) compared with no showering instruction (n = 57) for 114 patients. This study found that the povidone-iodine showers effectively reduced *Staphylococcus* colonization of the skin for clean plastic surgery procedures on the thorax and abdomen.[10] In an RCT studying healthy volunteers (n = 60) in the United Kingdom, Tanner et al[14] found that CHG preoperative body washes were more effective than soap for reducing microbial growth immediately and at six hours after the intervention, and that CHG had superior antibacterial activity in the groin area.

Evidence from two systematic reviews is inconclusive. A systematic review with meta-analysis of eight RCTs and eight quasi-RCTs found that routine preoperative whole-body bathing with CHG was not effective in preventing SSI.[13] Although the authors suggested that additional research in this area is needed, they also suggested that the low risk and low cost of preoperative bathing may be worth the marginal benefits of reducing SSI risk.[13] The second systematic review of 20 studies including RCTs, quasi-experimental studies, and nonexperimental studies found that antiseptic showers may reduce skin colonization and may prevent SSI, but data were inconclusive about which antiseptic was most effective.[12]

The number of preoperative baths or showers was the subject of another systematic review of 10 RCTs. Jakobsson et al[11] concluded that there was insufficient evidence to recommend a number of baths or showers to prevent SSI. The authors reverted to a previous recommendation of three to five showers until more evidence becomes available.[11]

There is a growing body of evidence supporting the use of 2% CHG-impregnated cloth products for preoperative bathing. Based on the collective evidence, this practice remains an unresolved issue and warrants additional generalizable, high-quality research to confirm the benefit of CHG-impregnated cloths. The results of studies involving the use of 2% CHG cloths for preoperative bathing conflict. Three RCTs,[15-17] six quasi-experimental studies,[18-23] and two organizational experiences[24,25] support the use of 2% CHG cloths for preoperative bathing. The limitations of two of the RCTs were that the studies were conducted in healthy volunteers and may not be generalizable to select patient populations.[16,17] Eight of these studies were conducted in patients undergoing orthopedic procedures and may also be limited in generalizability.[15,18,20-25]

A systematic review[26] and a literature review[27] also supported the practice of preoperative bathing with 2% CHG cloths, although the systematic review authors recommended additional studies to confirm their findings because of the observational nature of the studies and variations in the quality of data collection and analysis. One quasi-experimental study[28] refuted the use of 2% CHG cloths for preoperative bathing by finding no reduction in SSI with use of the cloths before total joint arthroplasty. Although many studies support the use of 2% CHG cloths for preoperative bathing, additional research is needed before a practice recommendation can be made.

I.a.1. The patient should be instructed to follow the product manufacturer's instructions for use. *[4: Benefits Balanced with Harms]*

I.a.2. After the preoperative bath or shower, the patient should be instructed not to apply
- alcohol-based hair or skin products,
- lotions,
- emollients, or
- cosmetics.

Patients should not apply deodorant for procedures involving the axilla. *[5: No Evidence]*

The collective evidence does not support or refute this recommendation. Alcohol-based products in the hair or on the skin at the surgical site may pose a fire hazard when an ignition source is used near the site. Lotions, emollients, cosmetics, and deodorants used at the surgical site may reduce the effectiveness of preoperative patient skin antiseptics or reduce the ability of patient monitors, adhesive surgical drapes, and adhesive dressings to adhere to the patient's skin.

I.a.3. For surgery on the hand or foot, the patient should be instructed that the nails on the operative extremity should be clean and natural, without artificial nail surfaces (eg, extensions, overlays, acrylic, silk wraps, enhancements).[29-31] *[2: Moderate Evidence]*

The evidence review found no cases of patient incision-site contamination related to the wearing of artificial nails or nail polish on the operative hand or foot. This is an unresolved issue that warrants additional research.

Two quasi-experimental studies evaluated the effect of health care personnel's wearing of artificial nails on surgical hand antisepsis. In these studies, researchers showed that the variety and amount of potentially pathogenic bacteria cultured from the fingertips of health care personnel wearing artificial nails was greater than for those with natural nails, both before and after hand washing.[30,31] With regard to nail polish, authors of a Cochrane systematic review found insufficient evidence to determine whether the fresh or chipped nail polish of health care personnel increased the risk of the patient developing an SSI.[29]

Although these studies showed nail contamination in health care personnel, these data may be extrapolated to the patient. Patients' wearing of artificial nails or nail polish at the surgical site may harbor microorganisms, which could contaminate the surgical site or reduce the effectiveness of preoperative patient skin antisepsis. Removal of artificial nails and nail polish that is near the surgical site may reduce contaminants on and under the nail.

I.a.4. The patient undergoing head or neck surgery should be instructed to shampoo his or her hair before surgery.[32] *[2: Moderate Evidence]*

The results from one RCT showed that shampooing with either 4% CHG or 7.5% povidone-iodine was effective in reducing resident flora on the scalp. No studies have compared other types of shampoo with antiseptics. The optimal preoperative shampoo product is an unresolved issue that warrants additional research.

Leclair et al[32] conducted an RCT of preoperative shampooing with a skin antiseptic by comparing scalp cultures, wound cultures, and SSI rates for 151 patients in four groups:
- preoperative shampoo and preoperative skin antisepsis with 4% CHG,
- no preoperative shampoo and preoperative skin antisepsis with 4% CHG,
- preoperative shampoo and preoperative skin antisepsis with 7.5% povidone-iodine, and
- no preoperative shampoo and preoperative skin antisepsis with 7.5% povidone-iodine.[32]

Patients randomly assigned to a shampoo group in the study were instructed to perform two preoperative shampoos with either CHG or povidone-iodine at least one hour apart during the two- to 24-hour period before surgery. All study patients had their hair clipped, scalp wetted with the assigned antiseptic, hair shaved with a razor, scalp scrubbed with the assigned antiseptic for a minimum of five minutes and blotted dry with a sterile towel, and an adherent plastic drape applied over the incision site. The researchers concluded that preoperative shampooing suppressed the emergence of resident flora on the scalp during neurosurgery and that CHG appeared to be superior to iodophors because of its residual antimicrobial activity.[32]

Prescribing 4% CHG shampoo is a medical decision. This practice contradicts the 4% CHG manufacturer's instructions for use, which state not to use the product on the head. The decision of the prescribing physician to order 4% CHG for preoperative shampooing constitutes off-label use. The benefits of a 4% CHG shampoo may not outweigh the potential harms of CHG causing injury by contact with the eyes, ears, or mouth.

I.b. A multidisciplinary team that includes perioperative RNs, physicians, and infection preventionists should develop a mechanism for evaluating and selecting products for preoperative patient bathing.[33] *[2: Moderate Evidence]*

Involvement of a multidisciplinary team allows input from personnel with clinical expertise.[33]

Recommendation II

Hair removal at the surgical site should be performed only in select clinical situations.

The collective evidence supports that hair at the surgical site should be left in place. When hair removal is necessary, clipping the hair may be associated with a lower risk of SSI development than hair removal with a razor.

The limitations of the evidence include that some studies had an inadequate sample size (ie, were underpowered) to determine the effect of hair removal on the development of SSI, the studies did not use a standardized definition of SSI, and the majority of the studies included in the systematic reviews are approximately 20 years old.

The benefits of leaving hair in place at the surgical site include preventing potential skin trauma from hair removal and potentially reducing the risk for SSI.[3] The harms of leaving the hair in place at the surgical site may include risk of fire.[34] The risk of fire may be minimized by confining the hair with a water-soluble gel and non-metallic ties or with braids for longer hair. No studies evaluated the use of alternative hair management techniques or products to reduce the risk of fire. The AORN Guideline for a Safe Environment of Care, Part 1 recommends coating facial hair with water-soluble gel for surgical procedures that involve the head and neck to minimize the risk of combustion.[34]

II.a. Hair at the surgical site should be left in place.[3-6,35,36] *[1: Strong Evidence]*

Removing hair at the surgical site has long been believed to be associated with an increased rate of SSI. In a landmark nonexperimental study of 23,649 surgical wounds, Cruse[5] found a 2.3% infection rate for surgical sites shaved with a razor, 1.7% for sites that were clipped, and 0.9% when no hair removal was performed. The researcher concluded that shaving should be kept to a minimum but did not suggest that hair should be left in place.[5]

Clinical practice guidelines from SHEA[6] and NICE[4] support the practice of leaving hair at the surgical site, unless the hair will interfere with the procedure. Conflicting evidence was examined in a Cochrane systematic review of 14 studies, including RCTs and quasi-RCTs, of a variety of procedure types. Tanner et al[3] concluded that the evidence sample sizes were too small and the studies were methodologically flawed, which prevented them from drawing strong conclusions that routine hair removal at the surgical site reduces the incidence of SSI.

A systematic review of 21 studies, including RCTs, quasi-experimental studies, and nonexperimental studies, found no evidence to suggest that hair should be routinely removed for neurosurgery procedures.[35] Another systematic review evaluated 18 studies and also determined that cranial surgeries should be performed without shaving.[36]

II.a.1. The patient should be instructed to leave hair in place at the surgical site before surgery.[37] *[2: Moderate Evidence]*

One nonexperimental study investigated patient compliance with not removing hair at the surgical site for cesarean deliveries. Ng et al[37] used an educational intervention campaign targeted toward prenatal patients to discourage pre-hospital hair removal after 36 weeks gestation. The researchers concluded that the patient education improved patient compliance with non-removal of hair at the surgical site from 41% to 27% in a three-year period.

Although the researchers noted that other evidence-based practices for reduction of SSI, including switching to an alcohol-based skin antiseptic, were implemented during the time of this investigation, they also saw a reduction in SSI rates for cesarean procedures and considered this educational campaign to be an important part of their multimodal approach to reducing SSI.[37] Additional research is needed to determine whether hair removal by the patient has an effect on risk for SSI.[37]

II.b. When necessary, hair at the surgical site should be removed by clipping or depilatory methods in a manner that minimizes injury to the skin.[3,4,6,7,35,38-40] *[1: Strong Evidence]*

When hair removal is necessary, hair removal by clippers may be associated with lower risk of SSI than when hair is removed by razors. No studies were found comparing clipping to depilatory methods. Additional research is needed to determine the most effective method of hair removal, the effect of hair removal on SSI development, and the optimal amount of time between hair removal at the surgical site and the surgical incision.

In a Cochrane systematic review, Tanner et al[3] concluded that although the patient sample size from the collective studies was too small to draw strong conclusions, use of clippers has been associated with lower SSI rates than use of razors. One of the RCTs included in this Cochrane review was a study of 789 spine procedures.[39] In this study, Celik and Kara[39] compared hair removal at the surgical site with a razor (n = 371) to no hair removal (n = 418) and found that shaving with a razor just before skin preparation increased the SSI rate. This study was limited by incomplete data because the researchers were not able to collect follow-up data on 47 shaved patients. In another systematic review of hair removal for neurosurgical procedures, Broekman et al[35] did not find any evidence that shaving decreased the incidence of SSIs, with a possibility that, conversely, shaving increased infections in neurosurgical patients. The authors recommended additional research in this area. A literature review also concluded that clipping and depilatory methods caused fewer SSIs than shaving with a razor.[38]

Studies involving removal of hair in the male genital area are limited and may conflict with recommendations to clip hair rather than shave hair with a razor, although additional research is needed. In an RCT of 217 procedures involving male genitalia, Grober et al[40] compared hair removal on the scrotum with clippers (n = 107) and razors (n = 108), with outcomes of quality of hair removal, skin trauma, and SSI events. The researchers concluded that hair removal by a razor on the scrotum prevented skin trauma and achieved better quality hair removal than clippers, with no apparent increase in infection rate.[40] The study did not describe whether wet or dry methods were used for either clipping or shaving and was limited by not being statistically powered to determine the effect on SSI.

There is consensus among professional associations to recommend hair removal with clipping or depilatory methods rather than shaving with a razor. The SHEA guidelines recommend removing hair by clipping or depilatory methods and specifically recommend not using a razor.[6] Guidelines from NICE advise removing hair with single-use clippers and also advise against using razors.[4] The NAON guidelines recommend using clippers for hair removal but do not address depilatory or shaving methods.[7] With regard to the timing of hair removal, the NAON guidelines recommend removing hair as close to the incision time as possible.[7]

II.b.1. The patient's hair should be removed in a location outside the operating or procedure room. *[4: Benefits Balanced with Harms]*

II.b.2. When removing hair outside the operating or procedure room is contraindicated (eg, by emergency, because of patient anxiety), the patient's hair should be removed in a manner that prevents dispersal of hair into the air of the operating or procedure room. Prevention of hair dispersal may be achieved by wet clipping, use of suction, or other methods. *[4: Benefits Balanced with Harms]*

II.b.3. Single-use clipper heads should be used and disposed of after each patient use. The reusable clipper handle should be disinfected after each use, in accordance with the manufacturer's instructions for use.[4] *[1: Strong Evidence]*

Guidelines from NICE recommend using single-use clipper heads to reduce the risk of cross-contamination of bloodborne pathogens between patients.[4]

II.b.4. When using depilatories for hair removal, the perioperative team member should follow the manufacturer's instructions for use, including testing skin for skin allergy and irritation reactions in an area away from the surgical site.[3] *[1: Strong Evidence]*

In a Cochrane systematic review, the authors discussed that depilatories may cause skin irritation and allergic reactions and recommended patch testing at least 24 hours before the cream is applied.[3]

II.b.5. The perioperative RN should document in the patient's health care record the hair removal method, time of removal, and area of hair removal. *[5: No Evidence]*

Recommendation III

A multidisciplinary team including perioperative RNs, physicians, and infection preventionists should select safe and effective antiseptic products for preoperative patient skin antisepsis.

The collective evidence indicates that there is no one antiseptic that is more effective than another for preventing SSI.

The limitations of the evidence review include that the literature has not determined which antiseptic is most effective for preoperative skin antisepsis because existing studies had inadequate sample sizes (ie, were underpowered) to determine the effect on SSI and are limited in quality. The evidence suggests that selection of a safe and effective preoperative skin antiseptic should be based on individual patient need.

III.a. The multidisciplinary team should develop a mechanism for product evaluation and selection of preoperative skin antiseptics.[33] *[2: Moderate Evidence]*

Involvement of a multidisciplinary team allows input from all departments in which the product will be used and from personnel with clinical expertise.[33]

III.a.1. The multidisciplinary team should select antiseptic skin preparation products based on a review of the current research literature. *[4: Benefits Balanced with Harms]*

No one antiseptic has been found to be better than another for preventing SSI, although alcohol-based antiseptics may be more effective than aqueous-based povidone-iodine when not contraindicated. This is an unresolved issue that warrants additional research. With a gap in the evidence to guide practice, decisions about which preoperative skin antiseptic to use in the practice setting are complex. A variety of products may be necessary to meet the needs of various patient populations. Input from a multidisciplinary team with diverse experience and knowledge of skin antiseptics is helpful during review of research, clinical guidelines, and literature from the manufacturers.

The evidence involving preoperative skin antiseptic selection conflicts. The NICE guidelines have no recommendation for skin antiseptic selection, citing a lack of evidence, although the document mentions that CHG and povidone-iodine are most suitable for preoperative skin antisepsis.[4] The NAON guidelines recommend using povidone-iodine, iodine-based alcohol, or CHG for preoperative skin antisepsis.[7] In a Cochrane systematic review of 13 RCTs, Dumville et al[1] concluded that the evidence for skin antisepsis was lacking in quality, and no determination could be made regarding the most effective skin antiseptic for clean surgery. One literature review recommended aqueous povidone-iodine for use on mucous membranes (eg, gynecological, genitourinary) and alcohol-based antiseptics for longer, open procedures.[41]

A nonexperimental study determined that iodine-based alcohol was an effective antiseptic for preoperative patient skin antisepsis.[42] In another paper describing the efficacy of skin antiseptics, a literature review supported the efficacy of CHG for reducing the risk of SSI.[43]

The evidence review also evaluated several studies that compared various skin antiseptic products, including aqueous povidone-iodine, CHG-alcohol, and iodine-based alcohol.

Some research studies support CHG-alcohol as more effective than aqueous povidone-iodine antiseptics.[44-47] A systematic review[48] and two literature reviews[49,50] found that CHG-alcohol was more effective than aqueous povidone-iodine.

Other evidence has indicated that CHG was more effective than povidone-iodine without accounting for the role of alcohol.[51,52] In a systematic review and meta-analysis, Maiwald and Chan[53] concluded that the role of alcohol has been overlooked in the literature and that studies showing a perceived efficacy of CHG actually demonstrate the effectiveness of CHG-alcohol.

Conversely, researchers who conducted an RCT involving 556 patients undergoing clean hernia surgeries compared aqueous 10% povidone-iodine (n = 285) to CHG-alcohol (n = 271) and concluded that there was no difference in reduction of bacterial counts.[54] A quasi-experimental cohort study also found that there was no difference in the rate of SSIs when either aqueous povidone-iodine (n = 29) or CHG-alcohol (n = 25) was used for cesarean delivery surgical site antisepsis.[55]

In an RCT involving 866 patients undergoing clean procedures, Berry et al[56] found there was no gold standard antiseptic for clean procedures and concluded that neither CHG-alcohol (n = 453) nor alcoholic povidone-iodine (n = 413) antiseptic was superior for reducing the risk of SSI. One

TABLE 1. US FOOD AND DRUG ADMINISTRATION CATEGORIES OF PATIENT PREOPERATIVE SKIN PREPARATIONS[1]

Active ingredient	Category
Benzalkonium chloride	IIIE
Chlorhexidine gluconate	"New drug"
Chloroxylenol	IIIE
Hexachlorophene	II
Iodine tincture USP	I
Iodine topical solution USP	I
Povidone-iodine 5% to 10%	I
Triclosan	IIIE
Iodine Povacrylex/Isopropyl Alcohol[2]	New drug[2]

E= Effectiveness

REFERENCES
1. US Food and Drug Administration. Tentative Final Monograph for Healthcare Antiseptic Drug Products proposed rule. Fed Regist. 1994;59(116):31402-31452.
2. US Food and Drug Administration. New Drug Application (NDA) #21-586.

RCT of 100 patients undergoing lumbar spine surgery also concluded that CHG-alcohol and iodine-based alcohol were equally effective for removing common pathogens at the surgical site.[57]

A systematic review of eight studies, including RCTs and quasi-RCTs, that compared foot and ankle surgery skin preparation techniques found that CHG-alcohol was more effective than iodine-based alcohol in reducing bacteria in the hallux nail fold area and that the antiseptics were equally effective at reducing bacterial counts in toe web spaces.[58] An RCT of 150 patients undergoing shoulder surgery found that CHG-alcohol was more effective than iodine-based alcohol and povidone-iodine for removing bacteria at the surgical site.[46] A conflicting quasi-experimental comparison of alcoholic iodine and CHG-alcohol products demonstrated that iodine-based alcohol antiseptics were more effective than CHG-alcohol antiseptics.[59]

Two RCTs compared preoperative skin antisepsis with aqueous two-step povidone-iodine products to skin antisepsis with one-step iodine-based alcohol products in cardiovascular procedures. These studies concluded that the iodine-based alcohol products were more effective than aqueous povidone-iodine solutions.[60,61]

III.a.2. The multidisciplinary team should select products for preoperative skin antisepsis that either meet US Food and Drug Administration (FDA) requirements as Category I in the Tentative Final Monograph (TFM) for Over-the-Counter (OTC) Healthcare Antiseptic Drug Products or are FDA-approved by the "New Drug Approval" (NDA) and "Abbreviated New Drug Approval" (ANDA) processes.[62] *[4: Benefits Balanced with Harms]*

The TFM approval process requires patient preoperative skin preparation drug products to be fast acting (ie, a 2-log reduction on the abdomen and 3-log reduction on the groin within 10 minutes), broad spectrum, and persistent (ie, no return to baseline flora count at six hours post application), and to significantly reduce the number of microorganisms on intact skin.[62] The FDA categorizes active ingredients in the TFM for patient preoperative skin preparation drug products as either Category I, II, or III. Category I means that the ingredient meets monograph conditions, and Category II or III means that the ingredient does not meet monograph conditions. In previous regulatory documents, Category I meant the product was generally recognized as safe, effective, and not misbranded; Category II meant that the product was not generally recognized as safe and effective or could be misbranded; and Category III meant that available data were insufficient to classify the product as safe and effective, and additional testing was required. Although the language in the TFM refers to monograph conditions, the document retains the previous concepts of the categories relating to safety and efficacy. Table 1 provides a summary of FDA categories for active ingredients in patient preoperative skin preparations. Table 2 provides a summary of the characteristics of commonly used skin antiseptics.

PATIENT SKIN ANTISEPSIS

Table 2. Activity and Considerations for Preoperative Patient Skin Antiseptics

	Aqueous iodine/ iodophors (10%)[1]	Chlorhexidine gluconate (CHG) (4%)[2]	*Alcohol (70%-91.3%)[3]	Alcoholic iodine/ iodophors[3]	CHG-alcohol[3]
Mechanism of action[1-3]	Oxidation/substitution with free iodine	Disrupts cell membrane	Denatures cell wall proteins, concentration determines effectiveness	See Aqueous Iodine/Iodophors and Alcohol	See CHG and Alcohol
Effectiveness against microorganisms[1-3]	Gram + and gram - bacteria, tubercle bacillus, fungi, and viruses	Gram + and gram - bacteria, yeasts, and some viruses	Gram + and gram - bacteria, mycobacteria, fungi, and viruses	See Aqueous Iodine/Iodophors and Alcohol	See CHG and Alcohol
Rapidity of action[1-3]	Moderate	Moderate	Most rapid	Rapid	Rapid
Residual activity[1-3]	Moderate	Excellent	None	Moderate	Excellent
Use on eyes, ears, or mouth[1,2,4]	Yes, ears and mouth. For eyes, use 5% ophthalmic solution.	No, eyes and ears. Can cause corneal damage or deafness if contacts middle ear. For mouth, use 0.12% CHG oral rinse.	Yes, ears. No, eyes and mouth. Can cause corneal damage or nerve damage.	No. Can cause corneal damage or nerve damage.	No. Can cause corneal damage. Can cause deafness if contacts middle ear.
Use in genital area[1,2,4]	Yes. Use with caution in patients susceptible to iodism.[5]	No[4]	No	No	No
Use internally[1,2,4]	No, external use only.	No, external use only. Do not use on wounds that involve more than superficial layers of skin.	No, external use only.	No, external use only. Do not use on open wounds.	No, external use only. Do not use on open wounds.
Contraindications[1,2,4]	Sensitivity or allergy to drug or any ingredients.	Sensitivity or allergy to drug or any ingredients. Do not use for lumbar puncture or in contact with meninges.	Sensitivity or allergy to drug or any ingredients.	Sensitivity or allergy to drug or any ingredients.	Sensitivity or allergy to drug or any ingredients. Do not use for lumbar puncture or in contact with meninges.
Cautions[1,2,4]	Use with caution in patients susceptible to iodism (eg, patients with burns, patients with thyroid disorders, neonates, pregnant women, lactating mothers). Prolonged exposure may cause irritation. Inactivated by blood.	Use with caution in premature infants or in infants younger than 2 months old, may cause chemical burns.	Flammable.	Flammable. Do not use in infants younger than 2 months old. Use with caution in nursing mothers. Use caution when removing adhesive drapes to avoid skin injury.	Flammable. Use with caution in premature infants or infants younger than 2 months old, may cause chemical burns.

*Isopropyl alcohol (70%-91.3%) is a classified as Category I for patient preoperative skin preparation for the limited indication of "for the preparation of the skin prior to an injection."[6(p31434)]

References
1. Zamora JL. Chemical and microbiologic characteristics and toxicity of povidone-iodine solutions. Am J Surg. 1986;151(3):400-406.
2. Lim K-S, Kam PCA. Chlorhexidine—pharmacology and clinical applications. Anaesth Intensive Care. 2008;36(4):502-512.
3. Reichman DE, Greenberg JA. Reducing surgical site infections: a review. Rev Obstet Gynecol. 2009;2(4):212-221.
4. DailyMed. US National Library of Medicine. http://dailymed.nlm.nih.gov/. Accessed July 14, 2014.
5. American College of Obstetricians and Gynecologists Women's Health Care Physicians, Committee on Gynecologic Practice. Committee Opinion No. 571: Solutions for surgical preparation of the vagina. Obstet Gynecol. 2013;122(3):718-720.
6. US Food and Drug Administration. Tentative Final Monograph for Healthcare Antiseptic Drug Products proposed rule. Fed Regist. 1994;59(116):31402-31452.

III.a.3. Selected products should be purchased in single-use containers.[63] *[1: Regulatory Requirement]*

In November 2013, the FDA issued a Drug Safety Communication requesting that manufacturers package antiseptics indicated for preoperative skin preparation in single-use containers to reduce the risk of infection from improper antiseptic use and contamination of products during use.[63]

III.a.4. Unless contraindicated (eg, antisepsis of split-thickness skin graft donor sites), the multidisciplinary team should select products for preoperative patient skin antisepsis that are colored or tinted (ie, not clear).[64] *[2: Moderate Evidence]*

Use of colored antiseptics was supported in a quasi-experimental study of skin preparation in upper-limb surgery.[64] This study showed that use of clear antiseptics resulted in more missed spots, mostly in finger areas, than did colored antiseptics.[64] Flammable clear antiseptics may also pose a fire or chemical burn hazard if unseen solution is allowed to drip or pool on or near the patient, although no evidence was found in the evidence review to evaluate the effect of visibility on reducing fire or chemical hazards.

III.b. The perioperative RN, in collaboration with the surgeon and anesthesia professional, should select a safe, effective, health care organization-approved preoperative antiseptic for the individual patient based on the patient assessment, the procedure type, and a review of the manufacturer's instructions for use and contraindications.[65,66] *[2: Moderate Evidence]*

Selection of a preoperative skin antiseptic based on individual patient assessment may reduce the risk for patient complications. One literature review discussed the various preoperative skin antiseptics and concluded that perioperative RNs should evaluate and select the most appropriate antiseptic for each patient.[65] Another literature review concluded that the patient assessment was critical to selection of the correct preoperative skin antiseptic.[66]

III.b.1. The perioperative RN should assess the patient for allergies and sensitivities to preoperative skin antiseptics.[67-78] *[2: Moderate Evidence]*

In an in vitro study, Quatresooz et al[67] found that the skin reacts differently to the action of chemicals in various anatomic sites of the body. These researchers found that, in the laboratory setting, povidone-iodine (100 mg/mL) produced less irritation in the stratum corneum than two other antiseptics (ie, povidone-iodine 70 mg/mL, chlorhexidine digluconate 50 mg/mL), but in in vivo settings the severity of skin irritation depends on individual susceptibility and the site of exposure.[67]

In a case report, Sanders and Hawken[68] described three cases of chemical skin reactions to CHG that provide an example of how anatomic location may cause the skin to react differently to chemicals. In this report, three patients undergoing shoulder arthroscopy developed partial thickness chemical burns on the shoulder from a CHG-alcohol preoperative skin antiseptic.[68] The authors determined that the occurrences of chemical skin injury were related to alteration of the skin at the shoulder from traction and to local swelling from the procedure.[68]

A 2004 position statement from the American Academy of Allergy Asthma and Immunology (AAAAI) asserted that fish or seafood allergies do not indicate allergy to iodine. According to the position statement, contact dermatitis related to topically applied iodine antiseptics does not indicate an iodine allergy; rather, this is a reaction to chemicals in the product. Anaphylaxis to topical iodine antiseptic solutions is exceedingly rare and not proven to be related to iodine.[69] The AAAAI posts this position statement for reference only, and it does not reflect the current position of the academy. Limited evidence was found describing the relationship between seafood and iodine allergies. One nonexperimental survey study[71] and one literature review[70] support the assertion in the AAAAI position statement that seafood allergy is not related to iodine allergy.

Two case reports describe patients who developed anaphylactic reactions to povidone-iodine solution: one is a report of a pediatric patient with broken skin[72] and one is a report of vaginal application of povidone-iodine to a hypersensitized patient.[73]

In a case report, Sivathasan and Goodfellow[74] discussed the potential dangers of chlorhexidine and recommended caution when using CHG as an antiseptic in patients with a history of contact dermatitis. They recommended that clinicians consider CHG allergy in the event of an allergic reaction.[74] Case reports of anaphylaxis from CHG have been reported in the literature.[75-77]

Although isopropyl alcohol is a rare allergen, there are reports of allergic reactions in the literature.[78] In a case report of a delayed hypersensitivity to isopropyl alcohol, Vujevich and Zirwas[78] recommended that clinicians consider alcohol as an allergen when contact dermatitis is suspected after a surgical procedure. The authors hypothesized that the combination of isopropyl alcohol application and alteration of the skin from a needle injection may have allowed isopropyl alcohol to penetrate the stratum corneum and cause an allergic reaction.[78]

III.b.2. The perioperative RN should assess the skin integrity at the surgical site before selecting a preoperative patient skin antiseptic. *[4: Benefits Balanced with Harms]*

III.b.3. The preoperative antiseptic product should be selected based on the procedure type. *[4: Benefits Balanced with Harms]*

Several studies evaluated the efficacy of preoperative patient skin antisepsis based on procedure type. The evidence involving the various procedure-specific preoperative skin antisepsis selection is limited, and this subject warrants additional research.

Several studies support preoperative eye antisepsis with 5% povidone-iodine ophthalmic solution irrigation to reduce rates of conjunctival bacterial load and risk of endophthalmitis from intraocular surgery.[79-83] Although researchers who conducted an RCT of 271 cataract surgeries concluded that 10% povidone-iodine was more effective than 1% or 5% povidone-iodine solutions for reducing bacterial load of the eye,[84] an international laboratory study in Taiwan warned of risk for corneal cell death by cytotoxicity from fixation during exposure to high concentrations of povidone-iodine (ie, 5% to 10%).[85] Researchers in Germany also discussed safety concerns regarding povidone-iodine and recommended use of 1.25% povidone-iodine for ocular antisepsis, citing concern for exacerbating untreated hyperthyroidism and that additional research is needed to evaluate the effect of ophthalmic povidone-iodine on thyroid function.[86,87]

The collective evidence indicates that povidone-iodine is commonly used for vaginal antisepsis in gynecological procedures. There are currently no FDA-approved antiseptic alternatives on the market for use in the vaginal vault when povidone-iodine is contraindicated (eg, by patient allergy). Two alternatives to vaginal povidone-iodine, sterile saline[88] and baby shampoo,[89] were discussed in the literature. Both studies suggested that these alternatives were as effective as povidone-iodine for preoperative vaginal antisepsis.

In a position statement from the American Congress of Obstetricians and Gynecologists (ACOG), the committee recommends off-label use of 4% CHG with low alcohol content (eg, 4%) as a safe and effective alternative for vaginal preparation when povidone-iodine is contraindicated or CHG is preferred by the surgeon.[90]

In an RCT of 1,570 abdominal hysterectomy procedures, Eason et al[91] compared preoperative vaginal antisepsis with a povidone-iodine gel (n = 780) to no gel (n = 790). The researchers found that the povidone-iodine gel group had a lower risk of developing abscesses, but there was no significant difference in infection rates.[91]

Performing preoperative antisepsis of the vagina for cesarean deliveries is supported in a Cochrane systematic review, although the reviewers concluded that evidence on the type of solution and method is lacking.[92] For cesarean procedures, two RCTs[93,94] and one quasi-experimental study[95] found that a vaginal preparation with povidone-iodine was effective for prevention of endometritis and SSI. One nonexperimental study suggested that abdomen preparation with CHG-alcohol was more effective than povidone-iodine.[47] A quasi-experimental study found that povidone-iodine and CHG-alcohol were equally effective in reducing SSI as preoperative abdominal skin antisepsis in cesarean procedures.[55] Authors of a Cochrane systematic review concluded that more research is needed to determine an ideal skin antiseptic for cesarean delivery incisions.[96]

Authors of a systematic review with meta-analysis[58] of eight RCTs and quasi-RCTs of foot and ankle surgery concluded that alcohol antiseptic solutions performed more effectively than aqueous iodine[97] for reducing bacterial load of the foot, and CHG-alcohol was more effective than iodine-based alcohol[98] for reducing foot flora. Researchers who conducted two small RCTs came to conclusions that conflict with this systematic review, including that alcohol gives no added benefit to antiseptic solutions[99] and that iodine-based alcohol is more effective at reducing bacterial load of the foot.[100]

Saltzman et al[46] conducted an RCT of 150 shoulder surgeries by comparing reduction of bacteria at the surgical site after skin antisepsis with three antiseptics: CHG-alcohol, iodine-based alcohol, and povidone-iodine. The researchers concluded that CHG-alcohol was most effective for reducing overall bacteria in the shoulder area and that povidone-iodine was the least effective for removing coagulase-negative *Staphylococcus* from the shoulder.[46]

In an RCT of 100 lumbar spine procedures, Savage et al[57] compared preoperative skin antisepsis with CHG-alcohol (n = 50) and iodine-based alcohol (n = 50). They concluded that the antiseptics were equally effective in removing bacterial pathogens at the surgical site. They also discussed that the skin flora of the lumbar spine differs from other locations of the body and that more research is needed to determine effective antiseptics for lumbar spine procedures.[57]

III.b.4. The perioperative RN should assess the surgical site for the presence of hair.[101] When an alcohol-based skin antiseptic is used for a procedure involving an ignition source, hair at the surgical site should be clipped before application of the antiseptic. *[4: Benefits Balanced with Harms]*

The presence of hair may contraindicate the use of flammable antiseptics according to manufacturers' instructions for use. A flammable antiseptic for preoperative skin antisepsis is contraindicated when the procedure involves an ignition source (eg, electrosurgical unit [ESU], laser) and the solution is unable to dry completely in hair. According to the Centers for Medicare & Medicaid Services (CMS), alcohol-based skin antiseptics that wick into the patient's hair result in prolonged drying times.[102,103] No evidence was found that describes the length or amount of hair that constitutes a fire risk during use of alcohol-based skin antiseptics.

In a case report, a patient described as having copious body hair was burned on the neck and shoulders while undergoing a tracheostomy.[101] After the patient's neck was prepared with an alcohol-based skin antiseptic, the surgical team allowed the solution to dry for three minutes before draping. Activation of electrocautery ignited the fire, which was fueled by the skin antiseptic and the patient's body hair and oxidized in an oxygen-enriched environment. The authors of the case report recommended that the alcohol-based skin antiseptic product not be used for a hirsute patient because the hair can impede drying of the solution.[101]

III.b.5. The perioperative RN should consult the physician when selecting iodine and iodophor-based preoperative patient skin antiseptics for patients susceptible to iodism (eg, patients with burns, patients with thyroid disorders, neonates, pregnant women, lactating mothers).[104] *[2: Moderate Evidence]*

Some patients are susceptible to iodism from preoperative skin antisepsis with iodine and iodophor-based antiseptics.

Three reports in the literature demonstrated that repeated application of povidone-iodine to the skin of burn patients may cause iodine absorption,[105] induced hyperthyroidism,[106] and metabolic acidosis.[107] A review explained that the amount of iodine absorption from polyvinylpyrrolidone-iodine in burn patients depends on the concentration applied, frequency of application, type and total surface area of the burn, and the patient's renal function.[104]

The author of a literature review concluded that most patients can tolerate excess quantities of iodine without negative effects, although iodine-induced hyperthyroidism may occur in patients with underlying hyperthyroidism or goiter.[104] In an RCT (n = 68), Tomoda et al[108] compared preoperative patient skin antisepsis with povidone-iodine (n = 47) to CHG (n = 21) in patients with thyroid carcinoma who were on an iodine-restricted diet and undergoing total thyroidectomy. The researchers demonstrated that iodism resulted from a single application of povidone-iodine for skin antisepsis. In this study, the patients' postoperative iodine levels in the urine were nearly seven times the preoperative levels. The researchers theorized that cutaneously absorbed iodine could potentially interfere with iodine therapy or cause thyroid dysfunction in susceptible patients.[108]

Researchers in Germany cautioned that ophthalmic application of povidone-iodine may cause thyroid disturbances, specifically exacerbation of untreated hyperthyroidism.[86,87] These researchers recommended additional research to evaluate the effect on the thyroid of administering ophthalmic povidone-iodine.

Several case reports and studies have demonstrated iodism in neonates[109] and advise cautious use of iodine-based antiseptics in neonates because of the risk for transient hypothyroidism[104,110,111] or iodine-induced hyperthyroidism.[112] A literature review recommended minimizing neonatal iodine exposure because of the risk of significant iodine overload and severe transient hypothyroidism, especially in premature neonates with increased skin permeability and immature thyroid glands.[113] The authors of the review recommended monitoring thyroid-stimulating hormone levels in neonates exposed to iodine skin antiseptics.[113] Two nonexperimental studies also recommended that iodine-based antiseptics be used with caution, including thyroid function monitoring, in premature infants who require repeated antiseptic applications, because transient thyroid alterations may be detrimental to neurologic development in this vulnerable population.[110,111]

A literature review recommended using iodine-based antiseptics with caution in pregnant mothers because iodine crosses the placental barrier.[104] In a Cochrane systematic review, Hadiati et al[96] discussed an abstract of one French RCT (n = 22) that compared CHG 0.5% with 70% alcohol to use of an antiseptic-impregnated adhesive incise drape and found a higher concentration of iodine in the cord blood of newborns in the antiseptic-impregnated adhesive incise drape group, but no significant difference in iodine of 48-hour urine or thyroid-stimulating hormone blood levels on the fifth day. The authors of the systematic review did not make a recommendation based on this abstract.

In a Cochrane systematic review that recommended the use of vaginal povidone-iodine immediately before cesarean deliveries, Haas et al[92] did not discuss any risk of iodism in either the mother or the newborn. In a nonexperimental study of nonpregnant women (n = 12), Vorherr et al[114] demonstrated iodism after a two-minute vaginal antisepsis with povidone-iodine. The researchers advised against treating vaginitis in pregnant women with repeated applications of povidone-iodine because of the risk for development of iodine-induced goiter and hypothyroidism in the fetus and newborn. They explained that this risk is especially high with repeated use of povidone-iodine.[114]

Manufacturer's instructions for use of one iodine-based alcohol skin antiseptic recommend caution when using the product for women who are lactating (ie, breast-feeding) because of potential transient hypothyroidism in the nursing newborn.[115] The evidence review found no research evidence on iodine application in lactating mothers.

III.b.6. The perioperative RN should consult with the physician when selecting CHG and alcohol-based preoperative patient skin antiseptics for neonates.[113,116-118] *[2: Moderate Evidence]*

Neonates, especially extremely premature neonates, are at an increased risk for skin irritation and chemical burns of the skin from both CHG and alcohol-based skin antiseptics. In a literature review, Afsar[113] recommended that alcohol antisepsis be avoided in neonates because alcohol can cause hemorrhagic necrosis and skin burns, especially in extremely low-birth-weight infants and suggested that CHG alone may be a safer alternative for antisepsis.

In one case report of an extremely premature infant with aqueous 2% CHG chemical burns, Lashkari et al[116] found that the chemical exposure could have been limited by immediately wiping excess CHG with normal saline to avoid burns. Another case report of two extremely premature neonates with severe chemical burns as a result of 70% isopropyl alcohol applications for skin antisepsis found that pressure and decreased perfusion also played a role in the skin injury.[117] The authors of this case report advised exercising extreme caution with use of alcohol for skin antisepsis in severely premature infants.[117]

In another case report, Harpin and Rutter[118] described cutaneous alcohol absorption and hemorrhagic skin necrosis in a 27-week gestation twin pre-term infant from skin antisepsis with methylated spirits (95% ethanol and 5% wood naphtha, which is 60% methanol). In this case, the extremely premature neonate died. Although the role of alcohol intoxication in the neonate's death was unknown because blood alcohol levels were not drawn until 18 hours after the alcohol application, the authors suspected that the maximum alcohol level from cutaneous alcohol absorption was in the potentially fatal range.[118]

III.b.7. When FDA-approved (ie, Category I, NDA, ANDA) antiseptic products are contraindicated, the perioperative team members should collaboratively evaluate the risks and benefits of using Class II or Class III FDA-approved antiseptics or other alternative solutions (eg, soaps, saline). *[4: Benefits Balanced with Harms]*

The evidence review found no literature regarding the efficacy of alternative antiseptic products. When a patient has an allergy or a condition such as a large open wound, all available Class I FDA-approved products for antisepsis might be contraindicated. In this situation, the perioperative team is challenged to select a safe, effective alternative for the individual patient. (See Recommendation III.a.)

Recommendation IV

Perioperative team members should apply the preoperative patient skin antiseptic in a safe and effective manner.

The collective evidence suggests that following the antiseptic manufacturer's instructions for use and applying preoperative patient skin antiseptics in a safe and effective manner may prevent patient harm (eg, inadequate skin antisepsis, fire, chemical injury).

The limitations of the evidence include the limited quality of existing studies and a lack of procedure-specific clinical research evaluating the effectiveness of various skin preparation and antisepsis techniques.

IV.a. Perioperative team members should confirm the surgical site before performing preoperative patient skin antisepsis.[119] *[2: Moderate Evidence]*

The evidence review found no research evidence to support or refute this recommendation. Performing preoperative skin antisepsis at the wrong surgical site may result in a cascade of events leading to wrong site surgery. Confirmation of the location of the surgical site before the time-out process increases communication and consistent documentation and may reduce the likelihood of error. The AORN Guideline for Transfer of Patient Care Information recommends verifying the surgical site as part of the time-out process.[119]

IV.a.1. The surgical site mark should remain visible after preoperative patient skin antisepsis.[120-124] *[2: Moderate Evidence]*

Marking the surgical site with a nonsterile permanent marker is a safe practice for identifying the surgical site. Two quasi-experimental studies, each of 20 healthy volunteers, evaluated the effect of site marking on the sterility of skin antisepsis.[120,121] The researchers concluded that skin marking with a nonsterile permanent marker did not effect the sterility of skin antisepsis with povidone-iodine, as evidenced by no culture growth at the treated areas.[120,121]

Researchers in a nonexperimental study investigated the potential for the surgical site marker to serve as reservoir for transmissible infections.[122] In this study, Wilson and Tate[122] compared two types of markers, water-based and alcohol-based, and determined that transmission of methicillin-resistant *Staphylococcus aureus* (MRSA) is feasible with water-based skin markers. They recommended against using water-based skin markers for multiple patients because of the theoretical risk of transmitting MRSA.[122]

The evidence review also evalutated studies that examined the erasure of the surgical site marking during preoperative patient skin antisepsis. In these experimental studies, each of which involved permanent, alcohol-based markers and had a sample size of 20, the researchers found that a CHG-alcohol antiseptic product erased more site markings than did an iodine-based alcohol antiseptic product.[123,124]

IV.b. The perioperative RN should assess the condition of the patient's skin at the surgical site[125] and prepare the skin for antisepsis. *[2: Moderate Evidence]*

The evidence review found no literature to support or refute this recommendation. Patient assessment before an intervention is a standard of perioperative nursing practice.[125]

IV.b.1. The skin at the surgical site should be free of soil, debris, emollients, cosmetics, and alcohol-based products. *[4: Benefits Balanced with Harms]*

The evidence review found no literature to support or refute this recommendation. Removal of superficial soil, debris, emollients, and cosmetics is generally accepted as a practice that may improve the effectiveness of preoperative patient skin antisepsis by decreasing the organic debris on the skin at the surgical site. Alcohol-based products on the skin or hair at the surgical site may pose a fire hazard if an ignition source will be used during the procedure.

IV.b.2. The patient's jewelry (eg, rings, piercings) at the surgical site should be removed before preoperative skin antisepsis.[29,126] *[4: Benefits Balanced with Harms]*

No literature was found regarding patients' wearing of jewelry and its effect on preoperative patient skin antisepsis. Jewelry at the surgical site may harbor microorganisms and trap these organisms on adjacent skin, which may contaminate the surgical site or reduce the effectiveness of preoperative patient skin antisepsis.

Two studies evaluated health care workers' wearing of jewelry on the effectiveness of surgical hand antisepsis. A Cochrane systematic review of health care workers wearing finger rings during surgical hand antisepsis found that no studies evaluated the effect of this practice on SSI, although there was a common theoretical concern that rings could harbor bacteria and reduce the effectiveness of surgical hand antisepsis.[29] In a quasi-experimental study of health care worker hand contamination, Trick et al[126] found that ring wearing increased the frequency of hand contamination with pathogens, although the levels of contamination were significantly reduced when alcohol-based hand rubs were used.

Although these studies showed hand contamination in health care personnel wearing rings, these data may be extrapolated to the patient. Patients' jewelry at the surgical site may harbor microorganisms, which could contaminate the surgical site or reduce the effectiveness of preoperative patient skin antisepsis. Removal of jewelry near the surgical site may reduce contaminants on the skin.

IV.b.3. If the patient did not bathe or shower preoperatively, the perioperative team member may wash the skin at the surgical site with soap or an antiseptic before performing preoperative skin antisepsis.[127] *[2: Moderate Evidence]*

Preoperative washing is supported by one prospective case-control study.[127] This quasi-experimental study demonstrated that patients undergoing emergency hip arthroplasty who had not followed preoperative bathing protocols were more likely to have more-abundant and different microbial flora at the surgical site before preoperative patient skin antisepsis.[127]

The presence of transient microorganisms has not been proven to be related to the development of SSI. There is a theoretical

PATIENT SKIN ANTISEPSIS

hypothesis that reducing the microbial load at the surgical site before antisepsis may lower the risk of a transient microorganism contaminating the surgical site. Preoperative washing also may remove gross soil, spores, and oils that may limit the effectiveness of the antiseptic. This is an unresolved issue that warrants additional research.

IV.b.4. Areas of greater contamination (ie, umbilicus, foreskin, under nails, intestinal or urinary stoma) in the surgical field should be cleansed before preoperative patient skin antisepsis is performed. *[4: Benefits Balanced with Harms]*

The evidence review found no literature to support or refute this recommendation. Some anatomic areas may contain more debris than other sites. Cleaning these areas before preoperative patient skin antisepsis may prevent contamination of the surgical site and allow the antiseptic to achieve its intended level of effectiveness.

Organic and inorganic material in the umbilicus (eg, detritus) may reduce the effectiveness of the skin antiseptic and contaminate the surgical site for abdominal procedures. Areas under nails (ie, subungual areas) also may harbor organic and inorganic material, including microorganisms, that could limit the effectiveness of antisepsis for procedures involving the hand or foot. Similarly, surgical sites including the penis may harbor microorganisms that accumulate in the area under the foreskin (ie, prepuce), if present, including organic material (ie, smegma). Intestinal or urinary stomas are also highly likely to contain organic material, such as mucin, that could render some antiseptics ineffective.

IV.b.5. Highly contaminated areas (eg, anus, colostomy) near the surgical site should be isolated with a sterile barrier drape. *[4: Benefits Balanced with Harms]*

IV.c. A nonscrubbed perioperative team member should apply the skin antiseptic using sterile technique. *[4: Benefits Balanced with Harms]*

The evidence review found no research evidence to support or refute this recommendation. The risk of contamination of a scrubbed perioperative team member's sterile gown and gloves may be high during preoperative patient skin antisepsis activities.

IV.c.1. The perioperative team member should perform hand hygiene before applying the preoperative patient skin antiseptic.[128] *[2: Moderate Evidence]*

IV.c.2. The perioperative team member should wear sterile gloves when performing preoperative patient skin antisepsis. Nonsterile gloves may be worn if the antiseptic applicator is of sufficient length to prevent contact of the gloved hand with the antiseptic solution and the patient's skin. *[4: Benefits Balanced with Harms]*

The evidence review found no literature to support or refute this recommendation. This is an unresolved issue that warrants additional research.

IV.c.3. The perioperative team member should wear surgical attire that covers his or her arms while performing preoperative patient skin antisepsis.[129] *[2: Moderate Evidence]*

IV.c.4. The perioperative team members should use sterile supplies to apply preoperative patient skin antiseptics. *[4: Benefits Balanced with Harms]*

One RCT compared povidone-iodine skin antisepsis using both clean and sterile kits and found no difference in microbial counts on patients' skin.[130] This study has not been replicated, and no similar studies were found in the evidence review. This is an unresolved issue that warrants additional research.

IV.c.5. Items that touch the patient's skin after preoperative skin antisepsis should be sterile to prevent introduction of microorganisms at the surgical site.[131] *[1: Strong Evidence]*

IV.d. Skin antiseptics should be applied using aseptic technique and according to the manufacturer's instructions for use. *[4: Benefits Balanced with Harm]*

The evidence review found no literature related to application technique. The benefit of using aseptic technique for applying preoperative skin antiseptics outweighs the harm of contaminating the surgical site.

Antiseptic manufacturers' instructions for use convey important safety and efficacy instructions to the user. Failure to adhere to manufacturers' instructions for use may result in patient harm or ineffectiveness of the preoperative patient skin antisepsis.

IV.d.1. The perioperative team member should apply the skin antiseptic to an area large enough to accommodate potential shifting of the surgical drapes, extension of the incision (eg, during conversion of a minimally invasive procedure to an open procedure), potential additional incisions, and all potential drain sites. *[4: Benefits Balanced with Harms]*

IV.d.2. The skin antiseptic should be applied starting at the incision site and moving away toward the periphery of the surgical site. The applicator should be discarded after contact with a peripheral or contaminated area. Another sterile applicator should be

IV.d.3. When the incision site is more highly contaminated than the surrounding skin (eg, anus, perineum, stoma, open wound, catheter, drain, axilla), the area with a lower bacterial count should be prepped first, followed by the area of higher contamination, as opposed to working from the incision toward the periphery. *[4: Benefits Balanced with Harms]*

The evidence review found no studies related to the sequence of skin antisepsis involving highly contaminated areas. This is an unresolved issue that warrants additional research.

IV.d.4. When using a pre-filled antiseptic applicator, the perioperative team member should follow the manufacturer's instructions for use (eg, maximum and minimum surface area per applicator) to apply the skin antiseptic with uniform distribution. *[4: Benefits Balanced with Harms]*

IV.d.5. The antiseptic should be applied with care (eg, gentle friction) on fragile tissue, burns, open wounds, or malignant areas.[66] *[2: Moderate Evidence]*

Fragile skin or tissue, burns, and open wounds are at a high risk for skin injury during preoperative patient skin antisepsis. Vigorous skin antisepsis in areas of malignancy may potentially spread cancer cells. The practice of using gentle friction when performing antisepsis in an area of malignancy is supported in one literature review.[66]

IV.d.6. For preoperative patient skin antisepsis with aqueous povidone-iodine, either scrub (ie, 7.5% povidone-iodine) and paint (ie, 10% povidone-iodine) or paint alone may be used.[132-136] *[2: Moderate Evidence]*

Literature related to the comparison of scrub versus paint application techniques for preoperative patient skin antisepsis conflicts. Some RCTs support[132-135] and one quasi-experimental study refutes[136] the benefits of scrubbing the patient's skin with 7.5% povidone-iodine before painting with 10% povidone-iodine. This issue is unresolved and warrants additional research.

IV.d.7. When performing preoperative skin antisepsis of the hand or foot, care should be taken to apply the antiseptic to all surfaces between fingers or toes.[58,137-140] *[2: Moderate Evidence]*

Antisepsis may be difficult in the areas between fingers and toes because of difficulty reaching all surfaces of the skin. The collective evidence did not reveal the most effective preparation techniques for the hands and feet, and this warrants additional research.

A systematic review of eight studies, including RCTs and quasi-RCTs, comparing skin preparation techniques for foot and ankle surgery found that although some studies did not clearly describe scrubbing techniques, the use of vigorous foot scrubbing may reduce fungal contamination of the foot.[58] In one RCT of 50 patients undergoing foot surgery, Brooks et al[137] compared the standard foot antisepsis technique of placing antiseptic solution between the toes (n = 24) to a method with additional cleansing of the toe clefts with an antiseptic-soaked gauze (n = 26). The researchers reported a significant reduction in bacterial recolonization of the foot for the method involving additional cleaning of the toe clefts (ie, 7.7% versus 20.8%).[137]

International studies from England, Australia, and New Zealand describe a preoperative patient skin antisepsis technique in which a sterile bag is used to apply 10% povidone-iodine solution to either the foot or hand.[138-140] Researchers have found the bag technique to be equally effective as painting techniques in reducing bacterial counts and more efficient (ie, 24 seconds versus 85 seconds).[138-140] One quasi-experimental study of the sterile bag application technique for antisepsis also discussed a potential benefit of reducing musculoskeletal injury for perioperative personnel who use the bag technique.[138]

IV.d.8. When performing preoperative patient skin antisepsis of the mouth, care should be taken to prevent patient aspiration of the antiseptic solution.[141] *[2: Moderate Evidence]*

In one case report, a patient developed povidone-iodine aspiration pneumonitis after treatment of the oral and nasal cavity with irrigation of a diluted povidone-iodine solution, even though a throat pack was in place. To prevent aspiration, the authors of this report advised against irrigating the oral cavity with povidone-iodine.[141]

IV.e. The antiseptic should be allowed to dry for the full time recommended in the manufacturer's instructions for use before sterile drapes are applied.[34,66,102,103,142-151] *[2: Moderate Evidence]*

Allowing the skin antiseptic to dry completely according to the manufacturer's instructions for use improves the safety and efficacy of preoperative patient skin antisepsis.

Several case reports of patients chemically injured by wet antiseptics dripping or pooling beneath them recommend allowing the skin antiseptic to dry fully before surgical draping to prevent these types of injury.[143-149]

Flammable skin antiseptics pose a risk for fire when dry times are not achieved. The CMS guidelines[102,103] and several clinical practice guidelines[34,150,151] advise allowing flammable skin antiseptics to dry completely in accordance with the manufacturer's instructions for use. (See Recommendation IV.g.)

In a nonexperimental study, Stinner et al[142] determined that application of 4% CHG for preoperative patient skin antisepsis required a two-minute dry time to achieve effectiveness, which was in accordance with the manufacturer's instructions for use. The manufacturer's instructions for use are the result of rigorous testing under specific conditions and contact times.[62] Compliance with contact times and allowing the skin antiseptic to dry facilitates effectiveness of the antiseptic.

IV.f. Protective measures should be taken to prevent prolonged contact with skin antiseptics.[143-149,152] *[2: Moderate Evidence]*

There are several case reports of patients experiencing chemical skin injury caused by prolonged contact with skin antiseptics.[143-149,152]

IV.f.1. Sheets, padding, positioning equipment, and adhesive tape should be protected from the dripping or pooling of skin antiseptics beneath and around the patient.[66,143,144] *[2: Moderate Evidence]*

Three case reports found that the dripping of antiseptic solution onto fabric and positioning equipment prevented the solution from drying, which prolonged patient skin contact with the wet solution and caused patient skin injury.[66,143,144]

V.f.2. Electrodes (eg, electrocardiogram [ECG], ESU dispersive electrode) and tourniquets should be protected from contact with skin antiseptics.[143,145,149,152] *[2: Moderate Evidence]*

There have been several case reports of injury caused by contact of electrodes and tourniquets with skin antiseptics. One review of multiple cases described patient injuries, including chemical and thermal burns, from skin antiseptic contact with electrodes and tourniquets.[143] Other case reports have described patient injury from skin antiseptic contact with an ESU dispersive electrode[145] and tourniquets.[149,152] Antiseptic contact between the skin and electrode increases impedance and the risk of skin injury or equipment malfunction. When tourniquets cuffs are in contact with antiseptics, compression and occlusion of the wet material against the patient's skin increases the likelihood of a chemical burn.

IV.f.3. A fluid-resistant pad should be placed under the patient's buttocks during preoperative patient skin antisepsis for patients in the lithotomy position.[146-148] The pad should be removed after the antiseptic is dry and before sterile drapes are applied. *[2: Moderate Evidence]*

There have been several case reports of patients sustaining chemical burn injury by prolonged contact with antiseptic solution that pooled beneath them while they were in the lithotomy position.[146-148] When a patient is in the lithotomy position, antiseptic solution dripping down the gluteal cleft may not be visible to perioperative team members.

IV.f.4. Any material near the patient that is in contact with the skin antiseptic solution, including electrodes (eg, ECG, ESU) and tourniquet materials (ie, cuff, padding), should be removed and replaced as necessary. *[4: Benefits Balanced with Harms]*

IV.g. Protective measures should be taken to minimize the risk of fire when flammable preoperative patient skin antiseptics are used.[34,102,103,150,151] *[1: Regulatory Requirement]*

Flammable skin antiseptics are a fuel source and pose a fire hazard. The prevention of pooling of flammable skin antiseptics and allowing for the complete drying of the antiseptic to minimize the fire hazard is supported by the CMS[102,103] and several clinical practice guidelines, including guidance from the National Fire Protection Association (NFPA),[151] the American Society of Anesthesiologists (ASA),[150] and the AORN Guideline for a Safe Environment of Care, Part 1.[34]

IV.g.1. Flammable skin antiseptics should be prevented from pooling or soaking into linens or the patient's hair by
- use of reusable or disposable sterile towels to absorb drips and excess solution during application,
- removal of materials that are saturated with the skin antiseptic before the patient is draped, and
- wicking of excess solution with a sterile towel to help dry the surgical prep area completely.[153-155]

[2: Moderate Evidence]

The practice of preventing pooling or soaking into linens or the patient's hair is supported by NFPA guidance[155] and the ECRI Institute.[153,154]

IV.g.2. Adequate time should be allowed for the flammable skin antiseptic to dry completely and for any fumes to dissipate before surgical drapes are applied or a potential ignition source is used.[150,153-156] *[1: Strong Evidence]*

The practice of allowing flammable skin antiseptics to dry completely and allowing any fumes to dissipate before applying surgical drapes is supported by guidelines from the ASA,[150] ECRI,[153,154] and the NFPA[155] and by a literature review.[156] Allowing adequate time for skin antiseptics to dry before applying drapes helps prevent the accumulation of volatile fumes beneath the drapes.[156] The volatile fumes are flammable and may ignite without a connection between the ignition source and the actual antiseptic solution.[153,154]

IV.g.3. Perioperative team members should communicate use of flammable skin antiseptics as part of the fire risk assessment involving the entire perioperative team before beginning a surgical procedure.[34,150,155] *[1: Strong Evidence]*

The NFPA,[155] the ASA,[150] and the AORN Guideline for a Safe Environment of Care, Part 1[34] support the importance of completing a fire risk assessment. Active communication regarding the use of flammable skin antiseptics alerts all perioperative team members to the inherent risks and allows appropriate precautions to be taken.

IV.g.4. Flammable skin antiseptics should not be heated. *[4: Benefits Balanced with Harms]*

The evidence review found no literature to support or refute this recommendation. Heating flammable antiseptics may pose a serious risk of fire. When the temperature of flammable chemicals increases, they become more unstable and may ignite easily.

IV.h. When lifting and holding the patient's extremity or head during preoperative patient skin antisepsis, the perioperative team member should minimize his or her muscle fatigue by using two hands for holding the extremity or head, obtaining assistance from another team member, using an assistive device, or using a combination of these methods.[157] *[2: Moderate Evidence]*

The evidence review found no literature to support or refute this recommendation. The AORN Guidance Statement: Safe Patient Handling and Movement in the Perioperative Setting supports this practice as part of an ergonomic tool that includes a chart outlining recommended holding techniques based on the patient's weight to help prevent muscle fatigue and musculoskeletal disorders.[157]

IV.i. At the end of the surgical procedure, the skin antiseptic should be removed from the patient's skin before application of an occlusive dressing or tape, unless otherwise indicated by the manufacturer's instructions for use.[66,144] *[2: Moderate Evidence]*

The removal of skin antiseptics from the skin at the end of the surgical procedure is supported by one literature review[66] and one case report of a chemical burn from povidone-iodine.[144] Residual skin antiseptics may cause skin irritation and contact dermatitis in sensitive individuals. Removing the solution as soon as possible after completion of the procedure minimizes the risk on ongoing irritation.

IV.j. The perioperative RN should assess the patient's skin for injury after surgery.[125] A thorough evaluation of the patient's skin may be postponed until the patient is transferred to the postoperative area, depending on the patient's condition. *[2: Moderate Evidence]*

No research evidence was found to support or refute this recommendation. Evaluating the patient's progress toward attaining outcomes after an intervention is a standard of perioperative nursing practice.[125] Reassessing the patient's skin after the procedure is an important method for evaluating the patient for injury.

IV.k. Preoperative patient skin antisepsis should be documented in the patient's record. Documentation should include the
- removal and disposition of any jewelry;
- condition of the skin at the surgical site (eg, presence of rashes, skin eruptions, abrasions, redness, irritation, burns);
- antiseptic used;
- person performing preoperative patient skin antisepsis;
- area prepped; and
- postoperative skin condition, including any skin irritation, hypersensitivity, or allergic response to preparation solutions.

[5: No Evidence]

Recommendation V

Perioperative team members should review and follow the skin antiseptic manufacturer's instructions for use and safety data sheets (SDSs) for handling, storing, and disposing of skin antiseptics.

The collective evidence found that following the antiseptic manufacturer's instructions for use and the SDS is the safest method for handling, storing, and disposing of skin antiseptics.

The evidence review identified a lack of research in the clinical setting for safe handling, storing, and disposing of skin antiseptics.

V.a. Skin antiseptics must be stored in the original, single-use container.[63,158-163] *[1: Regulatory Requirement]*

In November 2013, the FDA issued a drug safety communication requesting label changes and single-use packaging of over-the-counter topical antiseptic products to decrease risk of infection.[63] Topical antiseptics are not required by the FDA to be manufactured as sterile, although most are manufactured with a sterile process. Nonsterile antiseptics may be contaminated with bacteria during or after manufacturing.[63] As a result of reported outbreaks involving contaminated antiseptic products, the FDA requested that manufacturers package antiseptics for preoperative skin preparation in single-use containers, to be used only one time for one patient.

In several case reports and nonexperimental studies, antiseptics have been linked to patient infections from both intrinsic[159,160,162,163] and extrinsic[161] contamination. In a laboratory study, Anderson et al[158] found that *Pseudomonas cepacia* survived up to 29 weeks in the laboratory setting, which confirmed the plausibility of a case of *P cepacia* surviving in povidone-iodine for 68 weeks after contamination during manufacturing.

V.a.1. Skin antiseptics in single-use containers must be discarded after use and not refilled.[63] *[1: Regulatory Requirement]*

V.b. Skin antiseptics must not be diluted after opening.[63] *[1: Regulatory Requirement]*

In a drug safety communication, the FDA states that health care professionals should not dilute antiseptic products after opening them to reduce the possibility of these products becoming contaminated.[63]

V.c. Heating of nonflammable skin antiseptics should only be performed in accordance with the manufacturers' instructions for use.[164] *[2: Moderate Evidence]*

Heating may alter the chemical composition of the skin antiseptic and may alter the effectiveness of the antiseptic. In a 1985 expert opinion paper, Gottardi[164] described that the heating of povidone-iodine alters the equilibrium of the iodine content. No other evidence was found describing the effect of heating on antiseptics.

Heating antiseptics may also cause thermal or chemical burns. No case reports of injury were found in the evidence review.

V.c.1. Skin antiseptics should not be warmed in a microwave oven or autoclave. *[4: Benefits Balanced with Harms]*

The evidence review found no literature to support or refute this recommendation. The temperature of the skin antiseptic is uncontrolled when heated in a microwave or autoclave, and temperature extremes may result in a patient injury.

V.d. Safety data sheets for all skin antiseptics used must be readily available in the practice area.[165] *[1: Regulatory Requirement]*

The SDS provides information about the flammability of the antiseptic and the maximum safe storage temperature. The Occupational Safety and Health Administration requires that SDSs be available for all chemicals used in the practice setting.[165] These documents outline the hazards related to the chemicals and appropriate action to take in the event of a chemical exposure (eg, splash to the eyes).

V.e. Storage of flammable skin antiseptics must be in compliance with local, state, and federal regulations.[34,102,103,151,155] *[1: Regulatory Requirement]*

The NFPA has recommendations for storage of flammable solutions.[151,155] The CMS states in §482.41(c)(2) that "facilities, supplies, and equipment must be maintained to ensure an acceptable level of safety and quality," including storage in compliance with fire codes.[102,103] The AORN Guideline for a Safe Environment of Care, Part 1 also recommends following local and state fire regulations for storage of flammable liquids, such as alcohol-based skin antiseptic solutions.[34]

V.f. Disposal of unused flammable skin antiseptics must be handled in a manner to decrease the risk of fire and in accordance with local, state, and federal regulations.[102,103,166] *[1: Regulatory Requirement]*

Disposal of residual flammable antiseptics is regulated by the Environmental Protection Agency (EPA).[166] The CMS regulations state that trash must be stored and disposed of in accordance with federal, state, and local laws and regulations, including those from the EPA.[102,103] No reports of improper disposal of antiseptics were found. There is a risk that fires can occur when flammable antiseptics are discarded in nonhazardous trash, and incineration or autoclaving of biohazardous waste can rapidly ignite flammable antiseptics.

Glossary

Antiseptic: A product with antimicrobial activity applied to the skin to reduce the number of microbial flora.

Iodism: Poisoning by iodine, a condition marked by severe rhinitis, frontal headache, emaciation, weakness, and skin eruptions. Caused by the administration of iodine or one of the iodides.

Log reduction: The logarithmic death progression of microorganisms after exposure to a sterilant or antiseptic agent. The reduction difference between average surviving microbes for control and test carriers used as an efficacy parameter.

REFERENCES

1. Dumville JC, McFarlane E, Edwards P, Lipp A, Holmes A. Preoperative skin antiseptics for preventing surgical wound infections after clean surgery. *Cochrane Database Syst Rev.* 2013;3:CD003949. [IA]

2. Webster J, Osborne S. Preoperative bathing or showering with skin antiseptics to prevent surgical site infection. *Cochrane Database Syst Rev.* 2012;9:CD004985. [IA]

3. Tanner J, Norrie P, Melen K. Preoperative hair removal to reduce surgical site infection. *Cochrane Database Syst Rev.* 2011;11:CD004122. [IA]

4. Surgical site infection. National Institute for Health and Care Excellence. https://www.nice.org.uk/Guidance/QS49. Accessed July 14, 2014. [IVA]

5. Cruse PJ. A five-year prospective study of 23,649 surgical wounds. *Arch Surg.* 1973;107(2):206-210. [IIIA]

6. Anderson DJ, Kaye KS, Classen D, et al. Strategies to prevent surgical site infections in acute care hospitals. *Infect Control Hosp Epidemiol.* 2008;2(9 Suppl 1):51-61. [IVA]

7. Smith MA, Dahlen NR. Clinical practice guideline surgical site infection prevention. *Orthop Nurs.* 2013;32(5):242-248. [IVB]

8. Rotter ML, Larsen SO, Cooke EM, et al. A comparison of the effects of preoperative whole-body bathing with detergent alone and with detergent containing chlorhexidine gluconate on the frequency of wound infections after clean surgery. The European Working Party on Control of Hospital Infections. *J Hosp Infect.* 1988;11(4):310-320. [IA]

9. Veiga DF, Damasceno CA, Veiga-Filho J, et al. Randomized controlled trial of the effectiveness of chlorhexidine showers before elective plastic surgical procedures. *Infect Control Hospital Epidemiol.* 2009;30(1):77-79. [IB]

10. Veiga DF, Damasceno CA, Veiga Filho J, et al. Influence of povidone-iodine preoperative showers on skin colonization in elective plastic surgery procedures. *Plast Reconstr Surg.* 2008;121(1):115-118. [IA]

11. Jakobsson J, Perlkvist A, Wann-Hansson C. Searching for evidence regarding using preoperative disinfection showers to prevent surgical site infections: a systematic review. *Worldviews Evid Based Nurs.* 2011;8(3):143-152. [IIA]

12. Kamel C, McGahan L, Polisena J, Mierzwinski-Urban M, Embil JM. Preoperative skin antiseptic preparations for preventing surgical site infections: a systematic review. *Infect Control Hosp Epidemiol.* 2012;33(6):608-617. [IIA]

13. Chlebicki MP, Safdar N, O'Horo JC, Maki DG. Preoperative chlorhexidine shower or bath for prevention of surgical site infection: a meta-analysis. *Am J Infect Control.* 2013;41(2):167-173. [IIA]

14. Tanner J, Gould D, Jenkins P, Hilliam R, Mistry N, Walsh S. A fresh look at preoperative body washing. *J Infect Prev.* 2012;13(1):11-15. [IB]

15. Murray MR, Saltzman MD, Gryzlo SM, Terry MA, Woodward CC, Nuber GW. Efficacy of preoperative home use of 2% chlorhexidine gluconate cloth before shoulder surgery. *J Shoulder Elbow Surg.* 2011;20(6):928-933. [IA]

16. Edmiston Jr CE, Krepel CJ, Seabrook GR, Lewis BD, Brown KR, Towne JB. Preoperative shower revisited: can high topical antiseptic levels be achieved on the skin surface before surgical admission? *J Am Coll Surg.* 2008;207(2):233-239. [IB]

17. Edmiston CE Jr, Seabrook GR, Johnson CP, Paulson DS, Beausoleil CM. Comparative of a new and innovative 2% chlorhexidine gluconate-impregnated cloth with 4% chlorhexidine gluconate as topical antiseptic for preparation of the skin prior to surgery. *Am J Infect Control.* 2007;35(2):89-96. [IB]

18. Kapadia BH, Issa K, McElroy MJ, Pivec R, Daley JA, Mont MA. Advance pre-operative chlorhexidine preparation reduces periprosthetic infections following total joint arthroplasty. *Semin Arthroplasty.* 2013;24(2):83-86. [IIA]

19. Graling PR, Vasaly FW. Effectiveness of 2% CHG cloth bathing for reducing surgical site infections. *AORN J.* 2013;97(5):547-551. [IIB]

20. Johnson AJ, Kapadia BH, Daley JA, Molina CB, Mont MA. Chlorhexidine reduces infections in knee arthroplasty. *J Knee Surg.* 2013;26(3):213-218. [IIB]

21. Zywiel MG, Daley JA, Delanois RE, Naziri Q, Johnson AJ, Mont MA. Advance pre-operative chlorhexidine reduces the incidence of surgical site infections in knee arthroplasty. *Int Orthop.* 2011;35(7):1001-1006. [IIB]

22. Johnson AJ, Daley JA, Zywiel MG, Delanois RE, Mont MA. Preoperative chlorhexidine preparation and the incidence of surgical site infections after hip arthroplasty. *J Arthroplasty.* 2010;25(6 Suppl):98-102. [IIB]

23. Kapadia BH, Johnson AJ, Daley JA, Issa K, Mont MA. Pre-admission cutaneous chlorhexidine preparation reduces surgical site infections in total hip arthroplasty. *J Arthroplasty.* 2013;28(3):490-493. [IIB]

24. Kapadia BH, Johnson AJ, Issa K, Mont MA. Economic evaluation of chlorhexidine cloths on healthcare costs due to surgical site infections following total knee arthroplasty. *J Arthroplasty.* 2013;28(7):1061-1065. [VA]

25. Eiselt D. Presurgical skin preparation with a novel 2% chlorhexidine gluconate cloth reduces rates of surgical site infection in orthopaedic surgical patients. *Orthop Nurs.* 2009;28(3):141-145. [VA]

26. Karki S, Cheng AC. Impact of non-rinse skin cleansing with chlorhexidine gluconate on prevention of healthcare-associated infections and colonization with multi-resistant organisms: a systematic review. *J Hosp Infect.* 2012;82(2):71-84. [IIIA]

27. Edmiston CE Jr, Okoli O, Graham MB, Sinski S, Seabrook GR. Evidence for using chlorhexidine gluconate preoperative cleansing to reduce the risk of surgical site infection. *AORN J.* 2010;92(5):509-518. [VB]

28. Farber NJ, Chen AF, Bartsch SM, Feigel JL, Klatt BA. No infection reduction using chlorhexidine wipes in total joint arthroplasty. *Clin Orthop Relat Res.* 2013;471(10):3120-3125. [IIA]

29. Arrowsmith VA, Maunder JA, Sargent RJ, Taylor R. Removal of nail polish and finger rings to prevent surgical infection. *Cochrane Database Syst Rev.* 2001;4:CD003325. [IA]

30. Hedderwick SA, McNeil SA, Lyons MJ, Kauffman CA. Pathogenic organisms associated with artificial fingernails worn by healthcare workers. *Infect Control Hosp Epidemiol.* 2000;21(8):505-509. [IIB]

31. McNeil SA, Foster CL, Hedderwick SA, Kauffman CA. Effect of hand cleansing with antimicrobial soap or alcohol-based gel on microbial colonization of artificial fingernails worn by health care workers. *Clin Infect Dis.* 2001;32(3):367-372. [IIA]

32. Leclair JM, Winston KR, Sullivan BF, O'Connell JM, Harrington SM, Goldmann DA. Effect of preoperative shampoos on resident scalp flora. *Todays OR Nurse.* 1988;10(3):15-21. [IB]

33. Guideline for product selection. In: *Guidelines for Perioperative Practice.* Denver, CO: AORN, Inc; 2015:179-186. [IVB]

34. Guideline for a safe environment of care, part 1. In: *Guidelines for Perioperative Practice.* Denver, CO: AORN, Inc; 2015:239-263. [IVA]

35. Broekman ML, van Beijnum J, Peul WC, Regli L. Neurosurgery and shaving: what's the evidence? *J Neurosurg.* 2011;115(4):670-678. [IIIA]

36. Sebastian S. Does preoperative scalp shaving result in fewer postoperative wound infections when compared with no scalp shaving? A systematic review. *J Neurosci Nurs.* 2012;44(3):149-156. [IIIA]

37. Ng W, Alexander D, Kerr B, Ho MF, Amato M, Katz K. A hairy tale: successful patient education strategies to reduce prehospital hair removal by patients undergoing elective caesarean section. *J Hosp Infect.* 2013;83(1):64-67. [IIIB]

38. Jose B, Dignon A. Is there a relationship between preoperative shaving (hair removal) and surgical site infection? *J Perioper Pract.* 2013;23(1-2):22-25. [VB]

39. Celik SE, Kara A. Does shaving the incision site increase the infection rate after spinal surgery? *Spine*. 2007;32(15):1575-1577. [IA]

40. Grober ED, Domes T, Fanipour M, Copp JE. Preoperative hair removal on the male genitalia: clippers vs razors. *J Sex Med*. 2013;10(2):589-594. [IB]

41. Hemani ML, Lepor H. Skin preparation for the prevention of surgical site infection: which agent is best? *Rev Urol*. 2009;11(4):190-195. [VB]

42. Tschudin-Sutter S, Frei R, Egli-Gany D, et al. No risk of surgical site infections from residual bacteria after disinfection with povidone-iodine-alcohol in 1014 cases: A prospective observational study. *Ann Surg*. 2012;255(3):565-569. [IIIA]

43. Edmiston CE Jr, Bruden B, Rucinski MC, Henen C, Graham MB, Lewis BL. Reducing the risk of surgical site infections: does chlorhexidine gluconate provide a risk reduction benefit? *Am J Infect Control*. 2013;41(5 Suppl):S49-S55. [VB]

44. Darouiche RO, Wall MJ Jr, Itani KM, et al. Chlorhexidine-alcohol versus povidone-iodine for surgical-site antisepsis. *N Engl J Med*. 2010;362(1):18-26. [IA]

45. Nishihara Y, Kajiura T, Yokota K, Kobayashi H, Okubo T. Evaluation with a focus on both the antimicrobial efficacy and cumulative skin irritation potential of chlorhexidine gluconate alcohol-containing preoperative skin preparations. *Am J Infect Control*. 2012;40(10):973-978. [IB]

46. Saltzman MD, Nuber GW, Gryzlo SM, Marecek GS, Koh JL. Efficacy of surgical preparation solutions in shoulder surgery. *J Bone Joint Surg Am*. 2009;91(8):1949-1953. [IA]

47. Amer-Alshiek J, Alshiek T, Almog B, et al. Can we reduce the surgical site infection rate in cesarean sections using a chlorhexidine-based antisepsis protocol? *J Matern Fetal Neonatal Med*. 2013;26(17):1749-1752. [IIIB]

48. Lee I, Agarwal RK, Lee BY, Fishman NO, Umscheid CA. Systematic review and cost analysis comparing use of chlorhexidine with use of iodine for preoperative skin antisepsis to prevent surgical site infection. *Infect Control Hosp Epidemiol*. 2010;31(12):1219-1229. [IA]

49. Al Maqbali MA. Preoperative antiseptic skin preparations and reducing SSI. *Br J Nurs*. 2013;22(21):1227-1233. [VA]

50. Lim K-S, Kam PCA. Chlorhexidine—pharmacology and clinical applications. *Anaesth Intensive Care*. 2008;36(4):502-512. [VA]

51. Noorani A, Rabey N, Walsh SR, Davies RJ. Systematic review and meta-analysis of preoperative antisepsis with chlorhexidine versus povidone-iodine in clean-contaminated surgery. *Br J Surg*. 2010;97(11):1614-1620. [IIB]

52. Paocharoen V, Mingmalairak C, Apisarnthanarak A. Comparison of surgical wound infection after preoperative skin preparation with 4% chlorhexidine [correction of chlohexidine] and povidone iodine: a prospective randomized trial. *J Med Assoc Thai*. 2009;92(7):898-902. [IB]

53. Maiwald M, Chan ES-Y. The forgotten role of alcohol: a systematic review and meta-analysis of the clinical efficacy and perceived role of chlorhexidine in skin antisepsis. *PLoS One*. 2012;7(9):e44277. [IIA]

54. Sistla SC, Prabhu G, Sistla S, Sadasivan J. Minimizing wound contamination in a "clean" surgery: comparison of chlorhexidine-ethanol and povidone-iodine. *Chemotherapy*. 2010;56(4):261-267. [IA]

55. Menderes G, Athar Ali N, Aagaard K, Sangi-Haghpeykar H. Chlorhexidine-alcohol compared with povidone-iodine for surgical-site antisepsis in cesarean deliveries. *Obstet Gynecol*. 2012;120(5):1037-1044. [IIA]

56. Berry AR, Watt B, Goldacre MJ, Thomson JW, McNair TJ. A comparison of the use of povidone-iodine and chlorhexidine in the prophylaxis of postoperative wound infection. *J Hosp Infect*. 1982;3(1):55-63. [IB]

57. Savage JW, Weatherford BM, Sugrue PA, et al. Efficacy of surgical preparation solutions in lumbar spine surgery. *J Bone Joint Surg Am*. 2012;94(6):490-494. [IA]

58. Yammine K, Harvey A. Efficacy of preparation solutions and cleansing techniques on contamination of the skin in foot and ankle surgery: a systematic review and meta-analysis. *Bone Joint J*. 2013;95(4):498-503. [IB]

59. Swenson BR, Hedrick TL, Metzger R, Bonatti H, Pruett TL, Sawyer RG. Effects of preoperative skin preparation on postoperative wound infection rates: a prospective study of 3 skin preparation protocols. *Infect Control Hosp Epidemiol*. 2009;30(10):964-971. [IIB]

60. Segal CG, Anderson JJ. Preoperative skin preparation of cardiac patients. AORN J. 2002;76(5):821-828. [IA]

61. Roberts A, Wilcox K, Devineni R, Osevala M. Skin preparation in CABG surgery: a randomized control trial. *Comp Surg*. 1995;14(6):724, 741-744, 747. [IB]

62. US Food and Drug Administration. Tentative final monograph for healthcare antiseptic drug products proposed rule. *Fed Regist*. 1994;59(116):31402-31452.

63. Over-the-counter topical antiseptic products: drug safety communication—FDA requests label changes and single-use packaging to decrease risk of infection. http://www.fda.gov/safety/medwatch/safetyinformation/safetyalertsforhumanmedicalproducts/ucm374892.htm Accessed July 14, 2014.

64. Sullivan PJ, Healy CE, Hirpara KM, Hussey AJ, Potter SM, Kelly JL. An assessment of skin preparation in upper limb surgery. *J Hand Surg Eur* Vol. 2008;33(4):513-514. [IIB]

65. Digison MB. A review of anti-septic agents for pre-operative skin preparation. *Plast Surg Nurs*. 2007;27(4):185-189. [VB]

66. Murkin CE. Pre-operative antiseptic skin preparation. *Br J Nurs*. 2009;18(11):665-669. [VA]

67. Quatresooz P, Xhauflaire-Uhoda E, Pierard-Franchimont C, Pierard GE. Regional variability in stratum corneum reactivity to antiseptic formulations. *Contact Derm*. 2007;56(5):271-273. [IIIB]

68. Sanders TH, Hawken SM. Chlorhexidine burns after shoulder arthroscopy. *Am J Orthop* (Belle Mead NJ). 2012;41(4):172-174. [VB]

69. *Academy Position Statement: The Risk of Severe Allergic Reactions from the Use of Potassium Iodide for Radiation Emergencies*. February 2004. American Academy of Allergy Asthma and Immunology. https://www.aaaai.org/Aaaai/media/MediaLibrary/PDF%20Documents/Practice%20and%20Parameters/Potassium-iodide-in-radiation-emergencies-2004.pdf. Accessed July 14, 2014. [IVB]

70. Schabelman E, Witting M. The relationship of radiocontrast, iodine, and seafood allergies: a medical myth exposed. *J Emerg Med*. 2010;39(5):701-707. [VA]

71. Huang SW. Seafood and iodine: an analysis of a medical myth. *Allergy Asthma Proc*. 2005;26(6):468-469. [IIIC]

72. Yoshida K, Sakurai Y, Kawahara S, et al. Anaphylaxis to polyvinylpyrrolidone in povidone-iodine for impetigo contagiosum in a boy with atopic dermatitis. *Int Arch Allergy Immunol*. 2008;146(2):169-173. [VB]

73. Adachi A, Fukunaga A, Hayashi K, Kunisada M, Horikawa T. Anaphylaxis to polyvinylpyrrolidone after vaginal application of povidone-iodine. *Contact Dermatitis*. 2003;48(3):133-136. [VA]

74. Sivathasan N, Goodfellow PB. Skin cleansers: the risks of chlorhexidine. *J Clin Pharmacol.* 2011;51(5):785-786. [VA]

75. Garvey LH, Roed-Petersen J, Husum B. Anaphylactic reactions in anaesthetised patients - four cases of chlorhexidine allergy. *Acta Anaesthesiol Scand.* 2001;45(10):1290-1294. [VA]

76. Toomey M. Preoperative chlorhexidine anaphylaxis in a patient scheduled for coronary artery bypass graft: a case report. *AANA J.* 2013;81(3):209-214. [VA]

77. Khan RA, Kazi T, O'Donohoe B. Near fatal intraoperative anaphylaxis to chlorhexidine—is it time to change practice? *BMJ Case Rep.* 2011;2011. [VA]

78. Vujevich J, Zirwas M. Delayed hypersensitivity to isopropyl alcohol. *Contact Dermatitis.* 2007;56(5):287. [VC]

79. Baillif S, Roure-Sobas C, Le-Duff F, Kodjikian L. Aqueous humor contamination during phacoemulsification in a university teaching hospital. *J Fr Opthalmol.* 2012;35(3):153-156. [IIIB]

80. Quiroga LP, Lansingh V, Laspina F, et al. A prospective study demonstrating the effect of 5% povidone-iodine application for anterior segment intraocular surgery in Paraguay. *Arq Bras Oftalmol.* 2010;73(2):125-128. [IIA]

81. Ou JI, Ta CN. Endophthalmitis prophylaxis. *Ophthalmol Clin North Am.* 2006;19(4):449-456. [VA]

82. Wu PC, Li M, Chang SJ, et al. Risk of endophthalmitis after cataract surgery using different protocols for povidone-iodine preoperative disinfection. *J Ocul Pharmacol Ther.* 2006;22(1):54-61. [IIA]

83. Trinavarat A, Atchaneeyasakul LO, Nopmaneejumruslers C, Inson K. Reduction of endophthalmitis rate after cataract surgery with preoperative 5% povidone-iodine. *Dermatology.* 2006;212(Suppl 1):35-40. [IB]

84. Li B, Nentwich MM, Hoffmann LE, et al. Comparison of the efficacy of povidone-iodine 1.0%, 5.0%, and 10.0% irrigation combined with topical levofloxacin 0.3% as preoperative prophylaxis in cataract surgery. *J Cataract Refract Surg.* 2013;39(7):994-1001. [IA]

85. Chou SF, Lin CH, Chang SW. Povidone-iodine application induces corneal cell death through fixation. *Br J Ophthalmol.* 2011;95(2):277-283. [IIIB]

86. Below H, Behrens-Baumann W, Bernhardt C, Volzke H, Kramer A, Rudolph P. Systemic iodine absorption after preoperative antisepsis using povidone-iodine in cataract surgery—an open controlled study. *Dermatology.* 2006;212(Suppl 1):41-46. [IIB]

87. Razavi B, Zollinger R, Kramer A, et al. Systemic iodine absorption associated with the use of preoperative ophthalmic antiseptics containing iodine. *Cutan Ocul Toxicol.* 2013;32(4):279-282. [IIB]

88. Amstey MS, Jones AP. Preparation of the vagina for surgery. A comparison of povidone-iodine and saline solution. *JAMA.* 1981;245(8):839-841. [IIIB]

89. Lewis LA, Lathi RB, Crochet P, Nezhat C. Preoperative vaginal preparation with baby shampoo compared with povidone-iodine before gynecologic procedures. *J Minim Invasive Gynecol.* 2007;14(6):736-739. [IIA]

90. American College of Obstetricians and Gynecologists Women's Health Care Physicians, Committee on Gynecologic Practice. Committee Opinion No. 571: Solutions for surgical preparation of the vagina. *Obstet Gynecol.* 2013;122(3):718-720. [IVB]

91. Eason E, Wells G, Garber G, et al. Antisepsis for abdominal hysterectomy: a randomised controlled trial of povidone-iodine gel. *BJOG.* 2004;111(7):695-699. [IA]

92. Haas DM, Morgan S, Contreras K. Vaginal preparation with antiseptic solution before cesarean section for preventing postoperative infections. *Cochrane Database Systematic Rev.* 2013;1:CD007892. [IB]

93. Guzman Melissa A, Prien Samuel D, Blann David W. Post-cesarean related infection and vaginal preparation with povidone-iodine revisited. *Prim Care Update Ob Gyns.* 2002;9(6):206-209. [IB]

94. Haas DM, Pazouki F, Smith RR, et al. Vaginal cleansing before cesarean delivery to reduce postoperative infectious morbidity: a randomized, controlled trial. *Am J Obstet Gynecol.* 2010;202(3):310.e1-310.e6. [IB]

95. Asghania M, Mirblouk F, Shakiba M, Faraji R. Preoperative vaginal preparation with povidone-iodine on post-caesarean infectious morbidity. *J Obstet Gynaecol.* 2011;31(5):400-403. [IIA]

96. Hadiati DR, Hakimi M, Nurdiati DS. Skin preparation for preventing infection following caesarean section. *Cochrane Database Syst Rev.* 2012;9:CD007462. [IA]

97. Bibbo C, Patel DV, Gehrmann RM, Lin SS. Chlorhexidine provides superior skin decontamination in foot and ankle surgery: a prospective randomized study. *Clin Orthop Relat Res.* 2005;438:204-208. [IB]

98. Ostrander RV, Botte MJ, Brage ME. Efficacy of surgical preparation solutions in foot and ankle surgery. *J Bone Joint Surg Am.* 2005;87(5):980-985. [IA]

99. Hort KR, DeOrio JK. Residual bacterial contamination after surgical preparation of the foot or ankle with or without alcohol. *Foot Ankle Int.* 2002;23(10):946-948. [IB]

100. Becerro de Bengoa Vallejo R, Losa Iglesias ME, Alou Cervera L, Sevillano Fernandez D, Prieto Prieto J. Preoperative skin and nail preparation of the foot: comparison of the efficacy of 4 different methods in reducing bacterial load. *J Am Acad Dermatol.* 2009;61(6):986-992. [IB]

101. Weber SM, Hargunani CA, Wax MK. DuraPrep and the risk of fire during tracheostomy. *Head Neck.* 2006;28(7):649-652. [VA]

102. *State Operations Manual Appendix A—Survey Protocol, Regulations and Interpretive Guidelines for Hospitals.* Rev 89; 2013. Centers for Medicare & Medicaid Services. http://www.cms.gov/Regulations-and-Guidance/Guidance/Manuals/downloads/som107ap_a_hospitals.pdf. Accessed July 14, 2014.

103. *State Operations Manual Appendix L—Guidance for Surveyors: Ambulatory Surgical Centers.* Rev. 89; 2013. Centers for Medicare & Medicaid Services. http://www.cms.gov/Regulations-and-Guidance/Guidance/Manuals/downloads/som107ap_l_ambulatory.pdf. Accessed July 14, 2014.

104. Zamora JL. Chemical and microbiologic characteristics and toxicity of povidone-iodine solutions. *Am J Surg.* 1986;151(3):400-406. [VA]

105. Lavelle KJ, Doedens DJ, Kleit SA, Forney RB. Iodine absorption in burn patients treated topically with povidone-iodine. *Clin Pharmacol Ther.* 1975;17(3):355-362. [VB]

106. Rath T, Meissl G. Induction of hyperthyroidism in burn patients treated topically with povidone-iodine. *Burns Incl Therm Inj.* 1988;14(4):320-322. [VA]

107. Pietsch J, Meakins JL. Complications of povidone-iodine absorption in topically treated burn patients. *Lancet.* 1976;1(7954):280-282. [VA]

108. Tomoda C, Kitano H, Uruno T, et al. Transcutaneous iodine absorption in adult patients with thyroid cancer disinfected with povidone-iodine at operation. *Thyroid.* 2005;15(6):600-603. [IB]

109. Pyati SP, Ramamurthy RS, Krauss MT, Pildes RS. Absorption of iodine in the neonate following topical use of povidone iodine. *J Pediatr.* 1977;91(5):825-828. [IIB]

110. Linder N, Davidovitch N, Reichman B, et al. Topical iodine-containing antiseptics and subclinical hypothyroidism in preterm infants. *J Pediatr*. 1997;131(3):434-439. [IIIA]

111. Smerdely P, Lim A, Boyages SC, et al. Topical iodine-containing antiseptics and neonatal hypothyroidism in very-low-birthweight infants. *Lancet*. 1989;2(8664):661-664. [IIIB]

112. Bryant WP, Zimmerman D. Iodine-induced hyperthyroidism in a newborn. *Pediatrics*. 1995;95(3):434-436. [VB]

113. Afsar FS. Skin care for preterm and term neonates. *Clin Exp Derm*. 2009;34(8):855-858. [VA]

114. Vorherr H, Vorherr UF, Mehta P, Ulrich JA, Messer RH. Vaginal absorption of povidone-iodine. *JAMA*. 1980;244(23):2628-2629. [IIIC]

115. DailyMed. US National Library of Medicine. http://dailymed.nlm.nih.gov. Accessed July 14, 2014.

116. Lashkari HP, Chow P, Godambe S. Aqueous 2% chlorhexidine-induced chemical burns in an extremely premature infant. *Arch Dis Child Fetal Neonatal Ed*. 2012;97(1):F64. [VB]

117. Schick JB, Milstein JM. Burn hazard of isopropyl alcohol in the neonate. *Pediatrics*. 1981;68(4):587-588. [VB]

118. Harpin V, Rutter N. Percutaneous alcohol absorption and skin necrosis in a preterm infant. *Arch Dis Child*. 1982;57(6):477-479. [VA]

119. Guideline for transfer of patient care information. In: *Guidelines for Perioperative Practice*. Denver, CO: AORN, Inc; 2015: 583-588. [IVB]

120. Cronen G, Ringus V, Sigle G, Ryu J. Sterility of surgical site marking. *J Bone Joint Surg Am*. 2005;87(10):2193-2195. [IIB]

121. Rooney J, Khoo OKS, Higgs AR, Small TJ, Bell S. Surgical site marking does not affect sterility. *ANZ J Surg*. 2008;78(8):688-689. [IIB]

122. Wilson J, Tate D. Can pre-operative skin marking transfer methicillin-resistant Staphylococcus aureus between patients? A laboratory experiment. *J Bone Joint Surg Br*. 2006;88(4):541-542. [IIIA]

123. Mears SC, Dinah AF, Knight TA, Frassica FJ, Belkoff SM. Visibility of surgical site marking after preoperative skin preparation. *Eplasty* [Electronic Resource]. 2008;8:e35. [IIB]

124. Thakkar SC, Mears SC. Visibility of surgical site marking: a prospective randomized trial of two skin preparation solutions. *J Bone Joint Surg Am*. 2012;94(2):97-102. [IB]

125. Standards of perioperative nursing. In: *Perioperative Standards and Recommended Practices*. Denver, CO: AORN, Inc; 2014:3-18. [IVB]

126. Trick WE, Vernon MO, Hayes RA, et al. Impact of ring wearing on hand contamination and comparison of hand hygiene agents in a hospital. *Clin Infect Dis*. 2003;36(11):1383-1390. [IIA]

127. Bonnevialle N, Geiss L, Cavalie L, Ibnoulkhatib A, Verdeil X, Bonnevialle P. Skin preparation before hip replacement in emergency setting versus elective scheduled arthroplasty: bacteriological comparative analysis. *Orthop Traumatol Surg Res*. 2013;99(6):659-665. [IIA]

128. Guideline for hand hygiene. In: *Guidelines for Perioperative Practice*. Denver, CO: AORN, Inc; 2015:31-42. [IVB]

129. Guideline for surgical attire. In: *Guidelines for Perioperative Practice*. Denver, CO: AORN, Inc; 2015:97-120. [IVB]

130. Pearce BA, Miller LH, Martin MA, Roush DL. Efficacy of clean v sterile surgical prep kits. *AORN J*. 1997;66(3):464-470. [IB]

131. Guideline for sterile technique. In: *PGuidelines for Perioperative Practice*. Denver, CO: AORN, Inc; 2015:67-96. [IVA]

132. Cheng K, Robertson H, St Mart JP, Leanord A, McLeod I. Quantitative analysis of bacteria in forefoot surgery: a comparison of skin preparation techniques. *Foot Ankle Int*. 2009;30(10):992-997. [IB]

133. Ellenhorn JD, Smith DD, Schwarz RE, et al. Paint-only is equivalent to scrub-and-paint in preoperative preparation of abdominal surgery sites. *J Am Coll Surg*. 2005;201(5):737-741. [IC]

134. Gilliam DL, Nelson CL. Comparison of a one-step iodophor skin preparation versus traditional preparation in total joint surgery. *Clin Orthop Relat Res*. 1990;250:258-260. [IB]

135. Vagholkar Ketan, Julka Karan. Preoperative skin preparation: which is the best method? *Internet J Surg*. 2012;28(4):1-1. [IA]

136. Weed S, Bastek JA, Sammel MD, Beshara M, Hoffman S, Srinivas SK. Comparing postcesarean infectious complication rates using two different skin preparations. *Obstet Gynecol*. 2011;117(5):1123-1129. [IIA]

137. Brooks RA, Hollinghurst D, Ribbans WJ, Severn M. Bacterial recolonization during foot surgery: a prospective randomized study of toe preparation techniques. *Foot Ankle Int*. 2001;22(4):347-350. [IB]

138. Naderi N, Maw K, Thomas M, Boyce DE, Shokrollahi K. A quick and effective method of limb preparation with health, safety and efficiency benefits. *Ann R Coll Surg Engl*. 2012;94(2):83-86. [IIB]

139. Incoll IW, Saravanja D, Thorvaldson KT, Small T. Comparison of the effectiveness of painting onto the hand and immersing the hand in a bag, in pre-operative skin preparation of the hand. *J Hand Surg Eur Vol*. 2009;34(3):371-373. [IIB]

140. Chou J, Choudhary A, Dhillon RS. Comparing sterile bag rubbing and paint on technique in skin preparation of the hands. *ANZ J Surg*. 2011;81(9):629-632. [IIC]

141. Chepla KJ, Gosain AK. Interstitial pneumonitis after betadine aspiration. *J Craniofac Surg*. 2012;23(6):1787-1789. [VA]

142. Stinner DJ, Krueger CA, Masini BD, Wenke JC. Time-dependent effect of chlorhexidine surgical prep. *J Hosp Infect*. 2011;79(4):313-316. [IIIB]

143. Borrego L. Acute skin lesions after surgical procedures: a clinical approach. *Actas Dermo-Sifiliogr*. 2013;104(9):776-781. [VA]

144. Rees A, Sherrod Q, Young L. Chemical burn from povidone-iodine: case and review. *J Drugs Dermatol*. 2011;10(4):414-417. [VB]

145. Demir E, O'Dey DM, Pallua N. Accidental burns during surgery. *J Burn Care Res*. 2006;27(6):895-900. [IIIB]

146. Hodgkinson DJ, Irons GB, Williams TJ. Chemical burns and skin preparation solutions. *Surg Gynecol Obstet*. 1978;147(4):534-536. [IIIB]

147. Lowe DO, Knowles SR, Weber EA, Railton CJ, Shear NH. Povidone-iodine-induced burn: case report and review of the literature. *Pharmacotherapy*. 2006;26(11):1641-1645. [VA]

148. Murthy MB, Krishnamurthy B. Severe irritant contact dermatitis induced by povidone iodine solution. *Indian J Pharmacol*. 2009;41(4):199-200. [VB]

149. Chiang YC, Lin TS, Yeh MC. Povidone-iodine-related burn under the tourniquet of a child—a case report and literature review. *J Plast Reconstr Aesthet Surg*. 2011;64(3):412-415. [VA]

150. Apfelbaum JL, Caplan RA, Barker SJ, et al. Practice advisory for the prevention and management of operating room fires: an updated report by the American Society of Anesthesiologists Task Force on Operating Room Fires. *Anesthesiology.* 2013;118(2):271-290. [IVA]

151. *NFPA 101: Life Safety Code.* 2012 ed. Quincy, MA: National Fire Protection Association; 2012. [IVB]

152. Palmanovich E, Brin YS, Laver L, Nyska M, Kish B. Third-degree chemical burns from chlorhexidine local antisepsis. *Isr Med Assoc J.* 2013;15(6):323-324. [VA]

153. ECRI. New clinical guide to surgical fire prevention. Patients can catch fire—here's how to keep them safer. *Health Devices.* 2009;38(10):314-332. [VA]

154. ECRI. Fighting airway fires. *Healthc Risk Control.* 2010;4 (Surgery and Anesthesia):1-11. [IVC]

155. *Health Care Facilities Code Handbook.* 9th ed. Quincy, MA: National Fire Protection Association; 2012. [IVB]

156. Rinder CS. Fire safety in the operating room. *Curr Opin Anaesthesiol.* 2008;21(6):790-795. [VC]

157. AORN guidance statement: Safe patient handling and movement in the perioperative setting. In: *Perioperative Standards and Recommended Practices.* Denver, CO: AORN, Inc; 2014:615-634. [IVB]

158. Anderson RL, Vess RW, Panlilio AL, Favero MS. Prolonged survival of Pseudomonas cepacia in commercially manufactured povidone-iodine. *Appl Environ Microbiol.* 1990;56(11):3598-3600. [IIIB]

159. Berkelman RL, Lewin S, Allen JR, et al. Pseudobacteremia attributed to contamination of povidone-iodine with *Pseudomonas cepacia. Ann Intern Med.* 1981;95(1):32-36. [IIIB]

160. Craven DE, Moody B, Connolly MG, Kollisch NR, Stottmeier KD, McCabe WR. Pseudobacteremia caused by povidone-iodine solution contaminated with *Pseudomonas cepacia. N Engl J Med.* 1981;305(11):621-623. [IIIA]

161. O'Rourke E, Runyan D, O'Leary J, Stern J. Contaminated iodophor in the operating room. *Am J Infect Control.* 2003;31(4):255-256. [VA]

162. Panlilio AL, Beck-Sague CM, Siegel JD, et al. Infections and pseudoinfections due to povidone-iodine solution contaminated with *Pseudomonas cepacia. Clin Infect Dis.* 1992;14(5):1078-1083. [IIIA]

163. Parrott PL, Terry PM, Whitworth EN, et al. Pseudomonas aeruginosa peritonitis associated with contaminated poloxamer-iodine solution. *Lancet.* 1982;320(8300):683-685. [VA]

164. Gottardi W. The influence of the chemical behaviour of iodine on the germicidal action of disinfectant solutions containing iodine. *J Hosp Infect.* 1985;6(Suppl A):1-11. [VA]

165. 29 CFR 1910.1200: Occupational safety and health standards. Toxic and hazardous substances. Hazard communication. July 2013. Occupational Safety and Health Administration. https://www.osha.gov/pls/oshaweb/owadisp.show_document?p_table=standards&p_id=10099. Accessed July 14, 2014.

166. RCRA Online. US Environmental Protection Agency. http://www.epa.gov/epawaste/inforesources/online/index.htm. Accessed July 14, 2014.

Acknowledgements

LEAD AUTHOR
Amber Wood, MSN, RN, CNOR, CIC, CPN
Perioperative Nursing Specialist
AORN Nursing Department
Denver, Colorado

CONTRIBUTING AUTHOR
Ramona Conner, MSN, RN, CNOR
Manager Standards and Guidelines
AORN Nursing Department
Denver, Colorado

The authors and AORN thank Deborah S. Hickman, MS, RN, CNOR, CRNFA, Renue Plastic Surgery, Brunswick, Georgia; Melanie L. Braswell, DNP, RN, CNS, CNOR, Indiana University Health Arnett, Lafayette, Indiana; Judith R. Garcia, MHSS, MS, BSN, RN, CNOR, Perioperative Department, Ohio State University Wexner Medical Center James Cancer Hospital and Solove Research Institute, Columbus, Ohio; J. Hudson Garrett Jr, PhD, MSN, MPH, FNP-BC, Director, Clinical Affairs, PDI Healthcare, Atlanta, Georgia; and Lisa Spruce, DNP, RN, ACNS, ACNP, ANP, CNOR, Director of Evidence-based Perioperative Practice, AORN, Inc, Denver, Colorado, for their assistance in developing this guideline.

PUBLICATION HISTORY

Originally published May 1976, *AORN Journal,* as "Standards for preoperative skin preparation of patients." Format revision March 1978, July 1982.

Revised February 1983, November 1988, November 1992, June 1996. Published November 1996, *AORN Journal;* reformatted July 2000.

Revised November 2001; published January 2002, *AORN Journal.*

Revised 2007; published as "Recommended practices for preoperative patient skin antisepsis" in *Perioperative Standards and Recommended Practices,* 2008 edition.

Minor editing revisions made to omit PNDS codes; reformatted September 2012 for publication in *Perioperative Standards and Recommended Practices,* 2013 edition.

Revised July 2014 for online publication in *Perioperative Standards and Recommended Practices.*

Minor editing revisions made in November 2014 for publication in *Guidelines for Perioperative Practice,* 2015 edition.

GUIDELINE FOR STERILE TECHNIQUE

The Guideline for Sterile Technique was approved by the AORN Recommended Practices Advisory Board. It was presented as proposed recommendations for comments by members and others. The guideline is effective December 15, 2012. The recommendations in this guideline are intended to be achievable and represent what is believed to be an optimal level of practice. Policies and procedures will reflect variations in practice settings and/or clinical situations that determine the degree to which the guideline can be implemented. AORN recognizes the various settings in which perioperative nurses practice; therefore, this guideline is adaptable to various practice settings. These practice settings include traditional operating rooms (ORs), ambulatory surgery centers, physicians' offices, cardiac catheterization laboratories, endoscopy suites, radiology departments, and all other areas where surgery and other invasive procedures may be performed.

Purpose

This document provides guidance for establishing and maintaining a sterile field by following the principles and implementing the processes of sterile technique. Sterile technique involves the use of specific actions and activities to prevent contamination and maintain sterility of identified areas during operative and other invasive procedures. Implementing sterile technique when preparing, performing, or assisting with surgical and other invasive procedures is the cornerstone of maintaining sterility and preventing microbial contamination.

The creation and maintenance of a sterile field can directly influence patient outcomes.[1] All individuals who are involved in operative or other invasive procedures have a responsibility to provide a safe environment for patients. Perioperative team members must be vigilant in safeguarding the sterility of the field and ensuring that the principles and processes of sterile technique are followed and implemented. Perioperative leaders can promote a culture of safety by creating an environment where perioperative personnel are encouraged to identify, question, or stop practices believed to be unsafe without fear of repercussion.

The perioperative registered nurse (RN) uses ethical principles to make clinical decisions and act on them.[2] Adhering to the principles of and implementing the processes for sterile technique is a matter of individual conscience and an ethical obligation that applies to all members of the perioperative team. Perioperative team members should understand the professional responsibility to ensure that contamination of the sterile field is remedied immediately, and to make certain that any item for which sterility is in question is not used. Adhering to the principles of and implementing the processes for sterile technique and taking immediate action to protect the patient when breaks in sterile technique occur meets the maxim, "first, do no harm." The perioperative team serves as the protective intermediary between patients and personnel whose practices do not meet the highest standards of sterile technique. Perioperative nurses have a long-standing reputation of advocating for patients and working together with members of the health care team to provide a safe perioperative environment for patients undergoing operative or other invasive procedures.

Although these recommendations include several references to surgical attire (including surgical masks) and hand hygiene, the focus of this document is on sterile technique. Surgical attire and hand hygiene are outside the scope of these recommendations. The reader should refer to the AORN Guideline for Surgical Attire[3] and Guideline for Hand Hygiene[4] for additional guidance.

Evidence Review

A medical librarian conducted a systematic review of MEDLINE®, CINAHL®, Scopus®, and the Cochrane Database of Systematic Reviews for meta-analyses, randomized and nonrandomized trials and studies, systematic and nonsystematic reviews, and opinion documents and letters. Search terms included *sterile field, sterile technique, aseptic technique, aseptic practices, surgical drapes, double-gloving, assisted gloving, closed gloving, time-related sterilization, event-related sterilization, surgical attire, protective clothing, sterile supplies, sterile barriers, barrier precautions, body-exhaust suits, space suits, laminar air flow, bowel technique, (glove expansion and fluids), (glove perforation and electrosurgery), strikethrough, Spaulding's criteria, product packaging,* and *equipment contamination*.

The lead author and medical librarian identified and obtained relevant guidelines from government agencies, other professional organizations, and standards-setting bodies. The lead author assessed additional professional literature, including some that initially appeared in other articles provided to the author.

The initial search was confined to 2006 to 2011, but the time restriction was not considered in subsequent searches. The librarian also established continuing alerts on the topics included in this guideline and provided relevant results to the lead author.

Articles identified by the search were provided to the project team for evaluation. The team consisted of the lead author, two members of the Recommended Practices Advisory Board, and a member of the Research Committee. The lead author divided the search results into topics and assigned members of the team to review and critically appraise each article using the Johns Hopkins Evidence-Based Practice Model and the Research or Non-Research Evidence Appraisal Tools as appropriate. The literature was independently evaluated and appraised according to the strength and quality of the evidence. Each article was then assigned an appraisal score as agreed upon by consensus of the team. The appraisal score is noted in brackets after each reference, as applicable.

The collective evidence supporting each intervention within a specific recommendation was summarized and used to rate the strength of the evidence using the AORN Evidence Rating Model. Factors considered in review of the collective evidence were the quality of research, quantity of similar studies on a given topic, and consistency of results supporting a recommendation. The evidence rating is noted in brackets after each intervention.

Editor's note: MEDLINE is a registered trademark of the US National Library of Medicine's Medical Literature Analysis and Retrieval System, Bethesda, MD. CINAHL, Cumulative Index to Nursing and Allied Health Literature, is a registered trademark of EBSCO Industries, Birmingham, AL. Scopus is a registered trademark of Elsevier B.V., Amsterdam, Netherlands.

Recommendation I

Perioperative personnel should implement practices that reduce the spread of transmissible infections when preparing or working in the OR or invasive procedure room and when performing or assisting with operative or other invasive procedures.

Protecting patients and safeguarding health care providers from potentially infectious agent transmission is a key focus of perioperative nurses.[5] Hand hygiene has been recognized as a primary method of decreasing health care-associated infections.[4,6] Surgical attire and personal protective equipment (PPE) are worn to support cleanliness and hygiene, promote patient and health care provider safety, and aid in preserving the integrity of the sterile field within the perioperative environment.[3,5]

I.a. Perioperative personnel entering the OR or invasive procedure room for any reason (eg, stocking supplies, bringing procedural supplies and equipment into clean rooms) should wear clean
- scrub attire,[1] including a freshly laundered or single-use, long-sleeved jacket snapped closed with the cuffs down to the wrists, and
- surgical head covers or hoods that cover all hair and scalp skin, including facial hair, sideburns, and the hair at the nape of the neck.[1]

[1: Strong Evidence]

Surgical attire helps contain bacterial shedding and promotes environmental cleanliness.[1,3] Head coverings and hoods minimize microbial dispersal by containing hair and scalp skin.[1,3]

I.b. Perioperative personnel should perform hand hygiene before entering the OR or invasive procedure room and areas where sterile supplies have been opened. [1: Strong Evidence]

Following regular hand hygiene practices helps prevent transmission of infection and reduces health care-associated infections for patients and health care personnel.[4,6]

Prevention of health care-associated infections is a priority of all health care providers. Health care-associated infections can result in untoward outcomes such as increased morbidity and mortality, longer length of stay, increased pain and suffering, and escalating cost of care.[7] Hand hygiene, hand washing, and surgical hand scrubs are the most effective way to prevent and control infections and represent the least expensive means of achieving both.[4]

I.c. Perioperative personnel should wear a clean surgical mask that covers the mouth and nose and is secured in a manner to prevent venting when open sterile supplies are present[1] and when preparing, performing, or assisting with surgery and other invasive procedures, including
- central venous catheter (CVC) insertion, peripherally inserted central catheters (PICCs), and guidewire exchange[8-10];
- regional anesthesia procedures[11]; or
- high-risk spinal canal procedures (eg, myelogram, lumbar puncture, spinal anesthesia).[10,12-20]

[1: Strong Evidence]

A clean surgical mask helps protect the patient and procedure site from microbial contamination by organisms carried in the provider's mouth or nose.[1,3,10,21]

Researchers studied the effectiveness of surgical masks in reducing the dispersal of bacterial contamination from the upper airways of 25 volunteers. The volunteers were asked to speak directly at an agar plate for five minutes. A surgical mask was applied and the volunteers were instructed to speak at the agar plate for three additional periods of five minutes each. The results showed a marked reduction in the bacterial contamination of the agar plates while the volunteers were wearing surgical masks.[21]

In a study investigating the possibility that surgical masks increase vertical shedding of bacteria from the face during facial movement, volunteers were asked to speak for 20 minutes while moving their heads from side to side without a surgical mask for the first five minutes and then with a surgical mask for three additional five-minute periods. A blood agar plate was positioned 30 cm below the volunteers' faces. The results showed a statistically significant reduction in the number of colony-forming units on the agar plate when the volunteers were wearing surgical masks. The researchers recommended wearing a surgical mask, particularly when the perioperative team member's face is in close proximity to the procedural site and when the need for speaking during the procedure is anticipated.[22]

In a prospective, randomized, controlled trial of 221 patients, researchers assessed the need for surgical masks during cataract surgery. Patients were randomly assigned to group A, in which the surgeon wore a clean surgical mask, or group B, in which the surgeon did not wear a surgical mask. A settle plate was secured adjacent to the patient's head on the operative side within the sterile field during all procedures. The results showed a significant reduction of bacterial organisms falling on the operative side when the surgeon wore a surgical mask.[23]

In a study exploring the relationship between the use and position of a surgical mask during 30 cardiac catheterization procedures, researchers obtained bacterial samples within the draped, operative site adjacent to the femoral artery. Surgical masks were either not worn by perioperative team members, or worn in positions above and below the nose. The number of bacterial colonies recovered when no mask was worn was significantly greater than when a surgical mask was worn. Mask placement below the nose also was associated with a higher colony count than when the mask was worn above the nose. The researchers voluntarily discontinued the study after 30 patients in the interest of patient safety because of the high bacterial count associated with not wearing surgical masks.[24]

Surgical masks are effective in limiting the dispersal of oropharyngeal droplets[21,25] and are recommended by the Centers for Disease Control and Prevention (CDC) for the placement of CVCs, PICCs, and guidewire exchange.[8-10]

The American Society of Regional Anesthesia and Pain Medicine recommends the use of surgical masks during regional anesthesia as a method to reduce the likelihood of site contamination from microorganisms that may be present in the upper airway of providers.[11]

Oropharyngeal flora was found to be the source of contamination in a number of reported cases of bacterial meningitis after lumbar puncture, spinal and epidural anesthesia, and intrathecal chemotherapy.[12-19]

In 2004, the CDC investigated eight instances in which patients contracted meningitis after procedures that involved placing a catheter or injecting material into the spinal canal or epidural space. The cases involved blood or cerebrospinal fluid contaminated with streptococcal species or other pathogens consistent with oropharyngeal fluid. None of the clinicians wore surgical masks during the procedures. Equipment and products used during these procedures were excluded as sources of contamination.[10] In June 2007, the Healthcare Infection Control Practices Advisory Committee reviewed the cases and determined there was sufficient evidence to warrant the wearing of a surgical mask by the individual placing a catheter or injecting material into the spinal or epidural space.[10]

In September 2008, three cases of bacterial meningitis in postpartum women were reported to the New York State Department of Health. Two additional cases of meningitis were reported to the Ohio Department of Health in May 2009. All of the patients had received intrapartum spinal anesthesia. The investigators concluded that the New York incidents were associated with a single anesthesiologist. The anesthesiologist reported wearing a surgical mask; however, personnel reported that the presence of unmasked visitors in the procedure area was common. The Ohio incidents were found to be associated with a second anesthesiologist who did not wear a surgical mask. The findings underscore the need for adhering to aseptic practices and wearing surgical masks during spinal procedures.[20]

Recommendation II

Surgical gowns, gloves, and drape products for use in the perioperative setting should be evaluated and selected for safety, efficacy, and cost before purchase or use.

The safety and efficacy of surgical gowns, gloves, and drape products depends on the design of the item and the materials from which they are made.[26]

Quality, patient and worker safety, and cost containment are primary concerns for perioperative RNs when they participate in evaluating and selecting medical devices and products for use in practice settings.[27]

II.a. Surgical gowns, gloves, and drape products should be evaluated and selected for use in the perioperative setting according to
- product-specific requirements[27,28];
- procedure-related requirements[27];
- end-user requirements and preferences[27,28];
- patient-related requirements[27];
- environmental considerations[29];
- compliance with federal, state, and local regulatory agencies[5,30,31]; and
- compliance with standards-setting bodies.[32]

[2: Moderate Evidence]

Product-specific requirements include contractual agreements, compatibility with existing products, and implementation of new products of differing material or construction.[27,28]

Procedure-related requirements define what is necessary for the procedure where the surgical gowns, gloves, and drape products will be used, such as resistance to penetration by blood

STERILE TECHNIQUE

and other body fluids, or the presence of adhesive apertures.[27]

End-user requirements, such as the degree of protection from blood, body fluids, and other potentially infectious materials, and preferences, such as comfort, vary depending on how the surgical gowns, gloves, and drape products are used.[27]

Patient-related requirements define the ability of the product to meet the needs of the individual patient, such as being appropriately sized or able to conform to patient contours.[27]

Environmental considerations, such as the potential for recycling or reprocessing, may reduce waste, conserve resources, and decrease costs without compromising quality of care.[29]

Mandatory Occupational Safety and Health Administration regulations require that personal protective equipment such as surgical gowns and gloves do not permit blood or other potentially infectious material to "pass through to or reach the employee's work clothes, street clothes, undergarments, skin, eyes, mouth, or other mucous membranes under normal conditions of use and for the duration of time which the protective equipment will be used."[30(1910.1030(d)(3)(i))]

Surgical gowns and drape products are surgical devices, and as such are regulated by the US Food and Drug Administration (FDA).[31] Failure of these devices is subject to medical device reporting requirements according to the Safe Medical Devices Act of 1990 as amended in March 2000[33] and MedWatch: The FDA Safety Information and Adverse Event Reporting Program.[34]

The American National Standards Institute and Association for the Advancement of Medical Instrumentation standard PB70:2012, "Liquid barrier performance and classification of protective apparel and drapes intended for use in health care facilities," establishes a common system of classification and specifies labeling requirements for manufacturers of protective apparel and drapes used in health care facilities.[32] The classification system is based on standardized test methods for determining liquid barrier performance and compliance. The implementation of consistent classification and labeling requirements by the manufacturer aids in evaluation and selection of the most appropriate protective products for the health care organization.[32]

II.a.1. Surgical gowns, gloves, and drape products used during operative and other invasive procedures must provide a barrier[1,30,32] and should be resistant to tears, punctures, and abrasions.[28]

Tears, punctures, and abrasions may allow for the passage of microorganisms, particulates, and fluids between sterile and unsterile areas and expose patients and perioperative personnel to microbial contamination and bloodborne pathogens.

Abrasions may adversely affect barrier properties by weakening the material and causing it to tear or generate lint.[26]

In a study evaluating bacterial penetration of disposable, non-woven drapes used during total hip arthroplasty, six brands of drapes were tested after 30 and 90 minutes. The results showed that bacterial penetration was time dependent. Most of the drapes remained impenetrable or allowed passage of fewer than 100 colony forming units at 90 minutes; however, none of the drapes tested were completely impenetrable, and certain brands were more resistant to bacterial penetration than others.[35]

In another study considering the effects of moisture and physical stress on surgical draping materials, researchers found that materials differ dramatically in the ability to resist bacterial penetration.[36]

II.a.2. Seams and points of attachment of surgical gowns should minimize liquid penetration and passage of potential contaminants.[1,32]

Wicking or pressure on a seam or point of attachment may cause liquid transfer between sterile and unsterile surfaces, and one or both sides of the gown may become contaminated.

II.a.3. Surgical gowns, gloves, and drape products used during operative or other invasive procedures should be non-abrasive and non-toxic.[28]

Products that are abrasive and contain chemicals and other toxic materials may irritate tissue, damage the skin, and injure patients and perioperative personnel.[26]

II.a.4. Barrier materials used for surgical gowns and drape products should be as lint free as possible.[28]

Lint particles are disseminated into the environment where bacteria attach to them.[37] Bacteria-carrying lint may settle in surgical sites and wounds and may increase postoperative patient complications.

II.a.5. Surgical gowns and drape products should be functional and flexible.[28]

Gowns and drape products that do not adequately perform and are unable to conform to and closely cover the user's body or equipment may be difficult to use and may not provide protection from contamination by blood, body fluids, and other potentially infectious materials.[26]

II.b. Perioperative personnel should select surgical gowns, gloves, and drape products for the procedure according to the barrier performance class of the product as stated on the label and the anticipated degree of exposure to blood, body fluids, and other potentially infectious materials.[30,32] *[1: Regulatory Requirement]*

Surgical gowns and drapes are labeled by the manufacturer with the level of performance determined by the barrier properties of the area of the gown or drape where direct contact with blood, body fluids, and other potentially infectious materials is most likely to occur.[32]

Surgical gowns, gloves, and drape products are used to establish a barrier that minimizes the passage of microorganisms, body fluids, and particulate matter between sterile and unsterile areas.[1,30,32,38,39]

Surgical gloves are worn to protect patients and perioperative team members from transmission of pathogens. The process of surgery subjects gloves to mechanical stresses (eg, twisting, pulling, stretching) and exposure to fluids, fats, and chemical substances (eg, methyl methacrylate) that may affect the integrity of the glove barrier. The barrier properties of surgical gloves may be affected by the strength of the glove material and also may be compromised by hand and finger movements and other tasks (eg, holding retractors) that are required during invasive procedures.

In a study evaluating and comparing the barrier performance characteristics of latex, vinyl, and nitrile gloves under simulated use conditions, researchers tested a total of 2,000 gloves (800 latex, 800 vinyl, 400 nitrile) from seven different manufacturers. The gloves were purchased specifically for the study, taken directly from the packages, and immediately tested. A comparative baseline was established by leak-testing 100 gloves of each brand and type. The study gloves were consistently manipulated in a manner simulating patient care activities for a period of 20 minutes. The results showed that the barrier performance of latex and nitrile gloves is comparable, and both materials are much less susceptible to material breakdown and leakage than vinyl.[40]

To compare the frequency of glove defects in latex and nonlatex surgical gloves during routine surgery, researchers collected gloves at the end of 2,318 surgical procedures. They tested a total of 6,386 gloves used by 101 surgeons and residents representing 15 surgical services. Six brands of nonlatex and two brands of latex gloves were tested. The results showed that both latex and nonlatex gloves performed adequately during routine surgical use; however, nonlatex surgical gloves had a higher rate of defects than latex gloves. The data also indicated that nonlatex gloves were nearly twice as likely to fail when used in certain high-risk surgical specialties (eg, oral, dental, cardiac) that require fine motor movement, increased hand dexterity, or contact with hard surfaces and sharp bone.[41]

II.b.1. Factors that should be considered when selecting surgical gowns, gloves, and drape products for surgical or other invasive procedures include the
- anticipated blood loss;
- volume of irrigation fluid;
- potential for splash, spray, pooling, or soaking;
- duration of the procedure;
- potential for leaning or pressure;
- type of procedure (eg, minimally invasive versus open, superficial incision versus deep body cavity); and
- team member's role.[26]

II.c. Perioperative personnel should select surgical gowns of appropriate size and sleeve length. *[5: No Evidence]*

When a gown is of insufficient size or sleeve length to cover the perioperative team member's body, it may restrict movement, increase the potential for the scrubbed team member's unsterile skin or clothing to contact the sterile field, or fail to provide adequate coverage to prevent the scrubbed team member from exposure to blood, body fluids, or other potentially infectious materials.

When a gown is of excessive size or sleeve length, the extra gown material may brush against unsterile objects and surfaces.

II.c.1. Surgical gowns should be large enough to adequately wrap around the perioperative team member's body and completely cover the back.

In one study evaluating various combinations of surgical attire, the addition of a wrap-around gown reduced environmental microbial contamination by 51% when compared with scrub attire worn without a gown.[42]

II.c.2. Surgical gowns should be selected so the lower sleeves and gown cuffs
- conform to the shape of the wearer's arms,[32]
- are short enough to allow gloves to fully cover the cuffs and mate properly with the lower sleeves,[32] and
- are of sufficient length to prevent the gown cuffs from pulling out of the gloves when the wearer's arms are extended.[32]

Recommendation III

Perioperative personnel should use sterile technique when donning and wearing sterile gowns and gloves.

Implementing sterile technique when donning and wearing sterile gowns and gloves reduces the risk of wound contamination and surgical site infections that may result from direct contact of surgical team members' skin or clothing with the sterile field.[1]

STERILE TECHNIQUE

III.a. Perioperative team members should perform a surgical hand scrub before donning sterile gowns and gloves. *[1: Strong Evidence]*

Surgical hand antisepsis decreases transient and resident microorganisms on the skin, which may reduce health care-associated infections.[4,6] Prevention of health care-associated infections is a priority of all health care providers. Health care-associated infections can result in untoward outcomes, such as increased morbidity and mortality, greater pain and suffering, longer length of stay, and escalated cost of care.[7] Hand hygiene, hand washing, and surgical hand scrubs are the most effective way to prevent and control infections and represent the least expensive means of achieving both.[4]

III.b. Scrubbed team members should don sterile gowns and gloves in a sterile area away from the main instrument table and in a manner to prevent contamination of surgical attire. *[3: Limited Evidence]*

Donning gowns and gloves in a separate area may help prevent contamination of the main instrument table by droplets of water or skin antiseptic solution from the scrubbed team member's wet hands. Donning gowns and gloves in a separate area also may reduce the risk of contamination of the main instrument table from potential contact with the unprotected skin and clothing of the scrubbed team member as they don sterile gown and gloves.

In a non-experimental, two-part study with a small sample size, researchers cultured water droplets from 15 surgeons' arms after a five-minute standardized surgical hand scrub with 10% povidone-iodine followed by thorough rinsing with tap water. The water droplets from each of the surgeons' arms were collected and cultured. Pathogenic and environmental bacteria were recovered from the water droplets from the surgeons' scrubbed arms. In the second part of the study, the wrapping paper from two different brands of gloves was investigated for permeability and bacterial penetration. The paper packaging was found to be permeable. The researchers concluded that pathogenic bacteria could be transferred from the surgeons' arms to the gloves by water dropped on the glove packaging during the gowning and gloving process, and this represented a theoretical source of wound contamination.[43]

III.b.1. Sterile gloves should not be opened directly on top of the sterile gown that has been opened for donning by the scrubbed team member.

When the gown is retrieved, droplets of water or skin antiseptic solution from the scrubbed team member's wet hands may drip onto the glove wrapper and contaminate the sterile gloves.[43]

III.b.2. The scrubbed team member's hands and arms should be completely dry before donning a sterile gown.

Droplets of water or skin antiseptic solution from the scrubbed team member's wet hands and arms may drip onto the gown or gown wrapper and contaminate the sterile gown.[43]

III.b.3. Only the inside of the sterile gown should be touched when it is picked up for donning by the scrubbed team member.

Touching only the inside of the gown when picking it up prevents the scrubbed team member's hands from contaminating the front of the gown.

III.b.4. The sterile glove wrapper or gloves should not be touched until the sterile gown has been donned.

After donning the sterile gown, the scrubbed team member's hands are covered by the impervious gown sleeves, which prevents the scrubbed team member's unprotected hands from contaminating the glove wrapper and gloves.[43]

III.c. The front of a sterile gown should be considered sterile from the chest to the level of the sterile field. *[3: Limited Evidence]*

In a study evaluating the most sterile areas of surgical gowns, researchers obtained samples from 50 surgical gowns at the end of 29 spinal procedures. The samples were taken at six-inch increments beginning at the neck of the gown and ending at the bottom of the gown. An additional 50 gowns were swabbed immediately after donning and before entering the sterile field to serve as negative controls. When compared with the negative controls, the contamination rates of the gowns worn during the procedures were lowest in the section between the chest and the operative field. Bacterial growth was highest in the areas above the chest and below the OR table. The researchers theorized that the increased levels of bacterial growth in the areas above the chest were likely related to microbial shedding from the scrubbed team member's head or mask, whereas the portion of the gown below the operating table was likely contaminated by direct contact with unsterile objects below the level of the operative field. The researchers concluded the front of the gown between the chest and the sterile field to be the area of greatest sterility.[44]

III.c.1. The neckline, shoulders, and axillary regions of the surgical gown should be considered contaminated.

The neckline, shoulders, and axillary regions are areas of friction and may not provide effective microbial barriers.

III.c.2. The surgical gown back should be considered unsterile.

> The back of the gown cannot be constantly monitored.

III.d. Gown sleeves should be considered sterile from two inches above the elbow to the cuff, circumferentially. *[3: Limited Evidence]*

> From two inches above the elbow to the cuff, gown sleeves are adjacent to the area of the gown that is considered sterile (ie, the front of the gown from the chest to the level of the sterile field[44]). Circumferential sterility of the gown sleeves is necessary because the scrubbed team member's arms move across the sterile field.

III.d.1. Sleeve cuffs of the surgical gown should be considered contaminated when the scrubbed team member's hands pass through and beyond the cuff.

> Sleeve cuffs are not impervious and could allow for microbial transfer from the scrubbed team member's hand.[36]

III.d.2. Sleeve cuffs should be completely covered by sterile gloves and should not be exposed.

> Permeable sleeve cuffs that are not completely covered by sterile gloves may allow for microbial transfer and contact from the scrubbed team member's arms to the patient, and for contact with blood and body fluids from the patient to the scrubbed team member.

III.e. The closed assisted gloving method should be used to glove team members during initial gowning and gloving for operative or other invasive procedures (Figure 1). *[2: Moderate Evidence]*

> The risk for glove cuff contamination increases when open assisted gloving is used. In a blinded, randomized study comparing contamination of the inside of the glove cuff during open and closed assisted gloving, two surgeons were gloved 20 times after covering their fingers and hands with a fluorescent powder. One surgeon was gloved by the closed assisted method and the other by the open assisted method. The results showed that open assisted gloving led to significantly greater glove cuff contamination than the closed assisted gloving method.[45]

III.e.1. During closed assisted gloving, the gown cuff of the team member being gloved should remain at or beyond the fingertips. The glove to be donned should be held open by a scrubbed team member, and the team member being gloved should insert his or her hand into the glove with the gown cuff touching only the inside of the glove.

III.e.2. Open assisted gloving, where the team member's gown sleeve is pulled up so that the gown cuff is at wrist level, leaving the fingers and hand exposed, should be used when closed assisted gloving is not possible or practical (Figure 2).

III.f. Scrubbed team members should wear two pairs of surgical gloves, one over the other, during surgical and other invasive procedures with the potential for exposure to blood, body fluids, or other potentially infectious materials.[1,5] *[1: Strong Evidence]*

> To provide an effective sterile barrier and prevent microbial transfer from surgical team members' hands to the patient, and to protect surgical team members from blood, body fluids, and other potentially infectious materials from the patient, surgical gloves must be intact and without perforations. Wearing two pairs of gloves helps to reduce glove perforations to the inner glove.
>
> A systematic review of 31 randomized controlled trials measuring glove perforations showed that the addition of a second pair of surgical gloves significantly reduced perforations to

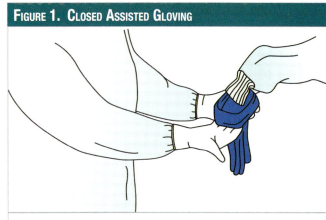

FIGURE 1. CLOSED ASSISTED GLOVING

During closed assisted gloving, the gown cuff should remain at or beyond the fingertips.
Illustration by Colleen Ladny.

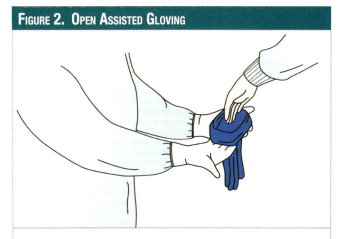

FIGURE 2. OPEN ASSISTED GLOVING

During open assisted gloving, the gown cuff is at wrist level, leaving the fingers and hand exposed.
Illustration by Colleen Ladny.

STERILE TECHNIQUE

the inner glove. Triple gloving, knitted outer gloves, and glove liners also significantly reduced perforations to the inner glove. More inner glove perforations were detected during surgery when perforation indicator systems were used.[46]

The CDC, the American College of Surgeons, and the American Academy of Orthopedic Surgeons support double gloving during invasive surgical procedures.[1,47,48]

III.f.1. When double gloves are worn, perforation indicator systems should be used.

A perforation indicator system is a double gloving system comprising a colored pair of surgical gloves worn beneath a standard pair of surgical gloves. When glove perforation occurs, moisture from the surgical field seeps through the perforation between the layers of gloves, allowing the site of perforation to be seen more easily (Figure 3).

A meta-analysis of five randomized, controlled trials with a combined sample size of 582 gloves showed significantly fewer perforations detected by scrubbed team members wearing standard double gloves compared with scrubbed team members using perforation indicator systems. When wearing standard double gloves, 21% of perforations were detected by the scrubbed team member. When wearing perforation indicator systems, 77% of perforations were detected.[46]

III.g. Scrubbed team members should inspect gloves for integrity after donning, before contact with the sterile field, and throughout use. *[2: Moderate Evidence]*

Careful inspection of glove integrity after donning and before contact with the sterile field may reveal holes and defects in the unused product that may have occurred during the manufacturing or donning process and could allow for the passage of microorganisms, particulates, and fluids between sterile and unsterile areas.

Careful inspection of glove integrity throughout the procedure may prevent unnoticed glove perforation. Unnoticed glove perforation during operative or other invasive procedures may present an increased risk for bloodborne pathogen transmission to perioperative team members related to prolonged exposure to blood, body fluids, or other potentially infectious materials, and also may increase the patient's risk for wound infection related to transfer of microorganisms from the hands of surgical team members.[1]

To investigate the frequency of undetected glove perforation, researchers studied glove perforations from 24 thoracoscopic and 23 open thoracotomy procedures and found that unnoticed glove perforation occurred in 25% of the gloves worn by the primary surgeon and in 12% of all gloves worn during the procedures.[49]

III.h. Surgical gloves worn during invasive surgical procedures should be changed
- after each patient procedure[6]; *[1: Strong Evidence]*
- when suspected or actual contamination occurs; *[5: No Evidence]*
- after touching surgical helmet system hoods and visors[50,51]; *[3: Limited Evidence]*
- after adjusting optic eyepieces on the operative microscope[52]; *[2: Moderate Evidence]*
- immediately after direct contact with methyl methacrylate[53-55]; *[1: Strong Evidence]*
- when gloves begin to swell, expand, and become loose on the hands as a result of the material's absorption of fluids and fats[56]; *[2: Moderate Evidence]*
- when a visible defect or perforation is noted or when a suspected or actual perforation from a needle, suture, bone, or other object occurs[1,57]; *[1: Strong Evidence]* and

FIGURE 3. PERFORATION INDICATOR SYSTEMS

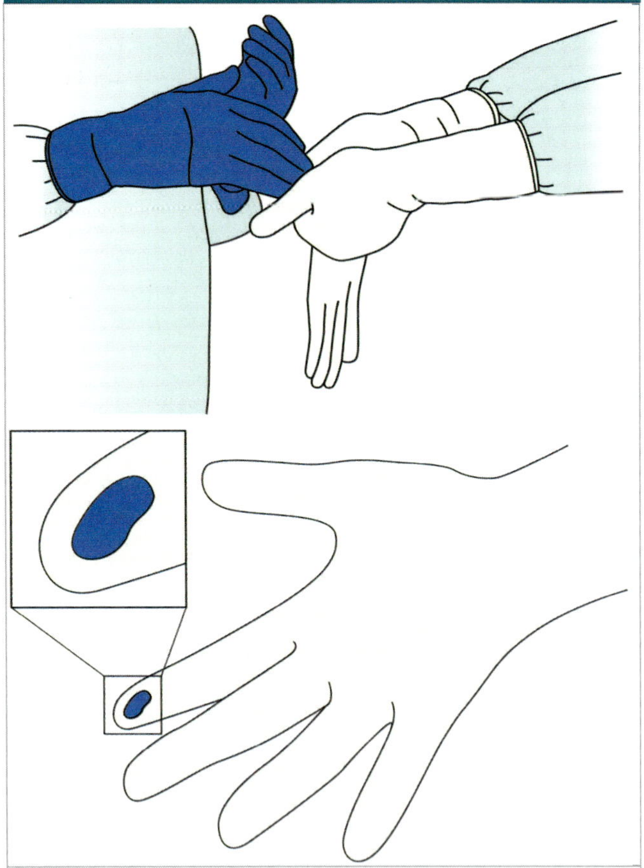

The use of perforation indicator systems may increase safety and reduce the potential for exposure to blood, body fluids, or other potentially infectious materials. When glove perforation occurs, the site of perforation can be more easily seen because of the colored gloves worn beneath the standard gloves.

Illustration by Colleen Ladny.

- every 90 to 150 minutes.[47,57-59] *[1: Strong Evidence]*

Failure to change gloves after each patient procedure may lead to transmission of microorganisms from one patient to another.[6]

Sterile gloves that have contacted unsterile items may transfer microorganisms or other unsterile particulates to the sterile field.

Surgical helmet systems consist of an unsterile reusable helmet with a built-in ventilation fan covered with a single-use disposable sterile visor mask hood. The unsterile helmet is donned before the surgical hand scrub is performed. The sterile visor mask hood that covers the unsterile helmet is applied during the gowning and gloving process (Figure 4).

In a study to evaluate the sterility of a surgical helmet system during six hip arthroplasty and 14 knee arthroplasty procedures, researchers sampled hoods at 30-minute intervals during, as well as at the end, of procedures. Although the small sample size was a limitation of the study, the results showed that 80% of the hoods were contaminated intraoperatively. The hoods were contaminated within 30 minutes of use and showed heavy growth of coagulase-negative *Staphylococcus aureus*. The researchers recommended avoiding direct contact with the surgical helmet hood system during surgical procedures or changing gloves if contact does occur.[50]

In another study evaluating microbial contamination of a surgical helmet system, researchers tested hoods used in 61 hip arthroplasty and 41 knee arthroplasty procedures. Samples were collected immediately after the hood was placed over the helmet and at the conclusion of the procedure. The contamination rate was 47%. The organisms found included coagulase-negative staphylococci, *Micrococcus*, methicillin-susceptible *S aureus*, and methicillin-resistant *S aureus*. The researchers recommended changing gloves if the hood or visor is touched or adjusted during the procedure.[51]

Researchers conducted a study to assess the contamination rates of sterile microscope drapes used during spine surgery. The study included 25 surgical spine procedures requiring the use of the operative microscope. The microscope drapes were swabbed immediately after application as negative controls. Postoperatively, the microscope drapes were sampled in seven different places. When compared with the negative controls, all of the sampled areas were found to be contaminated with bacteria. Four of the seven areas, including the shafts of the optic eyepieces, were found to have significant contamination rates. The regions above the eyepieces and the overhead portion of the drape also were contaminated. The researchers recommended avoiding contact with the upper portion of the drape and changing gloves after adjusting the optic eyepieces.[52]

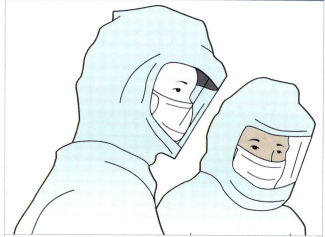

FIGURE 4. SURGICAL HELMET SYSTEMS

Surgical helmet systems consist of an unsterile reusable helmet covered with a single-use disposable sterile visor hood.

Illustration by Colleen Ladny and Kurt Jones.

Studies have demonstrated that surgical gloves are permeable to methyl methacrylate.[53,54] The amount of permeation depends on the type of glove and the duration it is worn.[53,54] A full discussion of methyl methacrylate is outside the scope of this document. The reader should refer to the AORN Guideline for a Safe Environment of Care, Part 1[55] for additional guidance.

Researchers studied the effectiveness of the barrier provided by latex surgical gloves and found that latex is subject to hydration (ie, the absorption of fluid molecules). Hydration rates are highly variable and depend on the properties of the individual glove product, the amount of perspiration from the scrubbed team member's hand, and the amount of body fluid exposure during the procedure. Hydrated gloves showed increased permeability and porosity and a significant reduction of electrical and mechanical resistance. The researchers concluded that latex is an effective barrier; however, the combined effects of the mechanical and biological stress to which the glove is subjected require careful monitoring by the user and changing gloves before the integrity of the glove is lost.[56]

Surgical gloves that are intact and without defects or perforations provide an effective sterile barrier and may prevent microbial transfer from perioperative team members' hands to the patient, and also protect the perioperative team members from transfer of blood, body fluids, and other potentially infectious materials from the patient.[1,57]

In a study measuring the concentration of bacteria passing through glove punctures under

STERILE TECHNIQUE

surgical conditions, 128 outer and 122 inner gloves used by surgical team members during 20 septic laparotomy procedures were tested. The rate of outer glove perforation averaged 15%; however, nearly 82% of the perforations went undetected. The frequency of perforation was directly correlated with the length of time the gloves were worn for both inner and outer gloves. Direct bacterial passage from the patient through a glove puncture occurred in almost 5% of all gloves worn. The researchers recommended a strict policy of changing gloves every 90 minutes.[57]

In a study measuring bacterial translocation through puncture holes in surgical gloves, 98 outer and 96 inner gloves worn by surgical team members during 20 consecutive surgical laparotomy procedures were examined. Ten outer gloves and one inner glove were perforated; however, seven of the perforations were detected because of the indicator glove system worn by surgical team members. Bacterial migration was demonstrated in five of the outer gloves and one of the inner gloves. The frequency of perforation increased with the length of time the gloves were worn. The researchers recommended double gloving and a change of gloves at least every 90 minutes.[58]

In another prospective study, researchers from one facility collected 898 consecutive pairs of surgical gloves used during all general surgery procedures during a nine-month period. There was a positive correlation between the rate of perforation and the duration of time the gloves were worn. Gloves worn for 90 minutes or less showed a perforation rate of 15%. Gloves worn for 91 to 150 minutes showed a perforation rate of 18%, while gloves worn longer than 150 minutes showed a perforation rate of 24%. There was no significant difference in the perforation rates of gloves worn by surgeons, first assistants, or scrub persons. Previously undetected perforations were found in 19% of the gloves worn by all team members. The researchers recommended that surgeons, first assistants, and scrub persons directly assisting at the operative field change gloves after 90 minutes of surgery.[59]

The American Academy of Orthopedic Surgeons recommends changing the outer pair of gloves at least every two hours to prevent skin exposure from perforations that may occur in the gloves with use over time.[47]

III.h.1. Perioperative team members should develop and implement strategies for changing gloves during operative and other invasive procedures and for identifying appropriate precautions to prevent microbial contamination and transmission of bloodborne pathogens.

The unique and critical factors associated with the immediate situation require thoughtful assessment and the application of informed clinical judgment.

Published literature does not provide conclusive evidence as to whether the outer gloves only or both the inner and outer gloves should be changed, or whether a surgical hand scrub should be performed each time gloves are changed. If the outer glove is contaminated by contact with an unsterile item (eg, surgical helmet hood), it may be sufficient to change only the outer gloves; however, if an outer glove has been perforated, the potential exists that the inner glove also may be perforated. In this case, the safest practice for both patient and surgical team member may be to remove gown and gloves, perform a surgical hand scrub, and don a clean gown and gloves.

III.i. Perioperative team members who must change their sterile gloves during operative or other invasive procedures should use the assisted gloving method. *[3: Limited Evidence]*

When using the assisted gloving method, one scrubbed team member touches only the outside of the new sterile glove when applying the glove to another scrubbed team member's hand.

Researchers evaluated glove donning techniques for microbial contamination by comparing open, closed, and assisted gloving techniques. After applying an ultraviolet luminescent cream to the tips of each of the fingers on both hands, 13 individuals were observed donning surgical gowns and gloves 20 times each. Contamination of the front and back cuff areas of the gown was noted in all 20 donning procedures using the open gloving method. Contamination of the back cuff areas of the gown was noted in all 20 donning procedures using the closed gloving method. No contamination of any areas of the gown was noted when using the assisted gloving method.[60]

III.i.1. If possible, the unscrubbed team member should remove the glove to be changed from the sterile team member without altering the position of the glove cuff (ie, pulling the cuff down over the scrubbed team member's hand).

III.i.2. When assisted gloving is not possible or practical, perioperative team members should change gowns and gloves using the closed gloving technique.

Recommendation IV

Sterile drapes should be used to establish a sterile field.

Sterile drapes provide a barrier that minimizes the passage of microorganisms from unsterile to sterile areas and reduces the risk of health care-associated infections.[1]

IV.a. Perioperative team members should place sterile drapes on the patient, furniture, and equipment in the sterile field and should handle them in a manner that prevents contamination.[1] *[1: Strong Evidence]*

In a randomized controlled trial comparing the use of maximal sterile barrier precautions (ie, sterile gown, sterile gloves, surgical cap, full body drape) with the use of only sterile gloves and a small drape during CVC insertion, results showed that maximal sterile barrier precautions led to fewer episodes of catheter colonization and catheter-related bloodstream infections.[61] One program that included using maximal sterile barriers during CVC insertion in 103 intensive care units in Michigan resulted in a 66% decrease in infection rates.[62]

The CDC recommends maximum sterile barrier precautions, including the use of a full body drape, during the placement of CVCs, PICCs, and guidewire exchanges.[8,9]

IV.a.1. Unsterile equipment (eg, Mayo stands) should be covered on the top, bottom, and sides with sterile barrier materials before being introduced to or brought over a sterile field. Sterile barrier material also should be applied to the portion of the equipment that will be positioned immediately adjacent to the sterile field.

IV.a.2. Sterile drapes should be handled as little as possible.

Rapid movement of draping materials creates air currents on which dust, lint, and other particles can migrate.[37]

IV.a.3. Draping materials should be held in a controlled manner that prevents the sterile drape from coming into contact with unsterile surfaces.

IV.a.4. During draping, gloved hands should be shielded by cuffing the drape material over the gloved hands.

Keeping the gloved hands beneath the cuff of the draping material may protect gloves from contact with unsterile items or areas.

Researchers tested 275 outer and inner gloves that were used during 10 total hip replacements for microbial contamination. The results indicated that contamination occurred most frequently on the outside of the gloves that were used exclusively for draping.[63]

IV.a.5. Surgical drapes should be placed in a manner that does not require scrubbed team members to lean across an unsterile area and prevents the front of the surgical gown from contacting an unsterile surface.

IV.a.6. Sterile drapes should be placed from the surgical site to peripheral areas.

IV.a.7. The portion of the surgical drape that establishes the sterile field should not be moved after it has been positioned.

IV.a.8. Only the top surface of a sterile, draped area should be considered sterile. Items that fall below the sterile area should be considered contaminated.

IV.b. Surgical equipment (eg, tubing, cables) should be secured to the sterile drapes with nonperforating devices. *[2: Moderate Evidence]*

Perforation of barrier materials may provide portals of entry and exit for microorganisms, blood, and other potentially infectious materials.[57]

IV.c. The upper portion of the C-arm drape should be considered contaminated. *[2: Moderate Evidence]*

In a prospective study evaluating the sterility of 25 C-arm drapes used during spinal surgery, researchers obtained samples postoperatively from five different locations on a standard fluoroscopic C-arm drape. The researchers also sampled the drapes preoperatively immediately after they were applied to establish a negative control. The results showed that bacterial contamination was present at all sampled locations; however, the samples at the top of the C-arm had the greatest degree of contamination when compared with the negative controls (ie, 56% at the top and 28% at the upper front of the receiver). Lower rates of contamination were observed on the lower front, receiver plate, and mid-portion of the C-arm drape (ie, 12% to 20%), but these were not considered significant. The researchers recommended the top portion of the C-arm drape be considered unsterile, and suggested that avoiding contact with these areas may decrease the risk of postoperative infection[64] (Figure 5).

IV.d. Plastic adhesive incise drapes should not be used for prevention of surgical site infection. *[1: Strong Evidence]*

In a systematic review of seven randomized, controlled studies involving 4,195 patients, researchers concluded there was no evidence to support the use of plastic adhesive incise drapes as a method for reducing infection, and that there was some evidence that infection rates may be increased when adhesive incise drapes are used. A meta-analysis of five studies included in the review, which included 3,082 participants, compared plain plastic adhesive incise drapes with no drape and showed a significantly higher number of patients developed a surgical site infection when the adhesive incise drape was used. There was no effect on surgical site infection rates according to a meta-analysis of two additional studies, including 1,113 participants, which compared iodine-impregnated plastic adhesive incise drapes

STERILE TECHNIQUE

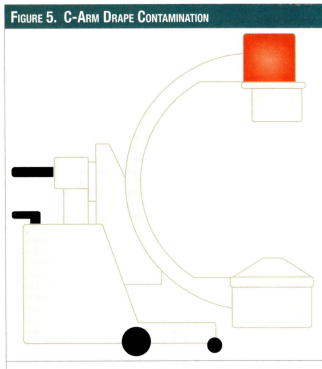

FIGURE 5. C-ARM DRAPE CONTAMINATION

Researchers found bacterial contamination was greatest at the top and upper front of the receiver.

Illustration by Colleen Ladny.

with no drape. The researchers theorized that the patient's skin is not likely to be a primary cause of surgical site infection if it is properly disinfected, and they concluded that attempting to isolate the skin from the surgical wound is of no benefit and may create increased moisture and bacterial growth under adhesive drapes.[65]

Recommendation V

A sterile field should be prepared for patients undergoing surgical or other invasive procedures.

Preparing a sterile field for patients undergoing surgical or other invasive procedures reduces the risk of microbial contamination and is a cornerstone of infection prevention. Failure to adhere to aseptic practices during invasive procedures has been associated with surgical site infections.[1]

V.a. The sterile field should be prepared in the location where it will be used and should not be moved. *[5: No Evidence]*

Moving the sterile field from one location to another increases the potential for contamination.

V.b. The sterile field should be prepared as close as possible to the time of use. *[1: Strong Evidence]*

The potential for bacterial growth and contamination increases with time because dust and other particles present in the ambient environment settle on horizontal surfaces. Particulate matter can be stirred up by personnel movement and can settle on opened sterile supplies.[1,37,66-70]

There is no specified amount of time that opened sterile supplies in an unused room can remain sterile. The sterility of an opened sterile field is event-related.[71]

V.c. Sterile supplies should be opened for only one patient at a time in the OR or other procedure room. *[4: Benefits Balanced With Harms]*

Opening sterile supplies for multiple patients in a single OR or other procedure room increases the risk of cross contamination.

V.d. One patient at a time should occupy the OR or other procedure room. *[1: Strong Evidence]*

Concurrent procedures performed on multiple patients in the same OR or other procedure room at the same time may expose patients to a variety of hazards and increase the risk of contamination and infection.

Infectious diseases may be transmitted by airborne, contact, and droplet methods.[10] The risk of cross contamination may be increased when two sterile fields, two surgical teams, and two open surgical wounds are confined to a single OR or other procedure room.

V.e. Perioperative personnel should perform a surgical hand scrub and don a sterile gown and gloves before setting up sterile supplies. *[1: Strong Evidence]*

Surgical hand hygiene decreases transient and resident microorganisms on the skin, which may reduce health care-associated infections.[4,6]

Donning a sterile gown and gloves before setting up sterile supplies minimizes the potential for wound contamination and reduces patient risks for surgical site infections that may result from contact with perioperative team members' skin or clothing.[1]

V.f. Only sterile items should come in contact with the sterile field. *[1: Strong Evidence]*

The creation and maintenance of a sterile field may influence patient outcomes.[1]

Using sterile items during invasive procedures minimizes the risk of infection and provides the highest level of assurance that procedural items are free of microorganisms.[72]

V.g. Sterile fields and instrumentation used during procedures that involve both the abdominal and perineal areas should be kept separate and should not be used interchangeably. *[2: Moderate Evidence]*

The perineal area has a higher microbial count than the abdominal area.[73] Placing instruments and other items that have been used in the perineal area into the abdominal area can transfer microorganisms from the perineum to the abdomen and cause an infection. Meticulous sterile technique is required during gynecologic laparoscopic procedures when transurethral instruments and catheters are passed to prevent infections of the urinary tract. These infections are the most common type of health care-associated infection reported to the National Healthcare Safety Network.[74]

The defense system of the peritoneum also may be negatively affected by the pneumoperitoneum used in laparoscopic procedures.[75] The mechanical distension changes the peritoneal microstructure, allowing passage of bacteria[76] to the bloodstream, lungs, and kidneys.[77] This is important because intra-abdominal infections often begin in the peritoneal cavity.[76] Systemic response coupled with the amount of tissue damage and the duration of the procedure may potentially lead to a higher risk for infection.[75]

V.h. Isolation technique should be used during bowel surgery. *[2: Moderate Evidence]*

Isolation technique, also known as bowel or contamination technique, is implemented to reduce the potential for microorganisms that exist in the bowel to be transferred into the abdominal cavity, tissues of the abdominal wall, and the surgical site. Isolation technique includes
- no longer using instruments or equipment that have contacted the inside of the bowel or the bowel lumen after the bowel lumen has been closed,
- using clean instruments to close the wound, and
- either removing contaminated instruments and equipment from the sterile field or placing them in a separate area that will not be touched by members of the sterile team.

The distal ileum is an area of transition between the small populations of bacteria in the proximal small intestine and the large numbers of bacteria and anaerobic microorganisms in the large bowel.[73,78-80] Only small numbers of bacteria are normally present in the duodenum and proximal jejunum.[73,78-80] Excessive colonization of bacteria in the small bowel is prevented by the destructive action of gastric acid and bile, digestion by proteolytic enzymes, and bacterial clearance by intestinal peristalsis.[73,78-80] Some gastrointestinal disorders that require surgical repair may be associated with an increase in the number of bacteria in the upper gastrointestinal tract (eg, obstruction, diverticula, fistula)[78-80] and may warrant the implementation of isolation technique.

In a study evaluating contamination of surgical instruments that have contacted bowel mucosa and whether isolation technique decreases contamination of the abdominal wall and peritoneal cavity, researchers compared contamination levels of instruments used during procedures involving the large bowel (ie, cecum, ascending, transverse, descending, and sigmoid colon, rectum) with contamination levels of instruments used during procedures involving the small bowel (ie, duodenum, jejunum, ileum). Researchers cultured the needle drivers used to grasp the needles that perforated mucosa when the bowel was anastomosed and the tissue forceps that were used to grasp the edge of the bowel during anastomosis from 20 procedures involving the large bowel. The same two types of instruments from 10 procedures involving the small bowel also were cultured. The study results showed that instruments that come into contact with the bowel lumen during bowel resection surgery become contaminated if they are not isolated, which increases the potential for contamination of the peritoneal cavity and abdominal wall from bowel organisms. The total number of organisms isolated was greater for the large bowel than for the small bowel, and the proportion of anaerobic organisms was greater in the large bowel group.[81]

In a prospective study assessing the risk factors for surgical site infection during gastrointestinal surgery, researchers conducted surveillance of 941 patients in 27 hospitals and found the overall infection rate was 15.5%; the incidence of infection after gastric surgery was 8%; and the incidence of infection after small bowel, colorectal, appendectomy, and stoma surgeries was as high as 20% to 30%. Researchers found that strict adherence to sterile technique and minimal blood loss were associated with a lower incidence of surgical site infection.[82]

V.h.1. The health care organization should develop and implement a standardized procedure for isolation technique.[81,83,84]

A standardized procedure for isolation technique (ie, following the same patterns and processes each time) assists in achieving accuracy, efficiency, and continuity among perioperative team members. Studies of human error have shown that many errors involve a deviation from routine practice.[85]

V.h.2. The use of isolation technique should begin when the gastrointestinal tract is transected and end when the anastomosis is closed.[83]

V.h.3. Isolation technique should be implemented using either a single setup or a dual setup.[83,84]

Single setup:
- Prepare one setup for the procedure, including anastomosis and closure.
- Before transection of the bowel, place clean sterile towels or a wound protector around the surgical site.
- Segregate all contaminated instruments and other items that have contacted the

STERILE TECHNIQUE

bowel lumen to a designated area (eg, Mayo stand, basin).
- Refrain from touching the sterile back table while the bowel is open.
- When the anastomosis is complete, remove the contaminated instruments, towel drapes, wound protector, and any other potentially contaminated items (eg, electrosurgical pencil, suction, light handles) from the sterile field, or place them in a separate area that will not be touched by perioperative team members.
- Irrigate the wound and apply moist counted sponges or towels to protect the tissue.
- Initiate team communication announcing the change to clean closure.
- One scrubbed team member should remain at the sterile field while all other team members change into clean gowns and gloves.
- The scrubbed team member who remained at the field should remove the moist counted sponges or towels and then change into a clean gown and gloves.
- Initiate accounting procedures.
- Apply clean light handles.
- Apply clean drapes to cover the existing drapes, which may be soiled with bowel contents.
- Secure a clean electrosurgical pencil and suction to the field.
- Proceed with wound closure using only clean instrumentation and other items.

Dual setup:
- Prepare one setup for the procedure and one for the closure.
- Before transection of the bowel, place clean sterile towels or a wound protector around the surgical site.
- When the anastomosis is complete, remove the contaminated instruments, towel drapes, wound protector, and any other potentially contaminated items (eg, electrosurgical pencil, suction, light handles) from the sterile field or return all contaminated instruments and other items to the procedure setup that will not be touched by perioperative team members.
- Irrigate the wound and apply moist counted sponges or towels to protect the tissue.
- Initiate team communication announcing the change to clean closure.
- One scrubbed team member should remain at the sterile field while all other team members change into clean gowns and gloves.
- The scrubbed team member who remained at the field should remove the moist counted sponges or towels and then change into a clean gown and gloves.
- Initiate accounting procedures.
- Apply clean light handles.
- Apply clean drapes to cover the existing drapes, which may be soiled with bowel contents.
- Secure a clean electrosurgical pencil and suction to the field.
- Proceed with wound closure using only instrumentation and other items from the closure setup.

V.i. Isolation technique should be used during procedures involving resection of metastatic tumors. *[2: Moderate Evidence]*

The use of isolation technique is a primary precaution to prevent the potential spread of cancer cells. There have been reports of local and distant implantation of tumor cells associated with the use of instrumentation used for both resection and closure or reconstruction.[86-88]

In one case, a 52-year-old man underwent a subtotal resection of a metastatic gliosarcoma in the right frontal region, a second surgery four months later, and a third surgery with complete resection five months after that. The dural defect that occurred as a result of the total resection was reconstructed using a tensor fascia lata graft from the right leg. Two months later, the patient presented with subcutaneous masses in the frontal and right temporal scalp and in the right upper leg in the area where the donor graft was taken. Pathologic examination of the excised masses verified the presence of cells identical to the primary tumor mass. The patient died two months later with multiple subcutaneous masses in the scalp. Implantation of tumor cells by the use of contaminated surgical instruments used for tumor resection was believed to be the cause of the development of local and distant recurrences.[86]

In another case, a 42-year-old man underwent sublabial transrhinoseptal incomplete resection of a clival chondroid chordoma and postoperative proton beam radiotherapy that resulted in stabilization of the residual tumor remnant. The patient experienced a painless loosening of an upper incisor 31 months later. Computerized tomography revealed a bone defect between the 11th and 12th teeth. Curettage biopsy and pathological examination showed a chondroid clival chordoma resembling the initial chordoma. The patient underwent two additional resections for intracranial recurrences and died at the age of 49 from infectious complications. Seeding during resection is believed to be the cause of the recurrence. The authors recommended removing resection instrumentation before closure and abundantly rinsing the surgical field.[87]

In another case, a 37-year-old woman who was diagnosed at age 10 with a low-grade oligoastrocytoma underwent craniotomy with surgical resection of the tumor at the time of diagnosis. The patient underwent a second craniotomy and surgical resection of the tumor followed by chemoradiation for progression of the tumor. Seven months later, the patient noticed an area of thickening in the scalp incision and underwent resection of the scar for what was believed to be poor wound healing. Pathological examination of the skin from the scalp revealed fibrosis and subcutaneous fat necrosis with chronic inflammation and foreign body giant cell reaction; however, the deep aspect of the subcutaneous tissue showed clusters and infiltrating cords of atypical cells morphologically similar to those of the resected tumor. The development of subcutaneous scalp involvement was believed to be from tumor implantation and seeding during surgical resection.[88]

Recommendation VI

Items introduced to the sterile field should be opened, dispensed, and transferred by methods that maintain the sterility and integrity of the item and the sterile field.

Sterile items that are not opened, dispensed, and transferred by methods that maintain sterility and integrity may contaminate the sterile field.

VI.a. Perioperative team members should inspect sterile items for proper processing, packaging, and package integrity immediately before presentation to the sterile field. *[1: Strong Evidence]*

Inspecting items before presentation to the sterile field helps verify that conditions required for sterility have been met and helps prevent microbial contamination that might occur if the integrity of the container has been breached and the item is placed on the sterile field.

Sterility is event-related and depends on maintenance of the integrity of the package.[71,89,90] The sterility of an item does not change with the passage of time but may be affected by particular events (eg, amount of handling) or environmental conditions (eg, humidity).

In a study of time-related contamination rates of sterilized dental instruments, researchers removed 25 sterilized examination mirrors from their packages and tested them for aerobic and anaerobic microbial contamination immediately after sterilization and at 31, 60, 90, and 124 days. Researchers found no contamination on any of the items at any time.[91]

In another study that evaluated whether storage time has any effect on the susceptibility of sterile packages to contamination under deliberate bacterial exposure, researchers prepared 700 packages containing six porcelain cylinders using four different types of packaging, including one cloth wrap, one paper wrap, and two peel pouches (ie, 175 of each packaging type). As a control group, 100 packages (ie, 25 of each packaging type) were immediately opened and tested for contamination. The outside of the remaining packages were deliberately contaminated with *Serratia marcescens* and opened at intervals of seven, 14, 28, 90, and 180 days. The packages were handled weekly and transferred from one container to another. The results showed no growth in the interior of any of the packages. Researchers concluded that the packages were able to protect the contents for up to six months, even with external contamination.[92]

Researchers tested 7,200 sterile packages to examine the effect of time on internal package sterility. The packages were tested immediately after sterilization and at monthly intervals during a 12-month period after storage in cabinet drawers in 24 different dental procedure rooms. No evidence of increased contamination over time was found for any of the packages. The researchers concluded that a 12-month or longer storage period is acceptable for sterile packages.[93]

To evaluate the sterility of packaged items in a variety of environmental conditions, researchers distributed 152 wrapped and packaged items to five different areas within a single hospital. Every three months over a two-year period, a number of items were removed from their packaging and tested for sterility. All of the tested items were found to be sterile. The results of this study demonstrated that unless the packaging is damaged, properly wrapped or packaged and sterilized items remain sterile. The researchers also concluded that although the study was conducted during a two-year period, there is no reason to suggest that this should be considered as a time limit for sterility.[94]

VI.a.1. If an expiration date is provided, perioperative team members should check the date before the package is opened and the contents are delivered to the sterile field. Items should not be used after the labeled expiration date.

VI.a.2. Perioperative team members should inspect the sterilization chemical indicator in the sterile package to verify the appropriate color change for the sterilization process used.[90]

VI.b. Items should be delivered to the sterile field in a manner that prevents unsterile objects or unscrubbed team members from leaning or reaching over the sterile field. *[1: Strong Evidence]*

STERILE TECHNIQUE

Microorganisms are shed from the skin of perioperative personnel.[1,37] Maintaining distance from the sterile field decreases the potential for contamination when items are passed from unsterile to sterile areas.

VI.c. Sterile items should be presented directly to the scrubbed team member or placed securely on the sterile field. *[5: No Evidence]*

Items tossed onto a sterile field may roll off the edge, create a hole in the sterile drape, or cause other items to be displaced, leading to contamination of the sterile field.

VI.c.1. Heavy items or items that are sharp and may penetrate the sterile barrier should be presented directly to the scrubbed team member or opened on a separate clean, dry surface.

VI.d. Perioperative personnel should open wrapped sterile supplies by opening
1. the farthest wrapper flap,
2. each of the side flaps, and
3. the nearest wrapper flap.

[5: No Evidence]

Opening the wrapper flap that is farthest away first prevents contamination that might occur from passing an unsterile arm over sterile items.

VI.d.1. Wrapper edges should be secured when supplies are opened and presented to the scrubbed team member or sterile field.[90]

Wrapper edges are considered contaminated. Securing the loose wrapper edges helps prevent them from contaminating sterile areas or items.

VI.d.2. Instrument tray wrappers should be visually inspected for moisture and integrity before the contents are placed on the sterile field.[90]

VI.e. Peel pouches should be presented to the scrubbed team member or opened onto the sterile field by pulling back the flaps without touching the inside of the package or allowing the contents to slide over the unsterile edges of the package. *[5: No Evidence]*

Touching the inside of the package or allowing the contents to slide over the unsterile edges may contaminate the contents of the package.

VI.f. Rigid sterilization containers should be inspected and opened on a clean, flat, and dry surface.[90] *[3: Limited Evidence]*

Opening rigid sterilization containers on a clean, flat, and dry surface facilitates removing sterile items from their containers without contaminating the items or sterile field.

VI.f.1. Perioperative team members should verify that external locks, latch filters, valves, and tamper-evident devices are intact before opening rigid sterilization containers.[90]

Ensuring container locks, latch filters, valves, and temper-evident devices are intact helps to verify there has not been a breach of the container seal.

VI.f.2. Perioperative team members should verify that the external chemical indicator has changed as appropriate before opening rigid sterilization containers.

Checking for the appropriate chemical indicator change verifies that the container has been through the sterilization process and reduces the potential for opening items that have not been sterilized.

VI.f.3. The rigid sterilization container should be opened according to the manufacturer's written instructions for use. The lid should be lifted up and toward the person opening the container and away from the container.
- The lid should be inspected for the integrity of the filter or valve and the integrity of the filter or valve and the gasket.[90]
- The container contents should be considered contaminated if the filter is damp or dislodged, or has holes, tears, or punctures.

Opening the container according to the manufacturer's written instructions for use facilitates aseptic removal of the contents.[90] Lifting the lid up and away from the container and toward the person removing the lid helps to prevent potential contamination from contact between the unsterile lid and the sterile inner rim, contents, and inside of the container system, and also helps to prevent the unscrubbed person from leaning over the sterile contents of the container.

VI.f.4. The scrubbed team member should avoid contacting the unsterile surfaces of the table or container while lifting the inner basket(s) out and above the container.[90] Before the instruments are placed on the sterile field, the internal chemical indicator should be examined for the appropriate color change and the inside surface of the container inspected for debris, contamination, or damage.[90]

VI.g. Medications and sterile solutions (eg, normal saline) should be transferred to and handled on the sterile field using sterile technique. *[2: Moderate Evidence]*

Transferring and handling medications and solutions on the sterile field poses increased risks for contamination of the medication, solution, sterile field, and surgical site because medications and solutions are removed from their original containers, stored on the sterile field, and passed from a scrubbed team member to a licensed practitioner for administration.[95] Using sterile technique helps prevent microbial contamination of the sterile field or medication.

VI.g.1. Medications and solutions should be visually inspected immediately before transfer to the sterile field and should not be used if the expiration date has passed or if there is any indication that the medication or solution has been compromised (eg, discoloration, particulate formation).[95]

Compromised and outdated medications and solutions may be contaminated or have reduced effectiveness.

VI.g.2. Sterile transfer devices (eg, sterile vial spike, filter straw, plastic catheter) should be used when transferring medications or solutions to the sterile field.[95]

Transfer devices are designed to reduce the potential for contamination of the sterile field by minimizing splashing and spilling and the need to reach over the sterile field.

VI.g.3. When solutions are dispensed to the sterile field, the entire contents of the container should be poured slowly into a solution receptacle that is placed near the sterile table's edge or is held by a scrubbed team member and labeled immediately.

Pouring the entire contents of the container slowly prevents splashing. Splashing may cause strike-through and splash-back from unsterile surfaces to the sterile field.

Placing the solution receptacle near the edge of the sterile table or having the scrubbed team member hold the receptacle reduces the potential for contamination of the sterile table and allows the unscrubbed team member to pour fluids without leaning over the sterile field.

VI.g.4. The edge of the container should be considered contaminated after the contents have been poured.

VI.g.5. The cap should not be replaced on opened medication or solution containers and any remaining fluids should be discarded.

The sterility of the contents of opened medication or solution containers cannot be ensured if the cap is replaced.

Reuse of open containers may contaminate solutions from drops contacting unsterile areas and then running back over container openings.

VI.g.6. Medications and solutions should be dispensed to the sterile field as close as possible to the time they will be used.[95]

VI.g.7. Stoppers should not be removed from vials for the purpose of pouring medications unless specifically designed for removal and pouring by the manufacturer.[95]

VI.g.8. Unused, opened irrigation or IV solutions should be discarded at the end of the procedure.[95]

Irrigation and IV containers and supplies are considered single-use. Using surplus volume from any irrigation or IV solution container or supplies for more than one patient increases the risk of cross-contamination.

Recommendation VII

Sterile fields should be constantly monitored.

The sterile field is subject to unrecognized contamination by personnel, vectors (eg, insects), or breaks in sterile technique if left unobserved.

VII.a. Once created, a sterile field should not be left unattended until the operative or other invasive procedure is completed. *[5: No Evidence]*

Observation increases the likelihood of detecting a breach in sterility.

VII.a.1. The doors to the OR or other procedure room should not be taped closed or otherwise secured as an alternative to monitoring the sterile field.

VII.b. When there is an unanticipated delay, or during periods of increased activity, a sterile field that has been prepared and will not immediately be used may be covered with a sterile drape. *[2: Moderate Evidence]*

To evaluate the contamination rate of sterile trays that have been opened in a controlled OR environment and the effect of traffic on the contamination rate, researchers opened 45 sterile trays in a positive air-flow OR and randomly assigned them to one of three groups:
- Trays were opened and left uncovered in a locked OR.
- Trays were opened and left uncovered in an OR with single-person traffic flowing in and out every 10 minutes from an unsterile corridor.
- Trays were opened, immediately covered with a sterile surgical towel, and left in a locked OR.

All trays were opened using sterile technique and were exposed for a total of four hours. Cultures of the trays were taken immediately after they were opened and every 30 minutes during the exposure period. The contamination rates for the uncovered trays were 4% at 30 minutes, 15% at 60 minutes, 22% at two hours, and 30% at four hours. There was no difference in the contamination rates between the uncovered trays in the room with traffic and those in the room without traffic. The covered trays had no contamination during the exposure period. The researchers recommended covering sterile trays that are not immediately used to minimize exposure to environmental contaminants.[96]

In a study of 41 total joint replacements (27 hip, 14 knee) that was conducted to evaluate the effectiveness of covering instruments, researchers found that covering the instruments during periods of increased activity (eg, patient transfer to the procedure bed, skin preparation) shortened the overall exposure time and shielded the instruments from bacterial dispersal, resulting in a 28-fold reduction of instrument contamination.[97]

VII.b.1. When sterile fields are covered, they should be covered in a manner that allows the cover to be removed without bringing the part of the cover that falls below the sterile field above the sterile field. When covering the sterile field, two sterile "cuffed" drapes should be used as follows:
- The first drape should be placed horizontally over the table or other area to be covered with the cuff at or just beyond the halfway point. The second drape should be placed from the opposite side of the table and the cuff positioned so that it completely covers the cuff of the first drape (Figure 6).
- The drapes should be removed by placing hands within the cuff of the top drape and lifting the drape up and away from the table and toward the person removing the drape. The second drape should be removed from the opposite side in a similar manner.

Removing the cover from the sterile field may result in a part of the cover that was below the sterile field being drawn above the sterile field, which may allow air currents to draw microorganisms and other contaminants (eg, dust, debris) from an unsterile area (eg, floor) and deposit them in sterile areas.[37]

VII.b.2. The health care organization should develop a standardized procedure in collaboration with infection prevention personnel for covering sterile fields to delineate the specific circumstances when sterile fields may be covered and to specify the method of covering and the length of time a sterile field may be covered.

Standardized procedures (ie, following the same patterns and processes each time) assist in achieving accuracy, efficiency, and continuity among perioperative team members. Studies of human error have shown that many errors involve a deviation from routine practice.[85]

VII.c. Perioperative personnel should observe for, recognize, and immediately correct breaks in sterile technique when preparing, performing, or assisting with operative or other invasive procedures and should implement measures to prevent future occurrences. *[1: Strong Evidence]*

Breaks in sterile technique may expose the patient to increased microbial contamination. The risk for infection increases with increased amounts of microbial contamination.[1] Preventing, observing for, recognizing, and taking immediate corrective action for breaks in sterile technique may prevent or reduce microbial contamination and help minimize the risk of surgical site infection.

VII.c.1. When a break in sterile technique occurs, corrective action should be taken immediately unless the patient's safety is at risk. When a break in sterile technique cannot be corrected immediately, corrective action should be taken as soon as it is safe for the patient.

The greater the length of time until the break in sterile technique is recognized, the more complex and difficult containment becomes and the more likely it becomes that full containment may not be possible.[98]

VII.d. If organic material (eg, blood, hair, tissue, bone fragments) or other debris (eg, bone cement, grease, mineral deposits) is found on an instrument or item in a sterile set, the entire set should be considered contaminated and perioperative team members should take corrective actions immediately. *[1: Strong Evidence]*

Organic and inorganic material that remains on a surgical instrument may be transferred to the surgical wound or other areas of the body, which increases the risk for surgical site infection or other postoperative complications.

FIGURE 6. COVERING A STERILE TABLE

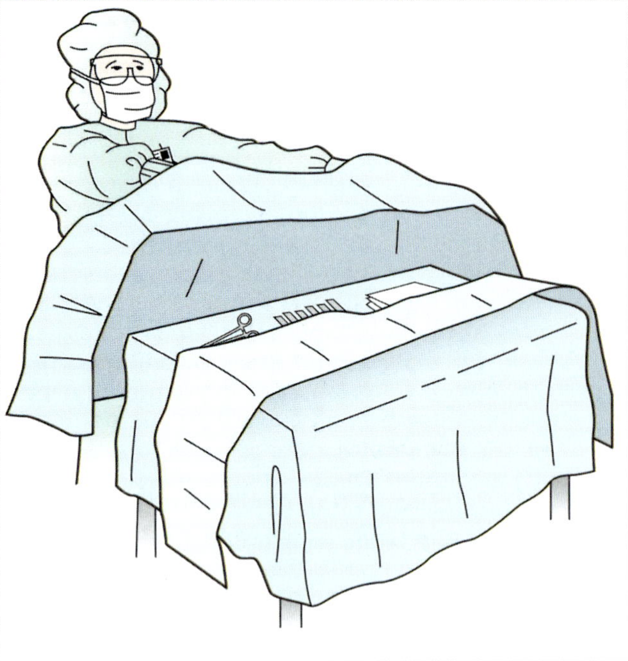

The first drape is placed with the cuff at the halfway point. The second drape is placed from the opposite side and completely covers the cuff of the first drape.
Illustration by Colleen Ladny and Kurt Jones.

Sterilization or high-level disinfection can only be achieved if all surfaces of an item have contacted the sterilizing agent or disinfectant under the appropriate conditions and for the appropriate amount of time. Organic materials and other debris may act as barriers that interfere with sterilization or high-level disinfection or may combine with and deactivate the sterilant or disinfectant.[71,89,90] If organic material or other debris is found on an instrument that has been through sterilization or high-level disinfection, there is no way to ensure that the sterilant or high-level disinfectant made contact with all surfaces of the item and with other items in the set. Sterility or high-level disinfection may not have been achieved; therefore, the sterility of the entire set is in question.

VII.d.1. Corrective actions should include, at a minimum, removing the entire set and any other items that may have come in contact with the contaminated item from the sterile field and changing the gloves of any team member who may have touched the contaminated item. Additional corrective actions may be required subject to thoughtful assessment and the application of informed clinical judgment based on the specific factors associated with the individual event.

VII.e. If an instrument in a sterile set is found assembled or clamped closed, the entire set should be considered contaminated and perioperative team members should take corrective actions immediately. *[1: Strong Evidence]*

Sterilization or high-level disinfection can only be achieved if all surfaces of an instrument have contacted the sterilizing or disinfecting agent under the appropriate conditions and for the appropriate amount of time.[71,89,90] If an instrument has not been correctly disassembled or is clamped closed before sterilization or high-level disinfection, there is no way to ensure that the sterilant or high-level disinfectant made contact with all surfaces of the item and with other items in the set. Sterility or high-level disinfection may not have been achieved; therefore, the sterility of the entire set is in question.

VII.e.1. Corrective actions should include, at a minimum, removing the entire set and any other instruments that may have come in contact with the contaminated instrument from the sterile field and changing the gloves of any team member who may have touched the contaminated item. Additional corrective actions may be required subject to thoughtful assessment and the application of informed clinical judgment based on the specific factors associated with the individual event.

Recommendation VIII

All personnel moving within or around a sterile field should do so in a manner that prevents contamination of the sterile field.

Airborne contaminants and microbial levels in the surgical environment are directly proportional to the amount of movement and the number of people in the OR or other procedure room.[37,66-70]

VIII.a. Scrubbed team members should remain close to the sterile field and touch only sterile areas or items. *[5: No Evidence]*

Walking outside the periphery of the sterile field or leaving and then returning to the OR or other procedure room in sterile attire increases the potential for contamination.

VIII.a.1. Scrubbed team members should not leave the sterile field to retrieve items from the sterilizer.

VIII.a.2. Scrubbed team members should wear protective devices (eg, lead aprons) that reduce radiological exposure so they are not required to leave the sterile field when x-rays are taken.[99]

VIII.b. Scrubbed team members should keep their hands and arms above waist level at all times. *[5: No Evidence]*

Keeping the hands and arms above waist level allows the perioperative team member to see them constantly. Contamination may occur when a perioperative team member moves his or her hands or arms below waist level.

VIII.b.1. Scrubbed team members' arms should not be folded with the hands in the axillary area.

The axillary area has the potential to become contaminated by perspiration, allowing for strike-through of the gown and potential contamination of the gloved hands. The axillary area of the gown is an area of friction and is not considered an effective microbial barrier.

VIII.c. Scrubbed team members should avoid changing levels and should be seated only when the entire procedure will be performed at that level. *[3: Limited Evidence]*

When scrubbed team members change levels, the unsterile portion of their gowns may come into contact with sterile areas.

To evaluate whether the surgical field could be contaminated by a perioperative team member stepping on and off of a footstool, researchers sprinkled starch powder on the portion of the drape below the level of the sterile field. A surgeon wearing a surgical gown made contact with the drape, and then stepped on and off a 6-inch footstool twice. The contamination level rose 6 inches with each movement. The researchers recommended that scrubbed team members reduce the number of times they step on a footstool.[100]

VIII.d. When changing position with each other, scrubbed team members should turn back to back or face to face while maintaining distance from each other, the sterile field, and unsterile areas. *[5: No Evidence]*

Contamination of sterile gowns and gloves and the sterile field may be prevented by scrubbed team members maintaining distance from each other and the sterile field when changing position, and by establishing patterns of movement that reduce the risk of contact with unsterile areas.

VIII.e. Unscrubbed personnel should face the sterile field on approach, should not walk between sterile fields or scrubbed persons, and should maintain a distance of at least 12 inches from the sterile field and scrubbed persons at all times. *[5: No Evidence]*

Contamination of the sterile field or scrubbed team members may be prevented by unscrubbed team members maintaining distance from the sterile field and scrubbed persons and establishing patterns of movement that reduce the risk of contact with sterile areas and scrubbed persons.

VIII.f. Conversations in the presence of a sterile field should be kept to a minimum. *[2: Moderate Evidence]*

Microorganisms are transported on airborne particles including respiratory droplets.[37]

Researchers studied the role of conversation in the OR by using small spherical particles of human albumin ranging in size from 10 to 35 micrometers in diameter to simulate particles that carry bacteria. Approximately 300,000 albumin particles were sprayed on the faces and in the nostrils beneath the surgical masks of the study participants. The participants read aloud continuously for periods of five, 10, 20, 30, 40, 50, and 60 minutes from a position 30 cm above a water bath simulating a surgical wound. The researchers collected particles from the water bath and processed them after each reading session. The results of the study showed that the longer the period of conversation, the greater the number of particles in the simulated wound. The effects of both time and conversation were found to be significant. The researchers concluded that conversation contributes to airborne contamination of surgical wounds.[68]

VIII.g. The number and movement of individuals involved in an operative or other invasive procedure should be kept to a minimum.[1,66,69] *[1: Strong Evidence]*

Bacterial shedding increases with activity. Air currents can pick up contaminated particles shed from patients, personnel, and drapes and distribute them to sterile areas.[37,67,70]

Researchers conducted a prospective, observational study in three pediatric ORs. During a two-week period, surgeons, anesthesia professionals, and perioperative team members were observed during 14 surgical procedures. A medical student observer recorded parameters, including the
- minimum and maximum numbers of personnel in the room during the procedure,
- number of personnel in the procedure room at each 30-minute interval, and
- number of personnel changes during the procedure.

There was a positive correlation between the length of the surgery and the number of personnel changes during the procedure, and a statistically significant increase in the number of personnel during spine procedures and procedures that lasted longer than 120 minutes. The researchers also noted a trend toward increased numbers of personnel during the middle of the procedure, especially during longer procedures. It was observed that personnel frequently entered the OR to check on the progress of the procedure, ask questions, or process paperwork. The researchers noted that these factors, in combination with frequent changes in personnel for breaks and shift changes, were a cause of distraction during the procedure, which could potentially lead to errors. Although this study was limited by its small sample size, the results support the need to limit the number of people and distractions in the OR during operative or other invasive procedures.[66]

In a study evaluating whether the behaviors and number of OR personnel can predict the density of airborne bacteria at the surgical site, researchers measured the number of airborne particulates and viable bacteria during 22 joint arthroplasty procedures with a range of five to 12 team members in the OR. The results indicated a relationship between the number and activity of team members present in the periphery of the OR and the number of particulates and colony forming units at the surgical site. The researchers recommended minimizing the number of team members who are present during the procedure.[101]

As part of a non-experimental study with two phases, researchers examined the levels of environmental contamination in ORs without personnel and the effect of unscrubbed persons on environmental contamination. The ORs without personnel showed a mean of 13.3 colony forming units per square foot per hour. When five persons wearing scrub suits, shoe covers, hoods, and masks were present, the number of colony forming units increased significantly to 447.3 per square foot per hour. The researchers concluded that people are the major source of environmental contamination in the OR.[67]

In response to an unexplained increase in surgical site infections at one facility, an observational study was conducted to monitor and record behaviors in the OR. Researchers theorized that the number of door openings increased in direct proportion to procedure length, but also had an exponential relationship with the number of team members in the OR. They randomly selected and audited 28 procedures in multiple services (eg, cardiac, orthopedic, neurosurgery, plastic, general). Data collection included the
- number of people entering and exiting the procedure room,
- role of the individuals, and
- reason for entering the room.

Researchers found that the number of door openings in some spinal procedures was as high as one door opening per minute, and there was an average rate of 40 door openings per hour during total joint procedures. With such high numbers of door openings, researchers noted that it was conceivable the door to the OR could remain open for as long as 15 to 20 minutes per hour. The greatest number of door openings occurred during the preincision period, and the most frequent reason for the door opening was requests for information. Personnel entering and exiting the room for breaks accounted for approximately 25% of door openings across every specialty. Retrieving and delivering supplies accounted for approximately 20% of door openings, and the RN circulator was responsible for 37% to 50% of door openings. The cumulative effect of increased door openings is the potential for increased numbers of microorganisms and other contaminants in the air and the surgical site. The researchers also noted that frequent door openings are distracting and have the potential to lead to errors.[102]

In another study of door openings, researchers used an electronic door counter and computer software to calculate and analyze the number of door openings during 46 cardiac procedures. Perioperative team members were blinded to the study. The total number of door openings was 4,273. After adjusting for procedure length and the time required for the door to close, it was found that the door to the OR was open approximately 11% of every hour. A direct correlation was found between the length of the procedure and the frequency of door openings. The data also indicated a trend toward surgical site infections with increased frequency of door openings and patients of advanced age. The researchers hypothesized that increased numbers of personnel and door openings are a distraction to the surgical team and may lead to surgical errors.[103]

Recommendation IX

Perioperative team members should receive initial and ongoing education and competency verification on their understanding of the principles of and performance of the processes for sterile technique.

It is the responsibility of the health care organization to provide initial and ongoing education and to verify the competency of perioperative team members to deliver safe care to patients undergoing operative or other invasive procedures.[2]

Initial and ongoing education of perioperative personnel on the principles and processes of sterile technique facilitates the development of knowledge, skills, and attitudes that affect safe patient care.

Periodic education programs provide the opportunity to reinforce the principles and processes of sterile technique and to introduce relevant new equipment or practices.

Competency verification measures individual performance and provides a mechanism for documentation, and may verify that perioperative personnel have an understanding of the principles and processes of sterile technique.

IX.a. Perioperative team members should receive education and competency verification that addresses specialized knowledge and skills related to the principles and processes of sterile technique. *[1: Regulatory Requirement]*

Specialized knowledge includes empirical knowledge (eg, technical understanding), practical knowledge (eg, clinical experience), and aesthetic knowledge (eg, patient advocacy).

Ongoing development of knowledge and skills and documentation of personnel participation is a regulatory and accreditation requirement for both hospitals and ambulatory settings.[104-114]

IX.a.1. Education regarding the principles and processes of sterile technique may include a review of the policies and procedures and protocols for
- surgical attire[3];
- surgical hand hygiene[4];
- preparation of ORs or other procedure rooms;
- selection and evaluation of surgical gowns, gloves, and drape products[27];
- assistance with operative or other invasive procedures;
- proper use of sterile gowns and gloves, including double gloving;
- proper use of sterile drape products;
- the use of sterile items during operative or other invasive procedures;
- preparation of a sterile field for patients undergoing operative or other invasive procedures;
- isolation technique;

STERILE TECHNIQUE

- how to introduce items to the sterile field, including the transfer of medications[95] and solutions;
- how to maintain a sterile field, including recognition and correction of breaks in sterile technique;
- movement within and around a sterile field;
- the number of people who are permitted in the procedure room; and
- operative or invasive procedure documentation,[115] including reporting of breaks in sterile technique.

IX.b. Perioperative personnel should receive education that addresses human factors related to the principles and processes of sterile technique. *[2: Moderate Evidence]*

Human factors includes the interpersonal and social aspects of the perioperative environment (eg, coordination of activities, teamwork, collaboration, communication). Effectively implementing the principles and processes of sterile technique requires that perioperative personnel demonstrate not only procedural knowledge and technical proficiency, but also demonstrate the ability to anticipate needs, coordinate a multitude of activities, work collaboratively with other team members, and communicate effectively.

In a synthesis of the literature on perioperative nursing competency published between 2000 and 2008, researchers identified two domains of perioperative competency:
- specialized knowledge, described as familiarity with standards and guidelines of perioperative practice, and
- human factors, described as interpersonal and social team interactions.

The researchers recognized teamwork and communication as important aspects of patient safety and indicators of perioperative competency.[116]

In a qualitative, focus group study exploring the perceptions of perioperative nurses on competency, researchers identified three themes:
- technical and procedural knowledge—the knowledge, psychomotor skills, and situational awareness required for competency in the perioperative setting;
- communication skills—the need for communication and team building skills, collegial support, and the ability to decipher and share complex clinical information; and
- managing and coordinating flow—the ability to anticipate needs, organize and prioritize resources, manage conflicts, and grasp the full perspective of the situation.

The findings of the study highlight the importance of human factors as a competency requirement for perioperative nurses.[117]

In a review of the literature exploring the cognitive and social skills used by scrub persons, researchers identified communication, teamwork, and situational awareness as the most valuable and relevant skills.
- Communication is vitally important because of the need to listen and interpret what is being said, to clarify any issues that are unclear, and to convey critical information accurately. The need to communicate using eye contact and nonverbal cues and to speak up when necessary while working at the sterile field was recognized as a required skill for the scrub person.
- Teamwork is an important skill because of the need for scrub persons to share information to aid the team and to establish good working relationships between team members.
- Situational awareness is an important skill that includes the ability of scrub persons to anticipate the actions of the surgeon and to make decisions regarding the need for additional supplies or actions that must be taken, and to anticipate future requirements of the procedure.[118]

IX.c. Relative to the principles and processes of sterile technique, the perioperative RN should
- participate in ongoing educational activities[2];
- identify personal learning needs[2];
- seek experiences to acquire, maintain, and augment personal knowledge and skill proficiency[2];
- share knowledge and skills[2];
- communicate pertinent information to perioperative team members[2];
- contribute to a healthy work environment by using appropriate and courteous verbal and nonverbal communication techniques[2]; and
- develop and implement conflict resolution skills to manage difficult behavior, promote positive working relationships, and advocate for patient safety.[2]

[2: Moderate Evidence]

Education, collegiality, and collaboration are standards of perioperative nursing and a primary responsibility of the perioperative RN who practices in the perioperative setting.[2,119]

Recommendation X

Nursing activities related to sterile technique should be documented in a manner consistent with health care organization policies and procedures and regulatory and accrediting agency requirements.

Documentation of nursing activities serves as the legal record of care delivery. Documentation of nursing activities is dictated by health care organization policy and regulatory and accrediting agency requirements and is necessary to inform other health care professionals involved in the patient's care. Highly reliable data collection is not only necessary to chronicle patient responses to nursing interventions, but also to demonstrate the health care organization's progress toward quality care outcomes.[115]

X.a. Significant or major breaks in sterile technique that are not immediately corrected should be documented or reported per organizational policy in consultation with infection prevention personnel. *[1: Regulatory Requirement]*

Perioperative documentation that accurately reflects the patient experience is essential for the continuity of outcome-focused nursing care and for effective comparison of realized versus anticipated patient outcomes.[115]

Effective management and collection of health care information that accurately reflects the patient's care, treatment, and services is a regulatory and accreditation requirement for both hospitals and ambulatory settings.[104,105,120-127]

Recommendation XI

Policies and procedures for the implementation of sterile technique should be developed, reviewed periodically, revised as necessary, and readily available in the practice setting.

Policies and procedures assist in the development of patient safety, quality assessment, and performance improvement activities. Policies and procedures establish authority, responsibility, and accountability within the organization. Policies and procedures also serve as operational guidelines that are used to minimize patient risk for injury or complications, standardize practice, direct perioperative personnel, and establish continuous performance improvement programs.

XI.a. Policies and procedures regarding the implementation of sterile technique should be developed. *[1: Regulatory Requirement]*

Policies and procedures that guide and support patient care, treatment, and services is a regulatory and accreditation requirement for both hospitals and ambulatory settings.[104,105,109,110,128-130]

XI.a.1. Policies and procedures regarding the principles and processes of sterile technique may include
- surgical attire[3];
- surgical hand hygiene[4];
- selection and evaluation of surgical gowns, gloves, and drape products[27];
- proper use of sterile gowns and gloves, including double gloving;
- proper use of sterile drape products;
- isolation technique;
- the numbers of people who are permitted in the OR or other procedure room; and
- reporting of breaks in sterile technique.

Recommendation XII

Perioperative personnel should participate in a variety of quality assurance and performance improvement activities that are consistent with the health care organization's plan to improve understanding of and compliance with the principles and processes of sterile technique.

Quality assurance and performance improvement programs assist in evaluating and improving the quality of patient care and formulating plans for corrective actions. These programs provide data that may be used to determine whether an individual organization is within benchmark goals and, if not, to identify areas that may require corrective actions.

XII.a. Performance improvement activities for sterile technique should include monitoring personnel for understanding of the principles of and compliance with the processes of sterile technique. *[1: Regulatory Requirement]*

Collecting data to monitor and improve patient care, treatment, and services is a regulatory and accreditation requirement for both hospitals and ambulatory settings.[104,105,108,131-135]

XII.a.1. Process monitoring for activities related to sterile technique may include monitoring compliance with policies and procedures for
- surgical attire[3];
- surgical hand hygiene[4];
- preparation of the OR or other procedure room;
- selection and evaluation of surgical gowns, gloves, and drape products[27];
- performance of or assistance with operative or other invasive procedures;
- proper use of sterile gowns and gloves, including double gloving;
- proper use of sterile drape products;
- isolation technique;
- introduction of items to the sterile field, including transfer of medications[95] and solutions;
- recognition and correction of breaks in sterile technique;
- movement within and around a sterile field;
- the number of people permitted in the OR or other procedure room; and
- reporting of breaks in sterile technique.

XII.a.2. The quality assurance and performance improvement program for sterile technique should include
- periodically reviewing and evaluating activities to verify compliance or to identify the need for improvement,
- identifying corrective actions directed toward improvement priorities, and
- taking additional actions when improvement is not achieved or sustained.

Reviewing and evaluating quality assurance and performance improvement activities may identify failure points that contribute to errors in sterile technique and help define actions for improvement and increased competency.

STERILE TECHNIQUE

Taking corrective actions may improve patient safety by enhancing understanding of the principles of and compliance with the processes for sterile technique.

XII.b. Perioperative RNs should participate in ongoing quality assurance and performance improvement activities related to sterile technique by
- identifying processes that are important for quality monitoring (eg, double gloving);
- developing strategies for compliance;
- establishing benchmarks to evaluate quality indicators;
- collecting data related to the levels of performance and quality indicators;
- evaluating practice based on the cumulative data that are collected;
- taking action to improve compliance; and
- assessing the effectiveness of the actions taken.

[2: Moderate Evidence]

Participating in ongoing quality assurance and performance improvement activities is a standard of perioperative nursing and a primary responsibility of the perioperative RN who is engaged in practice in the perioperative setting.[2]

Glossary

Aseptic: The absence of all pathogenic microorganisms. Synonym: sterile.

Aseptic practices: Patterns of behavior and processes that are implemented to prevent microbial contamination.

Assisted gloving: Technique used when changing a contaminated glove. One scrubbed team member assists another to don a new sterile glove by touching only the outside of the new sterile glove when applying the glove to another scrubbed team member's hand.

Barrier material: Material that minimizes or retards the penetration of microorganisms, particulates, and fluids.

Closed assisted gloving: Technique for donning sterile gloves during which the gown cuff of the team member being gloved remains at or beyond the fingertips. The glove to be donned is held open by a scrubbed team member, while the team member being gloved inserts his or her hand into the glove with the gown cuff touching only the inside of the glove.

Closed gloving: Technique used when donning surgical gloves. The scrubbed team member dons the gloves without assistance by keeping his or her hands inside the gown sleeves.

Colony forming unit: A measure of the number of viable bacterial cells in a sample.

Event-related sterility: Concept that the sterility of an item does not change with the passing of time but may be affected by particular events (eg, amount of handling), or environmental conditions (eg, temperature, humidity).

Invasive procedure: The surgical entry into tissues, cavities, or organs, or the repair of major traumatic injuries.

Isolation technique: Instruments and equipment that have contacted the inside of the bowel, or the bowel lumen, are no longer used after the lumen has been closed. Clean instruments are used to close the wound. The contaminated instruments and equipment are either removed from the sterile field or placed in a separate area that will not be touched by members of the sterile team. Synonyms: bowel technique, contamination technique.

Open assisted gloving: Technique for donning sterile gloves during which the gown sleeve of the team member being gloved is pulled up so that the gown cuff is at wrist level, leaving the fingers and hand exposed. The glove to be donned is held open by a scrubbed team member, while the team member being gloved inserts his or her hand into the glove without touching the outside of the glove.

Open gloving: Technique used to don sterile gloves without assistance. The cuff of each glove is everted to allow the team member to don sterile gloves by touching only the inner side of the glove with ungloved fingers and the outer sterile side of the glove with gloved fingers.

Perforation indicator system: A double gloving system comprising a colored pair of surgical gloves worn beneath a standard pair of surgical gloves. When a glove perforation occurs, moisture from the surgical field seeps through the perforation between the layers of gloves, allowing the site of perforation to be more easily seen.

Sterile: The absence of all living microorganisms. Synonym: aseptic.

Sterile field: The area surrounding the site of the incision or perforation into tissue, or the site of introduction of an instrument into a body orifice that has been prepared for an invasive procedure. The area includes all working areas, furniture, and equipment covered with sterile drapes and drape accessories, and all personnel in sterile attire.

Sterile technique: The use of specific actions and activities to prevent contamination and maintain sterility of identified areas during operative or other invasive procedures.

Surgical hand scrub: Antiseptic hand wash or antiseptic hand rub performed preoperatively by perioperative personnel to eliminate transient bacteria and reduce resident hand flora.

Surgical helmet system: An unsterile, reusable helmet with a built-in ventilation fan covered with a single-use, disposable sterile visor mask hood. The unsterile helmet is donned before the surgical hand scrub is performed. The sterile visor mask hood that covers the unsterile helmet is applied during the gowning and gloving process.

References

1. Mangram AJ, Horan TC, Pearson ML, Silver LC, Jarvis WR; Centers for Disease Control and Prevention (CDC) Hospital Infection Control Practices Advisory Committee.

Guideline for prevention of surgical site infection, 1999. *Am J Infect Control*. 1999;27(2):97-132. [IVA]

2. Standards of perioperative nursing. In: *Perioperative Standards and Recommended Practices*. Denver, CO: AORN, Inc; 2012:3-20. [IVB]

3. Guideline for surgical attire. In: *Guidelines for Perioperative Practice*. Denver, CO: AORN, Inc; 2015:97-120. [IVB]

4. Guideline for hand hygiene. In: *Guidelines for Perioperative Practice*. Denver, CO: AORN, Inc; 2015:31-42. [IVB]

5. Guideline for prevention of transmissible infections. In: *Guidelines for Perioperative Practice*. Denver, CO: AORN, Inc; 2015:419-451. [IVA]

6. Boyce JM, Pittet D; Healthcare Infection Control Practices Advisory Committee; HICPAC/SHEA/APIC/IDSA Hand Hygiene Task Force. Guideline for Hand Hygiene in Health-Care Settings. Recommendations of the Healthcare Infection Control Practices Advisory Committee and the HICPAC/SHEA/APIC/IDSA Hand Hygiene Task Force. Society for Healthcare Epidemiology of America/Association for Professionals in Infection Control/Infectious Diseases Society of America. *MMWR Recomm Rep*. 2002;51(RR-16):1-45. [IVA]

7. Graves PB, Twomey CL. Surgical hand antisepsis: an evidence-based review. *Periop Nurs Clin*. 2006;1(3):235-249. doi:10.1016/j.cpen.2006.06.002. [VA]

8. Weber DJ, Rutala WA. Central line-associated bloodstream infections: prevention and management. *Infect Dis Clin North Am*. 2011;25(1):77-102. [IVB]

9. O'Grady NP, Alexander M, Burns LA, et al; Healthcare Infection Control Practices Advisory Committee (HICPAC). *Guidelines for the Prevention of Intravascular Catheter-Related Infections, 2011*. Atlanta, GA: Centers for Disease Control and Prevention; 2011. [IVA]

10. Siegel JD, Rhinehart E, Jackson M, Chiarello L; Healthcare Infection Control Practices Advisory Committee. *2007 Guideline for Isolation Precautions: Preventing Transmission of Infectious Agents in Healthcare Settings*. Atlanta, GA: Centers for Disease Control and Prevention; 2007. http://www.cdc.gov/ncidod/dhqp/pdf/isolation2007.pdf. Accessed October 18, 2012. [IVA]

11. Hebl JR. The importance and implications of aseptic techniques during regional anesthesia. *Reg Anesth Pain Med*. 2006;31(4):311-323. [IVB]

12. Watanakunakorn C, Stahl C. Streptococcus salivarius meningitis following myelography. *Infect Control Hosp Epidemiol*. 1992;13(8):454. [VA]

13. Schlesinger JJ, Salit IE, McCormack G. Streptococcal meningitis after myelography. *Arch Neurol*. 1982;39(9):576-577. [VB]

14. Schlegel L, Merlet C, Laroche JM, Fremaux A, Geslin P. Iatrogenic meningitis due to Abiotrophia defectiva after myelography. *Clin Infect Dis*. 1999;28(1):155-156. doi:10.1086/517189. [VB]

15. Veringa E, van Belkum A, Schellekens H. Iatrogenic meningitis by *Streptococcus salivarius* following lumbar puncture. *J Hosp Infect*. 1995;29(4): 316-318. [VA]

16. Couzigou C, Vuong TK, Botherel AH, Aggoune M, Astagneau P. Iatrogenic *Streptococcus salivarius* meningitis after spinal anaesthesia: need for strict application of standard precautions. *J Hosp Infect*. 2003;53(4):313-314. [VA]

17. Torres E, Alba D, Frank A, Diez-Tejedor E. Iatrogenic meningitis due to Streptococcus salivarius following a spinal tap. *Clin Infect Dis*. 1993;17(3):525-526. [VB]

18. Schneeberger PM, Janssen M, Voss A. Alpha-hemolytic streptococci: a major pathogen of iatrogenic meningitis following lumbar puncture. Case reports and a review of the literature. *Infection*. 1996;24(1):29-33. [VB]

19. Yaniv LG, Potasman I. Iatrogenic meningitis: an increasing role for resistant viridans streptococci? Case report and review of the last 20 years. *Scand J Infect Dis*. 2000;32(6):693-696. [VB]

20. Centers for Disease Control and Prevention (CDC). Bacterial meningitis after intrapartum spinal anesthesia—New York and Ohio, 2008-2009. *MMWR*. 2010;59(3):65-69. [VA]

21. Philips BJ, Fergusson S, Armstrong P, Anderson FM, Wildsmith JA. Surgical face masks are effective in reducing bacterial contamination caused by dispersal from the upper airway. *Br J Anaesth*. 1992;69(4):407-408. [IIC]

22. McLure HA, Talboys CA, Yentis SM, Azadian BS. Surgical face masks and downward dispersal of bacteria. *Anaesthesia*. 1998;53(7):624-626. [IIB]

23. Alwitry A, Jackson E, Chen H, Holden R. The use of surgical facemasks during cataract surgery: is it necessary? *Br J Ophthalmol*. 2002;86(9):975-977. [IB]

24. Berger SA, Kramer M, Nagar H, Finkelstein A, Frimmerman A, Miller HI. Effect of surgical mask position on bacterial contamination of the operative field. *J Hosp Infect*. 1993;23(1):51-54. [IB]

25. Baer ET. Iatrogenic meningitis: the case for face masks. *Clin Infect Dis*. 2000;31(2):519-521. doi:10.1086/313991. [VB]

26. AAMI TI11: Selection and use of protective apparel and surgical drapes in health care facilities. Arlington, VA: Association for the Advancement of Medical Instrumentation; 2005. [IVC]

27. Guideline for product selection. In: *Guidelines for Perioperative Practice*. Denver, CO: AORN, Inc; 2015:179-186. [IVB]

28. Rutala WA, Weber DJ. A review of single-use and reusable gowns and drapes in health care. *Infect Control Hosp Epidemiol*. 2001;22(4):248-257. doi:10.1086/501895. [VA]

29. Position statement on environmental responsibility. AORN, Inc. http://www.aorn.org/WorkArea/DownloadAsset.aspx?id=21920. Accessed October 18, 2012. [IVB]

30. Occupational Safety and Health Standards, Toxic and Hazardous Substances: Bloodborne Pathogens, 29 CFR §1910.1030 (2012). Occupational Safety and Health Administration. http://www.osha.gov/pls/oshaweb/owadisp.show_document?p_table=STANDARDS&p_id=10051. Accessed October 18, 2012.

31. Medical Devices, General and Plastic Surgery Devices, 21 CFR §878 (2008).

32. AAMI PB70: Liquid barrier performance and classification of protective apparel and drapes intended for use in health care facilities. Arlington, VA: Association for the Advancement of Medical Instrumentation; 2012. [IVC]

33. Medical Device Reporting, 21 CFR §803 (2012).

34. MedWatch: the FDA safety information and adverse event reporting program. US Food and Drug Administration. http://www.fda.gov/Safety/MedWatch/default.htm. Accessed October 18, 2012.

35. Blom AW, Barnett A, Ajitsaria P, Noel A, Estela CM. Resistance of disposable drapes to bacterial penetration. *J Orthop Surg*. 2007;15(3):267-269. [IIIC]

36. Laufman H, Eudy WW, Vandernoot AM, Harris CA, Liu D. Strike-through of moist contamination by woven and nonwoven surgical materials. *Ann Surg*. 1975;181(6):857-862. [IIIC]

37. Edmiston CE Jr, Sinski S, Seabrook GR, Simons D, Goheen MP. Airborne particulates in the OR environment. *AORN J*. 1999;69(6):1169-72, 1175-7, 1179 passim. [IIB]

38. Surgical Apparel, 21 CFR §878.4040 (2000).

STERILE TECHNIQUE

39. Surgical Drape and Drape Accessories, 21 CFR §878.4370.

40. Rego A, Roley L. In-use barrier integrity of gloves: latex and nitrile superior to vinyl. *Am J Infect Control.* 1999;27(5):405-410. [IB]

41. Korniewicz DM, Garzon L, Seltzer J, Feinleib M. Failure rates in nonlatex surgical gloves. *Am J Infect Control.* 2004;32(5):268-273. doi:10.1016/j.ajic.2003.12.005. [IIB]

42. Ritter MA, Eitzen HE, Hart JB, French ML. The surgeon's garb. *Clin Orthop Relat Res.* 1980;153:204-209. [IIB]

43. Heal JS, Blom AW, Titcomb D, Taylor A, Bowker K, Hardy JR. Bacterial contamination of surgical gloves by water droplets spilt after scrubbing. *J Hosp Infect.* 2003;53(2):136-139. [IIIC]

44. Bible JE, Biswas D, Whang PG, Simpson AK, Grauer JN. Which regions of the operating gown should be considered most sterile? *Clin Orthop Related Res.* 2009;467(3):825-830. [IIC]

45. Jones C, Brooker B, Genon M. Comparison of open and closed staff-assisted glove donning on the nature of surgical glove cuff contamination. *ANZ J Surg.* 2010;80(3):174-177. [IIIB]

46. Tanner J, Parkinson H. Double gloving to reduce surgical cross-infection. *Cochrane Database Syst Rev.* 2009;3:CD003087. doi:10.1002/14651858.CD003087.pub2. [IA]

47. Information statement: preventing the transmission of bloodborne pathogens. American Academy of Orthopedic Surgeons, American Association of Orthopaedic Surgeons. http://www.aaos.org/about/papers/advistmt/1018.asp. Accessed October 18, 2012. [IVB]

48. ST-58: Statement on sharps safety. American College of Surgeons. http://www.facs.org/fellows_info/statements/st-58.html. Accessed October 18, 2012. [IVB]

49. Kojima Y, Ohashi M. Unnoticed glove perforation during thoracoscopic and open thoracic surgery. *Ann Thorac Surg.* 2005;80(3):1078-1080. [IIB]

50. Singh VK, Hussain S, Javed S, Singh I, Mulla R, Kalairajah Y. Sterile surgical helmet system in elective total hip and knee arthroplasty. *J Orthop Surg (Hong Kong).* 2011;19(2):234-237. [IIIC]

51. Kearns KA, Witmer D, Makda J, Parvizi J, Jungkind D. Sterility of the personal protection system in total joint arthroplasty. *Clin Orthop Relat Res.* 2011;469(11):3065-3069. doi:10.1007/s11999-011-1883-1. [IIIC]

52. Bible JE, O'Neill KR, Crosby CG, Schoenecker JG, McGirt MJ, Devin CJ. Microscope sterility during spine surgery. *Spine (Phila Pa 1976).* 2012;37(7):623-267. doi:10.1097/BRS.0b013e3182286129. [IIB]

53. Thomas S, Padmanabhan TV. Methyl methacrylate permeability of dental and industrial gloves. *N Y State Dent J.* 2009;75(4):40-42. [IIIB]

54. Waegemaekers TH, Seutter E, den Arend JA, Malten KE. Permeability of surgeons' gloves to methyl methacrylate. *Acta Orthop Scand.* 1983;54(6):790-795. [IIIB]

55. Guideline for a safe environment of care, part 1. In: *Guidelines for Perioperative Practice.* Denver, CO: AORN, Inc; 2015:239-263. [IVA]

56. Hentz RV, Traina GC, Cadossi R, Zucchini P, Muglia MA, Giordani M. The protective efficacy of surgical latex gloves against the risk of skin contamination: how well are the operators protected? *J Mater Sci Mater Med.* 2000;11(12):825-832. [IIB]

57. Harnoss JC, Partecke LI, Heidecke CD, Hubner NO, Kramer A, Assadian O. Concentration of bacteria passing through puncture holes in surgical gloves. *Am J Infect Control.* 2010;38(2):154-158. [IIA]

58. Hubner NO, Goerdt AM, Stanislawski N, et al. Bacterial migration through punctured surgical gloves under real surgical conditions. *BMC Infectious Diseases.* 2010;10:192. [IIIB]

59. Partecke LI, Goerdt AM, Langner I, et al. Incidence of microperforation for surgical gloves depends on duration of wear. *Infect Control Hosp Epidemiol.* 2009;30(5):409-414. [IA]

60. Newman JB, Bullock M, Goyal R. Comparison of glove donning techniques for the likelihood of gown contamination. An infection control study. *Acta Orthop Belg.* 2007;73(6):765-771. [IIIC]

61. Raad II, Hohn DC, Gilbreath BJ, et al. Prevention of central venous catheter-related infections by using maximal sterile barrier precautions during insertion. *Infect Control Hosp Epidemiol.* 1994;15(4 Pt 1):231-238. [IA]

62. Pronovost P, Needham D, Berenholtz S, et al. An intervention to decrease catheter-related bloodstream infections in the ICU. *N Engl J Med.* 2006;355(26):2725-2732. doi:10.1056/NEJMoa061115. [IIIB]

63. McCue SF, Berg EW, Saunders EA. Efficacy of double-gloving as a barrier to microbial contamination during total joint arthroplasty. *J Bone Joint Surg Am.* 1981;63(5):811-813. [IIB]

64. Biswas D, Bible JE, Whang PG, Simpson AK, Grauer JN. Sterility of C-arm fluoroscopy during spinal surgery. *Spine (Phila Pa 1976).* 2008;33(17):1913-1917. doi:10.1097/BRS.0b013e31817bb130. [IIB]

65. Webster J, Alghamdi A. Use of plastic adhesive drapes during surgery for preventing surgical site infection. *Cochrane Database Syst Rev.* 2011;1. [IA]

66. Parikh SN, Grice SS, Schnell BM, Salisbury SR. Operating room traffic: is there any role of monitoring it? *J Pediatr Orthop.* 2010;30(6):617-623. doi:10.1097/BPO.0b013e3181e4f3be. [IIC]

67. Ritter MA, Eitzen H, French ML, Hart JB. The operating room environment as affected by people and the surgical face mask. *Clin Orthop Relat Res.* 1975;111:147-150. [IIIC]

68. Letts RM, Doermer E. Conversation in the operating theater as a cause of airborne bacterial contamination. *J Bone Joint Surg Am.* 1983;65(3):357-362. [IIB]

69. Ritter MA. Operating room environment. *Clin Orthop Relat Res.* 1999;369:103-109. [IIB]

70. Howard JL, Hanssen AD. Principles of a clean operating room environment. *J Arthroplasty.* 2007;22(7 Suppl 3):6-11. doi:10.1016/j.arth.2007.05.013. [VB]

71. Guideline for sterilization. In: *Guidelines for Perioperative Practice.* Denver, CO: AORN, Inc; 2015:665-692. [IVA]

72. Spaulding EH, Cundy KR, Turner FJ, SS Block. Chemical disinfection of medical and surgical materials. In: SS Block, ed. *Disinfection, Sterilization, and Preservation.* 2nd ed. Philadelphia, PA: Lea & Febiger; 1977:654-684. [VB]

73. Gengelkirk P, Duben-Engelkirk J. Microbial ecology and microbial technology. In: Gengelkirk P, Duben-Engelkirk J, eds. *Burton's Microbiology for the Health Sciences.* 9th ed. 2011:158-170.

74. Healthcare-associated infections (HAIs): Catheter-associated urinary tract infections (CAUTI). Centers for Disease Control and Prevention. http://www.cdc.gov/HAI/ca_uti/uti.html. Accessed October 18, 2012. [IVA]

75. Ahmad A, Schirmir BD. Summary of intraoperative physiologic alterations associated with laparoscopic surgery. In: *The SAGES Manual of Perioperative Care in Minimally Invasive Surgery.* New York: Springer-Verlag; 2006:56-62. [VA]

76. Strickland AK, Martindale RG. The increased incidence of intraabdominal infections in laparoscopic procedures: potential causes, postoperative management, and prospective innovations. *Surg Endosc.* 2005;19(7):874-881. doi:10.1007/s00464-004-8211-8. [VA]

77. Ozmen MM, Col C, Aksoy AM, Tekeli FA, Berberoglu M. Effect of CO(2) insufflation on bacteremia and bacterial translocation in an animal model of peritonitis. *Surg Endosc.* 1999;13(8):801-803. [IIB]

78. Hao WL, Lee YK. Microflora of the gastrointestinal tract: a review. *Methods Mol Biol.* 2004;268:491-502. doi:10.1385/1-59259-766-1:491. [VA]

79. Bures J, Cyrany J, Kohoutova D, et al. Small intestinal bacterial overgrowth syndrome. *World J Gastroenterol.* 2010;16(24):2978-2990. [VA]

80. Husebye E. The pathogenesis of gastrointestinal bacterial overgrowth. *Chemotherapy.* 2005;51(Suppl 1):1-22. doi:10.1159/000081988. [VA]

81. Porteous J, Gembey D, Dieter M. Bowel technique in the O.R. Is it really necessary? *Can Oper Room Nurs J.* 1996;14(1):11-14. [IIA]

82. Watanabe A, Kohnoe S, Shimabukuro R, et al. Risk factors associated with surgical site infection in upper and lower gastrointestinal surgery. *Surg Today.* 2008;38(5):404-412. [IIIB]

83. Zach J. A review of the literature on bowel technique. *ACORN.* 2004;17(4):14-19. [VB]

84. Bruen E. Clean/dirty scrub technique. Is it worth the effort? *Br J Perioper Nurs.* 2001;11(12):532-537. [VA]

85. Reason J. Safety in the operating theatre—Part 2: human error and organisational failure. *Qual Saf Health Care.* 2005;14(1):56-60. [VA]

86. Bekar A, Kahveci R, Tolunay S, Kahraman A, Kuytu T. Metastatic gliosarcoma mass extension to a donor fascia lata graft harvest site by tumor cell contamination. *World Neurosurg.* 2010;73(6):719-721. doi:10.1016/j.wneu.2010.03.015. [VA]

87. Zemmoura I, Ben Ismail M, Travers N, Jan M, Francois P. Maxillary surgical seeding of a clival chordoma. *Br J Neurosurg.* 2012;26(1):102-103. doi:10.3109/02688697.2011.595844. [VB]

88. McLemore MS, Bruner JM, Curry JL, Prieto VG, Torres-Cabala CA. Anaplastic oligodendroglioma involving the subcutaneous tissue of the scalp: report of an exceptional case and review of the literature. *Am J Dermatopathol.* 2012;34(2):214-219. doi:10.1097/DAD.0b013e318230655c. [VA]

89. *Guideline for Disinfection and Sterilization in Healthcare Facilities, 2008.* Atlanta, GA: Centers for Disease Control and Prevention; 2008. [IVA]

90. ANSI/AAMI ST79:2010 & A1:2010 & A2:2011 (Consolidated Text). Arlington, VA: Association for the Advancement of Medical Instrumentation; 2011. [IVC]

91. Barker CS, Soro V, Dymock D, Fulford M, Sandy JR, Ireland AJ. Time-dependent recontamination rates of sterilised dental instruments. *Br Dent J.* 2011;211(8): E17. doi:10.1038/sj.bdj.2011.869; 10.1038/sj.bdj.2011.869. [IIB]

92. de Araújo Moriya GA, de Souza RQ, Gomes Pinto FM, Graziano KU. Periodic sterility assessment of materials stored for up to 6 months at continuous microbial contamination risk: laboratory study. *Am J Infect Control.* 2012;May 25. Epub ahead of print. doi:10.1016/j.ajic.2012.01.020. [IA]

93. Butt WE, Bradley DV Jr, Mayhew RB, Schwartz RS. Evaluation of the shelf life of sterile instrument packs. *Oral Surg Oral Med Oral Pathol.* 1991;72(6):650-654. [IA]

94. Webster J, Lloyd W, Ho P, Burridge C, George N. Rethinking sterilization practices: evidence for event-related outdating. *Infect Control Hosp Epidemiol.* 2003;24(8):622-624. doi:10.1086/502264. [IIB]

95. Guideline for medication safety. In: *Guidelines for Perioperative Practice.* Denver, CO: AORN, Inc; 2015:291-329. [IVB]

96. Dalstrom DJ, Venkatarayappa I, Manternach AL, Palcic MS, Heyse BA, Prayson MJ. Time-dependent contamination of opened sterile operating-room trays. *J Bone Joint Surg Am.* 2008;90(5):1022-1025. [IC]

97. Chosky SA, Modha D, Taylor GJ. Optimisation of ultraclean air. The role of instrument preparation. *J Bone Joint Surg Br.* 1996;78(5):835-837. [IB]

98. Hopper WR, Moss R. Common breaks in sterile technique: clinical perspectives and perioperative implications. *AORN J.* 2010;91(3):350-364. doi:10.1016/j.aorn.2009.09.027. [VB]

99. Guideline for reducing radiological exposure. In: *Guidelines for Perioperative Practice.* Denver, CO: AORN, Inc; 2015:335-344. [IVB]

100. Saito S, Kato W, Uchiyama M, Usui A, Ueda Y. Frequent stepping on and off the footstool contaminates the operative field. *Am J Infect Control.* 2007;35(1):68-69. doi:10.1016/j.ajic.2006.08.013. [IIIC]

101. Stocks GW, Self SD, Thompson B, Adame XA, O'Connor DP. Predicting bacterial populations based on airborne particulates: a study performed in nonlaminar flow operating rooms during joint arthroplasty surgery. *Am J Infect Control.* 2010;38(3):199-204. doi:10.1016/j.ajic.2009.07.006. [IIB]

102. Lynch RJ, Englesbe MJ, Sturm L, et al. Measurement of foot traffic in the operating room: implications for infection control. *Am J Med Qual.* 2009;24(1):45-52. doi:10.1177/1062860608326419. [IIIB]

103. Young RS, O'Regan DJ. Cardiac surgical theatre traffic: time for traffic calming measures? *Interac Cardiovasc Thorac Surg.* 2010;10(4):526-529. [IIIC]

104. Centers for Medicare & Medicaid Services. *State Operations Manual Appendix A—Survey Protocol, Regulations and Interpretive Guidelines for Hospitals.* Rev. 78; 2011.

105. Centers for Medicare & Medicaid Services. *State Operations Manual Appendix L: Guidance for Surveyors: Ambulatory Surgical Centers.* Rev. 76; 2011.

106. HR.01.05.03: Staff participate in ongoing education and training. In: *Comprehensive Accreditation Manual: CAMH for Hospitals.* Oakbrook Terrace, IL: The Joint Commission; 2012.

107. HR.01.05.03: Staff participate in ongoing education and training. In: *Comprehensive Accreditation Manual for Ambulatory Care.* Oakbrook Terrace, IL: Joint Commission; 2012.

108. Quality management and improvement. In: *2012 Accreditation Handbook for Ambulatory Health Care.* Skokie, IL: Accreditation Association for Ambulatory Health Care; 2012:34-39.

109. Personnel: personnel records. In: *Procedural Standards and Checklist for Accreditation of Ambulatory Surgery Facilities.* Version 3. Gurnee, IL: American Association for Accreditation of Ambulatory Surgery Facilities; 2011:77-79.

110. Personnel: personnel records; resumes. In: *Regular Standards and Checklist for Accreditation of Ambulatory Surgery Facilities.* Version 13. Gurnee, IL: American Association for Accreditation of Ambulatory Surgery Facilities; 2011:77-78.

111. Personnel: knowledge, skill & CME training. In: *Procedural Standards and Checklist for Accreditation of Ambulatory Surgery Facilities.* Version 3. Gurnee, IL:

American Association for Accreditation of Ambulatory Surgery Facilities; 2011:79.

112. Personnel: personnel safety. In: *Procedural Standards and Checklist for Accreditation of Ambulatory Surgery Facilities*. Version 3. Gurnee, IL: American Association for Accreditation of Ambulatory Surgery Facilities; 2011:79-80.

113. Personnel: knowledge, skill & CME training. In: *Regular Standards and Checklist for Accreditation of Ambulatory Surgery Facilities*. Version 13. Gurnee, IL: American Association for Accreditation of Ambulatory Surgery Facilities; 2011:78-79.

114. Personnel: personnel safety. In: *Regular Standards and Checklist for Accreditation of Ambulatory Surgery Facilities*. Version 13. Gurnee, IL: American Association for Accreditation of Ambulatory Surgery Facilities; 2011:80.

115. Guideline for perioperative health care information management. In: *Guidelines for Perioperative Practice*. Denver, CO: AORN, Inc; 2015:491-512. [IVB]

116. Gillespie BM, Hamlin L. A synthesis of the literature on "competence" as it applies to perioperative nursing. *AORN J*. 2009;90(2):245-258. doi:10.1016/j.aorn.2009.07.011. [VA]

117. Gillespie BM, Chaboyer W, Wallis M, Chang HY, Werder H. Operating theatre nurses' perceptions of competence: a focus group study. *J Adv Nurs*. 2009;65(5):1019-1028. [IIIB]

118. Mitchell L, Flin R. Non-technical skills of the operating theatre scrub nurse: literature review. *J Adv Nurs*. 2008;63(1):15-24. doi:10.1111/j.1365-2648.2008.04695.x. [VB]

119. Jordan C, Thomas MB, Evans ML, Green A. Public policy on competency: how will nursing address this complex issue? *J Contin Educ Nurs*. 2008;39(2):86-91. [VA]

120. RC.01.01.01: The hospital maintains complete and accurate medical records for each individual patient. In: *Hospital Accreditation Standards 2012*. Oakbrook Terrace, IL: Joint Commission on Resources; 2012.

121. RC.01.01.01: The organization maintains complete and accurate clinical records. In: *Standards for Ambulatory Care 2012 : Standards, Elements of Performance Scoring Accreditation Polices*. Oakbrook Terrace, IL: The Joint Commission; 2012.

122. Clinical records and health information. In: *2012 Accreditation Handbook for Ambulatory Health Care*. Skokie, IL: Accreditation Association for Ambulatory Health Care; 2012:40-42.

123. Medical records: procedure room records. In: *Procedural Standards and Checklist for Accreditation of Ambulatory Surgery Facilities*. Version 3. Gurnee, IL: American Association for Accreditation of Ambulatory Surgery Facilities; 2011:64-66.

124. Medical records: operating room records. In: *Regular Standards and Checklist for Accreditation of Ambulatory Surgery Facilities*. Version 13. Gurnee, IL: American Association for Accreditation of Ambulatory Surgery Facilities; 2011:64-66.

125. Medical records: general. In: *Procedural Standards and Checklist for Accreditation of Ambulatory Surgery Facilities*. Version 3. Gurnee, IL: American Association for Accreditation of Ambulatory Surgery Facilities; 2011:60-61.

126. Medical records: general. In: *Regular Standards and Checklist for Accreditation of Ambulatory Surgery Facilities*. Version 13. Gurnee, IL: American Association for Accreditation of Ambulatory Surgery Facilities; 2011:61.

127. Medical records: pre-operative medical record. In: *Regular Standards and Checklist for Accreditation of Ambulatory Surgery Facilities*. Version 13. Gurnee, IL: American Association for Accreditation of Ambulatory Surgery Facilities; 2011:62-63.

128. LD.04.01.07: The hospital has policies and procedures that guide and support patient care, treatment, and services. In: *Hospital Accreditation Standards 2012*. Oakbrook Terrace, IL: Joint Commission on Resources; 2012.

129. LD.04.01.07: The organization has policies and procedures that guide and support patient care, treatment, or services. In: *Standards for Ambulatory Care 2012: Standards, Elements of Performance Scoring Accreditation Polices*. Oakbrook Terrace, IL: The Joint Commission; 2012.

130. Governance. In: *2012 Accreditation Handbook for Ambulatory Health Care*. Skokie, IL: Accreditation Association for Ambulatory Health Care; 2012:20-27.

131. PI.03.01.01: The hospital improves performance on an ongoing basis. In: *Hospital Accreditation Standards 2012*. Oakbrook Terrace, IL: The Joint Commission; 2012.

132. PI.03.01.01: The organization improves performance. In: *Standards for Ambulatory Care 2012: Standards, Elements of Performance Scoring Accreditation Polices*. Oakbrook Terrace, IL: The Joint Commission; 2012.

133. Quality improvement/quality assessment: quality improvement. In: *Procedural Standards and Checklist for Accreditation of Ambulatory Surgery Facilities*. Version 3. Gurnee, IL: American Association for Accreditation of Ambulatory Surgery Facilities; 2011:67.

134. Quality assessment/quality improvement: quality improvement. In: *Regular Standards and Checklist for Accreditation of Ambulatory Surgery Facilities*. Version 13. Gurnee, IL: American Association for Accreditation of Ambulatory Surgery Facilities; 2011:67.

135. Quality assessment/quality improvement: unanticipated operative sequelae. In: *Regular Standards and Checklist for Accreditation of Ambulatory Surgery Facilities*. Version 13. Gurnee, IL: American Association for Accreditation of Ambulatory Surgery Facilities; 2011:69-71.

Acknowledgments

LEAD AUTHOR

Sharon A. Van Wicklin, MSN, RN, CNOR, CRNFA, CPSN, PLNC
Perioperative Nursing Specialist
AORN Nursing Department
Denver, Colorado

CONTRIBUTING AUTHOR

Ramona Conner, MSN, RN, CNOR
Manager, Standards and Guidelines
AORN Nursing Department
Denver, Colorado

The authors and AORN thank Paula J. Morton, MS, RN, CNOR, Director Perioperative Services, Sherman Health, Elgin, Illinois; Catherine M. Moses, RN, CNOR, CPHQ, QM Coordinator, Medical Arts Surgical Centers/BHSF, Miami, Florida; Christine Anderson, PhD, RN, Clinical Assistant Professor, University of Michigan School of Nursing, Ypsilanti, Michigan; and Annette Wasielewski, BSN, RN, CNOR, Senior

Consultant, Lodi, New Jersey, and Bariatric Coordinator, Hudson Valley Hospital Center, Cortlandt Manor, New York, for their assistance in developing this guideline.

PUBLICATION HISTORY

Originally published March 1978, *AORN Journal*, as "Recommended practices for aseptic technique." Format revision July 1982. Revised March 1987, October 1991.

Revised June 1996; published November 1996, *AORN Journal*.

Revised and reformatted; published February 2001, *AORN Journal*.

Revised November 2005; published as "Recommended practices for maintaining a sterile field" in *Standards, Recommended Practices, and Guidelines*, 2006 edition. Reprinted February 2006, *AORN Journal*.

Revised and reformatted December 2012 for online publication as "Recommended practices for sterile technique" in *Perioperative Standards and Recommended Practices*.

Evidence ratings revised 2013 to conform to the AORN Evidence Rating Model.

Minor editing revisions made in November 2014 for publication in *Guidelines for Perioperative Practice*, 2015 edition.

STERILE TECHNIQUE

GUIDELINE FOR SURGICAL ATTIRE

The Guideline for Surgical Attire has been approved by the AORN Guidelines Advisory Board. It was presented as a proposed guideline for comments by members and others. The guideline is effective November 15, 2014. The recommendations in the guideline are intended to be achievable and represent what is believed to be an optimal level of practice. Policies and procedures will reflect variations in practice settings and/or clinical situations that determine the degree to which the guideline can be implemented. AORN recognizes the many diverse settings in which perioperative nurses practice; therefore, this guideline is adaptable to all areas where operative and other invasive procedures may be performed.

Purpose

This document provides guidance for surgical attire including scrub attire, shoes, jewelry, head coverings, and masks worn in the semi-restricted and restricted areas of the perioperative practice setting. This document also provides guidance for personal items such as stethoscopes, backpacks, briefcases, cell phones, and tablets.

The human body and inanimate surfaces inherent in the surgical environment are major sources of microbial contamination and transmission.[1] Surgical attire and personal protective equipment (PPE) are worn to provide a high level of cleanliness and hygiene within the perioperative environment and to promote patient and worker safety. Reducing the patient's exposure to microorganisms that are shed from the skin and hair of perioperative personnel may reduce the patient's risk for surgical site infection (SSI). Patient safety is the primary consideration for perioperative personnel.

This document does not address patient clothing or linens used in health care facilities. A complete discussion of the use of PPE and sterile attire worn at the surgical field is outside the scope of this document. The reader should refer to the AORN Guideline for Sterile Technique,[2] Guideline for Prevention of Transmissible Infections,[3] and Guideline for Sharps Safety[4] for additional information. The use of nail polish, artificial nails, or other nail enhancements and the recommended fingernail length for perioperative personnel is outside the scope of this document. The reader should refer to the AORN Guideline for Hand Hygiene[5] for additional information. Ensuring and monitoring personnel compliance with policies and procedures for surgical attire and personal hygiene is a responsibility of the facility or health care organization administrators.

Evidence Review

On June 25 and June 27, 2013, a medical librarian conducted a systematic search of the databases MEDLINE® and CINAHL® and the Cochrane Database of Systematic Reviews for meta-analyses, systematic reviews, randomized controlled and non-randomized trials and studies, case reports, letters, reviews, and guidelines. The librarian also searched the Scopus database, although not systematically. The search was limited to literature published in English from January 2008 through June 2013.

Search terms included *surgical attire, clothing, personal protective equipment, protective gloves, respiratory protective devices, masks, eye protection, goggles, scrubs, surgical gown, jumpsuit, head covering, surgical cap, hoods, coveralls, bunny suit, textiles, bedding and linens, privacy curtain, hospital laundry service, laundering, laundry, washing machine, tie, backpack, fanny pack, fleece, briefcase, purse, stethoscope, lanyard, badge, patient attire, patient clothing, colonization, fomites, tattooing, body piercing, jewelry, ring, wedding band, fingernails, eyelashes, facial hair, beard, groin, armpit, scalp, skin, squames, dandruff, epithelial cells, seborrheic dermatitis, computers, mobile communication device, mobile phone, cell phone, cellular phone, tablet computer, smartphone, iPad, iPhone, text messaging, pollen, dust, fungi, mold, equipment contamination, nosocomial, cross infection, infectious disease transmission, surgical wound infection, bacterial load,* and *infection control.*

At the time of the search, the librarian established weekly alerts on the search topics and until March 2014, presented relevant results to the lead author.

Prior to the search, the medical librarian provided to the lead author the results of literature searches conducted for the 2010 edition of the AORN Recommended Practices for Surgical Attire. These articles had no time restriction. During the development of this edition, the authors also requested supplementary literature searches and additional literature that either did not fit the original search criteria or was discovered during the evidence-appraisal process. The time restriction was not considered in these subsequent searches. Relevant guidelines from government agencies and standards-setting bodies also were identified.

SURGICAL ATTIRE

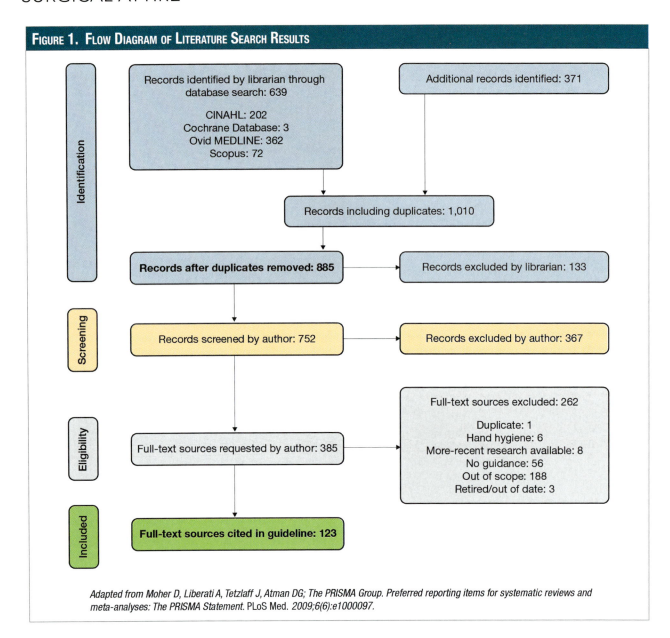

FIGURE 1. FLOW DIAGRAM OF LITERATURE SEARCH RESULTS

Adapted from Moher D, Liberati A, Tetzlaff J, Atman DG; The PRISMA Group. Preferred reporting items for systematic reviews and meta-analyses: The PRISMA Statement. PLoS Med. 2009;6(6):e1000097.

Inclusion criteria were research and non-research literature in English, complete publications, relevance to the key questions, and publication dates within the time restriction unless none were available. Excluded were non-peer-reviewed publications; literature that examined the use of sterile gowns, drapes, and masks worn for maintaining sterile technique; low-quality evidence when higher quality evidence was available; and literature outside the time restriction when literature within the time restriction was available. In total, 885 research and non-research sources of evidence were identified for possible inclusion, and of these, 123 were cited in the guidance document (Figure 1).

Articles identified by the search were provided to the project team. The team consisted of the lead author, a co-author, five members of the Guidelines Advisory Board, and two evidence appraisers. The lead author and the evidence appraisers reviewed and critically appraised each article using the AORN Research or Non-Research Evidence Appraisal Tools as appropriate. The literature was independently evaluated and appraised according to the strength and quality of the evidence. Each article was then assigned an appraisal score. The appraisal score is noted in brackets after each reference, as applicable.

Notably, much of the evidence related to surgical attire is not recent evidence. There are no randomized controlled trials (RCTs) or systematic reviews that show a direct causal relationship between surgical attire and SSI. There are many confounding variables that affect a patient's risk for SSI, and this makes it extraordinarily difficult to identify surgical attire as a singular source of SSIs. It is a well-accepted scientific principle that increased numbers of microorganisms in the perioperative environment will increase the patient's risk for SSI. It is unnecessary, and it may be unethical, for researchers to perform new studies for the sole purpose of demonstrating this recognized concept.

The methodology of the research and non-research evidence used to support this document was critically evaluated by the authors for validity and generalizability to current practice. The collective evidence supporting each intervention within a specific recommendation was summarized by the authors, and the AORN Evidence Rating Model was used to rate the strength of the evidence. Factors considered in the review of the collective evidence were the quality of evidence, the quantity of similar evidence on a given topic, and the consistency of evidence supporting a recommendation. The evidence rating is noted in brackets after each intervention.

Note: *The evidence summary table is available at http://www.aorn.org/evidencetables/.*

Editor's note: *MEDLINE is a registered trademark of the US National Library of Medicine's Medical Literature Analysis and Retrieval System, Bethesda, MD. CINAHL, Cumulative Index to Nursing and Allied Health Literature, is a registered trademark of EBSCO Industries, Birmingham, AL. Scopus is a registered trademark of Elsevier B.V., Amsterdam, The Netherlands. iPad and iPhone and registered trademarks of Apple, Inc, Cupertino, CA.*

Recommendation I

Clean surgical attire should be worn in the semi-restricted and restricted areas of the perioperative setting.

The collective body of evidence supports wearing clean surgical attire in the perioperative setting to reduce the number of microorganisms in the environment and the patient's risk for developing an SSI (Figure 2). Clean scrub attire has been laundered in a health care-accredited laundry facility and has not been previously worn.

The limitations of the evidence are that some research studies were underpowered, did not look at SSIs as an outcome, or did not control for factors contributing to SSIs (eg, antibiotic use, glucose levels). There was no clear definition of "tightly woven fabric."

The benefit of wearing clean surgical attire may include a reduction of microorganisms in the perioperative environment that may in turn lower the patient's risk for developing an SSI and reduce the potential for health care workers to transport microorganisms from the facility or health care organization into the home or community.

I.a. Fabrics used for scrub attire should be tightly woven, low linting, stain resistant, and durable. [2: Moderate Evidence]

One quasi-experimental[6] and four nonexperimental[7-10] studies compared airborne bacterial contamination levels when perioperative team members wore various types of scrub attire. The results of four of the studies indicated that tightly woven scrub attire was superior to other types of scrub attire in decreasing bacterial contamination of the air.[6-9] One study concluded that use of disposable scrub attire was better for achieving improved OR air quality.[10] Tammelin et al[6,8] defined conventional scrub attire as 50% cotton/50% polyester woven with 270 x 230 threads/10 cm and tightly woven scrub attire as 50% cotton/50% polyester woven with 560 x 395 threads/10 cm.

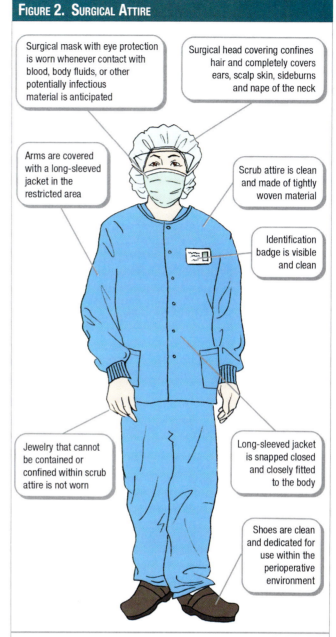

FIGURE 2. SURGICAL ATTIRE

- Surgical mask with eye protection is worn whenever contact with blood, body fluids, or other potentially infectious material is anticipated
- Surgical head covering confines hair and completely covers ears, scalp skin, sideburns and nape of the neck
- Arms are covered with a long-sleeved jacket in the restricted area
- Scrub attire is clean and made of tightly woven material
- Identification badge is visible and clean
- Jewelry that cannot be contained or confined within scrub attire is not worn
- Long-sleeved jacket is snapped closed and closely fitted to the body
- Shoes are clean and dedicated for use within the perioperative environment

Surgical attire and personal protective equipment are worn to provide a high level of cleanliness and hygiene within the perioperative environment, and to promote patient and worker safety.

Illustration by Kurt Jones.

SURGICAL ATTIRE

In a nonexperimental study conducted in a day surgery clinic at a university hospital after eight incidents of postoperative endophthalmitis, Andersen and Solheim[7] found there was a significant reduction of more than 50% of the bacterial load in the air when team members (N = 12) wore tightly woven polypropylene scrub attire (100% spunbond polypropylene [50 g/m³]) than when they wore traditional cotton scrub attire. No additional cases of endophthalmitis occurred when team members wore the tightly woven scrub attire. The researchers did not define thread counts for the traditional cotton scrub attire or the tightly woven polypropylene scrub attire.

Tammelin and colleagues conducted four studies of surgical scrub attire.[6,8-10] In the first, quasi-experimental study, conducted in a university hospital in 2000, Tammelin et al[6] examined methicillin-resistant *Staphylococcus epidermidis* (MRSE) shedding into the air to determine whether the amount of shedding could be reduced if team members wore tightly woven scrub attire. The scrubbed and non-scrubbed personnel (N = 40) participated in 33 surgical procedures while dressed in conventional scrub attire (ie, 50% cotton/50% polyester woven with 270 x 230 threads/10 cm) and in 32 surgical procedures while dressed in tightly woven scrub attire (ie, 50% cotton/50% polyester woven with 560 x 395 threads/10 cm). The researchers found that 25% of women and 43% of men dispersed MRSE that was shed into the air in the OR. The median number of colony-forming units (CFUs) dropped significantly from 14.5/m³ to 7.7/m³ when perioperative team members wore the tightly woven scrub attire. The researchers recommended wearing tightly woven scrub attire to decrease the risk of airborne bacterial transmission from shed skin squames.

In a second, nonexperimental study, conducted in a university hospital in 2001, Tammelin et al[8] examined whether team members wearing conventional scrub attire (ie, 50% cotton/50% polyester blend, 270 x 230 threads/10 cm) with shirts untucked (n = 33) or wearing scrub attire with a tighter weave (ie, 50% cotton/50% polyester blend, 560 x 365 threads/10 cm) with shirts tucked (n = 32) could reduce surgical wound contamination in patients undergoing cardiothoracic surgery. The investigators specifically investigated MRSE strains. They found that wearing the tightly woven scrub attire did not reduce the amount of MRSE in air samples compared with wearing conventional scrub attire.

In a third, nonexperimental study, conducted in 2012 in a hospital in which more than 6,000 orthopedic procedures were performed per year, Tammelin et al[9] compared levels of airborne bacterial contamination when 21 team members wore scrub attire made of one of three different types of fabric during orthopedic procedures in four operating rooms (ORs). The three fabrics were
- mixed material (69% cotton/30% polyester/1% carbon fiber, weight 150 g/m²),
- polyester material (99% polyester/1% carbon fiber, weight 100 g/m²), and
- polyester material (99% polyester/1% carbon fiber, weight 120 g/m²).

All team members wore scrub attire made from the same material during each procedure. The mean value of CFUs emitted by each team member was calculated for each of the three garments worn. The researchers found that wearing scrub attire made of either type of polyester material significantly reduced the number of CFUs/m³ emitted compared with wearing scrub attire made from mixed material. The results of this study indicated that airborne bacteria from the emitted skin flora of perioperative team members may reach the surgical site. The researchers emphasized the importance of having perioperative team members wear scrub attire that contains skin squames. The researchers recommended that additional studies be conducted to determine the protective efficacy of these materials.[9]

Tammelin et al[10] conducted a nonexperimental study in a 100-bed acute care hospital in 2013 that compared two types of scrub attire for bacterial dispersal levels:
- reusable scrub attire made of 69% cotton/30% polyester/1% carbon fiber, weight 150 g, washed 50 times (n = 32) and
- single-use scrub attire made of nonwoven, spun-bonded polypropylene, weight 35 g (n = 29).

Dispersal tests were conducted with team members wearing both types of scrub attire in a closed chamber and in an OR during 10 surgical procedures. Air sampling was conducted and CFUs were measured in both settings. The researchers found the number of CFUs was significantly lower when team members wore the single-use scrub attire compared with the reusable scrub attire in both the dispersal chamber and the OR. The researchers concluded that there can be a difference in protective capacity between different types of scrub attire.[10]

In a nonexperimental study, Noble et al[1] examined skin dispersal rates among men and women. The researchers found that the men had higher populations of skin organisms than the women. The researchers concluded that scrub attire made of tightly woven fabric is necessary to contain shed skin squames so they cannot pass through the pores of the fabric.

Lidwell et al[11] conducted a quasi-experimental study to determine the number of bacteria-carrying particles in the air during prosthetic joint surgery procedures in 15 hospitals. The researchers found coagulase-negative *Staphylococcus* in

51% of the air samples and *Staphylococcus aureus* in 39% of the air samples. Pulse-field gel electrophoresis showed the *S aureus* was identical to that carried by the study participants. There was a strong correlation between sepsis rates and the degree of bacterial air contamination. The researchers recommended limiting the number of persons present in the OR, avoiding unnecessary activity, and wearing closely woven fabrics with barrier qualities.

Wearing scrub attire that is lint-free may help prevent lint particles from being disseminated into the environment where bacteria may attach to them and settle in surgical sites and wounds and increase the potential for postoperative patient complications.[12] Scrub attire that is stain-resistant and durable promotes a professional appearance and is better able to withstand the rigorous laundering process necessary to maintain a high level of cleanliness.

I.a.1. Scrub attire may be made of antimicrobial fabric. *[2: Moderate Evidence]*

There is emerging evidence on the use of fabrics with antimicrobials incorporated into yarns during processing or during finishing to prevent bacteria and fungi from adhering to the fabric. Incorporating this technology into the material used for scrub attire and other garments worn by health care personnel may help to protect the patient from the risk of SSIs.[13-19] This issue warrants further research.

In a quasi-experimental study to examine whether antibacterial finishes on fabric could effectively reduce the presence of bacteria on fabric used for health care worker's uniforms, Chen et al[18] found that the antibacterial finishes provided a significant reduction of *Staphylococcus aureus* and *Klebsiella pneumoniae*. The researchers concluded that adding antibacterial finishes to fabric was an effective method of reducing bacterial contamination.

Mariscal et al[17] conducted a quasi-experimental study to evaluate the action of a commercially available antimicrobial textile (80% polyester/20% cotton containing silver [180 parts per million]) on 33 strains of bacteria. They found that the antimicrobial fabric significantly reduced the numbers of four reference microorganisms (ie, *Escherichia coli, Pseudomonas aeruginosa, Morganella morganii, Staphylococcus aureus*) compared with the numbers of reference microorganisms on the control fabric (80% polyester/20% cotton without silver).

Bearman et al[19] conducted an RCT to determine the effectiveness of antimicrobial fabric for reducing the bacterial burden on the hands of and scrub attire worn by health care workers in an intensive care unit (ICU) setting of an academic medical center. All study participants (N = 30) were randomly assigned to wear either traditional scrub attire or scrub attire made of antimicrobial fabric during a clinical shift during a four-week period. Each health care worker underwent unannounced weekly garment and hand cultures. Cultures taken at the beginning and end of the shifts included garment cultures taken from the abdominal and leg pockets of the scrub attire. The researchers did not specify the length of the clinical shifts.

The researchers found a significant difference (ie, a 4 to 7 mean log reduction) in the number of methicillin-resistant *Staphylococcus aureus* (MRSA) CFUs in both the leg and abdominal area of antimicrobial scrub attire and traditional scrub attire at the beginning and end of shifts. However, the researchers found no differences in the number of CFUs of vancomycin-resistant *Enterococcus* or gram-negative rods, and no difference was observed in the number or percentage of health care workers with positive hand cultures wearing either type of scrub attire.[19]

In a quasi-experimental study to evaluate the bactericidal effects of woven and nonwoven fabrics coated with a hydroxyapatite-binding silver/titanium dioxide ceramic composite, Kasuga et al[16] found that bacterial cell counts of *Staphylococcus aureus* and *Escherichia coli* on both the woven and nonwoven fabrics decreased to below 2-$\log_{10}$ CFU/mL within six hours and were undetectable at the end of the 18 hour incubation period. Bacterial cell counts of *Pseudomonas aeruginosa* could not be detected after three to six hours. The researchers found that bacterial counts on the coated woven fabric decreased more rapidly than counts on the coated nonwoven fabric. The bacterial counts on the uncoated woven and nonwoven fabric did not decrease during the 18-hour incubation period.

Sun et al[14] quantitatively and qualitatively evaluated 100% cotton and 35% cotton/65% polyester fabrics treated with antimicrobial chemicals in a nonexperimental study. The researchers found that even after 50 washings, the treated fabrics exhibited antibacterial properties against gram-negative (ie, *Escherichia coli*) and gram-positive (ie, *Staphylococcus aureus*) bacteria and fungi (ie, *Candida albicans*) within a two-minute contact time. Despite the biocidal properties of the antimicrobial fabric, the researchers found it was nontoxic to human skin. They concluded that antimicrobial fabrics were effective and suitable for medical use.

I.b. Personnel should don clean scrub attire daily. *[2: Moderate Evidence]*

SURGICAL ATTIRE

The primary source of bacteria dispersed into the air in the OR or procedure room comes from health care providers' skin.[20] Noble[20] reported that humans disseminate more than 10^7 skin particles every day. Approximately 10% of disseminated skin squames carry viable microorganisms that can pose a potential threat of SSI to perioperative patients.[20] Benediksdottir and Hambraeus[21] found that the highest density of bacteria was on the face and upper trunk of the health care worker and the highest yield of dispersed bacteria came from the lower trunk.

Weiner-Well et al[22] investigated the rate of potentially pathogenic organisms on 135 physicians' (n = 60) and nurses' (n = 75) uniforms in a nonexperimental study. The physicians and nurses reported that they changed attire daily, and 77% (n = 104) described their level of personal hygiene as fair to excellent. Sixty-three percent of the attire showed pathogenic organisms on at least one area (n = 85), and 20% (n = 17) of those were antibiotic-resistant organisms. The researchers did not determine whether these bacteria could be transmitted to patients and contribute to health care-associated infections (HAIs).

In an observational study conducted to determine the presence of bacteria in 10 locations on 30 sets of scrub attire worn by three orthopedic residents, Krueger et al[23] found that 41% of scrub attire had at least one bacterial species on it at the beginning of the work day; however, 89% of scrub attire had bacterial species on it at the end of the work day. The researchers did not specify the length of the residents' work day. Most of the organisms found were common skin flora and not multidrug-resistant microorganisms (MDROs). The researchers concluded that personnel should change into clean scrub attire before performing or assisting with surgical procedures, and they noted the need for further research to investigate how contaminated scrub attire contributes to SSIs.

I.b.1. Scrub attire should be donned in a designated dressing area before entry from the outdoors into the semi-restricted and restricted areas. *[4: Benefits Balanced with Harms]*

Changing from street apparel into clean or disposable scrub attire in a designated area assists in maintaining a clean environment and decreases the possibility of transferring microorganisms from street apparel to patients.

I.b.2. When donning scrub attire, perioperative team members should avoid contact of the clean attire with the floor or other potentially contaminated surfaces. *[4: Benefits Balanced with Harms]*

Scrub attire that contacts the floor could become a vehicle for transferring microorganisms from the floor to perioperative patients or surfaces.

I.b.3. When a two-piece scrub suit is worn, the top of the scrub suit should be secured at the waist or tucked into the pants or should fit close to the body. *[2: Moderate Evidence]*

Loose scrub tops may allow skin squames from the axilla and chest to disperse into the environment. A literature review by Ibrahimi et al[24] examined routes of bacterial transfer during surgery and found that one route that could potentially contribute to contamination of the air in the OR was skin cells dispersed through the openings of clothing by the bellows action of clothing that occurs with movement.

I.b.4. Scrub dresses may be worn over scrub pants or leggings that are laundered in a health care-accredited laundry facility after each daily use and when contaminated. *[4: Benefits Balanced with Harms]*

I.b.5. Personal clothing that cannot be contained within the scrub attire either should not be worn or should be laundered in a health care-accredited laundry facility after each daily use and when contaminated. *[4: Benefits Balanced with Harms]*

I.c. When in the restricted areas, all nonscrubbed personnel should completely cover their arms with a long-sleeved scrub top or jacket. *[2: Moderate Evidence]*

The collective body of evidence supports perioperative team members covering their arms to help contain skin squames.

Several studies have shown that human skin squames and bacteria are dispersed into the air.[1,11,21,25] A literature review by Noble[20] found 11 studies demonstrating that the skin is a source of multiple organisms and more than 10 million particles are shed from skin every day. The act of walking releases 1,000 skin scales per minute.[20]

In a nonexperimental study, May et al[25] examined dispersal of skin organisms. The results of this study demonstrated that skin squames were shed at varying rates from the test participants.

Benediktsdottir and Hambraeus[21] examined air dispersal of bacteria in a quasi-experimental study and determined that any organism present on the skin can be dispersed into the air. The dominant anaerobic bacteria dispersed were *Propionibacterium acnes*; however, *Propionibacterium avidum*, *Propionibacterium granulosum*, and gram-positive cocci also were isolated from the dispersal samples. The researchers did not determine the effect, if any, that the dispersed organisms had on the infection rates of patients.

Tammelin et al[6] conducted a quasi-experimental study to examine the dispersal of MRSE by personnel in a cardiothoracic operating suite. They found that dispersal of MRSE occurred in 25% of women and 43% of men. The researchers concluded that MRSE was a possible source of airborne contamination, and personnel should be covered by tightly woven scrub attire to help prevent dispersal of the organisms into the air.

Tammelin et al[9] conducted a nonexperimental study confirming that airborne bacteria from the skin flora of perioperative team members can reach the surgical site. The researchers emphasized the importance of surgical team members wearing scrub attire that contains skin squames.

In a literature review, Ibrahimi et al[24] found that the bacterial transfer of organisms during surgery included respiratory droplets, skin scales carried on air currents, direct contact with the perioperative team member's skin, and contaminated fomites (eg, clothing, identification badges, pens). The authors concluded that actions to decrease the bacterial load at the surgical site were prudent to reduce the risk of SSI. These actions included reducing the patient's exposure to the perioperative team member's skin.

I.c.1. The perioperative team member should wear scrub attire that covers the arms while performing preoperative patient skin antisepsis.[26] *[2: Moderate Evidence]*

Wearing long-sleeved attire helps contain skin squames shed from bare arms.[7] Performing the preoperative skin antisepsis without wearing a long-sleeved jacket may allow skin squames from the perioperative team member's bare arms to drop onto the area that is being prepped and may increase the patient's risk for an SSI.

For more information on preoperative patient skin antisepsis, the reader should refer to the AORN Guideline for Preoperative Patient Skin Antisepsis.[26]

I.c.2. The perioperative or sterile processing team member should wear scrub attire that covers the arms while preparing and packaging items in the clean assembly section of the sterile processing area. *[2: Moderate Evidence]*

Wearing long-sleeved attire helps contain skin squames shed from bare arms.[7] Not wearing a long-sleeved jacket while preparing and packaging items that will be used during operative or other invasive procedures may allow skin squames from the bare arm to drop onto the item that is being prepared or packaged and may increase the patient's risk for SSI. This organic material may be transferred to the surgical wound or other areas of the body and may increase the patients risk of SSI or other postoperative complications.[2]

I.c.3. Long-sleeved jackets and scrub attire tops should fit closely to the arms and torso to prevent the jacket or top from potentially contaminating the surgical site during preoperative patient skin antisepsis or other activities (eg, application of surgical dressings). *[4: Benefits Balanced with Harms]*

I.c.4. When a long-sleeved jacket is worn, it should be snapped closed or buttoned up the front. *[4: Benefits Balanced with Harms]*

Wearing the jacket snapped or buttoned closed helps prevent the edges of the front of the jacket from contaminating sterile areas.

I.d. Persons entering the semi-restricted or restricted areas of the surgical suite for a brief time (eg, law enforcement officers, parents, biomedical engineers) should don either clean scrub attire; single-use scrub attire; or a single-use jumpsuit (eg, coveralls, bunny suit) designed to completely cover personal apparel. *[4: Benefits Balanced with Harms]*

Donning clean scrub attire, single-use scrub attire, or single-use jumpsuits before entry into the semi-restricted and restricted areas may help to maintain a clean environment and decrease the possibility of transferring microorganisms from external areas and personal attire to perioperative surfaces and patients.

I.e. Health care personnel should change into street clothes whenever they go outside of the building. *[2: Moderate Evidence]*

Surgical attire may become contaminated by contact with the external environment. Changing into clean surgical attire before entering the semi-restricted area(s) decreases the possibility of contamination with microorganisms present in the external environment.

A prospective case control study by Sivanandan et al[27] compared the level and type of contamination of surgical attire worn inside and outside the perioperative suite within the facility. The researchers determined that there was no increased bacterial contamination of surgical attire worn in the facility; however, they did not evaluate contamination levels of surgical attire worn outside the facility. This is an unresolved issue that warrants further research.

A quasi-experimental study by Neeley and Maley,[28] and a nonexperimental study by Neeley and Orloff,[29] found that microorganisms such as enterococci and fungi can survive on fabrics and plastics for at least one day, and many can survive for as long as 90 days. These studies demonstrate that potentially pathogenic organisms can survive on many objects and fabrics. These pathogenic organisms may contaminate

SURGICAL ATTIRE

surgical attire when it is worn outside of the facility. When this contaminated attire is subsequently worn inside the facility, it could potentially increase the risk for SSIs via transfer of microorganisms from the contaminated attire to patients and surfaces within the perioperative environment. In addition, pathogenic microorganisms can be carried on contaminated surgical attire and transferred to a variety of external environments (eg, home, car, community).

I.f. Cover apparel (eg, lab coats) worn over scrub attire should be clean or be for single use. Reusable cover apparel should be laundered in a health care-accredited laundry facility after each daily use and when contaminated (Figure 3). *[2: Moderate Evidence]*

The collective evidence does not support wearing of cover apparel to protect scrub attire from contamination, and there is evidence that lab coats worn as cover apparel can be contaminated with large numbers of pathogenic microorganisms.[30-34] Researchers have found that cover apparel is not always discarded daily after use or laundered on a frequent basis.[30,31]

Kaplan et al[35] enrolled 75 participants in three groups for a quasi-experimental study to determine the effectiveness of cover apparel in preventing contamination of scrub attire.
- Group 1 participants wore a cover garment over their scrub attire,
- Group 2 participants wore scrub attire without a cover garment, and
- Group 3 participants wore scrub attire without a cover garment and also wore their scrub attire outdoors.

The researchers found there was no significant difference between the three groups, and they concluded that wearing cover apparel over scrub attire did not prevent contamination of scrub attire.[35]

A nonexperimental study conducted by Munoz-Price et al[31] examined the association between bacterial contamination of 119 health care workers' hands, lab coats, and scrub attire in five ICUs at a university medical center. Bacterial growth was detected on 104 hands; 13 grew *Staphylococcus aureus*, seven grew *Acinetobacter*, two grew enterococci, and 83 grew normal skin flora. The presence of pathogens on health care workers' hands was associated with an increased likelihood of the presence of pathogens on lab coats.

Loh et al[36] examined lab coats worn by 100 physicians in a nonexperimental study. *Staphylococcus aureus* was isolated from 25 of the lab coats, and the researchers found that the cuffs and pockets of the coats were the most contaminated areas.

In a nonexperimental study of 100 medical students' cover apparel, Banu et al[37] found microorganisms on the cuffs and side pockets of the cover apparel. Contamination was found on the dominant hand sleeve cuffs and the backs of the cover apparel 10 cm down from the collar. These areas were contaminated with *Staphylococcus* species on all cover apparel, *Acinetobacter* species on seven students' cover apparel, and diphtheroids on 12 students' cover apparel.

In a nonexperimental study, Munoz-Price et al[31] investigated the laundering practices of 160 health care providers related to scrub attire and

FIGURE 3. COVER APPAREL AND STETHOSCOPES

Reusable cover apparel should be laundered in a health care-accredited laundry facility after each daily use and when contaminated. Stethoscopes should not be worn around the neck and should be cleaned before and after each use with a low-level disinfectant.

Illustration by Kurt Jones.

lab coats. Overall, lab coats were washed every 12.4 days and scrub attire every 1.7 days. Ninety percent of respondents laundered their lab coats only once per month, and four people washed their lab coats only once every 90 days to 12 months. Water temperature used by health care providers to launder their lab coats included cold (11%), warm (21%), and hot (52%); 11% did not know the temperature used; and 6% dry-cleaned their lab coats. A total of 145 health care providers (90%) acknowledged that their lab coats were potentially contaminated with hospital pathogens. The researchers recommended that lab coats be laundered regularly (ie, at least once or twice per week) and whenever dirty or soiled with body fluids. The researchers also recommended that the lab coats be laundered in hot water with bleach to reduce or eliminate potential pathogens.

In a nonexperimental study of contamination levels of health care practitioners' cover apparel, Treakle et al[30] found that cover apparel in inpatient and outpatient areas, ICUs, administrative areas, and the OR was contaminated with *Staphylococcus aureus* that included both susceptible and resistant isolates. Two-thirds of the health care practitioners perceived their cover apparel to be dirty because it had not been washed in more than one week. Notably, health care personnel with contaminated cover apparel were more likely to have home laundered their cover apparel.

I.g. Perioperative personnel should wear clean shoes that are dedicated for use within the perioperative area. *[2: Moderate Evidence]*

In a quasi-experimental study, Amirfeyz et al[38] examined shoes worn outdoors and shoes worn only in the surgical suite (N = 120). The results of the study demonstrated that 98% of the outdoor shoes were contaminated with coagulase-negative staphylococci, coliform, and *Bacillus* species compared with 56% of the shoes worn only in the surgical suite. Bacteria on the perioperative floor may contribute up to 15% of CFUs dispersed into the air by walking. The researchers concluded that shoes worn only in the perioperative area may help to reduce contamination of the perioperative environment.

I.g.1. Shoes worn within the perioperative environment must have closed toes and backs, low heels, and nonskid soles and must meet Occupational Safety and Health Administration (OSHA) and the health care organization's safety requirements.[39] *[1: Regulatory Requirement]*

Shoes that enclose the foot with backs, low heels, and nonskid soles may reduce the risk for injury from slips and falls and from dropped items. The OSHA regulations require the use of protective footwear in areas where there is a danger of foot injuries from falling or rolling objects or objects piercing the sole. The employer is responsible for determining whether foot injury hazards exist and what, if any, protective footwear is required. The OSHA regulations mandate that employers perform a workplace hazard risk assessment and ensure that employees wear protective footwear to provide protection from identified potential hazards (eg, needle sticks, scalpel cuts, splashing from blood or other potentially infectious materials).[39]

Shoes that have holes or perforations may not protect health care workers' feet from exposure to blood, body fluids, or other liquids that may contain potentially infectious agents. Shoes made of cloth, that are open-toed, or that have holes on the top or sides do not offer protection against spilled liquids or sharp items that may be dropped or kicked.

In a quasi-experimental study, Barr and Seigel[40] examined 15 different types of shoes and tested them with an apparatus that measured resistance to penetration by scalpels. The materials of the shoes included leather, suede, rubber, and canvas. Sixty percent of the shoes sustained scalpel penetration through the shoe into a simulated foot. Only six materials prevented complete penetration. These materials included sneaker suede, suede with inner mesh lining, leather with inner canvas lining, non-pliable leather, rubber with inner leather lining, and rubber. Wearing shoes made of these materials could potentially prevent harm to the perioperative team member.

I.g.2. Shoe covers or boots must be worn in instances when gross contamination can reasonably be anticipated (eg, orthopedic surgery).[39] *[1: Regulatory Requirement]*

I.g.3. Single-use shoe covers worn as PPE must be removed immediately after use and discarded, and hand hygiene should be performed.[39] *[1: Regulatory Requirement]*

I.h. Surgical masks in combination with eye protection devices, such as goggles, glasses with solid side shields, or chin-length face shields, must be worn whenever splashes, spray, spatter, or droplets of blood, body fluids, or other potentially infectious materials may be generated and eye, nose, or mouth contamination can be reasonably anticipated.[41] *[1: Regulatory Requirement]*

Wearing surgical masks and face and eye protection is recommended by the Centers for Disease Control and Prevention (CDC)[42] and is a regulatory requirement.[41]

Surgical masks worn in the perioperative setting serve two purposes. First, they help protect

SURGICAL ATTIRE

the patient and environment from microbial contamination by organisms carried in the provider's mouth or nose. Second, they provide protection for the wearer from exposure to blood, body fluids, or other potentially infectious materials.

The results of an observational, descriptive, nonexperimental study conducted by White et al[43] involving 8,500 surgical procedures showed that 26% of exposures to blood were to the heads and necks of scrubbed personnel, and 17% of blood exposures were to circulating personnel outside the sterile field.

For additional information on surgical masks, the reader should refer to the AORN Guideline for Sterile Technique[2] and Guideline for Prevention of Transmissible Infections.[3]

I.h.1. Reusable eye protection devices worn with surgical masks, such as goggles, or personal glasses supplemented with solid side shields, should be cleaned according to the manufacturer's instructions for use before and after the health care worker performs or assists with each new procedure. *[4: Benefits Balanced with Harms]*

Reducing the number of microorganisms present on eye protection devices and glasses may protect patients from SSIs resulting from the transfer of microorganisms from the devices or hands of health care workers to patients or environmental surfaces.

I.h.2. The surgical mask should cover the mouth and nose and be secured in a manner that prevents venting at the sides of the mask (Figure 4). *[1: Strong Evidence]*

Masks with ear loops may not have been designed and intended for use as surgical masks and may not provide a secure facial fit that prevents venting at the sides of the mask. A mask that conforms to the perioperative team member's face decreases the risk that the health care worker will transmit nasopharyngeal and respiratory microorganisms to the patient or the sterile field.[42]

I.h.3. A fresh surgical mask should be donned before the health care worker performs or assists with each new procedure. The mask should be replaced and discarded whenever it becomes wet or soiled or has been taken down. *[4: Benefits Balanced with Harms]*

The filtering capacity of a surgical mask becomes compromised when it is wet or soiled. In a controlled, quasi-experimental study to determine whether filtration efficiency of surgical masks decreased with the length of time the mask was worn, Barbosa and Graziano[44] evaluated 32 individuals wearing surgical masks and 32 individuals without masks. The surgical masks used during the study had a bacterial filtration efficiency of 95%. Researchers took air samples from the surgical field at one, two, four, and six hours. The results of the study showed an increase in contamination of the filter portion of the mask after four hours. The researchers concluded that the microbial barrier of surgical masks decreased significantly after four hours.

FIGURE 4. SURGICAL MASKS

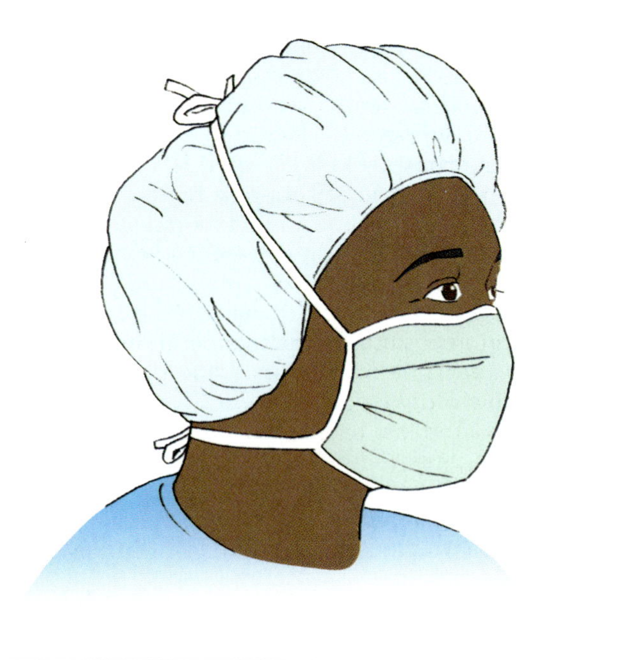

Surgical masks should cover the mouth and nose and be secured in a manner that prevents venting at the sides of the mask.
Illustration by Kurt Jones.

I.h.4. Surgical masks should not be worn hanging around the neck. *[4: Benefits Balanced with Harms]*

The filter portion of a surgical mask harbors bacteria collected from the nasopharyngeal airway. The contaminated mask may cross-contaminate the scrub attire top or long-sleeved jacket when the mask is worn hanging around the neck.

I.h.5. Surgical masks should be removed and discarded by handling only the mask ties. Hand hygiene should be performed after removal of masks.[42] *[1: Strong Evidence]*

The filter portion of the mask harbors bacteria collected from the nasopharyngeal airway. Removing masks by the ties prevents possible contamination of the hands from the filter portion of the mask.

I.i. Identification badges should be worn secured on the scrub attire top or long-sleeved jacket and should be visible. Lanyards should not be worn. Badges should be cleaned with a low-level disinfectant (eg, 70% isopropyl alcohol) regularly and when the badge becomes soiled. *[2: Moderate Evidence]*

Health care personnel as well as patients should be able to identify caregivers. Visible identification badges support security measures and assist in identifying persons authorized to be in the perioperative setting.

In a cross-sectional, quasi-experimental study, Kotsanas et al[45] examined the pathogenic contamination of identification badges and lanyards and found that the median bacterial load was tenfold greater for lanyards (3.1 CFUs/cm^2) than for identification badges (0.3 CFUs/cm^2). The microorganisms recovered from lanyards and identification badges were methicillin-sensitive *Staphylococcus aureus*, MRSA, *Enterococcus* species, and *Enterobacteriaceae*. The researchers concluded that identification badges should be clipped on and disinfected regularly and that lanyards should be changed frequently or not be worn.

I.j. Jewelry (eg, earrings, necklaces, bracelets, rings) that cannot be contained or confined within the scrub attire should not be worn in the semi-restricted or restricted areas. *[2: Moderate Evidence]*

Wearing earrings, watches, and rings was found to increase bacterial counts on skin surfaces both when the jewelry is in place and after its removal. The literature search did not find any research or non-research evidence related to bacterial contamination from necklaces. Four quasi-experimental studies[46-49] and three nonexperimental studies[50-52] collectively support the removal of rings, the removal or containment of watches, and the complete covering of ear and nose piercings with a surgical mask or head covering in the surgical setting.

A systematic review conducted by Arrowsmith and Taylor[53] determined there were no RCTs that compared ring wearing with the removal of rings in the prevention of SSIs.

In a quasi-experimental study, Trick et al[54] compared ring wearing to no ring wearing and determined that ring wearing was associated with a tenfold higher median skin organism count on the hands. The researchers recommended that all health care workers remove rings and perform hand hygiene before caring for patients.

Kelsall et al[49] found that finger rings increased skin surface bacterial counts in a quasi-experimental study. Although hand hygiene reduced bacterial skin counts, there were more bacteria under rings than on the adjacent skin or on the opposite hand. Pathogens identified by the researchers in this study included coagulase-negative staphylococci, gram-negative cocci, *Pseudomonas* species, *Staphylococcus aureus*, and other skin flora.

The results of a nonexperimental, retrospective, cohort study by Stein and Pankovich-Wargula[55] that compared SSI rates of a single surgeon over four years (ie, wearing a ring for two years versus not wearing a ring for two years) contradicted the results of other studies. The SSI rates were 19 infections in 987 surgeries in the no ring group (1.9%), and 6 infections in 1,140 surgeries in the ring group (0.53%)

I.k. Stethoscopes should not be worn around the neck and should be cleaned with a low-level disinfectant before and after each use. *[2: Moderate Evidence]*

Stethoscopes are one of the most commonly and frequently used medical devices in a health care facility. Stethoscopes come in direct contact with patients' skin and could provide an opportunity for transmission of microbes from patient to patient, from patient to health care worker, or from health care worker to patient.

The literature search found six quasi-experimental,[56-61] and 10 nonexperimental studies[62-71] of good or high quality that investigated stethoscope contamination. Contaminated stethoscope tubing and diaphragms may transmit pathogens such as MRSA by direct contact (eg, by using a contaminated stethoscope on a patient) or by indirect contact (eg, by wearing the stethoscope around the neck and contaminating the skin and scrub attire and subsequently transferring the microorganisms from the contaminated skin or attire to the patient). The collective evidence showed that hand hygiene and stethoscope cleaning by health care personnel decreased the possibility of transmitting pathogens to patients and environmental surfaces.

A quasi-experimental study by Denholm et al[60] examined the microbial contamination levels of the stethoscopes of 155 physicians and medical students and compared personal stethoscopes with facility-owned stethoscopes. The researchers isolated significantly more organisms from personal stethoscopes than from facility-owned stethoscopes; however, there was no significant relationship between the frequency of stethoscope cleaning and the degree of contamination. The researchers concluded that even regular cleaning of stethoscopes may be insufficient to prevent colonization with pathogenic organisms and that stethoscopes used for patients at high risk for HAIs should be restricted to single-patient use.

In a nonexperimental cross-sectional study, Campos-Murguia et al[68] examined the number of potentially pathogenic organisms present on stethoscopes by analyzing 112 stethoscopes from 12 hospital departments. At least 1 CFU was found on 106 stethoscopes (95%). Forty-eight stethoscopes (43%) had microorganisms that were potentially pathogenic. The results of this study showed that stethoscopes could be significant contributors to MRSA infections and that they should be routinely cleaned and disinfected before and after each patient use.

SURGICAL ATTIRE

I.k.1. Fabric stethoscope tubing covers should not be used. *[3: Limited Evidence]*

Fabric covers on stethoscope tubing may become contaminated with pathogenic microorganisms and subsequently act as fomites. In a nonexperimental study, Milam et al[72] isolated gram-positive aerobic bacteria, gram-negative aerobic bacteria, anaerobes, and yeast from 18 of 20 fabric stethoscope covers (90%) that had been used for one to 24 months. The researchers found that the average length of time between stethoscope cover laundering was 3.7 months, and some fabric covers were never laundered.

I.l. Briefcases, backpacks, and other personal items that are taken into the semi-restricted or restricted areas should be cleaned with a low-level disinfectant and should not be placed on the floor. *[2: Moderate Evidence]*

Items brought into the OR, such as briefcases, backpacks, and other personal items, may be difficult to clean and may harbor pathogens, dust, and bacteria. Maintaining a clean perioperative environment helps decrease the patient's risk of SSI.[73] Cleaning these items may help to decrease the transmission of potentially pathogenic microorganisms from external surfaces to perioperative surfaces and from perioperative surfaces to external surfaces.

Floors in the OR or procedure room are considered contaminated.[73] Items placed on the floor could become vehicles for transferring microorganisms from the floor to other perioperative or external surfaces.

The literature search did not find any literature that specifically examined the effect on SSIs associated with bringing backpacks, briefcases, or other personal items from an external environment into a surgical environment. Two quasi-experimental studies,[28,74] five nonexperimental studies,[29,75-78] and one literature review[79] addressed the survivability of microorganisms on fabrics, plastics, and other materials. The evidence did not suggest that these items should be prohibited in the health care setting; however, the collective evidence did support the need for thorough cleaning and disinfecting procedures.

In a quasi-experimental study, Neely and Maley[28] examined the ability of gram-positive bacteria (ie, vancomycin-sensitive and -resistant enterococci and methicillin-sensitive and -resistant staphylococci) to survive on five materials commonly found in health care facilities:
- smooth 100% cotton clothing,
- 100% cotton terry cloth towels,
- 60% cotton/40% polyester blend scrub attire and lab coats,
- 100% polyester privacy curtains, and
- 100% polypropylene plastic splash aprons.

The researchers found that all bacteria survived for at least one day, and some survived for more than 90 days. The researchers recommended meticulous cleaning to limit the spread of these bacteria.

Neely and Orloff[29] examined the ability of fungi to survive on seven materials commonly found in health care facilities:
- smooth 100% cotton clothing;
- 100% cotton terrycloth towels and washcloths;
- 60% cotton/40% polyester blend scrub attire, lab coats, and other clothing;
- 100% polyester privacy curtains;
- 25% spandex/75% nylon pressure garments;
- 100% polyethylene plastic splash aprons; and
- 100% polyurethane keyboard covers.

The researchers found that fungi associated with HAIs survived for at least one day, and some survived for weeks. The researchers recommended meticulous cleaning to reduce the potential for patient infection.

Four nonexperimental studies[75-78] and one literature review[79] supported the findings of Neeley and Maley[28] and Neely and Orloff.[29] Koca et al[76] conducted a nonexperimental study that demonstrated that bacteria and fungi survived for days to months on commonly used hospital fabrics. The researchers recommended that current national guidelines on disinfection and sterilization of fabrics be followed to minimize cross-infection and help prevent HAIs.

In a nonexperimental case control study to determine whether physician's purses were contaminated with microorganisms more frequently than the purses of women who were not physicians, Feldman et al[74] found that five of the 13 physicians' purses (38.5%) were colonized with bacteria compared with two of the 14 nonphysicians' purses (14%). The researchers concluded that there is a potential for physicians' purses to serve as a vector for disease transmission.

I.m. Cell phones, tablets, and other personal communication or hand-held electronic equipment should be cleaned with a low-level disinfectant according to the manufacturer's instructions for use before and after being brought into the perioperative setting. *[2: Moderate Evidence]*

The collective evidence demonstrates that cell phones, tablets, and other personal hand-held devices are highly contaminated with microorganisms, some potentially pathogenic. One RCT,[80] three quasi-experimental studies,[46,81,82] eight nonexperimental studies,[83-90] and one literature review[91] addressed cell phones and other electronic devices brought into the health care setting. All of the researchers recommended regular cleaning of these devices and implementing hand hygiene before and after use. Reducing the numbers of microorganisms present on the devices may protect patients from the risk of HAIs resulting from the transfer of microorganisms from the devices or hands of health care workers to patients.

Datta et al[80] conducted an RCT to investigate the rate of bacterial contamination of the mobile phones of health care workers employed in a tertiary health care teaching hospital and compared the contamination rate with that of a group of individuals not working in a health care environment. Of the 200 health care workers' mobile phones sampled, 144 (72%) were contaminated with bacteria, and 18% of those bacteria were MRSA. Of the 50 non-health care workers' mobile phones sampled, only five (10%) were contaminated with bacteria (ie, coagulase-negative staphylococci). The researchers concluded that simple measures such as regular cleaning of cell phones and other hand-held electronic devices and improving hand hygiene might help to decrease the risk of HAIs from bacteria carried on personal mobile devices.

Tekerekoglu et al[85] conducted a nonexperimental, cross-sectional study to determine the amount of bacterial colonization on the mobile phones of patients, patients' companions, health care workers, and visitors in a university medical center. Two hundred cell phones were tested, and the results showed a significantly higher rate of pathogenic organisms on the patients', patient companions', and visitors' phones than on those of the health care workers. The researchers concluded that the cleaning of phones brought into the health care setting by patients and others is just as important as cleaning the phones of health care workers.

Kilic et al[81] conducted a quasi-experimental study that tested the bacterial levels of 106 mobile phones carried by health care workers in three hospitals and compared them to bacterial levels of 30 phones carried by people who did not work in hospitals. Bacterial growth was observed in 65 of the 106 samples (61%) of the health care workers' phones; the most common pathogens were *Staphylococcus*, *Corynebacterium*, and *Escherichia coli*. Of the control phones carried by non-health care workers, 16 of the samples (53%) were colonized with *Staphylococcus epidermidis* and *Bacillus*.

During a nine-month period, White et al[89] conducted a nonexperimental study of microbial growth on smartphones used by students in the OR. Devices were sampled for two cohort groups (ie, nine devices on six occasions, and seven devices on three occasions), with a four- to five-hour period of use between sampling activity. No device was found to be free of growth. The devices demonstrated multiple species of microbial growth in all cases except one, which was contaminated solely with coagulase-negative *Staphylococcus* species.

Eighty-six percent of the smartphones had three or more types of bacteria on them; some had as many as seven types. The most common pathogen found was coagulase-negative *Staphylococcus*. Other pathogenic organisms found were MRSA, *Micrococcus* species, *Enterococcus* species, and coliforms. The researchers concluded that mobile phones are contaminated with significant numbers of pathogenic bacteria. They recommended cleaning mobile phones with 70% isopropyl alcohol in combination with frequent hand hygiene and other infection prevention measures to reduce the risk for infection from transmission of microorganisms found on mobile phones.[89]

Recommendation II

All individuals who enter the semi-restricted and restricted areas should wear scrub attire that has been laundered at a health care-accredited laundry facility or disposable scrub attire provided by the facility and intended for use within the perioperative setting.

The evidence regarding home laundering of scrub attire compared with health care-accredited laundering conflicts. Some evidence indicates there is a risk for pathogenic organisms to be carried on scrub attire laundered in the home.[92-95] These organisms can potentially put the patient at risk of infection or contaminate the home or community of the perioperative team member.

Limitations of the evidence are that some studies examined in-vitro conditions that may not be applicable to real-life conditions, and some evidence is not specific to the perioperative setting and therefore may not be generalizable to the perioperative environment. Except for one case report by Wright et al,[95] none of the authors considered SSI as an outcome.

The benefits of health care-accredited laundering compared with home laundering are that health care-accredited laundering may protect the patient from potential exposure to microorganisms that could contribute to an SSI and may protect the perioperative team member from contaminating the home or community with pathogenic organisms from the workplace. Health care-accredited laundering provides control of the laundering process and helps ensure that effective laundering standards have been met.

II.a. Scrub attire should be laundered in a health care-accredited laundry facility after each daily use and when contaminated. *[2: Moderate Evidence]*

The evidence regarding home laundering compared with health care-accredited laundering of surgical attire conflicts. Fijan and Turk[96] conducted a literature review of laundering practices of hospital textiles. The authors concluded that the available evidence is diverse and contradictory. Effective laundering of scrub attire is dependent on several factors including the duration, type of detergent and disinfectants, ratio of chemicals to water, and type of fabric being laundered.

Eight articles support health care-accredited laundering. In a quasi-experimental study to determine whether enteric and respiratory viruses could survive the wash, rinse, and drying cycles commonly used for home laundering, Gerba et al[92] concluded that common household laundering practices did not eliminate enteric and respiratory viruses from clothing.

In a literature review of laundering practices of nurses' uniforms, Halliwell[97] found a disparity between home and hospital laundering practices, inconsistency between laundering guidelines, and a lack of evidence that uniforms can act as a secondary source of HAIs. The results of the literature review revealed three important concepts:
- Nurses' uniforms become highly contaminated with microorganisms while they are worn.
- Contamination is higher on the areas of frequent hand contact, such as pockets, buttocks, and cuffs.
- Hands that touch the uniform also become contaminated.

The author concluded that nurses' uniforms could be considered "biological hazards" and suggested that legislation be implemented that requires employers to provide and launder uniforms for health care workers.

Lis et al[93] conducted a nonexperimental study to evaluate airborne *Staphylococcus aureus* in the homes of people who had contact with the hospital environment. The researchers found a significant difference in airborne multidrug-resistant *S aureus* strains in the homes of people who had contact with a hospital environment. The researchers suggested that the bacteria may have been transmitted to the home via clothing.

Nguyen et al[98] reported an outbreak of 22 sternal SSIs in a hospital in which approximately 400 open heart surgeries were performed per year. Of the 22 SSIs, four cases were *Gordonia* species. The authors found that antimicrobial dosing was often inadequate, cleaning practices were inadequate, personnel employed poor hand hygiene, there were inadequate environmental controls in place, and home laundered scrub attire was worn.

In a quasi-experimental study to determine whether hospital laundry facilities could adequately decontaminate enterococci from hospital linens, Orr et al[99] found that the organism was successfully decontaminated with a water temperature of 150° F (66° C) for 10 minutes and at a temperature of 160° F (71° C) for three minutes.

Sasahara et al[100] reviewed an outbreak of *Bacillus cereus* bacteremia and found that the hospital laundry and washing machines were highly contaminated with *B cereus*. The organism is resistant to heat and alcohol, and eliminating the organisms requires that laundry be washed at 176° F (80° C) for more than 10 minutes.

In a nonexperimental study to assess the bioburden associated with scrub attire, Twomey and Beitz[94] evaluated single-use, reusable, facility-laundered, third-party laundered, and home laundered scrub attire before and after wear. The researchers measured CFUs for each type of scrub attire. They found no differences in the mean microbial populations among the facility, third-party laundered, or single-use scrub attire before wear. Notably, the home laundered attire had a significantly greater microbial population before use. The home laundered scrub attire was as contaminated after laundering and before being worn as the facility-laundered and third-party laundered attire were at the end of a work day. The researchers concluded that home laundering is not as effective as facility- or third-party laundering for decontaminating scrub attire.

Wright et al[95] reported three cases of postoperative *Gordonia bronchialis* sternal infections after coronary artery bypass grafting surgery. *G bronchialis* was isolated from the scrub attire, axilla, hands, and purse of a nurse anesthetist and was implicated as the cause of the SSIs. Cultures taken from her roommate, who was also a nurse, showed the same microorganism. After notification of the culture results, the nurse anesthetist discarded her front-loading washing machine. During the next year, the nurse anesthetist and her roommate's scrub attire, hands, nares, and scalp tested negative for *G bronchialis*. The authors concluded that the home washing machine was the likely bacterial reservoir. Home laundering may not reliably kill all pathogens, and the pathogens may survive in the form of biofilms within the washing machine. Biofilms have been implicated in the malodor of washing machines. The author recommended that hospital-laundered scrub attire be implemented as a measure to reduce patients' risk of developing an SSI. This report is the first to demonstrate a causal relationship between home laundering and human disease.

Nine articles support home laundering. Al-Benna[101] conducted a literature review to explore home laundering of scrub attire and found there was little scientific evidence that facility laundering was better than home laundering; however, the author recommended the following guidelines for home laundering:
- Uniforms should be washed as the last laundry load of the day.
- Bleach should be used.
- Laundry should be totally submerged.
- Laundry personnel should wash their hands after handling laundry.

- The lid or door of the washer should be disinfected before clean laundry is removed to avoid contamination.
- Laundry should be dried at the highest temperature possible immediately after washing.
- Laundry should be transported in a manner that maintains cleanliness.

Belkin[102] noted the lack of evidence linking home laundering with SSI or HAIs in an expert opinion article and recommended the addition of a disinfecting agent, such as chlorine bleach to each load of laundry. In a second expert opinion article, Belkin[103] again noted the lack of evidence supporting facility laundering over home laundering and stated that no facilities have reported an increase in SSIs related to home laundering.

In a nonexperimental study to determine whether domestic laundry procedures were effective in eliminating viruses on clothing, Heinzel et al[104] used commercial powdered laundry detergent to test their virucidal performance. The researchers concluded that powdered detergents are able to decontaminate viruses from textiles in a common household laundering process.

Lakdawala et al[105] conducted a nonexperimental investigation of the effect of low-temperature washing cycles (140° F [60° C]) by assessing the amount of bioburden on health care workers uniforms before and after laundering. The researchers concluded that a washing cycle of 140° F (60° C) for 10 minutes was sufficient to decontaminate hospital uniforms and reduce the bacterial load by at least a 7-log reduction. The uniforms could become recontaminated after laundering, but the organisms could be easily removed by ironing.

In a nonexperimental study of OR surgical attire conducted as the result of an increase of MDROs and HAIs, Nordstrom et al[106] took swatches from unwashed, hospital-laundered, new cloth, and disposable scrub attire, and tested them for the presence of microorganisms. The researchers found that the home laundered scrub attire had a significantly higher total bacterial count than the facility laundered attire, and they found no significant difference in bacterial counts between hospital-laundered, unused, or disposable scrub attire. The researchers concluded that although it is not known how contaminated scrub attire contributes to the spread of HAIs, hospital administrators and infection preventionists should consider the potential for transmission of infection versus cost savings by the facility if home laundering is allowed. The researchers advised that health care workers should be made aware of the risks of home laundering and being provided with instructions for best methods for home laundering in order to reduce the risk of infection.

Patel et al[107] conducted a quasi-experimental study to determine the effectiveness of home laundering in removing *Staphylococcus aureus* from scrub attire. The researchers cut hospital laundered scrub attire into squares, inoculated them with *S aureus*, and washed them at a typical household laundry temperature of 104° F (40° C) and a higher temperature of 140° F (60° C). The researchers concluded that the lower 104° F (40° C) temperature did not remove *S aureus*; however, adding sequential tumble drying or ironing reduced the number of bacteria to an undetectable level. Washing at 140° F (60° C) produced a greater reduction in total viable organisms compared with the 104° F (40° C) temperature. The researchers concluded that scrub attire can be safely washed at 104° F (40° C) if tumble dried for 30 minutes or ironed.

Wilson et al[108] reviewed the literature related to health care workers uniforms as a vehicle for microbial transmission and to determine the efficacy of different laundry practices. The authors found limited evidence directly related to decontamination of health care workers' uniforms. They concluded that there was no strong evidence that home laundering of uniforms was inferior to industrial laundry practices; however, the authors recommended that if home laundering is performed, overloading of the machine should be avoided to ensure that a sufficient amount of water is present for adequate agitation and rinsing during the washing process.

In a nonexperimental study to determine the level of contamination of health care workers uniforms before and at the end of a work shift, Perry et al[109] found that the uniforms became progressively more contaminated the longer they were worn. The researchers questioned the ability of home laundering processes to adequately clean the uniforms. The researchers emphasized the importance of daily laundering, and also recommended that if home laundering is practiced, specific guidelines provided by the facility are necessary for standardized laundering, including the need for laundering uniforms separately from other household garments and at a water temperature sufficient to eliminate pathogenic organisms.

Using health care-accredited laundry facilities is recommended because they meet industry standards[110] including the following:
- Textile quality control procedures are defined and implemented.
- The inventory system is adequate to ensure supply.
- Soiled and contaminated textile areas are separated.
- The ventilation is controlled
  - with negative pressure in the soiled area,

SURGICAL ATTIRE

- with positive pressure from the clean textile area through the soiled textile area,
- at 6 to 10 air exchanges per hour, and
- with air vented to the outside.
◦ Clean textiles are stored at temperatures of 68° F to 78° F (20° C to 25.6° C) in an area free of vermin, dust, and lint.
◦ Storage shelves are 1 to 2 inches from the wall, the bottom shelf is 6 to 8 inches from the floor, and the top shelf is 12 to 18 inches below the ceiling.
◦ Hand washing facilities are located in all areas with soiled textiles; hand washing or antiseptic dispensers are in the clean textile area; and employees perform hand washing after glove removal and restroom use, before eating, and when hands are contaminated with blood, body fluids, or other potentially infectious materials.
◦ Work surfaces are clean and are disinfected if they become contaminated with blood, body fluids, or other potentially infectious materials.
◦ The OSHA Exposure Control Plan is in place and PPE is supplied, available, and worn.
◦ Quality control monitoring processes are in place.
◦ Personnel education and training is provided and documented.
◦ Safety data sheets are available for each chemical used.
◦ water quality is tested on a regular basis for hardness, alkalinity, iron content, and pH;
◦ Soiled health care textiles are handled, collected, and transported according to local, state, and federal regulations.
◦ Each laundry cycle is monitored and applicable data for each cycle are recorded, including pre-wash, wash, rinse, and final rinse times, water levels and usage, temperatures, and chemical usage.
◦ Water extraction and drying are performed using methods that preserve the integrity of the textiles and minimize bacterial growth.
◦ Cleaned textiles are packaged and stored in fluid-resistant bundles or fluid-resistant carts or hampers and are handled as little as possible.
◦ Carts used for transport or storage are kept clean and are well maintained.
◦ Clean textiles are stored and transported separately from soiled textiles.
◦ Vehicles used to transport textiles provide separation of clean and soiled textiles, and the vehicle interiors are cleaned on a regular basis.

The Healthcare Laundry Accreditation Council offers voluntary accreditation for those laundry facilities that process reusable health care textiles and that incorporate OSHA and CDC guidelines and professional association recommended practices.[110]

The benefit of health care-accredited laundering of surgical attire is that it may protect the patient from exposure to pathogenic organisms remaining on the health care worker's attire after home laundering and may prevent the health care worker from transmitting pathogenic organisms from the attire worn in the health care facility into the home or community. Health care-accredited laundering may reduce the potential for allergies to laundry detergents or other chemical additives because the rinsing process leaves little to no soap residue in the fabric.

The potential harm associated with home laundering is that it may not protect patients, health care workers, their family members, or the community from exposure to bloodborne pathogens or other infectious materials during handling and decontamination of scrub attire. To address health hazards posed by pathogens transported from the workplace to the home, the National Institute for Occupational Safety and Health published *Protecting Workers' Families: A Research Agenda*.[111] The authors emphasized that exposure to blood, body fluids, and potentially pathogenic organisms are possible threats for disease transmission that can be carried to the homes of workers on clothing and other objects that have been used in the workplace. To mitigate this risk, the authors recommended that employers institute engineering, administrative, and worker protection techniques, and that health care workers not bring objects used in the work setting into the home.

Home laundering is not monitored for quality, consistency, or safety. Home washing machines may not have the adjustable parameters or controls required to achieve the necessary thermal measures (eg, water temperature); mechanical measures (eg, agitation); or chemical measures (eg, capacity for additives to neutralize the alkalinity of the water, soap, or detergent) to reduce microbial levels in soiled scrub attire.

Scrub attire that is home laundered may not be protected from contaminants in the environment during transport to the practice setting.

II.a.1. Laundered scrub attire should be protected during transport to the practice setting.[112] *[3: Limited Evidence]*

Protecting clean scrub attire from contamination during transport from the laundry facility to the practice setting helps prevent physical damage and minimizes potential contamination from the external environment.[112]

II.a.2. Laundered scrub attire should be transported in enclosed carts or containers and in vehicles that are cleaned and disinfected regularly.[112] *[3: Limited Evidence]*

Carts, containers, and vehicles can be a source of contamination.

II.a.3. Laundered scrub attire should be stored in enclosed carts or cabinets that are cleaned and disinfected regularly.[112] *[3: Limited Evidence]*

Storing laundered surgical attire in clean enclosed carts or cabinets helps prevent contamination. Storing clean attire in a facility locker with personal items from outside of the facility may contaminate the clean scrub attire.

II.a.4. Laundered scrub attire may be stored in dispensing machines. Dispensing machines should be regularly cleaned and disinfected according to the manufacturer's instructions for use. *[4: Benefits Balanced with Harms]*

Scrub attire-dispensing machines may promote cost containment, help to facilitate an adequate supply of scrub attire, provide clean storage for scrub attire, and increase individual accountability.

II.b. Reusable scrub attire should be left at the health care facility for laundering. *[2: Moderate Evidence]*

Callaghan[113] conducted a nonexperimental study to evaluate the amount of bacterial contamination of nurses' uniforms during an eight-hour shift and found that at the end of the shift, the uniforms were highly contaminated with potentially pathogenic microorganisms.

II.b.1. Scrub attire that has been penetrated by blood, body fluids, or other potentially infectious materials must be removed immediately or as soon as possible and replaced with clean attire. When extensive contamination of the body occurs, the health care worker should take a shower or bath before donning fresh attire.[41,114] *[1: Regulatory Requirement]*

Changing contaminated, soiled, or wet attire may reduce the potential for contamination and protect personnel from exposure to potentially pathogenic microorganisms.

II.b.2. Scrub attire contaminated with visible blood or body fluids must remain at the health care facility for laundering or be sent to a health care-accredited laundry facility contracted by the health care organization.[41,111] *[1: Regulatory Requirement]*

Controlled laundering of attire contaminated by blood or body fluids reduces the risk of transferring pathogenic microorganisms from the health care facility to the home or community. Exposure to blood, body fluids, and potentially pathogenic organisms are potential threats to health care workers and their home environments.[111]

II.b.3. Wet or contaminated scrub attire must not be rinsed or sorted in the location of use.[41] *[1: Regulatory Requirement]*

Rinsing or sorting contaminated reusable attire may expose the health care worker to blood, body fluids, or other potentially infectious materials.

II.b.4. Reusable scrub attire that has been worn should not be stored in personal lockers for later use. *[2: Moderate Evidence]*

Scrub attire that has been worn may have bacterial colony counts that are even higher after the attire is removed, stored in a locker, and used again. Microbes have been shown to survive for long periods of time on fabrics.[28,29]

II.b.5. Reusable or single-use contaminated scrub attire should be placed in designated containers after use. *[4: Benefits Balanced with Harms]*

Recommendation III

Personnel entering the semi-restricted and restricted areas should cover the head, hair, ears, and facial hair.

Hair and skin can harbor bacteria that can be dispersed into the environment. The collective body of evidence supports covering the hair and ears while in the semi-restricted or restricted areas.

The limitations of the evidence are that some research studies had small sample sizes, were of low quality, or were conducted in laboratory settings that may not be generalizable to other settings.

The benefit of covering the head, ears, and hair is the reduction of the patient's exposure to potentially pathogenic microorganisms from the perioperative team member's head, hair, ears, and facial hair.

III.a. A clean surgical head cover or hood that confines all hair and completely covers the ears, scalp skin, sideburns, and nape of the neck should be worn. *[2: Moderate Evidence]*

There are several studies that show that hair can be a source of bacterial organisms.[1,115-117] The results of a nonexperimental study conducted by Noble et al[1] found that 10% of individuals had *Staphylococcus aureus* present in their hair. In a quasi-experimental study conducted by Summers et al,[115] the researchers cultured the hair of hospital personnel, inpatients, and outpatients, and found bacteria in the hair of all test participants. *S aureus* was the most common pathogen isolated. The researchers concluded that the exposed hair of health care workers is a potential source of patient infection. They recommended that health care workers cover all hair during even minor surgical procedures.

Dineen and Drusin[116] investigated two outbreaks of postoperative wound infections and found that the infections were directly related to personnel carrying *Staphylococcus aureus* in their hair. Mastro et al[117] investigated a prolonged outbreak of 20 postoperative SSIs caused by group A *Streptococcus*. Two case control studies and a review of records conducted by the researchers failed to identify the carrier. The researchers used bacterial settling plates to sample the air in the OR and identified the source of the outbreak as a surgical technologist who carried the identical type of group A *Streptococcus* on the scalp.

A literature review by McHugh et al[118] identified several conflicting studies related to the need for a surgical head covering. The authors concluded there was little evidence to suggest that covering the hair reduces SSI rates; however, they acknowledged that surgical team members wearing head coverings decreased bacterial contamination of the surgical field.

The results of a literature review conducted by Eisen[119] showed that hair is a potential vehicle for bacterial dispersal and that hair has been shown to carry *Staphylococcus aureus*. The author concluded that there is conflicting evidence about the effect of hair coverings on SSI rates.

Ibrahimi et al[24] conducted a literature review to examine SSIs and routes of bacterial transfer. The authors concluded that there was no convincing evidence that head coverings reduce SSI rates.

Mase et al[120] conducted a quasi-experimental study to determine whether staphylococci that were present on the hair could be removed by shampooing. The results of the study showed that staphylococci become firmly attached to the human hair surface and the edge of hair cuticles. Extensive treatment with neutral detergents did not remove the organism, suggesting that conventional shampooing has little effect on removing staphylococci from hair. Moreover, these neutral detergents had little bactericidal activity on staphylococci. These results suggest that hair could be a source of multidrug-resistant staphylococci in patient infections. The researchers concluded that hair could be a source of MRSA in HAIs.

A nonexperimental study conducted by McClure et al[121] examined dispersal of bacteria by men with and without beards and by women. The results of the study showed that there was significantly more bacterial shedding by bearded men than by clean-shaven men or by women, even when a mask was worn. The researchers suggested that beards may act as a reservoir for bacteria and dead organic material that can be dislodged when a face mask is removed. The researchers recommended that perioperative team members not wear beards.

Owers et al[122] conducted a nonexperimental study in which 20 OR team members had their foreheads, eyebrows, and ears cultured. The researchers found there was significantly more bacteria isolated from the ears than from the foreheads and eyebrows of the surgical team members. The researchers concluded that the ears should be covered by surgical head covers during surgery.

III.a.1. Personnel wearing scrub attire should not remove the surgical head covering when leaving the perioperative area. *[4: Benefits Balanced with Harms]*

The purpose of the head covering is to contain hair and minimize microbial dispersal. When the head covering is removed, hair and microbes may be shed onto scrub attire.

Head coverings commonly used in the perioperative setting (eg, bouffant caps) are worn for hair and skin containment and are not considered PPE. The Occupational Safety and Health Administration requires that PPE not permit blood, body fluids, or other potentially infectious materials to pass through or reach the employee's clothing, skin, eyes, or other mucous membranes under normal conditions of use.[123]

III.a.2. Personnel should remove surgical head coverings whenever they change into street clothes and go outside of the building. *[4: Benefits Balanced with Harms]*

Removing surgical head coverings when exiting the building decreases the possibility of contamination with microorganisms present in the external environment.

III.a.3. Used single-use head coverings should be removed at the end of the shift or when contaminated and should be discarded in a designated receptacle. *[4: Benefits Balanced with Harms]*

III.a.4. Reusable head coverings should be laundered in a health care-accredited laundry facility after each daily use and when contaminated (see Recommendation II.b). *[2: Moderate Evidence]*

Head coverings are part of the scrub attire.

Glossary

Fomite: An inanimate object which, when contaminated with a viable pathogen (eg, bacterium, virus), can transfer the pathogen to a host.

Health care-accredited laundry facility: An organization that processes health care linens and has successfully passed an inspection of its facility, policies and procedures, training programs, and relationships with customers.

Low-level disinfectant: An agent that destroys all vegetative bacteria, some fungi, and some viruses but not all bacterial spores.

Scrub attire: Nonsterile apparel designed for the perioperative practice setting that includes two-piece pantsuits, scrub dresses, long-sleeved cover jackets, and head coverings.

Squames: Flat, keratinized, dead cells shed from the outermost layer of stratified squamous epithelium.

Surgical attire: Nonsterile apparel designated for the perioperative practice setting that includes two-piece pantsuits, scrub dresses, cover jackets, head coverings, shoes, masks, and protective eyewear.

Surgical mask: A device worn over the mouth and nose by perioperative team members during surgical procedures to protect both the patient and perioperative team member from transfer of blood, body fluids, and other potentially infectious materials. Surgical masks prevent the transmission of large droplets (ie, greater than 5 microns). Surgical masks are evaluated for fluid resistance, bacterial filtration efficiency, differential pressure, and flammability.

References

1. Noble WC, Habbema JD, van Furth R, Smith I, de Raay C. Quantitative studies on the dispersal of skin bacteria into the air. *J Med Microbiol.* 1976;9(1):53-61. [IIIB]

2. Guideline for sterile technique. In: *Guidelines for Perioperative Practice.* Denver, CO: AORN, Inc; 2015:67-96. [IVA]

3. Guideline for prevention of transmissible infections. In: *Guidelines for Perioperative Practice.* Denver, CO: AORN, Inc; 2015:419-451. [IVA]

4. Guideline for sharps safety. In: *Guidelines for Perioperative Practice.* Denver, CO: AORN, Inc; 2015:365-388. [IVA]

5. Guideline for hand hygiene. In: *Guidelines for Perioperative Practice.* Denver, CO: AORN, Inc; 2015:31-42. [IVB]

6. Tammelin A, Domicel P, Hambraeus A, Stahle E. Dispersal of methicillin-resistant *Staphylococcus epidermidis* by staff in an operating suite for thoracic and cardiovascular surgery: relation to skin carriage and clothing. *J Hosp Infect.* 2000;44(2):119-126. [IIC]

7. Andersen BM, Solheim N. Occlusive scrub suits in operating theaters during cataract surgery: effect on airborne contamination. *Infect Control Hosp Epidemiol.* 2002;23(4):218-220. [IIIC]

8. Tammelin A, Hambraeus A, Stahle E. Source and route of methicillin-resistant *Staphylococcus epidermidis* transmitted to the surgical wound during cardiothoracic surgery. Possibility of preventing wound contamination by use of special scrub suits. *J Hosp Infect.* 2001;47(4):266-276. [IIIC]

9. Tammelin A, Ljungqvist B, Reinmüller B. Comparison of three distinct surgical clothing systems for protection from air-borne bacteria: a prospective observational study. *Patient Saf Surg.* 2012;6(1):23. [IIIC]

10. Tammelin A, Ljungqvist B, Reinmuller B. Single-use surgical clothing system for reduction of airborne bacteria in the operating room. *J Hosp Infect.* 2013;84(3):245-247. [IIIC]

11. Lidwell OM, Lowbury EJL, Whyte W, Blowers R, Stanley SJ, Lowe D. Airborne contamination of wounds in joint replacement operations: the relationship to sepsis rates. *J Hosp Infect.* 1983;4(2):111-131. [IIA]

12. Edmiston CE Jr, Sinski S, Seabrook GR, Simons D, Goheen MP. Airborne particulates in the OR environment. *AORN J.* 1999;69(6):1169-1179. [IIB]

13. Bauer J, Kowal K, Tofail SAM, Podbielska H. MRSA-resistant textiles. In: Tofail SAM, ed. *Biological Interactions with Surface Charge in Biomaterials.* Cambridge, England: RSC Publishing;2012:193-207. [VB]

14. Sun G, Qian L, Xu X. Antimicrobial and medical-use textiles. *Textile Asia.* 2001;32(9):33-35. [IIIB]

15. Rajendran R, Radhai R, Kotresh TM, Csiszar E. Development of antimicrobial cotton fabrics using herb loaded nanoparticles. *Carbohydr Polym.* 2013;91(2):613-617. [IIIA]

16. Kasuga E, Kawakami Y, Matsumoto T, et al. Bactericidal activities of woven cotton and nonwoven polypropylene fabrics coated with hydroxyapatite-binding silver/titanium dioxide ceramic nanocomposite "Earth-plus." *Int J Nanomed.* 2011;6:1937-1943. [IIB]

17. Mariscal A, Lopez-Gigosos RM, Carnero-Varo M, Fernandez-Crehuet J. Antimicrobial effect of medical textiles containing bioactive fibres. *Eur J Clin Microbiol Infect Dis.* 2011;30(2):227-232. [IIB]

18. Chen-Yu JH, Eberhardt DM, Kincade DH. Antibacterial and laundering properties of AMS and PHMB as finishing agents on fabric for health care workers' uniforms. *Clothing Text Res J.* 2007;25(3):258-272. [IIA]

19. Bearman GM, Rosato A, Elam K, et al. A crossover trial of antimicrobial scrubs to reduce methicillin-resistant *Staphylococcus aureus* burden on healthcare worker apparel. *Infect Control Hosp Epidemiol.* 2012;33(3):268-275. [IA]

20. Noble WC. Dispersal of skin microorganisms. *Br J Dermatol.* 1975;93(4):477-485. [VA]

21. Benediktsdottir E, Hambraeus A. Dispersal of non-sporeforming anaerobic bacteria from the skin. *J Hyg (Lond).* 1982;88(3):487-500. [IIA]

22. Wiener-Well Y, Galuty M, Rudensky B, Schlesinger Y, Attias D, Yinnon AM. Nursing and physician attire as possible source of nosocomial infections. *Am J Infect Control.* 2011;39(7):555-559. [IIIA]

23. Krueger CA, Murray CK, Mende K, Guymon CH, Gerlinger TL. The bacterial contamination of surgical scrubs. *Am J Orthoped.* 2012;41(5):e69-e73. [IIIA]

24. Ibrahimi OA, Sharon V, Eisen DB. Surgical-site infections and routes of bacterial transfer: Which ones are most plausible? *Dermatol Surg.* 2011;37(12):1709-1720. [VA]

25. May RK, Pomeroy NP, Hers JFP, Winkler KC. Bacterial dispersion from the body surface. In: Hers JFP, Winkler KC, eds. *Airborne Transmission and Airborne Infection.* Utrecht, The Netherlands: Oosthoek Publishing Company; 1973:426-432. [IIIB]

26. Guideline for preoperative patient skin antisepsis. In: *Guidelines for Perioperative Practice.* Denver, CO: AORN, Inc; 2015:43-66. [IVA]

27. Sivanandan I, Bowker KE, Bannister GC, Soar J. Reducing the risk of surgical site infection: a case controlled study of contamination of theatre clothing. *J Periop Pract.* 2011;21(2):69-72. [IIIB]

28. Neely AN, Maley MP. Survival of enterococci and staphylococci on hospital fabrics and plastic. *J Clin Microbiol.* 2000;38(2):724-726. [IIB]

29. Neely AN, Orloff MM. Survival of some medically important fungi on hospital fabrics and plastics. *J Clin Microbiol.* 2001;39(9):3360-3361. [IIIB]

30. Treakle AM, Thom KA, Furuno JP, Strauss SM, Harris AD, Perencevich EN. Bacterial contamination of

health care workers' white coats. *Am J Infect Control.* 2009;37(2):101-105. [IIIB]

31. Munoz-Price LS, Arheart KL, Lubarsky DA, Birnbach DJ. Differential laundering practices of white coats and scrubs among health care professionals. *Am J Infect Control.* 2013;41(6):565-567. [IIIA]

32. Munoz-Price LS, Arheart KL, Mills JP, et al. Associations between bacterial contamination of health care workers' hands and contamination of white coats and scrubs. *Am J Infect Control.* 2012;40(9):e245-e248. [IIIA]

33. Butler DL, Major Y, Bearman G, Edmond MB. Transmission of nosocomial pathogens by white coats: an in-vitro model. *J Hosp Infect.* 2010;75(2):137-138. [IIIC]

34. Henderson J. The endangered white coat. *Clin Infect Dis.* 2010;50(7):1073-1074. [VB]

35. Kaplan C, Mendiola R, Ndjatou V, Chapnick E, Minkoff H. The role of covering gowns in reducing rates of bacterial contamination of scrub suits. *Am J Obstet Gynecol.* 2003;188(5):1154-1155. [IIC]

36. Loh W, Ng VV, Holton J. Bacterial flora on the white coats of medical students. *J Hosp Infect.* 2000;45(1):65-68. [IIB]

37. Banu A, Anand M, Nagi N. White coats as a vehicle for bacterial dissemination. *J Clin Diag Res.* 2012;6(8):1381-1384. [IIIA]

38. Amirfeyz R, Tasker A, Ali S, Bowker K, Blom A. Theatre shoes—a link in the common pathway of postoperative wound infection? *Ann R Coll Surg Engl.* 2007;89(6):605-608. [IIB]

39. 29 CFR §1910.136: Personal protective equipment: Occupational foot protection. Occupational Safety and Health Administration. https://www.osha.gov/pls/oshaweb/owadisp.show_document?p_table=standards&p_id=9786. Accessed September 19, 2014.

40. Barr J, Siegel D. Dangers of dermatologic surgery: protect your feet. *Dermatol Surg.* 2004;30(12 Pt 1):1495-1497. [IIB]

41. Occupational Safety and Health Administration. Toxic and Hazardous Substances: Bloodborne Pathogens, 29 CFR §1910.1030 (2012). Occupational Safety and Health Administration. http://www.osha.gov/pls/oshawewb/owadisp.show_document?p_table=STANDARDS&p_id=10051. Accessed September 19, 2014.

42. Siegel JD, Rhinehart E, Jackson M, Chiarello L; the Healthcare Infection Control Practices Advisory Committee. 2007 Guideline for Isolation Precautions: Preventing Transmission of Infectious Agents in Healthcare Settings. 2007. http://www.cdc.gov/ncidod/dhqp/pdf/isolation2007.pdf. Accessed September 19, 2014. [IVA]

43. White MC, Lynch P. Blood contact and exposures among operating room personnel: a multicenter study. *Am J Infect Control.* 1993;21(5):243-248. [IIIA]

44. Barbosa MH, Graziano KU. Influence of wearing time on efficacy of disposable surgical masks as microbial barrier. *Braz J Microbiol.* 2006;37(3):216-217. [IIB]

45. Kotsanas D, Scott C, Gillespie EE, Korman TM, Stuart RL. What's hanging around your neck? Pathogenic bacteria on identity badges and lanyards. *Med J Aust.* 2008;188(1):5-8. [IIA]

46. Saxena S, Singh T, Agarwal H, Mehta G, Dutta R. Bacterial colonization of rings and cell phones carried by health-care providers: are these mobile bacterial zoos in the hospital? *Trop Doct.* 2011;41(2):116-118. [IIB]

47. Bartlett GE, Pollard TC, Bowker KE, Bannister GC. Effect of jewelry on surface bacterial counts of operating theatres. *J Hosp Infect.* 2002;52(1):68-70. [IIB]

48. Field EA, McGowan P, Pearce PK, Martin MV. Rings and watches: should they be removed prior to operative dental procedures? *J Dent.* 1996;24(1-2):65-69. [IIB]

49. Kelsall NKR, Griggs RKL, Bowker KE, Bannister GC. Should finger rings be removed prior to scrubbing for theatre? *J Hosp Infect.* 2006;62(4):450-452. [IIB]

50. Jeans AR, Moore J, Nicol C, Bates C, Read RC. Wristwatch use and hospital-acquired infection. *J Hosp Infect.* 2010;74(1):16-21. [IIIA]

51. Salisbury DM, Hutfilz P, Treen LM, Bollin GE, Gautam S. The effect of rings on microbial load of health care workers' hands. *Am J Infect Control.* 1997;25(1):24-27. [IIIB]

52. Khodavaisy S, Nabili M, Davari B, Vahedi M. Evaluation of bacterial and fungal contamination in the health care workers' hands and rings in the intensive care unit. *J Prev Med Hyg.* 2011;52(4):215-218. [IIIB]

53. Arrowsmith VA, Taylor R. Removal of nail polish and finger rings to prevent surgical infection. *Cochrane Database Syst Rev.* 2012;5:003325. [IA]

54. Trick WE, Vernon MO, Hayes RA, et al. Impact of ring wearing on hand contamination and comparison of hand hygiene agents in a hospital. *Clin Infect Dis.* 2003;36(11):1383-1390. [IIA]

55. Stein DT, Pankovich-Wargula AL. The dilemma of the wedding band. *Orthopedics.* 2009;32(2):86. [IIIC]

56. Wood MW, Lund RC, Stevenson KB. Bacterial contamination of stethoscopes with antimicrobial diaphragm covers. *Am J Infect Control.* 2007;35(4):263-266. [IIB]

57. Bernard L, Kereveur A, Durand D, et al. Bacterial contamination of hospital physicians' stethoscopes. *Infect Control Hosp Epidemiol.* 1999;20(9):626-628. [IIB]

58. Russell A, Secrest J, Schreeder C. Stethoscopes as a source of hospital-acquired methicillin-resistant Staphylococcus aureus. *J PeriAnesth Nurs.* 2012;27(2):82-87. [IIA]

59. Mehta AK, Halvosa JS, Gould CV, Steinberg JP. Efficacy of alcohol-based hand rubs in the disinfection of stethoscopes. *Infect Control Hosp Epidemiol.* 2010;31(8):870-872. [IIB]

60. Denholm JT, Levine A, Kerridge IH, Ashhurst-Smith C, Ferguson J, D'Este C. A microbiological survey of stethoscopes in Australian teaching hospitals: potential for nosocomial infection? *Aust Infect Control.* 2005;10(3):79. [IIA]

61. Waghorn DJ, Wan WY, Greaves C, Whittome N, Bosley HC, Cantrill S. Stethoscopes: a study of contamination and the effectiveness of disinfection procedures. *Br J Infect Control.* 2005;6(1):15-17. [IIB]

62. Gopinath KG, Stanley S, Mathai E, Chandy GM. Pagers and stethoscopes as vehicles of potential nosocomial pathogens in a tertiary care hospital in a developing country. *Trop Doct.* 2011;41(1):43-45. [IIIB]

63. Muniz J, Sethi RK, Zaghi J, Ziniel SI, Sandora TJ. Predictors of stethoscope disinfection among pediatric health care providers. *Am J Infect Control.* 2012;40(10):922-925. [IIIA]

64. Hyder O. Cross-sectional study of frequency and factors associated with stethoscope cleaning among medical practitioners in Pakistan. *East Mediterr Health J.* 2012;18(7):707-711. [IIIA]

65. Uneke CJ, Ogbonna A, Oyibo PG, Onu CM. Bacterial contamination of stethoscopes used by health workers: public health implications. *J Infect Develop Countries.* 2010;4(7):436-441. [IIIA]

66. Uneke CJ, Ogbonna A, Oyibo PG, Ekuma U. Bacteriological assessment of stethoscopes used by medical students in Nigeria: implications for nosocomial infection control. *World Health Popul.* 2008;10(4):53-61. [IIIB]

67. Bhatta DR, Gokhale S, Ansari MT, et al. Stethoscopes: a possible mode for transmission of nosocomial pathogens. *J Clin Diag Res.* 2012;5(6):1173-1176. [IIIB]

68. Campos-Murguia A, Leon-Lara X, Munoz JM, Macias AE, Alvarez JA. Stethoscopes as potential intrahospital carriers of pathogenic microorganisms. *Am J Infect Control.* 2013;42(1):82-83. [IIIB]

69. Worster AP, Srigley JA, Main CL. Examination of staphylococcal stethoscope contamination in the emergency department (pilot) study (EXSSCITED pilot study). *Can J Emerg Med.* 2011;13(4):239-244. [IIIB]

70. Williams C, Davis DL. Methicillin-resistant Staphylococcus aureus fomite survival. *Clin Lab Sci.* 2009;22(1):34-38. [IIIB]

71. Mitchell A, Dealwis N, Collins J, et al. Stethoscope or "staphoscope"? Infection by auscultation. *J Hosp Infect.* 2010;76(3):278-279. [IIIB]

72. Milam MW, Hall M, Pringle T, Buchanan K. Bacterial contamination of fabric stethoscope covers: the velveteen rabbit of health care? *Infect Control Hosp Epidemiol.* 2001;22(10):653-655. [IIIC]

73. Guideline for environmental cleaning. In: *Guidelines for Perioperative Practice.* Denver, CO: AORN, Inc; 2015:9-30. [IVA]

74. Feldman J, Feldman J, Feldman M. Women doctors' purses as an unrecognized fomite. *Del Med J.* 2012;84(9):277-280. [IIA]

75. Lankford MG, Collins S, Youngberg L, Rooney DM, Warren JR, Noskin GA. Assessment of materials commonly utilized in health care: implications for bacterial survival and transmission. *Am J Infect Control.* 2006;34(5):258-263. [IIIB]

76. Koca O, Altoparlak U, Ayyildiz A, Kaynar H. Persistence of nosocomial pathogens on various fabrics. *Eurasian J Med.* 2012;44(1):28-31. [IIIA]

77. Huang R, Mehta S, Weed D, Price CS. Methicillin-resistant Staphylococcus aureus survival on hospital fomites. *Infect Control Hosp Epidemiol.* 2006;27(11):1267-1269. [IIIC]

78. Malik YS, Allwood PB, Hedberg CW, Goyal SM. Disinfection of fabrics and carpets artificially contaminated with calicivirus: relevance in institutional and healthcare centres. *J Hosp Infect.* 2006;63(2):205-210. [IIIB]

79. McNeil E. Dissemination of microorganisms by fabrics and leather. *Dev Ind Microbiol.* 1964;5:30-35. [VB]

80. Datta P, Rani H, Chander J, Gupta V. Bacterial contamination of mobile phones of health care workers. *Indian J Med Microbiol.* 2009;27(3):279-281. [IB]

81. Kilic IH, Ozaslan M, Karagoz ID, Zer Y, Davutoglu V. The microbial colonisation of mobile phone used by healthcare staffs. *Pak J Biol Sci.* 2009;12(11):882-884. [IIA]

82. Albrecht UV, von Jan U, Sedlacek L, Groos S, Suerbaum S, Vonberg RP. Standardized, app-based disinfection of iPads in a clinical and nonclinical setting: comparative analysis. *J Med Internet Res.* 2013;15(8):e176. [IIA]

83. Al-Abdalall AH. Isolation and identification of microbes associated with mobile phones in Dammam in eastern Saudi Arabia. *J Family Community Med.* 2010;17(1):11-14. [IIIA]

84. Brady RR, Chitnis S, Stewart RW, Graham C, Yalamarthi S, Morris K. NHS connecting for health: healthcare professionals, mobile technology, and infection control. *Telemed J E-Health.* 2012;18(4):289-291. [IIIB]

85. Tekerekoglu MS, Duman Y, Serindag A, et al. Do mobile phones of patients, companions and visitors carry multidrug-resistant hospital pathogens? *Am J Infect Control.* 2011;39(5):379-381. [IIIA]

86. Sadat-Ali M, Al-Omran AK, Azam Q, et al. Bacterial flora on cell phones of health care providers in a teaching institution. *Am J Infect Control.* 2010;38(5):404-405. [IIIA]

87. Akinyemi KO, Atapu AD, Adetona OO, Coker AO. The potential role of mobile phones in the spread of bacterial infections. *J Infect Dev Countries.* 2009;3(8):628-632. [IIIB]

88. Basol R, Beckel J, Gilsdorf-Gracie J, et al. You missed a spot! Disinfecting shared mobile phones. *Nurs Manage.* 2013;44(7):16-18. [IIIC]

89. White S, Topping A, Humphreys P, Rout S, Williamson H. The cross-contamination potential of mobile telephones. *J Res Nurs.* 2012;17(6):582-595. [IIIB]

90. Ustun C, Cihangiroglu M. Health care workers' mobile phones: a potential cause of microbial cross-contamination between hospitals and community. *J Occup Environ Hyg.* 2012;9(9):538-542. [IIIB]

91. Singh A, Purohit B. Mobile phones in hospital settings: a serious threat to infection. *Occup Health Saf.* 2012;81(3):42-44. [VA]

92. Gerba CP, Kennedy D. Enteric virus survival during household laundering and impact of disinfection with sodium hypochlorite. *Appl Environ Microbiol.* 2007;73(14):4425-4428. [IIA]

93. Lis DO, Pacha JZ, Idzik D. Methicillin resistance of airborne coagulase-negative staphylococci in homes of persons having contact with a hospital environment. *Am J Infect Control.* 2009;37(3):177-182. [IIIB]

94. Twomey CL, Beitz H Johnson BJ. Bacterial contamination of surgical scrubs and laundering mechanisms: infection control implications. *Infection Control Today.* http://www.arta1.com/cms/uploads/Bacterial%20Contamination%20of%20Surgical%20Scrubs%20and%20Laundering%20Mechanisms_%20Infection%20Control%20Implications.pdf. Posted October 19, 2009. Accessed on September 23, 2014. [IIIB]

95. Wright SN, Gerry JS, Busowski MT, et al. Gordonia bronchialis sternal wound infection in 3 patients following open heart surgery: intraoperative transmission from a healthcare worker. *Infect Control Hosp Epidemiol.* 2012;33(12):1238-1241. [VA]

96. Fijan S, Turk SS. Hospital textiles, are they a possible vehicle for healthcare-associated infections? *Int J Environ Res Public Health.* 2012;9(9):3330-3343. [VA]

97. Halliwell C. Nurses' uniforms: off the radar. A review of guidelines and laundering practices. *Healthc Infect.* 2012;17(1):18-24. [VA]

98. Nguyen DB, Gupta N, Abou-Daoud A, et al. A polymicrobial outbreak of surgical site infections following cardiac surgery at a community hospital in Florida, 2011-2012. *Am J Infect Control.* 2014;42(4):432-435. [VB]

99. Orr KE, Holliday MG, Jones AL, Robson I, Perry JD. Survival of enterococci during hospital laundry processing. *J Hosp Infect.* 2002;50(2):133-139. [IIA]

100. Sasahara T, Hayashi S, Morisawa Y, Sakihama T, Yoshimura A, Hirai Y. Bacillus cereus bacteremia outbreak due to contaminated hospital linens. *Eur J Clin Microbiol Infect Dis.* 2011;30(2):219-226. [VB]

101. Al-Benna S. Laundering of theatre scrubs at home. *J Periop Pract.* 2010;20(11):392-396. [VA]

102. Belkin NL. Masks, barriers, laundering, and gloving: where is the evidence? *AORN J.* 2006;84(4):655-657. [VB]

103. Belkin NL. Laundry day: processing linens, textiles and uniforms. *Health Facil Manage.* 2010;23(3):36-38. [VC]

104. Heinzel M, Kyas A, Weide M, Breves R, Bockmühl DP. Evaluation of the virucidal performance of domestic laundry procedures. *Int J Hyg Environ Health.* 2010;213(5):334-337. [IIIB]

105. Lakdawala N, Pham J, Shah M, Holton J. Effectiveness of low-temperature domestic laundry on the decontamination of healthcare workers' uniforms. *Infect Control Hosp Epidemiol.* 2011;32(11):1103-1108. [IIIA]

106. Nordstrom JM, Reynolds KA, Gerba CP. Comparison of bacteria on new, disposable, laundered, and unlaundered hospital scrubs. *Am J Infect Control.* 2012;40(6):539-543. [IIIA]

107. Patel SN, Murray-Leonard J, Wilson AP. Laundering of hospital staff uniforms at home. *J Hosp Infect.* 2006;62(1):89-93. [IIA]

108. Wilson JA, Loveday HP, Hoffman PN, Pratt RJ. Uniform: an evidence review of the microbiological significance of uniforms and uniform policy in the prevention and control of healthcare-associated infections. Report to the Department of Health (England). *J Hosp Infect.* 2007;66(4):301-307. [VA]

109. Perry C, Marshall R, Jones E. Bacterial contamination of uniforms. *J Hosp Infect.* 2001;48(3):238-241. [IIIB]

110. *Accreditation Standards for Processing Reusable Textiles for Use in Healthcare Facilities.* 2011 ed. Frankfort, IL: Healthcare Laundry Accreditation Council; 2011.

111. Protecting Workers' Families—DHHS(NIOSH) Pub No. 2002-113. National Institutes for Occupational Safety and Health. http://www.cdc.gov/niosh/docs/2002-113/2002-113.html. Accessed September 19, 2014. [VB]

112. ANSI/AAMI. ST65 2008/(R) 2013: *Processing of Reusable Surgical textiles for Use in Health Care Facilities.* 2013. Arlington, VA: Association for the Advancement of Medical Instrumentation; 2013. [IVC]

113. Callaghan I. Bacterial contamination of nurses' uniforms: a study. *Nurs Stand.* 1998;13(1):37-42. [IIIB]

114. 29 CFR §1910.132: General requirements. Occupational Safety and Health Administration. https://www.osha.gov/pls/oshaweb/owadisp.show_document?p_id=9777&p_table=STANDARDS. Accessed September 19, 2014.

115. Summers MM, Lynch PF, Black T. Hair as a reservoir of staphylococci. *J Clin Path.* 1965;18(13):13-15. [IIB]

116. Dineen P, Drusin L. Epidemics of postoperative wound infections associated with hair carriers. *Lancet.* 1973;2(7839):1157-1159. [VA]

117. Mastro TD, Farley TA, Elliott JA, et al. An outbreak of surgical-wound infections due to group A streptococcus carried on the scalp. *N Engl J Med.* 1990;323(14):968-972. [IIIB]

118. McHugh SM, Corrigan MA, Hill AD, Humphreys H. Surgical attire, practices and their perception in the prevention of surgical site infection. *Surgeon.* 2014;12(1):47-52. [VA]

119. Eisen DB. Surgeon's garb and infection control: what's the evidence? *J Am Acad Dermatol.* 2011;64(5):960.e1-960.e20. [VA]

120. Mase K, Hasegawa T, Horii T, et al. Firm adherence of Staphylococcus aureus and Staphylococcus epidermidis to human hair and effect of detergent treatment. *Microbiol Immunol.* 2000;44(8):653-656. [IIB]

121. McLure HA, Mannam M, Talboys CA, Azadian BS, Yentis SM. The effect of facial hair and sex on the dispersal of bacteria below a masked subject. *Anaesthesia.* 2000;55(2):173-176. [IIIC]

122. Owers KL, James E, Bannister GC. Source of bacterial shedding in laminar flow theatres. *J Hosp Infect.* 2004;58(3):230-232. [IIIC]

123. Occupational exposure to bloodborne pathogens. OSHA Final rule. *Fed Regist.* 1991;56(235):64004-64182.

Acknowledgements

Lead Author
Lisa Spruce, DNP, RN, ACNS, ACNP, ANP, CNOR
Director of Evidence-based Perioperative Practice
AORN Nursing Department
Denver, Colorado

Co-author
Sharon A. Van Wicklin, MSN, RN, CNOR, CRNFA, CPSN, PLNC
Perioperative Nursing Specialist
AORN Nursing Department
Denver, Colorado

Contributing Author
Ramona L. Conner, MSN, RN, CNOR
Manager, Standards and Guidelines
AORN Nursing Department
Denver, Colorado

The authors and AORN thank Paula Berrett, BS, CRCST, Utah Valley Regional Medical Center, Provo, Utah, International Association of Healthcare Central Service Material Management liaison to the AORN Guidelines Advisory Board; Angela Hewett, MD, MS, University of Nebraska Medical Center, Omaha, Nebraska, Society for Healthcare Epidemiology of America liaison to the AORN Guidelines Advisory Board; Antonia B. Hughes, MA, BSN, RN, CNOR, Perioperative Education Specialist, Baltimore Washington Medical Center, Glen Burnie, Maryland; Deborah Mulloy, PhD, RN, CNOR, Brigham & Womens Hospital, Newtonville, Massachusetts; Janice A. Neil, RN, PhD, American Association of Colleges of Nursing Leadership Fellow, Associate Professor and Chair, Department of Undergraduate Nursing Science, East Carolina University College of Nursing, Greenville, North Carolina; and Marcia R. Patrick, MSN, RN, CIC, Association for Professionals in Infection Control and Epidemiology liaison to the AORN Guidelines Advisory Board and Independent Consultant, Tacoma, Washington, for their assistance in developing this guideline.

Publication History

Originally published March 1975, *AORN Journal*, as AORN "Standards for proper OR wearing apparel." Format revision March 1978, July 1982.

Revised March 1984, March 1990. Published as proposed recommended practices, August 1994.

Revised November 1998; published December 1998. Reformatted July 2000.

Revised November 2004; published in *Standards, Recommended Practices, and Guidelines*, 2005 edition. Reprinted February 2005, *AORN Journal.*

Revised October 2010 for online publication in *Perioperative Standards and Recommended Practices*.

Reformatted September 2012 for publication in *Perioperative Standards and Recommended Practices*, 2013 edition.

Revised September 2014 for online publication in *Perioperative Standards and Recommended Practices*.

Minor editing revisions made in November 2014 for publication in *Guidelines for Perioperative Practice*, 2015 edition.

SURGICAL ATTIRE

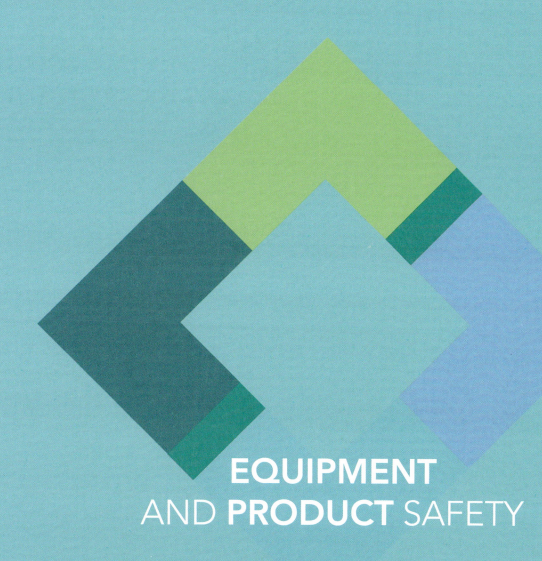

EQUIPMENT AND **PRODUCT** SAFETY

GUIDELINE FOR ELECTROSURGERY

The Guideline for Electrosurgery was developed by the AORN Recommended Practices Committee and was approved by the AORN Board of Directors. It was presented as proposed recommendations for comments by members and others. The guideline is effective July 1, 2009. The recommendations in the guideline are intended to be achievable and represent what is believed to be an optimal level of practice. Policies and procedures will reflect variations in practice settings and/or clinical situations that determine the degree to which the guideline can be implemented. AORN recognizes the various settings in which perioperative nurses practice; therefore, this guideline is adaptable to various practice settings. These practice settings include traditional operating rooms (ORs), ambulatory surgery centers, physicians' offices, cardiac catheterization laboratories, endoscopy suites, radiology departments, and all other areas where surgery and other invasive procedures may be performed.

Purpose

This document provides guidance to perioperative nurses in the use and care of electrosurgical equipment, including high frequency, ultrasound, and argon beam modalities. Proper care and handling of electrosurgical equipment are essential to patient and personnel safety. Electrosurgery, using high frequency (ie, radio frequency) electrical current, is used routinely to cut, coagulate, dissect, ablate, and shrink body tissue. Ultrasonic dissectors fragment tissue by vibration. Vessel sealing devices use a combination of pressure and heat to permanently fuse vessels and tissue. This guideline addresses all of these technologies and does not endorse any specific product.

Recommendation I

Personnel selecting new and refurbished electrosurgical units (ESUs) and accessories for purchase or use should make decisions based on safety features to minimize risks to patients and personnel.

ESUs and accessories are high-risk medical devices. Minimum safety standards for ESU systems have been developed by the Association for the Advancement of Medical Instrumentation (AAMI), approved by the American National Standards Institute (ANSI), and the International Electrotechnical Commission (IEC).[1]

I.a. ESUs and accessories should be selected based on safety features that minimize patient and personnel injury.[2]

Historically, the most frequently reported patient injury has been a skin injury (eg, burn) at the dispersive electrode site.[2] The risk of this type of injury has been minimized through advances in dispersive pad design and the use of return electrode contact quality monitoring.[2,3]

I.b. ESUs and accessories should be selected to include technology that minimizes the risk of alternate site injuries.

These injuries can result from use of ground-referenced (ie, spark-gap) ESUs that allow electrical current to seek alternate pathways to complete the circuit.[1,4] The use of isolated generator ESUs has minimized this risk.[5]

I.c. ESUs and accessories should be selected to include technology that minimizes or eliminates the risk of insulation failure and capacitive coupling injuries.

During minimally invasive procedures, alternate site injuries have resulted from insulation failure and capacitive coupling.[2,4,6-9] These injuries are far more serious than skin burns and have increased in number with the increased use of minimally invasive surgery.[10] Active electrode monitoring, active electrode insulation integrity testers, active electrode indicator shafts, and visual inspection minimize these risks.[7,9,11-14]

I.d. ESUs and accessories should be designed to minimize the risk of unintentional activation.

Unintentional activation has resulted in patient and personnel injuries. Unintentional ESU activation has been reported as the cause of 56% of alternate site injuries.[2,15] Audible activation tones minimize this risk.[1,15-17]

I.e. Electrosurgical accessories should be compatible with the ESU.

Injuries have resulted when an ESU accessory intended for bipolar use was inserted into monopolar connectors and subsequently activated.[1] Appropriate matching and use of accessories specific to the ESU minimizes this risk.

I.f. Health care organizations should attempt to standardize electrosurgical equipment used within the facility.

Equipment standardization reduces the risk of error.[18]

ELECTROSURGERY

Recommendation II

The ESU should be used in a manner that minimizes the potential for injuries.

Electrosurgical units are high-risk equipment.[1] Potential complications of electrosurgery include patient injuries, user injuries, fires, and electromagnetic interference with other medical equipment and internal electronic devices.[2] Electrosurgery safety is heightened by adhering to good practices.[18] Adverse events (eg, patient burns and fires) may be reduced by adhering to basic principles of electrosurgery safety.[15]

II.a. Instructions for ESU use, warranties, and a manual for maintenance and inspections should be obtained from the manufacturer and be readily available to users.[2,19]

Equipment manuals assist in developing operational, safety, and maintenance guidelines, as well as serve as a reference for appropriate use.[19]

II.a.1. Concise, clearly readable operating instructions specific for the device should be on or attached to each ESU.[19]

Readily available instructions reduce the risk of operator error.

II.b. The ESU should be securely mounted on a tip-resistant cart or shelf and should not be used as a shelf or table.

II.c. The ESU should be protected from liquids.[19]

Liquids entering the ESU can cause unintentional activation, device failure, or an electrical hazard.

II.c.1. Liquids should not be placed on top of the ESU.

II.c.2. Foot pedal accessories should be encased in a clean, impervious cover when there is potential for fluid spills on the floor.

II.d. Safety and warning alarms and activation indicators should be operational, audible, and visible at all times.[1,16-18,20]

Safety and warning alarms alert the operator to potential electrode failure.[5] The indicators and alarms immediately alert the perioperative team when the ESU is activated.[2,18]

II.e. The ESU should be visually inspected and the return electrode monitor tested according to manufacturer's instructions before use.[19,20]

The ESU will sound an alarm and not activate if the dispersive electrode is disconnected.[2,20]

II.f. Settings should be based on the operator's preference consistent with the intended application and the manufacturer's written instructions for patient size, active electrode type, and return electrode placement.

The ESU's power output capability is dependent on multiple variables related to the patient, generator, accessories, and the procedure.

II.f.1. The circulating nurse should confirm the power settings with the operator before activation of the ESU.

II.f.2. The ESU should be operated at the lowest effective power setting needed to achieve the desired tissue effect.[2,18,20-22]

The likelihood of arcing and capacitive coupling are increased when higher than necessary voltages are used.[22]

II.f.3. If the operator requests a continual increase in power, personnel should check the entire ESU and accessories circuit for adequate placement of the dispersive electrode and cord connections.[18,19,23]

Prolonged current at high power can cause patient injury. Common causes of ineffective coagulation and cutting are high impedance at the dispersive electrode, poor contact between the dispersive electrode and the patient, and use of an electrolytic irrigation/distention solution.[23,24]

II.f.4. The electrode tip should be visually inspected before each use and replaced if damaged.

A damaged active electrode tip may cause a buildup of eschar, creating increased resistance at the electrode tip. Cleaning a stainless steel tip with an abrasive pad or instrument may create grooves where eschar can collect.[22]

II.g. Perioperative registered nurses should be aware of potential patient safety hazards associated with specific internal implanted electronic devices (IEDs) and the appropriate patient care interventions required to protect the patient from injury.[25]

Electronic devices implanted in a patient may be affected by other IEDs or medical equipment with which a patient may come into contact in a health care facility. These devices may include cardiac pacemakers, implanted cardioverter defibrillators (ICDs), neurostimulators, implantable hearing devices, implantable infusion pumps, and osteogenic stimulators.[25]

II.h. After use, personnel should
- turn off the ESU;
- dispose of single use items;
- clean all reusable parts and accessories according to the manufacturer's directions; and
- inspect accessories and parts for damage, function, and cleanliness.

Following the manufacturer's cleaning and inspection instructions promotes safe and proper functioning of the equipment.

II.i. An ESU that is not working properly or is damaged should be removed from service immediately and reported to the designated individual

ELECTROSURGERY

responsible for equipment maintenance (eg, bio-engineering services personnel).[18,19,26]

Medical device users are required to report serious injury and death related to use of a device to the US Food and Drug Administration (FDA).[26]

Recommendation III

The electrical cords and plugs of the ESU should be handled in a manner that minimizes the potential for damage and subsequent patient and user injuries.

Improper handling of cords and plugs may result in breaks in the cord's insulation, fraying, and other electrical hazards.

III.a. The ESU's electrical cord should be adequate in length and flexibility to reach the electrical outlet without stress or the use of an extension cord.[19]

Tension on the electrical cord increases the risk that it will become disconnected, frayed, or move the equipment, which may result in injuries to patients and personnel.

III.a.1. The ESU should be placed near the sterile field, and the cord should reach the wall or column outlet without stress on the cord and without blocking a traffic path.[19]

Stress on the cord may cause damage to the cord, posing an electrical hazard.

III.a.2. The electrical cord should be free of kinks, knots, and bends.

Kinks, knots, and bends could damage the cord or cause leakage, current accumulation, and overheating of the cord's insulation.

III.a.3. The ESU plug, not the cord, should be held when it is removed from the outlet.

Pulling on the cord may cause cord breakage, which poses a fire hazard.

III.a.4. The ESU's cord should be kept dry.[19]

Fluids in or around the ESU connections and cord may cause an electrical hazard as a result of a short circuit.

III.b. The ESU's cord should be inspected or electrically tested for outer insulation damage.[19]

Cord failures can result in a fire or patient and personnel injuries.

III.b.1. The ESU should be removed from use if there is any evidence of breaks, nicks, or cracks in the outer insulation coating of the electrical cord.[19]

Recommendation IV

The active electrode should be used in a manner that minimizes the potential for injuries.

Incomplete circuitry, unintentional activation, and incompatibility of the active electrode to the ESU may result in patient and personnel injuries.[16,27]

IV.a. The active electrode should be visually inspected at the surgical field before use. Inspection should include but is not limited to
- identifying any apparent damage to the cord or hand piece (eg, impaired insulation),[19] and
- ensuring compatibility of the active electrode, accessories, the ESU, and the procedure.

Insulation failures allow an alternate pathway for current to leave the electrode and may result in an electrical shock or other injury.

IV.a.1. A damaged and/or incompatible active electrode, accessory, or ESU should be immediately removed from use.

IV.b. When not in use, the active electrode should be placed in a clean, dry, non-conductive safety holster.[2,15,22,28] A plastic or other non-conductive device should be used to secure the active electrode cord to the sterile drapes.[22]

Use of a non-conductive safety holster prevents the active electrode from falling off the sterile field and unintentional activation. Unintentional activation of the active electrode may cause burns of the patient, drapes, or personnel.[2,15]

IV.b.1. The protective cap of a battery-powered, hand-held cautery should be in place when the cautery is not in use.[29,30]

Application of the protective cap prevents unintended pressure on the activation button.[29,30]

IV.c. The electrode cord should be kept free of kinks and coils during use.

Kinks, knots, and bends could damage the cord, cause current leakage or accumulation, overheat the cord's insulation, or produce unanticipated changes in the surgical effect. "Hot spots" or field intensification are produced by coiling cables. Keeping the cords free of kinks and coils minimizes the risk of patient or personnel injury from conduction of stray current and capacitive current.[21]

IV.d. The active electrode should be connected directly into a designated receptacle on the ESU.

Incompatibility of the active electrode with the ESU may result in patient and personnel injuries.

IV.d.1. When needed, only adaptors approved by the manufacturers of both the ESU and the accessory should be used.

IV.e. Only the user of the active electrode should activate the device whether it is hand or foot controlled.[20,28]

Activation by the user of the active electrode prevents unintentional discharge of the device

123

ELECTROSURGERY

to minimize potential for patient and personnel injury.

IV.f. Active electrode tips should be used according to the manufacturer's instructions.

Failure to use the active electrode as outlined in the manufacturer's directions for use have resulted in patient injuries and surgical fires.[31-34]

IV.f.1. The active electrode tip
- should be compatible with the ESU,
- should be securely seated into the hand piece, and
- should not be altered.[34]

A loose electrode tip may cause a spark or burn tissue that comes in contact with the exposed, non-insulated section of the tip.[31,34] Bending the tip can damage the device and alter the desired function. Fires and patient injuries have resulted when insulating sheaths have been made from inappropriate material (eg, rubber catheters).[32,33]

IV.g. The active electrode tip should be cleaned away from the incision whenever there is visible eschar.[32]

Eschar buildup on the active electrode tip impedes the desired current flow, causing the entire unit to function less effectively and serving as a fuel source, which can lead to fires.[32] Debris on the electrode tip can tear tissue, cause re-bleeding, and serve as a foreign body when deposited in the wound.[22]

IV.g.1. Methods to remove debris from the active electrode tip should include but are not limited to
- a moistened sponge or instrument wipe to clean non-stick coated electrosurgical tips on the sterile field,[16,32] and
- abrasive electrode cleaning pads to remove eschar from non-coated electrodes on the sterile field.[32]

IV.g.2. The active electrode tip should not be cleaned with a scalpel blade.

Cleaning with a scalpel blade puts perioperative personnel at risk for a percutaneous injury.[35]

IV.h. If the active electrode becomes contaminated, it should be disconnected from the ESU and removed from the sterile field.

Disconnection of the contaminated active electrode minimizes the risk of unintentional activation and reduces the potential for patient and personnel injuries.[16]

IV.i. If an active monopolar electrode is being used in a fluid-filled cavity, the fluid used should be an electrically inert, near isotonic solution (eg, dextran 10, dextran 70, glycine 1.5%, sorbitol, mannitol) unless the equipment manufacturer's written directions for use instruct otherwise.[2,24]

Using an electrolyte solution instead of a nonconductive medium may render the active electrode less effective. Electrolyte solutions conduct and disperse the electrical current away from the intended site.[18,24]

IV.j. Fire safety measures should be followed when electrosurgery is in use according to local, state, and federal regulations.[36,37]

IV.j.1. Active electrodes should not be activated in the presence of flammable agents (eg, antimicrobial skin prep or hand antisepsis agents, tinctures, de-fatting agents, collodion, petroleum-based lubricants, phenol, aerosol adhesives, uncured methyl methacrylate) until the agents are dry and vapors have dissipated.[2,38-42]

Alcohol-based prep agents remain flammable until completely dry. Vapors occurring during evaporation also are flammable. Trapping of solution or vapors under incise or surgical drapes increases the risk of fire or burn injury. Alcohol-based skin prep agents are particularly hazardous because the surrounding hair or fabric can become saturated. Pooling can occur in body folds and crevices (eg, umbilicus, sternal notch). Ignition of flammable substances by active electrodes has caused fires and patient injuries. Flammable prep agents can be safely used by adhering to NFPA standards, local fire codes, and AORN recommendations and guidance statements. Use of nonflammable prep agents will minimize this risk.[16,42-46]

IV.j.2. Caution should be used during surgery on the head and neck when using an active electrode in the presence of combustible anesthetic gases.[2,44,47]

IV.j.3. Opened suture packets containing alcohol should be removed from the sterile field as soon as possible.[16]

Ignition of flammable substances by an active electrode has caused fires and patient injuries.[16,43]

IV.k. Sponges used near the active electrode tip should be moist to prevent unintentional ignition.[32,47,48]

Fires have resulted from ignition of dry sponges near the incision site.[16,49,50]

IV.l. When battery-powered, hand-held cautery units are used, the batteries should be removed before disposal of the cautery unit.[30]

Unintentional activation of a battery-powered, hand-held cautery unit after disposal has caused fires.[29,30]

IV.m. Electrosurgery should not be used in the presence of gastrointestinal gases.

ELECTROSURGERY

Gastrointestinal gases contain hydrogen and methane, which are highly flammable. Fires and patient injuries have occurred.[16,28,40,51,52]

IV.n. Electrosurgery should not be used in an oxygen-enriched environment.[28,32,53-55]

An oxygen-enriched environment lowers the temperature and energy at which fuels will ignite.[28,48] Fires, including airway fires, have resulted from the active electrode sparking in the presence of concentrated oxygen.[2,16,53,54]

IV.n.1. The lowest possible oxygen concentration that provides adequate patient oxygen saturation should be used.[47,48]

Mixing oygen with nonflammable gases such as medical air reduces the risk of fire.[16,47]

IV.n.2. Surgical drapes should be arranged to minimize the buildup of oxidizers (eg, oxygen and nitrous oxide) under the drapes, to allow air circulation, and to dilute the additional oxygen.[16,47,48]

IV.n.3. The active electrode should be used as far from the oxygen source as possible.

IV.o. Personnel should be prepared to immediately extinguish flames should they occur.[16,47]

A small fire can progress to a life threatening emergency of a large fire in seconds.[16] ESUs are a potential ignition source and a common cause of surgical fires and patient injury.[28]

IV.o.1. Nonflammable material (eg, wet towel, sterile saline, water) should be available on the sterile field to extinguish the fire.[16,28]

Recommendation V

When monopolar electrosurgery is used, a dispersive electrode should be used in a manner that minimizes the potential for injuries.

Patient skin injuries at the dispersive electrode site are the most reported ESU incidents.[2] Single-use dispersive electrode burns are decreasing with improved technology and the use of safety features. The reports of electrosurgical burns has decreased from 50 to 100 per month in the 1970s to one to two per month in 2007.[2]

V.a. The patient's skin condition should be assessed and documented before and after ESU use.

The most frequently reported patient injury from electrosurgery has been tissue damage (eg, burn) at the dispersive electrode site.[2] Preoperative and postoperative assessments are necessary to evaluate the patient's skin condition for possible injuries.

V.b. Return-electrode contact quality monitoring should be furnished on general purpose electrosurgery units.[18]

The technology of return-electrode contact quality monitoring inhibits the output of the ESU if the return electrode is not in contact with the patient and connected to the ESU. Return-electrode contact quality monitoring confirms that there is adequate contact between the return electrode and the patient. An audible alarm and visual indicator signals the user of a misconnection.[2,18]

V.b.1. Dual-foil return electrodes should be used.[18]

Dual-foil return electrodes are necessary for contact quality monitoring.[18] The return electrode contact quality monitoring system determines differences in impedance through patient's tissue between the two surfaces. If the impedance is too high as a result of poor contact, the alarm is triggered and the ESU stops functioning.[2]

V.c. Return-electrode continuity monitoring should be used if return-electrode contact quality monitoring is not available.

Return-electrode continuity monitoring detects breaks in the return-electrode cord or a misconnection (ie, the cord is not plugged into the ESU).[2,19]

V.c.1. If using return-electrode continuity monitoring, a single-foil electrode should be used.[2]

V.d. Dispersive electrodes should be compatible with the ESU.

Incompatibility of the electrosurgical unit and the dispersive electrode may result in patient injury.

V.e. A single-use dispersive electrode should be used once and discarded. If a single-use dispersive electrode must be repositioned, a new single-use electrode should be used.[23,56]

A reused single-use electrode may not adhere properly to the skin. Replacing the dispersive electrode provides an opportunity to examine the electrode and the patient's skin condition.

V.f. Dispersive electrodes should be an appropriate size for the patient (eg, neonate, infant, pediatric, adult) and not altered (eg, cut, folded).

Using the appropriately sized dispersive electrode reduces the concentration of current and minimizes the potential for electrosurgical injuries.

V.g. Before the application of a single-use dispersive electrode
- the manufacturer's expiration date should be verified and the dispersive electrode should not be used if it is past the manufacturer's expiration date[20];
- the package containing the dispersive electrode should be opened immediately before use[19]; and

ELECTROSURGERY

- the integrity of the dispersive electrode should be checked for flaws, damage, discoloration, adhesiveness, and dryness.[18,20,23,57]

Expired, damaged, or dry single-use dispersive electrodes may fail and lead to patient injury.

V.h. The conductive and adhesive surfaces of the single-use dispersive electrode should be placed on clean, dry skin over a large, well-perfused muscle mass on the surgical side and as close as possible to the surgical site according to the manufacturer's directions for use.[19,20]

Muscle is a better conductor of electricity than adipose tissue.[23]

V.h.1. Single-use electrodes should not be placed over bony prominences, scar tissue, hair, weight-bearing surfaces, potential pressure points, or areas distal to tourniquets.[5,18,19,23,58]

Fatty tissue, tissue over bone, scar tissue, and hair can impede electrosurgical return current flow.[59] High impedance leads to heating of the tissue, arcing to the tissue under the dispersive electrode, and subsequent burns. Adequate tissue perfusion cannot be assured if the dispersive electrode is placed distal to tourniquets or over scar tissue.[23]

V.h.2. Hair should be removed following recommended practices (ie, clipping) if it interferes with single-use electrode contact with the patient's skin.[18,20,60]

Burns have resulted when electrodes have been positioned over hairy surfaces. Hair can impede electrosurgical return current flow. Hair may interfere with adequate contact between the patient and the dispersive electrode.[23,58,61]

V.h.3. The single-use electrode should not be placed over an implanted metal prosthesis.

The tissue over prostheses contains scar tissue, which impedes return of the electric current. Although there has been no reported injury from superheating of the implant causing a tissue burn, this is a theoretical risk; therefore, it is prudent to avoid placing a dispersive electrode on the patient's skin over the site of a metal implant or prosthesis.

V.h.4. Placing the single-use dispersive electrode over a tattoo, many of which contain metallic dyes, should be avoided.

Although there have been no reported electrosurgery injuries from dispersive electrodes placed over tattoos, superheating of the tissue has occurred during magnetic resonance imaging. There is a theoretical possibility of this also happening with electrosurgery.[62-64]

V.i. Following application of the single-use dispersive electrode, uniform contact with the skin should be verified.

Injuries have been associated with inadequate adhesion of the dispersive electrode. Potential problems include tenting, gaping, and moisture, all of which interfere with adhesion to the patient's skin.[65-67]

V.i.1. Corrective measures for poor single-use dispersive electrode contact include, but are not limited to
- removing oil, lotion, moisture, or prep solution;
- removing excessive hair;
- changing sites; and
- applying a new pad.

V.i.2. Tape should not be used to hold the single-use dispersive electrode in place.

Taping the dispersive electrode may create localized pressure and increase the current concentration leading to a potential injury.[68]

V.j. The single-use dispersive electrode should be placed on the patient after final positioning.

Moving the patient after the application of the dispersive electrode may disrupt the contact to the patient's skin causing tenting, gapping, or moisture collection under the electrode. Injuries have been associated with inadequate contact of the dispersive electrode.[19,65-67]

V.j.1. If any tension is applied to the dispersive electrode cord, the perioperative registered nurse should reassess the integrity of the dispersive electrode, its contact with the patient's skin, and the connection to the ESU.

V.j.2. If the patient is repositioned, the perioperative registered nurse should verify that the dispersive electrode is in full contact with the patient's skin.

Inadequate contact of the dispersive electrode may result in a burn.[65-67]

V.k. The single-use dispersive electrode should be placed away from a warming device.[65,67]

The heat of a warming device may be cumulative with the heating of the dispersive electrode and may affect how the dispersive electrode adheres to the skin.[65,67]

V.l. Dispersive electrodes should be kept dry and protected from fluids seeping or pooling under the electrode.[23]

Liquids may prevent the electrode from adequately contacting the skin. These solutions also can cause skin injury and burns from prolonged skin exposure and concentration of electrical current.[57]

V.m. Contact between the patient and metal devices should be avoided.[69,70]

ELECTROSURGERY

Metal devices (eg, OR beds, stirrups, positioning devices, safety strap buckles) could offer a potential alternate return path for the electrical current.[69,70]

V.m.1. Patient's metal jewelry that is between the active and dispersive electrode should be removed.

Metallic jewelry, including body piercings, presents a potential risk of burn from directed current (ie, active electrode contact); heat conducted before an electrode cools; and leakage current. Eliminating metal near the activation site minimizes this risk. Jewelry that is left in place, particularly on the hands, has the potential to cause swelling at the site during surgery or recovery.[15]

V.m.2. Patient monitoring electrodes (eg, electrocardiogram, oximetry, fetal) should be placed as far away from the surgical site as possible.[21]

Alternate pathway burns have been reported at electrocardiogram (ECG) electrode sites and temperature probe entry sites with ground-referenced electrosurgery units.[19]

V.m.3. Needle electrodes for monitoring or nonsurgical functions should be avoided.[18,21]

Stray current may flow through the small contact area of the needle electrode causing a potential alternate pathway and risk of patient burn.[18,21,71,72]

V.m.4. When use of needle monitoring electrodes is medically necessary, alternate electrosurgery technologies (eg, bipolar, laser) should be considered.[18,73]

V.n. When multiple ESUs are used simultaneously during a surgical procedure, the compatibility of equipment and proper functioning of corresponding electrode monitoring systems should be verified with the manufacturer.

V.n.1. Separate single-use dispersive electrodes should be used for each ESU.

V.n.2. The dispersive electrodes should be placed as close as possible to their respective surgical sites and the single-use dispersive electrodes should not overlap.

V.o. During high-current, long-activation-time, radio-frequency (RF) ablations and other electrosurgical procedures (eg, tumor ablation, bulk tissue resection), considerations should include, but not be limited to

- identifying surgical procedures that require the use of high-current, long-activation-time RF ablation and electrosurgical techniques;
- taking inventory of RF generators that require special or multiple dispersive electrodes;
- following the manufacturer's recommendations for use of large-size dispersive electrodes or multiple dispersive electrodes;
- ensuring proper placement and full patient contact of the dispersive electrode;
- reviewing the manufacturer's directions for use and requirements for accessories;
- using and selecting the appropriate nonconductive, near-isotonic solution (eg, sorbitol, mannitol, dextran 10 or 70, glycine) for irrigation or distention unless contraindicated by manufacturer's directions; and
- using the lowest possible power settings and minimum activation time for obtaining the desired tissue effect.[2,24,74]

There is an increased risk of dispersive electrode site burns with high-current, long-activation-time procedures.[2,61,74-76]

V.o.1. When high current is not adequately dispersed by a single dispersive electrode and there are no specific manufacturer's directions, a second dispersive electrode with an adaptor or a return electrode with a larger conductive surface may be considered for use.[24,74]

A second dispersive electrode or a larger conductive surface increases the overall dispersive pad surface area for current to return to the generator.[74]

V.p. When removing the single-use dispersive electrode, the adjacent skin should be held in place and the dispersive electrode peeled back slowly.

Slowly removing the dispersive electrode will avoid denuding the surface of the skin. Skin injuries can result when the adhesive border pulls on the skin during electrode removal.[77]

V.q. Reusable, capacitive-coupled return electrode systems should be used according to manufacturers' written instructions for safe operation in conjunction with a compatible ESU.

V.q.1. Capacitive-coupling pads should be an appropriate size for the patient (ie, adult, pediatric).[78,79]

V.q.2. Skin preparation should not be performed unless otherwise recommended by the manufacturer's written directions.[78]

V.q.3. Adequate contact with the patient should be ensured by using minimal materials between the capacitive-coupled pad and patient.[79] The use of thick foam, gel pads, and extra linen between the patient and the capacitive-coupling pad should be avoided.

Distance and barriers (eg, positioning devices) between the patient and electrode may increase the risk of impedance, which can result in an alternate site injury when using a capacitive-coupling pad.[78]

V.q.4. An isolated generator should be used.[78]

ELECTROSURGERY

V.q.5. Use of a ground-referenced or grounded generators may cause a ground fault alarm.

V.q.5. The pad should be cleaned with the health care facility-approved and EPA-registered agent if contaminated with blood or body fluids in accordance with the manufacturer's directions. Acceptable cleaning solutions include a bleach solution diluted 1:10 and o-phenylphenol, o-benzyl-p-chlorophenol, or p-tertiary amylphenol.[78]

V.q.6. The integrity of the capacitive-coupled pad and cables should be checked for tears or breaks in the surface material before use, and
- pad cables should be replaced if damaged,
- surface damage may be repaired with the manufacturer's repair kit, and
- the pad should be replaced if superficial damage cannot be repaired.

V.q.7. When two ESUs are used, two capacitive-coupled pads or one capacitive-coupled pad with two cords should be used.

V.q.8. The pad should be replaced on its labeled expiration date.[78]

Recommendation VI

Personnel should take additional precautions when using electrosurgery during minimally invasive surgery.[18,80]

Minimally invasive surgery procedures using electrosurgery present unique patient safety risks, such as direct coupling of current, insulation failure, and capacitive coupling.

VI.a. Personnel should verify that the insufflation gas is nonflammable (ie, carbon dioxide).[81]

Carbon dioxide is noncombustible and will not ignite if the active electrosurgical electrode sparks.[81] Gases (eg, oxygen, nitrous oxide, air) are oxidizers that may support combustion. An oxidizer-enriched environment may enhance ignition and combustion.[28]

VI.b. Conductive trocar systems should be used.[7,8,11,82]

Conductive trocar cannulas provide a means for the electrosurgical current to flow safely between the cannula and the abdominal wall. This reduces high-density current concentration and heating of non-target tissue.[7,8,11,82]

VI.b.1. Hybrid trocar (ie, combination plastic and metal) systems should not be used.[8,82,83]

Each trocar and cannula can act as an electrical conductor inducing an electrical current from one to the other potentially causing a capacitive coupling injury.

VI.c. Minimally invasive surgery electrodes should be examined for impaired insulation before use.[11,83-85]

Insulation failure of electrodes caused by damage during use or reprocessing provides an alternate pathway for the electrical current to leave the active electrode. Some insulation failures are not visible. This has resulted in serious patient injuries.[4,7,8,11-13,85]

VI.c.1. Methods should be used to detect insulation failure, including but not limited to
- active electrode shielding and monitoring,[11,14]
- the use of active electrode indicator shafts that have two layers of insulation of different colors,[11] and
- the use of active electrode insulation integrity testers that use high DC voltage to detect full thickness insulation breaks.[11]

Active electrode shielding continuously monitors the endoscopic instruments to minimize the risks of insulation failure or capacitive-coupling injuries.[4,7-9,12-14,83]

The inner layer of the active electrode shaft of a different color is designed to show through the outer black layer if there is an insulation break.[11]

Testing of the electrode before the procedure identifies damaged electrodes that should be taken out of service. Testing of the electrode with the sterilizable probes and cables alerts the surgeon of an insulation break. The surgical field can be explored and treated if necessary.[11,85]

VI.c.2. The lowest power setting that achieves the desired result should be selected.[83]

Lower power settings for both cut and coagulation reduce the likelihood of insulation failure and capacitive-coupling injuries. Lower power settings also minimize damage from direct coupling when the active electrode is activated while in close proximity to another metal device inserted into an adjacent trocar port.[7]

VI.d. The active electrode should not be activated until it is in close proximity to the tissue.[7,8]

Activation only when in close proximity to the tissue minimizes the risk of current arcing and contacting unintended tissue.[7,8] Activating the electrode when it is not in very close proximity to the targeted tissue increases the risk of capacitive coupling. Capacitance is reduced during closed-circuit activation.

VI.e. Patients should be instructed to immediately report any postoperative signs or symptoms of electrosurgical injury. Patient postoperative care instructions should include symptoms to look for, including but not limited to,
o fever,
o inability to void,
o lower gastrointestinal bleeding,
o abdominal pain,
o abdominal distention,

- nausea,
- vomiting, and
- diarrhea.[8,86]

Symptoms of a minimally invasive electrosurgical injury can occur days after discharge from the perioperative setting and may include infection from an injured intestinal tract. Prompt reporting of electrosurgical injury symptoms ensures timely treatment and minimizes adverse outcomes.[8,84]

Recommendation VII

Bipolar active electrodes, including vessel occluding devices, should be used in a manner that minimizes the potential for injuries.

Unlike the monopolar ESU, bipolar technology incorporates an active electrode and a return electrode into a two-poled instrument, such as forceps or scissors.[6,19,53] Current flows only through the tissue contacted between two poles of the instruments; thus, the need for a dispersive electrode is eliminated.[19] This also eliminates the chance of stray or alternate pathways for current flow.[19] The bipolar ESU provides precise hemostasis or dissection at the surgical site with less potential stimulation or current spread to nearby body structures.[19]

VII.a. Molded, fixed-position pin placement bipolar cords should be used. Bipolar and monopolar plugs should be differentiated to prevent misconnections of active and return electrodes.[1,27]

Connection of a bipolar active electrode to a monopolar receptacle may activate current, causing a short circuit.

Recommendation VIII

Ultrasonic electrosurgical devices should be used in a manner that minimizes potential for injuries.

Ultrasonic devices have a generator that produces ultrasonic energy and mechanical vibrations rather than electrical energy. Ultrasonic instruments cut and coagulate by using the mechanical energy and heat that is generated to cause protein denaturation and the formation of a coagulum. A blade or probe can be used for sharp or blunt dissection, coagulation, or breaking apart of tissue without damaging adjacent tissues. Some ultrasonic dissectors incorporate an aspirator to remove tissue or fluids from the surgical field.[83,87]

VIII.a. When using an ultrasonic electrosurgical device, a dispersive electrode should not be used.

With an ultrasonic electrosurgical device, no electrical current enters the tissue; therefore, the current does not need to be returned to the generator by a dispersive electrode.[83,87]

VIII.b. Inhalation of aerosols generated by an ultrasonic electrosurgical hand piece should be minimized by implementing control measures, including but not limited to smoke evacuation systems and wall suction with an in-line ultra low penetration air (ULPA) filter.

Bio-aerosols are routinely produced by ultrasonic devices and pose a hazard to patients and perioperative professionals. Bio-aerosols contain odorless, toxic gases; vapors; dead and live cellular debris, including blood fragments; and viruses. These airborne contaminants can pose respiratory, ocular, dermatological, and other health-related risks, including mutagenic and carcinogenic potential, to patients and OR personnel. Wall suction with an in-line ULPA filter is only appropriate for a minimal amount of aerosol (ie, aerosols generated using ultrasonic electrosurgery are within the respirable range and include blood, blood by-products, and tissue).[88]

Recommendation IX

Argon enhanced coagulation (AEC) technology poses unique risks to patient and personnel safety and should be used in a manner that minimizes the potential for injury.

Each type of AEC has specific manufacturer's written operating instructions to be followed for safe operation of the unit.

IX.a. All safety measures for monopolar electrosurgery should be used when using AEC technology.

The AEC unit uses monopolar alternating current delivered to the tissue through ionized argon gas.[89] The risks of monopolar electrosurgery are present.

IX.b. Air should be purged from the argon gas line and electrode by activating the system before use, after moderate delays between activations, and between uses.[2,89,90]

Purging the argon gas line prevents delays in coagulation, minimizing the risk of gas embolism.[89] Activating without adequately purging may present the greatest risk of embolism when operating in an open cavity.[89]

IX.c. The argon gas flow should be limited to the lowest level possible that will provide the desired clinical effect.[2,90]

Argon gas flow is most likely to be directed to tissue without simultaneous coagulation when the initiation of ionization of the argon gas is delayed due to air bubbles in the argon gas line.[89]

IX.d. The active electrode should not be placed in direct contact with tissue and should be moved away from the patient's tissue after each activation.[89,90]

There is a risk of gas emboli when the active electrode is placed in direct contact with tissue.

ELECTROSURGERY

If argon gas pressure exceeds venous pressure in the circulating system and is applied to bleeding vessels, the result is a gas emboli in open surgical procedures.[2,90,91] The flow of argon gas could enter the open vessel and enter the heart.[2]

IX.e. When using the AEC unit during minimally invasive surgical procedures, personnel should follow all safety measures identified for AEC technology.

Patient injury and death have occurred as a complication of argon enhanced technology.[90]

IX.e.1. Endoscopic CO_2 insufflators should be equipped with audible and visual over-pressurization alarms that cannot be deactivated.[2,90]

The AEC acts as a secondary source of pressurized argon gas that can cause the patient's intra-abdominal pressure to rise rapidly and exceed venous pressure, possibly creating argon-enriched gas emboli formation. This has resulted in gas emboli.[90]

IX.e.2. The active electrode and argon gas line should be purged according to the manufacturer's recommendations.[2,90]

IX.e.3. The patient's intra-abdominal cavity should be flushed with several liters of CO_2 between extended activation periods.[90]

Flushing the intra-abdominal cavity with several liters of CO_2 between extended periods of deactivation reduces the potential for argon gas emboli formation.[90]

IX.f. Personnel using the AEC technology should be knowledgeable about signs, symptoms, and treatment of venous emboli.

There is a significant risk of gas embolism when AEC is used during laparoscopic procedures from abdominal over-pressurization and displacement of CO_2 by argon gas.[90]

IX.f.1. Patient monitoring should include devices that are considered effective for early detection of gas emboli (eg, end-tidal CO_2).[2,90]

Recommendation X

Potential hazards associated with surgical smoke generated in the practice setting should be identified, and safe practices established.

Surgical smoke (ie, plume) is generated from use of heat-producing instruments such as electrosurgical devices.[92,93] Airborne contaminants produced during electrosurgery have been analyzed. The electrosurgery plume contains toxic gas and vapors (eg, benzene, hydrogen cyanide, formaldehyde); bio-aerosols; dead and living cell material, including blood fragments; and viruses.[94-99] Many additional hazardous chemical compounds have been noted in surgical smoke.[95,99-102]

At some level, these contaminants have been shown to have an unpleasant odor, cause problems with visibility of the surgical site, cause ocular and upper respiratory tract irritation, and demonstrate mutagenic and carcinogenic potential.[94-96] The bacterial and/or viral contamination of smoke plume remains controversial, but has been highlighted by different studies.[103,104]

X.a. Surgical smoke should be removed by use of a smoke evacuation system in both open and minimally invasive procedures to prevent occupational exposure to airborne contaminants generated by electrosurgery.[94]

The National Institute for Occupational Safety and Health (NIOSH) recommends that smoke evacuation systems be used as the primary control to reduce potential acute and chronic health risks to health care personnel and patients.[95]

Local exhaust ventilation (LEV) is the primary means to protect health care personnel from occupational exposure to airborne contaminant generated by electrosurgery.[94] Potential health and liability risks may be reduced by the evacuation of surgical smoke.[96]

X.a.1. When surgical smoke is generated, an individual smoke evacuation unit with a 0.1 micron filter (eg, ultra-low particulate air [ULPA] or high efficiency particulate air [HEPA]) should be used to remove surgical smoke.[94,95]

During electrosurgery, cells are heated to a high temperature, which causes the cell membrane to rupture, releasing particles into the air. Electrosurgical procedures create particles approximately 0.7 microns in size.[99]

X.a.2. The capture device (eg, wand, nonflammable suction tip) of the smoke evacuation system should be positioned as close as possible, and no greater than 2 inches (5.08 cm), from the source of the smoke.[95,96,99]

Close proximity of the smoke evacuation wand maximizes particulate matter and odor capture and enhances visibility at the surgical site.[105]

X.a.3. Smoke evacuation units and accessories should be used according to manufacturers' written instructions.

Detectable odor during the use of a smoke evacuation system is a signal that
- smoke is not being captured at the site where the plume is being generated,
- inefficient air movement through the suction or smoke evacuation wand is occurring, or
- the filter has exceeded its usefulness and should be replaced.[96]

X.a.4. When a central suction system is used to evacuate smoke, a 0.1 micron in-line filter (eg, ULPA filter) should be used.[95,105,106] The in-line filter should be placed between the suction wall/ceiling connection and the suction canister.[94]

ELECTROSURGERY

Central suction units with an in-line 0.1 micron filter remove airborne contaminants.[95] Low suction rates associated with centralized suction units limit their efficiency in evacuating plume, making them suitable only for the evacuation of small amounts of plume.[96,106]

X.a.5. When a centralized system dedicated for smoke evacuation is available, the smoke evacuator lines should be flushed according to the manufacturer's instructions to prevent particulate matter buildup or contamination of the suction line.

X.b. Used smoke evacuator filters, tubing, and wands should be considered potentially infectious waste. These used devices should be handled using standard precautions and disposed of as biohazardous waste.[94-96]

Airborne contaminants produced during electrosurgical procedures have been analyzed and shown to contain gaseous toxic compounds, bioaerosols, and dead and living cell material.[95-97,99] Bacterial and/or viral contamination of smoke plume also has been identified.[103,104]

X.c. Personnel should wear respiratory protection (ie, fit-tested surgical N95 filtering face piece respirator, high-filtration surgical mask) during procedures that generate surgical smoke as secondary protection against residual plume that has escaped capture by LEV, the primary means of protection.[94,105,107,108]

Analysis of the airborne contaminants produced during electrosurgery has shown that the smoke plume contains toxic gas and vapors (eg, benzene, hydrogen cyanide, formaldehyde); bioaerosols; dead and living cell material, including blood fragments; and viruses.[95-97,99] Many additional hazardous chemical compounds have been identified in surgical smoke.[95,97,99-102]

X.c.1. Respiratory protection that is at least as protective as a fit-tested surgical N95 filtering face piece respirator should be considered for use in conjunction with LEV in disease transmissible cases (eg, human papillomavirus)[103,104,109] and during high-risk or aerosol transmissible disease procedures (eg, tuberculosis, varicella, rubeola).[110]

A fit-tested surgical N95 filtering face piece respirator is a personal protective device that is worn on the face, covers at least the nose and mouth, and is used to reduce the wearer's risk of inhaling hazardous airborne particles including infectious agents.[111] The NIOSH respirator approval regulation defines the term N95 as a filter class that removes at least 95% of airborne particles during "worse case" testing using a "most-penetrating" sized particle.[111] Filters meeting the criteria are given a 95 rating. Many filtering face piece respirators have an N95 class filter and those meeting this filtration performance are often referred to simply as "N95 respirators."[111]

X.c.2. High-filtration face masks should not be used as the first line of protection against surgical smoke inhalation or as protection from chemical or particulate contaminants found in surgical smoke plume.[108]

A surgical mask is intended to prevent the release of potential contaminants from the user into his or her immediate environment.[112] It also is used to protect the wearer from large droplets, sprays, and splashes of body fluids.[111,112] High-filtration face masks are specifically designed as barrier protection to filter particulate matter that is 0.1 micron in size and larger.[113] Surgical and high-filtration masks do not seal to the face and may allow dangerous contaminants to enter the health care worker's breathing zone.[107,111,114]

A high-filtration mask provides less protection than a fit tested N95 filtering face piece respirator.[115] Oberg and Brosseau evaluated nine different types of surgical masks for filtration performance and facial fit. The types included surgical, laser, and procedure masks that were cupped, flat, and duckbilled with ties and ear loops. The masks' filter efficiency varied widely from very low to high.[116] Facial fit was evaluated quantitatively and qualitatively. When filter performance and facial fit were evaluated, none of the surgical masks met the qualifications of respiratory protection devices.[116]

Research is pending to test the efficacy of high-filtration masks and the air quality and quantity of airborne contaminants resulting from varying energy devices (eg, laser, electrosurgery, ultrasonic).

Recommendation XI

Personnel should receive initial education and competency validation on procedures and should receive additional training when new equipment, instruments, supplies, or procedures are introduced.

Initial education on the underlying principles of electrosurgical safety provides direction for personnel in providing a safe environment. Additional, periodic educational programs provide reinforcement of principles of electrosurgery and new information on changes in technology, its application, compatibility of equipment and accessories, and potential hazards.

Electrosurgical equipment and accessories have been associated with numerous fires and patient injuries.[2,8,19,53] The National Fire Protection Association has identified ESUs as high-risk equipment, warranting training and retraining of personnel.[19]

XI.a. Personnel working with electrosurgery equipment should be knowledgeable about the principles of

ELECTROSURGERY

electrosurgery, risks to patients and personnel, measures to minimize these risks, and corrective actions to employ in the event of a fire or injury.[19]

Electrosurgical equipment and accessories have been associated with numerous fires and patient injuries.[2,8]

XI.b. Personnel should be instructed on the proper operation, care, and handling of the ESU and accessories before use.[19]

Incorrect use can result in serious injury to patients and personnel.

XI.b.1. If multiple types of electrosurgical equipment are used within the facility, training should be provided on all of the equipment.[18]

XI.c. Personnel should be instructed in the risks of electrosurgery during minimally invasive surgical procedures.

Direct coupling is the result of touching the laparoscopic active electrode to another anatomic structure. This can cause necrosis of underlying tissue. Insulation failure of the laparoscopic electrode can be caused by trauma during use or reprocessing. Current leaves the electrode through this alternate pathway. This can cause serious patient injury, particularly when the injury is internal. Capacitive-coupled RF currents can cause undetected burns to nearby tissue and organs outside the endoscope's viewing field. Severe patient injuries have resulted.[8]

XI.d. Perioperative registered nurses should be knowledgeable about the types of IEDs that may be encountered in the practice setting, and the precautions that must be taken when caring for patients with these devices.[25]

Electronic devices implanted in a patient may be affected by other IEDs or medical equipment with which a patient may come into contact in a health care facility.

XI.e. Administrative personnel should assess and document annual competency of personnel in the safe use of the ESU and accessories.

A competency assessment provides a record that personnel have basic understanding of electrosurgery, its risks, and appropriate corrective actions to take in the event of a fire or injury. This knowledge is essential to minimize the risks of misuse of the equipment and to provide a safe environment of care.

Recommendation XII

Documentation should be completed to enable the identification of trends and demonstrate compliance with regulatory and accrediting agency requirements.

Documentation of all nursing activities performed is legally and professionally important for clear communication and collaboration between health care team members and for continuity of patient care.

XII.a. Documentation using the PNDS should include a patient assessment, a plan of care, nursing diagnoses, identification of desired outcomes, interventions, and an evaluation of the patient's response to the care provided.

Documentation provides communication among all care providers involved in planning and implementing patient care.

XII.b. Documentation should be recorded in a manner consistent with health care organization policies and procedures and should include, but is not limited to
- electrosurgical system identification serial number[117];
- range of settings used;
- dispersive electrode placement;
- patient's skin condition before dispersive electrode placement;
- patient's skin condition after removal of dispersive electrode[117];
- adjunct electrosurgical devices used (eg, ultrasonic scalpel, bipolar forceps); and
- safety holster use.[18]

Recommendation XIII

Policies and procedures for electrosurgery should be developed, reviewed periodically, revised as necessary, and readily available in the practice setting.

Policies and procedures assist in the development of patient safety, quality assessment, and improvement activities. Policies and procedures establish authority, responsibility, and accountability within the facility. They also serve as operational guidelines that are used to minimize patient risk factors, standardize practice, direct staff members, and establish guidelines for continuous performance improvement activities.

XIII.a. The health care organization's policies and procedures for electrosurgery must be in compliance with the Safe Medical Devices Act of 1990, amended in March 2000.[26]

XIII.a.1. When patient or personnel injuries or equipment failures occur, the ESU should be removed from service and the active and dispersive electrodes retained if possible.[117]

Retaining the ESU, the active and dispersive electrodes, and packaging allows for a complete systems check to determine electrosurgical system integrity.[117]

XIII.a.2. Incidents of patient or personnel electrical injury or equipment failure should be reported as required by regulation to federal, state, and local authorities and to the equipment manufacturer.[117] Device identification, maintenance and service information, as well as adverse event information should be included in the report from the practice setting.

Documentation of details of the electrosurgical equipment and supplies allows for

ELECTROSURGERY

retrievable information for investigation into an adverse event.[117]

XIII.b. Policies and procedures for electrosurgery should include, but are not limited to the following:
- safety features required on ESUs;
- equipment maintenance programs;
- required supplemental safety monitors;
- equipment checks before initial use;
- reporting and impounding malfunctioning equipment;
- reporting of injuries;
- preoperative, intraoperative, and postoperative patient assessments;
- precautions during use;
- ESU sanitation; and
- documentation.

XIII.c. An introduction and review of policies and procedures for electrosurgery should be included in orientation and ongoing education of personnel to assist in the development of knowledge, skills, and attitudes that affect surgical patient outcomes.

Review of policies and procedures assists health care professionals in the development of knowledge, skills, and attitudes that affect patient outcomes.

XIII.d. A written fire prevention and management policy and procedure should be developed by a multidisciplinary group that includes all categories of perioperative personnel.[18,36]

Fire is a risk to both patients and health care workers in the perioperative setting.

XIII.d.1. The policy and procedure should describe processes to be implemented to safely manage different fire scenarios.

Recommendation XIV

A quality assurance/performance improvement process should be in place that measures patient, process, and structural (eg, system) outcome indicators.

A fundamental precept of AORN is that it is the responsibility of professional perioperative registered nurses to ensure safe, high-quality nursing care to patients undergoing surgical and invasive procedures.[118]

XIV.a. Structure, process, and clinical outcomes performance measures should be identified that can be used to improve patient care and that also monitor compliance with facility policy and procedure, national standards, and regulatory requirements.[119]

XIV.a.1. Process indicators may include, but are not limited to information about adverse patient outcomes and near misses associated with electrosurgery, which should be collected, analyzed, and used for performance improvement.[118]

XIV.b. Electrosurgical devices should be tested before initial use, inspected periodically, and receive preventive maintenance by a designated individual responsible for equipment maintenance (eg, biomedical engineering services personnel).[19]

Periodic preventative maintenance ensures continued safe operation of electrosurgical devices.[19]

XIV.c. Each ESU should be assigned an identification or serial number.

This number allows designated personnel to track function problems and document maintenance performed on individual ESUs.

XIV.d. Each health care organization should be responsible for staying abreast of evolving technology that may impact patient care and safety.

Electrosurgical technology continues to evolve, changing the way in which surgical hemostasis is achieved.

Glossary

Active electrode: The electrosurgical unit (ESU) accessory that directs current flow to the surgical site (eg, pencils, various pencil tips).

Active electrode indicator shaft: An active electrode composed of two layers of insulated material of different colors. The inner layer is a bright color, the outer layer is black. When the bright colored inner layer is evident upon visual inspection, a break in the insulation is indicated.

Active electrode insulation testing: Devices designed to test the integrity of the insulation surrounding the conductive shaft of laparoscopic electrosurgical active-electrode instruments. The devices detect full thickness breaks in the insulation layer.

Active electrode monitoring: A dynamic process of searching for insulation failures and capacitive coupling during monopolar surgery. If the monitor detects an unsafe level of stray energy, it signals the generator to deactivate.

Alternate site injury: Patient injury caused by an electrosurgical device that occurs away from the dispersive electrode site.

Argon-enhanced coagulation: Radio frequency coagulation from an electrosurgical generator that is capable of delivering monopolar current through a flow of ionized argon gas.

Bioengineering services personnel: Those individuals in an institution who are trained and qualified to check, troubleshoot, and repair medical equipment.

Bipolar electrosurgery: Electrosurgery in which current flows between two tips of a bipolar forceps that are positioned around tissue to create a surgical effect. Current passes from the active electrode of one tip of the forceps through the patient's desired tissue to the other dispersive electrode tip of the forceps—thus

ELECTROSURGERY

completing the circuit without entering another part of the patient's body.

Capacitance: Ability of an electrical circuit to transfer an electrical charge from one conductor to another, even when separated by an insulator.

Capacitive coupling: Transfer of electrical current from the active electrode through intact insulation to adjacent conductive items (eg, tissue, trocars).

Capacitively coupled return electrode: A large, nonadhesive return electrode placed close to and forming a capacitor with the patient, returning electrical current from the patient back to the electrosurgical unit (ESU).

Current: A movement of electrons analogous to the flow of a stream of water.

Direct coupling: The contact of an energized active electrode tip with another metal instrument or object within the surgical field.

Dispersive electrode: The accessory that directs electrical current flow from the patient back to the electrosurgical generator—often called the patient plate, return electrode, inactive electrode, or grounding pad.

Dual foil electrode: A dispersive return electrode that has two foil conductive surfaces on a single nonconductive adhesive pad. The two foil surfaces are connected independently through the same return electrode cord to the ESU. The dual foil design allows the return electrode quality monitor to detect impedance differences between the conductive surfaces. If a difference is detected between the two foil surfaces, the ESU will alarm and shut down. Dual foil electrodes are a necessary component of return electrode quality monitoring.

Electrosurgery: The cutting and coagulation of body tissue with a high-frequency (ie, radio-frequency) current.

Electrosurgical accessories: The active electrode with tip(s), dispersive electrode, adapters, and connectors to attach these devices to the electrosurgery generator.

Electrosurgical unit: The generator that produces a high-frequency current waveform that is delivered to tissues, the foot switch with cord (if applicable), the electrical plug, cord, and connections.

Endoscopic minimally invasive: Surgical techniques that use endoscopic approaches rather than dissection.

Eschar: Charred tissue residue.

Generator: The machine that produces radio-frequency waves (eg, ESU, power unit).

Ground-referenced electrosurgical unit: A system in which electrical current is sent to the patient and follows the path of least resistance back to the ground. This technology, which no longer is manufactured, produces high-frequency, high-voltage current and sometimes is referred to as a "spark gap" unit.

Insulator: A material that does not conduct electricity.

Insulation failure: Damage to the insulation of the active electrode that provides an alternate pathway for the current to leave that electrode as it completes the circuit to the dispersive electrode.

Isolated electrosurgical unit: A system in which electrical current is sent to the patient and selectively returns and is grounded through the generator.

Monopolar electrosurgery: Electrosurgery in which only the active electrode is in the surgical wound, and the electrical current is directed through the patient's body, received by the dispersive pad, and transferred back to the generator, completing the monopolar circuit.

Oxygen-enriched environment: Atmosphere containing more than 21% oxygen, frequently occurring in the oropharynx, trachea, lower respiratory tract, and near the head and neck during administration of oxygen to the patient.

Return electrode continuity monitor: A safety feature of a single foil dispersive electrode that detects an unconnected dispersive electrode or a break in the return electrode cord.

Return-electrode contact quality monitoring: A dynamic monitoring circuit measuring impedance of the dispersive return electrode. If the dispersive electrode becomes compromised, the circuit inhibits the ESU's output.

Ultra low particulate air (ULPA): Theoretically, a ULPA filter can remove from the air 99.9999% of bacteria, dust, pollen, mold, and particles with a size of 120 nanometers or larger.

Ultrasonic scalpel: A cutting/coagulation device that converts electrical energy into mechanical energy, providing a rapid ultrasonic motion.

Vessel sealing device: Bipolar technology that fuses collagen and elastin in the vessel walls and permanently obliterates the lumen of the vessel.

References

1. Association for the Advancement of Medical Instrumentation. *ANSI/AAMI HF18:2001. Electrosurgical Devices.* Arlington, VA: Association for the Advancement of Medical Instrumentation; 2001.
2. ECRI. Electrosurgery. Healthcare Risk Control Risk Analysis. 2007;4(Surgery and Anesthesia 16).
3. Electrosurgical units. *Health Devices.* 1998;27(3): 93-111.
4. Odell RC. Pearls, pitfalls, and advancements in the delivery of electrosurgical energy during laparoscopy. *Problems in General Surgery.* 2002;19(2):5-17.
5. Jones CM, Pierre KB, Nicoud IB, Stain SC, Melvin WV 3rd. Electrosurgery. *Curr Surg.* 2006;63(6):458-463.
6. ECRI. Laparoscopic electrosurgery risks. *Operating Room Risk Management.* 1999;2(Surgery 19):1-11.
7. Guidance section: ensuring monopolar electrosurgical safety during laparoscopy. *Health Devices.* 1995;24(1):20-26.
8. Wu MP, Ou CS, Chen SL, Yen EYT, Rowbotham R. Complications and recommended practices for electrosurgery in laparoscopy. *Am J Surg.* 2000/1;179(1):67-73.
9. Vilos GA, Newton DW, Odell RC, Abu-Rafea B, Vilos AG. Characterization and mitigation of stray radio-frequency currents during monopolar resectoscopic electrosurgery. *J Minim Invasive Gynecol.* 2006;13(2):134-140.
10. Physician Insurers Association of America. *Laparoscopic Injury Study.* Rockville, Md: Physician Insurers Association of America; 2000:1-5.
11. ECRI. Safety technologies for laparoscopic monopolar electrosurgery; devices for managing burn risks. *Health Devices.* 2005;34(8):259-272.
12. Evaluation of Electroscope Electroshield System. *Health Devices.* 1995;24(1):11-19.

13. Dennis V. Implementing active electrode monitoring: a perioperative call. *Ssm*. 2001;7(2):32, 34-38.

14. Harrell GJ, Kopps DR. Minimizing patient risk during laparoscopic electrosurgery. *AORN J*. 1998;67(6):1194-1196.

15. Electrosurgery safety issues. PA-PSRS Patient Safety Advisory. 2006;3(1):1-3.

16. ECRI. The patient is on fire! A surgical fires primer. http://www.mdsr.ecri.org/summary/detail.aspx?doc_id=8197. Accessed November 4, 2009.

17. Burns and fires from electrosurgical active electrodes. *Health Devices*. 1993;22(8-9):421-422.

18. Electrosurgical safety: conducting a safety audit. *Health Devices*. 2005;34(12):414-420.

19. Annex D. The safe use of high-frequency electricity in health care facilities. In: *Health Care Facilities Handbook*. 10th ed. Quincy, MA: National Fire Protection Association; 2005.

20. ECRI Institute. Electrosurgery checklist. *Operating Room Risk Management*. 2007;2(Surgery 10).

21. De Marco M, Maggi S. Evaluation of stray radiofrequency radiation emitted by electrosurgical devices. *Phys Med Biol*. 2006;51(14):3347-3358.

22. Massarweh NN, Cosgriff N, Slakey DP. Electrosurgery: history, principles, and current and future uses. *J Am Coll Surg*. 2006;202(3):520-530.

23. ESU burns from poor dispersive electrode site preparation. *Health Devices*. 1993;22(8-9):422-423.

24. Skin burns resulting from the use of electrolytic distention/irrigation media during electrosurgery with a rollerablation electrode. *Health Devices*. 1998;27(6):233-235.

25. AORN guidance statement: Care of the perioperative patient with an implanted electronic device. In: *Perioperative Standards and Recommended Practices*. Denver, CO: AORN, Inc; 2009:207-228.

26. Food and Drug Administration. Medical device reporting: Manufacturer reporting, importer reporting, user facility reporting, distributor reporting. *Fed Regist*. 2000;65:4112-4121.

27. Misconnection of bipolar electrosurgical electrodes. *Health Devices*. 1995;24(1):34-35.

28. ECRI Institute. Surgical fire safety. *Health Devices*. 2006;35(2):45-46.

29. Center for Devices and Radiological Health. Manufacturer and User Facility Device Experience (MAUDE) Database Adverse Event Report 421908. Reported October 9, 2002. http://www.accessdata.fda.gov/scripts/cdrh/cfdocs/cfMAUDE/Detail.CFM?MDRFOI__ID=421908. Accessed November 4, 2009.

30. Fire caused by improper disposal of electrocautery units. Health Devices. 1994;23(3):98.

31. Alternate-site burns from improperly seated electrosurgical pencil active electrodes. Health Devices. 2000;29(1):24-27.

32. Ignition of debris on active electrosurgical electrodes. Health Devices. 1998;27(9-10):367-370.

33. Center for Devices and Radiological Health. Manufacturer and User Facility Device Experience (MAUDE) Database Adverse Event Report 393590. Reported May 7, 2002. http://www.accessdata.fda.gov/scripts/cdrh/cfdocs/cfMAUDE/Detail.CFM?MDRFOI__ID=393590. Accessed November 4, 2009.

34. ECRI Institute. Hazard report. Improperly seated electrosurgical active electrodes can burn patients. *Health Devices*. 2007;36(10):337-339.

35. AORN guidance statement: sharps injury prevention in the perioperative setting. In: *Perioperative Standards and Recommended Practices*. Denver, CO: AORN, Inc; 2009:275-280.

36. Recommended practices for a safe environment of care. In: *Perioperative Standards and Recommended Practices*. Denver, CO: AORN, Inc; 2009:415-437.

37. AORN guidance statement: fire prevention in the operating room. In: *Perioperative Standards and Recommended Practices*. Denver, CO: AORN, Inc; 2009: 195-203.

38. *NFPA 99 Standard for Health Care Facilities*. Quincy, MA: National Fire Protection Association; 2002: Issue C.13.1.3.2.2:182.

39. A clinician's guide to surgical fires. How they occur, how to prevent them, how to put them out. *Health Devices*. 2003;32(1):5-24.

40. Beesley J, Taylor L. Reducing the risk of surgical fires: are you assessing the risk? *J Perioper Pract*. 2006;16(12):591-597.

41. Tentative interim amendment. In: *NFPA 99 Standard for Health Care Facilities*. Quincy, MA: National Fire Protection Association; 2005: 13.4.1.2.2-A-13.4.1.2.2.3.

42. Fire hazard created by the misuse of DuraPrep solution. *Health Devices*. 1998;27(11):400-402.

43. Center for Devices and Radiological Health. Manufacturer and User Facility Device Experience (MAUDE) Database Adverse Event Report 32071. Reported July 31, 1995. http://www.accessdata.fda.gov/scripts/cdrh/cfdocs/cfMAUDE/Detail.CFM?MDRFOI__ID=32071. Accessed November 4, 2009.

44. Barker SJ, Polson JS. Fire in the operating room: a case report and laboratory study. *Anesth Analg*. 2001;93(4):960-965.

45. Position statement on fire prevention. http://www.aorn.org/PracticeResources/AORNPositionStatements/Position_FirePrevention/. Accessed November 4, 2009.

46. *Standard for Health Care Facilities Tentative Interim Amendment: Germicides and Antiseptics*. Quincy, MA: National Fire Protection Association; 2005.

47. A Report by the American Society of Anesthesiologists Task Force on Operating Room Fires. Practice Advisory for the Prevention and Management of Operating Room Fires. *Anesthesiology*. 2008;108(5):786-801.

48. ECRI Institute. Surgical fires. *Operating Room Risk Management*. 2006;2(Safety 1):1-18.

49. Center for Devices and Radiological Health. Manufacturer and User Facility Device Experience (MAUDE) Database Adverse Event Report 441523. Reported August 23, 2002. http://www.accessdata.fda.gov/scripts/cdrh/cfdocs/cfMAUDE/Detail.CFM?MDRFOI__ID=441523. Accessed November 4, 2009.

50. Ortega RA. A rare cause of fire in the operating room. *Anesthesiology*. 1998;89(6):1608.

51. Soussan EB, Mathieu N, Roque I, Antonietti M. Bowel explosion with colonic perforation during argon plasma coagulation for hemorrhagic radiation-induced proctitis. *Gastrointestinal Endoscopy*. 2003/3;57(3):412-413.

52. Smith C. Home study program. Surgical fires—learn not to burn. *AORN J*. 2004;80(1):23-27, 29-31, 33-4.

53. Smith TL, Smith JM. Electrosurgery in otolaryngology-head and neck surgery: principles, advances, and complications. *Laryngoscope*. 2001;111(5):769-780.

54. Electrosurgical airway fires still a hot topic. *Health Devices*. 1996;25(7):260-262.

55. Manufacturer and User Facility Device Experience (MAUDE) Database. Adverse event report no. 837984: Electrosurgical unit. http://www.accessdata.fda.gov/scripts/cdrh/cfdocs/cfMAUDE/Detail.CFM?MDRFOI__ID=837984. Accessed November 4, 2009.

56. Manufacturer and User Facility Device Experience (MAUDE) Database. Adverse event report no. 767284: Dispersive electrode. http://www.accessdata.fda.gov/

scripts/cdrh/cfdocs/cfMAUDE/Detail.CFM?MDRFOI__ID=767284. Accessed November 4, 2009.

57. Demir E, O'Dey DM, Pallua N. Accidental burns during surgery. *J Burn Care Res.* 2006;27(6):895-900.

58. Center for Devices and Radiological Health. Manufacturer and User Facility Device Experience (MAUDE) Database Adverse Event Report 523194. Reported March 31, 2004. http://www.accessdata.fda.gov/scripts/cdrh/cfdocs/cfMAUDE/Detail.CFM?MDRFOI__ID=523194. Accessed November 4, 2009.

59. Manufacturer and User Facility Device Experience (MAUDE) Database Search. Adverse event report no. 115111: Dispersive electrode. http://www.accessdata.fda.gov/scripts/cdrh/cfdocs/cfMAUDE/Detail.CFM?MDRFOI__ID=115111. Accessed November 4, 2009.

60. Recommended practices for preoperative patient skin antisepsis. In: *Perioperative Standards and Recommended Practices.* Denver, CO: AORN, Inc; 2009:549-568.

61. Manufacturer and User Facility Device Experience (MAUDE) Database. Adverse event report no. 1021169: Grounding plate. http://www.accessdata.fda.gov/scripts/cdrh/cfdocs/cfMAUDE/Detail.CFM?MDRFOI__ID=1021169. Accessed November 4, 2009.

62. Ratnapalan S, Greenberg M, Armstrong D. Tattoos and MRI. *AJR Am J Roentgenol.* 2004;183(2):541.

63. Franiel T, Schmidt S, Klingebiel R. First-degree burns on MRI due to nonferrous tattoos. *AJR Am J Roentgenol.* 2006;187(5):W556.

64. Wagle WA, Smith M. Tattoo-induced skin burn during MR imaging. *Am J Roentgenol.* 2000;174(6):1795.

65. Center for Devices and Radiological Health. Manufacturer and User Facility Device Experience (MAUDE) Database Adverse Event Report 495428. Reported October 15, 2003. http://www.accessdata.fda.gov/scripts/cdrh/cfdocs/cfMAUDE/Detail.CFM?MDRFOI__ID=495428. Accessed November 4, 2009.

66. Center for Devices and Radiological Health. Manufacturer and User Facility Device Experience (MAUDE) Database Adverse Event Report 499965. Reported November 25, 2003. http://www.accessdata.fda.gov/scripts/cdrh/cfdocs/cfMAUDE/Detail.CFM?MDRFOI__ID=499965. Accessed November 4, 2009.

67. Center for Devices and Radiological Health. Manufacturer and User Facility Device Experience (MAUDE) Database Adverse Event Report 516905. Reported February 16, 2004. http://www.accessdata.fda.gov/scripts/cdrh/cfdocs/cfMAUDE/Detail.CFM?MDRFOI__ID=516905. Accessed November 4, 2009.

68. Manufacturer and User Facility Device Experience (MAUDE) Database. Adverse event report no. 851317: Dispersive electrode. http://www.accessdata.fda.gov/scripts/cdrh/cfdocs/cfMAUDE/Detail.CFM?MDRFOI__ID=851317. Accessed November 4, 2009.

69. Center for Devices and Radiological Health. Manufacturer and User Facility Device Experience (MAUDE) Database Adverse Event Report 286226. Reported July 6, 2002. http://www.accessdata.fda.gov/scripts/cdrh/cfdocs/cfMAUDE/Detail.CFM?MDRFOI__ID=286226. Accessed November 4, 2009.

70. Center for Devices and Radiological Health. Manufacturer and User Facility Device Experience (MAUDE) Database Adverse Event Report 396295. Reported May 16, 2002. http://www.accessdata.fda.gov/scripts/cdrh/cfdocs/cfMAUDE/Detail.CFM?MDRFOI__ID=396295. Accessed November 4, 2009.

71. Russell MJ, Gaetz M. Intraoperative electrode burns. *J Clin Monit Comput.* 2004;18(1):25-32.

72. Stecker MM, Patterson T, Netherton BL. Mechanisms of electrode induced injury. Part 1: theory. *Am J Electroneurodiagnostic Technol.* 2006;46(4):315-342.

73. Patterson T, Stecker MM, Netherton BL. Mechanisms of electrode induced injury. Part 2: Clinical experience. *Am J Electroneurodiagnostic Technol.* 2007;47(2):93-113.

74. ECRI Institute. Higher currents, greater risks: preventing patient burns at the return-electrode site during high-current electrosurgical procedures. *Health Devices.* 2005;34(8):273-279.

75. Manufacturer and User Facility Device Experience (MAUDE) Database. Adverse event report no. 1069874: REM PolyHesive II electrode, ESU, dispersive. http://www.accessdata.fda.gov/scripts/cdrh/cfdocs/cfMAUDE/Detail.CFM?MDRFOI__ID=1069874. Accessed November 4, 2009.

76. Manufacturer and User Facility Device Experience (MAUDE) Database. Adverse event report no. 907879: Generator. http://www.accessdata.fda.gov/scripts/cdrh/cfdocs/cfMAUDE/Detail.CFM?MDRFOI__ID=907879. Accessed November 4, 2009.

77. Skin lesions from aggressive adhesive on Valleylab electrosurgical return electrode pads. *Health Devices.* 1995;24(4):159-160.

78. MegaDyne Mega 2000 return electrode. *Health Devices.* 2000;29(12):445-460.

79. Center for Devices and Radiological Health. Manufacturer and User Facility Device Experience (MAUDE) Database Adverse Event Report 401617. Reported June 24, 2002. http://www.accessdata.fda.gov/scripts/cdrh/cfdocs/cfMAUDE/Detail.CFM?MDRFOI__ID=401617. Accessed November 4, 2009.

80. Recommended practices for endoscopic minimally invasive surgery. In: *Perioperative Standards and Recommended Practices.* Denver, CO: AORN, Inc; 2009:347-359.

81. Greilich PE, Greilich NB, Froelich EG. Intraabdominal fire during laparoscopic cholecystectomy. See comment. *Anesthesiology.* 1995;83(4):871-874.

82. Tucker RD, Voyles CR, Silvis SE. Capacitive coupled stray currents during laparoscopic and endoscopic electrosurgical procedures. Biomed Instrum Technol. 1992;26(4):303-311.

83. Wang K, Advincula AP. "Current thoughts" in electrosurgery. *Int J Gynaecol Obstet.* 2007;97(3):245-250.

84. Shirk GJ, Johns A, Redwine DB. Complications of laparoscopic surgery: how to avoid them and how to repair them. *J Minim Invasive Gynecol.* 2006;13(4):352-359.

85. Yazdani A, Krause H. Laparoscopic instrument insulation failure: the hidden hazard. *J Minim Invasive Gynecol.* 2007;14(2):228-232.

86. Brunner LS, Suddarth DS, Smeltzer SCO, Cheever K, eds. Management of patients with intestinal and rectal disorders. In: *Brunner & Suddarth's Textbook of Medical-Surgical Nursing.* 11th ed. Philadelphia, PA: Lippincott Williams & Wilkins; 2008:1231-1281.

87. McCarus SD. Physiologic mechanism of the ultrasonically activated scalpel. *J Am Assoc Gynecol Laparosc.* 1996;3(4):601-608.

88. Ott DE, Moss E, Martinez K. Aerosol exposure from an ultrasonically activated (Harmonic) device. *J Am Assoc Gynecol Laparosc.* 1998;5(1):29-32.

89. Matthews K. Argon beam coagulation. New directions in surgery. *AORN J.* 1992;56(5):885-889.

90. Fatal gas embolism caused by overpressurization during laparoscopic use of argon enhanced coagulation. *Health Devices.* 1994;23(6):257-259.

91. Veyckemans F, Michel I. Venous gas embolism from an Argon coagulator. *Anesthesiology.* 1996;85(2):443-444.

92. Bigony L. Risks associated with exposure to surgical smoke plume: a review of the literature. *AORN J.* 2007;86(6):1013-1020.

93. Brüske-Hohlfeld I, Preissler G, Jauch KW, et al. Surgical smoke and ultrafine particles. *J Occup Med and Toxicol.* 2008;3:31-45.

94. ANSI® Z136.3-2011: American National Standard for Safe Use of Lasers in Health Care. Washington, DC: American National Standards Institute; 2011.

95. NIOSH Hazard Control HC11: Control of smoke from laser/electric surgical procedures. http://www.cdc.gov/niosh/docs/hazardcontrol/hc11.html. Accessed May 22, 2012.

96. ECRI Institute. Smoke evacuation systems, surgical. *Healthcare Product Comparison System.* November 2007.

97. Al Sahaf OS, Vega-Carrascal I, Cunningham FO, McGrath JP, Bloomfield FJ. Chemical composition of smoke produced by high-frequency electrosurgery. *Ir J Med Sci.* 2007;176(3):229-232.

98. Baggish MS, Poiesz BJ, Joret D, Williamson P, Refai A. Presence of human immunodeficiency virus DNA in laser smoke. *Lasers Surg Med.* 1991;11(3):197-203.

99. Alp E, Bijl D, Bleichrodt RP, Hansson B, Voss A. Surgical smoke and infection control. *J Hosp Infect.* 2006;62(1):1-5.

100. Ulmer BC. The hazards of surgical smoke. *AORN J.* 2008;87(4):721-734.

101. Hoglan M. Potential hazards from electrosurgery plume—recommendations for surgical smoke evacuation. *Can Oper Room Nurs J.* 1995;13(4):10-16.

102. Occupational Safety and Health Administration, Hospital eTool: Surgical Suite—Use of Medical Lasers. http://www.osha.gov/SLTC/etools/hospital/surgical/lasers.html. Accessed May 22, 2012.

103. Garden JM, O'Banion MK, Shelnitz LS, et al. Papillomavirus in the vapor of carbon dioxide laser treated verrucae. *JAMA.* 1988;259(8):1199-1202.

104. Hallmo P, Naess O. Laryngeal papillomatosis with human papillomavirus DNA contracted by a laser surgeon. *Eur Arch Otorhinolaryngol.* 1991;248(7):425-427.

105. Houck PM. Comparison of operating room lasers: uses, hazards, guidelines. *Nurs Clin North Am.* 2006;41(2):193-218.

106. Canadian Standards Association. Z305.13-09. Plume Scavenging in surgical diagnostic, therapeutic, and aesthetic settings. Canadian Standards Association. Mississauga, Ontario, Canada. 2009.

107. International Social Society Association. *Surgical smoke: risks and preventive measures.* International Section of the ISSA on prevention of occupational risks in health services. D 22089 Hamburg, Pappelallee 33/35/37 Germany. 2011.

108. Part 8: Guidelines for the safe use of laser beams on humans. In: IEC TR 60825-8: *Safety of Laser Products.* 2nd ed. Geneva, Switzerland: International Electrotechnical Commission; 2006.

109. Garden JM, O'Banion MK, Bakus AD, Olson C. Viral disease transmitted by laser-generated plume (aerosol). *Arch Dermatol.* 2002;138(10):1303-1307.

110. Siegel JD, Rinehard E, Jackson M, Chiarello L; the Healthcare Infection Control Practices Advisory Committee. *2007 Guideline for Isolation Precautions: Preventing Transmission of Infectious Agents in Healthcare Settings.* Atlanta, GA: Centers for Disease Control and Prevention; 2007. http://www.cdc.gov/hicpac/pdf/isolation/Isolation2007.pdf. Accessed May 22, 2012.

111. Respirator trusted-source information page. National Institute for Occupational Safety and Health. http://www.cdc.gov/niosh/npptl/topics/respirators/disp_part/RespSource.html. Accessed May 22, 2012.

112. US Food and Drug Administration. Guidance for Industry and FDA Staff: High filtration surgical (laser) masks- Premarket notification [510(k)] Submissions; guidance for industry and FDA. http://www.fda.gov/MedicalDevices/DeviceRegulationandGuidance/GuidanceDocuments/ucm072549.htm. Accessed May 22, 2012.

113. OSHA Fact Sheet. Respiratory Infection Control: Respirators versus Surgical Masks. http://www.osha.gov/Publications/respirators-vs-surgicalmasks-factsheet.html Accessed May 22, 2012.

114. Rengasamy S, Miller A, Eimer BC, Shaffer RE. Filtration performance of FDA-cleared high filtration surgical (laser) masks. *JISRP.* 2009;26:54-70.

115. Derrick JL, Li PT, Tang SP, Gomersall CD. Protecting staff against airborne viral particles: in vivo efficiency of laser masks. *J Hosp Infect.* 2006;64(3):278-281.

116. Oberg T, Brosseau LM. Surgical mask filter and fit performance. *Am J Infect Control.* 2008;36(4):276-282.

117. ECRI Institute. Investigating device-related skin "burns." *Operating Room Risk Management.* 2(3):1-10.

118. Quality and performance improvement standards for perioperative nursing. In: *Perioperative Standards and Recommended Practices.* Denver, CO: AORN, Inc; 2009:65-74.

119. Improving organization performance. In: *Comprehensive Accreditation Manual for Hospitals: The Official Handbook.* Oakbrook Terrace, IL: Joint Commission on Accreditation of Healthcare Organizations; 2007:PI-8–PI-9.

Acknowledgments

LEAD AUTHOR
Mary Ogg, RN, MSN, CNOR
Perioperative Nursing Specialist
AORN Center for Nursing Practice
Denver, Colorado

CONTRIBUTING AUTHOR
Cecil A. King, MS, RN, CNOR
Perioperative Clinical Educator
Cape Cod Hospital
Hyannis, Massachusetts

PUBLICATION HISTORY

Originally published March 1985, *AORN Journal.* Revised April 1991; revised July 1993.

Revised November 1997; published January 1998, *AORN Journal.* Reformatted July 2000.

Revised November 2003; published February 2004, *AORN Journal.*

Revised November 2004; published in *Standards, Recommended Practices, and Guidelines,* 2005 edition. Reprinted March 2005, *AORN Journal.*

Revised July 2009 for online publication in *Perioperative Standards and Recommended Practices.*

Minor editing revisions made in November 2009 for publication in *Perioperative Standards and Recommended Practices,* 2010 edition.

Editorial revisions made July 2012. Recommendation X was revised and approved by the Recommended Practices Advisory Board. Reformatted September 2012 for publication in *Perioperative Standards and Recommended Practices,* 2013 edition.

Minor editing revisions made in November 2014 for publication in *Guidelines for Perioperative Practice,* 2015 edition.

ELECTROSURGERY

GUIDELINE FOR LASER SAFETY

The Guideline for Laser Safety was developed by the AORN Recommended Practices Committee and was approved by the AORN Board of Directors. It was presented as proposed recommendations for comments by members and others. The guideline is effective November 1, 2010. The recommendations in the guideline are intended to be achievable and represent what is believed to be an optimal level of practice. Policies and procedures will reflect variations in practice settings and/or clinical situations that determine the degree to which the guideline can be implemented. AORN recognizes the various settings in which perioperative nurses practice; therefore, this guideline is adaptable to various practice settings. These practice settings include traditional operating rooms (ORs), ambulatory surgery centers, physicians' offices, cardiac catheterization laboratories, endoscopy suites, radiology departments, and all other areas where operative and other invasive procedures may be performed.

Purpose

This document provides guidance to perioperative personnel in the use and care of laser equipment and to assist practitioners in providing a safe environment for patients and health care workers during use of laser technology. The guideline incorporates activities described in the American National Standards Institute's (ANSI's) *American National Standards for the Safe Use of Lasers in Health Care Facilities ANSI Z136.3*, which specifies standards for the use of class 3 and class 4 laser devices in the health care environment.[1] Health care facilities are encouraged to obtain *Safe Use of Lasers in Health Care Facilities ANSI Z136.3*[1] and ANSI's *American National Standard for Safe Use of Lasers ANSI Z136.1*[2] and to have them readily available in the practice environment.

Recommendation I

A laser safety program should be established for all owned, leased, or borrowed laser equipment in any location where lasers are used in the health care organization.[1,3,4]

Health care laser systems are classified by their relative hazard and the appropriate controls.[1] Class 3 and primarily class 4 lasers are used in the health care setting. Class 4 laser exposure may be hazardous to eyes and skin, and may pose a potential fire risk.[1] Class 3 lasers are potentially hazardous in the event of direct exposure or exposure to specular reflection (ie, mirror-like reflection of light).[1,4]

I.a. A formal laser safety program should include, but not be limited to,

- delegating authority and responsibility for supervising laser safety to a laser safety officer (LSO);
- establishing a multidisciplinary laser safety committee or safety committee[3];
- establishing usage criteria and authorized procedures for all health care personnel working in laser nominal hazard zones;
- identifying laser hazards and appropriate administrative, engineering, and procedural control measures;
- educating personnel (eg, operators) regarding the assessment and control of hazards; and
- managing and reporting accidents or incidents related to laser procedures, including creating action plans to prevent recurrences.[1]

A laser safety program may minimize potential laser hazards. A multidisciplinary laser safety committee is integral to establishing and monitoring laser safety.[3]

I.a.1. The multidisciplinary laser safety committee or safety committee may include
- the chief operating officer;
- the director of patient safety;
- the patent safety coordinator;
- the director of biomedical engineering and/or clinical/biomedical engineer[5];
- the LSO[5];
- the deputy laser safety officer;
- the chief of surgery;
- a physician representative from each specialty group using lasers[5];
- an anesthesia care provider[5];
- the perioperative services director[5];
- the perioperative educator;
- the director of medical staff education/credentialing;
- the environmental manager[5];
- the risk manager;
- a laser safety specialist (eg, nurse, technician)[5]; and/or
- the hazardous materials manager.[5]

I.a.2. The responsibilities of the laser safety committee or safety committee should include, but not be limited to,
- strategic planning (eg, technology assessment, cost analysis, product evaluation);
- credentialing;
- hazard assessment;
- laser safety program oversight;

LASER SAFETY

- laser-related policy and procedure development and enforcement; and
- laser-related education.

I.a.3. The laser safety committee or safety committee members should review activities including, but not limited to,
- acquisition of laser-related technology,[5]
- design of facilities where lasers are used,[5]
- marketing information from laser vendors,[5]
- credentialing education and competencies,
- education and training programs,[5]
- protocols,[5]
- policies and procedures,
- variance reporting,
- laser audits, and
- use of third-party laser systems.

I.a.4. The laser safety committee or safety committee should verify that any physician who operates the laser is credentialed to perform the procedure as defined by the health care organization's policy. Physician credentialing by the health care organization's medical board should include, but is not limited to,
- completing coursework in basic laser physics, laser tissue interaction, and clinical applications[3,5];
- training in the operation and safety of the specific laser for which privileges are sought[1,3,5]; and
- completing a preceptorship (ie, training, observation, mentoring).[1]

Lasers are highly technical medical devices with potential for harm. Laser experience among physicians varies depending on the degree that residency training programs incorporate lasers into their program.[1]

I.b. An LSO should be appointed as part of a laser safety program and should be authorized by the health care organization's administrators to monitor and oversee the control of laser hazards.[1]

The LSO helps to ensure the safety of patients and personnel where lasers are used.

I.b.1. The responsibilities of the LSO should include, but not be limited to,
- verifying the manufacturer's hazard classification label of all lasers and laser systems[1];
- performing a laser hazard evaluation before initial use[1];
- overseeing the implementation of the health care laser system manufacturer's control measures[1];
- developing policies and procedures for maintenance, service, and use of lasers[1];
- verifying that protective equipment is available, used correctly, and free of defects[1];
- ascertaining that warning signs and labels comply with the Federal Laser Product Performance Standard or international standards[1];
- approving equipment and installation according to the manufacturer's safety recommendations[1]; and
- coordinating laser safety and education programs.[1]

I.b.2. The LSO may fulfill multiple roles (eg, laser operator, laser safety specialist [LSS]) within the health care organization depending on the scope of services provided.

I.b.3. The LSO or an appointee should assess any rented or borrowed equipment for compliance with all federal, state, local, and facility requirements.[1]

The LSO is responsible for the monitoring and oversight of laser hazards control.[1]

I.b.4. The LSO should make certain that the terms of agreements with a third-party laser equipment provider and/or operator include, but are not limited to,
- laser operator credentials that meet the health care organization's policy;
- written validation of the laser's maintenance, service, and cleaning;
- documentation of data elements regarding each laser procedure performed that meets the health care organization's policy; and
- provision of safety orientation and training of the perioperative team associated with the laser procedure.

I.c. An LSS (eg, laser resource nurse) should be designated and approved by the LSO for each area when lasers are being used in multiple sites in a health care organization.

The LSS oversees the safe laser use in each area where a laser is used. An LSS may not be needed where the laser is used only in one location and the LSO is available.

I.c.1. The responsibilities of the LSS should include, but not be limited to,
- supervising laser usage in a specific area (eg, ambulatory surgery unit, eye clinic);
- acting as a liaison between the clinical laser users and the LSO;
- troubleshooting equipment problems[3];
- monitoring compliance with the health care organization's laser policies and procedures;
- reviewing laser-related documentation (eg, logs, laser manufacturer's directions);
- acting as a resource to staff members and laser users; and
- assessing needs for continuing education and training.

LASER SAFETY

Recommendation II

All personnel should know where lasers are being used and access to these areas should be controlled.[1,4]

Identifying the laser treatment area with laser warning signs and controlling access prevents unintentional exposure to the laser beam.

II.a. A nominal hazard zone (ie, the space in which the level of direct, reflected, or scattered radiation used during normal laser operation exceeds the applicable maximum permissible exposure) should be identified.[1]

 The nominal hazard zone usually is contained within the room but may extend through open doors and/or transparent windows, depending on the type of laser being used. Identification of the nominal hazard zone establishes the area where control measures are required.

II.a.1. The LSO should determine the nominal hazard zone by referencing ANSI Z136.1 and ANSI Z136.3, as well as the safety information supplied by the laser manufacturer.[1,2]

II.a.2. Personnel in the nominal hazard zone should be aware of all necessary laser safety precautions (eg, wearing appropriate eye protection) to avoid inadvertent exposure to laser hazards.[1]

II.b. Clearly marked laser signs should be placed at all entrances to laser treatment areas when lasers are in use.[3,4]

 Laser signs alert health care personnel to the areas where lasers are in use.

II.b.1. Recognizable warning signs specific to the type of laser being used should be designed according to the information described in ANSI Z136.3.[1,6]

II.b.2. Warning signs should be placed conspicuously to alert bystanders to potential hazards.[1]

II.b.3. Laser warning signs should be removed when the laser procedure is completed.[4]

II.c. Doors in the nominal hazard zone should remain closed and windows, including door windows, should be covered with a barrier that blocks transmission of a beam as appropriate to the type of laser being used.[1,4,6]

 Laser energy, except energy from carbon dioxide wavelength lasers, has the potential to pass through windows. Maintaining a blocking barrier stops the transmission of the laser beam.[7]

Recommendation III

Patients and health care personnel in the laser treatment area should be protected from unintentional laser beam exposure.[1]

Unintentional laser beam exposure may cause eye and skin damage.[1]

III.a. Procedures should be implemented to prevent accidental activation or misdirection of laser beams that include, but are not limited to, the following:
- access to laser keys should be restricted to authorized personnel who are skilled in laser operation[1,3,4,7];
- lasers should be placed in standby mode when not in active use[1,3,4,8];
- the laser foot switch should be placed in a position convenient to the operator with the activation mechanism identified; and
- the laser user should be the only one to activate the device with the foot pedal.[4,8]

 Accidental activation or misdirection of the laser beam may cause eye and skin injury to the patient and health care personnel.[9] Attention to proper placement of the foot switch and use of the standby setting can reduce unintended activation of the laser beam and potential injury to the patient and health care personnel. Control of activation by the laser user prevents unintentional discharge of laser energy to minimize the potential for patient or health care personnel injury.

III.b. The laser assistant (eg, RN, laser technician) should not have competing responsibilities that would require leaving the laser unattended during active use.

 Circulating responsibilities may preclude the ability to assume responsibility for laser operation. The laser assistant runs the laser console to control the laser parameters under the supervision of the laser user. The laser user operates the laser for its intended purpose within the user's scope of practice, education, and experience.[1]

III.b.1. Personnel assignments for a procedure during which a laser is used should be based on, but not limited to,
- patient assessment and acuity,
- the type of laser being used,
- the complexity and type of procedure,
- surgical site, and
- the experience and competency of the laser assistant and RN circulator.

III.c. The emergency shut off switch should be used to disable the laser in case of a component breakdown or untoward event.[1,7,10]

 Immediate shut down of the laser may prevent patient and health care personnel injury as well as equipment damage.

III.d. Reflective surfaces should be minimized during laser surgery.[1]

 The laser beam may refract off shiny surfaces, potentially causing skin or eye injury.[7]

LASER SAFETY

III.d.1. Anodized, dull, non-reflective, or matte-finished instruments should be used near the laser site.[3,4,7]

Anodized, dull, non-reflective, or matte-finished instruments decrease the reflectivity of laser beams.[1,3,4,7]

III.d.2. Instruments that have been coated (ie, ebonized) should be inspected regularly for damage to the integrity of the coating. Instruments with damaged coating should be removed from service and repaired or replaced.[7]

Damage or scratches to the coating may allow the laser beam to refract off shiny surfaces, potentially causing skin or eye injury.[7]

III.d.3. Reflective instruments that cannot be ebonized should be covered with saline-saturated materials (eg, towels, radiopaque sponges).

III.e. Exposed tissues around the surgical site should be protected with saline-saturated materials (eg, towels, sponges) when lasers with a thermal effect are being used.[1]

The solution (eg, saline) absorbs or disperses the energy of the laser beam in areas not intended for laser application.[4]

III.e.1. These materials should be remoistened periodically to prevent drying and becoming an ignition source.[7,11]

III.f. Backstops (eg, titanium rods, quartz rods) or guards should be used during CO_2 laser surgery to prevent the laser beam from striking normal tissue.[4,7]

The CO_2 laser beam continues to move through the tissue after it cuts or coagulates. A backstop or guard will prevent the laser beam from affecting non-targeted tissue.

III.f.1. Mirrors made of rhodium or stainless steel may be used as a backstop in hard-to-reach areas.

III.g. When a fiber is used to deliver laser energy through an endoscope, the end of the fiber should extend past the end of the endoscope and be in view at all times during active use.[1]

Activation of the laser fiber inside the endoscope may cause damage to the scope.

III.g.1. For rigid endoscopic delivery systems (eg, laryngoscopes, bronchoscopes, laparoscopes), care should be taken to avoid heating of the sheath wall by the laser beam.[1]

If the metallic tubular system is used improperly, the heat inside the endoscope will cause thermal damage to adjoining tissues.[1]

III.h. When using lasers with flexible endoscopic delivery systems, care should be taken to avoid laser beam exposure within the sheath.[1]

Flexible fiber-optic endoscopic sheaths may be damaged by heat. Flexible fiber-optic endoscope sheaths may be flammable.[1]

Recommendation IV

All people in the nominal hazard zone should wear appropriate eyewear selected and approved by the LSO.[1,3,4,10,12]

Scattered, diffused, and reflected laser beams, in addition to direct exposure from misdirected and damaged fibers, can cause eye injuries.[1,6]

IV.a. Selection of appropriate laser protective eyewear should be based on, but not limited to,
- the recommendations of the laser manufacturer[1] and
- the manufacturer's laser protective eyewear specifications.[1]

Laser protective eyewear protects the wearer from eye injury from direct or diffuse laser beams.[1]

IV.b. People in the nominal hazard zone must wear protective eyewear or use filters of specific wavelength and optical density for the laser in use.[1,6,12]

Eyes are vulnerable to injury from the laser beam. The part of the eye that is at risk depends on the wavelength of the laser used.[4] Color vision and/or night vision could be impaired or lost if the laser beam focuses on the retina.[6] Protective glasses are manufactured to specifications that will prevent damage to the eye by stopping the laser energy from penetrating the lens of the eye.[7] Lens filters protect the laser user from laser exposure.[1]

IV.b.1. Eyewear must be labeled with the appropriate optical density and wavelength for the laser in use.[1,4,12]

Optical density is the ability of laser protective eyewear to absorb a specific laser wavelength. The portion of the eye (eg, lens, cornea, retina) that may be injured by exposure to the laser beam depends on the laser's wavelength.[4]

IV.b.2. Correct laser wavelength and optical density eye protection should be available at the entrance to a room where a laser is in use.[1,6]

IV.b.3. Laser shutters or filters with the appropriate optical density should be used on microscopes to protect the laser user from laser exposure.[1]

Shutters and laser filters protect the laser user from laser exposure.[1]

IV.b.4. Laser filters with the appropriate optical density should be used on microscope accessory oculars. If filters are unavailable, personnel using accessory microscope view ports should wear protective eyewear.[1]

LASER SAFETY

Filters protect viewers using microscope accessory oculars from laser exposure.[1]

IV.b.5. Health care personnel in the nominal hazard zone should wear protective eyewear even when a microscope eye lens filter is in use unless the LSO has determined that protective eyewear is not needed in the nominal hazard zone.[1,6,7]

IV.b.6. A lens filter of the appropriate laser wavelength may be used over the top of an endoscope viewing port.[1,4]

IV.b.7. Protective eyewear should be carefully handled and stored to prevent scratches and damage.[4,7]

IV.b.8. Protective eyewear should be inspected for damage and scratches before use. Damaged eyewear should be removed from use and reported to the LSO or LSS.[1,7]

IV.c. Patients' eyes and eyelids should be protected from the laser beam.[1,3]

The laser beam may cause injury to the patient's eyes if they are unprotected. The part of the eye at risk depends on the wavelength of the laser being used.[4]

IV.c.1. Patients who remain awake during laser procedures should wear goggles or glasses designated for the type of laser being used.[3,4,7]

IV.c.2. Patients undergoing general anesthesia should be provided with appropriate protection, such as wet eye pads, laser-specific eye shields, or as approved by the LSO.[1,3,4]

IV.c.3. Patients undergoing laser treatments on or around the eyelids should have their eyes protected by metal corneal eye shields that are approved by the US Food and Drug Administration (FDA).[1,4,6,7]

IV.d. Medical surveillance (eg, baseline eye exam, post-procedure exposure exam) should be considered for health care personnel where class 3B and class 4 lasers are used, if requested by the employing health care organization.[1,4,7,13]

A baseline eye examination provides historical information in the event of a laser injury.[1,4]

IV.d.1. The baseline exam should be performed before working with lasers, as directed by the health care organization policy and procedure.[1,14]

IV.d.2. A medical eye exam should be performed at the time of a suspected or abnormal exposure to laser radiation.[1,13,14]

Recommendation V

Potential hazards associated with surgical smoke generated in the laser practice setting should be identified and safe practices established.

Surgical smoke (ie, plume) is generated from use of lasers.[1,15] Analysis of the airborne contaminants produced during laser surgery has shown that laser plume contains toxic gas and vapors (eg, benzene, hydrogen cyanide, formaldehyde); bioaerosols; dead and living cell material, including blood fragments; and viruses.[1,16-18]

Many additional hazardous chemical compounds have been noted in surgical smoke.[17-22] At some level, these contaminants have been shown to have an unpleasant odor, cause problems with visibility of the surgical site, cause ocular and upper respiratory tract irritation, and demonstrate mutagenic and carcinogenic potential.[1,17]

Bacterial and/or viral contamination of plume has been highlighted by different studies.[18,23,24] The National Institute for Occupational Safety and Health (NIOSH) recommends that smoke evacuation systems be used to reduce potential acute and chronic health risks to health care personnel and patients.[17] The Occupational Safety and Health Administration (OSHA) has no separate standard related to surgical smoke plume, but does address related safety hazards in the General Duty Clause and Bloodborne Pathogens Standard.[25,26]

V.a. Surgical smoke should be removed by use of a smoke evacuation system in both open and minimally invasive procedures to prevent occupational exposure to laser-generated airborne contaminants.[1]

Local exhaust ventilation (LEV) is the primary means to protect health care personnel from occupational exposure to laser-generated airborne contaminants.[1] Potential health and liability risks may be reduced by the evacuation of surgical smoke.[16]

V.a.1. When surgical smoke is generated, an individual smoke evacuation unit with a 0.1 micron filter (eg, ultra-low particulate air [ULPA] or high efficiency particulate air [HEPA]) should be used to remove surgical smoke.[1,17]

During laser surgery, the cells are heated to a high temperature causing the cell membrane to rupture, releasing particles into the air. Lasers create particles approximately 0.3 microns in size.[18]

V.a.2. The capture device (eg, wand, nonflammable suction tip) of the smoke evacuation system should be positioned as close as possible, but no greater than two inches (5.08 cm) from the source of the smoke.[16,17]

Close proximity of the smoke evacuation wand maximizes particulate matter and odor capture and enhances visibility at the surgical site.[1,4]

LASER SAFETY

V.a.3. Smoke evacuation units and accessories should be used according to manufacturers' written instructions.

V.a.4. When a central (wall) suction system is used to evacuate smoke, a 0.1 micron in-line filter (eg, ULPA filter) should be used.[4,17] The in-line filter should be placed between the suction connection and the suction canister.[1]

Central (ie, wall) suction units are designed to capture liquids and are used with an in-line 0.1 micron filter to remove airborne contaminants.[17] Low suction rates associated with centralized suction units limit their efficiency in evacuating plume, making them suitable only for the evacuation of small amounts of plume.[16]

V.a.5. When a centralized suction system dedicated for smoke evacuation is available, the smoke evacuator lines should be flushed according to the manufacturer's instructions to prevent particulate matter build up or contamination of the suction line.

V.b. Used smoke evacuator filters, tubing, and wands should be considered potentially infectious waste. These used devices should be handled using standard precautions and disposed of as biohazardous waste.[1,4,16,17]

Airborne contaminants produced during laser procedures have been analyzed and are shown to contain gaseous toxic compounds, bioaerosols, and dead and living cell material. At some level, these contaminants have been shown to have an unpleasant odor, cause visual problems for health care personnel, cause ocular and upper respiratory tract irritation, and demonstrate mutagenic and carcinogenic potential.[1] Bacterial and/or viral contamination of smoke plume also has been identified.[23,24]

V.c. Personnel should wear respiratory protection (ie, fit-tested surgical N95 filtering face piece respirator or high-filtration surgical mask) during procedures that generate surgical smoke as secondary protection against residual plume that has escaped capture by local exhaust ventilation.[4]

Local exhaust ventilation is the first line of protection from surgical smoke.[1,27]

Analysis of the airborne contaminants produced during laser surgery has shown that laser plume contains toxic gas and vapors (eg, benzene, hydrogen cyanide, formaldehyde); bioaerosols; dead and living cell material, including blood fragments; and viruses.[1,16-18]

Many additional hazardous chemical compounds have been noted in surgical smoke.[17-22]

V.c.1. High-filtration face masks should not be used as the first line of protection against surgical smoke inhalation or as protection from chemical or particulate contaminants found in surgical smoke plume.[1,27]

A surgical mask is intended to prevent the release of potential contaminants from the user into their immediate environment. It also is used to protect the wearer from large droplets, sprays, and splashes of body fluids.[28] High-filtration face masks are specifically designed to filter particulate matter that is 0.1 micron in size and larger. Virus particles range from about 0.01 to 0.3 micrometers.[19] Surgical and high filtration masks do not seal the face and may allow dangerous contaminants to enter the health care worker's breathing zone.[28]

A recent laboratory study of five surgical masks with bacterial filtration efficiency of 95% to 99% found that 80% to 100% of subjects failed an OSHA-accepted qualitative fit test using Bitrex (ie, a bitter tasting aerosol) and quantitative fit factors ranged from 4 to 8 (12% to 25% leakage) using a TSI Portacount.[29] In contrast, the least protective type of respirator (ie, negative pressure half mask) must have a fit factor (outside particle concentration divided by inside concentration) of at least 100 (1% leakage). A high-filtration mask provides less protection than a fit-tested N95 filtering face piece respirator.[30]

Research is pending to test the efficacy of high-filtration masks and the air quality and quantity of airborne contaminants resulting from varying energy devices (eg, laser, electrosurgery, ultrasonic).

V.c.2. Respiratory protection that is at least as protective as a fit-tested surgical N95 filtering face piece respirator should be considered for use in conjunction with LEV in disease transmissible cases (eg, human papillomavirus)[23,24,31] and during high-risk or aerosol transmissible disease procedures (eg, tuberculosis, varicella, rubeola).[32]

A fit-tested surgical N95 filtering face piece respirator is a personal protective device that is worn on the face, covers at least the nose and mouth, and is used to reduce the wearer's risk of inhaling hazardous airborne particles including infectious agents.[28] The NIOSH respirator approval regulation defines the term *N95* to refer to a filter class that removes at least 95% of airborne particles during "worse case" testing using a "most-penetrating" sized particle during NIOSH testing.[28] Filters meeting the criteria are given a 95 rating. Many filtering face piece respirators have an N95 class filter and those meeting this filtration performance are often referred to simply as N95 respirators.[28]

LASER SAFETY

Recommendation VI

All people in the laser treatment area should be protected from electrical hazards associated with laser use.

Lasers may use high voltage electrical current.[7] Electrocutions and accidental shock of personnel have been reported.[3]

VI.a. The LSO should approve laser systems and equipment after they are evaluated for electrical hazards and before they are placed in service.

  The LSO is responsible for administration and oversight of laser hazards.[1]

VI.b. The manufacturer's directions for laser installation, operation, and maintenance should be followed.

  Some laser systems require special utilities (eg three-phase, 208 VAC, 50 ampere service).[3]

VI.b.1. The manufacturer's recommendations for electrical plugs and outlets should be followed.[3,4]

VI.c. The electrical cord and plugs of the laser should be handled in a manner that minimizes the potential for damage and subsequent patient and health care personnel injuries.

  Improper handling of cords and plugs may result in breaks in the cord's insulation, fraying, and other electrical hazards.

VI.c.1. The electrical cord should be free of kinks, knots, and bends.

  Kinks, knots, and bends damage the cord and cause current leakage, current accumulation, and overheating of the cord's insulation.

VI.c.2. The laser plug, not the cord, should be held when it is removed from the outlet.

  Pulling on the cord may cause cord breakage, which poses a fire hazard.

VI.c.3. The laser cord and plug should be kept dry.[3]

  Fluids in or around the laser connection and cord may cause an electrical hazard as a result of a short circuit.

VI.c.4. The laser's cord should be inspected before use or electrically tested for outer insulation damage.[3]

  Cord failures can result in electrical shock, sparking, or a fire, which could injure the patient or health care personnel.

VI.d. Liquids should not be placed on laser units.[4,7]

  Lasers are high-voltage equipment that should be protected against short circuiting associated with spillage or splatter.[4,7]

VI.e. Laser service and preventive maintenance in accordance with the manufacturer's guidelines should be performed on a regular basis by trained personnel who have knowledge of laser systems.[3]

  Periodic preventive maintenance helps to support continued safe operation of laser devices.[1]

VI.e.1. The laser safety officer should review maintenance documents before allowing any laser to be reentered into service.

Recommendation VII

All people in the laser treatment area should be protected from flammable hazards associated with laser use.

Fire is a potential hazard of laser use.[3,4,8,11,33-35] The intense heat of laser beams can ignite combustible or flammable solids, liquids, and gases.[34] The presence of increased oxygen concentrations enhances combustion and leads to the rapid spread of flames.

VII.a. Fire safety measures should be followed when lasers are in use according to local, state, and federal regulations.[36,37]

  Lasers are a potential ignition and fire source in the perioperative environment.[11]

VII.a.1. The laser should not be activated in the presence of flammable agents (eg, antimicrobial skin prep or hand antisepsis agents, tinctures, de-fatting agents, collodion, petroleum-based lubricants, phenol, aerosol adhesives, uncured methyl metharylate) until the agents are dry and vapors have dissipated.[11,33,38-41]

  Alcohol-based prep agents remain flammable until they are completely dry. Vapors occurring during evaporation also are flammable. Trapped solution or vapors under clear, adhesive, or surgical drapes increases the risk of fire or burn injury.[40] Alcohol-based skin prep agents are particularly hazardous because the surrounding hair or fabric can become saturated.

  Pooling can occur in body folds and crevices (eg, umbilicus, sternal notch).

  Ignition of flammable substances by lasers has caused fires and patient injuries. Flammable prep agents can be safely used by adhering to National Fire Protection Agency standards, local fire codes, and AORN recommendations and guidance statements.

  Use of nonflammable prep agents will minimize this risk.[20,37,38,41]

VII.a.2. Caution should be used when using a laser in the presence of combustible anesthetic gases during surgery on the head, face, neck, and upper chest.[11,34,39,42]

  The intense heat of laser beams can ignite combustible or flammable solids, liquids, and gases.[34] The presence of increased oxygen concentrations enhances combustion and leads to the rapid spread of flames.[42]

LASER SAFETY

VII.a.3. When using a laser, sponges and drapes near the surgical site should be kept moist.[3,4,11,27,33,35,43,44]

In an oxygen-enriched environment, the high energy delivery of a laser will burn anything combustible or flammable.[11,44] The fire triangle requires an ignition source (eg, the laser); an oxidizer (eg, the oxygen enriched environment); and fuel (eg, surgical drapes). Moistening draping materials decreases the potential for fire.[4]

VII.a.4. During perineal surgery, moistened radiopaque sponges may be used for rectal packing or covering the anus.[1,4,7]

Moist packing prevents the release of methane gas from the rectum. Methane gas is highly flammable and potentially explosive.[3,4,7]

VII.b. Laser surgery should not be performed in an oxygen-enriched environment.[11,34]

An oxygen-enriched environment lowers the temperature and energy at which fuels will ignite.[8,33,40,42] Fires, including airway fires, have resulted from the laser sparking in the presence of concentrated oxygen.[8]

VII.b.1. The lowest possible oxygen concentration that provides adequate patient oxygen saturation should be used.[1,4,33,35,38,43,45-47]

Mixing oxygen with nonflammable gases such as medical air or helium reduces the risk of fire.[1,11,47,48]

VII.b.2. Surgical drapes should be arranged to minimize the buildup of oxidizers (eg, oxygen, nitrous oxide) under the drapes.[11,33-35,42,43]

VII.c. Personnel should be prepared to immediately extinguish flames should they occur.[11]

A small fire can progress to a life-threatening emergency in seconds. Lasers are a potential ignition source and a common cause of surgical fires and patient injury.[11]

VII.c.1. Wet towels and saline should be available on the sterile field to extinguish a fire should one occur.[4,6]

VII.d. Fuel risks should be minimized.[11]

Many of the materials and solutions used in the perioperative setting are potential fuel sources (eg, prepping agents, linens, dressings, ointments, anesthesia components).[11]

VII.d.1. Flammable prep solution should have enough time to evaporate before drapes are applied.[11,43]

Prep solutions can be absorbed into linens and body fibers (eg, hair). Alcohol-based skin prep vapors can become trapped under drapes and coverings, and the volatility of these vapors can increase the risk of surgical drape fires.[11]

VII.d.2. Pooled solutions should be removed or patted dry.[4,11]

VII.e. The LSO should determine the type of extinguisher needed for each specific laser based on manufacturers' suggestions.[44]

VII.e.1. Fire extinguishers and saline should be immediately available where lasers are used.[1,4,7]

Immediate action can reduce the magnitude of injury.[1]

VII.f. Laser-resistant endotracheal tubes should be used to minimize the potential for fire during laser procedures involving the patient's airway or aerodigestive tract.[1,7,8,10,11,34,35,42,43,49]

Polyvinylchloride (PVC), silicone, and red rubber endotracheal tubes are combustible.[1,4,8,34,49] Burned PVC produces hydrochloric acid and harmful vapors.[1,42] Burned red rubber tubes produce carbon monoxide.[1] An airway fire may result in damage to the trachea and lungs, severe injury, and death.[8,49]

VII.f.1. Endotracheal tube cuffs should be inflated with normal saline during laser procedures involving the patient's airway or aerodigestive tract.[1,4,8,11,43,49,50]

VII.f.2. Saline with dye (eg, methylene blue) in the endotracheal tube cuff should be used to enhance the detection of a cuff puncture.[4,8,11,42,43,49,50]

Using saline with dye in the endotracheal tube cuff helps perioperative personnel recognize punctures and take immediate action.[43,49,50] The saline also provides a means of heat transfer and fire suppression.[50]

VII.f.3. Moistened packs may be placed around the endotracheal tube. These packs should be kept moist throughout the procedure.[1,11,43]

VII.f.4. Health care personnel should be aware of other flammable items associated with endotracheal tube use during laser procedures. These include, but are not limited to,
- plastic items (eg, breathing circuit, airway, suction catheter)[11,34,49];
- adhesive tape[11]; and
- ointment or lubricant.[11,34,49]

VII.g. The airway fire management procedure should be posted in laser treatment areas.[49]

Immediate action is required if an airway fire occurs. An airway fire can damage a patient's lungs almost immediately.[49]

VII.h. Surgical fires should be reported as a sentinel event to the appropriate agency (eg, FDA, state health department, certifying body, local fire department, ECRI).[43,51]

Reporting surgical fires raises awareness about hazards and adds to the body of prevention knowledge.[52]

LASER SAFETY

Recommendation VIII

Personnel working in laser environments should demonstrate competency commensurate with their responsibilities. Education programs should be specific to laser systems used and procedures performed in the facility.

Initial education on the underlying principles of laser safety and laser biophysics provides direction for personnel in providing a safe environment. Additionally, periodic educational programs provide reinforcement of principles of laser technology and new information on changes in technology, its application, compatibility of equipment and accessories, and potential hazards.

VIII.a. Personnel working in a laser environment should have knowledge of the established laser safety program.

The laser safety education program should provide health care personnel with a thorough understanding of laser procedures and the technology required for establishing and maintaining a safe environment during laser procedures. Laser education and training gives direction for personnel working in or near laser use areas and provides a safe environment for the patient and health care personnel.

VIII.a.1. Program criteria and content should be in accordance with applicable standards; the facility's policies and procedures; and federal, state, and local regulations.

VIII.a.2. Personnel should be required to demonstrate laser competency periodically and when new laser equipment, accessories, or safety equipment is purchased or brought into the practice environment.

VIII.a.3. The laser safety program should provide participants with a thorough understanding of laser procedures and the technology required for establishing and maintaining a safe environment during laser procedures.

VIII.b. The LSO should be qualified through education and experience to administer the laser safety program.[1]

Laser education and training gives direction for the LSO to provide a safe environment for the patient and health care personnel.

VIII.b.1. The LSO should have education and experience in laser operations, clinical applications, and safety.[5]

VIII.b.2. Laser safety officer education and preparation should include, but not be limited to,
- completion of a formal medical laser safety course,
- completion of a formal medical laser safety officer course,
- certification as a medical laser safety officer, and
- previous laser operator work experience.

VIII.c. The LSS and laser assistant (eg, laser nurse, technician) should be qualified by education and training.[1]

Laser education and training gives direction for the laser operator to provide a safe environment for patients and health care personnel.

VIII.c.1. Laser assistant training should include, but not be limited to,
- laser operation principles[5];
- laser biophysics;
- clinical applications[5];
- potential risks to the patient and health care personnel[5];
- safety procedures[3,5];
- care of the laser, safety equipment, and accessories[5]; and
- hands-on use of the laser (eg, set-up, testing, control panel use).[5]

VIII.d. Personnel using lasers should be knowledgeable about the fire hazards associated with laser use.[34]

Fire is a potential hazard of laser use.[8,11,33,35] The intense heat of laser beams can ignite combustible or flammable solids, liquids, and gases.[34] The presence of increased oxygen concentrations during surgery enhances combustion and leads to the rapid spread of flames.

Flammable and combustible items in the laser environment include
- liquids (eg, alcohol-based skin prep solutions)[11,44];
- ointments (eg, petroleum- or oil-based lubricants)[11,44];
- gases (eg, oxygen, methane, anesthetic agents, alcohol vapor)[11];
- plastics[44];
- paper or gauze materials[8];
- surgical drapes[4,11,44];
- foam positioning devices;
- adhesive tape[11]; and
- endotracheal tubes.[8,11,34,44]

VIII.d.1. Emergency fire drills should be performed at least once a year with the entire perioperative team, including anesthesia care providers.[43,44] Airway fire management should be included in fire drills.[49] Fire extinguisher training should be included as part of the health care organization's fire plan.[44]

VIII.e. Administrative personnel should assess and document initial and annual competency of personnel in the safe use of lasers and the accessories for each type of laser used.[4]

A competency assessment provides a record that personnel have a basic understanding of laser technology, its risks, and appropriate corrective actions to take in the event of a fire or injury. This knowledge is essential to minimize the risks of equipment misuse and to provide a safe environment of care.

LASER SAFETY

Recommendation IX

Policies and procedures for laser surgery should be developed, reviewed periodically, revised as necessary, and readily available in the practice setting.[5]

Policies and procedures assist in the development of patient safety protocols, as well as quality assessment and improvement activities. Policies and procedures establish authority, responsibility, and accountability within the facility. They also serve as operational guidelines that are used to minimize patient risk factors, standardize practice, direct staff members, and establish guidelines for continuous performance improvement activities.

IX.a. Policies and procedures for laser safety should be developed with regard to individual practice settings, applicable standards, and federal and state regulations.

Policies and procedures define administrative, engineering, and procedural control measures for beam and non-beam hazards.[1]

IX.a.1. Policies and procedures for laser use should include, but not be limited to, the following:
- equipment checks before initial use,[1]
- equipment maintenance schedules,
- safety features required on the laser,
- reporting and impounding malfunctioning equipment,[9]
- injury reporting,
- precautions during use,
- fire safety,
- laser sanitation, and
- documentation of laser procedure.

IX.b. The health care organization's policies and procedures for laser surgery must be in compliance with the Safe Medical Devices Act of 1990, as amended in March 2000.[5,53]

The Safe Medical Device Act requires personnel at the facility where the device is used to report deaths and serious injuries caused or contributed by a device, to establish and maintain adverse event files, and to submit follow-up and summary reports to the FDA.[53]

IX.b.1. Incidents of patient or personnel laser injury or equipment failure should be reported as required by regulation to federal, state, and local authorities and to the equipment manufacturer.[9] Device identification, maintenance and service information, and adverse event information should be included in the practice setting report.

Documentation of details of the laser equipment allows for retrievable information for investigation into an adverse event.[9]

IX.c. A written fire prevention and management policy and procedure should be developed by a multidisciplinary group that includes all categories of perioperative personnel.[37]

Fire is a risk to both patients and health care workers in the perioperative setting. Fire is a potential hazard of laser use.[4,8,11,33-35] The intense heat of laser beams can ignite combustible or flammable solids, liquids, and gases.[34] The presence of increased oxygen concentrations during surgery enhances combustion and leads to the rapid spread of flames.

IX.c.1. The policy and procedure should describe processes to be implemented to safely manage different fire scenarios.

IX.c.2. The policy and procedure should include the roles and responsibilities of the perioperative team responding to fire.[11,44]

IX.d. A health care organization-specific policy and procedure should be developed by a multidisciplinary team to describe actions to take in the event of an airway fire.[4,7,51]

Airway fires are life-threatening emergencies.[7] Quick action may minimize consequences.

IX.d.1. The airway fire policy and procedure should include, but not be limited to, the following actions:
- removing the endotracheal tube while simultaneously disconnecting the breathing circuit[7,11,43];
- turning off the oxygen[7,11,43];
- pouring saline into the airway[43];
- removing all flammable and burning substances from the airway[43,50];
- re-establishing the airway initially using air and then switching to oxygen when the anesthesia care provider determines there is no burning in the airway[11];
- assessing the airway for damage with a bronchoscope[7,11];
- performing a tracheostomy if the patient cannot be reintubated or as necessitated by the patient's condition[7];
- assessing the patient for follow-up care (eg, admission to an intensive care unit for observation and further evaluation)[7,43]; and
- saving all involved materials for investigation.[11]

Recommendation X

Documentation should be completed to enable the identification of trends and demonstrate compliance with regulatory and accrediting agency requirements.

Documentation of all nursing activities performed is legally and professionally important for clear communication and collaboration between health care team members and for continuity of patient care.

X.a. Documentation data elements regarding the laser procedure should include, but not be limited to, the following:
- patient information[1];

LASER SAFETY

- type of laser used (eg, wavelength, serial or biomedical number);
- laser settings and parameters[1];
- safety measures implemented during laser use[1];
- surgical procedure[1];
- on/off laser activation and de-activation times for head, neck, and chest procedures; and
- patient protection (eg, eyewear, eye shield).[1]

Documentation provides communication among all care providers involved in planning and implementing patient care.

X.b. A laser safety checklist should be used.[1,5,7]

A laser safety checklist helps ensure that all safety measures have been implemented.[1,5,7]

X.b.1. A laser safety checklist includes, but is not limited to, the following activities:
- performing a laser self-test check before the patient is brought into the room,
- calibrating the laser if needed,
- conducting a test fire of the laser,
- posting "laser in use" signs at all entrances of the procedure room,
- providing appropriate eyewear,
- covering the windows of the procedure room as needed,[1]
- checking the availability of saline at the surgical field, and
- checking the appropriate type of fire extinguisher for the laser being used.

X.c. A laser log may be used as an adjunct to the perioperative documentation.

The laser log may serve as a reporting mechanism for
- collecting statistics,
- tracking types of procedures,
- identifying deviations from policies and procedures,[1,7] and
- usage trends.

X.c.1. Data that may be tracked with a laser log can include the
- individual patient's identification information;
- type of laser, its model number, serial number, and health care organization biomedical number;
- procedures performed with laser surgery;
- names of the personnel in the room;
- completed laser safety checklists;
- number of joules used;
- total energy used; and
- wattage used.[1,7]

X.d. Service and maintenance activities should be documented.

Documentation of actions taken to ensure the reliability and safe operation of lasers assists the LSO in maintaining a safe laser environment. Recurring problems can be detected and solved with appropriate follow-up.[1]

Recommendation XI

A quality assurance and performance improvement process should be in place to measure patient, process, and structural (eg, system) outcome indicators.

A fundamental precept of AORN is that it is the responsibility of professional perioperative RNs to provide safe, high-quality nursing care to patients undergoing operative and invasive procedures.[54]

XI.a. A laser safety audit of the health care organization and safety equipment should be completed at least annually or more frequently as determined by the LSO.[1]

A laser safety audit validates the testing of the equipment and the presence of protective safety measures (eg, glasses, smoke/plume evacuation, warning signs).[1]

XI.a.1. The safety audit should include, but not be limited to,
- examining all laser-related equipment and safety features (eg, eyewear, warning signs, smoke plume evacuation equipment, inspection stickers);[1]
- examining laser use areas;
- assessing staff members' knowledge of laser safety; and
- observing laser practices for compliance with the health care organization's written policies and procedures.

XI.a.2. The safety audit should be documented according to health care organizational policy.[1] The written report should include identified deficits and describe a proposed correction plan.

XI.b. A medical surveillance program should be established for health care personnel participating in laser use.

A medical surveillance program provides a baseline of visual acuity and documents physical changes that occurred after an abnormal exposure.[1]

XI.b.1. A physician should perform an examination of the affected body part as soon as possible after a suspected or confirmed laser-induced injury.[1]

XI.c. Incidents of failure to follow the health care organization's laser safety policy, laser and related equipment failure, and patient or personnel injury should be reported to the LSO and reviewed by the laser safety or safety committee.[1,9]

All laser accidents require reporting and follow-up.[1,53]

XI.d. Laser devices should be tested or assessed before initial use, inspected periodically, and undergo preventive maintenance by a designated, trained individual who is responsible for

LASER SAFETY

laser equipment maintenance (eg, biomedical engineering services personnel).[3]

Periodic preventive maintenance helps support continued safe operation of laser devices.[3,44]

Glossary

American National Standards Institute: Organization that provides guidance for the safe use of lasers for diagnostic and therapeutic uses in health care facilities. ANSI facilitates the development of consensus US standards and administers a system that assesses conformance to standards such as the ISO 9000 (quality) and ISO 14000 (environmental).

Anodized: A matte finish applied to metal surgical instruments to decrease reflectivity.

Authorized laser operator: A person educated and trained in laser safety and approved by the facility to operate the laser.

Class 3 laser: Lasers that are potentially hazardous for direct exposure to specular (ie, mirror-like) reflection.

Class 4 laser: Lasers that present significant skin and fire hazards. Most surgical lasers are class 4 lasers.

Controlled access area: The area where the laser is to be used. Access to this area is restricted to laser team members and/or those given permission to enter the area. Access is granted only to those who have been approved by the laser safety officer.

Corneal eye shield: A device placed over the eye to protect the cornea from self-induced trauma, such as rubbing, pressure, or excessive use.

Ebonized: A black finish applied to metal surgical instruments to decrease reflectivity.

Fire/flame retardant: A substance that by chemical or physical action reduces flammability of combustibles.

Health care laser system: A system used in health care applications that includes a delivery apparatus to direct the output of the laser, a power supply with control and calibration functions, a mechanical house with interlocks, and associated fluids and gases required for the operation of the laser.

High-efficiency particulate air filter (HEPA): Filters composed of a material of randomly arranged fibres having a filtration rating of 0.3 microns at 99.7% efficiency.

High filtration masks: Masks having a filtering capacity of particulate matter at 0.3 microns to 0.1 microns in size.

Laser: A device that produces an intense, coherent, directional beam of light by stimulating electronic or molecular transitions to lower energy levels. An acronym for "light amplification by stimulated emission of radiation."

Laser assistant: The person who sets up the laser and runs the laser console to control the laser parameters under the supervision of the laser user.

Laser-generated airborne contaminants: Particles, toxins, and steam produced by vaporization of target tissues.

Laser safety officer: Person responsible for effecting the knowledgeable evaluation of laser hazards and authorized and responsible for monitoring and overseeing the control of such laser hazards.

Laser safety specialist: The designated person responsible for oversight of safe laser use in each area where a laser is used. Synonym: laser resource nurse.

Laser treatment area: Area in which the laser is being operated.

Laser user: The person employing the laser for its intended purpose within the user's scope of practice, education, and experience. Synonym: laser operator.

Limiting-exposure duration: The length of time for which tissue can be exposed to the laser beam. This duration is determined by the design and/or intended use of the laser.

Maximum permissible exposure: The level of laser radiation to which a person may be exposed without hazardous effects of adverse biologic changes in his or her eyes or skin.

Nominal hazard zone: The space in which the level of direct, reflected, or scattered radiation used during normal laser operation exceeds the applicable maximum permissible exposure. Exposure levels beyond the boundary of the nominal hazard zone should be below the appropriate maximum permissible exposure level of the laser. Special eye and skin precautions must be enforced in the nominal hazard zone.

Optical density: Ability to absorb a specific laser wavelength.

Oxygen-enriched environment: Atmosphere containing more than 21% oxygen, frequently occurring in the oropharynx, trachea, lower respiratory tract, and near the head and neck during administration of oxygen to the patient.

Ultra low particulate air (ULPA) filter: Theoretically, a ULPA filter can remove from the air 99.9999% of bacteria, dust, pollen, mold, and particles with a size of 120 nanometers or larger.

References

1. *Z136.3-2005: Safe Use of Lasers in Health Care Facilities*. Washington, DC: American National Standards Institute; 2005.

2. *Z136.1-2007: Safe Use of Lasers*. Washington, DC: American National Standards Institute; 2007.

3. Annex D. The safe use of high-frequency electricity in health care facilities. In: *Health Care Facilities Handbook*. 10th ed. Quincy, MA: National Fire Protection Association; 2005.

4. Houck PM. Comparison of operating room lasers: uses, hazards, guidelines. *Nurs Clin North Am*. 2006; 41(2):193-218, vi.

5. ECRI. Laser safety. *Healthcare Risk Control*. 2008;1(January):1-14.

6. Baxter DA. Laser safety in the operating room. *Insight*. 2006;31(4):13-14.

7. Andersen K. Safe use of lasers in the operating room—what perioperative nurses should know. *AORN J.* 2004;79(1):171-188.

8. Patient Safety Authority. Airway fires during surgery. *PA-PSRS Patient Safety Advisory.* 2007;4(1):1, 4-6.

9. ECRI. Investigating device-related skin "burns." *ORRM.* 2006;2(Quality Assurance/Risk Management 3):1, 3-10.

10. Muller GJ, Berlien P, Scholz C. The medical laser. *Medical Laser Application.* 2006;21:99-108.

11. New clinical guide to surgical fire prevention. *Health Devices.* 2009;38(10):314-332.

12. Occupational Health and Safety Administration. 29 CFR § 1910.132-134: General requirements; eye and face protection; respiratory protection; 2008.

13. Medical surveillance (rationale). In: *Environmental Health Criteria 23: Lasers and Optical Radiation.* Geneva, Switzerland: World Health Organization;1982:132.

14. Suess MJ, Benwell-Morrison DA. *Nonionizing Radiation Protection.* 2nd ed. Copenhagen; Albany, N.Y.: World Health Organization, Regional Office for Europe; distributed by WHO Publications Centre USA; 1989.

15. Bigony L. Risks associated with exposure to surgical smoke plume: a review of the literature. *AORN J.* 2007;86(6):1013-1020; quiz 1021-1024.

16. ECRI Institute. Smoke evacuation systems, surgical. *Healthcare Product Comparison System.* November 2007.

17. NIOSH Hazard Control HC11: Control of smoke from laser/electric surgical procedures. http://www.cdc.gov/niosh/hc11.html. Accessed October 6, 2010.

18. Alp E, Bijl D, Bleichrodt RP, Hansson B, Voss A. Surgical smoke and infection control. *J Hosp Infect.* 2006;62(1):1-5.

19. Ulmer BC. The hazards of surgical smoke. *AORN J.* 2008;87(4):721-734, quiz 735-738.

20. Barker SJ, Polson JS. Fire in the operating room: a case report and laboratory study. *Anesth Analg.* 2001;93(4):960-965.

21. Hoglan M. Potential hazards from electrosurgery plume—recommendations for surgical smoke evacuation. *Can Oper Room Nurs J.* 1995;13(4):10-16.

22. Occupational Safety and Health Administration, Hospital eTool: Surgical Suite—Use of Medical Lasers. http://www.osha.gov/SLTC/etools/hospital/surgical/lasers.html. Accessed October 5, 2010.

23. Garden JM, O'Banion MK, Shelnitz LS, et al. Papillomavirus in the vapor of carbon dioxide laser-treated verrucae. *JAMA.* 1988;259(8):1199-1202.

24. Hallmo P, Naess O. Laryngeal papillomatosis with human papillomavirus DNA contracted by a laser surgeon. *Eur Arch Otorhinolaryngol.* 1991;248(7):425-427.

25. Occupational Safety and Health Act of 1970, S 2193, 91st Cong (1970). Pub L No. 91-596, 84 Stat 1590. Amended January 1, 2004.

26. Safety and health topics: laser hazards. http://www.osha.gov/SLTC/laserhazards. Accessed October 6, 2010.

27. Part 8: Guidelines for the safe use of laser beams on humans. In: *IEC TR 60825-8: Safety of Laser Products.* 2nd ed. Geneva, Switzerland: International Electrotechnical Commission; 2006.

28. Respirator trusted-source information page. National Institute for Occupational Safety and Health. http://www.cdc.gov/niosh/npptl/topics/respirators/disp_part/RespSource.html. Accessed October 6, 2010.

29. Oberg T, Brosseau LM. Surgical mask filter and fit performance. *Am J Infect Control.* 2008;36(4):276-282.

30. Derrick JL, Li PT, Tang SP, Gomersall CD. Protecting staff against airborne viral particles: in vivo efficiency of laser masks. *J Hosp Infect.* 2006;64(3):278-281.

31. Garden JM, O'Banion MK, Bakus AD, Olson C. Viral disease transmitted by laser-generated plume (aerosol). *Arch Dermatol.* 2002;138(10):1303-1307.

32. Siegel JD, Rinehard E, Jackson M, Chiarello L; the Healthcare Infection Control Practices Advisory Committee. *2007 Guideline for Isolation Precautions: Preventing Transmission of Infectious Agents in Healthcare Settings.* Atlanta, GA: Centers for Disease Control and Prevention; 2007. http://www.cdc.gov/hicpac/pdf/isolation/Isolation2007.pdf. Accessed October 6, 2010.

33. ECRI. Top 10 health technology hazards. *Health Devices.* 2008;November:343-350.

34. Rinder CS. Fire safety in the operating room. *Curr Opin Anaesthesiol.* 2008;21(6):790-795.

35. Daane SP, Toth BA. Fire in the operating room: principles and prevention. *Plast Reconstr Surg.* 2005;115(5):73e-75e.

36. AORN guidance statement: Fire prevention in the operating room. In: *Perioperative Standards and Recommended Practices.* Denver, CO: AORN, Inc; 2009: 195-203.

37. Recommended practices for a safe environment of care. In: *Perioperative Standards and Recommended Practices.* Denver, CO: AORN, Inc; 2010: 217-240.

38. Environment of care. In: *Comprehensive Accreditation Manual for Hospitals.* Oakbrook Terrace, IL: The Joint Commission; 2010.

39. Beesley J, Taylor L. Reducing the risk of surgical fires: are you assessing the risk? *J Perioper Pract.* 2006;16(12):591-597.

40. A clinician's guide to surgical fires. How they occur, how to prevent them, how to put them out. *Health Devices.* 2003;32(1):5-24.

41. *NFPA 99 Standard for Healthcare Facilities.* Quincy, MA: National Fire Protection Association; 2005: 13.4.1.2.2-A.

42. Sheinbein DS, Loeb RG. Laser surgery and fire hazards in ear, nose, and throat surgeries. *Anesthesiol Clin.* 2010;28(3):485-496.

43. American Society of Anesthesiologists Task Force on Operating Room Fires, Caplan RA, Barker SJ, et al. Practice advisory for the prevention and management of operating room fires. *Anesthesiology.* 2008;108(5):786-801, quiz 971-972.

44. National Fire Protection Association. *NFPA 115: Standard for Laser Fire Protection.* 2008 ed. Quincy, MA: National Fire Protection Association; 2008.

45. ECRI. Surgical fires. *ORRM.* 2006;2(Safety 1):1-18.

46. Bielen RP; National Fire Protection Association. Annex C: additional explanatory notes to chapters 1-20. In: *Health Care Facilities Handbook.* Quincy, MA: National Fire Protection Association; 2005:567-568.

47. Podnos Y, Irving CA, Williams R; American College of Surgeons Committee on Perioperative Care. Fires in the operating room. http://www.facs.org/about/committees/cpc/oper0897.html. Accessed October 5, 2010.

48. McHenry CR, Berguer R, Ortega RA, Yowler CJ. Recognition, management, and prevention of specific operating room catastrophes. *J Am Coll Surg.* 2004; 198(5):810-821.

49. ECRI. Fighting airway fires. *Healthcare Risk Control.* 2010;4(Surgery and Anesthesia 10):1-5.

50. ECRI. Selecting laser-resistant tracheal tubes [Membership required]. https://members2.ecri.org/Componénts/HRC/Pages/SurgAnPol27.aspx. Accessed April 22, 2010.

51. Beyea SC. Preventing fires in the OR. *AORN J.* 2003;78(4):664-666.

52. The Joint Commission. Preventing surgical fires. *Sentinel Event Alert.* June 24, 2003;29. http://www.jointcommission.org/SentinelEvents/SentinelEventAlert/sea_29.htm. Accessed October 5, 2010.

53. US Food and Drug Administration. Medical device reporting: manufacturer reporting, importer reporting, user facility reporting, distributor reporting. *Fed Regist.* 2000;654112-4121.

54. Quality and performance improvement standards for perioperative nursing. In: *Perioperative Standards and Recommended Practices.* Denver, CO: AORN, Inc; 2010: 783-792.

Acknowledgments

Lead Authors

Mary Ogg, MSN, RN, CNOR
Perioperative Nursing Specialist
AORN Center for Nursing Practice
Denver, Colorado

Evangeline Dennis, RN, CNOR, CMLSO
Clinical Manager for Procedural Service
Gwinnett Medical Center
Duluth, Georgia

Contributing Authors

Carla M. McDermott, RN, CNOR
Staff Nurse
South Florida Baptist Hospital
Lakeland, Florida

David L. Feldman, MD, MBA, CPE, FACS
American College of Surgeons
Vice President Perioperative Services
Maimonides Medical Center
Brooklyn, New York

Publication History

Originally published November 1989, *AORN Journal.*

Revised November 1993.

Revised November 1997; published January 1998, *AORN Journal.*

Reformatted July 2000.

Revised November 2003; published in *Standards, Recommended Practices, and Guidelines*, 2004 edition.

Reprinted April 2004, *AORN Journal.*

Revised October 2010 for online publication in *Perioperative Standards and Recommended Practices.*

Reformatted September 2012 for publication in *Perioperative Standards and Recommended Practices,* 2013 edition.

Minor editing revisions made in November 2014 for publication in *Guidelines for Perioperative Practice,* 2015 edition.

GUIDELINE FOR CARE OF PATIENTS UNDERGOING PNEUMATIC TOURNIQUET-ASSISTED PROCEDURES

The following Guideline for Care of Patients Undergoing Pneumatic Tourniquet-Assisted Procedures has been approved by the AORN Recommended Practices Advisory Board. It was presented as proposed recommendations for comments by members and others. The guideline is effective June 15, 2013. The recommendations in this guideline are intended to be achievable and represent what is believed to be an optimal level of practice. Policies and procedures will reflect variations in practice settings and/or clinical situations that determine the degree to which the guideline can be implemented. AORN recognizes the various settings in which perioperative nurses practice; therefore, this guideline is adaptable to various practice settings. These practice settings include traditional operating rooms (ORs), ambulatory surgery centers, physicians' offices, cardiac catheterization laboratories, endoscopy suites, radiology departments, and all other areas where surgery and other invasive procedures may be performed.

Purpose

Pneumatic tourniquets are used to occlude blood flow, obtain a near bloodless field for extremity surgery, and confine a bolus of anesthetic in an extremity for intravenous regional anesthesia. Serious patient injuries related to the use of pneumatic tourniquets are uncommon, but risk is present. The Norwegian Orthopedic Society conducted a survey of 398 surgeons working in 71 health care organizations who performed an estimated 63,484 procedures involving a pneumatic tourniquet. The response rate was 67% (265 surgeons). The researchers determined the incidence of complications was one in 2,442 procedures. Of the 26 complications reported, 15 were nerve injuries; three were blistering or skin necrosis; six were compartment syndrome or deep vein thrombosis (DVT), although these complications may have related more to the injury or surgical procedure than the tourniquet; and two were excluded from the study because of limited specific information. Specific to nerve injuries, the researchers determined the incidence of complications was one in 6,155 procedures involving tourniquets applied to upper limbs and one in 3,752 procedures involving tourniquets applied to lower limbs.[1]

The Arthroscopy Association of North America conducted a national survey and reported 930 complications in 118,590 arthroscopic procedures (0.8%). Sixty-three of the complications were neurological injuries and 80% of those were related to tourniquet use.[2] Researchers from the University of British Columbia sent an e-mail survey to 1,908 active fellows of the American College of Foot and Ankle Surgeons in the United States and Canada. The response rate was 19% (317 respondents) based on the 1,665 surveys that were successfully delivered. Nerve injury and DVT were listed as the most common concerns of using a tourniquet (ie, cited by 25% of the 73 respondents on tourniquet-related hazards). However, 28 respondents with eight to 31 years of clinical practice commented that complications were rare or had never been encountered (ie, 38% of the 73 respondents on tourniquet-related hazards).[3]

Pain from the tourniquet is one of the most common complications related to pneumatic tourniquet use.[4] Other complications that patients may experience include cardiovascular, respiratory, cerebral circulatory, and hematological effects related to the metabolic changes that result from ischemia caused by the pneumatic tourniquet applied to the extremity during surgery. Temperature changes, prolonged postoperative swelling of the affected limb, and arterial injury are other complications that may occur when a pneumatic tourniquet is used.[4,5]

In reports compiled by the Pennsylvania Patient Safety Authority from December 2004 through December 2009, 140 reported events were associated with pneumatic tourniquet use. The data revealed that 41% of the events were related to limb redness, bruising, or swelling, 19% were related to skin tears or blisters, and more than 40% were related to equipment or safety issues.[6]

This document provides guidance to perioperative team members on the use of pneumatic tourniquets. The guideline provides information about testing, applying, and cleaning pneumatic tourniquet equipment, and the patient care associated with the safe use of this equipment. Pneumatic tourniquet equipment consists of a pressure regulator with display, connective tubing, and an inflatable cuff. The guideline provides general recommendations for developing policies and procedures for safe use of a pneumatic tourniquet in the practice setting. Due to the variety and complexity of pneumatic tourniquet equipment, policies and procedures that reflect considerations for specific pneumatic tourniquet systems are beyond the scope of this guideline. Finger tourniquets and tourniquets used for phlebotomy or traumatic bleeding are outside the scope of this document.

Evidence Review

A medical librarian conducted searches of the databases MEDLINE®, CINAHL®, Scopus®, and the

PNEUMATIC TOURNIQUET

Cochrane Database of Systematic Reviews for meta-analyses, systematic reviews, randomized controlled and non-randomized trials, guidelines, and case reports. Search terms included *pneumatic tourniquet, tourniquet safety, tourniquet, surgical hemostasis, surgical procedures, nursing care, perioperative care, patient positioning, compartment syndromes, arm injuries, leg injuries, hand injuries, pain measurement, peripheral nervous system, peripheral nervous system diseases, nerve palsy, metabolic phenomena, metabolic changes, metabolic effects, vital signs, respiration, carbon dioxide, intracranial pressure, oxygen consumption, cardiac output, acidosis, hyperemia, venous congestion, blood pressure, lactic acid, hemodynamics, pulse, hypothermia, hyperthermia, systemic inflammatory response, Esmarch bandage, Urias bag, Pomidor roll-cuff, bandage, elastic wrap, intravenous regional anesthesia, Bier block, ankle block, conduction anesthesia, bloodless field, occlusion pressure, ischemia,* and *reperfusion injury.*

The search was limited to articles published in English between January 2006 and February 2012. The search was expanded to include articles published before 2006 when the original search did not identify more recent literature on a particular topic. The librarian established continuing alerts on the pneumatic tourniquet topics. The lead author and librarian identified relevant guidelines from government agencies and standards-setting bodies.

Articles identified in the search were provided to the lead author and a doctorally prepared evidence appraiser for evaluation. Each article was reviewed and critically appraised using the Johns Hopkins Evidence-Based Practice Model and the Research or Non-Research Evidence Appraisal Tools as appropriate. The literature was independently evaluated and appraised according to the strength and quality of the evidence. Each article was then assigned an appraisal score as agreed upon by consensus of the lead author and evidence appraiser. The appraisal score is noted in brackets after each reference, as applicable.

The collective evidence supporting each intervention within a specific recommendation was summarized and used to rate the strength of the evidence using the AORN Evidence Rating Model. Factors considered in review of the collective evidence were the quality of research, quantity of similar studies on a given topic, and consistency of results supporting a recommendation. The evidence rating is noted in brackets after each intervention.

Editor's note: MEDLINE is a registered trademark of the US National Library of Medicine's Medical Literature Analysis and Retrieval System, Bethesda, MD. CINAHL, Cumulative Index to Nursing and Allied Health Literature, is a registered trademark of EBSCO Industries, Birmingham, AL. Scopus is a registered trademark of Elsevier B.V., Amsterdam, Netherlands.

Recommendation I

The perioperative registered nurse (RN) should assess the patient preoperatively for risks and potential contraindications related to the use of a pneumatic tourniquet.

Risks related to the use of a pneumatic tourniquet include nerve injuries,[1-3] skin injuries (eg, blistering, bruising, necrosis),[1,6] compartment syndrome,[1] DVT,[1,3] and pain.[4] When a pneumatic tourniquet is used on a patient's extremity, the patient may experience systemic responses (eg, changes in temperature or blood pressure) related to reperfusion upon cuff deflation.[4,5] Using a pneumatic tourniquet on patients who have preoperative conditions that predispose them to these risks may result in a cumulative effect.

I.a. The perioperative RN should not assume routine use of a pneumatic tourniquet for all extremity procedures. The RN should confirm in the surgeon's or anesthesia professional's plan of care whether a pneumatic tourniquet will be used. *[1: Strong Evidence]*

The surgeon or anesthesia professional determines whether to use a tourniquet based on the risks and benefits to the patient. There is debate in the medical community regarding the use of a pneumatic tourniquet for surgical procedures. Based on the evidence, routine use of a pneumatic tourniquet for limb occlusion can no longer be assumed. Findings from an e-mail survey sent to 1,665 foot and ankle surgeons in North America revealed that 11 respondents (3.4%) rarely or never used a tourniquet.[3]

One researcher used a randomized controlled study to explore tourniquet use in patients undergoing arthroscopic knee surgery. Comparing the outcomes of 56 patients who were assigned either to the control group or the intervention group, the researcher found no significant differences related to operative times, technical difficulties, identification of intra-articular structures, postoperative pain, or postoperative complications when a tourniquet was not used. The researcher suggested the use of a tourniquet may be unnecessary for arthroscopic knee surgery.[7]

Findings from another prospective randomized controlled trial also revealed that knee arthroscopy could be performed successfully without the use of a tourniquet. In this study, tourniquets were applied to all of the 109 patients who participated, with 58 patients assigned to a group that had the tourniquet inflated and the other 51 assigned to a group that did not have the tourniquet inflated. The operative view was rated poor by the surgeon in four procedures (7.8% of procedures performed) in the uninflated tourniquet group, requiring those tourniquets to be inflated for 5% to 60% of the procedure time. The mean procedure time was 27 minutes for the inflated tourniquet group (ie, range 10 minutes to 80 minutes) and 30 minutes for the uninflated tourniquet group (ie, range 10 minutes to 87 minutes). The researchers did not report significant differences between the two groups when measuring the operative view, duration of the procedure, pain scores, analgesic requirements, or complications.[8]

A prospective double-blind randomized clinical trial involved 120 patients who were having routine arthroscopies. Sixty-one patients were randomly assigned to the inflated tourniquet group and 59 patients were assigned to the uninflated tourniquet group. Intraoperatively, for the inflated tourniquet group, surgeons reported they had better ability to see and experienced less technical difficulty; however, the findings revealed that the mean operative time was similar; the average operative time for the inflated tourniquet group was 30.5 minutes compared to an average of 31.1 minutes for the uninflated tourniquet group. The study was designed to be blinded, but the surgeon was able to tell whether the tourniquet cuff was inflated or deflated in all but five of the procedures, thus introducing a potential bias. The researchers discussed the need for further study to determine whether using an infusion pump in combination with intermittent tourniquet inflation would improve the ability to see during procedures on the uninflated tourniquet group. They reported an increase in postoperative pain in the inflated tourniquet group when the tourniquet was inflated for more than 30 minutes.[9]

Researchers conducted a meta-analysis and identified nine studies to compare outcomes of arthroscopic knee procedures in which a tourniquet was used and arthroscopic knee procedures in which a tourniquet was not used. With the exception of the ability to see the operative field, there were no significant differences for all other outcome measures. The researchers reported that there was limited evidence to suggest that a tourniquet assists in arthroscopic knee surgery.[10]

Tourniquet use for total knee replacements was the focus of a study involving 100 patients. Patients were randomly assigned to group A, which involved epinephrine-augmented hypotensive epidural anesthesia, or group B, which involved normotensive epidural anesthesia with use of a tourniquet. The researchers measured perioperative hemoglobin values and transfusion rates postoperatively and for six days after the procedure. They determined that the patients in group A did not experience detrimental effects on their perioperative hemoglobin values or transfusion rates. They also reported that when epinephrine-augmented hypotensive epidural anesthesia was used, it was an effective method to avoid the use of a tourniquet during total knee arthroplasty. The average surgery time for group A was 1.53 hours and for group B was 1.58 hours.[11]

Researchers conducted a meta-analysis and identified 15 studies to compare outcome measures and parameters of 1,040 total knee replacements in 991 patients. The researchers reported a trend for greater complications in the patients who had a tourniquet applied compared to the patients who did not have a tourniquet applied. They also reported that patients who underwent surgeries without a tourniquet had significantly greater intraoperative blood loss compared to patients who underwent tourniquet-assisted surgery; however, they did not identify a significant difference between the two groups for total blood loss or transfusion rate. There was no difference between the groups for any other outcome measure assessed; therefore, the researchers concluded that there was no advantage to using a tourniquet in knee replacement surgery for reduction of transfusion requirements.[12]

In another meta-analysis, researchers explored the correlation between 318 tourniquet-assisted total knee arthroplasties and the risks of complications when compared to 316 non-tourniquet-assisted total knee arthroplasties. They included eight randomized controlled trials and three high-quality prospective studies in the analysis. They reported that the evidence suggests that using a tourniquet in total knee arthroplasty may increase the risk of thromboembolic complications and that use of a tourniquet may save the surgeon time but it may not reduce the patient's blood loss.[13]

Researchers conducted a meta-analysis and identified four studies comparing outcomes of tourniquet-assisted ankle and foot surgery to non-tourniquet-assisted ankle and foot surgery. The analysis concluded that hospital length of stay was significantly shorter and that the postoperative period was less painful, with reduced swelling from the fifth postoperative day in surgeries undertaken without a tourniquet compared to tourniquet-assisted procedures. There may be a greater incidence of wound infection and DVT in tourniquet-assisted foot and ankle procedures. Because of methodological limitations of the reviewed studies, the researchers recommended further study to determine whether a tourniquet should be used during ankle or foot procedures.[14]

Researchers conducted a systematic review and meta-analysis to compare the patient outcomes when a tourniquet was used for orthopedic surgery on upper limbs to the patient outcomes when a tourniquet was not used. In 849 citations, they found only two studies that met their criteria. These two studies involved 55 patients and assessed the surgeon's ability to see, the patient's pain, and the total operative time. From the analysis, the researchers suggested that

PNEUMATIC TOURNIQUET

technical difficulties during upper limb surgery may have been reduced when tourniquets were used. However, they were not able to determine whether pain perception or operative time was influenced by the use of a tourniquet. They recommended further studies with stronger methodology.[15]

In another study, researchers followed 138 patients for at least one year after their surgical procedures to repair tibial fractures. The patients were randomly assigned to one of two groups (ie, with or without tourniquet use). The researchers reported that use of a tourniquet did not influence the infection rate or the healing time. They did report that patients' perceptions of pain decreased when a tourniquet was not used. They suggested that a tourniquet may not be necessary when plating tibial fractures because the surgical repair can be a short procedure that does not typically involve severe bleeding.[16]

I.b. The perioperative RN should assess the patient for considerations related to tourniquet use, including
- planned location of the tourniquet,
- condition of skin under and distal to the planned cuff site,
- size and shape of the extremity, and
- peripheral pulses distal to the cuff.

[2: Moderate Evidence]

Preoperative skin assessment provides a baseline to evaluate skin injuries that may occur at the site of the tourniquet cuff because of pressure necrosis or friction burns. Applying the tourniquet cuff to the proximal portion of the limb in an area of the limb where there is the most soft tissue can help to decrease the risk of injury to underlying nerves and vessels.[5]

Preoperative patient assessment facilitates planning for tourniquet cuff selection. There is a direct correlation between the circumference of the limb at the site of cuff application and the cuff pressure required to suppress circulation. Large limb circumferences indicate a higher tourniquet pressure will be necessary to achieve vessel occlusion.[17] Patients with small limb circumferences (eg, children younger than two years, small adults) will require a tourniquet cuff specifically designed for this patient population.[18,19]

Preoperative assessment of the limb shape also helps to plan for the selection of a properly fitting tourniquet cuff (eg, straight-cylindrical versus wide-contour cuff).[20] The risk of the tourniquet cuff shifting may be increased when the patient is obese or has limb tissue that is loose.[21]

Preoperative assessment of the patient's circulatory system including a baseline measurement of peripheral pulses helps to evaluate the risk of applying a tourniquet to the patient's limb. Indicators of poor circulatory nutrition include brittle, dry nails; shining or scaly skin; and extremity hair loss. Other indicators for circulatory considerations include capillary filling time and the presence of varicose veins.[22]

I.c. The nursing assessment should include screening for potential contraindications for tourniquet use, including
- venous thromboembolism,[2,3,23-27]
- impaired circulation or peripheral vascular compromise,[17,27-29]
- previous revascularization of the extremity,[22,30]
- extremities with dialysis access (eg, arteriovenous grafts, fistulas),[22]
- acidosis,[31]
- hemoglobinopathy (eg, sickle cell anemia),[17,28,32-34]
- extremity infection,[17]
- tumor distal to the tourniquet,[17]
- medications (eg, antihypertensives)[35,36] and supplements (eg, creatine),[37]
- history of pain[38] or weakness[39] in muscles or bones in extremities,
- open fracture, and
- increased intracranial pressure.[23,28]

[2: Moderate Evidence]

Risk of complications may be higher for certain patient populations. Using a 17-item questionnaire delivered by e-mail, researchers conducted an investigation to determine current practice patterns among members of the American College of Foot and Ankle Surgeons. A total of 317 respondents reported that the most commonly listed contraindications to tourniquet use included vascular disease or previous bypass and DVT.[3]

Researchers conducting a prospective comparison study examined the outcomes of 48 consecutive patients undergoing total knee arthroplasty and reported that the incidence of DVT was high (81.3%) with or without the use of a tourniquet. The first group of 21 patients underwent the surgical procedure without a tourniquet, and the next 27 patients underwent a tourniquet-assisted procedure. The researchers concluded that the use of a tourniquet decreased perioperative blood loss and did not increase the risk of DVT. They identified symptomatic pulmonary embolism in 1.7% of the patients and emphasized the importance of prevention and early detection of DVT to decrease the risk of fatal pulmonary thromboembolism.[24]

Twenty patients participated in a prospective study to determine whether extramedullary guided total knee arthroplasty decreased the severity of embolic showers after tourniquet deflation. The researchers reported that 14 patients experienced large venous emboli and six patients experienced small venous emboli. The researchers concluded that the thrombogenic effect of the tourniquet may be the cause of venous emboli rather than the manipulation of the marrow cavity because they did not find a difference in the incidence of venous emboli with extramedullary guided total knee arthroplasty when compared to the results of previous studies reporting the incidence of venous emboli with intramedullary guided total knee arthroplasty.[25]

Researchers conducted a randomized comparison study to determine the incidence of large venous emboli in 23 patients who underwent total knee arthroplasty procedures (ie, either intramedullary or extramedullary guided) without pneumatic tourniquet inflation. Their findings suggest a 5.33-fold greater risk of experiencing a large emboli for patients who have a knee arthroplasty with a tourniquet inflated, based on comparison with historical controls from a previous investigation.[26]

Patients who have arterial calcification, abnormal clotting times, diabetes, sickle cell trait, tumor, infection, or hypertension may have a higher risk of experiencing negative outcomes when a tourniquet is used.[17] Venous stasis and tissue hypoxia occur with use of a tourniquet, increasing the risk for exaggerated clotting cascade responses and poor wound healing.[23] A case study analysis of a patient with peripheral vascular disease and a femoral artery stent reported the patient developed an asymptomatic thrombosis in the stent between the time the surgeon last saw the patient in the clinic and the day of surgery. The authors recommended that the surgeon obtain a preoperative pedal pulse and perform a vascular examination immediately before marking the surgical site to identify recent changes in vascularity before initiating tourniquet-induced vein occlusion and tissue ischemia.[30]

Using a tourniquet on a limb that has arthrosclerotic vessels increases the risk for poor wound healing and sepsis. When a limb has an arterial prosthesis, there may be insufficient implant elasticity and impaired collateral circulation that cannot accommodate the sudden increased blood flow after tourniquet deflation.[22] One case has been reported in which calcification of an underlying artery may have caused tourniquet failure.[29]

Patients who have cardiopulmonary conditions, renal compromise, or clinically significant acid-base imbalance also have a higher risk of complications with application of a tourniquet.[31] Diabetic patients may already be at a higher risk for poor peripheral circulation, delayed healing, and prolonged infections in distal extremities.

Patients with sickle cell trait are at a higher risk for complications because of the hemostasis, hypoxia, and acidosis that occur beneath the tourniquet cuff and that provide ideal conditions to promote red cell sickling.[28,32] Researchers reviewed four studies that included 96 patients with sickle cell traits or hemoglobinopathies who underwent surgical procedures with tourniquet inflation. Ten patients who had tourniquet surgery on a lower extremity experienced complications compared to one patient with a complication after tourniquet surgery on an upper extremity. Therefore, the researchers suggested that a stronger correlation may exist between patients with sickle cell trait or hemoglobinopathies who undergo lower extremity tourniquet procedures than those who undergo upper extremity tourniquet procedures.[32] Based on findings from this review and an earlier case study, there is limited evidence to suggest that tourniquets may be safe to use for patients with sickle cell indicators when effective perioperative management is implemented.[32,33] Another case study in which surgeons used a tourniquet safely during a total knee replacement for an 82-year-old woman who was a Jehovah's Witness with sickle cell trait supports this finding.[34]

One case study reported a severe drop in blood pressure followed by myocardial depression at the time of tourniquet deflation. The authors attributed the severe reaction to the patient's preoperative dose of oral clonidine. They recommended using caution when using tourniquets on patients who are taking antihypertensives.[35] After investigating 75 patients who were having elective surgical procedures on their lower limbs, other researchers found that preoperative clonidine was an effective way to prevent systemic arterial pressure increases related to tourniquet use for patients under general anesthesia.[36]

Preoperative assessment is important for young adults as well as older adults. Two case studies have been reported involving younger people undergoing orthopedic procedures. The first case report involved a 21-year-old athlete who experienced rhabdomyolysis and acute renal failure after arthroscopic knee surgery. The authors suggested the patient's risk of tourniquet-related skeletal muscle injury was increased because of the patient's use of creatine supplements.[37]

The second case study did not relate to medications, but highlights the importance of the preoperative interview to reveal a history of pain. A 35-year-old patient undergoing a tourniquet-assisted open reduction-internal fixation of an ankle fracture developed symptoms of anterior compartment syndrome 10 hours after surgery. Preoperatively, the patient stated he had experienced pain in his legs previously while playing football and the pain continued afterward. The authors believed the tourniquet may have contributed to the development of the compartment syndrome. Retrospectively, they also believed that the patient may have had a predisposition to an exercise-induced compartment syndrome and that postoperative pain medications contributed to the delay in diagnosis. They encouraged the assessment of pre-injury pain when patients are injured during sporting activities and suggested using tourniquets with caution.[38]

Risks may be higher when a tourniquet is applied to an extremity of a patient who has a condition that causes muscle weakness (eg, myasthenia gravis). Authors of one case study advised caution when using bilateral tourniquets and prolonged tourniquet application in patients who have myasthenia gravis because of the risk of exacerbated symptoms in spite of regional anesthesia and the avoidance of muscle relaxants.[39]

Recommendation II

The perioperative RN should collaborate with the surgeon and anesthesia professional to develop and confirm the plan of care related to the use of a tourniquet.

Variations in patient conditions or the planned procedure influence perioperative plans relating to the use of a tourniquet. Because of these variations, the whole perioperative team should be in alignment. For example, administration of the preoperative antibiotic may be adjusted to coordinate with the timing of tourniquet inflation with the intent of increasing tissue concentrations.[40,41] Anesthesia professionals may plan to implement preconditioning or adjust their anesthetic plan to reduce oxidative stress resulting from tourniquet-induced ischemia-reperfusion.[42-44]

Anesthesia professionals may adjust their anesthesia plan of care (eg, preconditioning, supplementing regional anesthetic with ketamine) to reduce pain or rhabdomyolysis.[45,46] Intravenous regional anesthesia may be planned for upper extremity surgeries, requiring the perioperative nurse to anticipate the need for equipment and medications and be prepared for adverse events including those associated with intravenous regional anesthesia.[47-49]

Findings from the preoperative assessment may provide information that influences the size or shape of the tourniquet cuff to be used to obtain effective vessel occlusion with the lowest possible pressure.[50]

II.a. The timing of preoperative prophylactic antibiotic administration, when ordered, should be based on the health care organization's policy and procedure with a goal of achieving optimal tissue concentration. *[2: Moderate Evidence]*

Efficacy of prophylactic antibiotics requires tissue perfusion of the surgical site. In studies published in 1994 and 1995, researchers reported that optimal tissue concentrations were found when antibiotics were administered preoperatively, 20 minutes before tourniquet inflation.[51,52]

In a more recent study, researchers conducted a single-center randomized double-blind study of 908 patients who underwent total knee arthroplasty procedures to determine the importance of a "tourniquet-release" dose of antibiotics. One group of patients (n = 442) received the standard regimen (ie, receiving antibiotics before tourniquet inflation); the other group (n = 466) did not receive antibiotics before inflation but received a "tourniquet release dose" of the same dose of the antibiotic 10 minutes before release of the tourniquet. Both groups received a postoperative dose of the same antibiotic six hours after the procedure. The researchers speculated that the standard regimen (ie, administering antibiotics before tourniquet inflation) may result in a lower serum antibiotic concentration at the end of the surgical procedure and that is when the highest concentrations of antibiotics are needed to prevent growth of microorganisms during the 12 to 24 hours after the surgery. They found the "tourniquet-release" dose was more effective than the standard regimen, but there was not a statistically significant difference. The primary limitation to this study was that more patients were needed to determine statistical significance because the researchers' initial predictions about the difference in infection rate between both groups was higher than what occurred in the study.[41]

In another recent study, researchers measured outcomes for 106 patients, with 54 patients receiving antibiotics before tourniquet inflation and 52 patients receiving antibiotics one minute after tourniquet inflation. More than 70% of the procedures involved open reduction and internal fixation of fractures on lower extremities. The researchers concluded that administering an antibiotic shortly after inflation of the tourniquet did not produce an inferior outcome when compared to administering an antibiotic before exsanguination and inflation of a lower extremity tourniquet.[40]

II.b. The perioperative nurse should collaborate with the surgeon and the anesthesia professional to address DVT risk factors identified during the patient's preoperative assessment.[53] *[2: Moderate Evidence]*

Researchers in one study hypothesized that systemic thrombin generation begins after tourniquet deflation in total knee arthroplasty procedures. However, they also acknowledged that a tourniquet may damage endothelial vessels and create venous stasis in the extremity, which may increase thrombogenic and fibrinolytic activity. The participating patients were treated preoperatively with thromboprophylaxis. However, the researchers found that the patients' coagulation systems were activated 10 minutes after surgery. They recommended additional studies to explore correlations between preoperative and postoperative thromboprophylaxis and fibrinolytic system activities. Their data indicated that vein occlusion caused by tourniquets may contribute to thrombosis formation during surgery on lower extremities. However, the researchers did not believe the tourniquet inflation alone activated a systemic formation of the thrombosis.[54]

In another study, researchers confirmed that cellular interactions that augment blood coagulability were increased in the perioperative period for patients who underwent total knee arthroplasty. They also concluded that these responses were more prominent during tourniquet-assisted total knee procedures.[55]

II.c. The perioperative nurse should collaborate with the surgeon and anesthesia professional to address considerations related to the plan for anesthesia or ischemic preconditioning.[53] *[2: Moderate Evidence]*

The purpose of ischemic preconditioning is to increase the tolerance of tissue to a longer period of ischemia by initiating brief periods of ischemia[56] or influencing skeletal muscle tolerance with anesthetic regimens.[57] Several studies have investigated the correlation between various anesthesia or preconditioning techniques and oxidative stress related to ischemia and reperfusion that occurs after the release of a tourniquet.[42-44,56-64]

To reduce oxidative stress related to tourniquet inflation, preconditioning techniques may be planned to initiate short intervals of temporary ischemia (eg, three cycles of five minutes, followed by five minutes of reperfusion just before tourniquet inflation).[42,44,59,61] Perioperative nurses may participate in activities related to preconditioning (eg, retrieving medications, setting up equipment, coordinating the timing of skin preparation, documenting intervals of inflation). By collaborating with the surgeon and anesthesia professional, the nurse will be better prepared to assist in preconditioning-related activities.[53]

II.d. Before the patient enters the OR, a pneumatic tourniquet cuff should be selected using the following considerations.
  o The width of the tourniquet cuff should be as wide as possible without inhibiting surgical site exposure.[50,65]
  o Contoured tourniquet cuffs should be used for patient extremities in which there is a tapering of the extremity between the upper and lower edge of the cuff.[23,50,65]
  o The length of the tourniquet cuff should be sufficient to provide bladder overlap on the limb and full engagement of the hook-and-loop fasteners.

[2: Moderate Evidence]

Confirming that a tourniquet with the appropriate cuff size and shape is available before the patient enters the OR decreases the risk of using the wrong cuff size or shape or causing a delay to search for the appropriately sized cuff while the patient is under anesthesia.

Improper tourniquet cuff application may lead to skin injuries (eg, pressure necrosis, friction burns).[5] The risk of injury to tissue and nerves increases when more pressure is required for vessel occlusion. The ratio of the cuff width to the limb circumference has an inverse relationship with limb occlusion pressure (eg, wider cuffs require lower tourniquet pressures, narrower cuffs require higher tourniquet pressures).[20] Choosing the wrong cuff size or shape could lead to unnecessarily higher pressures and increase the risk for injury.

Wider cuffs minimize the risk for injury to underlying tissue by dispersing pressure over a greater surface area. In clinical trials, using a wider cuff has been found consistently to occlude blood flow at a lower pressure in adult patients.[50,65-67] Similar results were found using wider cuffs in children.[18] Contoured tourniquet cuffs have been found in clinical trials to occlude arterial flow at lower pressures than straight tourniquet cuffs of equal width. Contoured tourniquet cuffs minimize the risk of excessive pressure on one edge of the cuff, migration of the cuff, and a shearing injury to underlying tissue.[23,50,65]

II.e. A sterile cuff should be used when the cuff will be very close to the sterile field. A single-use cuff should be used when adequate protection of the cuff from contamination cannot be assured. *[3: Limited Evidence]*

Researchers conducted a study at two hospitals to assess microbial colonization on reusable tourniquet cuffs versus sterile single-use disposable tourniquets. They found that 23 of the 34 reusable tourniquet cuffs were contaminated before surgical application. Although they did not follow the patients to find out the incidence of surgical site infection in the 23 patients who had contaminated cuffs applied, the researchers concluded that sterile single-use tourniquet cuffs are preferred to decrease the bacterial load when the cuff is placed in close proximity to the surgical site.[68]

II.f. Potential risks for patient injuries and complications associated with dual-bladder cuffs used for intravenous regional anesthesia should be identified and safe practices should be established. *[3: Limited Evidence]*

Reports indicate that complications associated with intravenous regional anesthesia include local anesthetic toxicity, seizures, cardiac arrests, compartment syndrome, thrombophlebitis, discoloration, or widespread petechiae.[47] When using intravenous regional anesthesia, there is a risk for local anesthetic toxicity caused by accidental tourniquet failure or leakage around the tourniquet due to high venous pressure.[49,69] Complications can also occur that are related to tubings and misconnections (eg, attaching to distal versus proximal cuffs) when using dual cuffs for intravenous regional anesthesia.[70,71]

PNEUMATIC TOURNIQUET

II.f.1. Based on the preoperative patient assessment, the perioperative nurse should identify medication allergies, especially sensitivities to local anesthetics, and communicate with the anesthesia professional to clarify the plan for intravenous regional anesthesia before the tourniquet is applied.

II.f.2. The perioperative RN should confirm that
- a dual-bladder tourniquet cuff and extra connective tubing will be used,
- the planned location on the extremity is wide enough to accommodate the additional width of the dual-bladder tourniquet cuff, and
- a higher pressure is planned to compensate for the narrow size of each cuff bladder.[17]

Although intravenous regional anesthesia is more common in upper extremities, dual tourniquet cuffs and injection of local anesthetics have been used for lower extremities.[72] Variation in cuff sizes and the need for dual cuffs versus two separate cuffs will depend on the size of the patient's extremity and the location planned for the regional block.

II.f.3. Members of the perioperative team should clearly communicate with each other about the inflation-deflation sequence when using a dual-bladder cuff and when using two single-bladder cuffs together for intravenous regional anesthesia.

II.f.4. The proximal and distal cuffs and the respective tubing should be clearly identified.

Recommendation III

Patient safety should be the primary consideration when using a pneumatic tourniquet and its accessories.

Patient injury related to pneumatic tourniquet use has been reported. For example, one case report found that if the cuff that is applied to a patient's extremity has a bladder that is bent, folded, or crushed, adequate pressure may be compromised, resulting in bleeding at the surgical site.[73] Excessive pressure from the tourniquet may cause limb redness, bruising, swelling, or nerve injury.[6]

III.a. The tourniquet's tubing and connectors should be incompatible with other tubing (eg, intravenous) or labeled to clearly identify that they are part of the tourniquet system.[70,71] *[3: Limited Evidence]*

Although reports of misconnections involving tourniquet tubing are not common, misconnections of other types of tubing and connectors (eg, blood pressure tubing, Luer connections) have been reported.[70,71]

III.b. Before each use, the perioperative nurse should verify that the entire tourniquet system is complete, clean, and functioning according to the manufacturer's instructions for use.
- The pneumatic tourniquet regulator should be compatible with all associated components, and the connections should be secure.[17]
- The cuff, tubing, connectors, and o-rings should be inspected for cracks, leaks, and other damage.[17]
- The tourniquet should be tested for integrity and function.[17]
- The integrity of the hook-and-loop fasteners and tie ribbons should be inspected.[17]
- A full battery power charge should be confirmed, if applicable.[17]

[3: Limited Evidence]

Ensuring that the tourniquet functions properly before a procedure reduces the risk of pressure loss and patient injury.[17]

Unintentional pressure loss can result from loose tubing connectors, deteriorated tubing, or cuff bladder leaks and may result in patient injury.

III.c. A pneumatic tourniquet that is not working properly or is damaged should be removed from service immediately, along with all its accessories, and reported to the designated individual responsible for equipment maintenance (eg, biomedical engineering personnel).[74] *[2: Moderate Evidence]*

III.d. The perioperative RN should verify the correct surgical site before application of the tourniquet cuff and verify the tourniquet inflation pressure during the time-out process.[75] *[2: Moderate Evidence]*

Placing a tourniquet on the wrong limb may result in a cascade of events leading to wrong site surgery. Confirmation of the location of the tourniquet and its pressure setting during the time-out process increases communication and consistent documentation and reduces the likelihood of error.

III.e. Safety practices should be implemented when applying tourniquet cuffs to the verified operative extremity. *[2: Moderate Evidence]*

When the tourniquet cuff is inflated, nerves and blood vessels are compressed. This poses a potential risk to superficial nerves that are in unprotected areas during cuff placement.[4,23]

Proper application of the cuff decreases the risk for injury or pressure variances.[5,17,76-80] For example, a loose fitting cuff may shift after placement, causing a friction burn on the skin.[5] Higher pressures also may be needed if the cuff is applied too loosely.[17] Patients who are obese or others who have loose skin and adipose tissue at the site of the tourniquet cuff are at risk for the skin folding or puckering beneath the tourniquet cuff. This increases the risk for uneven pressure on vessels and skin injury.[17]

PNEUMATIC TOURNIQUET

III.e.1. Tourniquet cuffs should be applied snugly to the verified operative extremity[50] and in a position on the extremity that creates a minimal amount of ischemia.[27]

In one quasi-experimental study of 50 patients undergoing surgery for carpal tunnel syndrome under local anesthesia, researchers recommended placement of the tourniquet on the upper arm. They reported that there were not significant differences for patients tolerating tourniquets placed on the upper arm versus the forearm when the tourniquet time was shorter than 20 minutes. In addition, the patient's fingers may curl up and the tourniquet cuff may interfere with the surgical incision when it is placed at the forearm.[81] Researchers have found that patients undergoing foot surgery with local anesthesia have less pain when the cuff is placed at the ankle.[82-84]

III.e.2. When applying the tourniquet cuff to the small limb of a child where space is limited, the perioperative RN should evaluate the size, shape, and fit of the tourniquet to avoid its movement during the procedure. Sterile tourniquets should be considered for use if the tourniquet must be positioned close to the surgical site.[76]

Children's extremities can present unique challenges related to the size of the limb (eg, no space for the tourniquet, acute taper of a young child's thigh). If the tourniquet is not the right shape or is not applied tightly enough, it may slide toward the surgical wound, risking loss of compression or interference at the surgical site.[76]

III.e.3. The cuff should be applied in its final position. If at any time a cuff position change is necessary, the cuff should be removed and reapplied.

Moving a cuff after placement may cause shearing of underlying tissues and subsequent injury.

III.e.4. A low-lint, soft padding (eg, limb protection sleeve, two layers of stockinette) should be placed around the limb according to the cuff manufacturer's instructions for use. The padding should be wrinkle-free and should not pinch the skin.

In two clinical trials, the overall skin complication rate was lower when padding was used.[77,78] However, higher pressures may be needed if a cuff is applied over a thick layer of loose padding.[17]

Avoiding padding materials that may shed fibers (eg, cotton cast padding, sheet padding) will decrease linting. When lint from padding materials becomes embedded in the hook-and-loop fasteners of a tourniquet, it may reduce the effectiveness of the fasteners and potentially lead to an unexpected release of the cuff during a procedure.

III.e.5. The patient's skin under the tourniquet cuff should be protected to prevent fluid accumulation (eg, skin prep solutions, irrigation) under the cuff.

Underpadding and tourniquet cuffs can harbor moisture, resulting in skin breakdown if protective interventions are not taken. Two cases have been reported in which patients had to undergo burn wound excision and skin grafting because of chemical burns caused by pooling of the prep solution under a tourniquet.[80]

III.e.6. Reusable tourniquet cuffs should be protected from contamination by fluid, blood, and other potentially infectious material during surgery. Tourniquet protectors (eg, U-shaped drapes, adhesive drapes, tourniquet covers) should be used to minimize soiling.

Reusable tourniquet cuffs that are not protected from fluid, blood, and other potentially infectious material can be a source of cross contamination.

III.e.7. The cuff tubing should be positioned on or near the lateral aspect of the extremity.

Lateral placement of the cuff tubing may help avoid pressure on nerves of the extremity and prevent kinking of the tubing.

III.f. Procedures involving pneumatic tourniquet control on two extremities should have the tourniquet tubing labeled to clearly identify which tubing belongs to which cuff and which is associated with which components of the tourniquet system(s). The perioperative RN, surgical team members, and anesthesia professionals should confirm the respective placement of the tourniquets and plans for inflation during the time-out process.[75] *[2: Moderate Evidence]*

The risk for complications and the systemic effects of tourniquet use may increase when ischemia and reperfusion occur in two extremities. However, in one published expert opinion, the authors suggested that the delay between the sequential deflation of the first cuff and inflation of the second cuff allows time for caregivers to assess the systemic response and accommodate for the lactic acid released from the first procedure before the second cuff is inflated. If the patient does not tolerate the reperfusion or if complications occur in the first procedure, the option of aborting the second procedure may be a better choice than performing simultaneous bilateral procedures.[85]

The use of two tourniquet cuffs increases the number of tubings and connections which can increase the opportunity for errors of misconnections or inflation or deflation of the wrong cuff. Labeling the tubing to each cuff

PNEUMATIC TOURNIQUET

minimizes the risk of inflating or deflating the wrong cuff.[70,71]

Recommendation IV

Inflation of the tourniquet cuff should be done under the direction of the surgeon and coordinated with the anesthesia professional.

After limb exsanguination and cuff inflation, there is an increase in blood volume to vital organs and a subsequent increase in systolic blood pressure.[28] Healthy adults may experience only minor hemodynamic changes when a tourniquet is inflated. However, patients who are elderly or have cardiac conditions (eg, cardiac failure, cardiac enlargement) may experience intraoperative hypertension or other complications related to the increased blood volume (eg, 800 mL of blood may be added when exsanguinating a leg).[4,5] Coordination with the anesthesia professional facilitates management of the patient during this rapid physiologic change.

Several cases of fatal complications immediately or within 30 minutes following exsanguination of the operative leg have been reported.[86] Patients who are older than 50 years or who have not been mobile or whose preoperative cardiovascular evaluation suggests higher risk factors for DVT (eg, smoking, obesity, cardiac arrhythmias) are at higher risk for complications during or following exsanguination of the lower limb.[86]

IV.a. The extremity should be exsanguinated before inflation of the tourniquet. *[2: Moderate Evidence]*

When a limb is exsanguinated, an elastic wrap (eg, an Esmarch bandage) compresses superficial blood vessels, forcing blood out of the extremity. Use of an elastic bandage for exsanguination enhances the bloodless field and may minimize the pain associated with tourniquet use.

The surgeon or anesthesia professional determines appropriate use of an elastic wrap, taking into consideration the risks and benefits to the patient. Exsanguination using an elastic wrap may not be appropriate following traumatic injury or if the extremity has been in a cast. In these instances, thrombi in blood vessels may become dislodged, resulting in emboli. Fatal pulmonary emboli have been reported following exsanguination of such extremities.[86]

In a randomized trial, 100 patients were assigned to one of three groups to compare the effectiveness of exsanguination methods (ie, limb elevation, squeezing the limb hand over hand starting distally and moving proximally with the limb elevated, and mechanical exsanguination with a sterile elastic bandage). The researchers concluded that the "squeeze" method and the elastic bandage methods were more effective at providing a bloodless surgical field than the elevation method.[87] However, elevating the extremity may be the preferred method for exsanguination when a patient has an infection or a malignant tumor in the operative extremity and using an elastic wrap for exsanguination is contraindicated.[88,89] Elevation also may be a preferred exsanguination method to reduce the risk for additional tissue damage when the patient has an unstable fracture in the operative extremity or when the patient has a latex allergy and a latex-safe elastic wrap is not available.[89]

IV.a.1. An elastic wrap should be available for exsanguination.

IV.a.2. The extremity should be elevated to allow venous blood to exit the limb.

IV.a.3. If the patient has an infection, malignant tumor, or fractures in the operative extremity, exsanguination should be accomplished by extremity elevation alone.[88,89]

IV.a.4. The anesthesia professional should be alerted before the extremity is wrapped.

Notification of the anesthesia professional facilitates monitoring for potential complications.

IV.b. Tourniquet inflation pressure should be determined by the surgeon[17] or anesthesia professional[4] based on the patient's systolic blood pressure and limb circumference. Inflation should be kept to the minimum effective pressure.[90-94] *[1: Strong Evidence]*

Overpressurization may cause pain at the tourniquet cuff site; muscle weakness; compression injuries to blood vessels, nerves, muscles, or skin; or extremity paralysis. Underpressurization may result in blood in the surgical field, passive congestion of the limb, shock, and hemorrhagic infiltration of a nerve. Sustaining adequate tourniquet pressure decreases the risk for poor visualization at the surgical field and engorgement of the limb or compartment syndrome related to arterial flow entering the limb.[65] Applying lower pressure has been found to result in less postoperative pain.[90,95,96]

Although many surgeons assume that standard tourniquet pressures are appropriate in all cases, researchers have shown that lower pressures than those typically used are effective.[65,94,95,97-100] Standard settings for tourniquet pressures have been identified as 300 mm Hg to 350 mm Hg in lower limbs and 200 mm Hg to 250 mm Hg in upper limbs.[4] In a retrospective study of 3,115 patient records for podiatry procedures, tourniquet pressures for cuffs applied at the ankle averaged 310.52 mm Hg, with 325 mm Hg as the pressure used most often. For tourniquet cuffs applied to the thigh, the average pressure was 398.39 mm Hg, and 400 mm Hg was the most common pressure setting.[27]

A web-based survey was distributed to 350 academic or community-based orthopedic surgeons in the United States to identify the tourniquet pressures surgeons routinely used and whether the surgeons based their decision on findings from the literature. There was a response rate of 57% (n = 199), which was further divided into responses for lower extremity (n = 151) or upper extremity (n = 141). For the lower extremity, the mean and the median pressures were 300 mm Hg (range 145 mm Hg to 400 mm Hg). Thirty surgeons (20.5%) reported being able to cite evidence to support the decision. For the upper extremity, the mean tourniquet pressure was 242 mm Hg and the median was 250 mm Hg (range 150 mm Hg to 300 mm Hg). Twenty-five surgeons (17.7%) reported being able to cite evidence to support the decision. The researchers recommended increasing surgeons' awareness through training and daily practice to encourage them to use lower pressures and base their practice on findings in the literature.[93]

In another study of surgeon's practice, 253 surveys were mailed to members of the American Orthopaedic Foot and Ankle Society. The response rate was 55%, with 140 surgeons returning completed surveys. Nine percent of the respondents based their pressure settings on limb occlusion pressure (LOP); however, 73% of the respondents evaluated the patient's blood pressure as a factor to determine the cuff pressure, 65% evaluated the patient's limb size, and 43% evaluated both blood pressure and limb size in their determinations of pressure. Of the responding surgeons, 49% said they applied tourniquet cuffs to the thigh and reported their most common pressures to be 301 mm Hg to 350 mm Hg. For procedures in which a calf or ankle tourniquet cuff was applied, 52% of the surgeons who used calf cuffs and 66% of those who used ankle cuffs reported their most common pressures to be above 201 mm Hg to 250 mm Hg. However, 41% of the surgeons who used calf cuffs and 19% of those who used ankle cuffs reported they often used pressure above 250 mm Hg. The researchers concluded that more surgeons might adopt lower pressures and base their determinations on LOP if there were more explicit recommendations for using LOP.[101]

Research studies have shown that occlusion can be achieved using a lower pressure when an LOP method is used in conjunction with a wide tourniquet cuff in adult patients.[65,67,91,95,98,100] The same was found when studying pediatric patients.[18] Some tourniquet systems are designed to determine LOP automatically and add a safety margin to allow for fluctuations in blood pressure intraoperatively.

When using a wide contoured thigh cuff for patients older than 18 years, the cuff pressure setting researchers have suggested is determined by adding a safety margin to the LOP as follows:
- add 40 mm Hg to 50 mm Hg for LOP less than 130 mm Hg,
- add 60 mm Hg to 75 mm Hg for LOP between 131 mm Hg and 190 mm Hg, and
- add 80 mm Hg to 100 mm Hg for LOP greater than 190 mm Hg.[65,100]

For pediatric patients, the cuff pressure setting should be adjusted by adding 50 mm Hg to the LOP.[19]

IV.b.1. The baseline systolic blood pressure or LOP measurement should be taken when the patient's blood pressure is stabilized to the level expected during surgery and may be taken before or after induction of anesthesia.

IV.b.2. Before inflating the cuff, members of the perioperative team should confirm the setting to be used.

IV.c. Members of the perioperative team should confirm the positioning of the patient's extremity before inflating the tourniquet. *[3: Limited Evidence]*

For a lower extremity, if the invasive procedure is related to the quadriceps muscles, the surgeon may want the knee in a flexed position when inflating the tourniquet to avoid "tethering" of the underlying structures. The surgeon may prefer the knee extended if the invasive procedure involves the hamstring muscles.[102] In a comparative study of 30 patients to determine whether the position of the knee at the time of tourniquet inflation had a correlation with postoperative knee range of motion, researchers found a statistically significant difference in the range of motion between the two groups (ie, knee flexed at the time of inflation, knee extended at the time of inflation) but they did not find the statistical difference to be clinically significant.[102]

IV.d. Pneumatic tourniquets should be inflated under the direction of the surgeon and the anesthesia professional. *[2: Moderate Evidence]*

Inflation of the tourniquet cuff may be associated with hemodynamic changes (eg, hypertension, complications related to increased blood volume after exsanguination).[4,5]

IV.e. Activation indicators and pressure displays should be visible and audible alarms should be sufficiently loud to be heard above other sounds in the OR.[103] *[2: Moderate Evidence]*

Equipment alarms alert personnel to a change in pressure, equipment failure, or lapse of a designated duration of inflation time.

When the pressure gauge or digital display is clearly visible while the tourniquet cuff is inflated, the perioperative team can monitor for excessive fluctuation.

PNEUMATIC TOURNIQUET

Because nerve damage may result from excessive tourniquet pressure and rhabdomyolysis has been reported with the tourniquet pressure set at an extreme pressure (ie, 520 mm Hg) even though the application time was relatively short (ie, 45 minutes), alarms are necessary to warn about conditions that may cause patient harm.[104,105]

Recommendation V

Tourniquet inflation time and patient condition should be monitored while the tourniquet cuff is inflated.

Tourniquet inflation time has a direct correlation to tourniquet-related complications (ie, increased inflation time increases the risk for injury). The patient's systemic response to ischemia is dependent on both tissue type and tourniquet time.[20] While cardiac muscle has a higher demand for oxygen, skeletal muscle is considered highly susceptible to ischemia.[106,107] This is because of the higher volumes of skeletal muscle mass releasing toxic substances into the circulatory system when reperfusion occurs, which can then lead to a severe inflammatory response.[107,108] Excessive tourniquet inflation time (ie, two to three hours) may result in metabolic changes; muscle damage; impaired pulmonary, hepatic, or renal function; neurological complications; or pain.[108-113]

To determine the efficacy and safety of distally placed pneumatic tourniquets, researchers initiated a retrospective study to review 3,027 procedures during which the surgeons used ankle tourniquets. Following a chart review, the researchers determined that the duration of ankle ischemia was as short as four minutes to as long as 139 minutes. Tourniquet failure was reported in 50 cases. Clinically, five complications were determined (ie, three post-tourniquet syndrome, one sickle cell-related problem, one DVT) and all eventually resolved. Based on the study, the authors concluded that an upper limit of two hours resulted in fewer complications.[27]

In a prospective study of awake patients, researchers investigated tolerance of intraoperative tourniquet pain. The study was designed to include 1,000 patients undergoing elective foot surgery with a local block, but 12 patients were excluded because the surgeon chose not to use a tourniquet. This left a sample size of 988 patients. The researchers found that 31 patients (3.1%) expressed pain during the procedure and eight of those experienced symptoms (eg, breakthrough bleeding from reduced tourniquet pressure, oversedation, excessive restlessness) that required the surgeon to interrupt the procedure. Of those eight patients, the anesthesia professional converted four patients to general anesthesia. The maximum tourniquet inflation time was 90 minutes (ie, range two to 90 minutes, median 18 minutes). The researchers concluded that for foot procedures with local blocks and ankle tourniquets, a tourniquet time of up to 30 minutes is tolerated by patients younger than 70 years tof age, but 1% of the patients will report pain for each 11 minutes beyond 30 minutes. They recommended caution when administering local anesthesia to patients older than 70 years, especially if the tourniquet inflation time is expected to be longer than 30 minutes.[84]

In a retrospective review of more than 1,000 patients who had total knee arthroplasties (ie, primary and revision knee replacements), researchers set out to identify risk factors that contribute to neurological complications. All patients had tourniquet times greater than 120 minutes. The researchers reported that 90 patients (7.7%) experienced 129 peroneal and/or tibial nerve palsies. They concluded that extended tourniquet times, the patient's age (ie, postoperative neurological dysfunction was associated with younger age), and the presence of preoperative flexion contractures were contributing factors to neurological complications. The authors also reported that total tourniquet time and a reperfusion interval only modestly decreased the risk of nerve injuries.[111]

Twenty-six patients undergoing arthroscopic anterior cruciate ligament repairs participated in a prospective open randomized study that compared metabolic effects of using wide, curved tourniquet cuffs at a pressure of 250 mm Hg in one group and narrow, straight cuffs at a pressure of 350 mm Hg in the other. The researchers reported a significant correlation between femoral vein lactate levels and tourniquet time. They found the test parameters for measuring muscle injuries and anaerobic metabolism were the same between the two groups for the first hour of tourniquet inflation, but the metabolic changes increased as the tourniquet time increased.[110]

V.a. Pneumatic tourniquet inflation time should be kept to a minimum. *[2: Moderate Evidence]*

Even with relatively short tourniquet inflation times (ie, 26 minutes ± eight minutes), researchers have found significant markers of systemic inflammatory response when they were measured 15 minutes after tourniquet deflation.[106] Inflation times of 60 minutes for an upper extremity and 90 minutes for a lower extremity have been identified as a general guideline for inflation duration.[17] However, some sources indicate that two hours is a safe time limit for tourniquet inflation.[20,31] In pediatric patients, inflation times of less than 75 minutes for lower extremities has been recommended.[114]

Irreversible skeletal muscle damage is thought to begin after three hours of ischemia and is extensive at six hours.[115] Allowing intermittent reperfusion restores oxygenation and releases toxins.[31] Deflating the tourniquet every two hours with at least a 10-minute reperfusion time has been identified as a strategy to consider to decrease the risk for tissue damage.[28] Another approach is to release the tourniquet after 90 minutes for at least 10 to 15 minutes for the first reperfusion period, then 15 to 20 minutes for each subsequent reperfusion period.[17] However, it has also been reported that implementing reperfusion periods after

60 to 90 minutes of ischemia can contribute to muscle injury.[23]

V.a.1. The surgeon should be informed of the tourniquet inflation time at regular, established intervals.[28]

V.a.2. When the duration of tourniquet inflation is longer than two hours, the RN circulator should confer with the surgeon and anesthesia professional about deflating the tourniquet for 10 to 15 minutes to allow tissue reperfusion.[17,28]

V.b. The patient should be monitored for physiological responses to tourniquet cuff inflation. *[2: Moderate Evidence]*

Patients may experience pain or anxiety accompanied by an increase in heart rate and blood pressure when the tourniquet is inflated.[28,116-118] An increase in core body temperature has been reported in both pediatric and adult patients after tourniquet inflation.[119-121]

V.b.1. Care should be exercised to avoid overheating the patient while the tourniquet cuff is inflated, particularly for pediatric patients.[120,122]

V.c. The perioperative nurse should collaborate with the anesthesia professional to prepare for potential patient injuries and complications associated with the inflation rotation sequence used with dual-bladder tourniquet cuffs during intravenous regional anesthesia.[53] *[2: Moderate Evidence]*

Adverse reaction to local anesthetic agents is a potential complication of intravenous regional anesthesia. A bolus of local anesthesia entering the general circulation can occur when there is an unplanned sudden deflation of the tourniquet soon after injection of local anesthetic or when the bolus is released too rapidly at the end of the procedure.[49]

Recommendation VI

The perioperative RN should collaborate with the surgeon and anesthesia professional to implement safe practices when deflating the pneumatic tourniquet.

Physiologic changes resulting from deflation of the tourniquet are dependent on the relative size of the extremity, duration of tourniquet time, and overall physiologic status of the patient. A decrease in blood pressure occurs as blood is shunted back to the extremity.[28] A significant decrease in core body temperature occurs after deflation of a lower extremity cuff.[121,123] Studies measuring emboli released after tourniquet cuff deflation have revealed that the highest number of emboli were released within one minute of deflation.[124,125]

Products of anaerobic metabolism (eg, lactate, hyperkalemia) enter the systemic circulation when the tourniquet cuff is deflated and cause acidosis.[4,28,108] This can result in severe myocardial depression and possibly cardiac arrest.[35]

Ischemia-reperfusion injury also can cause an increase in intracranial pressure. Three studies have investigated the effect of different anesthetics (eg, isoflurane, sevoflurane, propofol) on the degree of cerebral vasodilation.[126-128] The findings from one study revealed an increase in the velocity of blood flow in the middle cerebral artery for five minutes after tourniquet deflation, with a greater degree of increased flow when isoflurane was used.[126] A study using hyperventilation to decrease the risk of increased cerebral blood flow after tourniquet deflation reported a greater increase in flow with isoflurane when compared to sevoflurane and propofol.[128]

Coordination among members of the perioperative team can facilitate management of the patient's physiologic status during this period of rapid change.

VI.a. Pneumatic tourniquets should be deflated under the direction of the surgeon and anesthesia professional. *[2: Moderate Evidence]*

Hemodynamic changes may occur when the tourniquet is deflated. One prospective, randomized study found that the rate of acute systemic metabolic changes were reduced and there was greater hemodynamic stability when the tourniquet deflation was staggered (ie, deflated for 30 seconds, reinflated, and then repeated twice at three minute intervals).[129]

VI.a.1. The cuff and skin protection (eg, sleeve, padding) should be removed from the extremity after deflation of the tourniquet.

The padding or a deflated cuff may hinder venous return, resulting in congestion and pooling of blood at the surgical site.[17]

VI.b. Timing of the deflation of the pneumatic tourniquet should be coordinated based on the surgical procedure and the anesthesia plan of care. *[1: Strong Evidence]*

A meta-analysis of 11 randomized controlled trials revealed that the tourniquet may be deflated before wound closure (ie, early release) as a strategy to control bleeding during the surgical procedure. There was a significantly higher risk for early postoperative complications when the tourniquet was deflated after wound closure (ie, late release). However, researchers identified a wide diversity in methodologies and clinical strategies and concluded that larger studies are needed to clarify how the timing of tourniquet deflation correlates with the risk of postoperative complications.[130]

In a randomized clinical trial involving 84 patients and 96 total knee arthroplasty procedures, researchers compared blood loss and operative time when no tourniquet was used, when the tourniquet was deflated after implant insertion and cautery was used for hemostasis before closing, and when the tourniquet was deflated after wound closure and application of compression dressings. They did not identify

PNEUMATIC TOURNIQUET

any significant differences in blood loss or blood transfusions between the three groups, but they did report a significant increase in operative time when no tourniquet was used (ie, an average of 115 minutes without a tourniquet compared to an average of 82 minutes with intraoperative deflation and an average of 77 minutes with deflation after wound closure).[131] Another study evaluated 939 patients who had total knee replacements. The findings revealed that when the surgeon released the tourniquet after wound closure, there was a significantly higher degree of perioperative blood loss than when the surgeon released the tourniquet intraoperatively.[132]

The anesthesia professional may choose to increase IV fluids immediately before deflating the tourniquet cuff.[35] Hyperventilation before tourniquet cuff deflation also has been recommended to reduce the risk of severe increases in intracranial pressure.[126,128,133]

VI.c. When tourniquets are used on two extremities, the perioperative RN should confirm the sequence and timing of the deflation of each of the tourniquets. *[2: Moderate Evidence]*

The risk of complications and the systemic effects of tourniquet use may be increased when two tourniquets are applied at the same time. Tourniquet inflation causes anaerobic metabolism, which produces lactic acid and other metabolites.[115] Tourniquet deflation returns blood flow into the extremity and also releases the toxins that have built up in the extremity. Systemic responses related to tourniquet deflation on the first limb could occur during the second limb procedure.

A study of 15 healthy children ages six months to 15 years found that systolic blood pressure decreased 8 mm Hg to 10 mm Hg for five to 10 minutes after tourniquet deflation and a greater decrease in pH occurred with simultaneous deflation of bilateral tourniquets.[114]

VI.c.1. The first tourniquet cuff inflated should be completely deflated (and the cuff and limb protection removed, if possible) to assess circulation in the first limb while the procedure on the second limb is being completed.[85]

Sequential deflation lessens the potential for adverse patient reactions from simultaneous release of metabolic by-products from both extremities.[85] Researchers studied 35 patients who underwent bilateral total knee replacements and found the blood pressure changes were more evident after deflation of the tourniquet cuff on the second extremity than after the deflation of the tourniquet cuff on the first extremity.[134]

Respondents from a survey reported one case in which an amputation of the primary limb became necessary because of severe ischemia related to the primary tourniquet cuff remaining inflated unintentionally throughout the secondary procedure.[19]

VI.c.2. The surgeon or anesthesia professional may choose to stagger the tourniquet deflations 30 to 45 minutes apart.[17]

Staggering the tourniquet deflations may reduce the rapid simultaneous release of large amounts of metabolic by-products from both limbs into the vascular system.[17]

VI.d. When dual-bladder tourniquet cuffs are used with intravenous regional anesthesia, the tourniquet should be deflated as determined by the anesthesia professional. *[2: Moderate Evidence]*

As the tourniquet cuff deflates, the anesthetic agent may be released into the circulatory system, causing systemic effects.[135-137] Various techniques for deflation of the tourniquet after intravenous regional anesthesia have been reported.[135,136,138] One case study was reported in which a 21-year-old woman undergoing an open reduction and fixation of a fractured finger with intravenous regional anesthesia experienced temporary bilateral blindness after a member of the perioperative team deflated the tourniquet cuff without consulting the anesthesia professional. The authors of the case study concluded that the bilateral blindness occurred as a result of a toxic overdose of lidocaine. The patient's blindness resolved within 10 minutes postoperatively, and she did not have residual visual symptoms at the one month postoperative examination.[137]

Recommendation VII

The perioperative RN should evaluate the outcome of patient care after the tourniquet has been deflated.

The patient's blood pressure may be low for the first hour after tourniquet cuff deflation because of blood that is shunted to reperfuse the tissue. This is also related to bleeding at the surgical site and reactive vasodilatation and microvascular permeability.[23]

Systemic responses occur in relation to ischemia when a tourniquet is inflated and reperfusion when the tourniquet has been deflated.[139] The amount of time it takes the patient's body to clear the anaerobic metabolites depends on the patient's physiologic status, the extremity involved, and the duration of tourniquet inflation.

During the reperfusion phase, free radicals often are released into the circulatory system resulting in oxidative stress.[107] Several researchers have studied the biochemical mechanisms that contribute to ischemia-reperfusion injury and the appropriate pharmacological interventions to effectively reduce the patient's systemic response to oxidative stress.[42,139-143] In a study of 16 elderly patients undergoing bilateral total knee arthroplasty, researchers evaluated whether the administration of an antioxidant (eg, ascorbic acid, tocopherol, coenzyme Q10) could prevent the decreased vascular compliance and cardiac injury caused by oxidative stress. The researchers found that the administration of a high dose of vitamin C during bilateral total knee arthroplasties could play a part in protecting the myocardium because it prevents the production of oxygen free radicals and lowers arterial oxygen tension and the mean blood pressure caused by ischemia-reperfusion injury.[107] A case report indicated that younger people also can be affected by cardiac ischemia related to tourniquet inflation. A 25-year-old man exhibited respiratory and electrocardiogram changes 20 minutes after the tourniquet had been deflated. His laboratory reports revealed increased serum potassium and metabolic acidosis, which the clinicians believed caused coronary vasospasm. The patient's electrocardiogram and laboratory values reflected resolution of the systematic response to the ischemia-reperfusion injury three hours after surgery.[144]

Other researchers studied cell damage resulting from tourniquet-induced ischemia. Their findings revealed that the highest level of cell damage was measured immediately after reperfusion and that the markers of cell damage remained one hour after tourniquet deflation.[145]

A decrease in core body temperature may occur when a tourniquet cuff that is placed on a lower extremity is deflated.[123] In a randomized single-blind study of 24 older adults undergoing general anesthesia for unilateral total knee arthroplasties, researchers reported that intraoperative forced-air warming prevented hypothermia when the tourniquet was deflated.[146]

VII.a. The perioperative RN should include a report on pressure settings, duration of the pneumatic tourniquet inflation, and patient outcomes when transferring the care of the patient to other caregivers. *[2: Moderate Evidence]*

Transfer of care reports facilitate continuity in care.[75]

VII.b. The patient should be monitored for systemic responses and blood loss after the pneumatic tourniquet cuff has been deflated. *[1: Strong Evidence]*

Patients may experience a drop in blood pressure immediately after tourniquet cuff deflation and for an extended time after surgery.[23,121] Systemic responses to anaerobic metabolites and pulmonary emboli may occur after the tourniquet is deflated.[125,139,147]

Postoperative blood loss will vary after tourniquet-assisted procedures. Inflating a pneumatic tourniquet may decrease the blood loss intraoperatively, but researchers in one study found that patients who undergo tourniquet-assisted total knee arthroplasties may have more hidden blood loss and may not be able to participate in rehabilitation exercises as early as those who have the same surgery without a tourniquet.[148] In another study, researchers set out to determine whether postoperative drainage following knee replacement would be reduced if the release of suction drains was delayed by an hour, thereby allowing tamponade. A total of 100 patients participated in the study and were randomly assigned to either a group in which the drains were released immediately after deflation of the tourniquet or a group in which the drains were clamped until one hour after the tourniquet was deflated. The findings revealed that the group with the clamped drains had a statistically significant reduction in postoperative bleeding and required fewer postoperative transfusions. Furthermore, the researchers reported that one patient in the "immediate release" group experienced a pulmonary embolus, and two in the "clamped" group experienced DVT.[149]

Some researchers have undertaken studies to investigate how medications administered intraoperatively influence postoperative blood loss in total knee arthroplasty procedures. In one study of 84 patients, researchers infused a low dose of norepinephrine (dilution 1:200,000) into the knees of 29 patients before the tourniquets were released. Researchers reported a significant reduction in perioperative blood loss in the group of patients that received the norepinephrine irrigation. They attributed this to the hemostatic effect that norepinephrine had on peak blood flow 20 to 30 minutes after the tourniquet cuff was deflated. The control group patients (n = 55) received a saline wash. The researchers reported that no patients in either group experienced DVT or skin edge necrosis.[150] A different study was designed to explore the effectiveness of tranexamic acid in inhibiting the fibrinolytic system to reduce blood loss without resulting in an increase of DVT. The researchers concluded that there was a significant decrease in the "amount of blood loss in the early postoperative period" when they injected 15 mg/kg of tranexamic acid at the time of cementing the knee implant, before tourniquet deflation. They did not find an increase in thromboembolic complications related to the use of tranexamic acid.[151]

VII.b.1. The postoperative evaluation should include
- vital signs, including oxygen saturation;
- temperature;
- skin condition under the tourniquet (eg, temperature, color, integrity);
- pulses distal to the tourniquet cuff;
- surgical wound site (eg, dressings, drains); and
- blood loss.

VII.c. Complications should be reported to the surgeon and anesthesia professional and discussed during the hand off of care to other caregivers. *[2: Moderate Evidence]*

PNEUMATIC TOURNIQUET

Pulmonary emboli have been reported to occur after tourniquet cuff deflation.[28,124,152-157] Postoperative neurological complications related to tourniquet use also have been reported.[111,158] Although unusual, compartment syndrome related to tourniquet use has also been reported.[159-161]

Recommendation VIII

The pneumatic tourniquet and accessories should be cleaned after each use according to the manufacturer's written instructions.

Studies have reported microbial growth after culturing of reusable tourniquet cuffs.[162-164] In a limited study, researchers cultured 10 reusable tourniquet cuffs and 10 exsanguinators and compared the findings with microbes found in infected fracture wounds. They found that all 10 of the exsanguinators and eight of the tourniquet cuffs grew pathogens. *Staphylococcus aureus* and *Acinetobacter* were among the pathogens that were isolated, and coagulase-negative staphylococcus was the most commonly cultured pathogen. *Staphylococcus epidermidis* was the coagulase-negative pathogen found in two wound site infections out of 24 ankle fractures. Although the researchers found all of the exsanguinators and the majority of the cuffs they cultured to be contaminated, they could not identify evidence linking exsanguinators and tourniquet cuffs to surgical site infections. Despite this, the researchers recommended autoclaving tourniquet cuffs and using a clean exsanguinator for each procedure.[164]

VIII.a. After use, personnel should turn off the pneumatic tourniquet and clean and inspect it according to the manufacturer's written instructions. *[1: Strong Evidence]*

Cleaning between procedures prevents cross contamination.[165,166] Inspecting equipment after use helps to identify issues that can be handled before the equipment is used again.

VIII.a.1. Single-use cuffs should be discarded in an appropriate receptacle.

VIII.b. Between uses on patients, reusable cuffs and bladders should be cleaned using an Environmental Protection Agency-registered hospital disinfectant and then rinsed and dried.[162-166] *[1: Strong Evidence]*

Rinsing removes residue that may cause skin irritation, increase the chance of allergic reaction, and decrease the life of the cuff and bladder.[17]

VIII.b.1. If a reusable cuff is unable to be cleaned adequately, it should be discarded in an appropriate receptacle.

Recommendation IX

Perioperative team members should receive initial and ongoing education and competency verification on the use of the pneumatic tourniquet and on their understanding of the physiologic responses that influence the care of a patient undergoing pneumatic tourniquet-assisted operative or invasive procedures.

Health care organizations have a responsibility to provide initial and ongoing education and to evaluate the competency of perioperative team members to deliver safe care to patients undergoing pneumatic tourniquet-assisted operative or invasive procedures.[53,167] Every nurse is personally accountable for maintaining competency.[53,168]

Initial and ongoing development of knowledge and skills and documentation of personnel participation is a regulatory and accreditation requirement for both hospitals and ambulatory settings.[169-174]

Two studies evaluating the knowledge of perioperative personnel who used tourniquets identified the need for education on the application of tourniquet cuffs and the use of pneumatic tourniquets to prevent injuries and complications.[164,175] In one study, researchers distributed questionnaires to assistants and orthopedic specialists in the OR from five different hospitals. A total of 54 questionnaires were returned and analyzed. The mean score for the orthopedic specialists was 41.3% (standards deviation 6.85%; range 29.0% to 54.8%). The mean score for the assistants was 46.7% (standard deviation 9.64%; range 23.3% to 62.9%). The researchers concluded that there is a need for standard guidelines on tourniquet use.[175] In another study, researchers distributed a questionnaire to OR personnel who used exsanguinators and pneumatic tourniquets. A total of 74 questionnaires were returned and analyzed. The respondents included eight porters, 12 nurses, 10 senior house officers, 38 registrars, and six consultants. The nursing group had the highest mean score of 38.8%. The other mean scores were reported as 36.1% for the specialist registrars, 33.6% for the consultants, 32.8% for the registrars, 25.5% for the senior house officers, and 11.9% for the porters. The researchers identified the need for providing education to provide the best patient care.[164]

IX.a. Perioperative team members should receive education and competency verification that addresses the care of patients undergoing pneumatic tourniquet-assisted operative or other invasive procedures.[169-174] The education should address
- differentiating indications and contraindications for tourniquet use,
- identifying risks to patients and precautions to minimize these risks,
- selecting appropriate tourniquet cuffs based on patient assessment,
- following specific manufacturers' instructions for use,
- operating the tourniquet regulator according to the manufacturer's recommendations,
- measuring LOP,
- identifying physiologic changes during and after tourniquet use,
- implementing proper care and handling of the tourniquet and its accessories,

PNEUMATIC TOURNIQUET

- documenting and communicating tourniquet information and its affects during hand offs to facilitate continuity in patient care, and
- employing corrective actions in the event of a patient injury.

[1: Regulatory Requirement]

Tourniquets and accessories have been associated with patient injuries.[106,108,112,113] Education provides a foundation to guide safe patient care and minimize these risks.[111]

Competency verification confirms that personnel have knowledge regarding the use of the pneumatic tourniquet and appropriate corrective action to be taken in the event of a patient injury.[176-179]

IX.b. Perioperative personnel should receive education that addresses human factors related to the management of patient care for patients undergoing pneumatic tourniquet-assisted operative or other invasive procedures. *[2: Moderate Evidence]*

Human factors include the interpersonal and social aspects of the perioperative environment (eg, coordination of activities, teamwork, collaboration, communication).

In a synthesis of the literature on perioperative nursing competency published between 2000 and 2008, researchers identified two domains of perioperative competency:
- specialized knowledge, described as familiarity with standards and guidelines of perioperative practice, and
- human factors, described as interpersonal and social team interactions.

The researchers recognized teamwork and communication as important aspects of patient safety and indicators of perioperative competency.[176]

In a qualitative focus group study exploring the perceptions of perioperative nurses on competency, researchers identified three themes as competency requirements:
- technical and procedural knowledge—the knowledge, psychomotor skills, and situational awareness required for competency in the perioperative setting;
- communication skills—the need for communication and team building skills, collegial support, and the ability to decipher and share complex clinical information; and
- managing and coordinating flow—the ability to anticipate needs, organize and prioritize resources, manage conflicts, and grasp the full perspective of the situation.

The findings of the study highlight the importance of human factors as a competency requirement for perioperative nurses.[180]

Education, collegiality, and collaboration are standards of perioperative nursing and primary responsibilities of the perioperative RN who practices in the perioperative setting.[53,179]

Recommendation X

Documentation should reflect activities related to the care of the patient undergoing pneumatic tourniquet-assisted operative or other invasive procedures.

Documentation is a professional medicolegal standard. Documentation of nursing activities is dictated by the health care organization's policy and regulatory and accrediting agency requirements and is necessary to inform other health care professionals involved in the patient's care. Highly reliable data collection is not only necessary to chronicle patient responses to nursing interventions, but also to demonstrate the health care organization's progress toward quality care outcomes.[181]

X.a. Patient assessments, the plan of care, interventions implemented, and evaluation of care related to use of a pneumatic tourniquet should be documented. *[1: Regulatory Requirement]*

At the patient care level, documentation facilitates continuity of patient care through clear communication and supports collaboration among health care team members.

Perioperative documentation that accurately reflects the patient experience is essential for the continuity of outcome-focused nursing care and for effective comparison of realized versus anticipated patient outcomes.[181]

Effective management and collection of health care information that accurately reflects the patient's care, treatment, and services provided is a regulatory and accreditation requirement for both hospitals and ambulatory settings.[169,170,182-187]

X.a.1. Documentation should include
- pneumatic tourniquet system identification,
- limb occlusion pressure,
- cuff pressure,
- skin protection measures,
- location of the tourniquet cuff,
- skin integrity under the cuff before and after use of the pneumatic tourniquet,
- the person placing the tourniquet cuff,
- time of inflation and deflation,
- assessment and evaluation of the entire extremity including preoperative and postoperative pulses distal to the tourniquet, and
- systemic reactions to ischemia and reperfusion.

X.b. The perioperative RN should include information about pressure settings, the duration of the pneumatic tourniquet inflation, and patient outcomes when transferring the care of the patient to other caregivers. *[2: Moderate Evidence]*

Transfer of care reports facilitate continuity in care.[75]

PNEUMATIC TOURNIQUET

X.b.1. Complications should be reported to the surgeon and anesthesia professional and included in documentation communicated during the hand off of care to other caregivers.

X.c. The perioperative RN should document all postoperative patient instructions given to the patient and his or her support person(s) related to pneumatic tourniquet-assisted operative or other invasive procedures.[181] *[2: Moderate Evidence]*

Postoperative limb swelling and neurological complications (eg, compression paralysis, cutaneous sensory loss) have been reported to occur in relation to tourniquet use.[158,188,189] Patients and their support person(s) are better prepared to alert the surgeon or surgical facility about unusual symptoms if they have received adequate postoperative and discharge instructions.

X.d. Documentation of tourniquet testing should reflect the biomedical equipment identification number or serial number, date of inspection, preventive maintenance, and status of all equipment.[74] *[2: Moderate Evidence]*

Records of equipment failure and preventative maintenance assist in identifying equipment performance problems or hazards and minimize risk of patient injury and equipment failure.

Recommendation XI

Policies and procedures for use of pneumatic tourniquets should be developed, reviewed periodically, revised as necessary, and readily available in the practice setting.

Policies and procedures assist in the development of patient safety, quality assessment, and performance improvement activities. Policies and procedures establish authority, responsibility, and accountability within the health care organization. Policies and procedures also serve as operational guidelines that are used to minimize patient risk for injury or complications, standardize practice, direct perioperative personnel, and establish continuous performance improvement programs.

XI.a. Policies and procedures for the pneumatic tourniquet should include
- preoperative, intraoperative, and postoperative patient assessments;
- the timing of prophylactic antibiotic administration;
- guidelines for cuff selection (eg, sterile, reusable, width, length, shape) and fit;
- equipment checks before initial use, including cuff compatibility with the regulator and appropriate power or gas source;
- reporting and impounding of malfunctioning equipment[190];
- equipment maintenance programs and intervals for evaluation by designated personnel;
- responsibility for exsanguination;
- responsibility for cuff application;
- precautions during use;
- the interval for reporting tourniquet inflation time to the physician;
- safe parameters for tourniquet inflation times;
- safe parameters for tourniquet inflation pressures;
- parameters for reperfusion following extended inflation times;
- reporting of injuries;
- care and cleaning of the tourniquet and cuffs after use; and
- documentation.

[1: Regulatory Requirement]

Policies and procedures that guide and support patient care, treatment, and services are a regulatory and accreditation requirement for both hospitals and ambulatory settings.[169,170,173,191-193]

XI.b. The pneumatic tourniquet manufacturer's written instructions for cleaning, operation, and maintenance should be reviewed and reflected in policies and procedures. *[5: No Evidence]*

As new technologies are introduced for use in perioperative practice settings, it is imperative that health care personnel strictly follow manufacturers' written instructions for the operation and maintenance of equipment and be aware of the hazards that the equipment may pose to patients.

XI.b.1. User manuals for pneumatic tourniquets should be readily available and retained for the life of the equipment.

Recommendation XII

Perioperative personnel should participate in quality assurance and performance improvement activities that are consistent with the health care organization's plan to improve understanding of the physiologic responses that influence the care of a patient undergoing pneumatic tourniquet-assisted operative or other invasive procedures and compliance with safe practices when using pneumatic tourniquets.

Quality assurance and performance improvement programs assist in evaluating and improving the quality of patient care and formulating plans for corrective actions. These programs provide data that may be used to determine whether an individual organization is within benchmark goals and, if not, to identify areas that may require corrective actions. Participating in ongoing quality assurance and performance improvement activities is a standard of perioperative nursing and a primary responsibility of the RN who is engaged in practice in the perioperative setting.[53]

Complications related to equipment failure and pneumatic tourniquet use have been reported.[1,2,6]

XII.a. The pneumatic tourniquet system should be evaluated for safe use by designated personnel (eg, biomedical engineering personnel) within the health care organization and at intervals consistent with the manufacturer's written instructions and policies of the health care organization. *[2: Moderate Evidence]*

Periodic preventative maintenance supports continuous safe operation of pneumatic tourniquets.[74]

XII.b. The quality management program should include processes to monitor compliance with patient safety considerations when a pneumatic tourniquet and accessories are used in perioperative settings. Considerations should include
- that tourniquet cuffs are decontaminated after each use,
- that the tourniquet cuff chosen is the right size and shape for the patient's extremity,
- tourniquet inflation times that exceed the health care organization's specified parameters, and
- tourniquet inflation pressures that exceed the health care organization's specified parameters.

[1: Strong Evidence]

Collecting data to monitor and improve patient care, treatment, and services is a regulatory and accreditation requirement for both hospitals and ambulatory settings.[194-197]

Monitoring cleaning and disinfection practices to ensure adherence can help control transmission of multidrug-resistant organisms and other pathogens that may be residing in the environment.[165,166,198] The information obtained from assessments can be used to develop focused administrative and educational interventions that incorporate ongoing feedback to the environmental services personnel to improve cleaning and disinfection practices in health care institutions.[199] Compliance and adjunct monitoring after terminal cleaning can help prevent cross-contamination of areas that have or have had patients with multidrug-resistant organisms.[198,200]

XII.c. When compliance issues are identified, quality indicators should be developed to measure improvement in compliance with safe practices related to pneumatic tourniquets. *[1: Strong Evidence]*

Quality indicators are measurable and demonstrate that facilities are using specific interventions to provide safe patient care.[201]

According to the Agency for Healthcare Research and Quality, "An adequate quality indicator must have a sound clinical or empirical rationale for its use. It should measure an important aspect of quality that is subject to provider or healthcare system control."[201(p3)] Quality indicators are one response to the need for multidimensional, accessible, quality measures that can be used to gauge performance in health care. The quality indicators are evidence-based and can be used to identify variations in the quality of care provided on both an inpatient and outpatient basis.

XII.d. The health care organization's quality management program should include investigation of adverse events and near misses associated with use of a pneumatic tourniquet.[202,203] *[1: Regulatory Requirement]*

Reporting and investigating adverse events and near misses facilitates identification of trends and patterns and evaluation of the quality of patient care to assist in the formulation of plans for corrective actions.

XII.d.1. If a patient injury or equipment failure occurs, the pneumatic tourniquet system (eg, regulator, tubing, cuff) must be handled in accordance with the Safe Medical Devices Act of 1990, amended in March 2000.[190]

XII.d.2. Device identification, maintenance and service information, and adverse event information should be included in the report from the practice setting. Retaining the regulator, tubing, and cuff allows for a complete systems check to determine the tourniquet system integrity.

Glossary

Compartment syndrome: A pathologic condition caused by the progressive development of arterial compression and consequent reduction of blood supply. Clinical manifestations include swelling, restriction of movement, vascular compromise, and severe pain or lack of sensation.

Contoured tourniquet cuffs: Pneumatic tourniquet cuffs with a distal edge shorter than the proximal edge, creating a funnel-like shape when applied to an extremity.

Exsanguination: The process of forcible expulsion of blood from an extremity before pneumatic tourniquet use.

Limb occlusion pressure (LOP): The pneumatic tourniquet cuff pressure required to occlude arterial flow in the limb.

Preconditioning: Techniques used to reduce oxidative stress and increase skeletal muscle ischemia tolerance related to tourniquet inflation by initiating anesthetic regimens or short intervals of temporary ischemia.

Shearing: A sliding movement of skin and subcutaneous tissue that leaves the underlying muscle stationary.

References

1. Odinsson A, Finsen V. Tourniquet use and its complications in Norway. *J Bone Joint Surg Br.* 2006;88(8):1090-1092. [IIIB]

2. Complications of arthroscopy and arthroscopic surgery: results of a national survey. Committee on Complications of Arthroscopy Association of North America. *Arthroscopy.* 1985;1(4):214-220. [IIIC]

3. Kalla TP, Younger A, McEwen JA, Inkpen K. Survey of tourniquet use in podiatric surgery. *J Foot Ankle Surg.* 2003;42(2):68-76. [IIIC]

4. Aziz ES. Tourniquet use in orthopaedic anaesthesia. *Curr Anaesth Crit Care.* 2009;20(2):55-59. [VC]

5. Klenerman L. Effect of a tourniquet on the limb and the systemic circulation. In: *The Tourniquet Manual: Principles and Practice.* London, UK: Springer; 2003:13-38. [VA]

6. Strategies for avoiding problems with the use of pneumatic tourniquets. *Pa Patient Saf Advis.* 2010;7(3):97-101. [VA]

7. Tibrewal SB. The pneumatic tourniquet in arthroscopic surgery of the knee. *Int Orthop.* 2001;24(6):347-349. [IB]

8. Johnson DS, Stewart H, Hirst P, Harper NJ. Is tourniquet use necessary for knee arthroscopy? *Arthroscopy.* 2000;16(6):648-651. [IA]

9. Kirkley A, Rampersaud R, Griffin S, Amendola A, Litchfield R, Fowler P. Tourniquet versus no tourniquet use in routine knee arthroscopy: a prospective, double-blind, randomized clinical trial. *Arthroscopy.* 2000;16(2):121-126. [IA]

10. Smith TO, Hing CB. A meta-analysis of tourniquet assisted arthroscopic knee surgery. *Knee.* 2009;16(5):317-321. [IIB]

11. Kiss H, Raffl M, Neumann D, Hutter J, Dorn U. Epinephrine-augmented hypotensive epidural anesthesia replaces tourniquet use in total knee replacement. *Clin Orthop Relat Res.* 2005;(436):184-189. [IA]

12. Smith TO, Hing CB. Is a tourniquet beneficial in total knee replacement surgery? A meta-analysis and systematic review. *Knee.* 2010;17(2):141-147. [IIB]

13. Tai TW, Lin CJ, Jou IM, Chang CW, Lai KA, Yang CY. Tourniquet use in total knee arthroplasty: a meta-analysis. *Knee Surg Sports Traumatol Arthrosc.* 2011;19(7):1121-1130. [IB]

14. Smith TO, Hing CB. The efficacy of the tourniquet in foot and ankle surgery? A systematic review and meta-analysis. *Foot Ankle Surg.* 2010;16(1):3-8. [IIIB]

15. Smith TO, Hing CB. Should tourniquets be used in upper limb surgery? A systematic review and meta-analysis. *Acta Orthop Belg.* 2009;75(3):289-296. [IIIC]

16. Saied A, Zyaei A. Tourniquet use during plating of acute extra-articular tibial fractures: effects on final results of the operation. *J Trauma.* 2010;69(6):E94-E97. [IA]

17. McEwen JA. Tourniquet use and care. http://www.tourniquets.org/use_care.php. Accessed May 4, 2013. [VC]

18. Lieberman JR, Staheli LT, Dales MC. Tourniquet pressures on pediatric patients: a clinical study. *Orthopedics.* 1997;20(12):1143-1147. [IIB]

19. Tredwell SJ, Wilmink M, Inkpen K, McEwen JA. Pediatric tourniquets: analysis of cuff and limb interface, current practice, and guidelines for use. *J Pediatr Orthop.* 2001;21(5):671-676. [IIIC]

20. Noordin S, McEwen JA, Kragh JF Jr, Eisen A, Masri BA. Surgical tourniquets in orthopaedics. *J Bone Joint Surg Am.* 2009;91(12):2958-2967. [VB]

21. Krackow KA. A maneuver for improved positioning of a tourniquet in the obese patient. *Clin Orthop Relat Res.* 1982;(168):80-82. [VC]

22. Klenerman L. Complications. In: *The Tourniquet Manual: Principles and Practice.* London, UK: Springer; 2003:61-75. [VA]

23. Estebe JP, Davies JM, Richebe P. The pneumatic tourniquet: mechanical, ischaemia-reperfusion and systemic effects. *Eur J Anaesthesiol.* 2011;28(6):404-411. [VB]

24. Fukuda A, Hasegawa M, Kato K, Shi D, Sudo A, Uchida A. Effect of tourniquet application on deep vein thrombosis after total knee arthroplasty. *Arch Orthop Trauma Surg.* 2007;127(8):671-675. [IIIC]

25. Parmet JL, Horrow JC, Pharo G, Collins L, Berman AT, Rosenberg H. The incidence of venous emboli during extramedullary guided total knee arthroplasty. *Anesth Analg.* 1995;81(4):757-762. [IIIB]

26. Parmet JL, Horrow JC, Berman AT, Miller F, Pharo G, Collins L. The incidence of large venous emboli during total knee arthroplasty without pneumatic tourniquet use. *Anesth Analg.* 1998;87(2):439-444. [IIB]

27. Derner R, Buckholz J. Surgical hemostasis by pneumatic ankle tourniquet during 3027 podiatric operations. *J Foot Ankle Surg.* 1995;34(3):236-246. [IIIA]

28. Kam PC, Kavanagh R, Yoong FF. The arterial tourniquet: pathophysiological consequences and anaesthetic implications. *Anaesthesia.* 2001;56(6):534-545. [VB]

29. Barr L, Iyer US, Sardesai A, Chitnavis J. Tourniquet failure during total knee replacement due to arterial calcification: case report and review of the literature. *J Perioper Pract.* 2010;20(2):55-58. [VC]

30. Garabekyan T, Oliashirazi A, Winters K. The value of immediate preoperative vascular examination in an at-risk patient for total knee arthroplasty. *Orthopedics.* 2011;34(1):52. [VB]

31. Wakai A, Winter DC, Street JT, Redmond PH. Pneumatic tourniquets in extremity surgery. *J Am Acad Orthop Surg.* 2001;9(5):345-351. [VB]

32. Fisher B, Roberts CS. Tourniquet use and sickle cell hemoglobinopathy: how should we proceed? *South Med J.* 2010;103(11):1156-1160. [VB]

33. Fanning R, O'Donnell B, Lynch B, Stephens M, O'Donovan F. Anesthesia for sickle cell disease and congenital myopathy in combination. *Paediatr Anaesth.* 2006;16(8):880-883. [VB]

34. Siddiqui FM, Slater RM, Razzaq I, Atkinson M, Ryan K. Tourniquet use during total knee replacement in a Jehovah's Witness with sickle cell trait: a case report. *Eur J Anaesthesiol.* 2010;27(6):581-582. [VC]

35. Gupta K, Aggarwal N, Rao M, Verma UC, Anand R. Re-emphasizing the importance of tourniquet time: severe myocardial depression following tourniquet deflation. *Acta Anaesthesiol Scand.* 2008;52(6):873. [VC]

36. Honarmand A, Safavi MR. Preoperative oral dextromethorphan vs. clonidine to prevent tourniquet-induced cardiovascular responses in orthopaedic patients under general anaesthesia. *Eur J Anaesthesiol.* 2007;24(6):511-515. [IB]

37. Sheth NP, Sennett B, Berns JS. Rhabdomyolysis and acute renal failure following arthroscopic knee surgery in a college football player taking creatine supplements. *Clin Nephrol.* 2006;65(2):134-137. [VB]

38. Seyahi A, Uludag S, Akman S, Demirhan M. Unrecognized anterior compartment syndrome following ankle fracture surgery: a case report. *J Am Podiatr Med Assoc.* 2009;99(5):438-442. [VB]

39. Brodsky MA, Smith JA. Exacerbation of myasthenia gravis after tourniquet release. *J Clin Anesth.* 2007;19(7):543-545. [VC]

40. Akinyoola AL, Adegbehingbe OO, Odunsi A. Timing of antibiotic prophylaxis in tourniquet surgery. *J Foot Ankle Surg.* 2011;50(4):374-376. [IB]

41. Soriano A, Bori G, Garcia-Ramiro S, et al. Timing of antibiotic prophylaxis for primary total knee arthroplasty performed during ischemia. *Clin Infect Dis.* 2008;46(7):1009-1014. [IB]

42. Koca K, Yurttas Y, Cayci T, et al. The role of preconditioning and N-acetylcysteine on oxidative stress resulting from tourniquet-induced ischemia-reperfusion in

43. Mas E, Barden AE, Corcoran TB, Phillips M, Roberts LJ 2nd, Mori TA. Effects of spinal or general anesthesia on F-isoprostanes and isofurans during ischemia/reperfusion of the leg in patients undergoing knee replacement surgery. *Free Radic Biol Med.* 2011;50(9):1171-1176. [IIIB]

44. Lin LN, Wang LR, Wang WT, et al. Ischemic preconditioning attenuates pulmonary dysfunction after unilateral thigh tourniquet-induced ischemia-reperfusion. *Anesth Analg.* 2010;111(2):539-543. [IC]

45. Viscomi CM, Friend A, Parker C, Murphy T, Yarnell M. Ketamine as an adjuvant in lidocaine intravenous regional anesthesia: a randomized, double-blind, systemic control trial. *Reg Anesth Pain Med.* 2009;34(2):130-133. [IIC]

46. Orban JC, Levraut J, Gindre S, et al. Effects of acetylcysteine and ischaemic preconditioning on muscular function and postoperative pain after orthopaedic surgery using a pneumatic tourniquet. *Eur J Anaesthesiol.* 2006;23(12):1025-1030. [IC]

47. Guay J. Adverse events associated with intravenous regional anesthesia (Bier block): a systematic review of complications. *J Clin Anesth.* 2009;21(8):585-594. [VC]

48. Kol IO, Ozturk H, Kaygusuz K, Gursoy S, Comert B, Mimaroglu C. Addition of dexmedetomidine or lornoxicam to prilocaine in intravenous regional anaesthesia for hand or forearm surgery: a randomized controlled study. *Clin Drug Investig.* 2009;29(2):121-129. [IB]

49. Singh R, Bhagwat A, Bhadoria P, Kohli A. Forearm IVRA, using 0.5% lidocaine in a dose of 1.5 mg/kg with ketorolac 0.15 mg/kg for hand and wrist surgeries. *Minerva Anestesiol.* 2010;76(2):109-114. [IC]

50. Graham B, Breault MJ, McEwen JA, McGraw RW. Occlusion of arterial flow in the extremities at subsystolic pressures through the use of wide tourniquet cuffs. *Clin Orthop Relat Res.* 1993;(286):257-261. [IIIB]

51. Dounis E, Tsourvakas S, Kalivas L, Giamacellou H. Effect of time interval on tissue concentrations of cephalosporins after tourniquet inflation. Highest levels achieved by administration 20 minutes before inflation. *Acta Orthop Scand.* 1995;66(2):158-160. [IIB]

52. Papaioannou N, Kalivas L, Kalavritinos J, Tsourvakas S. Tissue concentrations of third-generation cephalosporins (ceftazidime and ceftriaxone) in lower extremity tissues using a tourniquet. *Arch Orthop Trauma Surg.* 1994;113(3):167-169. [IIIB]

53. Standards of perioperative nursing. In: *Perioperative Standards and Recommended Practices.* Denver, CO: AORN, Inc; 2012:20. [IVB]

54. Reikeras O, Clementsen T. Time course of thrombosis and fibrinolysis in total knee arthroplasty with tourniquet application. Local versus systemic activations. *J Thromb Thrombolysis.* 2009;28(4):425-428. [IIIC]

55. Kageyama K, Nakajima Y, Shibasaki M, Hashimoto S, Mizobe T. Increased platelet, leukocyte, and endothelial cell activity are associated with increased coagulability in patients after total knee arthroplasty. *J Thromb Haemost.* 2007;5(4):738-745. [IB]

56. Van M, Olguner C, Koca U, et al. Ischaemic preconditioning attenuates haemodynamic response and lipid peroxidation in lower-extremity surgery with unilateral pneumatic tourniquet application: a clinical pilot study. *Adv Ther.* 2008;25(4):355-366. [IC]

57. Carles M, Dellamonica J, Roux J, et al. Sevoflurane but not propofol increases interstitial glycolysis metabolites availability during tourniquet-induced ischaemia-reperfusion. *Br J Anaesth.* 2008;100(1):29-35. [IC]

58. Budic I, Pavlovic D, Kocic G, et al. Biomarkers of oxidative stress and endothelial dysfunction after tourniquet release in children. *Physiol Res.* 2011;60(Suppl 1):S137-S145. [IIIC]

59. Murphy T, Walsh PM, Doran PP, Mulhall KJ. Transcriptional responses in the adaptation to ischaemia-reperfusion injury: a study of the effect of ischaemic preconditioning in total knee arthroplasty patients. *J Transl Med.* 2010;8:46. [IC]

60. Erturk E, Cekic B, Geze S, et al. Comparison of the effect of propofol and N-acetyl cysteine in preventing ischaemia-reperfusion injury. *Eur J Anaesthesiol.* 2009;26(4):279-284. [IB]

61. Sullivan PJ, Sweeney KJ, Hirpara KM, Malone CB, Curtin W, Kerin MJ. Cyclical ischaemic preconditioning modulates the adaptive immune response in human limb ischaemia-reperfusion injury. *Br J Surg.* 2009;96(4):381-390. [IB]

62. Yagmurdur H, Ozcan N, Dokumaci F, Kilinc K, Yilmaz F, Basar H. Dexmedetomidine reduces the ischemia-reperfusion injury markers during upper extremity surgery with tourniquet. *J Hand Surg Am.* 2008;33(6):941-947. [IB]

63. Turan R, Yagmurdur H, Kavutcu M, Dikmen B. Propofol and tourniquet induced ischaemia reperfusion injury in lower extremity operations. *Eur J Anaesthesiol.* 2007;24(2):185-189. [IIC]

64. Memtsoudis SG, Valle AG, Jules-Elysse K, et al. Perioperative inflammatory response in total knee arthroplasty patients: impact of limb preconditioning. *Reg Anesth Pain Med.* 2010;35(5):412-416. [IB]

65. Younger AS, McEwen JA, Inkpen K. Wide contoured thigh cuffs and automated limb occlusion measurement allow lower tourniquet pressures. *Clin Orthop Relat Res.* 2004;(428):286-293. [IB]

66. Moore MR, Garfin SR, Hargens AR. Wide tourniquets eliminate blood flow at low inflation pressures. *J Hand Surg Am.* 1987;12(6):1006-1011. [IIIB]

67. Pedowitz RA, Gershuni DH, Botte MJ, Kuiper S, Rydevik BL, Hargens AR. The use of lower tourniquet inflation pressures in extremity surgery facilitated by curved and wide tourniquets and an integrated cuff inflation system. *Clin Orthop Relat Res.* 1993;(287):237-244. [IB]

68. Thompson SM, Middleton M, Farook M, Cameron-Smith A, Bone S, Hassan A. The effect of sterile versus non-sterile tourniquets on microbiological colonisation in lower limb surgery. *Ann R Coll Surg Engl.* 2011;93(8):589-590. [IIC]

69. Guedj MP. Sudden deflation of a tourniquet caused by lowering of the operating table. *Ann Fr Anesth Reanim.* 2007;26(2):174. [VC]

70. Simmons D, Phillips MS, Grissinger M, Becker SC; USP Safe Medication Use Expert Committee. Error-avoidance recommendations for tubing misconnections when using Luer-tip connectors: a statement by the USP Safe Medication Use Expert Committee. *Jt Comm J Qual Patient Saf.* 2008;34(5):293-296, 245. [VC]

71. Paparella S. Inadvertent attachment of a blood pressure device to a needleless IV "Y-site": surprising, fatal connections. *J Emerg Nurs.* 2005;31(2):180-182. [VC]

72. Arslan M, Canturk M, Ornek D, et al. Regional intravenous anesthesia in knee arthroscopy. *Clinics (Sao Paulo).* 2010;65(9):831-835. [IIC]

73. US Food and Drug Administration. Pneumatic tourniquet cuffs, with the tourniquet systems. *Medical Product Safety News.* 2007;7(1):24. http://www.fda.gov/MedicalDevices/Safety/AlertsandNotices/TipsandArticlesonDeviceSafety/ucm070189.htm. Accessed May 4, 2013. [VB]

PNEUMATIC TOURNIQUET

74. ECRI. Optimizing an IPM program. *Healthc Risk Control.* 2009;3(Risk Analysis Medical Technology 9). [VB]

75. Guideline for transfer of patient care information. In: *Guidelines for Perioperative Practice.* Denver, CO: AORN, Inc; 2015:583-588. [IVB]

76. Eidelman M, Katzman A, Bialik V. A novel elastic exsanguination tourniquet as an alternative to the pneumatic cuff in pediatric orthopedic limb surgery. *J Pediatr Orthop B.* 2006;15(5):379-384. [IIIC]

77. Olivecrona C, Tidermark J, Hamberg P, Ponzer S, Cederfjall C. Skin protection underneath the pneumatic tourniquet during total knee arthroplasty: a randomized controlled trial of 92 patients. *Acta Orthop.* 2006;77(3):519-523. [IB]

78. Din R, Geddes T. Skin protection beneath the tourniquet. A prospective randomized trial. *ANZ J Surg.* 2004;74(9):721-722. [IC]

79. Guo S. Is Velband still a safe and cost effective skin protection beneath the tourniquet in hand surgery? *Hand Surg.* 2011;16(1):5-8. [IIIB]

80. Hubik DJ, Connors A, Cleland H. Iatrogenic chemical burns associated with tourniquet use and prep solution. *ANZ J Surg.* 2009;79(10):762. [VC]

81. Odinsson A, Finsen V. The position of the tourniquet on the upper limb. *J Bone Joint Surg Br.* 2002;84(2):202-204. [IIC]

82. Finsen V, Kasseth AM. Tourniquets in forefoot surgery: less pain when placed at the ankle. *J Bone Joint Surg Br.* 1997;79(1):99-101. [IIC]

83. Lichtenfeld NS. The pneumatic ankle tourniquet with ankle block anesthesia for foot surgery. *Foot Ankle.* 1992;13(6):344-349. [IIIB]

84. Rudkin AK, Rudkin GE, Dracopoulos GC. Acceptability of ankle tourniquet use in midfoot and forefoot surgery: audit of 1000 cases. *Foot Ankle Int.* 2004;25(11):788-794. [IIIA]

85. Branson JJ, Goldstein WM. Sequential bilateral total knee arthroplasty. *AORN J.* 2001;73(3):610-635; quiz 637-642. [VB]

86. Darmanis S, Papanikolaou A, Pavlakis D. Fatal intraoperative pulmonary embolism following application of an Esmarch bandage. *Injury.* 2002;33(9):761-764. [VB]

87. Blond L, Jensen NV, Soe Nielsen NH. Clinical consequences of different exsanguination methods in hand surgery. a double-blind randomised study. *J Hand Surg Eur Vol.* 2008;33(4):475-477. [IIB]

88. Iyer S, Pabari A, Branford OA. Refinement of a simple technique with new relevance for exsanguination of the upper limb. *Tech Hand Up Extrem Surg.* 2011;15(2):82-83. [VC]

89. Angadi DS, Blanco J, Garde A, West SC. Lower limb elevation: useful and effective technique of exsanguination prior to knee arthroscopy. *Knee Surg Sports Traumatol Arthrosc.* 2010;18(11):1559-1561. [IIIC]

90. Estebe JP, Le Naoures A, Chemaly L, Ecoffey C. Tourniquet pain in a volunteer study: effect of changes in cuff width and pressure. *Anaethesia.* 2000;55(1):21-26. [IIC]

91. McEwen JA, Kelly DL, Jardanowski T, Inkpen K. Tourniquet safety in lower leg applications. *Orthop Nurs.* 2002;21(5):55-62. [IIIB]

92. Tuncali B, Karci A, Tuncali BE, et al. A new method for estimating arterial occlusion pressure in optimizing pneumatic tourniquet inflation pressure. *Anesth Analg.* 2006;102(6):1752-1757. [IIIB]

93. Tejwani NC, Immerman I, Achan P, Egol KA, McLaurin T. Tourniquet cuff pressure: The gulf between science and practice. *J Trauma.* 2006;61(6):1415-1418. [IIIC]

94. Ishii Y, Noguchi H, Matsuda Y, Takeda M, Higashihara T. A new tourniquet system that determines pressures in synchrony with systolic blood pressure in total knee arthroplasty. *J Arthroplasty.* 2008;23(7):1050-1056. [IIB]

95. Newman RJ, Muirhead A. A safe and effective low pressure tourniquet. A prospective evaluation. *J Bone Joint Surg Br.* 1986;68(4):625-628. [IA]

96. Worland RL, Arredondo J, Angles F, Lopez-Jimenez F, Jessup DE. Thigh pain following tourniquet application in simultaneous bilateral total knee replacement arthroplasty. *J Arthroplasty.* 1997;12(8):848-852. [IB]

97. Tuncali B, Karci A, Bacakoglu AK, Tuncali BE, Ekin A. Controlled hypotension and minimal inflation pressure: a new approach for pneumatic tourniquet application in upper limb surgery. *Anesth Analg.* 2003;97(5):1529-1532. [IB]

98. Younger AS, Manzary M, Wing KJ, Stothers K. Automated cuff occlusion pressure effect on quality of operative fields in foot and ankle surgery: a randomized prospective study. *Foot Ankle Int.* 2011;32(3):239-243. [IA]

99. Reilly CW, McEwen JA, Leveille L, Perdios A, Mulpuri K. Minimizing tourniquet pressure in pediatric anterior cruciate ligament reconstructive surgery: a blinded, prospective randomized controlled trial. *J Pediatr Orthop.* 2009;29(3):275-280. [IB]

100. Olivecrona C, Ponzer S, Hamberg P, Blomfeldt R. Lower tourniquet cuff pressure reduces postoperative wound complications after total knee arthroplasty: a randomized controlled study of 164 patients. *J Bone Joint Surg Am.* 2012;94(24):2216-2221. [IA]

101. Younger AS, Kalla TP, McEwen JA, Inkpen K. Survey of tourniquet use in orthopaedic foot and ankle surgery. *Foot Ankle Int.* 2005;26(3):208-217. [IIIB]

102. Zura RD, Adams SB Jr, Mata BA, Pietrobon R, Olson SA. Does knee position at the time of tourniquet inflation affect knee range of motion? *J Surg Orthop Adv.* 2007;16(4):171-173. [IIIC]

103. Guideline for a safe environment of care, part 1. In: *Guidelines for Perioperative Practice.* Denver, CO: AORN, Inc; 2015:239-263. [IVB]

104. Hodgson AJ. A proposed etiology for tourniquet-induced neuropathies. *J Biomech Eng.* 1994;116(2):224-227. [IIIB]

105. Lee YG, Park W, Kim SH, et al. A case of rhabdomyolysis associated with use of a pneumatic tourniquet during arthroscopic knee surgery. *Korean J Intern Med.* 2010;25(1):105-109. [VC]

106. Wakai A, Wang JH, Winter DC, Street JT, O'Sullivan RG, Redmond HP. Tourniquet-induced systemic inflammatory response in extremity surgery. *J Trauma.* 2001;51(5):922-926. [IB]

107. Lee JY, Kim CJ, Chung MY. Effect of high-dose vitamin C on oxygen free radical production and myocardial enzyme after tourniquet ischaemia-reperfusion injury during bilateral total knee replacement. *J Int Med Res.* 2010;38(4):1519-1529. [IC]

108. Gourdin MJ, Bree B, De Kock M. The impact of ischaemia-reperfusion on the blood vessel. *Eur J Anaesthesiol.* 2009;26(7):537-547. [VB]

109. Kim JG, Lee J, Roe J, Tromberg BJ, Brenner M, Walters TJ. Hemodynamic changes in rat leg muscles during tourniquet-induced ischemia-reperfusion injury observed by near-infrared spectroscopy. *Physiol Meas.* 2009;30(7):529-540. [IIB]

110. Kokki H, Vaatainen U, Penttila I. Metabolic effects of a low-pressure tourniquet system compared with a

high-pressure tourniquet system in arthroscopic anterior crucial ligament reconstruction. *Acta Anaesthesiol Scand.* 1998;42(4):418-424. [IIB]

111. Horlocker TT, Hebl JR, Gali B, et al. Anesthetic, patient, and surgical risk factors for neurologic complications after prolonged total tourniquet time during total knee arthroplasty. *Anesth Analg.* 2006;102(3):950-955. [IIIA]

112. Jacobson MD, Pedowitz RA, Oyama BK, Tryon B, Gershuni DH. Muscle functional deficits after tourniquet ischemia. *Am J Sports Med.* 1994;22(3):372-377. [IB]

113. Yassin MM, Harkin DW, Barros D'Sa AA, Halliday MI, Rowlands BJ. Lower limb ischemia-reperfusion injury triggers a systemic inflammatory response and multiple organ dysfunction. *World J Surg.* 2002;26(1):115-121. [IB]

114. Lynn AM, Fischer T, Brandford HG, Pendergrass TW. Systemic responses to tourniquet release in children. *Anesth Analg.* 1986;65(8):865-872. [IIIC]

115. Blaisdell FW. The pathophysiology of skeletal muscle ischemia and the reperfusion syndrome: a review. *Cardiovasc Surg.* 2002;10(6):620-630. [VB]

116. Sunder RA, Toshniwal G. An atypical presentation of tourniquet pain. *Acta Anaesthesiol Scand.* 2006;50(4):525-526. [VC]

117. Burg A, Tytiun Y, Velkes S, Heller S, Haviv B, Dudkiewicz I. Ankle tourniquet pain control in forefoot surgery: a randomized study. *Foot Ankle Int.* 2011;32(6):595-598. [IB]

118. Rastogi S, Brady WJ. Trousseau's sign related to upper arm tourniquet following brachial plexus blockade. *Anaesthesia.* 2011;66(9):846-847. [VB]

119. Goodarzi M, Shier NH, Ogden JA. Physiologic changes during tourniquet use in children. *J Pediatr Orthop.* 1992;12(4):510-513. [IIIB]

120. Bloch EC, Ginsberg B, Binner RA Jr, Sessler DI. Limb tourniquets and central temperature in anesthetized children. *Anesth Analg.* 1992;74(4):486-489. [IIB]

121. Estebe JP, Le Naoures A, Malledant Y, Ecoffey C. Use of a pneumatic tourniquet induces changes in central temperature. *Br J Anaesth.* 1996;77(6):786-788. [IC]

122. Bloch EC. Hyperthermia resulting from tourniquet application in children. *Ann R Coll Surg Engl.* 1986;68(4):193-194. [IIIC]

123. Sanders BJ, D'Alessio JG, Jernigan JR. Intraoperative hypothermia associated with lower extremity tourniquet deflation. *J Clin Anesth.* 1996;8(6):504-507. [IIIC]

124. Hirota K, Hashimoto H, Kabara S, et al. The relationship between pneumatic tourniquet time and the amount of pulmonary emboli in patients undergoing knee arthroscopic surgeries. *Anesth Analg.* 2001;93(3):776-780. [IIIB]

125. Hirota K, Hashimoto H, Tsubo T, Ishihara H, Matsuki A. Quantification and comparison of pulmonary emboli formation after pneumatic tourniquet release in patients undergoing reconstruction of anterior cruciate ligament and total knee arthroplasty. *Anesth Analg.* 2002;94(6):1633-1638. [IIIC]

126. Kadoi Y, Kawauchi CH, Ide M, Saito S, Mizutani A. Differential increases in blood flow velocity in the middle cerebral artery after tourniquet deflation during sevoflurane, isoflurane or propofol anaesthesia. *Anaesth Intensive Care.* 2009;37(4):598-603. [IIC]

127. Hinohara H, Kadoi Y, Takahashi K, Saito S, Kawauchi C, Mizutani A. Time course of changes in cerebral blood flow velocity after tourniquet deflation in patients with diabetes mellitus or previous stroke under sevoflurane anesthesia. *J Anesth.* 2011;25(3):409-414. [IIC]

128. Hinohara H, Kadoi Y, Ide M, Kuroda M, Saito S, Mizutani A. Differential effects of hyperventilation on cerebral blood flow velocity after tourniquet deflation during sevoflurane, isoflurane, or propofol anesthesia. *J Anesth.* 2010;24(4):587-593. [IIB]

129. van der Velde J, Serfontein L, Iohom G. Reducing the potential for tourniquet-associated reperfusion injury. *Eur J Emerg Med.* 2012. [IB]

130. Rama KR, Apsingi S, Poovali S, Jetti A. Timing of tourniquet release in knee arthroplasty. Meta-analysis of randomized, controlled trials. *J Bone Joint Surg Am.* 2007;89(4):699-705. [IA]

131. Yavarikia A, Amjad GG, Davoudpour K. The influence of tourniquet use and timing of its release on blood loss in total knee arthroplasty. *Pak J Biol Sci.* 2010;13(5):249-252. [IA]

132. Bell TH, Berta D, Ralley F, et al. Factors affecting perioperative blood loss and transfusion rates in primary total joint arthroplasty: a prospective analysis of 1642 patients. *Can J Surg.* 2009;52(4):295-301. [IIIB]

133. Conaty KR, Klemm MS. Severe increase of intracranial pressure after deflation of a pneumatic tourniquet. *Anesthesiology.* 1989;71(2):294-295. [VC]

134. Huang CH, Wang MJ, Chen TL, et al. Blood and central venous pressure responses after serial tourniquet deflation during bilateral total knee replacement. *J Formos Med Assoc.* 1996;95(6):496-499. [IIIB]

135. Sukhani R, Garcia CJ, Munhall RJ, Winnie AP, Rodvold KA. Lidocaine disposition following intravenous regional anesthesia with different tourniquet deflation technics. *Anesth Analg.* 1989;68(5):633-637. [IIIB]

136. Rodola F, Vagnoni S, Ingletti S. An update on intravenous regional anaesthesia of the arm. *Eur Rev Med Pharmacol Sci.* 2003;7(5):131-138. [VB]

137. Sawyer RJ, von Schroeder H. Temporary bilateral blindness after acute lidocaine toxicity. *Anesth Analg.* 2002;95(1):224-226. [VB]

138. Barry LA, Balliana SA, Galeppi AC. Intravenous regional anesthesia (Bier block). *Tech Reg Anesth Pain Manag.* 2006;10(3):123-131. [VB]

139. Budic I, Pavlovic D, Cvetkovic T, et al. The effects of different anesthesia techniques on free radical production after tourniquet-induced ischemia-reperfusion injury at children's age. *Vojnosanit Pregl.* 2010;67(8):659-664. [IIIC]

140. Wang L, Wang W, Zhao X, et al. Effect of Shenmai injection, a traditional Chinese medicine, on pulmonary dysfunction after tourniquet-induced limb ischemia-reperfusion. *J Trauma.* 2011;71(4):893-897. [IB]

141. Laisalmi-Kokki M, Pesonen E, Kokki H, et al. Potentially detrimental effects of N-acetylcysteine on renal function in knee arthroplasty. *Free Radic Res.* 2009;43(7):691-696. [IB]

142. Hughes SF, Hendricks BD, Edwards DR, Middleton JF. Tourniquet-applied upper limb orthopaedic surgery results in increased inflammation and changes to leukocyte, coagulation and endothelial markers. *PLoS One.* 2010;5(7):e11846. [IIIC]

143. Lin L, Wang L, Bai Y, et al. Pulmonary gas exchange impairment following tourniquet deflation: a prospective, single-blind clinical trial. *Orthopedics.* 2010;33(6):395. [IIC]

144. Broom MA, Rimmer C, Parris MR. Tourniquet-associated cardiac ischaemia in a healthy patient undergoing trauma hand surgery. *Eur J Anaesthesiol.* 2007;24(8):729-730. [VB]

145. Lialiaris T, Kouskoukis A, Tiaka E, et al. Cytogenetic damage after ischemia and reperfusion. *Genet Test Mol Biomarkers.* 2010;14(4):471-475. [IIIC]

146. Kim YS, Jeon YS, Lee JA, et al. Intra-operative warming with a forced-air warmer in preventing

hypothermia after tourniquet deflation in elderly patients. *J Int Med Res.* 2009;37(5):1457-1464. [IC]

147. Townsend HS, Goodman SB, Schurman DJ, Hackel A, Brock-Utne JG. Tourniquet release: systemic and metabolic effects. *Acta Anaesthesiol Scand.* 1996;40(10):1234-1237. [IIIC]

148. Li B, Wen Y, Wu H, Qian Q, Lin X, Zhao H. The effect of tourniquet use on hidden blood loss in total knee arthroplasty. *Int Orthop.* 2009;33(5):1263-1268. [IA]

149. Roy N, Smith M, Anwar M, Elsworth C. Delayed release of drain in total knee replacement reduces blood loss. A prospective randomised study. *Acta Orthop Belg.* 2006;72(1):34-38. [IA]

150. Gasparini G, Papaleo P, Pola P, Cerciello S, Pola E, Fabbriciani C. Local infusion of norepinephrine reduces blood losses and need of transfusion in total knee arthroplasty. *Int Orthop.* 2006;30(4):253-256. [IIB]

151. Orpen NM, Little C, Walker G, Crawfurd EJ. Tranexamic acid reduces early post-operative blood loss after total knee arthroplasty: a prospective randomised controlled trial of 29 patients. *Knee.* 2006;13(2):106-110. [IB]

152. Asakura Y, Tsuchiya H, Nieda Y, Yano T, Kato T, Takagi H. Deep vein thrombosis: how long will it remain? *J Anesth.* 2010;24(3):490-491. [VC]

153. McGrath BJ, Hsia J, Boyd A, et al. Venous embolization after deflation of lower extremity tourniquets. *Anesth Analg.* 1994;78(2):349-353. [IIIC]

154. Bharti N, Mahajan S. Massive pulmonary embolism leading to cardiac arrest after tourniquet deflation following lower limb surgery. *Anaesth Intensive Care.* 2009;37(5):867-868. [VB]

155. Cohen JD, Keslin JS, Nili M, Yosipovitch Z, Gassner S. Massive pulmonary embolism and tourniquet deflation. *Anesth Analg.* 1994;79(3):583-585. [VB]

156. Watanabe S, Terazawa K, Matoba K, Yamada N. An autopsy case of intraoperative death due to pulmonary fat embolism—possibly caused by release of tourniquet after multiple muscle-release and tenotomy of the bilateral lower limbs. *Forensic Sci Int.* 2007;171(1):73-77. [VB]

157. Sinicina I, Bise K, Hetterich R, Pankratz H. Tourniquet use in childhood: a harmless procedure? *Paediatr Anaesth.* 2007;17(2):167-170. [VC]

158. Maguina P, Jean-Pierre F, Grevious MA, Malk AS. Posterior interosseous branch palsy following pneumatic tourniquet application for hand surgery. *Plast Reconstr Surg.* 2008;122(2):97e-99e. [VC]

159. Kort NP, van Raay JJ, van Horn JR. Compartment syndrome and popliteal vascular injury complicating unicompartmental knee arthroplasty. *J Arthroplasty.* 2007;22(3):472-476. [VB]

160. O'Neil D, Sheppard JE. Transient compartment syndrome of the forearm resulting from venous congestion from a tourniquet. *J Hand Surg Am.* 1989;14(5):894-896. [VC]

161. Kerrary S, Schouman T, Cox A, Bertolus C, Febrer G, Bertrand JC. Acute compartment syndrome following fibula flap harvest for mandibular reconstruction. *J Craniomaxillofac Surg.* 2011;39(3):206-208. [VC]

162. Ahmed SM, Ahmad R, Case R, Spencer RF. A study of microbial colonisation of orthopaedic tourniquets. *Ann R Coll Surg Engl.* 2009;91(2):131-134. [IIIB]

163. Walsh EF, Ben-David D, Ritter M, Mechrefe A, Mermel LA, DiGiovanni C. Microbial colonization of tourniquets used in orthopedic surgery. *Orthopedics.* 2006;29(8):709-713. [IIIB]

164. Daruwalla ZJ, Rowan F, Finnegan M, Fennell J, Neligan M. Exsanguinators and tourniquets: do we need to change our practice? *Surgeon.* 2012;10(3):137-142. [IIIC]

165. Guideline for environmental cleaning. In: *Guidelines for Perioperative Practice.* Denver, CO: AORN, Inc; 2015:9-30. [IVB]

166. Guideline for prevention of transmissible infections. In: *Guidelines for Perioperative Practice.* Denver, CO: AORN, Inc; 2015:419-451. [IVA]

167. Meeting the Ongoing Challenge of Continued Competence. 2005. National Council of State Boards of Nursing. https://www.ncsbn.org/Continued_Comp_Paper_TestingServices.pdf. Accessed May 4, 2013. [VC]

168. Sportsman S. Competency education and validation in the United States: what should nurses know? *Nurs Forum.* 2010;45(3):140-149. [VA]

169. Centers for Medicare & Medicaid Services. State Operations Manual Appendix A: Survey Protocol, Regulations and Interpretive Guidelines for Hospitals. Rev. 78; 2011. http://www.cms.gov/Regulations-and-Guidance/Guidance/Manuals/downloads/som107ap_a_hospitals.pdf. Accessed May 4, 2013.

170. Centers for Medicare & Medicaid Services. State Operations Manual Appendix L: Guidance for Surveyors: Ambulatory Surgical Centers. Rev. 76; 2011. http://www.cms.gov/Regulations-and-Guidance/Guidance/Manuals/downloads/som107ap_l_ambulatory.pdf. Accessed May 4, 2013.

171. The Joint Commission. HR.01.05.03: Staff participate in ongoing education and training. *Comprehensive Accreditation Manual for Ambulatory Care.* Oakbrook Terrace, IL: Joint Commission Accreditation; 2012.

172. The Joint Commission. HR.01.05.03: Staff participate in ongoing education and training. In: *Comprehensive Accreditation Manual: CAMH for Hospitals.* Oakbrook Terrace, IL: Joint Commission Accreditation; 2012.

173. American Association for Accreditation of Ambulatory Surgery Facilities. Personnel: personnel records; resumes. In: *Regular Standards and Checklist for Accreditation of Ambulatory Surgery Facilities.* Version 13 ed. Gurnee, IL: American Association for Accreditation of Ambulatory Surgery Facilities; 2011: 77-78.

174. American Association for Accreditation of Ambulatory Surgery Facilities. Personnel: knowledge, skill & CME training. In: *Regular Standards and Checklist for Accreditation of Ambulatory Surgery Facilities.* Version 13 ed. Gurnee, IL: American Association for Accreditation of Ambulatory Surgery Facilities; 2011: 78-79.

175. Sadri A, Braithwaite IJ, Abdul-Jabar HB, Sarraf KM. Understanding of intra-operative tourniquets amongst orthopaedic surgeons and theatre staff—a questionnaire study. *Ann R Coll Surg Engl.* 2010;92(3):243-245. [IIIC]

176. Gillespie BM, Hamlin L. A synthesis of the literature on "competence" as it applies to perioperative nursing. *AORN J.* 2009;90(2):245-258. [VA]

177. Kak N, Burkhalter B, Cooper M-A. Measuring the Competence of Healthcare Providers. Operations Research Issue Paper 2(1). Bethesda, MD: Quality Assurance Project for the US Agency for International Development; 2001. http://www.hciproject.org/sites/default/files/Measuring%20the%20Competence%20of%20HC%20Providers_QAP_2001.pdf. Accessed May 4, 2013. [VA]

178. Ringerman E, Flint LJ, Hughes DE. An innovative education program: the peer competency validator model. *J Nurses Staff Dev.* 2006;22(3):114-123. [VB]

179. Jordan C, Thomas MB, Evans ML, Green A. Public policy on competency: how will nursing address this complex issue? *J Contin Educ Nurs.* 2008;39(2):86-91. [VA]

180. Gillespie BM, Chaboyer W, Wallis M, Chang HY, Werder H. Operating theatre nurses' perceptions

of competence: a focus group study. *J Adv Nurs.* 2009;65(5):1019-1028. [IIIB]

181. Guideline for perioperative health care information management. In: *Guidelines for Perioperative Practice.* Denver, CO: AORN, Inc; 2015:491-512. [IVB]

182. RC.01.01.01: The hospital maintains complete and accurate medical records for each individual patient. In: *Hospital Accreditation Standards 2012.* Oakbrook Terrace, IL: Joint Commission Resources; 2012.

183. RC.01.01.01: The organization maintains complete and accurate clinical records. In: *Standards for Ambulatory Care 2012: Standards, Elements of Performance Scoring Accreditation Polices.* Oakbrook Terrace, IL: The Joint Commission; 2012.

184. Clinical records and health information. In: *2012 Accreditation Handbook for Ambulatory Health Care.* Skokie, IL: Accreditation Association for Ambulatory Health Care; 2012:40-42.

185. American Association for Accreditation of Ambulatory Surgery Facilities. Medical records: general. In: *Regular Standards and Checklist for Accreditation of Ambulatory Surgery Facilities.* Version 13 ed. Gurnee, IL: American Association for Accreditation of Ambulatory Surgery Facilities; 2011:61.

186. American Association for Accreditation of Ambulatory Surgery Facilities. Medical records: pre-operative medical record. In: *Regular Standards and Checklist for Accreditation of Ambulatory Surgery Facilities.* Version 13 ed. Gurnee, IL: American Association for Accreditation of Ambulatory Surgery Facilities; 2011:62-63.

187. American Association for Accreditation of Ambulatory Surgery Facilities. Medical records: operating room records. In: *Regular Standards and Checklist for Accreditation of Ambulatory Surgery Facilities.* Version 13 ed. Gurnee, IL: American Association for Accreditation of Ambulatory Surgery Facilities; 2011:64-66.

188. Silver R, de la Garza J, Rang M, Koreska J. Limb swelling after release of a tourniquet. *Clin Orthop Relat Res.* 1986;(206):86-89. [IIIC]

189. Subramanian S, Lateef H, Massraf A. Cutaneous sensory loss following primary total knee arthroplasty. A two years follow-up study. *Acta Orthop Belg.* 2009;75(5):649-653. [IIIC]

190. 65 FR 4112. Medical device reporting: manufacturer reporting, importer reporting, user facility reporting, distributor reporting. US Government Printing Office. http://www.gpo.gov/fdsys/granule/FR-2000-01-26/00-1785/content-detail.html. Accessed May 4, 2013.

191. Governance. In: *2012 Accreditation Handbook for Ambulatory Health Care.* Skokie, IL: Accreditation Association for Ambulatory Health Care; 2012:20-27.

192. LD.04.01.07: The hospital has policies and procedures that guide and support patient care, treatment, and services. In: *Hospital Accreditation Standards 2012.* 2012 ed. Oakbrook Terrace, IL: Joint Commission Resources; 2012.

193. LD.04.01.07: The organization has policies and procedures that guide and support patient care, treatment, or services. In: *Standards for Ambulatory Care 2012: Standards, Elements of Performance Scoring Accreditation Polices.* Oakbrook Terrace, IL: The Joint Commission; 2012.

194. PI.03.01.01: The hospital improves performance on an ongoing basis. In: *Hospital Accreditation Standards 2012.* 2012 ed. Oakbrook Terrace, IL: Joint Commission Resources; 2012.

195. American Association for Accreditation of Ambulatory Surgery Facilities. Quality assessment/quality improvement: quality improvement. In: *Regular Standards and Checklist for Accreditation of Ambulatory Surgery Facilities.* Version 13 ed. Gurnee, IL: American Association for Accreditation of Ambulatory Surgery Facilities; 2011:67.

196. American Association for Accreditation of Ambulatory Surgery Facilities. Quality assessment/quality improvement: unanticipated operative sequelae. In: *Regular Standards and Checklist for Accreditation of Ambulatory Surgery Facilities.* Version 13 ed. Gurnee, IL: American Association for Accreditation of Ambulatory Surgery Facilities; 2011:69-71.

197. Quality management and improvement. In: *2012 Accreditation Handbook for Ambulatory Health Care.* Skokie, IL: Accreditation Association for Ambulatory Health Care; 2012:34-39.

198. Carling PC, Bartley JM. Evaluating hygienic cleaning in health care settings: what you do not know can harm your patients. *Am J Infect Control.* 2010;38(5 Suppl 1): S41-S50. [IIB]

199. Carling PC, Parry MF, Von Beheren SM; Healthcare Environmental Hygiene Study Group. Identifying opportunities to enhance environmental cleaning in 23 acute care hospitals. *Infect Control Hosp Epidemiol.* 2008;29(1):1-7. [IIIB]

200. Siegel JD Rhinehart E Jackson M Chiarello L; Healthcare Infection Control Practices Advisory Committee. *2007 Guideline for Isolation Precautions: Preventing Transmission of Infectious Agents in Healthcare Settings.* Atlanta, GA: Centers for Disease Control and Prevention; 2006. [IVA]

201. Farquhar M. AHRQ quality indicators. In: Hughes RG, ed. *Patient Safety and Quality: An Evidence-based Handbook for Nurses.* (Prepared with support from the Robert Wood Johnson Foundation). AHRQ Publication No. 08-0043. Rockville, MD: Agency for Healthcare Research and Quality; 2008. http://www.ahrq.gov/professionals/clinicians-providers/resources/nursing/resources/nurseshdbk/nurseshdbk.pdf. Accessed May 4, 2013. [IA]

202. 42 CFR 416: Ambulatory surgical services. 2011. US Government Printing Office. http://www.gpo.gov/fdsys/granule/CFR-2011-title42-vol3/CFR-2011-title42-vol3-part416/content-detail.html. Accessed May 4, 2013.

203. 42 CFR 482: Conditions of participation for hospitals. US Government Printing Office. http://www.gpo.gov/fdsys/granule/CFR-2011-title42-vol5/CFR-2011-title42-vol5-part482/content-detail.html. Accessed May 4, 2013.

Acknowledgements

Lead Author
Bonnie Denholm, MS, BSN, RN, CNOR
Perioperative Nursing Specialist
AORN Nursing Department
Denver, Colorado

Contributing Authors
Ramona Conner, MSN, RN, CNOR
Manager, Standards and Guidelines
AORN Nursing Department
Denver, Colorado

Rodney W. Hicks, PhD, RN, FNP-BC, FAANP, FAAN
Professor
Western University of Health Sciences
Pomona, California

PNEUMATIC TOURNIQUET

The authors and AORN thank Janice A. Neil, PhD, RN, Associate Professor and Chair, Department of Undergraduate Nursing Science, College of Nursing, East Carolina University, Greenville, NC; Jim McEwen, PhD, DSc, PEng, Adjunct Professor, Departments of Orthopaedics & Electrical and Computer Engineering, University of British Columbia, Vancouver, Canada; and Lisa Spruce, DNP, RN, ACNS, ACNP, ANP, CNOR, Director of Evidence-based Perioperative Practice, AORN, Inc, Denver, CO, for their assistance in developing this guideline.

Publication History

Originally published April 1984, *AORN Journal*. Revised November 1990.

Published as proposed recommended practices March 1994. Revised November 1998; published December 1998. Reformatted July 2000.

Revised November 2001; published February 2002, *AORN Journal*.

Revised 2006; published in *Standards, Recommended Practices, and Guidelines*, 2007 edition.

Minor editing revisions made to omit PNDS codes; reformatted September 2012 for publication in *Perioperative Standards and Recommended Practices*, 2013 edition.

Revised April 2013 for online publication in *Perioperative Standards and Recommended Practices*.

Evidence ratings revised 2013 to conform to the AORN Evidence Rating Model.

Minor editing revisions made in November 2014 for publication in *Guidelines for Perioperative Practice*, 2015 edition.

GUIDELINE FOR PRODUCT SELECTION

The Guideline for Product Selection was developed by the AORN Recommended Practices Committee and was approved by the AORN Board of Directors. It was presented as proposed recommendations for comments by members and others. The guideline is effective March 1, 2010. The recommendations in the guideline are intended to be achievable and represent what is believed to be an optimal level of practice. Policies and procedures will reflect variations in practice settings and/or clinical situations that determine the degree to which the guideline can be implemented. AORN recognizes the various settings in which perioperative RNs practice; therefore, this guideline is adaptable to various practice settings. These practice settings include traditional operating rooms (ORs), ambulatory surgery centers, physicians' offices, cardiac catheterization laboratories, endoscopy suites, radiology departments, and all other areas where operative and other invasive procedures may be performed.

Purpose

This document provides guidance for evaluating and purchasing medical devices and other products used in perioperative settings. Patient and worker safety, quality, and cost containment are primary concerns of perioperative RNs as they participate in evaluating and selecting medical devices and products for use in practice settings.[1] In this document, the term *product(s)* is used to refer to all products, medical devices, and capital equipment unless otherwise stated.

Recommendation I

A mechanism for product selection should be developed.

A mechanism for product selection assists with consistently selecting functional and reliable products that are safe, cost-effective, and environmentally friendly; promote quality care; and prevent duplication or rapid obsolescence.

I.a. A multidisciplinary product evaluation and selection committee should be established.

Involvement of a multidisciplinary committee allows input from all departments where the product will be used and from personnel with expertise beyond clinical end-users (eg, infection control, finance, materials management/purchasing).[2,3]

I.a.1. The members of a multidisciplinary product evaluation and selection committee should be based on the size of the health care organization, the type of product, and the affected end-users consisting of, but not limited to,[3,4]
- RNs;
- physicians;
- scrub personnel;
- central/sterile processing personnel;
- anesthesia care providers;
- infection preventionists;
- pharmacists;
- nurse educators; and
- material management/purchasing agents;

and, as applicable, liaisons from
- environmental services,
- administration,
- biomedical engineering,
- risk management,
- radiology,
- finance, and
- laboratory.

Adjusting the composition of the committee will allow health care organizations of various sizes to appoint a responsible individual with the competency and authority to fulfill more than one role (eg, perioperative RN functioning as an infection preventionist and nurse educator). There may be products that do not affect all departments, in which case only the specific end-users or representatives from directly affected departments would need to be involved.

I.b. Perioperative RNs should have an integral role in the evaluation and selection of surgical products.

The perioperative RN has a professional responsibility to consider "factors related to safety, effectiveness, efficiency, and the environment, as well as the cost in planning, delivering, and evaluating patient care."[1(p19)] Perioperative RNs play a crucial role in providing practical insight and expertise in the use and evaluation of surgical products.[5,6]

Recommendation II

The multidisciplinary committee should develop a process to guide product selection.

A standardized product selection process assists in the selection of functional and reliable products that are safe, cost-effective, and environmentally friendly and that promote quality care, as well as decrease duplication or rapid obsolescence.[3,7,8]

PRODUCT SELECTION

II.a. The committee should gather information about new or existing products from professional resources and the manufacturer.

Manufacturers' representatives have access to information concerning products currently on the market. Manufacturers' representatives can provide both clinical and technical data related to product research, processing, packaging, disinfection, sterilization, and environmental conservation.[3]

II.b. Consistent requirements should be identified for each product under evaluation.

The health care organization's multidisciplinary product evaluation and selection committee identifies the written objective, generic criteria specific to the desired product, and its ability to function as desired. Consistency in process requirements provide a reliable and valid means of evaluating the end results.[5,9]

- II.b.1. Product-specific requirements should include, but not be limited to,
  - contractual agreements (eg, warranties and maintenance agreements)[5];
  - required compatibility with new or existing products;
  - compatibility with existing disposal methods;
  - compatibility with existing reprocessing methods;
  - procedure-related requirements (eg, for a drape: resistance to penetration by blood and other body fluids, size, presence of adhesive apertures, low linting);
  - end-user preference and requirements (eg, for a surgical gown: comfort, degree of protection from blood and body fluids, size, absence of toxic ingredients/allergens; for an instrument: ease of use, performance, the type of decontamination and sterilization process necessary);
  - patient-related requirements (eg, the size of the patient, presence of allergies or infectious diseases);
  - compliance with federal, state, and local regulatory agencies such as the Occupational Safety and Health Administration (OSHA) or the US Food and Drug Administration (FDA)[10-13]; and
  - compliance with standards-setting bodies.

Contractual agreements are documents such as warranties and maintenance agreements that are stipulated before the time of evaluation assisting the manufacturer to be aware of the requirements of the health care organization.

Defining compatibility requirements assists in ensuring that the new product will be compatible with an existing product or if it is not compatible will clarify the need for additional adapters or other products.

The disposal method is considered to determine the effect of disposing of the product on the existing methods and to ensure the correct disposal method is available. For example, if the product is considered a hazardous material, consider whether a method exists for disposing of hazardous materials, including appropriate labeling and a company to remove the waste.

The list of products which the reprocessing company has obtained clearance to reprocess may not contain the product under consideration. An additional company may be required for reprocessing the product, if the product is on the FDA list of approved products to be reprocessed.[14]

Procedure-related requirements define what is required for the procedure or multiple procedures for which the product will be used. Some of these requirements can be determined by using a scale such as the ANSI/AAMI barrier performance scale.[15,16]

End-user–related requirements will vary depending on how the product is used and, when addressed, increase the compliance by the end-user.

Patient-related requirements define the ability of the product to adapt to individual patients.

Most standards-setting bodies use research to create standards, and some of the standards may be adopted for enforcement by regulatory agencies.[15,17-20]

II.c. A financial impact analysis should be performed on each product to be purchased.

A financial impact analysis can be used to clarify a choice between two different products with equivalent functionality.[3,5]

- II.c.1. The financial impact analysis should include
  - direct costs (eg, cost of the product, replacement strategy, associated equipment);
  - indirect costs (eg, utilities, waste disposal, processing, training, storage, energy utilization, depreciation, retrofitting to existing equipment)[5];
  - reimbursement potential; and
  - group purchasing organization (GPO) contract pricing.

When a product is being replaced, the replacement strategy is a direct cost resulting from the need to dispose of the existing stock of the product being replaced. If the new product is being phased in and will replace the existing product after the current inventory is exhausted, then there

PRODUCT SELECTION

will be no additional direct cost. The indirect costs are the costs associated with the use of the product after purchase. These costs may include electricity, decontamination and sterilization method, and disposal. The sum of the direct and indirect costs incurred over the product's lifetime is the complete cost for the product.[3,21] An example of a large indirect cost is energy, on which hospitals spend approximately $8.3 billion annually.[22]

The reimbursement potential is used in determining the impact on the profit margin of each procedure and will vary with each product.

Group purchasing organization contract pricing may determine the direct cost of the product by defining the quantities required, applicable time frames, and pricing on other products purchased.[5]

II.c.2. As appropriate, other health care organizations should be contacted based on contract terms and affiliations or working relationships regarding
- purchasing partial quantities of infrequently used supplies or
- creating a shared inventory.

Purchasing partial quantities of infrequently used supplies or using a shared inventory may assist with decreasing the amount of infrequently used inventory in stock, direct costs, and the amount of waste generated.

II.c.3. Vendors should be contacted regarding
- return of unopened, expired products;
- creation of a consigned inventory; and
- lowest unit of purchase.

Returning unopened, expired products may decrease the amount of infrequently used inventory in stock and the amount of waste generated. Expenses may be reduced based on the cost associated with restocking and freight for the return shipment. The upfront expense for consigned inventory may be less because the product is paid for at the time of use, and the product is frequently only a portion of the total inventory consigned. If the product was not consigned, the entire inventory would need to be purchased before use. Vendors may be willing to ship in small quantities to meet the needs of the health care organization that requires a low inventory because of low usage.

II.d. An interdepartmental and intradepartmental standardization initiative and plan should be developed and reviewed to determine the applicability for each product being evaluated.

Reports indicate that standardization can reduce costs and may improve inventory control and use of storage space. Standardization also decreases end-user training and errors related to unfamiliarity with the product.[3,5,6,9] The perioperative RN is a qualified person to assist with standardization because of familiarity with the use of many products.

II.d.1. The plan should include a list of products requiring standardization and a process for determining which products will be standardized.

II.e. The product's environmental impact should be assessed by addressing the following criteria:
- Can the product be recycled?
- Is the product made of recycled materials?
- What method is used for disposal?

Using any or all of these criteria can help decrease the 6,600 tons of waste generated daily by US health care facilities.[23] Considering only one of the environmental impact criteria may not reveal other environmental benefits or negative effects of the product.[24] It is estimated that only 10% to 25% of hospital waste is regulated waste; the remainder is equivalent to household waste and can be recycled.[23,25,26] Recycling noninfectious waste materials has environmental and financial benefits that may include, but are not limited to,
- providing materials for remanufacture;
- limiting the expansion of landfills and incinerator use, thereby decreasing air and water pollution;
- conserving energy;
- preserving resources for future generations; and
- decreasing the cost of waste removal.[22,27,28]

The method of disposal is assessed to determine if the product can be disposed of by a method currently being used or if a new method needs to be introduced. For example, if the health care organization has never handled hazardous waste such as chemotherapy products, a method to dispose of this type of waste would be necessary before the product is introduced.

Products manufactured from recycled materials decrease the amount of waste created and natural resources utilized in creation of the product.[29]

Resources are available (eg, sample policies and procedures, contract language, a listing of environmentally friendly products) to assist in determining the environmental impact of products.[30]

II.f. The following criteria should be considered when determining whether to purchase a single-use, reposable, or reusable product:
- the useful life of the product;
- the estimated use of the product;
- the availability of required decontamination and sterilization processes;
- if single-use, whether the product can be reprocessed;
- inventory required;
- storage facilities;

PRODUCT SELECTION

- knowledge of health care workers who use, maintain, and reprocess instruments and other equipment; and
- maintenance, repair, or restoration programs for instruments and equipment.

Purchasing reusable products demonstrates the health care organization's commitment to supply conservation and fiscal responsibility through conservation of resources and energy, optimization of resources, and reduction of the pollution that occurs with waste disposal. Health care organizations have reported a large reduction in the amount of waste generated annually by reusing, repairing, and refurbishing products.[22,31]

Pollution is reduced when a health care organization purchases a reposable or reusable product or reprocesses a single-use product because the final disposal of the product is delayed. Health care organizations have reported large monetary savings when using reusable products.[2,32] There are reports of original equipment manufacturers increasing the cost of products because a single-use product was reprocessed, which caused a decrease in the number of new products being purchased.[2]

Projecting the useful life of the product assists in maintaining an adequate inventory to allow for completion of scheduled maintenance and to reduce frequency of reprocessing and wear. When the product has a short life span, it may be more economical to consider a disposable option because the product may become outdated before use.

When a product has a very low usage, purchasing a disposable product may be more economical when compared to a reusable product that requires repeated sterilizations and other maintenance.

If the required decontamination and sterilization processes, including proper containment devices, are not available, the cost per use may increase.[33] Proper sterilization processes are required because to achieve a sterile product, the sterilizing agent must contact all surfaces.[34]

The amount of inventory directly affects the amount of storage space required, and reusable items may require less inventory and storage space.

If health care workers who use, maintain, and reprocess instruments and other equipment are knowledgeable of the processes involved, the life of the product will be extended.

Regular maintenance, repair, or remanufacturer programs for instruments and equipment will reduce malfunction and maintain function.[4]

II.g. When determining if a product labeled as a single-use device (SUD) should be reprocessed, consider
- whether the product is listed on the FDA list of products approved for reprocessing,
- the financial effect of the reprocessing program, and
- whether the health care organization can accomplish the reprocessing with existing internal or external resources.

Certain SUDs are listed by the FDA as being acceptable for reprocessing.[14] The financial effect is determined by weighing the cost savings against the cost of initiating and maintaining the program. Some facilities report a cost savings from reprocessing some SUDs, a major reason for initiating a reprocessing program. The amount of cost savings depends on the size of the health care organization, the number of devices reprocessed, staff education, labor costs, and the health care organization's commitment to the program.[35,36] The FDA requires health care organizations and third parties that reprocess SUDs to adhere to the same regulations as the original equipment manufacturers. These regulations include
- quality system regulations,[37]
- medical device reporting,[38]
- registration and listing,[39]
- labeling,[40]
- premarket approval and premarket notification,[41-43]
- medical device corrections and removals,[44] and
- medical device tracking.[45]

These regulations lead many health care organizations to hire a third-party reprocessor.[2,35]

II.h. An evaluation process should be developed based on objective criteria specific to the product.

Using a consistent evaluation process assists with obtaining an objective review and analysis.[3,5,46]

II.h.1. A multidisciplinary evaluation team of end-users and representatives from other departments affected by a product (eg, infection control, sterile processing) should be developed to participate in the clinical evaluation process.

Involvement of a multidisciplinary team allows input from departments with varying needs to select the most appropriate products to meet those needs.[2] Including all clinical areas in the evaluation process provides direct feedback from staff members whose practices will be affected by the product.[3,27] The team concept also allows input from departments that are not end-users but can provide expert advice beyond the scope of the end-users (eg, infection preventionists).

II.h.2. A product-specific evaluation tool should be developed using unique product-specific criteria, which may include, but is not limited to,
- safety;
- performance;
- quality;
- efficiency;
- ease of use;
- compatibility with other products;

PRODUCT SELECTION

- effect on quality patient care and clinical outcomes;
- evidence-based efficacy;
- financial impact analysis;
- compliance with GPO agreements;
- sterilization/reprocessing parameters including degree of difficulty;
- liability (eg, for investigational products);
- federal, state, and local regulatory requirements;
- standardization;
- compatibility with new and existing products;
- environmental impact;
- availability and quality of service after purchase;
- amount of personnel training required; and
- the quality of the manufacturer's instructions.

Careful selection of criteria ensures the reliability and validity of trial evaluation results. A product-specific written or electronic evaluation tool facilitates an objective review and analysis.[46]

II.h.3. Limits should be placed on the scope of the clinical evaluation. These limitations should include, but not be limited to,
- the number of users;
- cost;
- the number of products to be evaluated;
- time span;
- the number of departments and clinical areas involved;
- desired patient outcomes; and
- follow-up patient data, if indicated.

Placing limits on product evaluations increases the usefulness of user feedback. Allowing unlimited time to evaluate products may result in decreased evaluator input and enthusiasm.[5]

II.h.4. The amount of end-user education required regarding the use of the product being evaluated should be determined.

The amount of time required for education may differ between products based on the familiarity of personnel with one of the products compared to the other. The time required for education will affect the indirect cost of the product and the start time of the evaluation.

II.h.5. Evaluation data should be analyzed to determine product purchase recommendations based on actual clinical performance compared to the predetermined, unique, product-specific criteria.

This information facilitates efficient and consistent decisions based on previously established criteria and an evidence-based product assessment.[5]

II.i. After a product has been selected, a comprehensive plan for introduction and use should be developed and implemented to include, but not be limited to,
- education required to complete the end-users' competencies in all departments involved,
- physician credentialing required before use,
- projected date of first use, and
- replacement strategy.

The development of a comprehensive plan for the introduction of a product will facilitate smooth implementation. The development of a replacement strategy also assists in decreasing inventory and dual educational needs. This strategy also may reduce the risk of making an unsatisfactory product selection.

Recommendation III

Perioperative RNs should demonstrate competency related to product evaluation and selection.

Ongoing competency validation and education provides the perioperative RN with the information required to take an active role and effectively influence the evaluation process and product selection.

III.a. Educational programs should be provided regarding
- specific steps required for product selection;
- safe care and handling of products;
- selection of products;
- the environmental effects of health care, new environmental conditions, and appropriate green responses[27];
- governmental regulations regarding purchasing and product requirements;
- reprocessing, repair, recycling, and refurbishing initiatives of the health care organization[2,47]; and
- how to evaluate and provide objective input on the product's appropriateness and effectiveness.

Staff members should be educated about manufacturers' various methods of designating specific product characteristics, such as using color-coded labels to signify a sterile gown's level of protection.[48,49]

Education increases the perioperative RN's active participation in decreasing the environmental impact of health care.[27,47]

III.b. Demonstration and instruction on the use of the products should be conducted before the clinical evaluation and before initiating general use.

Instructing all individuals involved in the clinical evaluation facilitates safe clinical practice and helps establish validity of the product evaluation.[5]

PRODUCT SELECTION

Recommendation IV

The product selection process and any product-specific information should be documented.

Documentation of this information provides retrievable records to answer potential questions regarding the justification for purchasing a specific product and for future purchasing decisions.

IV.a. Documentation of the product-selection process using a specific product-related evaluation tool[5] or meeting minutes should include, but not be limited to,
- the names of the committee participants,
- generic product performance requirements,
- requirements for standardization,
- the environmental impact,
- results of the financial impact analysis,
- evaluation methods to include the tools and the results of the evaluations,
- a comparative listing of products evaluated,
- justification for purchasing single-use versus reusable products,
- an implementation plan, and
- the final decision.

Recommendation V

Policies and procedures for evaluating and selecting products should be developed, reviewed periodically, revised as necessary, and readily available in the practice setting.

Policies and procedures assist in the development of patient and worker safety, quality assessment, and improvement activities. Policies and procedures establish authority, responsibility, and accountability within the facility. They also serve as operational guidelines that are used to minimize patient and worker risk factors, standardize practice, direct staff members, and establish guidelines for continuous performance improvement activities.

V.a. Policies and procedures should encompass all aspects of the product selection process to include
- the composition of the multidisciplinary committee members,
- product performance requirements to include patient and worker safety requirements,
- standardization process,
- the environmental impact assessment,
- the financial impact assessment,
- utilization of evaluation methods,
- components of an implementation plan,
- authorization and approval process,
- how products are introduced and the role of the health care industry representative,
- the role and responsibility of the health care industry representative,[50]
- the process to request and initiate a product review, and
- steps to take if an injury occurs during trial or use as described in the Safe Medical Devices Act of 1990.[51]

Recommendation VI

A quality assurance/performance improvement process should be established to measure product performance to include post-purchase cost effectiveness and user satisfaction.

This evaluation helps to ensure that new products are meeting expected performance criteria (eg, cost-effectiveness, product life span) and that the pre-selection evaluation process has met its objectives.

VI.a. New product performance and user satisfaction should be evaluated at planned intervals.

Establishing intervals for measurement assists in ensuring all products are evaluated and inventories can be adjusted as necessary to eliminate ineffective products.

VI.b. Quality programs should include monitoring of reprocessing and recycling efforts to include review of additional opportunities to minimize environmental impact.

Monitoring of reprocessing and recycling efforts provides the data to assess operational errors and noncompliance, quality and effectiveness of the product, and financial impact.[2]

VI.c. The quality program must describe required actions necessary for compliance with the Safe Medical Devices Act of 1990.[51]

VI.d. After a product has been selected, a comprehensive plan for evaluation of the product should be developed and implemented to include, but not be limited to, frequency and criteria for reevaluation.

Glossary

Process: "A goal-directed, interrelated series of actions, events, mechanisms, or steps. An interrelated series of events, activities, actions, mechanisms, or steps that transforms inputs into outputs." Source: Joint Commission on Accreditation of Healthcare Organizations. Glossary. In: *Hospital Accreditation Standards*. Oakbrook Terrace, IL: Joint Commission on Accreditation of Healthcare Organizations; 2002:331, 346, 354, 360.

Reposable: An instrument that has limited use or an instrument with a combination of reusable and disposable components.

Reprocessing: Includes all operations to render a contaminated reusable or single-use device patient ready. Single-use devices to be reprocessed may be either used or unused. Reprocessing steps include cleaning, decontamination, functional testing, repackaging, relabeling, and sterilization/disinfection.

Reusable: Any product or piece of equipment intended by the manufacturer for multiple uses. As appropriate to each item, the manufacturer is to provide instructions for reprocessing, care, and/or maintenance of the item.

Reuse: The repeated or multiple uses of any medical device whether marketed as reusable or single-use. Repeated/multiple use may be on the same patient or on different patients with applicable reprocessing of the device between uses.

Useful life: Length of time, as determined by the manufacturer, for which a product maintains acceptable safety and performance characteristics. The manufacturer should provide data to support useful life of the material. Useful life is affected by the number of sterilization processing and washing cycles a product can endure and yet maintain an acceptable barrier capability.

REFERENCES

1. Standards of perioperative nursing. In: *Perioperative Standards and Recommended Practices*. Denver, CO: AORN, Inc; 2010:9-62.
2. Flynn AB, Knishinsky R. A matter of reprocessing. *Mater Manag Health Care.* 2005;14(10):32-35.
3. Barlow RD. Infusing value analysis in contracting strategies: it's not just a pricing or product evaluation and selection game. *Healthc Purchasing News.* 2008; 32(10):62.
4. DeMeo M. Understanding the elements of reprocessing surgical instrumentation for clinically safer and financially sound outcomes. *Infection Control Today.* 2009;13(5):24-26.
5. Halvorson CK, Chinnes LF. Collaborative leadership in product evaluation. *AORN J.* 2007;85(2):334-352.
6. Greene J. Value analysis team guides OR purchasing. *OR Manager.* 2006;22(11):19, 21.
7. Adler S, Scherrer M, Ruckauer KD, Daschner FD. Comparison of economic and environmental impacts between disposable and reusable instruments used for laparoscopic cholecystectomy. *Surg Endosc.* 2005; 19(2):268-272.
8. Howes BW. The reliability of laryngoscope lights. *Anaesthesia.* 2006;61(5):488-491.
9. Hupp D. A strategy for review of new products. *OR Manager.* 2005;21(11):23-24.
10. Medical gloves and gowns. US Food and Drug Administration Center for Devices and Radiological Health. http://www.fda.gov/MedicalDevices/Products andMedicalProcedures/MedicalToolsandSupplies/Per sonalProtectiveEquipment/ucm056077.htm. Accessed February 10, 2010.
11. Siegel JD, Rhinehart E, Jackson M, Chiarello L; the Healthcare Infection Control Practices Advisory Committee. *2007 Guideline for Isolation Precautions: Preventing Transmission of Infectious Agents in Healthcare Settings.* http://www.cdc.gov/hicpac/2007IP/2007isolation Precautions.html. Accessed February 10, 2010.
12. FDA-cleared surgical drapes. US Food and Drug Administration Center for Devices and Radiological Health, 2003-2008. http://www.accessdata.fda.gov/scripts/cdrh/devicesatfda/index.cfm. Accessed February 10, 2010.
13. US Occupational Health and Safety Administration. Bloodborne pathogens. 29 CFR 1910.1030. Revised July 1, 2009. http://edocket.access.gpo.gov/cfr_2009/jul-qtr/pdf/29cfr1910.1030.pdf. Accessed February 10, 2010.
14. FDA's web site for cleared reprocessed single-use devices. US Department of Health and Human Services. http://www.fda.gov/MedicalDevices/DeviceRegulation andGuidance/ReprocessingofSingle-UseDevices /ucm121197.htm. Accessed February 10, 2010.
15. AAMI. *Technical Information Report 11: Selection and Use of Protective Apparel and Surgical Drapes in Health Care Facilities.* Arlington, VA: Association for the Advancement of Medical Instrumentation; 2005.
16. AAMI. *PB70:2003: Liquid Barrier Performance and Classification of Protective Apparel and Drapes Intended for Use in Health Care Facilities.* Arlington, VA: Association for the Advancement of Medical Instrumentation; 2003.
17. ANSI. *Z136.3-2005: Safe Use of Lasers in Health Care Facilities.* New York, NY: American National Standards Institute; 2005.
18. Recommended practices for laser safety in practice settings. In: *Perioperative Standards and Recommended Practices.* Denver, CO: AORN, Inc; 2010:133-138.
19. Recommended practices for electrosurgery. In: *Perioperative Standards and Recommended Practices.* Denver, CO: AORN, Inc; 2010:105-126.
20. *ASTM International. ASTM F2407: Standard Specification for Surgical Gowns Intended for Use in Healthcare Facilities.* West Conshohocken, PA: ASTM International; 2006.
21. Carter S. How to evaluate and justify the implementation of disposal products in your facility. *Infection Control Today.* 2009;13(6):80.
22. Serb C. Think green. *Hosp Health Netw.* 2008; 82(8):22-6, 35.
23. Waste management. Practice Greenhealth. http://www.practicegreenhealth.org/educate/operations /waste. Accessed February 10, 2010.
24. Davis MR. Environmental impacts of surgical draping and gowning systems: results of a Life Cycle Analysis. *ACORN.* 2005;18(4):16-17, 21-24.
25. Chaerul M, Tanaka M, Shekdar AV. A system dynamics approach for hospital waste management. *Waste Manag.* 2008;28(2):442-449.
26. Cheng YW, Sung FC, Yang Y, Lo YH, Chung YT, Li KC. Medical waste production at hospitals and associated factors. *Waste Manag.* 2009;29(1):440-444.
27. McGain F, Clark M, Williams T, Wardlaw T. Recycling plastics from the operating suite. *Anaesth Intensive Care.* 2008;36(6):913-914.
28. Ogden J. Blue wrap recycling: it can be done! *AORN J.* 2009;89(4):739-743.
29. Environmentally preferable purchasing. Environmental Protection Agency. http://www.epa.gov/epp/. Accessed February 10, 2010.
30. Environmental purchasing. Practice Greenhealth. http://www.practicegreenhealth.org/educate/purchasing. Accessed February 10, 2010.
31. Birk S. An issue that can't be contained. *Mater Manag Health Care.* 2008;17(5):42-44.
32. Texas health system identifies numerous cost-savings opportunities. *Hosp Mater Manage.* 2007;32(4):1-3.
33. Recommended practices for sterilization in the perioperative practice setting. In: *Perioperative Standards and Recommended Practices.* Denver, CO: AORN, Inc; 2010:457-480.
34. AAMI. *ST65: Processing of Reusable Surgical Textiles for Use in Health Care Facilities.* Arlington, VA: Association for the Advancement of Medical Instrumentation; 2000.
35. Follow expert insight to launch a successful reprocessing program. *Hosp Mater Manage.* 2008;33(3):1-4.
36. DiConsiglio J. Reprocessing SUDs reduces waste, costs. *Mater Manag Health Care.* 2008;17(9):40-42.

PRODUCT SELECTION

37. US Food and Drug Administration. Definitions. 21 CFR 820.3. Revised April 1, 2008. http://edocket.access.gpo.gov/cfr_2008/aprqtr/pdf/21cfr820.3.pdf. Accessed February 10, 2010.

38. How to report a problem (medical devices). US Food and Drug Administration. http://www.fda.gov/cdrh/mdr/mdr-general.html. Accessed February 10, 2010.

39. US Food and Drug Administration. 21 CFR 807. Establishment registration and device listing for manufacturers and initial importers of devices. Revised April 1, 2008. http://www.access.gpo.gov/nara/cfr/waisidx_08/21cfr807_08.html. Accessed February 10, 2010.

40. US Food and Drug Administration. Labeling. 21 CFR 801. Revised April 1, 2008. http://www.access.gpo.gov/nara/cfr/waisidx_08/21cfr801_08.html. Accessed February 10, 2010.

41. US Food and Drug Administration. Exemptions for device establishments. 21 CFR 807.65. Revised April 1, 2008. http://edocket.access.gpo.gov/cfr_2008/aprqtr/pdf/21cfr807.65.pdf. Accessed February 10, 2010.

42. US Food and Drug Administration. Premarket approval of medical devices. 21 CFR 814. Revised April 1, 2008. http://www.access.gpo.gov/nara/cfr/waisidx_08/21cfr814_08.html. Accessed February 10, 2010.

43. US Food and Drug Administration. Investigational device exemptions. 21 CFR 812. Revised April 1, 2008. http://www.access.gpo.gov/nara/cfr/waisidx_08/21cfr812_08.html. Accessed February 10, 2010.

44. US Food and Drug Administration. Definitions. 21 CFR 806.2. Revised April 1, 2008. http://edocket.access.gpo.gov/cfr_2008/aprqtr/pdf/21cfr806.2.pdf. Accessed February 10, 2010.

45. US Food and Drug Administration. Medical device reporting. 21 CFR 803. Revised April 1, 2009. http://www.access.gpo.gov/nara/cfr/waisidx_09/21cfr803_09.html. Accessed February 10, 2010.

46. Akridge J. Softer, stronger fabrics enhance gowns and drapes. *Healthc Purchasing News.* 2009;33(4):14-19.

47. Topf M. Psychological explanations and interventions for indifference to greening hospitals. *Healthc Manage Rev.* 2005;30(1):2-8.

48. Williamson JE. New gown, drape features have O.R. staff covered. *Healthc Purchasing News.* 2005;29(9):22, 24, 26 assm.

49. Akridge J. Task-specific surgical apparel balances comfort with protection. *Healthc Purchasing News.* 2008;32(10):28.

50. AORN guidance statement: The role of the health care industry representative in the perioperative setting. In: *Perioperative Standards and Recommended Practices.* Denver, CO: AORN, Inc; 2010:657-660.

51. Medical device reporting: manufacturer reporting, importer reporting, user facility reporting, distributor reporting. Food and Drug Administration, HHS. Final rule. *Fed Regist.* 2000;65(17):4112-4121.

Acknowledgments

Lead Authors

Byron Burlingame, MS, RN, CNOR
Perioperative Nursing Specialist
AORN Center for Nursing Practice
Denver, Colorado

George Allen, PhD, RN, CNOR, CIC
Director of Infection Control
Downstate Medical Center
Brooklyn, New York

Contributing Authors

Josette Coicou-Brioche, MSN, RN, CNOR
Associate Director of Perioperative Services
Kings County Hospital Center
Brooklyn, New York

Nancy B. Bjerke, RN, MPH, CIC
Health Care Consultant
San Antonio, Texas

Publication History

Originally published April 1989, *AORN Journal.* Revised August 1993.

Revised November 1997; published January 1998, *AORN Journal.* Reformatted July 2000.

Revised November 2003; published in *Standards, Recommended Practices, and Guidelines,* 2004 edition. Reprinted March 2004, *AORN Journal.*

Revised January 2010 for online publication in *Perioperative Standards and Recommended Practices.*

Reformatted September 2012 for publication in *Perioperative Standards and Recommended Practices,* 2013 edition.

Minor editing revisions made in November 2014 for publication in *Guidelines for Perioperative Practice,* 2015 edition.

PATIENT AND **WORKER** SAFETY

GUIDELINE FOR AUTOLOGOUS TISSUE MANAGEMENT

The Guideline for Autologous Tissue Management has been approved by the AORN Guideline Advisory Board. It was presented as a proposed guideline for comments by members and others. The guideline is effective November 15, 2014. The recommendations in the guideline are intended to be achievable and represent what is believed to be an optimal level of practice. Policies and procedures will reflect variations in practice settings and/or clinical situations that determine the degree to which the guideline can be implemented. AORN recognizes the many diverse settings in which perioperative nurses practice; therefore, this guideline is adaptable to all areas where operative and other invasive procedures may be performed.

Purpose

This document provides guidance to perioperative personnel for managing autologous tissue in the perioperative setting, including avulsed teeth, cranial bone flaps, parathyroid glands, skin, veins, and dropped autografts. Guidance is provided for transferring tissue from the sterile field, packaging and labeling, transporting and storing, and handling autologous tissue for delayed replantation or autotransplantation within the same facility. Guidance for managing autologous adipose tissue is not provided. Currently, adipose aspirates can only be used for immediate autologous fat grafting at the time of recovery, and there is no reliable method for preserving and storing adipose tissue for delayed autotransplantation.[1,2] Recommendations related to processes for intraoperative storage and cryopreservation of autologous tissue are outside the scope of this document.

A facility that handles autologous tissue for delayed replantation or autotransplantation into the same patient and within the same facility is not required to register with the US Food and Drug Administration (FDA) as a tissue establishment (ie, tissue bank) that manufactures human cells, tissues, and cellular and tissue-based products, nor to follow requirements of 21 CFR Part 1271 (ie, the FDA regulations for these products).[3,4] Facilities or health care organizations that handle autologous tissue are required to recover, process, package, label, store, track, and replant or autotransplant the tissue in a manner that minimizes microbial growth, prevents mix-ups, and reduces the risk for errors.[3] Although the regulation defines manufacturing to include recovery, processing, storage, labeling, packaging, or distribution of any human cell or tissue,[3,5] the FDA considers most procedures related to autologous tissue to be a single procedure encompassed within the element of storage. The reader can refer to section 1271.15(b), in which storage of autologous tissue is exempt if replantation or autotransplantation will occur in the facility where the recovery took place.[4] Similarly, packaging and labeling of autologous tissue can be encompassed within the exception for storage.[4] Freezing autologous tissue as a method of storage does not, in itself, require registration and listing with the FDA as a tissue establishment.[4]

In addition, the FDA has interpreted the "same surgical procedure" language in its final rule to include recovery and storage before replantation or autotransplantation.[3] Retaining autologous tissue to be used in a subsequent application for the same patient is exempt from registration because the two applications are essentially a single, continuous procedure.[4]

The facility is required to register with the FDA if autologous tissue handling includes steps to process the autograft when any step requires specific manufacturing controls to decontaminate the tissue (ie, subjecting the autograft to a steam sterilization process).[4] If autologous tissue-handling functions are expanded to include distribution of the autograft to another facility located at a different address, registration and listing with the FDA using Form FDA 3356 is required.[3]

Whether or not facility registration is required, the federal regulations described in 21 CFR Part 1271 provide good practices for preventing the introduction, transmission, or spread of communicable disease and enhancing patient safety related to autologous tissue management.[3,5]

The reader can also refer to the standards of the American Association of Tissue Banks (AATB), which reflect the collective expertise and efforts of tissue bank professionals to provide a comprehensive foundation to support tissue banking activities, including practices for managing autologous tissue.[6]

Evidence Review

On January 24 and January 27, 2014, a medical librarian conducted a systematic search of the databases MEDLINE®, CINAHL®, and the Cochrane Database of Systematic Reviews for meta-analyses, systematic reviews, randomized controlled and non-randomized trials and studies, case reports, letters, reviews, and guidelines. The librarian also searched Scopus®, although not systematically. Search terms included *autologous transplantation, tissue preservation, organ transplantation, preservation, storage, storage solution, saline solution, isotonic saline, potassium chloride, N-acetylhistidine, ice, cold temperature, bone flap, bone transplantation, skull, bone and bones, surgical flap, saphenous vein, radial artery, renal artery, mammary artery,* and *thoracic artery*. During the development of this document, the lead author also requested supplementary

AUTOLOGOUS TISSUE MANAGEMENT

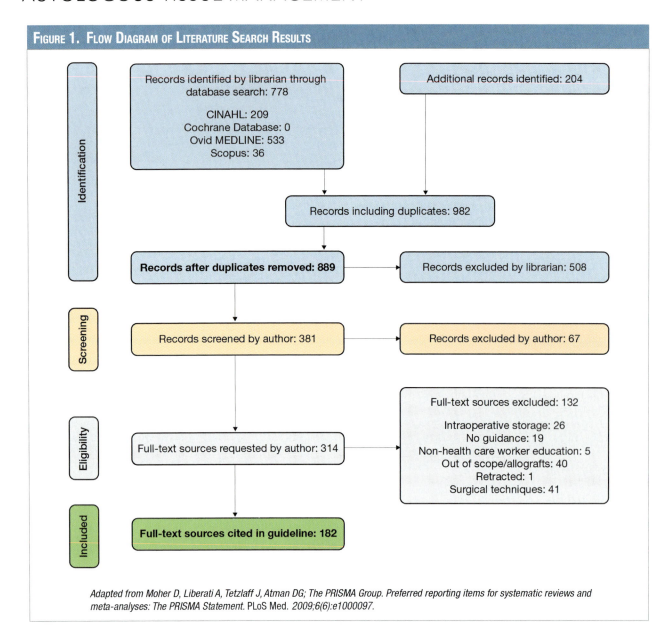

Figure 1. Flow Diagram of Literature Search Results

Adapted from Moher D, Liberati A, Tetzlaff J, Atman DG; The PRISMA Group. Preferred reporting items for systematic reviews and meta-analyses: The PRISMA Statement. PLoS Med. 2009;6(6):e1000097.

searches on the topics of storage media, preservation of avulsed teeth, and the use of swab cultures.

The initial search was limited to literature published in English since January 2006; however, the time restriction was not considered in subsequent searches. At the time of the initial search, the librarian also established weekly alerts on the topics included in the initial search. The librarian later added terms from subsequent supplementary searches to the alerts and, until May 2014, presented relevant results to the lead author.

The lead author reviewed search results from the medical librarian's literature search for the AORN Guideline for Specimen Management to identify literature specific to management of other tissues and the preservation of avulsed teeth. During the development of the document, the lead author requested additional articles and other literature that either did not fit the original search criteria or was discovered during the evidence appraisal process. Finally, the lead author and the medical librarian identified relevant guidelines from government agencies and standards-setting bodies. In total, 889 research and non-research sources of evidence were identified for possible inclusion, and of these, 182 were cited in the guidance document (Figure 1).

Excluded were non-peer-reviewed or retracted publications; evidence specific to organ transplantations, processes for cryopreservation, and surgical techniques and treatment protocols; and some evidence related to allografts, intraoperative storage of autologous tissue, and educational needs surrounding traumatic dental injuries not specific to health care workers.

Articles identified in the search were provided to the lead author and the assigned evidence reviewer for review and critical appraisal using the AORN Research or Non-Research Evidence Appraisal Tools as appropriate. The literature was independently evaluated and appraised by the lead author and the evidence reviewer according to the strength and quality of the evidence. Each article was then assigned an appraisal score determined by consensus. The appraisal score is noted in brackets after each reference, as applicable. Various articles also were provided to an expert member of the project team for consideration regarding relevance and application of the evidence for determining practice guidelines.

The evidence supporting each intervention and activity statement within a specific recommendation was summarized, and the AORN Evidence-Rating Model was used to rate the strength of the collective evidence. Factors considered in the review of the collective evidence were the quality of the evidence, the quantity of similar evidence on a given topic, the consistency of evidence supporting a recommendation, and the potential benefits and harms. The assigned evidence rating is noted in brackets after each intervention and activity statement.

Note: The evidence summary table is available at http://www.aorn.org/evidencetables/.

Editor's note: MEDLINE is a registered trademark of the US National Library of Medicine's Medical Literature Analysis and Retrieval System, Bethesda, MD. CINAHL, Cumulative Index to Nursing and Allied Health Literature, is a registered trademark of EBSCO Industries, Birmingham, AL. Scopus is a registered trademark of Elsevier B.V., Amsterdam, The Netherlands.

Recommendation I

Avulsed teeth that cannot be immediately replanted in the patient at the time of avulsion should be placed in a storage medium to help maintain periodontal ligament (PDL) cell viability.

Tooth avulsion is characterized by a complete displacement of the tooth from the alveolar socket.[7-14] The avulsion causes a rupture in the PDL tissue as shown in Figure 2. A portion of the PDL tissue remains on the walls of the alveolar socket, and a portion remains attached to the root surface of the avulsed tooth.[15] The PDL cells attached to the alveolar wall maintain viability; however, the PDL cells attached to the root surface are at risk for necrosis[12,16-18] or infection.[9] Neurovascular supply to the tooth is compromised and may result in loss of tooth pulp vitality.[7,8,13,19-22]

The collective evidence indicates that the ability to successfully replant an avulsed tooth often depends on measures taken at the time of the avulsion and immediately afterward.[23-25] Immediate replantation of the tooth at the site of the avulsion injury is the preferred treatment.[8-20,22,25-41] When immediate replantation is not possible, storing the tooth in an effective storage medium can help to maintain the viability of the PDL cells.[7-24,27,32,34-36,38-47] Numerous types of media have been recommended for storage of avulsed teeth. The most effective media to support PDL cell viability are Hank's Balanced Salt Solution (HBSS) or milk. Table 1 provides a list of recommended storage media

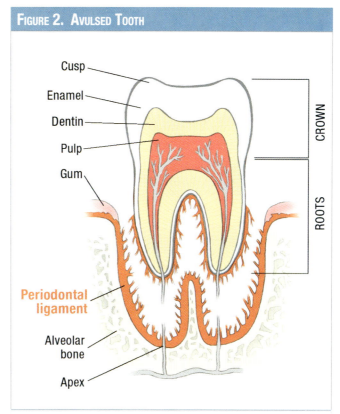

FIGURE 2. AVULSED TOOTH

Avulsion causes a rupture in the periodontal ligament (PDL). A portion of the PDL tissue remains on the walls of the alveolar socket, and a portion remains attached to the root surface of the avulsed tooth. Neurovascular supply to the tooth is compromised and may result in loss of tooth pulp vitality.

Illustration by Kurt Jones.

for avulsed teeth, and Table 2 provides information related to the characteristics of various types of storage media.

The limitations of the evidence are that some of the recommended storage media are not likely to be immediately available at the site of the avulsion injury or where treatment of the injury will occur. Some research studies were conducted in laboratory settings, and the results may not be generalizable to settings outside of the laboratory.

The benefit of immediate replantation or storage of avulsed teeth in a medium that will help to maintain PDL cell viability is that it increases the chances for successful replantation of an avulsed tooth. The harms associated with immediate replantation are that the tooth replantation may be performed incorrectly. Replantation of a tooth that is contaminated with debris may increase the patient's risk for infection. There are no harms associated with storing avulsed teeth in a medium that will maintain PDL cell viability.

In a nonexperimental study, Karayilmaz et al[24] reviewed patient records from a university dental health and treatment center during a nine-year period and found that 5.9% of all traumatic dental injuries treated (66 of 1,124) were avulsion injuries. Notably, 64.5% of avulsed teeth (60 of 93) were lost as a result of panic and a lack of knowledge of the individuals at

189

AUTOLOGOUS TISSUE MANAGEMENT

Table 1. Recommended Storage Media for Avulsed Teeth

Researchers/authors	CLS	CW	Egg white	Formula	Gatorade®	GTE	HBSS	Milk	Mulberry[a]	NaCl	ORS	Pedialyte®	Probiotic[b]	Propolis	Ricetral	Sage[c]	Saliva	Soymilk	ViaSpan®	Water
Ahangari et al (2013)[47]														+						
Al-Nazhan and Al-Nasser (2006)[30]	+																			
American Association of Endodontists (2013)[53]							+													
Andersson (2012)[25]							+	+		+							+			−
Andreasen et al (1995)[31]										+										+
Ballal and Jothi (2011)[54]	−					+							+							
Brullmann et al (2010)[11]							+			+							+			−
Caglar (2010)[26]							+	+		+			+							
Ceallaigh et al (2007)[29]								+									+			
Chamorro et al (2008)[48]	−				−															
Chen and Huang (2012)[9]						+														
de Sousa et al (2008)[39]			+					+									+			
de Souza et al (2010)[52]							+													−
Doshi (2009)[21]							+													
Eskandarian et al (2013)[34]												+								
Gjertsen et al (2011)[10]														+						
Gopikrishna et al (2008)[13]		+																		
Huang et al (1996)[46]							+	+												
Hwang et al (2011)[37]							+													
Jung et al (2011)[51]						+														
Karayilmaz et al (2013)[24]							+	+												
Khademi et al (2008)[12]				+			+													
Koca et al (2010)[56]																	+			
Krasner (2010)[15]																				
Lin et al (2007)[22]							+	+		+										
Macway-Gomez and Lallier (2013)[35]		+																		
Malhotra (2011)[27]							+	+		−			+				−		+	−
Moazami et al (2012)[19]					+		+											+		
Moradian et al (2013)[16]								+												
Moreira-Neto et al (2009)[38]								+												
Moura et al (2012)[36]																	+			
Mousavi et al (2010)[50]							+				+									−
Ozan et al (2007)[20]												+								
Ozan et al (2008)[41]								+												
Ozan et al (2008)[40]																+				
Rajendran et al (2011)[44]							+	−												
Royal College of Surgeons (2004)[43]								+		+										
Sanghavi et al (2013)[7]			+									+								
Saxena et al (2011)[28]								+				+								
Sigalas et al (2004)[14]	+				+		+	+												−
Silva et al (2013)[33]							+	+									+			
Sonoda et al (2008)[55]																	+			
Souza et al (2010)[32]								+												
Souza et al (2011)[18]								+						+						
Subramaniam et al (2011)[45]																				
Thomas et al (2008)[8]			+				+													
Udoye et al (2012)[17]								+												

Abbreviations: CLS = contact lens solution; CW = coconut water; GTE = green tea extract; HBSS = Hank's Balanced Salt Solution; NaCl = sodium chloride (saline) solution; ORS = oral rehydration solution.
[a] Morus rubra (Red Mulberry) [b] Lactobacillis reuteri [c] Salvia officinalis
+ Recommended   − Not recommended   ■ Most recommended storage media

Editor's note: Gatorade is a registered trademark of Stokely-Van Camp, Inc, Chicago, IL. Pedialyte is a registered trademark of Abbott Laboratories, Inc, Abbott Park, IL. ViaSpan is a registered trademark of Barr Laboratories, Inc, Champaign, IL.

the scene of the accident regarding the need to store the avulsed tooth in an effective storage medium for future replantation.

I.a. Avulsed teeth should be replanted at the time of avulsion. [2: Moderate Evidence]

The longer an avulsed tooth is outside of the mouth, the greater the potential for root resorption and reduced pulpal healing.[7,9,10,12-14,17,22,24,28,30,33,35-39,43-45,47,48]

The International Association for Dental Traumatology recommends

AUTOLOGOUS TISSUE MANAGEMENT

Table 2. Characteristics of Types of Storage Media for Avulsed Teeth

Storage medium	Characteristics
Contact lens solution	May be an effective storage medium.[46] The presence of preservatives in contact lens solution may be harmful to periodontal ligament (PDL) cell viability.[17,23,30]
Coconut water	May be effective as a storage medium due to the amino acids, proteins, vitamins and minerals present in coconut water.[7,8,13,23,26] It is an isotonic solution[8,9] that resembles intracellular fluid.[13] Coconut water supports PDL viability and helps to reduce bacterial growth.[35] Coconut water has a pH of 4.1 that may be detrimental for cell metabolism.[17,38]
Egg white	May be an effective storage medium due to osmolality of 251-298 mOsm/Kg that promotes cell growth.[12,23]
Formula	May be as effective as milk as a storage medium, does not require refrigeration, and has a long shelf life.[23]
Gatorade®	Low pH (2.91) may be harmful to PDL cell viability.[17,50] Gatorade is a hypotonic solution that may cause the PDL cells to lose water.[23]
Green tea extract	May be effective as a storage medium due to anti-inflammatory and antioxidant properties that help to preserve tissues and cells.[3,5,9,30] Adding green tea extract to the storage medium may allow for storage periods longer than 14 days.[5]
Hank's Balanced Salt Solution	Contains nutrients and salts that can sustain and reconstitute the cellular components of PDL cells.[4,22] Considered the gold standard of storage mediums.[26,27,32,40] May be effective for an extended time (ie, as long as 48 hours).[26]
Milk	Significantly better than other storage media. Its osmolality, pH, and physiologic properties are compatible with PDL cells.[21,22] Milk also provides nutritional substances, such as amino acids, carbohydrates, and vitamins.[14,22,23,26,27] Chilled milk is preferred over milk at room temperature.[26] The antigens in milk may interfere with the PDL cell reattachment process.[26] The time period during which PDL cell viability is maintained when stored in milk is controversial.[27] Skim milk is not as effective in preserving cell viability as whole milk.[36]
Mulberry (*Morus rubra*)	May be an effective storage medium due to its antioxidant properties.[41]
Sodium chloride (NaCl)	Osmolality of 280 mOsm/Kg is compatible with PDL cells; however, NaCl lacks essential nutrients (eg, glucose, calcium, magnesium) necessary to maintain the metabolic needs of PDL cells.[17,23,26] May only be effective for a brief period of time (ie, < 2-3 hours).[17,22,26]
Oral rehydration solution	May be an effective storage medium due to its ability to preserve cell viability and its potential regenerative effect.[34]
Pedialyte®	May be an effective storage medium due to its ability to support PDL cell survival and reduce bacterial growth.[35]
Probiotic (*Lactobacillis reuteri*)	May be as effective as milk, Hank's Balanced Salt Solution (HBBS), or saline as a storage media.[5,23]
Propolis	May be an effective storage medium. Propolis maintains PDL cell viability and is antimicrobial, anti-inflammatory, and antioxidant.[10,17,23,26,28,47,54] Propolis also decreases apoptosis of PDL fibroblasts.[10]
Ricetral	May be effective as a storage medium due to concentrations of glucose and vital salts that are adequate for cell metabolism.[30]
Sage (*Salvia officinalis*)	May be an effective storage medium due to its antimicrobial properties.[40]
Saliva	Effective for a short period of time (ie, < 60 minutes).[17] Low osmolality of 60-80 mOsm/Kg may increase the harmful effects of bacteria.[8,10,22,23,26,32,39] Saliva is a hypotonic solution that may lead to lysis of the PDL cells.[8,17,26,40]
Soymilk	May be an effective storage medium due to its ability to maintain cell viability at similar levels as milk and HBSS.[19,33,36]
Viaspan	May be an effective long-term storage medium due to pH of 7.4 that is ideal for cell growth.[8,23,26] Viaspan contains a hydrogen ion buffer that may help to maintain pH. Viaspan also contains adenosine which is necessary for cell division and may improve vitality of PDL cells by preventing cell swelling.[32] Requires refrigeration.[17]
Water	One of the least effective storage mediums. It is a hypotonic medium that may lead to rapid lysis of the PDL cells.[5,17,23,26,39,40,43,48] Water has a low osmolality and may contain chlorine.[40]

Editor's note: Gatorade is a registered trademark of Stokely-Van Camp, Inc, Chicago, IL. Pedialyte is a registered trademark of Abbott Laboratories, Inc, Abbott Park, IL. ViaSpan is a registered trademark of Barr Laboratories, Inc, Champaign, IL.

- picking up the tooth by the crown and not touching the root,[15,25,29]
- washing the tooth[29] under cold running water for no longer than 10 seconds,[11,25]
- replanting the tooth if possible and holding it in place,[11,25,29]
- placing the tooth in a glass of milk or other storage medium (eg, HBBS) if immediate replantation is not possible,[25,29] and
- seeking emergency treatment as soon as possible.[25]

AUTOLOGOUS TISSUE MANAGEMENT

The patient's teeth and mouth may be covered in debris that may require removal by gentle washing[29] with a physiologic solution.[15] Lin et al[49] recommended immediate fixation of the tooth by suturing as a method to initiate pulpal and periodontal healing and improve long-term prognosis and stabilization of the tooth.

I.a.1. Members of the health care team should record the events leading to the tooth avulsion in the patient's health record and conduct a thorough patient examination as soon as possible after the event occurs (eg, during intubation) or when the patient arrives at the facility. This
- an examination for head injury and facial fracture,[11,22,25,43]
- an examination for signs of external injury (eg, laceration),[22]
- an oral examination[22] that includes accounting for all of the patient's teeth to ensure they have not been inhaled,[29] and
- a review of the patient's tetanus vaccination history.[29]

[2: Moderate Evidence]

I.b. Avulsed teeth that cannot be immediately replanted should be placed in a storage medium. [2: Moderate Evidence]

The storage medium should
- maintain viability of the PDL cells,[7,33,38,41,46]
- facilitate repopulation of the denuded root surface and prevent root resorption,[7]
- provide physiological osmolality (230 mOsm/Kg to 400 mOsm/Kg)[8,38] and pH (7.0)[38] to allow optimal cell growth and survival,[7,10,21] and
- be available and readily accessible at the location of the avulsion injury.[7,33-36,38,46]

Successful replantation of avulsed teeth is directly related to PDL cell viability.[8,13-15,17,20,21,23,28,30,37,38,41,44,45,48,50,51] Prolonged drying of the tooth reduces the viability of the PDL cells[27,30,44] and leads to dehydration of the tooth pulp.[31,43] Patients with avulsed teeth may have suffered other serious injuries that require immediate treatment. In these cases, it may be necessary to store the avulsed tooth in a medium that will help prevent dehydration and maintain PDL viability until the tooth can be replanted.[7,8,11,13,24,25,33,34,46,49,52,51]

When immediate replantation of the avulsed tooth is not possible, the American Association of Endodontists recommends storing an avulsed tooth in HBBS, milk, normal saline solution, or saliva.[53] The Royal College of Surgeons recommends storing the tooth in cold milk, normal saline solution, or saliva.[43] The International Association for Dental Traumatology recommends placing the tooth in milk, HBSS, or another storage medium.[25]

I.b.1. Avulsed teeth that will not be immediately replanted should be stored in HBSS or milk. [2: Moderate Evidence]

Hank's Balanced Salt Solution is an effective medium for maintaining the viability of PDL cells at room temperature[17,27,46] and is considered the gold standard for storage of avulsed teeth.[12,14,18-20,22,24,32,35,40,41,47,49,54] It is often used as a comparison medium for determining the effectiveness of other storage media.[27,40]

Hank's Balanced Salt Solution is available commercially as an emergency tooth preserving system[20,40] that allows the avulsed tooth to be suspended in a basket that helps wash debris off the tooth while preventing damage to the PDL cells.[17,43] The system also allows the tooth to be removed from the basket without being touched by forceps or fingers.[23] The unopened product has a three-year shelf life,[17,27] but it cannot be stored at temperatures above 104° F (40° C).[11] The German Dental Association recommends that all kindergartens, schools, sports centers, dental practices, and medical institutions keep a supply of tooth rescue kits readily available for tooth avulsion injuries.[11]

Milk has been widely accepted as a suitable storage medium for avulsed teeth.[12,14,17,18,20,22,24,26,28-30,32,36,38,42,46,47,54] Milk has a physiological osmolality (230 mOsm/Kg to 270 mOsm/Kg), has a slightly acidic pH (6.5 to 6.8), and contains nutrients and growth factors that support the PDL cells.[22,28,42,47] Moradian et al[16] reported successful replantation of an avulsed maxillary central incisor after 12 hours of storage in milk. The tooth was stable and remained functional and aesthetically acceptable after three years. Storing the avulsed tooth in milk at a cool temperature (32° F to 39° F [0° C to 4° C])[27] may help reduce cell metabolism, limit bacterial growth, and prevent the milk from spoiling.[42]

In a nonexperimental study to assess the viability of PDL cells at room temperature and on ice, Sigalas et al[14] concluded that storage on ice was more beneficial than storage at room temperature. In a quasi-experimental study to investigate apoptosis in PDL cells, Chamorro et al[48] found that storage on ice inhibited cell death.

de Souza et al[42] conducted a quasi-experimental study to determine whether the renewal of milk used as a storage medium with fresh milk every 24 hours for up to 120 hours would improve viability of PDL fibroblasts. They found that, regardless of the temperature, renewal of the milk did not affect the viability of PDL fibroblasts.

In a quasi-experimental study, Moura et al[36] investigated the efficacy of soy milk in maintaining the viability of PDL fibroblasts compared with different cow milks. The researchers found that soy milk was an adequate storage medium for avulsed teeth, but skim milk was not as effective in preserving PDL cell viability.

I.b.2. Avulsed teeth that will not be immediately replanted may be temporarily stored in the patient's saliva if a more effective type of storage medium is not available. *[2: Moderate Evidence]*

The availability of saliva at the moment of avulsion allows for its use as a temporary storage medium until the tooth can be replanted or placed into a more effective medium. Sonoda et al[55] reported the case of a 30-year-old woman with an accidentally avulsed permanent incisor that was kept in her oral cavity from the moment of trauma until its replantation 90 minutes later. Three years later, clinical and radiographic findings showed no root absorption or mobility of the tooth.

Koca et al[56] reported the case of an eight-year-old boy whose avulsed left upper central incisor was kept in his oral cavity in direct contact with saliva for five hours, from the moment of trauma until its replantation. Two years later, clinical and radiographic findings showed no root resorption or mobility of the replanted tooth.

I.b.3. Avulsed teeth that will not be immediately replanted should not be stored in water, unless the only alternative is dry storage. *[2: Moderate Evidence]*

It is not advisable to store an avulsed tooth in water[8,11,17,19,25,27,32,37,39,43,50]; however, dry storage of a tooth is not recommended.[14,23,29,38,43,50] Ize-Iyamu and Saheeb[57] reported two cases of successful replantation of avulsed teeth that occurred after 72 hours of dry storage. In a nonexperimental study that examined pulpal healing of 400 avulsed and replanted teeth, Andreasen et al[31] found an increasing negative effect on pulp healing with increasing periods of dry storage. However, the researchers still recommended replanting teeth that had been kept dry for a long period of time. In a literature review conducted by Goswami et al,[23] the authors concluded that moist storage optimizes PDL cell survival, but no storage medium is ideal, and further research is warranted.

I.c. Education and competency verification activities related to best practices for the management of avulsed teeth should be provided for perioperative or other health care personnel who may be involved in caring for patients who have sustained traumatic tooth avulsion. *[2: Moderate Evidence]*

The collective evidence supports providing education to health care workers and others involved in the care of patients who have sustained traumatic tooth avulsion. The limitations of the evidence are that some studies may not be generalizable outside of the geographic area in which the study was conducted, and some research studies used surveys, so the responses may be subjective and not representative of the broader population.

The benefit of providing education to perioperative or other health care personnel involved in caring for patients who have sustained traumatic tooth avulsion is that it may increase the likelihood of successful replantation of avulsed teeth for patients treated within the facility or health care organization. The benefit will be even greater if parents, school teachers, athletic coaches, and the general public also receive education regarding the protocols for managing traumatic tooth avulsion injuries and if tooth rescue kits are available in schools, sporting facilities, and health care facilities.[21,24,25,27,49] There are no harms associated with providing education and competency verification activities for perioperative and other health care personnel involved in caring for patients who have sustained traumatic tooth avulsion.

In a nonexperimental study conducted to evaluate the knowledge of treatment of tooth avulsion injuries among 50 school nurses in Bialystok, Poland, Baginska and Wilczynska-Borawska[58] found that the nurses had knowledge about the need for an effective storage medium for the avulsed tooth and that they understood the critical need for keeping the time to treatment at a minimum to achieve successful replantation of an avulsed tooth. The researchers found a significant correlation between the level of the nurses' knowledge and the receipt of previous education related to dental trauma.

Ulusoy et al[59] surveyed 69 emergency physicians from one university and 10 public hospitals in Samsun, Turkey, to evaluate their knowledge related to treatment of traumatic tooth avulsion injuries and found that the majority of physicians could not provide correct answers to the survey questions. The researchers concluded there was a need for education of emergency physicians related to treatment of traumatic tooth avulsion injuries.

In a nonexperimental study conducted to investigate dentists' knowledge of procedures for managing traumatic dental injuries in children, Yeng and Parashos[60] surveyed 693 dentists in Victoria, Australia, and found that the respondents demonstrated only a moderate level of knowledge. The researchers concluded that professional education programs on the management of dental trauma in children were needed to improve practice.

Kargul and Welbury[61] conducted a retrospective observational study of the patient records of 75 children with 120 avulsed teeth treated in a dental hospital trauma clinic in Istanbul, Turkey. They found that only 42.5% of avulsed teeth (n = 51) were placed in an effective storage medium before replantation. The researchers determined public education was needed to improve successful tooth replantation in patients treated for avulsion injuries.

To assess the level of dental practitioners' knowledge of recommended guidelines for treatment of tooth avulsion injuries, de Vasconcellos et al[62] surveyed 264 dental practitioners from public and private dental schools in São José dos Campos, Brazil. The results of the study showed that the participants exhibited knowledge of the correct procedures for treatment of traumatic tooth avulsion. However, the results also showed a lack of communication regarding treatment guidelines for avulsion injuries by the dental practitioners to those at risk for avulsion injury (eg, individuals who participate in contact sports).

Zhao and Gong[63] conducted a study to evaluate the knowledge of dentists (N = 258) working in urban and suburban areas of Beijing, China, related to the management and treatment of dental emergencies. The results of the study showed that 87.2% of participants (n = 225) recommended immediate replantation of the avulsed tooth; however, only 15.9% of the participants (n = 41) were able to correctly identify the most effective storage media, and only 55.8% (n = 144) had received any education related to emergency management of avulsed teeth.

Loh et al[64] surveyed 167 dental therapists (formerly known as school dental nurses) in Singapore to gather information on their knowledge related to the management of traumatic dental injuries. The majority of respondents (54.5%; n = 91) were not aware of the most effective storage media for avulsed teeth, and a very high percentage (94.6%; n = 158) indicated there was a need for more education.

In a nonexperimental study, Hugar et al[65] assessed the knowledge of 300 nurses and prospective nurses from a university hospital in Belgaum, India, about emergency management of traumatic dental injuries. The researchers found that only 2.3% (n = 7) were aware of effective storage media for avulsed teeth, and 49.7% (n = 149) had received no education related to the management of traumatic dental injuries. The researchers emphasized the need for education for nurses, as they may be the first health care personnel to provide patient care.

In a survey of Massachusetts emergency department directors (n = 16) and physicians (n = 56), Needleman et al[66] investigated the physicians' knowledge of traumatic dental injury management. The researchers found that none of the emergency departments had a formal, written protocol in place for managing traumatic dental injuries. Most of the physicians who responded to the survey (45 of 56; 80.4%) had received education related to managing traumatic dental injuries during their residency; however, their knowledge of the correct treatment for dental fractures was poor, as indicated by correct responses of only 55.4% or lower to survey questions. The responding physicians scored higher on questions related to management of dislocated or avulsed teeth, with correct responses ranging between 61% and 89%. Physicians who specialized in pediatric emergency medicine were more likely to answer the questions correctly than were emergency medicine physicians. Physicians at hospitals with an academic affiliation scored significantly better than those at nonacademic-affiliated hospitals. The researchers concluded that educational campaigns were needed to improve physicians' knowledge of managing traumatic dental injuries and that education would enhance the long-term outcomes for patients who sustain dental trauma and who present to the emergency department for treatment.

Choi et al[67] conducted a survey of 100 randomly selected public and private school nurses in New York City. The researchers found that 87% of the nurses (n = 87) had not received education in managing traumatic dental injuries in children. Sixty-eight percent of the nurses either thought that the tooth should not be replanted (52%; n = 52), or did not know whether the tooth should be replanted (16%; n = 16). Although school nurses were often the first persons to provide emergency treatment for children with avulsed teeth, they had limited knowledge, resources, and experience to provide the correct treatment. The researchers concluded there was a need to provide educational programs for school nurses to improve the management of traumatic dental injuries in children.

Recommendation II

The patient's autologous cranial bone flap may be preserved and replanted.

The collective evidence indicates that decompressive craniectomy with removal of cranial bone and subsequent replantation with the patient's preserved bone flap or with artificial material is a widely used technique for the management of refractory intracranial hypertension after traumatic brain injury or extensive cerebral infarctions or brain tumors.[68-76] The evidence supports replanting the autologous cranial bone flap compared with using artificial materials for cranial reconstruction.[73,75-82] Autologous bone, such as rib and iliac crest, also may be used for cranial reconstruction; however, it is difficult to shape into the desired configuration, may not be large enough to fill the cranial defect, and may necessitate additional incisions.[81,82] Using autologous bone rather than artificial materials may increase the patient's risk for infection and bone resorption,[68,70,71,79,83] and there may be potential for infection related to the nonviability of the cranial bone flap.[70]

Artificial materials most suitable for use in reconstructive cranioplasty procedures are those that are resistant to infection, radiolucent, protective, thermally nonconductive, non-ionizing, and noncorrosive, and provide aesthetically pleasing results.[79] Artificial materials used for cranioplasty include methyl methacrylate, hydroxyapatite-based ceramics, titanium, and polypropylene polyester.[69,79] Methyl methacrylate is not suited to modeling large areas or reproducing the curved shape of the cranium,[79,84] and using it to reconstruct the cranium may increase the patient's risk for infection compared with using titanium.[83] Hydroxyapatite-based ceramics are expensive, may crack during drilling, and do not allow for the use of screws for fixation.[79] The organic nature and macroporosity of hydroxyapatite allows for osseointegration; however, this process takes several months and does not provide strong protection for the cranium during the early postoperative period.[75] Artificial materials used for cranioplasty may be rejected as foreign bodies even after they have remained in the patient for many years.[81]

The limitations of the evidence are that some research studies had small sample sizes and limited availability of cranial bone; some studies lacked controls; different methods (eg, storage time, storage temperature) may have achieved different results; and the results of the studies may not be generalizable to all settings where autologous cranial bone grafts are replanted.

The benefits of using the patient's autologous bone for cranial reconstruction compared with artificial materials include improved appearance[68,69,71,74,77,79,80,82,85]; increased potential for bone engrafting, remodeling, and growth[68,69,74,82]; reduced potential for immunoreaction or disease transmission[69,71,74,77,79,82]; improved heat conduction[69]; reduced cost[68,69,74,79]; and reduced operating time.[85] The harms associated with the use of autologous bone for reconstructive cranioplasty include the potential for infection from contaminated cranial bone grafts, and bone nonviability and resorption,[68,70,71,79,83] particularly in pediatric patients.[74]

II.a. Cranial bone flaps to be replanted may be frozen or cryopreserved. *[2: Moderate Evidence]*

The collective evidence indicates that freezing and cryopreservation are common methods of preserving excised cranial bone for replantation at a later date[70-72,79,86]; however, the optimal storage temperature has not been determined.[68,72,74] There are gaps in the literature related to best practices for managing frozen or cryopreserved autologous cranial bone flaps. To date, there are no consistent guidelines for preserving cranial bone flaps relative to temperature settings, length of storage, packaging method, or treatment of the excised flap with antibiotic or antiseptic solutions before storage or replantation.[68,74]

Likewise, the effect of freezing on the biological properties of skull bone and the process of autograft incorporation after replantation of frozen cranial bone warrant further research.[70,72] Understanding the viability of frozen bone cells may have significant ramifications for clinical practice in trauma, orthopedic, plastic and reconstructive, and neurosurgery.[70] Research to determine cell viability after storage of cranial bone flaps under various conditions may help provide insight into the most effective storage methods for improving graft revascularization and incorporation and reducing infection and bone resorption.[70,74]

However, maintaining cell viability in a bone autograft may not be necessary. For replantation success, provision of a suitable bone matrix for partial repopulation by autologous cells may suffice for osteoconduction, osteoinduction, and osseointegration[87] because similar success has been experienced with transplants involving nonviable bone allografts.[88-93] The evidence review did not reveal any evidence that addressed the effect of apoptotic autologous cells on undesirable replantation outcomes, such as resorption. Steps taken to maintain viable cells may also increase the risk that microorganisms will survive if the autograft becomes contaminated because of patient trauma or steps taken in handling or packaging the autologous cranial bone for storage.

The limitations of the evidence are that some research studies had a small sample size, and the results of the studies may not be generalizable to all settings where frozen or cryopreserved autologous cranial bone grafts are used.

The benefits of frozen or cryopreserved storage of autologous cranial bone flaps are that it may preserve the autograft for replantation at a later date and does not require additional surgical time or incisions. The harms associated with frozen or cryopreserved storage of autologous cranial bone flaps are that the autograft may be contaminated during storage or during the recovery or replantation procedure. The process of cryopreservation and long-term storage may lead to mechanical instability (eg, crack formation) of the bone or surface abrasiveness that facilitates bacterial adhesion and colonization.[72] Long-term storage of autologous tissue carries with it the potential for mix-ups if autograft labeling methods are inadequate (eg, smudging of identifiers during cold storage, labels separating from the package), and contamination or cross-contamination if the graft's packaging material is not validated for use at the storage temperature selected.

During a seven-month period, Bhaskar et al[74] surveyed 25 neurosurgical centers in public and teaching hospitals in Australia to obtain information related to cranial bone flap preparation after craniectomy, temperature and duration of frozen storage of cranial bone flaps, infection prevention protocols, methods for detecting contamination in the flaps, and procedures for cranial replantation. The results of the study were the following:

- Neurosurgeons preferred using frozen autologous cranial bone flaps over synthetic materials (96%; n = 24).
- Cranial bone flaps were prepared for storage by double- or triple-bagging under dry, sterile conditions (88%; n = 22).
- Cranial bone flaps were irrigated with normal saline solution containing antibiotics or povidone-iodine before cryopreservation (16%; n = 4).
- Biopsies or cultures were obtained from the cranial bone flaps before cryopreservation to determine contamination levels (68%; n = 17).
- Cranial bone flaps were cryopreserved at temperatures of -0.4° F to -117.4° F (-18° C to -83° C) for varying time intervals (eg, six months, until the patient died).
- Cranial bone flaps were stored in facility freezers (52%; n = 13) or in commercial bone banks (48%; n = 12).
- Some facilities used specific thawing procedures involving immersion of the frozen cranial flap in lactated Ringer's solution, povidone-iodine, or both (24%; n = 6).
- Biopsies or cultures were obtained from the cranial bone flaps before replantation to determine contamination levels (12%; n = 3).
- Maximum duration of storage before designation as biohazardous waste and disposal varied between five years (56%; n = 14), two years (8%; n = 2), nine months (4%; n = 1), six months (16%; n = 4), until the patient was deceased (4%; n = 1), and no time limit (12%; n = 3).

The researchers concluded that practices for cryopreservation and storage of autologous cranial bone flaps were highly variable in neurosurgical centers throughout Australia. They also concluded that there was a need for further research to determine the biological and biomechanical effects of frozen storage conditions on cranial bone and to verify best practices for cranial bone flap management.

In a quasi-experimental study to assess whether viable bone cells could be cultured from cranial bone flaps that had been cryopreserved without cryoprotectants for more than six months, Bhaskar et al[70] examined bone cultures from 27 cranial bone flaps harvested from patients who had undergone decompressive craniectomies for intractable intracranial hypertension at a university medical center. The flaps had been stored at -22° F (-30° C) for 7.6 to 41.8 months. The researchers found that the control samples showed abundant growth of osteoblasts, whereas samples taken from the cryopreserved cranial bone flaps showed no osteoblasts. The researchers concluded that cranial bone flaps cryopreserved without cryoprotectants for longer than six months were not viable.

In a nonexperimental study to evaluate the surface structure of cryopreserved cranial bone flaps, Beez et al[72] used scanning electron microscopy to examine cranial bone flaps removed from five patients during decompressive craniectomy and then stored for six to eight months at -112° F (-80° C) in a university neurosurgical center freezer. During morphological analysis of the bone flaps, the researchers found that two of the flaps had smooth bone surfaces, two had mixed surfaces (ie, smooth and abrasive), and one had an abrasive surface. The researchers found no correlation with any patient variables, such as age, or with the length of the cryopreservation; they determined that the differences in bone surface were reflective of differences in individual human anatomy. The researchers concluded that cryopreservation for as long as eight months did not alter the physiological surface of the skull bone, and they theorized that cryopreservation for longer periods would not harm the surface structure of the bone.

Elwatidy et al[73] conducted a nonexperimental study to evaluate the microbiological and histological characteristics of 14 cranial bone flaps preserved at -0.4° F (-18° C) for two months to five years at a university hospital. The bone flaps were prepared for storage by removal of soft tissue and bone spicules and washing with 1 L normal saline solution containing 80 mg gentamicin followed by 1 L normal saline solution containing 1 g vancomycin. The bone flaps were then dried, wrapped in sterile towels, and placed into two layers of sterile plastic bags. The packages were labeled with the patient's name, identification number, and the date of removal and were stored in the freezer.

On the day of the cranioplasty procedure, the researchers removed the cranial bone flap from its package and obtained swab cultures and histology specimens from the flap. They washed the bone in 1 L normal saline solution containing 80 mg gentamicin followed by 1 L normal saline solution containing 1 g vancomycin and then replanted it. The results of microbiology and histology examination showed no bacterial contamination in any of the cranial bone flaps. All of the flaps were viable except one. The viability of the bone was proportional to the duration of preservation in the freezer. The specimen that showed no viability had been stored in the freezer for five years.[73]

One patient developed a superficial wound infection that resolved after treatment with antibiotics. A second patient experienced partial bone resorption that resolved with spontaneous bone growth a few months later. The researchers concluded that preservation of cranial bone flaps by storage in a freezer at -0.4° F (-18° C) maintained sterility and viability for as long as 12 months. Notably, the swab culture method used by the researchers could not determine graft sterility. The results obtained when using such a method can only be deemed "swab culture negative."

Prolo et al[76] conducted a nonexperimental study in a university medical center to examine and analyze the repair of membranous skull after cranioplasty with frozen preservation of autologous cranial bone flaps. The researchers examined three groups of cranial bone flaps.

For Group 1, fresh cranial bone flaps were obtained from five patients who required a second craniectomy of the same area of the skull where the original craniectomy procedure had been performed 1.25 to 19 years earlier. The researchers examined the flaps visually and microscopically and found that in all patients, the replanted cranial bone flap was grossly thinner than the adjacent skull. They also found variable numbers of osteocytes in the bone flaps. The researchers concluded that segmental portions of skull removed and then replaced during cranioplasty regained viability.

For Group 2, the researchers visually and microscopically examined fragments from 12 excised cranial bone flaps that had been soaked for one to three hours in a bacitracin solution (500 units/mL), frozen in the solution at -4° F (-20° C), and then stored frozen for three to 35 months. They found no bacterial or fungal growth in any of the samples and found variable numbers of osteocytes in the bone flaps. There was no correlation between the length of time the bone flap had been stored and the number of osteocytes present. The researchers concluded that cranial bone removed aseptically during craniectomy and frozen in bacitracin solution for as long as three years was culture negative and not visually or microscopically altered in morphology.

For Group 3, 53 patients who underwent decompressive craniectomy and subsequent cranioplasty with autologous cranial bone flaps soaked in bacitracin (500 units/mL) and stored frozen at either -4° F (-20° C; n = 28) or -94° F (-70° C; n = 25) for a period of three weeks to 19 months were followed postoperatively for one to nine years. The researchers found there was some resorption of the bone in all patients, causing the graft to diminish in size over a period of years. In two children, ages seven months and two years, the amount of bone resorption was considerable; however, in all cases, the graft was functional and retained a cosmetically acceptable appearance. Two grafts were removed because of infection, and two patients died from causes unrelated to the autologous cranioplasty. The researchers concluded that the skull bone was intensely active after replantation and was the ideal material for cranioplasty. The researchers also concluded that freezing cranial bone flaps after decompressive craniectomy was an effective method of preservation for patients from the latter part of the first decade of life through adulthood.

Iwama et al[79] conducted a retrospective study in a university medical center to evaluate the use of frozen autologous cranial bone flaps for delayed cranioplasty in 49 patients during a 12-year period. The cranial bone flaps removed during the initial craniectomy procedure were wiped to remove all blood, sealed in three sterile vinyl bags, and stored at -31° F (-35° C) (n = 37) or -119.2° F (-84° C) (n = 12) for four to 168 days.

On the day of the cranioplasty procedure, the cranial bone flap was removed from the package, thawed at room temperature, and washed in 500 mL normal saline solution supplemented with 60 mg tobramycin. Forty-seven patients (96%) experienced no complications. The clinical and aesthetic results were satisfactory. Bone resorption was observed in one 12-year-old boy, and a 14-year-old boy developed an infection. Both patients underwent a second cranioplasty procedure with ceramic plates. The researchers concluded that delayed cranioplasty using frozen autologous cranial bone flaps achieved satisfactory clinical and aesthetic results.

Grossman et al[71] prospectively reviewed and reported the results of 12 cases of decompressive craniectomy followed by reconstructive cranioplasty performed during a nine-year period at a university medical center. A protocol was developed to prepare the excised cranial bone flaps for replantation. The autologous bone flaps were excised and transferred to the tissue bank within six hours. They were gently rinsed with 1 L to 3 L normal saline solution supplemented with neomycin (926 mg/L), wrapped in two layers of sterile plastic, and preserved at -112° F (-80° C) for 0.25 to 27 months.

On the day of the reconstructive procedure, the cranial bone flap was removed from the freezer and transferred to the OR in an icebox. The flap was allowed to thaw and was then removed from the package and washed with normal saline solution. All of the cranial bone flaps were replanted. The researchers found no bone flap resorption or infection, and the aesthetic results were satisfactory. The researchers concluded that freezing at -112° F (-80° C) was an effective method of preserving autologous cranial bone flaps.

Tahir et al[68] conducted a retrospective review of infection rates in 88 patients who had undergone autologous cranioplasty procedures at a busy neurotrauma center in a university hospital during a 10-year period. The patients' excised cranial bone flaps were wrapped in two layers of sterile, waterproof paper and placed in a close-fitting, sterile, air-tight plastic bag. This package was placed into a second, larger, sterile, air-tight plastic bag. All packages were labeled with the patient's identification and placed into an OR freezer maintained at a constant temperature of -14.8° F (-26° C) for a mean of 78.05 ± 66.7 days.

To minimize exposure time during the replantation procedure, the frozen cranial bone flaps were not removed from the packaging until after the subgaleal pocket was created. The bone flaps were cleaned of bone dust, attached soft tissue, and loose fragments and then immersed in povidone-iodine solution for 10 minutes, followed by irrigation with a solution of equal parts hydrogen peroxide (H_2O_2) and normal saline. The flaps were rinsed with an antibiotic solution immediately before replantation.

Three patients (3.4%) developed infections after the cranioplasty procedure. Two patients developed superficial wound infections, and one patient developed a deep wound infection involving the subgaleal space. The two patients with superficial infections were treated with antibiotics. The patient with the deep wound infection required wound exploration and irrigation and treatment with oral antibiotics. All the postoperative infections resolved completely. The researchers did not provide the formulation for "antibiotic solution" or the strength of the povidone-iodine and H_2O_2 solutions. The researchers concluded that frozen storage of autologous cranial bone flaps at a temperature of -14.8° F (-26° C) was safe, and the risk for infection was low.

To investigate whether cranial bone flaps preserved by freezing could survive and regenerate after autologous replantation, Lu et al[69] followed 16 patients undergoing cranioplasty procedures with replantation of autologous cranial bone flaps in a university hospital during a 16-month period. The bone flaps had been excised and sealed in a double-layer sterile plastic bag under sterile conditions, labeled with the patient's identification, and subsequently frozen at -112° F (-80° C) for 63 to 289 days.

On the day of the reconstructive procedure, the frozen autologous bone graft was thawed for 60 minutes, immersed in 3% povidone-iodine solution for 30 minutes, and then rinsed twice with normal saline solution before replantation. After surgery, the researchers used cranial bone tomography to examine the replanted bone at two-week, three-month, and 12-month periods. The researchers found that the frozen cranial bone was able to survive and regenerate new blood vessels and osteoblasts. They concluded that frozen autologous cranial bone could survive and regenerate after autologous replantation.

II.a.1. Facilities recovering, packaging, labeling, and freezing or cryopreserving autologous cranial bone for storage and replantation within the same facility are not required to register with the FDA as a tissue establishment. *[1: Regulatory Requirement]*

The facility would meet the exception from registration described in section 1271.15(b), in which storage of tissue for autologous use is exempt as long as no other manufacturing controls are performed (ie, subjecting the autograft to the steam sterilization process, distributing the autograft to another facility).[3,4]

II.b. The cranial bone flap to be replanted may be stored in a subcutaneous pocket within the patient in an anatomical location determined by the physician. *[2: Moderate Evidence]*

The collective evidence indicates there are two primary methods for preserving autologous cranial bone flaps: preserving the flap in the patient's body and storing the flap outside of the body.[53,71,86,94] The most commonly used preservation methods are frozen storage or storage in a subcutaneous pocket, most often in the lower abdominal wall, anterolateral thigh, or scalp.

The limitations of the evidence are that some research studies had small sample sizes, and the results of the studies may not be generalizable to all settings where cranial bone grafts are replanted.

The benefits of subcutaneous storage of autologous cranial bone flaps are that it may offer a sterile,[95] physiological storage environment that reduces graft devitalization,[75,78,80] and the autograft cannot be lost when stored within the patient.[95] The benefits of subgaleal storage are that it avoids an abdominal scar and may be less time consuming to perform than subcutaneous abdominal storage.[96]

The harms associated with subcutaneous storage of autologous cranial bone flaps are that the procedure requires additional surgical time and may require an additional surgical incision, and the graft may be contaminated during recovery, during storage, or during the replantation procedure. Patients may experience discomfort from the stored autograft, and osteoclast activity may cause the autograft to diminish in size during subcutaneous storage.[75,78,97]

Zingale and Albanese[86] conducted a meta-analysis of the literature to investigate the best methods for preserving autologous cranial bone flaps for delayed replantation. Statistical analysis showed no significant difference between frozen storage and subcutaneous storage relative to the frequency of postoperative complications (ie, bone resorption, infection). However, the researchers opined that frozen storage was superior to subcutaneous storage because it requires no additional surgical time, and the frozen bone flap may be stronger than the fresh flap. The researchers concluded there was a need for more research in this area.

In a retrospective study to investigate whether differences in the storage method of cranial bone flaps affected the incidence of postoperative surgical site infection (SSI), Inamasu et al[98] compared the incidence of SSI in 70 patients undergoing decompressive craniectomy and subsequent cranioplasty with autologous cranial bone during a nine-year period in a tertiary trauma referral center. Bone flaps for 39 patients were stored subcutaneously in the patient's abdominal wall. Bone flaps for the remaining 31 patients were immersed in 10% povidone-iodine solution immediately after recovery, wrapped in sterile gauze, and stored in the facility freezer at -94° F (-70° C). The frozen bone flaps were thawed at room temperature immediately before cranioplasty. Two patients from the subcutaneous storage group (5.1%), and five patients from the frozen storage group (16.1%) developed an SSI. The difference was not statistically significant. The researchers concluded that subcutaneous storage and frozen storage of cranial bone flaps were equally efficacious storage methods, but subcutaneous storage may be the better method.

Sultan et al[99] conducted a prospective study to compare frozen and subcutaneous storage of cranial bone grafts in rats. The cranial bone grafts (N = 30) were stored in a surgically created subcutaneous pocket in the animals' abdominal walls (n = 15) or wrapped in sterile saline-soaked gauze, placed in a 50 cm3 conical tube, and frozen at -112° F (-80° C) (n = 15). After 10 days of storage, the grafts were either replanted (subcutaneous, n = 3; frozen, n = 3), or analyzed (subcutaneous, n = 12; frozen, n = 12). The researchers found no microbial growth after culturing the frozen bone grafts and found normal skin flora after culturing the subcutaneous grafts. After 12 weeks, the researchers found there was limited bony union and considerable bone resorption in all the replanted grafts. The researchers concluded that neither storage method maintained bone graft viability, but subcutaneous storage might provide a small advantage compared with frozen storage.

In a retrospective study, Shoakazemi et al[77] reviewed the medical records of 100 consecutive patients who underwent decompressive craniectomy, storage of the excised cranial bone flap in a subcutaneous pocket in the abdominal wall, and subsequent replantation at a regional hospital neuroscience unit between 2000 and 2005. The researchers analyzed patient outcomes one year after the replantation procedure. They found eight patients had died before replantation of the stored cranial bone flap, and data were missing for three patients. Of the 89 patients who had their cranial bone flaps replanted, the bone flaps were removed for seven patients (7.8%) because of infection (n = 5; 5.6%) or for cosmetic reasons associated with bone flap resorption (n = 2; 2.2%) and were successfully replanted in 82 patients (92%). The researchers concluded that storage of the excised cranial bone flap in a subcutaneous pouch in the patient's abdominal wall produced a favorable long-term outcome.

Movassaghi et al[78] conducted a retrospective study of 53 of 65 consecutive patients who underwent emergency decompressive craniectomy with autologous cranial bone placement in the abdominal wall for 15 to 388 days. The study was conducted in a medical school general hospital during a six-year period. Clinical outcome after autograft replantation was determined by the ability of the stored cranial bone to achieve a satisfactory cosmetic result, the incidence of infection, and the need for additional surgery.

The researchers found that 49 of the 53 patients (92%) achieved a satisfactory reconstruction. In eight patients (15%), it was necessary to supplement the graft with alloplastic material to achieve the desired contour. One patient (2%) required a secondary procedure to improve the cranial contour. Three patients (6%) developed infections, including one patient whose graft was found to be infected when retrieved from the abdominal pocket.[78]

The researchers also histologically evaluated the bone viability of two autografts after subcutaneous storage and assessed the extent of autograft revascularization using bone scans one year after graft replantation in two patients. They found a mixture of necrotic and newly formed bone during the histological examinations. The bone scans showed that the osteoblast activity of the replanted cranial graft was almost identical to that of the adjacent bone. The researchers concluded that subcutaneous storage preserved the viability of the excised cranial bone graft and that cranioplasty performed with subcutaneously preserved cranial bone graft had low infection and revision rates.[78]

Baldo and Tacconi[75] conducted a prospective pilot study during a one-year period in a university hospital in Trieste, Italy, to assess the effectiveness and safety of reconstructing a cranial bone defect using an autologous cranial bone flap stored subcutaneously in the patient's abdominal wall. The researchers evaluated the infection rate and the need for revision in 12 of 15 consecutive patients who had undergone decompressive craniectomy and subsequent cranioplasty with autologous cranial bone flap stored in the patient's abdominal wall for 15 to 180 days.

To assess the viability of the bone, a bone biopsy was taken at the time the cranial flap was placed into the subcutaneous abdominal pocket and also when the cranial flap was removed for replantation. Cultures were taken from the subcutaneous site where the cranial bone had been stored and also from the site of replantation. A computed tomography (CT) scan was performed a few days after replantation and at six months after surgery to quantify the degree of bone gapping. Technetium bone scans were performed in four patients one year after replantation to assess the extent of graft revascularization. Hospital nurses subjectively assessed cosmetic appearance as good, satisfactory, or poor on postoperative day one, three, five, and seven and at three, six, nine, and 12 months.[75]

Among the 15 consecutive patients, two died and one patient was diagnosed with a malignant brain tumor that prevented replantation of the autologous cranial bone flap. Among the remaining 12 patients, two died from complications not related to the procedure, and one patient was not available for follow up. None of the patients developed an infection, and in all cases, the nurses had rated the patient's overall cosmetic appearance as good. All of the bone samples had a normal histological appearance.[75]

The CT scans showed no significant bone resorption. The technetium bone scans showed an insignificant reduction in perfusion. The researchers concluded that subcutaneous storage of an autologous cranial bone flap was a feasible option that preserved the viability of the autograft, provided good cosmetic results, and resulted in low infection rates.[75]

In 75 cases of cranioplasty with subcutaneously preserved cranial autografts in Kosova during an eight-year period, Morina et al[80] placed the excised cranial bone graft in the patient's left abdomen with the convex part of the autograft on the upper side to prevent interference with potential future appendectomy or cholecystectomy procedures and to prevent skin injury from the bone edges. The duration of subcutaneous abdominal storage ranged from 14 to 232 days. The authors reported that 66 patients (88%) achieved a satisfactory cosmetic result, whereas nine patients (12%) required augmentation of the replanted cranial bone flap with methyl methacrylate to achieve a satisfactory result.

Two patients (2.7%) developed postoperative infections requiring removal of the graft and subsequent replacement with methyl methacrylate after six months. Two patients (2.7%) complained of abdominal pressure. The authors concluded that storage of autologous cranial bone flaps in a subcutaneous pocket of the patient's abdominal wall was a safe and effective method for preserving the cranial bone graft and achieved satisfactory cosmetic results.[80]

Flannery and McConnell[95] described their experience with 20 patients who underwent decompressive craniectomy with subcutaneous placement of the autologous cranial bone graft during an 11-month period at a busy regional trauma center. The autografts were stored subcutaneously in the patient's abdominal wall for a period of six weeks to three months. The authors noted that for patients in whom the autograft was stored for a longer period of time, there was some difficulty in removal as a result of the granulation tissue that had formed around the graft.

The authors reported that all of the cranial bone flaps appeared visually normal after removal from the abdomen. All of the cranioplasty and abdominal wounds healed without any procedure-related complications or evidence of bone resorption, with the exception of one patient who developed a wound infection and one patient who required removal of a loose screw. The authors suggested that preservation of the excised cranial bone flap in a subcutaneous pocket of the patient's abdominal wall provided superior cosmetic results and might represent the best option for the patient.[95]

Krishnan et al[96] described their experience using a technique for preserving excised cranial bone flaps in a subgaleal pocket created over the noninvolved side of the cranium. The authors prospectively analyzed 74 consecutive cases of decompressive craniectomy procedures performed at a national neurosciences center during a two-year period. The cranial bone flap was preserved in a subgaleal pocket in 55 patients (74%), was preserved in a subcutaneous abdominal pocket in nine patients (12%), and was not preserved in 10 patients (14%).

To decrease the potential for abrasion of the overlying skin, the sharp edges of the excised cranial bone were removed before the autograft was placed in the abdominal or subgaleal space. The cranial bone flaps were stored from six weeks to eight months before replantation. After removal from the abdominal or subgaleal pocket, the authors examined the flaps and did not find any macroscopic evidence of bone resorption.[96]

The authors encountered complications in two cases. One patient developed a skin breakdown caused by a sharp bone spicule on the graft, and one patient developed a skin necrosis caused by the storage pocket being too small. The authors suggested that subgaleal preservation of the patient's cranial bone flap provided better physiological and cosmetic results than other methods of storage.[96]

Pasaoglu et al[81] described their experience managing 27 patients undergoing decompressive craniectomy with subgaleal preservation of the autologous cranial bone flap at a university school of medicine during a 30-month period. The cranial bone flaps were stored in a subgaleal pocket for a period of 14 to 98 days before replantation. The macroscopic appearance of the autografts removed from the subgaleal space in preparation for replantation was normal. The authors encountered no bone resorption, infection, or complaints of discomfort during the 26-month follow-up period and found that cosmetic results were excellent.

In a literature review of 18 articles related to subcutaneous storage of excised cranial bone flaps under the scalp (ie, subgaleal) and in the abdominal wall, Joaquim et al[94] concluded that it was not possible to state with certainty that one method was superior to another. They concluded that further research was warranted, and the method of storage should be determined based on factors specific to the patient and situation.

II.c. Autologous bone should not be subjected to the steam sterilization process unless there is a clinical indication to do so. *[2: Moderate Evidence]*

The collective evidence suggests that subjecting excised cranial bone flaps to the steam sterilization process may denature bone protein and severely damage the bone structure and increase the potential for bone resorption and infection[84]; however, steam sterilization may also destroy and prevent recurrence of tumor cells.[82,85] There are gaps in the literature related to best practices for management of autologous cranial bone flaps removed for treatment of brain tumors and subjected to steam or other sterilization processes. Further research is warranted.

The limitations of the evidence are that some research studies had small sample sizes, and the results of the studies may not be generalizable to all settings in which autologous cranial bone grafts are used.

The benefits of subjecting autologous cranial bone flaps to the steam sterilization process are that it may destroy tumor cells and may allow for reuse of the patient's autologous cranial bone for cranioplasty after tumor removal.[82,85] The harms associated with subjecting autologous cranial bone flaps to the steam sterilization process are that it denatures bone protein and may severely damage the bone structure and increase the potential for bone resorption and infection.[84] The steam sterilization process has not been validated for use with human tissue for transplantation. A significantly high rate of postoperative graft infection was found when cranial bone grafts subjected to the steam sterilization process were used for cranial reconstruction.[83]

Osawa et al[100] described their experience with 27 cases of cranioplasty performed with autologous cranial bone flaps that had been frozen and then subjected to a steam sterilization process before replantation. The excised cranial bone flaps were wrapped in sponges that had been soaked in a solution supplemented with either gentamicin 10 mg or amikacin 200 mg. The researchers did not specify the amount of irrigation solution or how many bone flaps were soaked in each antibiotic. The bone flaps were then sealed in a sterile plastic bag, and stored at -112° F (-80° C) in a facility freezer for 19 to 79 days. The day before the replantation procedure, the bone flaps were thawed and subjected to a steam sterilization process at 270° F (132° C) for 20 minutes. The researchers did not provide information as to the type of cycle that was used (ie, gravity or prevacuum) or whether any dry time was applied.

The authors took samples of the cranial bone flaps and performed histological examination when the cranial bone flap was removed from the patient, after storage at -112° F (-80° C) for seven days, and after the steam sterilization process. The patients were followed for a period of four months to two years. During this time, the authors performed skull radiographs to evaluate the amount of bone resorption. There were no serious complications except in two patients who developed small areas of bone resorption and in one patient who developed an epidural abscess that required removal of the autologous cranial bone flap. The histological examination showed only minimal effects on bone structure from the freezing and steam sterilization process. The authors suggested that subjecting the cranial bone flap to the steam sterilization process did not increase the risk of postoperative complications, such as bone resorption or infection.[100]

In a nonexperimental study to investigate the effects of the steam sterilization process on bone morphology, Vanaclocha et al[82] examined the excised cranial bone flaps of 62 patients undergoing craniectomy procedures for treatment of 64 tumors (meningiomas, n = 35; bone tumors, n = 16; scalp tumors, n = 8; metastasis, n = 5) in a university medical center during a six-year period. The researchers contended that bone flaps infiltrated by tumor cells could not be replanted because of the propensity of the tumor cells to invade and destroy the bone; however, they theorized that although the steam sterilization process destroys living cells and damages bone structure, the remaining bone scaffolding might allow for repopulation of the bone and the creation of new bone through the remodeling process.

The researchers cleaned the excised cranial bone flaps, and subjected them to the steam sterilization process at 273° F (134° C) for 20

201

minutes. The bone flaps were soaked for 15 minutes in normal saline solution supplemented with rifampicine, rinsed with sterile normal saline solution, and then replanted into the patient. The researchers did not provide information as to the type of cycle that was used (ie, gravity or prevacuum) or whether any dry time was applied, nor did they specify the amount of rifampicine or the amount of normal saline used for the soaking solution.[82]

The researchers followed the patients for 10 to 58 months; in addition to conducting the postoperative clinical examinations, they took radiographs and photographs at each follow-up visit. The thickness of the bone flap was assessed by CT scan as needed. In six patients, bone biopsies of the replanted flaps were taken during a second surgical procedure.[82]

The cosmetic appearance was satisfactory in all patients, there were no postoperative infections, and none of the cranial bone flaps had to be removed because of infection. The histological examination showed complete cellular destruction and preservation of the mineral matrix with severe damage to the protein structure of the bone flap. The radiographs and CT scans showed slow but progressive revitalization of the cranial bone grafts. The researchers observed partial bone resorption in 12 patients (19.4%) and some loss of bone volume manifested as bone thinning in 35 patients (56.5%). A second surgery was required for six patients (9.7%) because of a recurrence of the original tumor. The researchers concluded that

- the steam sterilization process destroyed tumor cells in excised cranial bone flaps and helped to prevent tumor recurrence;
- the steam sterilization process severely damaged the bone structure of cranial bone flaps, but the replanted bone flap was progressively revitalized by the adjacent bone; and
- bone resorption was a common occurrence in cranial bone flaps subjected to the steam sterilization process, but it did not lead to bad cosmetic results.[82]

Wester[85] reported the results of 25 cranioplasty procedures. In six patients, the excised cranial bone graft was macroscopically infiltrated with tumor tissue (meningiomas, n = 5; prostate cancer metastasis, n = 1). The cranial bone flaps were removed, cleaned of all osseous material, subjected to the steam sterilization process at 273° F (134° C) for 20 minutes, and replanted. In nine patients, the excised cranial bone grafts were removed, cleaned of all osseous material, subjected to the steam sterilization process at 273° F (134° C) for 20 minutes, preserved in a freezer for three to six months, subjected to the steam sterilization process at 273° F (134° C) for 20 minutes, washed with normal saline solution supplemented with penicillin, and replanted. The researchers did not specify the temperature of the freezer, the amount of penicillin, or the amount of normal saline solution, nor did they provide information as to the type of cycle that was used for the steam sterilization process (ie, gravity or prevacuum) or whether any dry time was applied.

In 10 patients, the excised cranial bone graft was unavailable for storage and replantation, and a reinforced acrylic prosthesis was used for the cranioplasty. All patients were followed for three months to eight years. The researchers found no tumor recurrence in any of the six patients with tumor-infiltrated cranial bone flaps subjected to the steam sterilization process and replanted. One patient required a second surgery for a recurrence of the intracranial malignant tumor. During the procedure, the researchers found that the bone flap was viable and there was no sign of tumor infiltration. The patient lived for another two years and then died from the intracranial malignant tumor. At the time of the patient's death, there was still no sign of tumor infiltration of the cranial bone flap.[85]

There were no postoperative complications in any of the nine patients replanted with autologous cranial bone grafts. Radiographs and CT scans showed revitalization of all bone flaps without bone resorption. The researchers concluded that cranial bone flaps could be revitalized and safely replanted after being subjected to the steam sterilization process, and that the steam sterilization process effectively killed tumor cells in the bone. The researchers also concluded that there was no difference in infection rates between patients who received autologous cranial bone versus those who received cranial grafts made of artificial material; however, the patient's autologous bone provided a satisfactory cosmetic result with a shorter operative time, and for this reason, the researchers recommended replanting autologous bone whenever possible.[85]

Schultke et al[84] conducted a quasi-experimental study to evaluate different methods for disinfecting cranial bone grafts. In the first part of the experiment, the researchers excised 20 palm-sized cranial flaps immediately after craniectomy. The grafts were cleaned of all adherent tissue, washed in 3% H2O2 solution, placed into a sterile double-layer package, placed in a sterile plastic bag, and stored at -5.8° F (-21° C). After storage for various periods of time, the bone flaps were removed, thawed, and boiled in normal saline solution for 30 minutes. The researchers did not provide details regarding the length of time the grafts were stored or the thawing or boiling process that was used. The researchers examined the boiled bone flaps and found a bacterial contamination rate of 20%.

In the second part of the experiment, the researchers compared three methods for disinfecting autologous cranial bone grafts to be replanted. After disinfection as described in the first part of the experiment, eight bone flaps from patients who did not survive their stroke or brain injury were divided into 84 sterile bone pieces. The bone pieces were artificially contaminated with virulent strains of *Serratia marcescens*, *Enterococcus faecium*, or *Staphylococcus aureus*. The pieces from each contamination group were divided, frozen at -5.8° F (-21° C), thawed, and disinfected by boiling in normal saline solution for 15 minutes, boiling in normal saline solution for 30 minutes, immersing in 3% H_2O_2 solution for 60 minutes, or heating at 167° F (75° C) for 20 minutes in a prevacuum steam sterilizer. The researchers did not provide information regarding the length of time the grafts were stored, the thawing or boiling process that was used, or whether any dry time was applied during the sterilization process.[84]

The researchers examined the bone pieces from each group for bacterial contamination and found no bacterial strains in the group treated in the prevacuum steam sterilizer. The researchers concluded that steam disinfection at 167° F (75° C) for 20 minutes in a prevacuum steam sterilizer was an effective method for disinfecting autologous cranial bone grafts before replantation.[84]

To evaluate the effectiveness of using ethylene oxide (ETO) and room temperature storage of excised autologous cranial bone flaps, Jho et al[97] conducted a retrospective review of 103 consecutive patients who underwent decompressive craniectomy and subsequent cranioplasty with autologous cranial bone flap in a university medical center between March 1999 and July 2005. After craniectomy, the excised cranial bone flaps were cleaned of any remaining soft tissue. The flaps were air dried for 72 hours and then placed into two sealed sterilization pouches, one pouch inside of the other. Both pouches were labeled with patient identification information.

The sealed packages were subjected to an ETO sterilization process and aerated for 16 hours to remove residual ETO from the bone flap and packaging. The packaged bone flaps were then stored in a locked cabinet maintained at a temperature of 68° F (20° C) for nine days to 15 months before replantation into the patient. The researchers followed the patients for one to 63 months after the procedure.[97]

Aesthetic and functional results of the cranioplasty procedure were assessed by CT scans and cosmetic appearance. The researchers found that 95 patients (92.2%) had excellent cosmetic and functional results. Eight patients (7.8%) developed postoperative infections requiring removal of the flap and subsequent reconstruction with methyl methacrylate with satisfactory results. A preservation time longer than 10 months was associated with a significantly increased risk of infection. The researchers concluded that subjecting the excised cranial bone flap to the ETO sterilization process and storing at room temperature was simple and effective; however, they suggested that bone flaps preserved beyond 10 months be discarded or reprocessed before use.[97]

II.c.1. Facilities or health care organizations that subject autologous bone to steam or other sterilization processes that require manufacturing controls must register with the FDA as a tissue establishment that manufactures human cells, tissues, and cellular and tissue-based products and must follow applicable requirements of 21 CFR Part 1271.[3,5] *[1: Regulatory Requirement]*

Subjecting tissue to mechanisms for sterilization, such as the steam sterilization process, for the purpose of inactivating or removing adventitious agents is considered processing under section 1271.3(ff), and under section 1271.220(c), would require manufacturing controls to validate that the correct time, temperature, and pressure has been achieved with each load.[3,5]

Recommendation III

The patient's parathyroid tissue may be cryopreserved and autotransplanted.

The collective evidence suggests there is an indication for autotransplantation of cryopreserved autologous parathyroid tissue in cases of postoperative hypoparathyroidism resulting from the unintentional removal or injury of parathyroid glands during thyroid and parathyroid surgery.[101-103]

A standard protocol for the cryopreservation of parathyroid tissue does not exist.[104] The cryopreservation process may impair cellular function and viability and lead to cell necrosis.[101] Autograft functionality may depend on storage time and may decrease with storage times longer than 22 months.[101] Further research is warranted to determine the optimal process of cryopreservation to enhance cell viability.[105,106]

The limitations of the evidence are that there was an inadequate amount of literature addressing this practice issue. The research studies had small sample sizes, and there was no uniform assessment of cell viability. Although one study included samples that had been cryopreserved for as long as 15 years, there was no controlled method of cryopreservation for the samples included in that study.[105]

The benefits of cryopreservation and autotransplantation of the patient's parathyroid tissue are that it permits storage of parathyroid tissue for later transplantation without compromising cellular integrity or function[107] and also allows the clinician to determine whether any residual parathyroid tissue will recover function or whether a delayed autotransplantation will be required.[101] Autotransplantation of cryopreserved parathyroid tissue can eliminate or minimize the requirements for calcium and vitamin D supplementation required for patients who have lost thyroid function.[105]

The harms associated with cryopreservation and autotransplantation of patients' parathyroid tissue include the need for a secondary surgery, increased cost, and the increased potential for infection from transplanting contaminated or nonviable autologous parathyroid tissue. There is an increased risk of autograft failure with cryopreserved tissue compared with fresh tissue.[106] Parathyroid tissue may be destroyed by the cryopreservation process or degraded to the extent that insufficient parathyroid hormone is released after autotransplantation.[106] Long-term storage of autologous tissue carries with it the potential for mix-ups if autograft labeling methods are inadequate (eg, smudging of identifiers during cold storage, labels separating from the package), and contamination or cross-contamination if the graft's packaging material is not validated for use at the storage temperature selected.

III.a. Parathyroid tissue may be cryopreserved for delayed autotransplantation for as long as 24 months. *[2: Moderate Evidence]*

Agarwal et al[107] described the cryopreservation technique and storage methods used for autologous parathyroid glands in a university medical center since 2002. Within 15 minutes of excision, fragments of parathyroid tissue removed from the patient were minced into 30 to 40 uniform small pieces (ie, 2 mm), suspended in sterile normal saline solution, and drawn into a 1 mL tuberculin syringe. The syringe was capped and labeled, placed into a plastic bag labeled as biohazardous, surrounded by ice, and immediately transported by perioperative personnel to the laboratory where the autologous parathyroid segments were preserved in cryopreservation media and stored in liquid nitrogen.

To prevent storage of cancerous or nonparathyroid tissue, the pathologist histologically confirmed the tissue to be normal parathyroid tissue by frozen section before the cryopreservation process was initiated. Perioperative personnel collected approximately 5 mL to 10 mL of the patient's blood in tubes that contained no additives. The tubes were labeled and transported to the laboratory where the blood was

---

Overview of Parathyroid Cryopreservation and Autotransplantation

Parathyroid cryopreservation is performed to provide a source of viable parathyroid tissue that can be autotransplanted at a later date to treat permanent hypoparathyroidism that may occur after thyroid or parathyroid surgery.[1-3] The risk of hypoparathyroidism is greatest after subtotal or total parathyroidectomy, thyroid resection, nodal dissection for large thyroid cancers, and reoperative neck procedures.[4] Permanent hypoparathyroidism is defined as persistent hypocalcemia requiring calcium and vitamin D supplements six months after surgery.[5] Effective management of hypoparathyroidism requires lifelong medication and frequent laboratory testing and may necessitate frequent hospital admissions.[5] The absence of parathyroid hormone has long-term systemic effects on the body, including the development of osteoporosis, premature cataracts, cardiac dysfunction, and neurologic dysfunction.[5] Hypoparathyroidism that persists longer than six months after parathyroid or thyroid surgery is commonly treated with autotransplantation of cryopreserved autologous parathyroid tissue if it is available.[5]

Intraoperative preparation of parathyroid tissue for cryopreservation most often involves removing the tissue surgically and then dissecting it into small segments approximately 1 mm x 1 mm x 1 mm.[4] The segments are placed into a sterile container, positioned on ice, and transported to the laboratory for cyropreservation.[4] On the day of the autotransplantation procedure, the parathyroid tissue to be transplanted is removed from storage and placed in a warm water bath until thawed.[4] The tissue segments may be rinsed in a serial fashion to remove any cryoprotectant residue or contaminants that may be present on the tissue.[4] Pockets are created in the brachioradialis muscle of the nondominant arm,[4] sternocleidomastoid muscle, thigh muscles, or muscles of the anterior chest or abdominal wall.[5] One to three parathyroid tissue segments are placed into each muscle pocket until a total of 20 to 40 segments has been transplanted.[4] It is important to prevent excess bleeding, because an intramuscular hematoma may compromise graft function.[4]

Success of the autotransplantation is measured by sampling blood from both the grafted and nongrafted arms to determine parathyroid hormone levels at both sites.[4] Transplanted parathyroid segments may require as long as six months to resume adequate function.[5] The autograft is considered to be fully functional when the patient remains asymptomatic and is no longer dependent on calcium and vitamin D supplements.[4] The success of the autotransplantation may depend on the cryopreservation process used, the amount of storage time, and the amount and size of the parathyroid segments transplanted.[5]

References

1. Guerrero MA. Cryopreservation of parathyroid glands. Int J Endocrinol. 2010;2010:829540. Epub December 8, 2010.
2. Stotler BA, Reich-Slotky R, Schwartz J, et al. Quality monitoring of microbial contamination of cryopreserved parathyroid tissue. Cell Tissue Bank. 2011;12(2):111-116.
3. Cohen MS, Dilley WG, Wells SA Jr, et al. Long-term functionality of cryopreserved parathyroid autografts: a 13-year prospective analysis. Surgery. 2005;138(6):1033-1040.
4. Agarwal A, Waghray A, Gupta S, Sharma R, Milas M. Cryopreservation of parathyroid tissue: an illustrated technique using the Cleveland Clinic protocol. J Am Coll Surg. 2013;216(1):e1-e9.
5. Guerrero MA, Evans DB, Lee JE, et al. Viability of cryopreserved parathyroid tissue: when is continued storage versus disposal indicated? World J Surg. 2008;32(5):836-839.

used to prepare the cryopreservation media. The cryopreservation process took approximately one to two hours. The tissue was stored for a minimum of two years.[107]

Laboratory personnel were notified the day before the autotransplantation procedure in order to allow sufficient time to thaw the desired quantity of parathyroid tissue. The tissue was gradually thawed and delivered to the operating room (OR) either at room temperature or on ice, based on the surgeon's preference. Perioperative personnel transferred the tissue to a sterile specimen cup and diluted it with sterile normal saline solution.[107]

The surgeon transplanted the parathyroid tissue into several small muscular pockets of the patient's nondominant arm, with one to two fragments transplanted into each pocket. The surgeon determined the amount of parathyroid tissue to be replanted, which was generally an amount equal to two normal-sized parathyroid glands. After surgery, the surgeon closely monitored the patient's serum calcium and parathyroid hormone levels. The authors noted that parathyroid function may take several weeks to manifest as levels detectable with blood samples.[107]

Stotler et al[102] described a university medical center's quality monitoring protocol for detecting the presence of bacterial contamination in parathyroid tissue intended for autotransplantation. Laboratory personnel performed bacterial cultures on all parathyroid tissue immediately before processing of the tissue and at the completion of the cryopreservation process; cultures were also performed on the corresponding cryopreservation medium. If the culture result was positive, they performed a Gram stain and subcultured the samples in cell media. Bacterial identification and antimicrobial susceptibility testing were performed.

Between January 2005 and October 2008, a total of 47 parathyroid tissues were cryopreserved for potential future autotransplantation. The authors found bacterial contamination in 23% of cases (n = 11). Contamination was present before tissue processing in 91% of the contaminated samples (n = 10). In 27% of the contaminated samples (n = 3), contamination was present both before and after processing. In 9% (n = 1), contamination was found only after processing. Of the 11 contaminated samples, 55% (n = 6) grew *Staphylococcus epidermidis*. The authors concluded there is a need to monitor the contamination levels of resected parathyroid tissue that will be cryopreserved and replanted into a patient.[102]

In a study conducted to determine the viability of cryopreserved autologous parathyroid tissue in relation to the length of time in storage and to define the most effective time frame for tissue transplantation and disposal, Guerrero et al[105] identified all parathyroid autografts cryopreserved at -112° F (-80° C) between 1991 and 2006 at a major medical college. From the 501 cryopreserved parathyroid autografts, four to 12 samples from each year were randomly selected for the study (N = 106).

The researchers assessed cell viability using a hemacytometer to count viable and nonviable cells. Of the 106 autografts, only 11 (10.3%) were found to be viable. The researchers found that one autograft was viable for 120 months, but none of the autografts were viable for longer than 120 months. Of the autografts cryopreserved for 24 months or less, 71.4% (10 of 14) were viable, compared with only 1.1% of autografts (one of 92) stored for more than 24 months. The single autograft with evidence of viability beyond 24 months had only 2% viable cells.[105]

The researchers concluded that the viability of the cryopreserved parathyroid cells was associated with the duration of storage and that parathyroid tissue preserved for longer than 24 months was unlikely to be viable. They recommended limiting the preservation time for parathyroid tissue to 24 months. The researchers noted that knowing the viability of cryopreserved autologous parathyroid tissue could help to minimize ethical concerns and enable more objective decision-making related to establishing time frames for discarding autologous parathyroid tissue.[105]

Alvarez-Hernandez et al[108] conducted a quasi-experimental study to test the viability and functionality of fresh and cryopreserved parathyroid tissue. Small fragments of 18 parathyroid glands removed from 18 patients with secondary hyperparathyroidism were cultured immediately after excision and again after cryopreservation at -112° F (-80° C) for a maximum of 18 months. The researchers found that cell viability at both the beginning and end of the testing period was greater than 85% and concluded there were no differences in viability or functionality between the fresh and cryopreserved parathyroid tissue.

In a prospective study to determine the amount of time that human parathyroid tissue can be stored before cryopreservation, Barreira et al[109] evaluated parathyroid tissue from 11 patients undergoing total parathyroidectomy in a university medical center between April and October 2009. Immediately after surgical resection, the researchers cut the parathyroid tissue intended for pathology examination into 2-mm segments. The resected tissue was equally divided into five groups and examined immediately after resection and after storage at 39.2° F (4° C) in Dulbecco's modified Eagle's medium for two, six, 12, and 24 hours.

The researchers found that 10 (90.9%) of the parathyroid tissue samples maintained structural integrity at the molecular level for up to

12 hours. At 24 hours, all of the samples showed degenerative changes in cell cytoplasm and mitochondria. Two samples (18.2%) showed cellular changes consistent with apoptosis and cell death. The researchers concluded that molecular structural integrity was maintained in the parathyroid tissue segments stored for as long as 12 hours in culture medium at 39.2° F (4° C).[109]

Cohen et al[103] conducted a study of 29 patients who underwent 34 parathyroid autotransplantation procedures in a university medical center between November 1991 and November 2004. After surgical resection, the researchers divided the parathyroid tissue into 30 to 40 segments approximately 1 mm x 1 mm x 3 mm. The fragments were placed in a sterile medicine cup filled with normal saline solution and then placed on ice and submitted to laboratory personnel for cryopreservation. In addition to the parathyroid tissue, perioperative personnel drew 10 mL of the patient's blood and submitted it to the laboratory to prepare autologous serum. The parathyroid tissue was stored in a liquid nitrogen freezer at -274° F (-170° C) for as long as 11 months.

On the day of the procedure, perioperative personnel removed the samples from storage and placed them in a 98.6° F (37° C) water bath. The surgeons placed approximately 20 to 25 pieces of parathyroid tissue (approximately 50 mg to 75 mg) into five to 10 pockets created in the brachioradialis muscle of the patient's forearm. Patients were followed for two months to 11 years, with an average follow-up time of 24 months. Outcomes were determined based on peripheral parathyroid hormone levels. Parathyroid autograft function was defined as

- completely functional (ie, normal parathyroid hormone and calcium levels with no supplements required),
- partially functional (ie, normal parathyroid hormone levels and mild hypocalcemia requiring calcium supplementation), or
- nonfunctional (ie, low parathyroid hormone levels and dependence on calcium and vitamin D supplementation).[103]

Of the 29 patients, prospective data were available for 26 patients undergoing 30 parathyroid autotransplantation procedures. The researchers found that 12 of the 26 patients (46%) had completely functional autografts, six patients (23%) had partially functional autografts, and eight patients (31%) had nonfunctional autografts. The researchers found the duration of cryopreservation was a significant indicator of graft failure.[103]

The 18 functional grafts had an average cryopreservation time of 7.9 months. The eight nonfunctional grafts had an average cryopreservation time of 15.3 months. No autograft was observed to be functional beyond 22 months of cryopreservation, suggesting that shorter cryopreservation times may result in an improved functional outcome. None of the patients experienced recurrent hyperparathyroidism. The researchers concluded that delayed replantation of cryopreserved parathyroid tissue is beneficial for patients who have permanent postoperative hypoparathyroidism.[103]

de Menezes Montenegro et al[110] reported successful results with autotransplantation of parathyroid tissue cryopreserved for 21 months. The patient was a 40-year-old woman with renal hyperparathyroidism who underwent total parathyroidectomy with cryopreservation of parathyroid tissue. After 21 months of follow up, she was hypocalcemic and had an undetectable parathyroid hormone level. Approximately 45 cryopreserved parathyroid segments were thawed and transplanted into her forearm. After autotransplantation, the patient's clinical condition improved. Within 18 months, her parathyroid hormone levels were normal, and she did not require any calcium or vitamin D supplements. The authors recommended cryopreservation of excised parathyroid tissue for all cases of hyperparathyroidism should the need to correct postoperative hypoparathyroidism arise.

Saxe et al[106] reported on 12 patients who underwent parathyroid autotransplantation with cryopreserved parathyroid tissue in the forearm between August 1975 and March 1981 in a national cancer institute. The surgeons divided the excised parathyroid tissue into 1 mm x 1 mm x 1 mm segments in the OR in chilled normal saline solution or Roswell Park Memorial Institute 1640 culture medium. Perioperative personnel transported the tissue to the laboratory where it was cryopreserved for two to 18 months.

Two hours before the autotransplantation procedure, perioperative personnel thawed the tissue in a 107.6° F (42° C) water bath. The surgeons placed 20 to 30 segments in an equal number of muscular pockets in the brachioradialis muscle of the nondominant arm. Follow-up ranged from four to 66 months. Because all patients had been dependent on calcium supplements before the autotransplantation procedure, the authors considered freedom from calcium therapy to be the best evidence of autograft function. Six patients (50%) no longer required calcium supplementation and in one patient (8%), the dose was reduced. The researchers concluded that further research was warranted regarding the optimal procedures for cryopreservation of human parathyroid tissue.[106]

To evaluate their experience with parathyroid autotransplantation and analyze the role of cryopreservation and delayed autotransplantation of parathyroid tissue in the treatment of patients with renal hyperparathyroidism, Schneider et al[104] reviewed a university medical center database of 883 patients with renal hyperparathyroidism. They found that 15 patients (1.7%) had undergone delayed parathyroid autotransplantation with parathyroid tissue cryopreserved for one to 86 months between 1976 and 2011. The standardized process used for cryopreservation included first having the pathologist verify parathyroid origin of the excised tissue by histological examination. The surgeons then divided the tissue into 1 mm x 1 mm x 1 mm segments, and perioperative personnel transported the segments to the laboratory in cold normal saline solution.

On the day of the autotransplantation procedure, the pathologist estimated viability of the tissue by histological examination to determine the number of necrotic and viable cells in a sample of the tissue. Laboratory personnel tested the tissue to be autotransplanted for microbial contamination. If the amount of cell necrosis was found to be less than 50% and the sample showed no sign of microbial contamination, laboratory personnel thawed the remaining tissue in a 98.6° F (37° C) water bath, rinsed it, and preserved it on ice during transport to the OR.[104]

During surgery, the surgeons placed approximately 30 segments of parathyroid tissue into muscular pockets in the brachioradialis muscle of the patient's nondominant or non-shunt-bearing arm. The researchers reviewed the histopathology reports and found no necrosis of the tissue in 14 patients (93.3%) and 70% necrosis of the tissue in one patient (6.7%).[104]

The patients' serum calcium and parathyroid hormone levels were closely monitored by the researchers during the follow-up period. The autotransplantation procedure raised serum calcium and parathyroid hormone levels to normal levels in all patients during the 78-month follow-up period. The researchers theorized that the high success rate of the autotransplantation procedure could be explained by the microbiological and histological examinations conducted before autotransplantation because only tissues with low levels of necrosis and no microbial contamination were replanted. They also noted that the time from resection to cryopreservation was always less than one hour. The researchers concluded that the success of the procedure was high; however, because of the low number of patients requiring delayed autotransplantation of parathyroid tissue, the practice of cryopreserving and storing tissue for every patient should be questioned.[104]

III.a.1. Facilities recovering, packaging, labeling, or cryopreserving autologous parathyroid tissue for storage and autotransplantation within the same facility are not required to register with the FDA as a tissue establishment. *[1: Regulatory Requirement]*

The facility would meet the exception from registration described in section 1271.15(b), in which storage of tissue for autologous use is exempt as long as no other manufacturing controls are performed (ie, subjecting the autograft to the steam sterilization process, distributing the autograft to another facility).[3,4]

Recommendation IV

The patient's autologous skin may be preserved and autotransplanted.

The collective evidence indicates that refrigerated storage of split-thickness skin grafts for delayed autotransplantation is a common practice.[111,112] The use of a storage medium may improve and extend the viability of the stored human skin autograft compared with storage in normal saline solution.[113,114] Skin grafts may also be stored at the donor site for delayed autotransplantation.[112] There are gaps in the literature regarding histological changes that occur in stored autologous skin and the optimal storage methods, storage media, storage temperatures, and acceptable length of storage for human skin. Further research is warranted.

Human skin is sometimes meshed before storage. Meshing the skin graft allows the surgeon to stretch the skin graft to cover a larger area and also allows fluid to drain from the underlying wound; however, meshing the skin exposes it to mechanical trauma that may compromise cellular function.[115]

The limitations of the evidence are that only a small amount of literature addressed this practice issue, and the research studies had small sample sizes. One research study did not provide sufficient detail regarding the methods used to prepare human skin autografts for storage, the storage temperatures used, or the time required to thaw frozen autografts.[116]

The benefits of storing autologous skin for delayed autotransplantation include reduced cost and the potential elimination of a secondary donor site. The benefits of storing autologous skin at the donor site for delayed autotransplantation are that it allows the skin graft placement to be performed at the patient's bedside after the initial swelling at the recipient site has gone down.[112] This delayed placement increases the potential for the graft to be accepted by reducing stress on the graft that might occur from its being stretched and pulled over swollen tissue and also helps ensure there is no fluid collection at the recipient site that could collect under the graft, increase tension, and prevent adherence of the graft to the graft site. Storing the patient's skin autograft at the donor site also may prevent the need for an additional surgical procedure.

The harms associated with storing autologous skin for delayed autotransplantation include the increased potential for infection from contaminated or nonviable autologous skin grafts. Long-term storage of autologous tissue carries with it the potential for mix-ups if autograft labeling methods are inadequate (eg, smudging of identifiers during cold storage, labels separating from the package) and for contamination or cross-contamination if the graft's packaging material is not validated for use at the storage temperature selected.

AUTOLOGOUS TISSUE MANAGEMENT

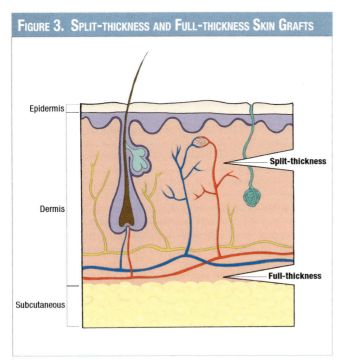

FIGURE 3. SPLIT-THICKNESS AND FULL-THICKNESS SKIN GRAFTS

A split-thickness skin graft includes the epidermis and part of the dermis. A full-thickness skin graft includes the epidermis and all of the dermis.

Illustration by Kurt Jones.

IV.a. Autologous skin for delayed autotransplantation may be refrigerated and stored in normal saline solution or in a storage medium or may be cryopreserved. *[2: Moderate Evidence]*

In a retrospective review conducted between January 1991 and December 1995 in the burn institute of a general hospital and medical school, Sheridan et al[116] found that human skin autografts had been autotransplanted to 42 open wounds in 28 patients. The autografts consisted of remnants of unused skin from the initial split-thickness skin grafting procedure (Figure 3). The remnants of skin had been stored from four to 117 days in one of two ways:

○ If the interval to anticipated autotransplantation was anticipated to be fewer than seven days, the autograft was refrigerated.
○ If the interval to autotransplantation was anticipated to be more than seven days, the skin was treated with 15% glycerol solution; frozen; and stored in a sealed, labeled, plastic envelope.

None of the refrigerated grafts were autotransplanted. The frozen skin was thawed by placing it in room-temperature normal saline solution before replantation. The researchers did not provide information as to the refrigerator or freezer storage temperatures, the method of storage preparation of the refrigerated autografts, the cryopreservation process, or the length of time required to thaw the frozen autografts. Notably, the researchers found documentation of the rate of successful engraftment of the frozen skin in 12 cases. In these cases, the amount of successful engraftment averaged 70%. The researchers recommended autologous skin banking as a method to preserve unused portions of human skin grafts for delayed autotransplantation to minimize the need for obtaining additional tissue from new donor sites.[116]

Sterne et al[115] obtained skin grafts from six patients undergoing abdominoplasty to provide a qualitative description of the histological changes that occurred in split-thickness skin grafts wrapped in saline-soaked gauze and stored at 39.2° F (4° C) during a four-week period. The researchers divided the tissue into two groups of four grafts:

○ unmeshed skin, rolled (ie, folded in half longitudinally with the dermal surfaces contacting each other and rolled);
○ unmeshed skin, flat (ie, folded in half and placed in a sterile plastic cassette and covered with saline-moistened filter paper);
○ meshed skin, rolled; or
○ meshed skin, flat.

The skin grafts were placed on tulle gras, wrapped in saline-soaked gauze, placed into a sterile specimen container, and stored in one of two refrigerators at 39.2° F (4° C). A tissue sample was sent for histological examination at the time of initial storage and after one, seven, 14, 21, and 28 days of refrigeration. The researchers found variability in the size and shape of the cells and cell nuclei beginning at day seven. The meshed skin showed greater swelling and more acute variability in the shape of the cells and cell nuclei. From day 14 through day 21, the structure of the dermal collagen became progressively degraded. From day 21 through day 28, the researchers found extensive separation of the epidermis from its vascular supply. They concluded that the viability of the stored grafts was greatest when the grafts were stored as an unmeshed roll at 39.2° F (4° C) for fewer than seven days.[115]

Titley et al[117] conducted a quantitative and qualitative study of 102 consecutive split-thickness skin grafts to

○ identify the organisms colonizing split-thickness skin grafts at the time of recovery and after three weeks of refrigerated storage,
○ relate the number of organisms on fresh skin to the percentage of successful engraftment, and
○ compare the number of organisms contaminating skin grafts.

The study was conducted in a plastic surgery unit of a regional hospital. The researchers took tissue samples of all skin autografts. The grafts were placed on tulle gras, wrapped in saline-moistened gauze, placed into a sterile specimen container, and stored in the facility refrigerator at 42.8° F to 51.8° F (6° C to 11° C) for as long as three weeks.[117]

When the stored skin was autotransplanted, the researchers took a second sample of the graft. *Staphylococcus aureus* and coagulase-negative staphylococci were the organisms most commonly isolated from the initial skin sample. There was no growth in 56.9% of the grafts (n = 58), but more than one organism was grown from 10.8% of the grafts (n = 11). At three weeks, the remaining stored skin was submitted for microbial examination. The researchers found that coagulase-negative staphylococci were still the predominant organisms on the grafts; however, there was an increase in the number of *Acinetobacter* and *Pseudomonas* species. The researchers also found more organisms on the skin grafts of male patients than of female patients. They theorized that because men have more body hair than women, there may be more preoperative shaving of the male donor sites. The shaving may have caused microscopic wounds that increased bacterial proliferation, particularly if the patient was shaved several hours before the procedure.[117]

During the first dressing change, the researchers recorded the percentage of the graft that had successfully engrafted. They found the percentage of successful engraftment was inversely proportional to the number of microorganisms on the grafts (ie, as the number of microorganisms increased, the percentage of engraftment decreased). Notably, the researchers found a spike in temperature (57° F [13.9° C]) whenever the refrigerator door was opened. The researchers concluded that storage of human skin autografts in refrigerators allowed for significant bacterial proliferation during a three-week storage period. The researchers also concluded there was a need for strict temperature monitoring of refrigerators used for storage of human skin autografts. They suggested that the temperature of the refrigerator be maintained at 39.2° F (4° C) or colder to help prevent bacterial proliferation.[117]

DeBono et al[111] conducted a quasi-experimental study to assess the efficacy of McCoy's 5A medium for human skin storage and to assess whether supplying supplementary oxygen (O_2) to the medium would improve survival of the graft. The researchers stored two 3-mm discs of split-thickness human skin obtained from a single patient in 40 sterile sealable containers in one of four solutions:

- 4.4 mL normal saline solution plus 80 mg gentamicin,
- 4 mL McCoy's 5A medium plus 80 mg gentamicin,
- 4 mL McCoy's 5A medium plus 80 mg gentamicin supplemented with carbon dioxide (CO_2) at 2 L/minute for 30 seconds repeated every seven days, or
- 4 mL McCoy's 5A medium plus 80 mg gentamicin supplemented with O_2 at 2 L/minute for 30 seconds repeated every seven days.

The sealed containers were stored in a temperature-monitored refrigerator at 39.2° F (4° C). A tissue culture of the stored skin was taken every seven days to assess the viability of the stored skin. The researchers found that the skin stored in McCoy's 5A medium supplemented with CO_2 was viable for less than one week. The skin stored in normal saline solution was viable for only one week. The skin stored in McCoy's 5A medium or in McCoy's 5A medium supplemented with O_2 was viable for four weeks. The researchers noted that oxygenating the medium did not improve the viable storage time, and they theorized that the extended skin viability was caused by the nutrients and buffers present in the medium. The researchers concluded that McCoy's 5A medium was an acceptable storage medium that prolonged the viability of the stored skin for as long as four weeks.[111]

IV.a.1. Facilities recovering, packaging, labeling, and refrigerating autologous skin for storage and autotransplantation within the same facility are not required to register with the FDA as a tissue establishment. *[1: Regulatory Requirement]*

The facility would meet the exception from registration described in section 1271.15(b), in which storage of tissue for autologous use is exempt as long as no other manufacturing controls are performed (ie, subjecting the autograft to the steam sterilization process, distributing the autograft to another facility).[3,4]

IV.b. Human skin for delayed autotransplantation may be stored on the patient's donor site. *[2: Moderate Evidence]*

Mardini et al[112] described their experience with 10 patients undergoing voice reconstruction surgery using jejunal and ileocolonic flaps between January and July 2006. Delayed autotransplantation from the thigh to the neck was carried out at the patient's bedside during the third to eighth postoperative day, using skin that had been recovered from and stored at the patients' thighs during the initial reconstructive surgery. Elevation of the stored graft was well tolerated, and there was greater than 95% engraftment in all cases. The authors found all grafts were completely healed during the five- to 12-month follow-up period. They recommended storage of the skin autograft at the donor site for as long as eight days as a reliable technique with diverse clinical applications when traditional skin banking is not feasible.

AUTOLOGOUS TISSUE MANAGEMENT

Recommendation V

The patient's autologous vein may be preserved and autotransplanted.

The collective evidence indicates that storing unused segments of autologous vein grafts after cardiac surgery for delayed autotransplantation in the event of a graft failure is common,[118,119] especially for older patients.[120] The autologous saphenous vein is the most commonly used conduit in cardiac surgery.[118,120] Storing vein grafts in a manner that prevents epithelial injury and maintains vessel function is important for successful autotransplantation.[120] Endothelial injury resulting from storage of autologous veins may promote vessel thrombosis, vessel wall inflammation, and graft failure.[119] Normal saline and lactated Ringer's solutions have commonly been used for storage of autologous vein grafts; however, using culture media may be a better option for maintaining vessel function.[120] Cryopreservation maintains the elastic properties of the vein[118] but destroys the integrity of the endothelial layer of the vessel, and for this reason, it is not considered to be an effective storage mechanism for autologous vein grafts.[118,120]

The limitations of the evidence are that only a small amount of literature addressed this practice issue, and the research studies had small sample sizes.

The benefits of storing the patient's autologous vein for delayed autotransplantation include reduced cost and the potential elimination of a secondary donor site. The harm associated with storing the patient's autologous vein for delayed autotransplantation is the increased potential for infection from contaminated or nonviable autologous vein grafts.

V.a. Autologous veins for delayed autotransplantation may be refrigerated and stored in normal saline or lactated Ringer's solution or in a storage medium. *[2: Moderate Evidence]*

To identify alterations in the functional, morphologic, and molecular level of blood vessels after cold storage, Ebner et al[119] examined 2-mm segments of mouse aorta placed in TiProtec® solution and stored at 39.2° F (4° C) after two hours and one, two, four, and seven days. The researchers found significant genetic alterations in the vessel segments within the first two hours of storage. They theorized that these molecular alterations could affect graft function. The researchers also found impairment of vessel function after cold storage for two days; however, they did not find any histologic changes in the structure of the vessel segments. The researchers concluded that storage beyond two days impaired vessel function, but further research was warranted to determine whether any comorbidities are associated with the impaired vessel function.

To investigate the effect of storing saphenous vein segments in normal saline solution compared with TiProtec solution, Wilbring et al[120] isolated 19 saphenous vein segments from patients undergoing coronary artery bypass grafting with autologous saphenous veins in a university heart center between October 2008 and March 2010. The veins were extracted without the use of electrocoagulation. Each vein segment was divided into two parts and placed in either normal saline solution or TiProtec. The vein segments were stored at 39.2° F (4° C) for 96 hours and then examined.

The researchers found that the vessel function was significantly reduced after 24 hours of cold storage in normal saline solution. After 96 hours of storage in normal saline solution, there was minimal to no vessel function remaining. Vascular function of the vein segments stored in TiProtec was significantly better preserved. The researchers concluded that cold storage of venous grafts was feasible for as long as 96 hours when the grafts were stored in TiProtec solution; however, storage of venous grafts in normal saline solution was not recommended beyond 24 hours.[120]

Molnar et al[118] conducted a quasi-experimental study to investigate the passive and active biomechanical properties of 72 saphenous vein segments remaining after coronary bypass grafting from 32 patients in a university medical center. The vein segments were divided into eight testing groups:

- fresh, examined immediately after recovery;
- stored in normal Krebs-Ringer solution at 32° F to 39.2° F (0° C to 4° C), examined one week after recovery;
- stored in normal Krebs-Ringer solution at 32° F to 39.2° F (0° C to 4° C), examined two weeks after recovery;
- stored in X-Vivo 10® at 32° F to 39.2° F (0° C to 4° C), examined one week after recovery;
- stored in X-Vivo 10 at 32° F to 39.2° F (0° C to 4° C), examined two weeks after recovery;
- stored in X-Vivo 10 at 32° F to 39.2° F (0° C to 4° C), examined three weeks after recovery;
- stored in X-Vivo 10 at 32° F to 39.2° F (0° C to 4° C), examined four weeks after recovery; or
- cryopreserved at -220° F (-140° C), examined three weeks after recovery.

The cryopreserved samples were thawed by immersion in warm (98.6° F; 37° C) Krebs-Ringer solution. The biomechanical testing showed that the vein segments stored in Krebs-Ringer solution lost their ability to dilate and contract within one week. The segments stored in X-Vivo 10 preserved their contractility after one week, and it only slowly decreased during the four-week study period. There was a slight decrease in vessel wall thickness, but the lumen diameter was not affected. The elastic parameters were almost identical to the fresh segments. The cryopreserved segments narrowed, the vessel wall thickened, and contractility diminished. The researchers concluded that storage in X-Vivo 10 helped to preserve the passive and active biomechanical properties of human saphenous vein segments. They also concluded that maintaining these properties could be expected to improve stored autologous vein graft viability.[118]

Baumann et al[121] used light transmission and scanning electron microscopy to investigate the effects of various methods of vein preparation on endothelial and smooth muscle cells in dog cephalic veins. The researchers removed the veins, divided them into 10-cm segments (N = 10), and placed them in one of three solutions (ie, autologous blood [n = 3], Plasma-Lyte® [n = 2], or Plasma-Lyte with 0.6 mg/mL papaverine [n = 5]) containing heparin 10,000 units/L, and then stored them at 50° F (10° C) for either five minutes or one hour.

The researchers found the vein wall was extremely sensitive to dissection, manipulation, or introduction of fixative solutions and reacted to such stimulations with severe contraction that not only diminished the luminal diameter but also resulted in protrusion of endothelial cells into the lumen and the formation of cytoplasmic extensions of medial smooth muscle cells. The veins stored in autologous blood demonstrated the greatest amount of vessel wall contraction and endothelial cell loss. Veins stored in Plasma-Lyte for five minutes showed few contractions; however, after one hour, there were contractions and some endothelial cell loss. Veins stored in Plasma-Lyte supplemented with papaverine had the most relaxed appearance and minimal endothelial cell loss. The researchers recommended mitigating damaging vein graft contractions by

- using gentle surgical dissection to avoid vein spasm;
- instituting and intermittently repeating (ie, every two to three minutes) gentle perfusion with a solution of Plasma-Lyte supplemented with papaverine immediately after exposure of the distal end of the vein and while the rest of the vein is removed;
- avoiding the use of autologous blood for vein immersion, storage, or distention; and
- monitoring the pressure used to check vein grafts for leaks at less than 100 mmHg.[121]

The researchers concluded that attention to the details of vein dissection, preparation, and storage medium could lead to a significant improvement in endothelial preservation and subsequent patency rates after cardiac bypass procedures.[121]

V.a.1. Facilities recovering, packaging, labeling, and refrigerating autologous veins for storage and autotransplantation within the same facility are not required to register with the FDA as a tissue establishment. *[1: Regulatory Requirement]*

The facility would meet the exception from registration described in section 1271.15(b), in which storage of tissue for autologous use is exempt as long as no other manufacturing controls are performed (ie, subjecting the autograft to the steam sterilization process, distributing the autograft to another facility).[3,4]

Recommendation VI

A multidisciplinary team consisting of the surgeon, perioperative RN, and infection preventionist should conduct a risk assessment to consider the benefits and potential harms associated with replantation or autotransplantation of a contaminated autograft compared with other treatment options (eg, discarding the graft and using artificial material).

The collective evidence indicates there are instances in which autologous grafts necessary for replantation or autotransplantation are contaminated or dropped on the OR floor. The collective evidence also indicates that the infection rate associated with replantation or autotransplantation of contaminated grafts is low.[122-124] Various processes for decontaminating the graft have been implemented; however, there is no consistent protocol for managing the event when this occurs.[122-124] Further research is warranted on best practices for decontaminating contaminated autologous tissue, defining the specifications for low-pressure and high-pressure pulsatile lavage, and determining methods to prevent the graft from being dropped or otherwise contaminated.

The limitations of the evidence are that the long-term risk of SSI related to replantation or autotransplantation of contaminated autologous tissue is unknown. The results of surveys related to management of this event may be subjective and may not reflect the true number of incidents in the broader population. One survey had a low response rate (223 of 1,900; 12%) and therefore cannot be construed as representative of all members of the group surveyed.[124] Some research studies had no negative control. Some studies were conducted in controlled laboratory conditions, and the results of these studies may not be generalizable to settings outside of the laboratory.

The benefits of replantation or autotransplantation of contaminated autologous grafts include reduced cost, surgical time, and need for a secondary procedure and may include improved cosmetic appearance. The harm associated with replantation or autotransplantation of contaminated autologous grafts is the increased potential for the patient to develop an SSI.

In a retrospective review of 15,157 craniectomy procedures during a 16-year period in three health care facilities, Jankowitz and Kondziolka[122] assessed when bone grafts were dropped and how these events were managed. They also conducted a survey of 50 neurosurgeons in the United States to determine their experiences and protocols for managing dropped bone grafts.

AUTOLOGOUS TISSUE MANAGEMENT

In their review, the researchers found 14 instances of dropped cranial bone grafts. The cranial bone flaps were dropped
- during elevation of the bone flap from the cranium (n = 4; 28.6%),
- during movement of the bone flap from the surgical field to the back table (n = 4; 28.6%),
- during plating of titanium hardware (n = 4; 28.6%), and
- for unknown reasons (n = 2; 14.3%).[122]

Management of the dropped cranial bone flaps included
- soaking the flap in povidone-iodine or antibiotic solution and replanting (n = 8; 57.1%),
- subjecting the flap to the steam sterilization process and replanting (n = 2; 14.3%),
- discarding the flap and using artificial materials (n = 3; 21.4%), and
- using unknown methods (n = 1; 7.1%).[122]

According to the survey (N = 50), recommendations for managing dropped cranial bone flaps included
- soaking the flap in povidone-iodine solution and replanting (n = 11; 22%),
- soaking the flap in povidone-iodine and antibiotic solution and replanting (n = 16; 32%),
- subjecting the flap to the steam sterilization process and replanting (n = 18; 36%), and
- discarding the flap and using artificial materials to reconstruct the cranium (n = 9; 18%).[122]

After reviewing the records from 2004 and 2005, the researchers found there were 693 and 692 craniectomy procedures, respectively, that involved excising a cranial bone flap with the intention of replanting it. During this time period, a total of five cranial bone flaps were dropped, resulting in an incidence of 3.6 drops per 1,000 craniotomies (0.36%). The results of the survey showed that 66% of the polled neurosurgeons (n = 33) had experienced a dropped cranial bone graft, and 83% (n = 45 of 54) would replant the dropped graft after implementing a method of disinfection (eg, irrigation with antibiotic solution). There was a greater number of responses than polled surgeons because some surgeons reported their treatment of multiple incidents. The patients were followed for two to 176 months. There were no postoperative infections and no long term complications in any of the patients. The researchers concluded that disinfection of a dropped cranial bone graft and replantation is an acceptable option for treatment.[122]

Kang et al[123] conducted a survey of orthopedic surgeons who routinely performed orthopedic trauma surgery to determine how often autologous bone was dropped on the floor during orthopedic trauma surgery and the decontamination protocols that were implemented on these occasions. A total of 104 orthopedic surgeons responded to the survey. Forty surgeons (38%) reported that they had experienced at least one case in which the autologous bone was dropped from the sterile field during surgery. Methods used by the surgeons for decontaminating the dropped autologous bone included
- irrigating the bone with low-pressure pulsatile lavage (n = 36; 90%),
- soaking the bone in bacitracin solution (n = 28; 70%),
- soaking the bone in povidone-iodine solution (n = 26; 65%),
- soaking the bone in H_2O_2 solution (n = 4; 10%),
- subjecting the bone to the steam sterilization process (n = 7; 18%), and
- using other unspecified methods (n = 27; 68%).[123]

The researchers did not provide a definition for "low-pressure" lavage, the formulation for "bacitracin solution," or the strength of the povidone-iodine and H_2O_2 solutions used. None of the surgeons reported that replantation or autotransplantation of the contaminated autograft resulted in an SSI. The results of the survey showed that approximately one in three surgeons had experienced at least one instance in which autologous bone was dropped from the sterile field during surgery and that multiple methods were used for decontamination of the dropped bone, reflecting a lack of consensus on best practices. The researchers concluded that further research was warranted to determine the best procedures for decontamination of autologous bone after exposure to potential contamination and that guidelines reflecting best practices would be helpful for mitigating risk to patients.[123]

Centeno et al[124] conducted an online survey of 1,900 American Society for Aesthetic Plastic Surgery members to determine their practices for managing contaminated autologous grafts and received 223 responses (12%). The survey was designed to obtain information related to frequency of contamination, treatment preferences, clinical outcomes, and patient disclosure. Surgeons were asked whether they had witnessed or experienced a graft contamination. Thirty-three percent of respondents (n = 52 of 156) reported two occurrences, and 26% (n = 40 of 156) reported four or more contaminated autologous graft incidents. The researchers allowed multiple responses for many survey questions to capture a fuller range of experience for each question.

Reasons provided by the surgeons for graft contamination (ie, for 312 contamination incidents reported by 160 respondents) included
- the graft falling on the floor (75%),
- the graft being exposed to a nonsterile part of the drape (44.3%),
- the graft being exposed to a nonsterile part of the surgical field (28.7%),
- the graft being discarded in the trash (28.1%),
- the graft being exposed to a nonsterile specimen container (16.9%), and
- unknown reasons (1.9%).[124]

The anatomical areas involved (ie, for 246 contamination incidents reported by 158 respondents) included
- craniofacial (n = 104; 65.8%),
- lower extremity (n = 43; 27.2%),
- breast (n = 40; 25.3%),
- trunk (n = 28; 17.7%),
- upper extremity (n = 27; 17.1%), and
- genitourinary (n = 4; 2.5%).[124]

The types of contaminated autologous grafts (ie, for 284 contamination incidents reported by 158 respondents) included
- skin (n = 97; 61.4%),
- cartilage (n = 62; 39.2%),
- nipple-areolar complex (n = 35; 22.2%),
- bone (n =34; 21.5%),
- composite (n = 20; 12.7%),
- muscle (n = 18; 11.4%),
- fascia (n = 12; 7.6%), and
- fat (n = 6; 3.8%).[124]

Management of the contaminated autologous grafts (ie, based on responses from 160 respondents, with multiple responses allowed) included
- decontaminating and using the graft (n = 151; 94.4%),
- harvesting a graft from another site (n = 11; 6.9%),
- using another reconstructive technique (n = 6; 3.5%),
- using an alloplastic material or implant (n = 3; 1.9%), and
- discarding the graft and ending the surgery (n = 0).[124]

Solutions and methods used for decontaminating the contaminated autologous graft (ie, based on responses from 157 respondents, with multiple responses allowed) included
- povidone-iodine solution (n = 85; 54.1%),
- antibiotic solution (n = 79; 50.3%),
- normal saline solution with a bulb syringe (n = 67; 42.7%),
- normal saline solution with pulsatile lavage (n = 18; 11.5%),
- chlorhexidine gluconate (CHG) solution (n = 1; 0.6%), and
- no decontamination (n = 4; 3.2%).[124]

More than 98% of plastic surgeons responding to the survey (n = 154) who had experienced a contaminated autologous graft and replanted or autotransplanted the graft responded that its use did not lead to an infection. Only three patients with decontaminated grafts (1.9%) were reported to have developed an infection. Notably, 60% of respondents (n = 96 of 160) did not disclose the incident to the patient.[124]

VI.a. If a decision is made to replant or autotransplant the contaminated autograft, the following steps should be taken:
  ○ Rinse the contaminated graft in sterile normal saline solution to remove surface debris and contaminants.
  ○ Use pulsatile lavage at low-pressure settings (eg, 6 lb to 14 lb per square inch [psi])[125,126] and use sterile normal saline solution for more thorough cleansing of contaminated bone grafts if indicated (eg, adherent debris).
  ○ Use a separate sterile field for decontaminating the dropped graft and exercise care to prevent splashing onto the primary sterile field.
  ○ Implement corrective actions as necessary to maintain the sterility of the primary sterile field (eg, changing gowns and gloves after pulsatile lavage of the contaminated graft).
  ○ Change the wound classification to Class III, Contaminated.[127]
  ○ Document the event in a variance report.
  ○ Conduct a debriefing session and a root cause analysis with members of the surgical team and other individuals who may be helpful in providing a critical analysis and determining the factors that contributed to the event and methods to prevent its recurrence.

[2: Moderate Evidence]

Rinsing the dropped autograft in normal saline solution may be sufficient to remove surface debris and contaminants. In a randomized controlled trial (RCT) conducted to determine the amount of contamination that occurred when a bone graft was dropped on the floor, Presnal and Kimbrough[128] collected bone samples that were to be discarded during 50 orthopedic and neurosurgical procedures. Two bone samples of similar size were collected from each procedure. The first sample was placed directly into a culture tube under sterile conditions. The second sample was dropped on the OR floor near the operating table. The researchers chose this location because it was a high traffic area and also the most likely place that a bone graft would be dropped.

The bone sample was left on the floor for one minute and then retrieved using sterile technique and placed directly into a culture tube. Perioperative personnel then transported both samples to the laboratory for culture studies. No changes were made to the procedures for cleaning the OR floors, and the team members responsible for cleaning the floors were blinded to the study. Samples were obtained from random ORs at various times during the day. The results showed no positive cultures from either study group. The researchers concluded that replanting a dropped bone graft was acceptable without extensive and potentially damaging efforts to disinfect the graft.[128]

Pulsatile lavage may be useful for removing soil or microorganisms that are difficult to kill or remove with rinsing, such as heavy contamination and debris embedded in the tissue (eg, from a traumatic accident). There is no agreement in the literature as to the absolute definition of low-pressure versus high-pressure lavage.[125] Bhandari et al[129] found that high-pressure lavage (ie, 70 psi) may damage the bone and carry surface contaminants deeper into the bone. In another study, Bhandari et al[125] found that low-pressure lavage (ie, 14 psi) was as effective as high-pressure lavage (ie, 70 psi) in removing adherent bacteria from bone and preserved the bony architecture when applied within three hours of contamination. However, the researchers found that after six hours of contamination, low-pressure pulsatile lavage may not effectively remove adherent bacteria from cortical bone.

In a study to investigate the contamination rate of fresh frozen bone allografts after treatment with different decontamination methods, Hirn et al[126] contaminated 103 bone grafts harvested from healthy donors during primary total hip arthroplasty procedures. The researchers contaminated the bone grafts by rubbing them against the OR floor and leaving them on the floor for 60 minutes. The researchers also cultured the OR floor to determine the microorganisms present on the floor. Both coagulase-negative staphylococci and Bacillis species were cultured from the floor. The researchers cultured 23 bone grafts after contamination on the OR floor as a control group and found that 22 (96%) of the grafts were culture positive. The remaining 80 contaminated grafts were divided into groups of 20 grafts:
- Group 1 grafts were rinsed with 3 L normal saline solution.
- Group 2 grafts were rinsed with 3 L normal saline supplemented with 3 g cefuroxime.
- Group 3 grafts were rinsed with 3 L normal saline supplemented with 1.2 g rafampicin solution.
- Group 4 grafts were rinsed with 1 L normal saline using low-pressure lavage (6 psi).

The researchers cultured all grafts after treatment. The results showed that two grafts from Group 1 were culture negative (10%); seven grafts from Group 2 were culture negative (35%); 12 grafts from Group 3 were culture negative (60%); and 14 grafts from Group 4 were culture negative (70%). The researchers concluded that low-pressure lavage with sterile normal saline solution decreased bioburden on the contaminated graft, avoided the potential negative effects on bone that may arise with high-pressure lavage, and was effective when compared with the antibiotic solutions tested.[126]

Using a separate sterile field may help prevent contamination of the primary sterile field by microorganisms on the contaminated autograft and from droplets caused by rinsing or irrigation fluid used to decontaminate the graft. Implementing corrective actions to maintain the sterility of the surgical field may prevent or reduce microbial contamination and help minimize the patient's risk of SSI.

Replantation or autotransplantation of a contaminated autograft constitutes a major break in sterile technique. According to the Centers for Disease Control and Prevention surgical wound classification system, a surgical wound with a major break in sterile technique is classified as Class III, Contaminated.[127]

Variance reports document the steps taken during the event and provide a mechanism for alerting infection preventionists to the need for surveillance. Variance reports can also be useful for quality improvement activities. Implementing a process of debriefing and root cause analysis after the event has occurred may help prevent future incidents by examining underlying factors and system flaws that may have contributed to the event and may be responsive to analysis and correction.[130]

VI.a.1. The following actions may be taken:
- Add antibiotics or antiseptics to the solution used to rinse the autograft.
- Take cultures before and after decontamination of the graft to determine the identity of the contaminating microorganism and the level of contamination.
- Consult with an infection preventionist to assess the benefits versus harms of implementing postoperative broad-spectrum antibiotic prophylaxis therapy.
- Send the autograft to a tissue bank for decontamination and processing.

[2: Moderate Evidence]

Adding antibiotics or antiseptics to the irrigation solution may be unnecessary or potentially harmful. Antibiotics and antiseptics may not have been validated for use in irrigation solutions and may therefore pose a risk to the patient. Tissue proteins may inhibit effectiveness of the antibiotics.[131] Some antibiotics, such as bacitracin,[132] have not been found to be effective for eliminating bone contaminants, whereas others, such as rifamycin,[133] have been found to be effective for decontaminating contaminated bone grafts. Antiseptic solutions are intended for external use and may be ineffective or toxic when used internally. Povidone-iodine solution has been found to provide effective bone decontamination[134]; however, the antibacterial activity of 10% povidone-iodine solution is directly related to the level of contamination and the duration of exposure to the contaminated bone.[135]

Lacey[136] found that the antibacterial effect of povidone-iodine solution was inactivated in the presence of blood. Kaysinger et al[137] found that 0.5%, 5%, and 50% povidone-iodine solutions and 1.5% and 3% H_2O_2 solutions were cytotoxic to osteoblasts. Bhandari et al[125] found that povidone-iodine solution and bacitracin decreased the number of osteoclasts and impaired osteoblast function. When used to disinfect explanted bone, Schultke et al[84] found that H_2O_2 was ineffective.

Chlorhexidine gluconate has been found to be both effective[134] and ineffective[133] for decontaminating contaminated bone grafts and has also been found to be toxic to bone cells, even at very low concentrations (ie, 1%).[132] Using chemical disinfectants (eg, glutaraldehyde) on bone may cause tissue damage, or they may be difficult to remove. The steam sterilization process denatures bone protein and may severely damage bone structure and increase the potential for bone resorption and infection.[84]

Bhandari et al[132] conducted a two-part quasi-experimental study to compare the effects of various irrigating solutions on the number and function of osteoblasts and osteoclasts in bone and to examine the effectiveness of these solutions in removing adherent bacteria from bone. In Part 1, the researchers isolated calvarial cells from newborn mice and exposed the cells to equivalent concentrations of
- 1% ethanol,
- 10% ethanol,
- 1% povidone-iodine,
- 10% povidone-iodine,
- 1% soap (10 mL liquid soap/1 L normal saline),
- 10% soap (100 mL liquid soap/1 L normal saline),
- 1% CHG,
- 4% CHG,
- 1% antimicrobial (50 units bacitracin/L normal saline),
- 10% antimicrobial (500 units bacitracin/L normal saline), and
- normal saline solution

for two, 10, and 20 minutes. The researchers found that all of the irrigation solutions decreased the number of viable osteoblasts and osteocytes. The 10% povidone-iodine and 4% CHG solutions caused the most cell destruction. The 1% soap solution provided the least amount of cell destruction and the greatest amount of cell preservation.

In Part 2, the researchers contaminated canine cortical tibias with *Staphylococcus aureus* for six hours, and then subjected them to the same irrigating solutions used in Part 1 of the study with and without low-pressure lavage (ie, 14 psi). The researchers found the fewest number of bacteria on the contaminated tibias after exposure to 1% and 10% povidone-iodine, 1% and 4% CHG, and 1% and 10% soap. Low-pressure pulsatile lavage with 1% soap solution removed the most bacteria from the contaminated tibias. The antimicrobial solutions were the least effective at eliminating bacteria from the tibial samples.[132]

The researchers noted that the optimal technique for bone debridement should maximize the removal of adherent bacteria while preserving the structure and function of bone. They concluded that low-pressure lavage is as effective as high-pressure lavage in removing bacteria from the bone with significantly less macroscopic and microscopic bone damage.[132]

Bruce et al[134] conducted a three-phase quasi-experimental investigation to establish an intraoperative protocol for the management of contaminated autologous bone that will be replanted in the patient.
- Phase 1 of the study was performed to quantify the rate of contamination and the microbial profile of 162 bone fragments dropped on the OR floor. The results showed a contamination rate of 70%, with coagulase-negative staphylococcus being the most commonly cultured organism.
- Phase 2 of the study was performed to assess the feasibility and determine the optimal method of decontaminating 340 bone fragments contaminated with bacteria identified in Phase 1 of the study and decontaminated by methods and with cleansing solutions commonly available in an OR. The researchers tested 10% povidone-iodine, 4% CHG, 70% alcohol/2% CHG, and 0.9% normal saline solutions. The results showed the most effective solutions for decontaminating the bone fragments were 10% povidone-iodine and 4% CHG. Increasing exposure time to the decontaminating solutions from five to 10 minutes did not make a significant difference in contamination levels; however, mechanical scrubbing of the bone provided superior results to irrigating with a bulb syringe.
- Phase 3 of the study was performed to histologically assess the viability of the chondrocyte cells of 101 bone fragments after each decontamination process. The results showed that the bone samples treated with 10% povidone-iodine solution and normal saline solution maintained the greatest number of live cells.

The researchers concluded that five minutes of cleansing with 10% povidone-iodine solution followed by rinsing with normal saline solution provided the optimal balance between effective decontamination and maintaining cellular viability of the bone.[134]

In a systematic review conducted to explore intraoperative anterior cruciate ligament (ACL) graft decontamination, Khan et al[138] analyzed six experimental studies conducted between 1991 and 2012. The experimental groups from the studies included 328 allograft samples composed of fresh-frozen human Achilles tendocalcaneal grafts (n = 15), fresh-frozen human patellar tendon bone grafts (n = 30), excess hamstring graft from ACL reconstructions (n = 90), live human ACLs (n = 150), human cadaveric ACLs (n = 10), and human cadaveric patellar tendons (n = 33).

AUTOLOGOUS TISSUE MANAGEMENT

The allograft samples were contaminated by the researchers using various methods, such as dropping the tissue samples onto the OR floor or directly contaminating the samples with common pathogens (ie, *Staphylococcus aureus*, *Staphylococcus epidermidis*, *Pseudomonas aeruginosa*, *Klebsiella pneumoniae*, diphtheroids, micrococcus species). The researchers decontaminated the allografts using a variety of antiseptic and antibiotic solutions, including 2% and 4% CHG, normal saline solution, antibiotic solutions of polymyxin B and bacitracin or polymyxin B and neomycin, and 10% povidone-iodine. The decontamination protocols included seven to eight minutes of irrigation, mechanical agitation, serial dilution, pulsatile lavage, soaking for a variable duration of time, or a combination of rinsing and soaking. The researchers did not provide a definition for mechanical agitation or serial dilution, nor did they provide information as to the exact composition of the antiseptic and antibiotic solutions used in the studies included in the review.[138]

The researchers found that seven to eight minutes of irrigation with 3 L of 2% CHG and mechanical agitation and serial dilution with a polymyxin B-bacitracin solution provided 100% microbial decontamination (n = 10 of 10 samples). In two studies, they found that soaking the allograft in 4% CHG for 90 seconds provided 98% microbial decontamination (n = 49 of 50 samples) and 97% microbial decontamination (n = 29 of 30 samples), respectively. Soaking the grafts in bacitracin solution provided 97% microbial contamination (n = 29 of 30 samples), and soaking them in a combined solution of neomycin and polymyxin B provided 94% microbial decontamination (n = 47 of 50). Soaking the allografts in normal saline solution provided 70% microbial decontamination (n = 21 of 30). The results from two pooled studies showed that pulsatile lavage with normal saline solution provided 40% microbial decontamination (n = 6 of 15 samples). A combined solution of bacitracin and polymyxin B provided 57% microbial decontamination (n = 17 of 30 samples). Combined data from two studies showed that the least effective microbial decontamination (48%) occurred after soaking the allografts in 10% povidone-iodine (n = 40 of 84 samples).[138]

The researchers concluded the optimal antiseptic for decontaminating a contaminated allograft was CHG. However, they pointed out that the evidence included in the review was laboratory based and might not accurately reflect clinical conditions.

They recommended interpreting the findings of the systematic review with caution.[138]

Tissue cultures may be helpful in determining whether the dropped autograft was contaminated before or after decontamination measures were implemented. The results of the cultures may be useful in guiding treatment after replantation.

Some tissue banks provide services to decontaminate autologous bone skull flaps when contamination is suspected (ie, dropped autograft, head trauma, positive culture result). When sending an autograft to a tissue bank for decontamination and processing, the sending facility is not required to register with the FDA.

VI.a.2. The contaminated graft should not be subjected to the steam sterilization process. *[2: Moderate Evidence]*

The steam sterilization process denatures bone protein and may severely damage the bone structure and increase the potential for bone resorption and infection.[84] The steam sterilization process has not been validated for use with human tissue. A significantly high rate of postoperative graft infection has been found when cranial bone grafts subjected to the steam sterilization process were used for cranial reconstruction.[83]

VI.b. Perioperative team members should develop and implement measures to prevent dropped autografts. *[2: Moderate Evidence]*

In their review of 15,157 craniectomy procedures, Jankowitz and Kondziolka[122] found no consistent association between the dropping of the bone and the type of procedure, location of the surgical site, position of the patient, or activity being performed. To help prevent dropped cranial bone grafts, the researchers recommended that

- surgeons keep one hand on the flap and use the other hand to detach the dura from the bone with an instrument;
- surgeons elevate the bone by positioning themselves on the side exposed to the floor in order to direct the force of the elevation towards the surgical field and allow the excised cranial bone graft to fall onto the sterile drapes rather than the floor;
- surgeons complete the bone plating on a large surface area, such as the back table, while an assistant holds the bone;
- surgical assistants hold the flap with an instrument or position themselves to catch the cranial flap; and
- surgical team members place the bone flap directly onto the Mayo stand or back table rather than handing it to another team member.

Based on a review of the literature, Centeno et al[124] provided the following recommendations

for managing contaminated autologous grafts used in plastic surgery:
- Alert all team members during the preoperative briefing or mandatory time out that an autologous graft will be obtained, and ask that all team members be vigilant of the location of the graft at all times during the procedure.
- Place the autologous graft in a labeled container, preferably a lidded container, and keep the labeled container on the largest table in the sterile field (eg, the back table), and away from instruments and the edge of the table.
- Limit handling and exchanging of the autologous graft between personnel as much as possible.
- Include the location of the autograft in the transfer-of-care report when surgical team members are relieved during the procedure.
- Do not discard any tissue without confirmation from the surgeon.
- Include the potential for autograft contamination and replantation or autotransplantation of a decontaminated autologous graft in the informed consent. If the autologous graft is contaminated during the procedure, provide full disclosure to the patient.

Recommendation VII

Autologous tissue that will be stored within the facility or health care organization for delayed replantation or autotransplantation should be transferred from the sterile field in a manner that maintains the sterility and integrity of the tissue and prevents exposure of health care personnel to blood, body fluids, or other potentially infectious materials.

The collective evidence review found gaps in the literature related to best practices for transferring autologous tissue from the sterile field. No research studies were found that compared different methods of transferring autologous tissue from the sterile field. Further research is warranted.

The benefits associated with transferring autologous tissue from the sterile field in a manner that maintains the sterility and integrity of the tissue and prevents exposure of health care personnel to blood, body fluids, or other potentially infectious materials are the reduced potential for compromise and contamination of the tissue that could lead to replantation or autotransplantation failure or infection, and the reduced potential for exposure of health care personnel to blood, body fluids, or other potentially infectious materials. There are no harms associated with transferring autologous tissue from the sterile field in the manner recommended in this document.

VII.a. Autologous tissue that will be stored within the facility or health care organization for delayed replantation or autotransplantation should be passed off the sterile field as soon as possible. *[5: No Evidence]*

Passing the tissue off the sterile field as soon as possible reduces the potential for the integrity of the tissue to be compromised or for the tissue to be misplaced or lost.

VII.b. Autologous tissue that will be kept on the sterile field before transfer should be sequestered, identified, and monitored.[139] *[5: No Evidence]*

Isolating, identifying, and monitoring autologous tissue kept on the sterile field reduces the possibility for the tissue to be contaminated, compromised, or lost.[139]

VII.c. Autologous tissue should be kept moist until transfer from the sterile field and should not be placed on dry, absorbent surfaces or materials. *[2: Moderate Evidence]*

Air exposure can lead to desiccation of tissue.[140] Dry, absorbent surfaces or materials may adhere to the tissue.[140] Keeping tissue moist helps prevent drying of the tissue before packaging and storage.[141]

VII.d. Patient and tissue identification should be verified before tissue is transferred from the sterile field. *[2: Moderate Evidence]*

Autologous tissue transferred from the sterile field should be verbally identified by the surgeon and verified by the perioperative RN using a "write down, read back" technique.[142]

Verifying patient and tissue identification using a "write down, read back" technique during the transfer process helps prevent misidentification of the patient or tissue and minimizes the potential for labeling errors.[142]

VII.e. Perioperative personnel should use standard precautions when transferring autologous tissue from the sterile field. *[1: Strong Evidence]*

Using standard precautions represents the minimum infection prevention strategy to be applied during all patient care activities (regardless of the suspected or confirmed infection status of the patient) in any setting in which health care is delivered.[143] Implementing standard precautions when autologous tissue is transferred from the sterile field helps prevent exposure of personnel to blood, body fluids, or other potentially infectious materials.[143]

VII.f. Autologous tissue should be transferred from the sterile field by personnel using sterile technique. *[4: Benefits Balanced with Harms]*

Using sterile technique when autologous tissue is transferred from the sterile field helps to prevent microbial contamination of the tissue.[139]

VII.g. The cellular structure of the tissue should be maintained during the transfer process by not crushing, twisting, or otherwise damaging the integrity of the tissue.[139] *[4: Benefits Balanced with Harms]*

Maintaining the cellular structure of the tissue reduces the potential for replantation failure

AUTOLOGOUS TISSUE MANAGEMENT

or infection associated with tissue viability and integrity.

Recommendation VIII

Autologous tissue that will be stored within the facility or health care organization for delayed replantation or autotransplantation should be packaged and labeled in a manner that protects and secures the autograft; prevents cross-contamination and mix-ups during storage; facilitates tissue tracking; and prevents exposure of health care personnel to blood, body fluids, or other potentially infectious materials.

The collective evidence review found gaps in the literature related to best practices for packaging and labeling autologous tissue. No research studies were found that compared different packaging materials and methods of packaging and labeling autologous tissue. Further research is warranted.

The benefits associated with packaging and labeling autologous tissue are the reduced potential for mix-ups if autograft labeling methods are inadequate (eg, smudging of identifiers during cold storage, labels separating from the package) and contamination or cross-contamination if the graft's packaging material is not validated for use at the storage temperature selected. Donors of autologous tissue are usually not screened or tested for communicable diseases (eg, HIV, hepatitis B, hepatitis C, syphilis). If the packaging that contains the autograft sufficiently secures the autograft, the potential for cross-contamination of other packages stored with the autograft is reduced. There are no harms associated with packaging and labeling autologous tissue in the manner recommended in this document.

A full discussion of the requirements for packaging systems for sterilization is outside the scope of these recommendations. The reader should refer to the AORN Guideline for Selection and Use of Packaging Systems for Sterilization[144] for additional guidance related to packaging for sterilization.

VIII.a. Autologous tissue intended for delayed replantation or autotransplantation should be contained and labeled immediately after transfer from the sterile field.[139] *[2: Moderate Evidence]*

Containing and labeling autologous tissue immediately after transfer from the sterile field helps preserve the quality and integrity of the tissue and prevent contamination, damage, or loss of the autograft.[139] Correctly labeling the autologous tissue may also prevent transplantation of the tissue into an unintended recipient.

VIII.b. Packaging materials for autologous tissue must be
- leak proof and punctures resistant[145] and
- designed to prevent the introduction, transmission, or spread of communicable diseases.[3]

[1: Regulatory Requirement]

Using packaging materials and containers that are leak proof, puncture resistant,[145] and designed to prevent the introduction, transmission, or spread of communicable diseases[3] is a regulatory requirement.

VIII.c. Packaging materials for autologous tissue should be validated to meet the anticipated storage conditions and should
- maintain the integrity and stability of the autograft[139] throughout
  - preparation (eg, exposure to antibiotics or other chemicals),
  - processing (eg, cryopreservation),
  - storage (eg, -148° F [-100° C]), and
  - thawing procedures, if the autograft will be thawed in its package[6];
- not produce toxic residues;
- be large enough and of the correct size to secure the tissue[139]; and
- remain impervious to microorganisms and microscopic particles.

[2: Moderate Evidence]

Using packaging materials that are validated to meet the anticipated storage conditions is an AATB standard.[6] Validated packaging materials help maintain the tissue at the correct temperature.[146]

Verifying that containers are of the correct size to fully secure the tissue may help prevent damage to the autograft. This can also prevent leakage and help protect perioperative personnel or others who handle the container or its contents from unnecessary exposure to blood, body fluids, or other potentially infectious materials.[139]

Using packages or containers that maintain integrity and prevent contamination of the autograft helps prevent compromise of the autograft that could lead to an SSI[139] or the inability to replant or autotransplant the tissue.

VIII.c.1. Packages or containers used for storage of autologous tissue that will be frozen or cryopreserved should be able to withstand temperatures of -4° F (-20° C) or colder.[6,131] *[3: Limited Evidence]*

Frozen storage requires a packaging material that will not become brittle or break when exposed to extremely low temperatures. The minimum acceptable temperature for short-term storage of autologous tissue is -4° F (-20° C) or colder.[6,131] Long-term storage (ie, longer than six months) occurs at temperatures of -40° F (-40° C) or colder.

VIII.d. Autologous bone should not be packaged or stored in solution. *[3: Limited Evidence]*

Packaging and storing autologous bone while it is still wet or in solution may be harmful to the bone.[131]

During freezing, the graft is biologically inactive. Antibiotic solutions have no effect on bacteria.[126]

AUTOLOGOUS TISSUE MANAGEMENT

VIII.e. When autologous tissue is placed into a storage container, the perioperative RN should confirm and document
- the patient's identity using two unique identifiers (eg, patient name and medical record number) according to the facility or health care organization policy[139];
- the originating source of the tissue including laterality, if applicable;
- the type of tissue;
- the clinical diagnosis; and
- any additional pertinent clinical information.[139]

[3: Limited Evidence]

Maintaining a procedure to verify the accuracy of labels when labeling human tissue is a regulatory requirement for good tissue practice[3] and an AATB standard.[6]

VIII.f. The autograft package must be labeled
- "For Autologous Use Only,"[3,5,6]
- "Not Evaluated for Infectious Substances" (if infectious disease testing has not been performed),[3,5,6,131] and
- "Biohazard" (if infectious disease testing was performed and any results were positive, or if donor screening was performed and risk factors were identified).[3,5,145]

The package should also be labeled with an expiration date.[3,6] *[1: Regulatory Requirement]*

Autologous tissue may not have undergone culturing to detect contaminating microorganisms, and the autologous donor was likely not tested for communicable diseases. Labeling to communicate "For Autologous Use Only" and "Not Evaluated for Infectious Substances" (if infectious disease testing has not been performed),[3] biohazard information,[145] and the expiration date[3,6] are regulatory requirements. Failure to communicate biohazard information could result in exposure or injury to personnel who handle the tissue or to an unintended tissue recipient. Failure to communicate the expiration date could result in expired tissue being replanted into a patient.

VIII.g. The autograft package label should include the
- facility- or health care organization-defined unique patient identifiers (eg, patient name and medical record number)[6,131,139];
- donor classification statement "Autologous Donor"[6];
- procedure, date of recovery, and name of the surgeon[131];
- tissue type and site, including laterality if applicable[131,139];
- identity of the person who packaged and labeled the autograft[131];
- date of tissue recovery[131];
- time the autograft was placed into storage and the identity of the person placing it into storage[131];
- method of preservation, if applicable[6];
- recommended storage temperature and acceptable storage temperature range[6];
- method of decontamination and identification of any potential processing or solution residues (eg, antibiotics) if used[6]; and
- manner in which the tissue was recovered and prepared (eg, under aseptic conditions).[6]

[3: Limited Evidence]

Labeling in the manner described here is an AATB standard.[6,131] Accurate and detailed labeling may help prevent autologous tissue from being transplanted into a recipient other than the original donor.

VIII.h. Dark indelible ink should be used on autograft package labels.[131,139] *[3: Limited Evidence]*

Using dark ink improves visibility on both handwritten and electronic labels.[139] Using indelible ink helps prevent ink from being removed from the label.[139]

VIII.i. A bar-code labeling system should be used and a bar-code label applied to the package or container if the technology is available.[3] *[2: Moderate Evidence]*

Bar-code labeling systems may reduce identification errors by facilitating improved accuracy in matching tissue to the desired recipient[147,148] and may also improve the accuracy of facility or health care organization records. Bar-code labeling also may enhance tissue tracking records.

Implementing a procedure to verify the accuracy of labels for human tissue is a regulatory requirement for good tissue practice.[3]

VIII.j. Identification labels should be securely affixed to the outside of both the inner and outer package or container[131] and should not be secured to a container lid.[148] *[3: Limited Evidence]*

Labels should adhere to the packaging material under all anticipated storage conditions for the shelf-life of the tissue.[6]

Labeling the autograft package in a manner that minimizes the risk for errors is a regulatory requirement for good tissue practice[3] and an AATB standard.[6] Using both an internal and external label is recommended because the outer label may fall off or become unreadable during frozen storage (eg, smudged from condensation).[131] Placing the label on the container instead of the lid may help prevent loss of autograft information after the lid is removed from the container or if the lid becomes detached from the container.[148]

VIII.k. Autograft tissue identification and labeling should be confirmed among surgical team members during the debriefing at the end of the operative or other invasive procedure.[139] Confirmation should include
- visual confirmation that the autograft is in the container and

AUTOLOGOUS TISSUE MANAGEMENT

○ verification that the patient and autograft information on the label is correct and legible, including laterality as applicable.[139]

[4: Benefits Balanced with Harms]

Management of autologous tissue is a multidisciplinary process. Postprocedure confirmation of the autograft identification and labeling can improve communication among team members and may help to reduce or eliminate errors[130] in autologous tissue management.

Recommendation IX

Autologous tissue should be transported in a manner that protects and secures the autograft; maintains the integrity of the tissue; prevents exposure of health care personnel to blood, body fluids, or other potentially infectious materials; and ensures the confidentiality of protected patient information.

The collective evidence review found gaps in the literature related to best practices for transporting autologous tissue. No research studies were found that compared different methods of transporting autologous tissue. Further research is warranted.

The benefits associated with transporting autologous tissue in a manner that protects and secures the autograft; maintains the integrity of the tissue; prevents exposure of health care personnel to blood, body fluids, or other potentially infectious materials; and ensures the confidentiality of protected patient information are the reduced potential for compromising and contaminating the tissue that could lead to replantation or autotransplantation failure or infection; the reduced potential for exposing health care personnel to blood, body fluids, or other potentially infectious materials; and the reduced potential for violating the confidentiality of the patient's protected information. There are no harms associated with transporting autologous tissue in the manner recommended in this document.

IX.a. Autologous tissue must be transported in a manner that prevents exposure of health care personnel to blood, body fluids, or other potentially infectious materials.[145] [1: Regulatory Requirement]

Transporting tissue in a manner that prevents exposure of health care personnel to blood, body fluids, or other potentially infectious materials is a regulatory requirement.[145]

IX.b. Autologous tissue must be transported in a manner that ensures the confidentiality of protected patient information.[149] [1: Regulatory Requirement]

Ensuring the confidentiality of protected health information is a regulatory requirement and a standard of perioperative nursing care.[149-151]

IX.c. Autologous tissue must be transported in a manner that maintains the required temperature and minimizes the risk of degradation or contamination of the autograft.[3,5] [1: Regulatory Requirement]

Transporting autologous tissue in a manner that minimizes the risk of degradation or contamination of the autograft is a regulatory requirement for good tissue practice.[3,5]

Maintaining the tissue at the required temperatures during transport reduces the potential for the autograft to become degraded or contaminated. Degradation of the autograft may increase the potential for an adverse reaction and unexpected outcome for the patient.

IX.d. Devices intended for transport of specimens must be labeled with biohazard information.[145] [1: Regulatory Requirement]

Labeling to communicate biohazard information is a regulatory requirement.[145] Failure to communicate biohazard information could result in exposure of personnel handling the autograft package to blood, body fluids, or other potentially infectious materials.

Recommendation X

Autologous tissue intended for delayed replantation or autotransplantation should be stored in a manner that protects and secures the autograft, prevents cross-contamination and mix-ups during storage, and prevents exposure of health care personnel to blood, body fluids, or other potentially infectious materials.

The collective evidence review found gaps in the literature related to best practices for storage of autologous tissue. No research studies were found that compared different storage methods for autologous tissue. Further research is warranted.

The benefits of storing autologous tissue in a manner that protects and secures the autograft, prevents cross-contamination and mix-ups during storage, and prevents exposure of health care personnel to blood, body fluids, or other potentially infectious materials are the reduced potential for compromise and contamination of the tissue that could lead to replantation or autotransplantation failure or infection; the reduced potential for distributing the tissue to an unintended recipient; and the reduced potential for exposing health care personnel to blood, body fluids, or other potentially infectious materials. There are no harms associated with storing autologous tissue in the manner recommended in this document.

X.a. Autologous tissue intended for delayed replantation or autotransplantation must be stored in a manner that prevents exposure of health care personnel to blood, body fluids, or other potentially infectious materials.[145] [1: Regulatory Requirement]

Preventing exposure of health care personnel to blood, body fluids, or other potentially infectious materials is a regulatory requirement.[145]

X.b. Autologous tissue that will be stored within the facility or health care organization for delayed

AUTOLOGOUS TISSUE MANAGEMENT

replantation or autotransplantation must be stored in an area that is controlled to prevent mix-ups, contamination, and cross-contamination of tissue and the potential for tissue to be incorrectly distributed.[3,5,6] *[1: Regulatory Requirement]*

Storing tissue in a controlled area that reduces the potential for tissue contamination or incorrect distribution is a regulatory requirement for good tissue practice[3,5] and an AATB standard.[6]

X.c. Tissue from two or more donors must not be comingled.[3,5,6] *[1: Regulatory Requirement]*

Combining tissue from two or more donors in the same package or container increases the potential for introducing, transmitting, or spreading communicable diseases.

X.d. Autologous tissue should be separated from allografts.[6] *[3: Limited Evidence]*

Tissue from an autologous donor is usually not tested for contaminating microorganisms, and autologous donors are usually not screened or tested for communicable diseases. Separating autologous tissue from allografts minimizes the potential for autologous tissue to be transplanted into a patient who is not the donor.

X.d.1. Autografts and allografts may be stored in the same refrigerator or freezer if
- they are stored separately (eg, allografts stored on the upper shelves and autografts stored on the lower shelves, allografts and autografts placed in separate storage bins),
- they are packaged using validated packaging materials,
- they are prominently labeled, and
- the correct storage conditions exist for all items in the refrigerator or freezer.

[5: No Evidence]

Using separate storage areas or bins and providing prominent, easy-to-identify labels helps perioperative personal distinguish between the containers and reduces the potential for error.

Using validated packaging materials and ensuring the correct storage conditions exist for all items in the refrigerator or freezer helps ensure the tissue is maintained in optimal condition for replantation or autotransplantation.

X.e. The number of autografts in storage should be inventoried according to an established schedule, and autografts should be removed and discarded by the expiration date. *[4: Benefits Balanced with Harms]*

Inventorying the number of autografts in storage and removing and discarding expired autografts helps ensure autografts are maintained in optimal storage conditions for successful replantation or autotransplantation and helps prevent replantation or autotransplantation of potentially compromised tissue.

X.f. Autologous tissue that may have been compromised should be removed from storage[152,153] and discarded and should not be replanted or autotransplanted. *[4: Benefits Balanced with Harms]*

Removing from storage and discarding autologous tissue that may have been compromised (eg, exposed to incorrect storage temperatures) helps ensure potentially compromised tissue is not replanted or autotransplanted into a patient. Replanting or autotransplanting compromised tissue could lead to serious patient injury.

X.g. Autologous tissue must be stored at temperatures that will prevent contamination or degradation of the tissue.[3,5] Storage temperatures
○ must be maintained and periodically reviewed to ensure that temperatures are within acceptable limits[3,5,6] and
○ should be established in accordance with federal and state regulations and AATB standards.[6]

[1: Regulatory Requirement]

Maintaining storage temperatures within recommended parameters helps ensure that autografts are maintained in optimal condition for successful replantation or autotransplantation.

X.h. Autologous bone should be stored at -4° F (-20° C) or colder for six months or less.[6] *[3: Limited Evidence]*

Autologous bone may be stored at -40° F (-40° C) or colder for up to five years; however, this is considered long-term storage and may require registering with the FDA as a tissue establishment.[6,131]

Storage at -40° F (-40° C) or colder is preferred because tissue enzymes may be active at temperatures warmer than -40° F (-40° C) and may negatively affect tissue if it is stored for an extended time. Temperatures of -94° F (-70° C) or colder may prevent enzymatic destruction of tissue.[131]

Maintaining the storage temperature below -40° F (-40° C) may also be a "buffer" that provides additional time before critical temperatures are reached in the event of a freezer malfunction.[131]

X.i. Autologous skin should be stored between 32° F to 50° F (0° C to 10° C) for no longer than 14 days.[6] *[2: Moderate Evidence]*

Refrigerated skin should be submerged in a storage medium, and the storage medium should be changed every 72 hours.[113]

Refrigeration retards autolysis and helps prevent bacterial proliferation.[117] Keeping the skin submerged helps prevent dehydration of the tissue. Changing the storage medium every 72 hours may help to prevent microbial growth and improve skin autograft viability.[113,114]

Cram and Domayer[114] stored split-thickness autologous skin grafts from 32 patients in 100 mL Roswell Park Memorial Institute 1640 culture medium supplemented with 25 units/mL penicillin and 25 mcg/mL streptomycin. The skin grafts were stored in a refrigerator at 39.2° F (4° C) for 22 days. The storage medium was changed every three to four days during the storage period. The grafts were rinsed with normal saline solution before autotransplantation. The authors found that 75% of the grafts (n = 24) were successfully engrafted. They concluded that skin autografts could be stored up to 22 days using this technique.

In a quasi-experimental study conducted to evaluate the effects of storage solutions, temperature and the changing of storage media on skin graft anatomy as an indicator of graft viability, Robb et al[113] retrieved split-thickness human skin grafts from cadaveric donors and grafted them to circumferential, full-thickness skin wounds on mice. After three months, samples of the human skin (N = 149) were recovered from the mice and divided into four groups:

- Group 1: normal saline solution,
- Group 2: normal saline solution changed every three days,
- Group 3: Eagle's minimum essential medium, and
- Group 4: Eagle's minimum essential medium changed every three days.

All sample groups were stored at either room temperature, or in a refrigerator at 39.2° F (4° C) for five, 10, or 21 days. The results showed that skin stored in Eagle's minimum essential medium maintained better histological anatomy than skin stored in normal saline solution. There was also better preservation of skin anatomy after storage at room temperature for 21 days with media changes every three days when compared with changed and unchanged media stored at 39.2° F (4° C). The researchers concluded that storage at room temperature and the increased nutrients in the Eagle's minimum essential medium maintained increased viability of the human skin samples; however, despite replenishment of storage media every three days, the skin samples were no longer viable after 21 days.

X.j. Autologous veins should be stored between 32° F to 50° F (0° C to 10° C) for no longer than 14 days. *[2: Moderate Evidence]*

Refrigerated veins should be submerged in storage medium, and the storage medium should be changed every 72 hours.

Keeping the veins submerged helps prevent dehydration of the tissue. Changing the storage medium every 72 hours may help to prevent microbial growth and improve autograft viability.[114,113]

X.k. Autografts that are to be frozen should be frozen within a few hours of recovery.[131] *[3: Limited Evidence]*

Warm tissue is a medium for bacterial growth. Freezing the tissue within a few hours of recovery helps decrease the potential for microbial contamination that may lead to an SSI.

X.l. Autologous tissue that will not be immediately transported to the storage area should be temporarily stored in a manner that maintains autograft integrity. *[3: Limited Evidence]*

Equipment (eg, refrigerators, freezers) or devices used for transport or temporary storage (eg, coolers) should maintain tissue at the AATB recommended temperature.[6]

Maintaining optimal integrity of autologous tissue and ensuring the autograft is maintained at the recommended temperature may help prevent degradation of the autograft.

X.m. Documentation should be provided when autologous tissue is placed into the refrigerator or freezer for storage. Documentation should include

- the facility- or health care organization-defined unique identifiers (eg, patient name and medical record number);
- the procedure, date of the procedure, and name of the surgeon[131];
- the date and time of tissue storage and the identity of the person placing it into storage[131];
- whether the tissue was cultured[131]; and
- any additional pertinent clinical information (eg, increased potential for autograft contamination because of trauma).[131]

[3: Limited Evidence]

Documentation as described here is recommended by the AATB.[131]

X.n. Equipment and devices used for storage of autologous tissue must be cleaned, sanitized, and maintained according to an established schedule to prevent malfunctions, contamination or cross-contamination, or other events that may result in the introduction, transmission, or spread of communicable diseases.[3,5,6] *[1: Regulatory Requirement]*

Cleaning, sanitizing, and maintaining equipment and devices used for storage of autologous tissue is a regulatory requirement[3,5] and an AATB standard.[6]

X.n.1. Records of cleaning and sanitation, including cleaning and sanitation methods used, cleaning schedule, and personnel responsible for cleaning and sanitation, must be retained for three years after the record is created.[3,5] *[1: Regulatory Requirement]*

Retaining cleaning and sanitation records for three years after the record is created is a regulatory requirement.[3,5]

AUTOLOGOUS TISSUE MANAGEMENT

X.o. Refrigerators and freezers used for storage of autologous tissue must have regular calibration checks in accordance with the manufacturer's written instructions for use.[3,5] *[1: Regulatory Requirement]*

Performing regular calibration checks on equipment used for storage of autologous tissue is a regulatory requirement[3,5] and an AATB standard.[6] Performing regular calibration checks helps ensure that tissue is being stored at the correct temperatures.[146]

X.o.1. Maintenance, calibration, and other activities performed on refrigerators and freezers used for storage of autologous tissue must be documented, and the records must be readily available.[3,5] *[1: Regulatory Requirement]*

Documentation and availability of records related to maintenance and calibration of refrigerators and freezers used for storage of autologous tissue is a regulatory requirement.[3,5]

X.p. Freezers and refrigerators used for storage of autologous tissue should provide continuous temperature monitoring[6,131,152,153] and should
- be monitored regularly with daily temperature checks recorded[152,153];
- have an alert or alarm system[131,152,153] that notifies personnel when the temperature is not within the acceptable range; and
- have an emergency power system.

[3: Limited Evidence]

Daily temperature checks of refrigerators and freezers used for storage of autologous tissue is an accreditation standard.[152,153] Maintaining the recommended temperatures for storage of tissue helps ensure tissue integrity. Temperature fluctuations outside of the recommended temperature range may render the tissue unsafe for replantation or autotransplantation.

X.p.1. The alert or alarm system should
- sound in an area where an individual is present at all times to initiate corrective action or
- notify personnel who are available to respond.

[4: Benefits Balanced with Harms]

Temperature fluctuations outside of the recommended temperature range may require rapid corrective action to prevent compromise or degradation of tissue intended for replantation or autotransplantation.

X.q. Processes should be established for
- maintaining the temperature and integrity of stored autologous tissues in the event of a refrigerator or freezer malfunction (eg, transferring tissue to another storage unit)[6,152,153] and
- responding to a malfunction of the refrigerator or freezer that occurs when the facility is closed or when the area where the tissue is stored is unoccupied.

[3: Limited Evidence]

Maintaining the recommended temperatures for storage of tissue helps ensure the tissue is not compromised. Temperature fluctuations outside of the recommended temperature range may render the tissue unsafe for replantation or autotransplantation.

X.q.1. Autologous tissue should not be stored on-site if the facility or health care organization does not have the capability of monitoring storage conditions when the facility is closed or when the area where the tissue is stored is unoccupied. *[4: Benefits Balanced with Harms]*

Temperature fluctuations outside of the recommended temperature range may require rapid corrective action to prevent compromise or degradation of tissue intended for replantation or autotransplantation.

Recommendation XI

Autologous tissue intended for replantation or autotransplantation should be handled using sterile technique and in a manner that protects and secures the autograft from damage or contamination.

The collective evidence review found gaps in the literature related to best practices for handling autologous tissue. No research studies were found that compared different protocols for handling autologous tissue. Further research is warranted.

The benefits of handling autologous tissue using sterile technique and in a manner that protects and secures the autograft are that it may help prevent compromise or contamination that may render the autograft unacceptable for replantation or autotransplantation and may decrease the patient's risk for SSI. There are no harms associated with handling autologous tissue in the manner recommended in this document.

XI.a. Autologous tissue management should be assessed and planned among surgical team members during the preoperative briefing before operative or other invasive procedures. *[2: Moderate Evidence]*

Management of autologous tissue is a multidisciplinary process. Collaborative preprocedural assessment and planning may improve efficiency and communication among team members and may help to reduce or eliminate errors[154] in autologous tissue management.

XI.b. Autologous tissue must be released only for replantation or autotransplantation in the donor.[3,6] *[1: Regulatory Requirement]*

Autologous tissue is not tested for infectious organisms or diseases, so release to another recipient could cause serious injury.

XI.b.1. The facility- or health care organization-defined unique identifiers (eg, patient name

AUTOLOGOUS TISSUE MANAGEMENT

and medical record number) should be used to verify autologous donor identity for release of autologous tissue. *[4: Benefits Balanced with Harms]*

Using unique identifiers to verify donor identity may help to reduce the potential for errors in donor patient identification.

XI.b.2. Bar-coding technology should be used if available.[3] *[2: Moderate Evidence]*

Bar-code labeling systems may reduce identification errors by facilitating improved accuracy in matching tissue to the desired recipient[147,148] and may also improve the accuracy of facility or health care organization and patient records.

XI.b.3. Removal of the autograft from storage should be documented. *[3: Limited Evidence]*

Documentation should include the date and time of removal and the identity of the person removing the tissue.[131] Documentation as described here is recommended by the AATB.[131]

XI.c. Autologous tissue should not be released for replantation or autotransplantation until all handling criteria (ie, processing, labeling, storage, cultures) have been verified and determined to be satisfactory for release. *[4: Benefits Balanced with Harms]*

Verifying criteria for release helps minimize the potential for errors.

XI.c.1. Autologous tissue that does not meet the release criteria should be considered compromised and should not be used. *[4: Benefits Balanced with Harms]*

Replantation or autotransplantation of compromised tissue could cause serious injury.

XI.d. The perioperative RN should review the culture results for stored autografts before the autograft is replanted or autotransplanted.[131] *[2: Moderate Evidence]*

Collecting health data relevant to the patient's situation is necessary to inform other health care professionals involved in the patient's care.[150]

XI.d.1. If the culture result is positive, a multidisciplinary team consisting of the surgeon, perioperative RN, and infection preventionist should determine whether or not the autograft will be replanted or autotransplanted. *[3: Limited Evidence]*

Chiang et al[155] conducted a prospective cohort study in a university hospital to identify the prevalence of bone flaps with positive cultures and to assess the risk of SSI after replantation of bone flaps with positive cultures. Nursing personnel swabbed all surfaces of the cranial bone flaps of 372 neurosurgery patients undergoing craniectomy procedures between November 1, 2007, and November 30, 2008, and submitted the swab cultures for aerobic and anaerobic testing before soaking the flap in 500 mL normal saline solution supplemented with 50,000 units bacitracin. The bone flaps were then either replanted during the same procedure or wrapped in a sterile towel, labeled with the patient's identifiers, placed into a sterile freezer bag, and cryopreserved at -94° F (-70° C) or colder until the time of replantation. The researchers did not specify how long the bone flaps were soaked before replantation or packaging for cryopreservation and storage.

The researchers found that 50% of the bone flaps were contaminated with microorganisms (n = 186). The microorganisms were primarily skin flora such as *Propionibacterium acnes*, coagulase negative staphylococci, and *Staphylococcus aureus*. Replanting the bone flaps with positive culture results did not increase the patient's risk for infection. The researchers concluded that cranial bone flaps with low numbers of skin flora contaminants could be safely replanted. The researchers did not specify what were considered "low numbers of skin flora." The researchers also found that the risk of SSI increased when the preoperative skin antiseptics were not allowed to dry, and they concluded that operative factors were more important than low numbers of skin flora contaminating the cranial bone flap in the pathogenesis of SSI after craniectomy procedures.[156]

XI.d.2. If a decision is made to replant or autotransplant the tissue, the multidisciplinary team should determine whether any disinfection measures (eg, prophylactic antibiotics, extensive rinsing with or without pulsatile lavage) will be applied to the autograft.[131] *[3: Limited Evidence]*

Autologous tissue management is a multidisciplinary process. Collaborative discussion and decision making may improve patient outcomes.

XI.e. Frozen bone autografts should be removed from the freezer after the surgeon has confirmed the autograft will be replanted or autotransplanted.[131] *[3: Limited Evidence]*

Removing the frozen autograft after the surgeon has confirmed it will be replanted or autotransplanted helps prevent unnecessary thawing and refreezing of autografts.

XI.f. The perioperative RN and a scrubbed team member should verify the contents of the autologous tissue package, patient and tissue identification, expiration date, and other pertinent information

AUTOLOGOUS TISSUE MANAGEMENT

before the tissue is transferred to the sterile field. *[4: Benefits Balanced with Harms]*

Verifying identification of the autologous tissue during the transfer process minimizes opportunities for error and helps prevent misidentification of the autograft.

XI.g. Frozen bone autografts should be removed from their packages using sterile technique and placed into
- a sterile basin filled with warm (ie, 98.6° F to 105.8° F [37° C to 41° C]), sterile normal saline or lactated Ringer's solution for 15 to 20 minutes or
- an empty sterile basin and allowed to thaw at room temperature for a minimum of 30 minutes before replantation or autotransplantation.[131]

[3: Limited Evidence]

Using sterile technique to remove autografts from their packages may help to prevent contamination of the autograft. Complete thawing of the frozen autograft reduces bone brittleness.[131] Antibiotics added to the irrigation fluid may not be effective because the autograft contains lipids, red blood cells, and other proteins that may neutralize the intended activity of the antibiotics.[131]

XI.h. Before replantation or autotransplantation, the autograft should be rinsed at least three times with sterile normal saline or lactated Ringer's solution.[131] *[3: Limited Evidence]*

The volume of fluid used should be at least 10 times the volume of the autograft.[131]

Rinsing may remove surface contamination. Rinsing as described here is recommended by the AATB.[131]

XI.i. The date and time of replantation or autotransplantation, the procedure used to prepare the autograft, and the names and titles of all individuals involved in preparing the autograft should be documented in the patient's record.[131] *[3: Limited Evidence]*

Documentation as described here is recommended by the AATB.[131]

XI.j. Autologous bone grafts may be refrozen if necessary (eg, an autograft thawed for replantation that is then not replanted).[131] *[3: Limited Evidence]*

A multidisciplinary team consisting of the surgeon, perioperative RN, and infection preventionist should conduct a risk assessment to consider the benefits and potential harms associated with replanting refrozen bone compared with other treatment options (eg, discarding the graft and using artificial material) and to determine the number of acceptable freeze-thaw cycles.

Refreezing autologous bone may allow it to be used for cranioplasty; however, additional freeze-thaw cycles may increase the patient's risk for SSI.[131]

XI.j.1. If a decision is made to refreeze the bone graft, cell remnants and nonviable cells within the thawed bone graft should be removed using pulsatile lavage followed by a series of 30-minute soaks in a warm, sterile isotonic solution at a volume 10 times that of the autograft and then rinsing.[131] *[3: Limited Evidence]*

Bone marrow and red blood cell remnants and nonviable cells may be present within the cancellous bone of an autologous bone graft that has been thawed after frozen storage.[131] The cell remnants and nonviable cells may be recognized by the donor's immune system at the time of replantation or autotransplantation and may increase the potential for an inflammatory or immune system response.[131]

XI.k. In the event the autograft is not replanted or autotransplanted and is transferred to another facility or discarded, documentation must be provided so that the autograft can be traced to its final disposition.[3,5,6] *[1: Regulatory Requirement]*

Traceability of the autograft to its final disposition and retention of records related to disposition of autologous tissue are regulatory requirements[3,5] and AATB standards.[6]

XI.l. If it becomes necessary to transfer the autograft to another facility, an AATB-accredited tissue source facility should be contacted for assistance with packaging and shipping.[131] *[3: Limited Evidence]*

Personnel at an AATB-accredited tissue bank can offer expert assistance with packaging and shipping autologous tissue.

XI.l.1. Facilities or health care organizations that distribute autologous tissue to another facility at a different address are required to register with the FDA as a tissue establishment that manufactures human cells, tissues, and cellular and tissue-based products and to follow applicable requirements of 21 CFR Part 1271.[3,5] *[1: Regulatory Requirement]*

Transferring tissue to another facility is considered distribution. The requirement for registration as a tissue establishment exists even if distribution occurs only rarely.[3,5]

XI.m. Autologous human tissue must be treated as biohazardous waste and disposed of in accordance with local and state regulations.[145] *[1: Regulatory Requirement]*

Local and state regulations related to disposal of human tissue vary. Disposal of human tissue as biohazardous waste helps prevent exposure of health care personnel to blood, body fluids, or other potentially infectious materials.

XI.m.1. A multidisciplinary team consisting of surgeons, perioperative RNs, pathology laboratory representatives, infection preventionists,

AUTOLOGOUS TISSUE MANAGEMENT

risk management personnel, and other involved stakeholders should develop a plan for disposal of autologous tissue that addresses the need to contact the patient or patient's legal representative, the patient's cultural preferences, and any requests for release of autologous tissue for burial or cremation before disposal. *[4: Benefits Balanced with Harms]*

Management of autologous tissue is a multidisciplinary process. Collaborative discussion and decision making may improve outcomes.

XI.m.2. Facilities that distribute autologous tissue for burial or cremation are not required to register with the FDA as a tissue establishment.

The facility would meet the exception from registration described in section 1271.15(b), in which storage of tissue for autologous use is exempt as long as no other manufacturing controls are performed (ie, subjecting the autograft to the steam sterilization process, distributing the autograft to another facility).[3,4]

Recommendation XII

Policies and procedures for managing autologous tissue must be developed, reviewed periodically, revised as necessary, and readily available in the practice setting.[3,5,6,152,153,156]

Establishing and maintaining policies and procedures for managing autologous tissue is a regulatory requirement[3,5] and an AATB[6] and accreditation agency standard.[152,153,156]

Policies and procedures assist in the development of patient safety, quality assessment, and performance improvement activities. Policies and procedures establish authority, responsibility, and accountability within the organization. Policies and procedures also serve as operational guidelines used to minimize patient risk for injury or complications, standardize practice, direct perioperative personnel, and establish continuous performance improvement programs.

XII.a. Policies and procedures for autologous tissue management must designate personnel responsible for oversight of autologous tissue and with authority and accountability for all activities performed.[3,5,6,152,153] *[1: Regulatory Requirement]*

Centralized oversight of all aspects of autologous tissue management helps ensure that tissue is
- safe for replantation or autotransplantation;
- managed in compliance with regulatory requirements;
- monitored on an ongoing basis;
- packaged, transported, stored, and handled according to standardized processes; and
- able to be traced to the original source and recalled, if necessary.

Review and approval of all procedures related to autologous tissue management and designation of the personnel responsible for oversight is a regulatory requirement[3,5] and an AATB[6] and accreditation standard.[152,153]

XII.a.1. A physician or medical advisory committee should be available to provide direction for medical decisions.[6] *[3: Limited Evidence]*

The AATB recommends that a medical director be appointed for oversight.[6]

XII.b. Policies and procedures for managing autologous tissue must be designed to decrease the risk of introducing, transmitting, or spreading communicable diseases (ie, diseases transmitted by viruses, bacteria, fungi, parasites, and transmissible spongiform encephalopathy agents).[3,5] *[1: Regulatory Requirement]*

Developing policies and procedures for tracking, storing, and handling autologous tissue and investigating adverse reactions is a regulatory requirement[3,5] and an AATB[6] and accreditation agency standard.[152,153,156]

XII.c. Policies and procedures for autologous tissue management should be developed by a multidisciplinary team that includes infection preventionists, risk management personnel, pathology laboratory representatives, perioperative RNs, and other stakeholders (eg, surgeons who replant or autotransplant tissue). *[4: Benefits Balanced with Harms]*

Management of autologous tissue is a multidisciplinary process. Collaborative discussion and decision making may improve patient outcomes.

XII.c.1. Policies and procedures related to autologous tissue management may include processes for
- providing care for patients who have sustained traumatic tooth avulsion injuries, including immediate replantation or storage of the tooth in a storage medium;
- providing care for patients who may be undergoing recovery, replantation, or autotransplantation of autologous tissue;
- transferring autologous tissue from the sterile field;
- packaging and labeling autologous tissue;
- transporting autologous tissue;
- preserving and storing autologous tissue;
- determining the maximum storage duration of autologous tissue and ensuring tissue is not replanted or autotransplanted beyond its expiration date;
- cleaning and sanitizing equipment or devices used to transport or store autologous tissue;
- maintaining and monitoring equipment used to store autologous tissue;
- responding to alarms and malfunction of equipment used to store autologous tissue and designating the personnel who are responsible for responding;

- monitoring temperatures of stored autologous tissue;
- maintaining tissue at required temperatures during storage equipment malfunction or a power outage;
- handling autologous tissue using sterile technique;
- culturing autologous tissue;
- thawing frozen autologous tissue;
- determining whether or not contaminated autologous tissue will be replanted or autotransplanted;
- refreezing autologous bone;
- transferring or releasing autologous tissue to another facility or a funeral home[131];
- discarding autologous tissue[131];
- documenting activities related to autologous tissue management;
- responding to and investigating adverse reactions related to autologous tissue[152,153]; and
- determining individual roles and responsibilities.

[4: Benefits Balanced with Harms]

Developing and maintaining policies and procedures that guide and support patient care, treatment, and services is a regulatory requirement[157,158] and an accreditation agency standard[159-162] for both hospitals and ambulatory settings.

Recommendation XIII

Perioperative team members should receive initial and ongoing education and complete competency verification activities on the principles and processes of autologous tissue management.

It is the responsibility of the health care organization to provide initial and ongoing education and to evaluate the competency of perioperative team members to deliver safe care to patients undergoing operative or other invasive procedures.[151]

Initial and ongoing education of perioperative personnel related to autologous tissue management facilitates the development of knowledge, skills, and attitudes that affect safe patient care. Periodic education programs provide the opportunity to reinforce the principles and processes of autologous tissue management and to introduce relevant new equipment or practices. Competency verification measures individual performance, provides a mechanism for documentation, and helps verify that perioperative personnel have an understanding of the principles and processes of autologous tissue management.

XIII.a. Education related to autologous tissue management may include a review of the policies and procedures for
- providing care for patients who have sustained traumatic tooth avulsion injuries, including immediate replantation or storage of the tooth in an effective storage medium;
- providing care for patients who may be undergoing recovery, replantation, or autotransplantation of autologous tissue;
- transferring autologous tissue from the sterile field;
- packaging and labeling autologous tissue;
- transporting autologous tissue;
- preserving and storing autologous tissue;
- determining maximum storage duration of autologous tissue and ensuring tissue is not replanted or autotransplanted beyond its expiration date;
- cleaning and sanitizing equipment or devices used to transport or store autologous tissue;
- maintaining and monitoring equipment used to store autologous tissue;
- responding to alarms and malfunction of equipment used to store autologous tissue;
- monitoring temperatures of stored autologous tissue;
- maintaining tissue at required temperatures during storage equipment malfunction or power outage;
- handling autologous tissue using sterile technique;
- culturing autologous tissue;
- thawing frozen autologous tissue;
- determining whether or not contaminated autologous tissue will be replanted or autotransplanted;
- refreezing autologous bone;
- transferring or releasing autologous tissue to another facility or a funeral home[131];
- discarding autologous tissue[131];
- documenting activities related to autologous tissue management;
- responding to and investigating adverse reactions related to autologous tissue[152,153]; and
- determining individual roles and responsibilities.

[4: Benefits Balanced with Harms]

Ongoing development of knowledge and skills and documentation of personnel participation is a regulatory requirement[157,158] and an accreditation agency standard[163-166] for both hospitals and ambulatory settings.

Recommendation XIV

Nursing activities related to autologous tissue management should be documented in a manner consistent with facility or health care organization policies and procedures, regulatory requirements,[3,5] AORN guidelines,[150] and accreditation agency[152,153,156] and AATB standards.[6]

Documentation of nursing activities serves as the legal record of care delivery. Documentation of nursing activities is dictated by facility or health care organization policy, regulatory requirements, accreditation agency standards, and professional guidelines. Documentation is necessary to inform other health care professionals involved in the patient's care. Perioperative documentation that accurately reflects the patient's

AUTOLOGOUS TISSUE MANAGEMENT

experience is essential for the continuity of outcome-focused nursing care and for effective comparison of realized versus anticipated patient outcomes.[150] Highly reliable data collection is not only necessary to chronicle patient responses to nursing interventions, but also to demonstrate the facility or health care organization's progress toward quality care outcomes.[150]

XIV.a. Nursing activities related to autologous tissue management must be documented.[3,5] *[1: Regulatory Requirement]*

Maintaining records related to autologous tissue management is a regulatory requirement[3,5] and an accreditation agency[152,153,156] and AATB standard.[6]

XIV.a.1. Tracking of autologous tissue from its source to its final destination must be included in documentation related to autologous tissue management.[3,5,6,152,153] *[1: Regulatory Requirement]*

Traceability of the autograft to its final disposition and retention of records related to disposition of autologous tissue are regulatory requirements[3,5] and AATB standards.[6]

XIV.a.2. Documentation related to autologous tissue management should include
- a listing of all autologous tissue stored and used[152,153];
- records of informed consent;
- information on
  - recovery,
  - processing,
  - preservation,
  - labeling,
  - storage,
  - tissue culture results, and
  - release or transfer of autologous tissue[152,153];
- dates and times of autologous tissue preparation and the identities of personnel preparing the tissue for preservation;
- dates and times of autologous tissue storage and retrieval and the identities of personnel storing and retrieving tissue;
- quality assurance records; and
- information about transfer or disposal of tissue.

[4: Benefits Balanced with Harms]

Effective management and collection of health care information that accurately reflects the patient's care, treatment, and services is a regulatory requirement[157,158] and an accreditation agency standard[167-170] for both hospitals and ambulatory settings.

XIV.a.3. Records related to autologous tissue must be maintained for a minimum of 10 years after the tissue is dispensed or expired, whichever is longer.[3,5] *[1: Regulatory Requirement]*

Maintaining records related to autologous tissue for 10 years is a regulatory requirement[3,5] and an AATB[6] and accreditation agency standard.[152,153]

Recommendation XV

Perioperative personnel should participate in a variety of quality assurance and performance improvement activities that are consistent with the facility or health care organization plan to improve understanding of and compliance with the principles and processes of autologous tissue management.

Quality assurance and performance improvement programs assist in evaluating and improving the quality of patient care and formulating plans for corrective actions. These programs provide data that may be used to determine whether an individual organization is within benchmark goals and, if not, to identify areas that may require corrective actions.

XV.a. A quality assurance program must be maintained to prevent the introduction, transmission, or spread of communicable disease during every step of the autologous tissue management process.[3] *[1: Regulatory Requirement]*

Maintaining a quality assurance program to prevent the introduction, transmission, or spread of communicable disease during every step of the autologous tissue management process is a regulatory requirement[3] and an AATB[6] and accreditation agency standard.[152,153]

XV.a.1. The quality assurance program should prevent contamination, avoid mix-ups, and promote tissue tracking and investigation and reporting of adverse reactions.[6] *[3: Limited Evidence]*

Maintaining a quality improvement program to prevent contamination, avoid mix-ups, and promote tissue tracking and investigation and reporting of adverse reactions is an AATB standard.[6]

XV.a.2. The quality assurance program for autologous tissue management should
- establish a multidisciplinary committee to perform a baseline assessment of the processes (eg, to verify alignment with federal regulations and AATB and accreditation agency standards)[152,153];
- provide at least annual program reviews to monitor ongoing compliance with regulations and safe autologous tissue management processes[152,153];
- identify quality indicators including
  - tissue-handling protocols,
  - labeling procedures,
  - storage requirements,
  - criteria for release of tissue,
  - verification processes, and
  - record maintenance;
- measure compliance with established policies and procedures; and

- mandate investigation and reporting of adverse reactions and events.

[4: Benefits Balanced with Harms]

Collecting data to monitor and improve patient care, treatment, and services is a regulatory requirement[157,158] and an accreditation agency standard[171-174] for both hospitals and ambulatory settings.

XV.a.3. Performance improvement activities for autologous tissue management should include
- monitoring personnel for compliance with safe practices for autologous tissue management,
- periodically reviewing and evaluating activities to identify the need for improvement,
- identifying corrective actions directed toward improvement priorities, and
- taking additional actions when improvement is not achieved or sustained.

[4: Benefits Balanced with Harms]

Reviewing and evaluating quality assurance and performance improvement activities may identify failure points that contribute to errors in autologous tissue management and help define actions for improvement and increased competency.

Taking corrective actions may improve patient safety by enhancing understanding of and compliance with safe practices for autologous tissue management.

XV.b. Perioperative personnel who may be involved in culturing autologous tissue should participate in quality assurance and performance improvement activities related to effective methods of culturing autologous tissue. [2: Moderate Evidence]

The collective evidence indicates that autologous tissue culture results may identify tissue that is not acceptable for replantation or autotransplantation and also provide a baseline for evaluation of processing and storage; however, there is a need to optimize and standardize quality monitoring of autologous tissue and culture methods and protocols.[102] Swab cultures are commonly used to determine the level and identity of microbial growth on a surface. They are convenient and easy to use; however, they may pose potential problems when used for identifying and determining the number of microorganisms on autologous tissue.

Surface swab cultures may have limited sensitivity and specificity even when transferred to culture media for incubation.[175] A negative culture result does not mean the autograft is sterile; likewise, a positive culture does not necessarily indicate that the autograft cannot be replanted.[155] Swab cultures are prone to error as a result of variation in the way the swab is manipulated.[175] It is possible that all of the microorganisms on the surface of the tissue being cultured will not be collected by the swab.[175] In addition, some of the microorganisms that are collected may become trapped in the matrix of the swab itself, not transferred to the culture medium, and not detected.[175]

The ability of the swab to recover microorganisms is dependent on its ability to pick up viable microorganisms from the surface of the item being swabbed and to release those microorganisms from the swab into the culture medium.[176] The swab tip may be relatively small compared with the surface area of an autograft. If the existing amount of bioburden is low, it reduces the potential for the swab to collect all microorganisms on the surface.[177]

Liquid culture methods involving a tissue wash may be more effective. The tissue is submerged in solution, and a portion of the solution is aspirated and incubated in culture medium for a defined period of time.[178] Further research is warranted on best methods for determining microbial presence on autologous tissue and the implications of microorganisms on autologous tissue that will be replanted or autotransplanted into the patient.

The limitations of the evidence are that using different methods of culturing or culturing different tissues may have resulted in different outcomes.

The benefit of culturing tissue to determine the level and identity of microbial growth on autologous tissue surfaces is that it may allow for more effective and directed antibiotic therapy to prevent or treat infection. The harm associated with culturing tissue to determine the level and identity of microbial growth on autologous tissue surfaces is that the patient may receive unnecessary antibiotics or other treatments to prevent infection.

Aggarwal et al[179] prospectively compared the effectiveness of tissue and swab cultures in diagnosing periprosthetic joint infections. The samples were collected during a consecutive series of 156 septic and aseptic arthroplasty revisions from October 2011 through April 2012. Three tissue and three swab cultures were taken in a standardized manner from identical regions of the joint. The tissue samples, approximately 1 cm3 in size, were obtained using sterile instruments and placed directly into sterile specimen containers. The researchers found that
- the tissue cultures were positive in 28 of 30 septic cases (93%),
- the swab cultures were positive in 21 of 30 septic cases (70%),
- the tissue cultures were positive in two of 87 aseptic cases (2%), and
- the swab cultures were positive in 10 of 87 aseptic cases (11%).

The researchers concluded that tissue samples demonstrated higher sensitivity for diagnosing periprosthetic joint infections than swab cultures. The swab cultures had more false-negative and false-positive results than the tissue cultures. The researchers recommended against the use of swab cultures for intraoperative tissue cultures because they posed a higher risk of not identifying or of incorrectly identifying infective organisms.[179]

In a quasi-experimental study, Dennis et al[178] evaluated allograft tissue from 78 musculoskeletal donors by concurrently testing for microorganisms using liquid and swab culture methods. The swab cultures were obtained using a single swab from the surface of the long bones, medullary canal, and joint soft tissue. The liquid cultures were obtained by immersion of the tissue in 4,000 mL of sterile normal saline solution for 10 minutes and then shaking for one minute. A portion of the rinse solution (10 mL) was then injected into a culture medium. The results showed that the swab method detected four of 20 organisms (20%) while the liquid culture method detected 18 of 20 organisms (90%). The researchers concluded that the liquid culture method was superior to the swab method; however, further research was warranted to determine the best method for obtaining optimal culture results when using the liquid culture method.

Ronholdt and Bogdansky[176] conducted an RCT to evaluate the suitability of using swab cultures as a method for determining microbial contamination of allograft tissues. The researchers compared two swab-culturing systems using 168 human allograft tissues sterilized by radiation and then inoculated with low levels of multiple bacterial and fungal microorganisms (ie, *Staphylococcus aureus*, *Pseudomonas aeruginosa*, *Bacillus subtillus*, *Candida albicans*, *Aspergillus niger*, *Clostridium sporogenes*). The inoculated allograft tissues were swabbed in a "zigzag" pattern to ensure that the greatest surface area of the allograft was swabbed, and then streaked onto the culture medium three times while the culture plate was turned 120 degrees clockwise each time, for a total of 360 degrees. The swab tip was also rotated 120 degrees each time the plate was turned to ensure the entire surface of the swab contacted the entire surface of the culture medium, thus increasing the likelihood of recovering the challenge microorganisms.

The researchers calculated the average amount of challenge microorganism recovery for each swab system. The results showed that both swab-culturing systems tested exhibited low and variable microorganism recovery from the allograft tissues, and there was not a statistically significant difference between the two systems. No organisms were recovered in 73.8% of cultures (n = 124).

The researchers noted an interesting trend in that the soft tissue allografts (ie, tissues used to repair and reconstruct tendons and ligaments [eg, fascia, Achilles tendon]) (n = 84) had more positive cultures compared with the cut tissue allografts (ie, load-bearing tissues [eg, tricortical wedges, femoral heads]) (n = 84). The researchers theorized that this was because the microorganisms resided on the surface of the soft tissue and were more easily recovered, whereas the porous nature of the cut tissue allowed the microorganisms to be absorbed into the interior of the tissue, making recovery more difficult.

In addition, the researchers noted that a moist swab was more likely to capture and retain microorganisms than was a dry swab. The researchers concluded that swab-culturing methods may not have the sensitivity or reproducibility necessary to be used for final release of allograft tissues. They recommended that alternative, validated microbial detection methods be evaluated and implemented for tissue cultures.

XV.b.1. Microbiologic culture testing should be performed in a laboratory that is either certified under the Clinical Laboratory Improvement Amendments of 1988 (CLIA-88)[180] or is certified or accredited by another laboratory-accrediting organization that has deemed status for CLIA-88.[6] *[4: Benefits Balanced with Harms]*

Using a certified laboratory for microbiologic culture testing is an AATB standard.[6]

XV.b.2. Cultures obtained for determining the level and identity of microbial growth on autologous tissue should
- be obtained before the tissue is treated with antibiotics or cleansing agents[131] and
- include testing to detect bacteria (ie, aerobic and anaerobic) and fungi.[6]

[3: Limited Evidence]

Using antibiotics or other cleansing agents may inhibit the culture method used to detect viable organisms and may result in a false-negative culture result. Obtaining cultures to detect bacteria and fungi may help to identify tissue that is contaminated and may be unacceptable for replantation.

XV.c. Perioperative personnel must investigate any adverse reaction or event involving a communicable disease related to replanted or autotransplanted autologous tissue.[3,5] An adverse reaction or event involving a communicable disease must be reported if it
◦ is life-threatening or fatal;
◦ results in permanent impairment of a body function or permanent damage to a body structure; or

- necessitates medical or surgical intervention, including hospitalization.[3,5,181]

[1: Regulatory Requirement]

Reporting adverse reactions and events related to replanted or autotransplanted tissue is a regulatory requirement[3,5,181] and an AATB[6] and accreditation agency standard.[152,153] [1: Regulatory Requirement]

XV.c.1. Reports should be submitted through MedWatch: The FDA Safety Information and Adverse Event Reporting Program.[182]

Editor's note: *TiProtec is a registered trademark of Dr. Franz Köhler Chemie GmbH, Bensheim, Germany. X-Vivo 10 is a registered trademark of BioWhittaker Molecular Applications, Rockland, ME. Plasma-Lyte is a registered trademark of Baxter International, Deerfield, IL.*

Glossary

Adverse reaction: Related to replanted or autotransplanted autologous tissue, a harmful and unintended response to human cells or tissue for which there is a reasonable probability that the human cells or tissue caused the event.

Allograft: A graft taken from a living or nonliving donor for transplantation to a different individual.

American Association of Tissue Banks (AATB): A nonprofit organization that defines the standards for tissue banking.

Apoptosis: A sequence of events leading to cell death by fragmentation of cell particles that are engulfed by other cells.

Autograft: Tissue recovered from an individual for implantation or transplantation exclusively on or in the same individual.

Autologous: Cells or tissues obtained from the same individual.

Autotransplantation: Transplantation of tissue from one site to another in the same individual.

Avulsed tooth: A tooth separated by a traumatic action from the socket in which the roots of the tooth are embedded.

Cancellous bone: Bone with a lattice-like or spongy structure typically found at the ends of long bones, proximal to joints, and within the interior of vertebrae.

Chondrocyte: A cartilage cell.

Computed tomography (CT): A three-dimensional radiograph generated by computer synthesis of multiple cross-sectional images made along an axis.

Craniectomy: Surgical removal of a portion of the skull.

Cranioplasty: Surgical repair of a defect or deformity of the skull.

Cryopreservation: A process for maintaining the viability of resected tissue or organs by storing them at very low temperatures without causing damage from the formation of ice that may occur during freezing.

Cryoprotectant: A chemical substance used to protect biological tissue from damage due to ice formation during the cryopreservation process.

Cytotoxic: A substance that is poisonous to living cells.

Dulbecco's modified Eagle's medium: A modified version of Eagle's minimum essential medium that contains iron, phenol red, four times the amount of vitamins and amino acids, and two to four times as much glucose.

Eagle's minimum essential medium: A cell and culture medium that contains amino acids, salts, glucose, and vitamins.

Engrafting: A process that occurs when a piece of tissue (eg, skin) that has been surgically transplanted begins to function normally.

Fibroblasts: Star-shaped cells capable of forming collagen fibers.

Hank's Balanced Salt Solution: A solution composed of inorganic salts and bicarbonate ions designed to maintain physiological acid-base balance and osmotic pressure necessary for cell growth.

Hemacytometer: A device used to count cells.

Isotonic: Having the same solute concentration as a reference solution.

Krebs-Ringer solution: A balanced salt solution and physiological buffer used to maintain structural integrity of cells in culture.

Lactobacillis reuteri: A Gram-positive, rod-shaped, nonpathogenic bacteria that inhabits the intestinal tract of mammals.

McCoy's 5A medium: A sterile nutrient medium made up of amino acids, vitamins, minerals, antibiotics, and buffers.

Meshed skin: A skin graft with multiple cuts that allow it to be stretched to cover a larger area.

Mitochondria: Structures located in cell cytoplasm that are responsible for energy production.

Morus rubra: A mulberry tree, also known as red mulberry.

Oral rehydration solution: A solution made of water with small amounts of sugar and salt that is used to prevent or correct dehydration.

Osmolality: A measurement of the concentration of chemical particles found in a fluid. The greater the concentration of dissolved particles, the higher the osmolality.

Osseointegration: The structural and functional connection that develops between living bone and the surface of an implant.

Osteoblasts: Large cells responsible for synthesis and mineralization of bone during bone formation and regeneration. Osteoblasts are the major cellular component of bone.

Osteoclasts: Large multinuclear bone cells that resorb bone tissue.

Osteoconduction: Growth of bone tissue into an implant or graft.

Osteocytes: Bone cells located within the bone matrix.

Osteoinduction: Acceleration of new bone formation.

Periodontal ligament: Connective tissue that surrounds the tooth root.

Plasma-Lyte®: An isotonic solution that closely resembles human plasma in its electrolyte content, osmolality, and pH.

Pulsatile lavage: A method of delivering irrigation under pressure with pulsation. Used to remove microorganisms and debris from the surface of a wound.

Replantation: Replacement of an organ or body part (eg, avulsed tooth) into its original site and reestablishing its circulation.

Roswell Park Memorial Institute 1640 culture medium: A cell and culture medium enriched with amino acids and vitamins that contains a bicarbonate buffering system.

Salvia officinalis: An evergreen shrub also known as garden sage or common sage.

Storage medium: A physiologic solution that closely replicates conditions that help to preserve the viability of cells.

Subgaleal: The space between the skin and the skull.

TiProtec®: A sterile, hypothermic solution enriched with potassium chloride and N-acetyl histidine used for long-term protection and storage of tissue.

Tissue bank: A facility that participates in procuring, processing, preserving, or storing human cells and tissue for transplantation.

Tooth pulp: Soft tissue in the center of the tooth that contains blood vessels, connective tissue, and nerves.

Transmissible spongiform encephalopathy agents: Abnormal protein particles known as prions that are believed to be the cause of a group of diseases that affect the brain and nervous system. The development of tiny holes in the brain give it a sponge-like appearance, hence the term *spongiform*.

Tulle gras: A fine-meshed gauze impregnated with vegetable oil or soft paraffin.

X-Vivo 10®: A serum-free, cell media containing human proteins, phenol red, and gentamicin that supports the formation of blood or blood cells.

References

1. Pu LL, Cui X, Fink BF, Cibull ML, Gao D. Long-term preservation of adipose aspirates after conventional lipoplasty. *Aesthet Surg J.* 2004;24(6):536-541. [IB]
2. Pu LLQ. Cryopreservation of adipose tissue. *Organogenesis.* 2009;5(3):138-142. [VA]
3. §21 CFR 1271: Human cells, tissues, and cellular and tissue-based products. April;2013. US Food and Drug Administration. http://www.accessdata.fda.gov/scripts/cdrh/cfdocs/cfcfr/CFRSearch.cfm?CFRPart=1271. Accessed September 26, 2014.
4. Human Cells, Tissues, and Cellular and Tissue-Based Products; Establishment Registration and Listing. *Fed Regist.* 2001;66(13):5447-5469. http://www.gpo.gov/fdsys/pkg/FR-2001-01-19/pdf/01-1126.pdf. Accessed September 26, 2014.
5. *Current Good Tissue Practice (CGTP) and Additional Requirements for Manufacturers of Human Cells, Tissues, and Cellular and Tissue-Based Products (HCT/Ps).* Silver Spring, MD: US Food and Drug Administration; 2012.
6. *Standards for Tissue Banking.* McLean, VA: American Association of Tissue Banks; 2012. [IVC]
7. Sanghavi T, Shah N, Parekh V, Singbal K. Evaluation and comparison of efficacy of three different storage media, coconut water, propolis, and oral rehydration solution, in maintaining the viability of periodontal ligament cells. *J Cons Dentistry.* 2013;16(1):71-74. [IIB]
8. Thomas T, Gopikrishna V, Kandaswamy D. Comparative evaluation of maintenance of cell viability of an experimental transport media "coconut water" with Hank's balanced salt solution and milk, for transportation of an avulsed tooth: an in vitro cell culture study. *J Conserv Dentistry.* 2008;11(1):22-29. [IIB]
9. Chen H, Huang B. (-)-Epigallocatechin-3-gallate: a novel storage medium for avulsed teeth. *Dent Traumatol.* 2012;28(2):158-160. [IB]
10. Gjertsen AW, Stothz KA, Neiva KG, Pileggi R. Effect of propolis on proliferation and apoptosis of periodontal ligament fibroblasts. *Oral Surg Oral Med Oral Pathol Oral Radiol Endod.* 2011;112(6):843-848. [IIB]
11. Brullmann D, Schulze RK, d'Hoedt B. The treatment of anterior dental trauma. *Dtsch Arztebl Int.* 2010;108(34-35):565-570. [VB]
12. Khademi AA, Saei S, Mohajeri MR, et al. A new storage medium for an avulsed tooth. *J Contemp Dent Pract.* [Electronic Resource]. 2008;9(6):25-32. [IB]
13. Gopikrishna V, Thomas T, Kandaswamy D. A quantitative analysis of coconut water: a new storage media for avulsed teeth. *Oral Surg Oral Med Oral Pathol Oral Radiol Endod.* 2008;105(2):e61-e65. [IB]
14. Sigalas E, Regan JD, Kramer PR, Witherspoon DE, Opperman LA. Survival of human periodontal ligament cells in media proposed for transport of avulsed teeth. *Dent Traumatol.* 2004;20(1):21-28. [IIIC]
15. Krasner P. Treatment of avulsed teeth by oral and maxillofacial surgeons. *J Oral Maxillofac Surg.* 2010;68(11):2888-2892. [VB]
16. Moradian H, Badakhsh S, Rahimi M, Hekmatfar S. Replantation of an avulsed maxillary incisor after 12 hours: three-year follow-up. *Iranian Endod J.* 2013;8(1):33-36. [VB]
17. Udoye CI, Jafarzadeh H, Abbott PV. Transport media for avulsed teeth: a review. *Austr Endod J.* 2012;38(3):129-136. [VB]
18. Souza BD, Luckemeyer DD, Reyes-Carmona JF, Felippe WT, Simoes CM, Felippe MC. Viability of human periodontal ligament fibroblasts in milk, Hank's balanced salt solution and coconut water as storage media. *Int Endod J.* 2011;44(2):111-115. [IIB]
19. Moazami F, Mirhadi H, Geramizadeh B, Sahebi S. Comparison of soymilk, powdered milk, Hank's balanced salt solution and tap water on periodontal ligament cell survival. *Dent Traumatol.* 2012;28(2):132-135. [IIB]
20. Ozan F, Polat ZA, Er K, Ozan U, Deger O. Effect of propolis on survival of periodontal ligament cells: new storage media for avulsed teeth. *J Endod.* 2007;33(5):570-573. [IIB]
21. Doshi D. Bet 3. Avulsed tooth brought in milk for replantation. *Emerg Med J.* 2009;26(10):736-737. [VB]
22. Lin S, Zuckerman O, Fuss Z, et al. New emphasis in the treatment of dental trauma: avulsion and luxation. *Dent Traumatol.* 2007;23(5):297-303. [VB]
23. Goswami M, Chaitra T, Chaudhary S, Manuja N, Sinha A. Strategies for periodontal ligament cell viability: an overview. *J Conserv Dent.* 2011;14(3):215-220. [VB]
24. Karayilmaz H, Kirzioglu Z, Erken Gungor O. Aetiology, treatment patterns and long-term outcomes of tooth avulsion in children and adolescents. *Pakistan J Med Sci.* 2013;29(2):464-468. [IIIB]
25. Andersson L, Andreasen JO, Day P, et al. International Association of Dental Traumatology guidelines for

the management of traumatic dental injuries: 2. Avulsion of permanent teeth. *Dent Traumatol.* 2012;28(2):88-96. [IVB]

26. Caglar E, Sandalli N, Kuscu OO, et al. Viability of fibroblasts in a novel probiotic storage media. *Dent Traumatol.* 2010;26(5):383-387. [IIC]

27. Malhotra N. Current developments in interim transport (storage) media in dentistry: an update. *Br Dent J.* 2011;211(1):29-33. [VB]

28. Saxena P, Pant VA, Wadhwani KK, Kashyap MP, Gupta SK, Pant AB. Potential of the propolis as storage medium to preserve the viability of cultured human periodontal ligament cells: an in vitro study. *Dent Traumatol.* 2011;27(2):102-108. [IIB]

29. Ceallaigh PO, Ekanaykaee K, Beirne CJ, Patton DW. Diagnosis and management of common maxillofacial injuries in the emergency department. Part 5: dentoalveolar injuries. *Emerg Med J.* 2007;24(6):429-430. [VB]

30. Al-Nazhan S, Al-Nasser A. Viability of human periodontal ligament fibroblasts in tissue culture after exposure to different contact lens solutions. *J Contemp Dent Pract.* [Electronic Resource]. 2006;7(4):37-44. [IIC]

31. Andreasen JO, Borum MK, Jacobsen HL, Andreasen FM. Replantation of 400 avulsed permanent incisors. 4. Factors related to periodontal ligament healing. *Endod Dent Traumatol.* 1995;11(2):76-89. [IIIB]

32. Souza BD, Luckemeyer DD, Felippe WT, Simoes CM, Felippe MC. Effect of temperature and storage media on human periodontal ligament fibroblast viability. *Dent Traumatol.* 2010;26(3):271-275. [IIB]

33. Silva EJ, Rollemberg CB, Coutinho-Filho TS, Krebs RL, Zaia AA. Use of soymilk as a storage medium for avulsed teeth. *Acta Odontol Scand.* 2013;71(5):1101-1104. [IIB]

34. Eskandarian T, Badakhsh S, Esmaeilpour T. The effectiveness of oral rehydration solution at various concentrations as a storage media for avulsed teeth. *Iranian Endod J.* 2013;8(1):22-24. [IIB]

35. Macway-Gomez S, Lallier TE. Pedialyte promotes periodontal ligament cell survival and motility. *J Endod.* 2013;39(2):202-207. [IIB]

36. Moura CC, Soares PB, Reis MV, Fernandes Neto AJ, Soares CJ. Soy milk as a storage medium to preserve human fibroblast cell viability: an in vitro study. *Braz Dent J.* 2012;23(5):559-563. [IIB]

37. Hwang JY, Choi SC, Park JH, Kang SW. The use of green tea extract as a storage medium for the avulsed tooth. *J Endod.* 2011;37(7):962-967. [IIB]

38. Moreira-Neto JJ, Gondim JO, Raddi MS, Pansani CA. Viability of human fibroblasts in coconut water as a storage medium. *Int Endod J.* 2009;42(9):827-830. [IIB]

39. de Sousa HA, de Alencar AH, Bruno KF, Batista AC, de Carvalho AC. Microscopic evaluation of the effect of different storage media on the periodontal ligament of surgically extracted human teeth. *Dent Traumatol.* 2008;24(6):628-632. [IIB]

40. Ozan F, Polat ZA, Tepe B, Er K. Influence of storage media containing *Salvia officinalis* on survival of periodontal ligament cells. *J Contemp Dent Pract.* [Electronic Resource]. 2008;9(6):17-24. [IIB]

41. Ozan F, Tepe B, Polat ZA, Er K. Evaluation of in vitro effect of *Morus rubra* (red mulberry) on survival of periodontal ligament cells. *Oral Surg Oral Med Oral Pathol Oral Radiol Endod.* 2008;105(2):e66-e69. [IIB]

42. de Souza BD, Luckemeyer DD, Felippe WT, Alves AM, Simoes CM, Felippe MC. Effect of milk renewal on human periodontal ligament fibroblast viability in vitro. *Dent Traumatol.* 2012;28(3):214-216. [IIB]

43. *Treatment of Avulsed Permanent Teeth in Children.* Rev. 2004. Royal College of Surgeons. http://www.rcseng.ac.uk/fds/publications-clinical-guidelines/clinical_guidelines/documents/avulsed_permanent_treatment.pdf/view. Accessed September 26, 2014. [IVB]

44. Rajendran P, Varghese NO, Varughese JM, Murugaian E. Evaluation, using extracted human teeth, of Ricetral as a storage medium for avulsions—an in vitro study. *Dent Traumatol.* 2011;27(3):217-220. [IC]

45. Subramaniam P, Eswara U, Girish Babu KL, Vardhan B. Oral rehydration salt-liquid as an alternative storage medium—a preliminary study. *J Clin Pediatr Dent.* 2011;35(4):393-395. [IC]

46. Huang SC, Remeikis NA, Daniel JC. Effects of long-term exposure of human periodontal ligament cells to milk and other solutions. *J Endod.* 1996;22(1):30-33. [IIB]

47. Ahangari Z, Alborzi S, Yadegari Z, Dehghani F, Ahangari L, Naseri M. The effect of propolis as a biological storage media on periodontal ligament cell survival in an avulsed tooth: an in vitro study. *Cell J.* 2013;15(3):244-249. [IIB]

48. Chamorro MM, Regan JD, Opperman LA, Kramer PR. Effect of storage media on human periodontal ligament cell apoptosis. *Dent Traumatol.* 2008;24(1):11-16. [IIC]

49. Lin S, Emodi O, Abu El-Naaj I. Splinting of an injured tooth as part of emergency treatment. *Dent Traumatol.* 2008;24(3):370-372. [VB]

50. Mousavi B, Alavi SA, Mohajeri MR, Mirkheshti N, Ghassami F, Mirkheshti N. Standard oral rehydration solution as a new storage medium for avulsed teeth. *Int Dent J.* 2010;60(6):379-382. [IB]

51. Jung IH, Yun JH, Cho AR, Kim CS, Chung WG, Choi SH. Effect of (-)-epigallocatechin-3-gallate on maintaining the periodontal ligament cell viability of avulsed teeth: a preliminary study. *J Periodontal Implant Sci.* 2011;41(1):10-16. [IIB]

52. de Souza BD, Bortoluzzi EA, da Silveira Teixeira C, Felippe WT, Simoes CM, Felippe MC. Effect of HBSS storage time on human periodontal ligament fibroblast viability. *Dent Traumatol.* 2010;26(6):481-483. [IIC]

53. *Recommended Guidelines of the American Association of Endodontists for the Treatment of Traumatic Dental Injuries.* 2013. American Association of Endodontists. http://www.nxtbook.com/nxtbooks/aae/traumaguidelines/. Accessed September 26, 2014. [IVC]

54. Ballal V, V J. Storage media. *Br Dent J.* 2011;211(4):153. [VB]

55. Sonoda CK, Poi WR, Panzarini SR, Sottovia AD, Okamoto T. Tooth replantation after keeping the avulsed tooth in oral environment: case report of a 3-year follow-up. *Am Assoc Endod.* 2008;24(3):373-376. [VB]

56. Koca H, Topaloglu-Ak A, Sutekin E, Koca O, Acar S. Delayed replantation of an avulsed tooth after 5 hours of storage in saliva: a case report. *Dent Traumatol.* 2010;26(4):370-373. [VB]

57. Ize-Iyamu IN, Saheeb B. Reimplantation of avulsed dry permanent teeth after three days: a report of two cases. *Nigerian J Clin Pract.* 2013;16(1):119-122. [VC]

58. Baginska J, Wilczynska-Borawska M. Knowledge of nurses working at schools in Bialystok, Poland, of tooth avulsion and its management. *Dent Traumatol.* 2012;28(4):314-319. [IIIB]

59. Ulusoy AT, Onder H, Cetin B, Kaya S. Knowledge of medical hospital emergency physicians about the first-aid management of traumatic tooth avulsion. *Int J Paed Dent.* 2012;22(3):211-216. [IIIB]

60. Yeng T, Parashos P. An investigation into dentists' management methods of dental trauma to maxillary

permanent incisors in Victoria, Australia. *Dent Traumatol.* 2008;24(4):443-448. [IIIB]

61. Kargul B, Welbury R. An audit of the time to initial treatment in avulsion injuries. *Dent Traumatol.* 2009;25(1):123-125. [IIIB]

62. de Vasconcellos LG, Brentel AS, Vanderlei AD, de Vasconcellos LM, Valera MC, de Araujo MA. Knowledge of general dentists in the current guidelines for emergency treatment of avulsed teeth and dental trauma prevention. *Dent Traumatol.* 2009;25(6):578-583. [IIIB]

63. Zhao Y, Gong Y. Knowledge of emergency management of avulsed teeth: a survey of dentists in Beijing, China. *Dent Traumatol.* 2010;26(3):281-284. [IIIB]

64. Loh T, Sae-Lim V, Yian TB, Liang S. Dental therapists' experience in the immediate management of traumatized teeth. *Dent Traumatol.* 2006;22(2) 66-70. [IIIB]

65. Hugar SM, Suganya M, Kiran K, Vikneshan M, More VP. Knowledge and awareness of dental trauma among Indian nurses. *Int Emerg Nurs.* 2013;21(4):252-256. [IIIB]

66. Needleman HL, Stucenski K, Forbes PW, Chen Q, Stack AM. Massachusetts emergency departments' resources and physicians' knowledge of management of traumatic dental injuries. *Dent Traumatol.* 2013;29(4):272-279. [IIIC]

67. Choi D, Badner VM, Yeroshalmi F, Margulis KS, Dougherty NJ, Kreiner-Litt G. Dental trauma management by New York City school nurses. *J Dent Child.* 2012;79(2):74-78. [IIIB]

68. Tahir MZ, Shamim MS, Sobani ZA, Zafar SN, Qadeer M, Bari ME. Safety of untreated autologous cranioplasty after extracorporeal storage at -26 degree celsius. *Br J Neurosurg.* 2013;27(4):479-482. [IIIB]

69. Lu Y, Hui G, Liu F, Wang Z, Tang Y, Gao S. Survival and regeneration of deep-freeze preserved autologous cranial bones after cranioplasty. *Br J Neurosurg.* 2012;26(2):216-221. [IIIC]

70. Bhaskar IP, Yusheng L, Zheng M, Lee GY. Autogenous skull flaps stored frozen for more than 6 months: do they remain viable? *J Clin Neurosci.* 2011;18(12):1690-1693. [IIB]

71. Grossman N, Shemesh-Jan HS, Merkin V, Gideon M, Cohen A. Deep-freeze preservation of cranial bones for future cranioplasty: nine years of experience in Soroka University Medical Center. *Cell Tissue Bank.* 2007;8(3):243-246. [VB]

72. Beez T, Sabel M, Ahmadi SA, Beseoglu K, Steiger H-J, Sabel M. Scanning electron microscopic surface analysis of cryoconserved skull bone after decompressive craniectomy. *Cell Tissue Bank.* 2013;15(1):85-88. [IIIC]

73. Elwatidy S, Elgamal E, Jamjoom Z, Habib H, Raddaoui E. Assessment of bone flap viability and sterility after long periods of preservation in the freezer. *Pan Arab J Neurosurg.* 2011;15(1):24-28. [IIIC]

74. Bhaskar IP, Zaw NN, Zheng M, Lee GYF. Bone flap storage following craniectomy: A survey of practices in major Australian Neurosurgical centres. *ANZ J Surg.* 2011;81(3):137-141. [IIIC]

75. Baldo S, Tacconi L. Effectiveness and safety of subcutaneous abdominal preservation of autologous bone flap after decompressive craniectomy: a prospective pilot study. *World Neurosurg.* 2010;73(5):552-556. [IIIB]

76. Prolo DJ, Burres KP, McLaughlin WT, Christensen AH. Autogenous skull cranioplasty: fresh and preserved (frozen), with consideration of the cellular response. *Neurosurgery.* 1979;4(1):18-29. [IIIB]

77. Shoakazemi A, Flannery T, McConnell RS. Long-term outcome of subcutaneously preserved autologous cranioplasty. *Neurosurgery.* 2009;65(3):505-510. [IIIB]

78. Movassaghi K, Ver Halen J, Ganchi P, Amin-Hanjani S, Mesa J, Yaremchuk MJ. Cranioplasty with subcutaneously preserved autologous bone grafts. *Plast Reconstr Surg.* 2006;117(1):202-206. [IIIC]

79. Iwama T, Yamada J, Imai S, Shinoda J, Funakoshi T, Sakai N. The use of frozen autogenous bone flaps in delayed cranioplasty revisited. *Neurosurgery.* 2003;52(3):591-596. [IIIB]

80. Morina A, Kelmendi F, Morina Q, et al. Cranioplasty with subcutaneously preserved autologous bone grafts in abdominal wall—experience with 75 cases in a post-war country Kosova. *Surg Neurol Int.* 2011;2:72. [VB]

81. Pasaoglu A, Kurtsoy A, Koc RK, et al. Cranioplasty with bone flaps preserved under the scalp. *Neurosurg Rev.* 1996;19(3):153-156. [IIIC]

82. Vanaclocha V, Saiz-Sapena N, Garcia-Casasola C, De Alava E. Cranioplasty with autogenous autoclaved calvarial bone flap in the cases of tumoural invasion. *Acta Neurochir (Wien).* 1997;139(10):970-976. [IIIC]

83. Matsuno A, Tanaka H, Iwamuro H, et al. Analyses of the factors influencing bone graft infection after delayed cranioplasty. *Acta Neurochir (Wien).* 2006;148(5):535-540. [IIIB]

84. Schultke E, Hampl JA, Jatzwauk L, Krex D, Schackert G. An easy and safe method to store and disinfect explanted skull bone. *Acta Neurochir (Wien).* 1999;141(5):525-528. [IIB]

85. Wester K. Cranioplasty with an autoclaved bone flap, with special reference to tumour infiltration of the flap. *Acta Neurochir (Wien).* 1994;131(3-4):223-225. [VB]

86. Zingale A, Albanese V. Cryopreservation of autogeneous bone flap in cranial surgical practice: what is the future? A grade B and evidence level 4 meta-analytic study. *J Neurosurg Sci.* 2003;47(3):137-139. [IC]

87. Albrektsson T, Johansson C. Osteoinduction, osteoconduction and osseointegration. *Eur Spine J.* 2001;10(Suppl 2):S96-S101. [VA]

88. Gibson S, McLeod I, Wardlaw D, Urbaniak S. Allograft versus autograft in instrumented posterolateral lumbar spinal fusion: a randomized control trial. *Spine (Phila Pa 1976).* 2002;27(15):1599-1603. [IB]

89. Yazici M, Asher MA. Freeze-dried allograft for posterior spinal fusion in patients with neuromuscular spinal deformities. *Spine (Phila Pa 1976).* 1997;22(13):1467-1471. [VB]

90. Bridwell KH, O'Brien MF, Lenke LG, Baldus C, Blanke K. Posterior spinal fusion supplemented with only allograft bone in paralytic scoliosis. Does it work? *Spine (Phila Pa 1976).* 1994;19(23):2658-2666. [IIIC]

91. Gill K, O'Brien JP. Observations of resorption of the posterior lateral bone graft in combined anterior and posterior lumbar fusion. *Spine (Phila Pa 1976).* 1993;18(13):1885-1889. [IIIC]

92. Nasca RJ, Whelchel JD. Use of cryopreserved bone in spinal surgery. *Spine (Phila Pa 1976).* 1987;12(3):222-227. [IIIB]

93. Wimmer C, Krismer M, Gluch H, Ogon M, Stockl B. Autogenic versus allogenic bone grafts in anterior lumbar interbody fusion. *Clin Orthop Relat Res.* 1999;(360)(360):122-126. [IIIB]

94. Joaquim AF, Mattos JP, Neto FC, Lopes A, de Oliveira E. Bone flap management in neurosurgery. *Revi Neuroci.* 2009;17(2):133-137. [VB]

95. Flannery T, McConnell RS. Cranioplasty: why throw the bone flap out? *Br J Neurosurg.* 2001;15(6):518-520. [VB]

96. Krishnan P, Bhattacharyya AK, Sil K, De R. Bone flap preservation after decompressive craniectomy—experience with 55 cases. *Neurol India.* 2006;54(3):291-292. [VC]

97. Jho DH, Neckrysh S, Hardman J, Charbel FT, Amin-Hanjani S. Ethylene oxide gas sterilization: a simple technique for storing explanted skull bone. Technical note. *J Neurosurg*. 2007;107(2):440-445. [IIIB]

98. Inamasu J, Kuramae T, Nakatsukasa M. Does difference in the storage method of bone flaps after decompressive craniectomy affect the incidence of surgical site infection after cranioplasty? Comparison between subcutaneous pocket and cryopreservation. *J Trauma-Inj Infect Crit Care*. 2010;68(1):183-187. [IIIB]

99. Sultan SM, Davidson EH, Butala P, et al. Interval cranioplasty: Comparison of current standards. *Plast Reconstr Surg*. 2011;127(5):1855-1864. [IIB]

100. Osawa M, Hara H, Ichinose Y, Koyama T, Kobayashi S, Sugita Y. Cranioplasty with a frozen and autoclaved bone flap. *Acta Neurochir (Wien)*. 1990;102(1-2):38-41. [VB]

101. Guerrero MA. Cryopreservation of parathyroid glands. *Int J Endocrinol*. 2010;2010:829540. [VA]

102. Stotler BA, Reich-Slotky R, Schwartz J, et al. Quality monitoring of microbial contamination of cryopreserved parathyroid tissue. *Cell Tissue Bank*. 2011;12(2):111-116. [VB]

103. Cohen MS, Dilley WG, Wells SA Jr, et al. Long-term functionality of cryopreserved parathyroid autografts: a 13-year prospective analysis. *Surgery*. 2005;138(6):1033-1040. [IIIB]

104. Schneider R, Ramaswamy A, Slater EP, Bartsch DK, Schlosser K. Cryopreservation of parathyroid tissue after parathyroid surgery for renal hyperparathyroidism: does it really make sense? *World J Surg*. 2012;36(11):2598-2604. [IIIB]

105. Guerrero MA, Evans DB, Lee JE, et al. Viability of cryopreserved parathyroid tissue: when is continued storage versus disposal indicated? *World J Surg*. 2008;32(5):836-839. [IIIB]

106. Saxe AW, Spiegel AM, Marx SJ, Brennan MF. Deferred parathyroid autografts with cryopreserved tissue after reoperative parathyroid surgery. *Arch Surg*. 1982;117(5):538-543. [IIIC]

107. Agarwal A, Waghray A, Gupta S, Sharma R, Milas M. Cryopreservation of parathyroid tissue: an illustrated technique using the Cleveland Clinic protocol. *J Am Coll Surg*. 2013;216(1):e1-e9. [VA]

108. Alvarez-Hernandez D, Gonzalez-Suarez I, Carrillo-Lopez N, Naves-Diaz M, Anguita-Velasco J, Cannata-Andia JB. Viability and functionality of fresh and cryopreserved human hyperplastic parathyroid tissue tested in vitro. *Am J Nephrol*. 2008;28(1):76-82. [IIC]

109. Barreira CE, Cernea CR, Brandão LG, Custodio MR, Caldini ET, de Menezes Montenegro FL. Effects of time on ultrastructural integrity of parathyroid tissue before cryopreservation. *World J Surg*. 2011;35(11):2440-2444. [IIC]

110. de Menezes Montenegro FL, Custodio MR, Arap SS, et al. Successful implant of long-term cryopreserved parathyroid glands after total parathyroidectomy. *Head Neck*. 2007;29(3):296-300. [VB]

111. DeBono R, Rao GS, Berry RB. The survival of human skin stored by refrigeration at 4 degrees C in McCoy's 5A medium: does oxygenation of the medium improve storage time? *Plast Reconstr Surg*. 1998;102(1):78-83. [IIB]

112. Mardini S, Agullo FJ, Salgado CJ, Rose V, Moran SL, Chen HC. Delayed skin grafting utilizing autologous banked tissue. *Ann Plast Surg*. 2009;63(3):311-313. [VB]

113. Robb EC, Bechmann NRVT, Plessinger RT, Boyce ST, Warden GD, Kagan RJ. Storage media and temperature maintain normal anatomy of cadaveric human skin for transplantation to full-thickness skin wounds. *J Burn Care Rehabil*. 2001;22(6):393-396. [IIB]

114. Cram AE, Domayer MA. Short-term preservation of human autografts. *J Trauma*. 1983;23(10):872-873. [VC]

115. Sterne GD, Titley OG, Christie JL. A qualitative histological assessment of various storage conditions on short term preservation of human split skin grafts. *Br J Plast Surg*. 2000;53(4):331-336. [IIC]

116. Sheridan R, Mahe J, Walters P. Autologous skin banking. *Burns*. 1998;24(1):46-48. [IIIC]

117. Titley OG, Cooper M, Thomas A, Hancock K. Stored skin--stored trouble? *Br J Plast Surg*. 1994;47(1):24-29. [IIIB]

118. Molnar GF, Nemes A, Kekesi V, Monos E, Nadasy GL. Maintained geometry, elasticity and contractility of human saphenous vein segments stored in a complex tissue culture medium. *Eur J Vasc Endovasc Surg*. 2010;40(1):88-93. [IB]

119. Ebner A, Poitz DM, Augstein A, Strasser RH, Deussen A. Functional, morphologic, and molecular characterization of cold storage injury. *J Vasc Surg*. 2012;56(1):189-198.e3. [IIB]

120. Wilbring M, Tugtekin SM, Zatschler B, et al. Preservation of endothelial vascular function of saphenous vein grafts after long-time storage with a recently developed potassium-chloride and N-acetylhistidine enriched storage solution. *Thorac Cardiovasc Surg*. 2013;61(8):656-662. [IIIB]

121. Baumann FG, Catinella FP, Cunningham JN Jr, Spencer FC. Vein contraction and smooth muscle cell extensions as causes of endothelial damage during graft preparation. *Ann Surg*. 1981;194(2):199-211. [IIB]

122. Jankowitz BT, Kondziolka DS. When the bone flap hits the floor. *Neurosurgery*. 2006;59(3):585-589. [IIIB]

123. Kang L, Mermel LA, Trafton PG. What happens when autogenous bone drops out of the sterile field during orthopaedic trauma surgery. *J Orthop Trauma*. 2008;22(6):430-431. [IIIB]

124. Centeno RF, Desai AR, Watson ME. Management of contaminated autologous grafts in plastic surgery. *Eplasty*. April 22, 2008;8:e23. [IIIB]

125. Bhandari M, Schemitsch EH, Adili A, Lachowski RJ, Shaughnessy SG. High and low pressure pulsatile lavage of contaminated tibial fractures: an in vitro study of bacterial adherence and bone damage. *J Orthop Trauma*. 1999;13(8):526-533. [IIB]

126. Hirn M, Laitinen M, Pirkkalainen S, Vuento R. Cefuroxime, rifampicin and pulse lavage in decontamination of allograft bone. *J Hosp Infect*. 2004;56(3):198-201. [IIB]

127. Mangram AJ, Horan TC, Pearson ML, Silver LC, Jarvis WR. Guideline for Prevention of Surgical Site Infection, 1999. Centers for Disease Control and Prevention (CDC) Hospital Infection Control Practices Advisory Committee. *Am J Infect Control*. 1999;27(2):97-132; quiz 133-4; discussion 96. [IVA]

128. Presnal BP, Kimbrough EE. What to do about a dropped bone graft. *Clin Orthop Relat Res*. 1993;Nov;(296):310-311. [IB]

129. Bhandari M, Adili A, Lachowski RJ. High pressure pulsatile lavage of contaminated human tibiae: an in vitro study. *J Orthop Trauma*. 1998;12(7):479-484. [IIB]

130. Makary MA, Holzmueller CG, Sexton JB, et al. Operating room debriefings. *Jt Comm J Qual Patient Saf*. 2006;32(7):407-410, 357. [VB]

131. *Sample Procedure: Handling Autologous Bone Skull Flaps*. Version 14. McLean, VA: American Association of Tissue Banks; 2012. [IVC]

132. Bhandari M, Adili A, Schemitsch EH. The efficacy of low-pressure lavage with different irrigating solutions

AUTOLOGOUS TISSUE MANAGEMENT

to remove adherent bacteria from bone. *J Bone Joint Surg Am.* 2001;83-A(3):412-419. [IIB]

133. Yaman F, Unlu G, Atilgan S, Celik Y, Ozekinci T, Yaldiz M. Microbiologic and histologic assessment of intentional bacterial contamination of bone grafts. *J Oral Maxillofac Surg.* 2007;65(8):1490-1494. [IIB]

134. Bruce B, Sheibani-Rad S, Appleyard D, et al. Are dropped osteoarticular bone fragments safely reimplantable in vivo? *J Bone Joint Surg Am.* 2011;93(5):430-438. [IIB]

135. Soyer J, Rouil M, Castel O. The effect of 10% povidone-iodine solution on contaminated bone allografts. *J Hosp Infect.* 2002;50(3):183-187. [IB]

136. Lacey RW. Antibacterial activity of povidone iodine towards non-sporing bacteria. *J Appl Bacteriol.* 1979;46(3):443-449. [IIB]

137. Kaysinger KK, Nicholson NC, Ramp WK, Kellam JF. Toxic effects of wound irrigation solutions on cultured tibiae and osteoblasts. *J Orthop Trauma.* 1995;9(4):303-311. [IIB]

138. Khan M, Rothrauff BB, Merali F, Musahl V, Peterson D, Ayeni OR. Management of the contaminated anterior cruciate ligament graft. *Arthroscopy.* 2014;30(2):236-244. [IA]

139. Guideline for specimen management. In: *Guidelines for Perioperative Practice.* Denver, CO: AORN, Inc; 2015:389-418. [IVA]

140. Lagios MD. Pathology procedures for evaluation of the specimen with potential or documented ductal carcinoma in situ. *Semin Breast Dis.* 2000;3:42-49. [VB]

141. Wolff AC, Hammond ME, Hicks DG, et al. Recommendations for human epidermal growth factor receptor 2 testing in breast cancer: American Society of Clinical Oncology/College of American Pathologists clinical practice guideline update. *Arch Pathol Lab Med.* 2014;138(2):241-256.

142. Greenberg CC, Regenbogen SE, Studdert DM, et al. Patterns of communication breakdowns resulting in injury to surgical patients. *J Am Coll Surg.* 2007;204(4):533-540. [IIIB]

143. Siegel JD, Rhinehart E, Jackson M, Chiarello L, Health Care Infection Control Practices Advisory Committee. 2007 Guideline for Isolation Precautions: Preventing Transmission of Infectious Agents in Health Care Settings. *Am J Infect Control.* 2007;35(10 Suppl 2):S65-S64. [IVA]

144. Guideline for selection and use of packaging systems for sterilization. In: *Guidelines for Perioperative Practice.* Denver, CO: AORN, Inc; 2015:651-664. [IVA]

145. Occupational Safety and Health Administration. Toxic and Hazardous substances: Bloodborne pathogens, 29 CFR §1910.1030 (2012). Occupational Safety and Health Administration. https://www.osha.gov/pls/oshaweb/owadisp.show_document?p_id=10051&p_table=STANDARDS. Accessed September 26, 2014.

146. Benner J. Establish a transparent chain-of-custody to mitigate risk and ensure quality of specialized samples. *Biopreserv Biobank.* 2009;7(3):151-153. [VB]

147. Valenstein PN, Sirota RL. Identification errors in pathology and laboratory medicine. *Clin Lab Med.* 2004;24(4):979-96, vii. [VB]

148. College of American Pathologists. When a rose is not a rose: the problem of mislabeled specimens. *Lab Med DirecTIPs.* http://www.cap.org/apps/portlets/content-Viewer/show.do?printFriendly=true&contentReference=practice_management%2Fdirectips%2Fmislabeled_specimens.html. Updated February 23, 2010. Accessed October 14, 2014. [VB]

149. 45 CFR Parts 160 and 164. Modifications to the HIPAA Privacy, Security, Enforcement, and Breach Notification Rules Under the Health Information Technology for Economic and Clinical Health Act and the Genetic Information Nondiscrimination Act; Other Modifications to the HIPAA Rules; Final Rule. *Fed Regist.* 2013;78(17):5566-5702.

150. Guideline for perioperative health care information management. In: *Guidelines for Perioperative Practice.* Denver, CO: AORN, Inc; 2015:491-512. [IVB]

151. Standards of perioperative nursing practice. In: *Perioperative Standards and Recommended Practices.* Denver, CO: AORN, Inc; 2014:3-42. [IVB]

152. Joint Commission. Transplant safety. In: *Comprehensive Accreditation Manual for Hospitals E-dition.* Washington, DC: The Joint Commission; March 2014.

153. Joint Commission. Transplant safety. In: *Comprehensive Accreditation Manual for Ambulatory Care E-dition.* Washington, DC: The Joint Commission; March 2014.

154. Makary MA, Holzmueller CG, Thompson D, et al. Operating room briefings: working on the same page. *Jt Comm J Qual Patient Saf.* 2006;32(6):351-355. [VB]

155. Chiang HY, Steelman VM, Pottinger JM, et al. Clinical significance of positive cranial bone flap cultures and associated risk of surgical site infection after craniotomies or craniectomies. *J Neurosurg.* 2011;114(6):1746-1754. [IIIA]

156. Surgical and related services. In: *Accreditation Handbook for Ambulatory Health Care.* Skokie, Ill.: Accreditation Association for Ambulatory Health Care; 2014:52-55.

157. Centers for Medicare & Medicaid Services. State Operations Manual Appendix A Survey Protocol, Regulations and Interpretive Guidelines for Hospitals. Rev. 105; 3/21/14. Baltimore, MD: Centers for Medicare & Medicaid; 2014.

158. Centers for Medicare & Medicaid Services. State Operations Manual Appendix L: Guidance for Surveyors: Ambulatory Surgical Centers. Rev. 99; 1/31/14. Baltimore, MD: Centers for Medicare & Medicaid; 2014.

159. LD.04.01.07: The hospital has policies and procedures that guide and support patient care, treatment, and services. In: *Hospital Accreditation Standards 2014.* 2014 ed. Oakbrook Terrace, IL: Joint Commission Resources; 2014.

160. LD.04.01.07: The organization has policies and procedures that guide and support patient care, treatment, or services. In: *Standards for ambulatory care 2014: Standards, Elements of Performance, Scoring, Accreditation Polices.* Oakbrook Terrace, IL: Joint Commission Resources; 2014.

161. Governance. In: *2014 Accreditation Handbook for Ambulatory Health Care.* Skokie, IL: Accreditation Association for Ambulatory Health Care; 2014:19-26.

162. SS.1: Organization. In: *NIAHO Interpretive Guidelines and Surveyor Guidance.* 10.1 ed. Milford, OH: DNV Healthcare Inc; 2012:70-71.

163. HR.01.05.03: Staff participate in ongoing education and training. In: *Comprehensive Accreditation Manual: CAMH for Hospitals.* 2014 ed. Oakbrook Terrace, Ill.: Joint Commission Resources; 2014.

164. HR.01.05.03: Staff participate in ongoing education and training. In: *Comprehensive Accreditation Manual: CAMAC for Ambulatory Care.* 2014 ed. Oakbrook Terrace, Ill.: Joint Commission Resources; 2014.

165. Quality management and improvement. In: *2014 Accreditation Handbook for Ambulatory Health Care.* Skokie, IL: Accreditation Association for Ambulatory Health Care; 2014:32-36.

166. MS.10 Continuing education. In: *NIAHO Interpretive Guidelines and Surveyor Guidance*. 10.1 ed. Milford, OH: DNV Healthcare Inc; 2012:24.

167. RC.01.01.01: The hospital maintains complete and accurate medical records for each individual patient. In: *Hospital Accreditation Standards 2014*. 2014 ed. Oakbrook Terrace, IL: Joint Commission Resources; 2014.

168. RC.01.01.01: The organization maintains complete and accurate clinical records. In: *Standards for ambulatory care 2014: Standards, Elements of Performance Scoring Accreditation Polices*. Oakbrook Terrace, IL: Joint Commission Resources; 2014.

169. Clinical records and health information. In: *2014 Accreditation Handbook for Ambulatory Health Care*. Skokie, IL: Accreditation Association for Ambulatory Health Care; 2014:37-39.

170. MS.16 Medical record maintenance. In: *NIAHO Interpretive Guidelines and Surveyor Guidance*. 10.1 ed. Milford, OH: DNV Healthcare Inc; 2012:29.

171. PI.03.01.01: The hospital improves performance on an ongoing basis. In: *Hospital Accreditation Standards 2014*. 2014 ed. Oakbrook Terrace, IL: Joint Commission Resources; 2014.

172. PI.03.01.01: The organization improves performance. In: *Standards for ambulatory care 2014: Standards, Elements of Performance, Scoring, Accreditation Polices*. Oakbrook Terrace, IL: Joint Commission Resources; 2014.

173. Quality management and improvement. In: *2014 Accreditation Handbook for Ambulatory Health Care*. Skokie, IL: Accreditation Association for Ambulatory Health Care; 2014:32-36.

174. Quality management system. In: *NIAHO Interpretive Guidelines and Surveyor Guidance*. 10.1 ed. Milford, OH: DNV Healthcare Inc; 2012:10-16.

175. International Organization for Standardization. *Sterilization of Medical Devices: Microbiological Methods*. Part 1. Geneva, Switzerland: International Organization for Standardization; 2006. [IVC]

176. Ronholdt CJ, Bogdansky S. The appropriateness of swab cultures for the release of human allograft tissue. *J Industr Microbiol Biotechnol*. 2005;32(8):349-354. [IB]

177. Nguyen H, Morgan DA, Cull S, Benkovich M, Forwood MR. Sponge swabs increase sensitivity of sterility testing of processed bone and tendon allografts. *J Ind Microbiol Biotechnol*. 2011;38(8):1127-1132. [IIB]

178. Dennis JA, Martinez OV, Landy DC, et al. A comparison of two microbial detection methods used in aseptic processing of musculoskeletal allograft tissues. *Cell Tissue Bank*. 2011;12(1):45-50. [IIB]

179. Aggarwal VK, Higuera C, Deirmengian G, Parvizi J, Austin MS. Swab cultures are not as effective as tissue cultures for diagnosis of periprosthetic joint infection. *Clin Orthopaed Rel Res*. 2013;471(10):3196-3203. [IIIB]

180. 42 CFR §493 - Condition of participation: Laboratory Requirements. Washington, DC: Government Printing Office; 2012.

181. Vaccines, Blood and Biologics. Guidance for Industry: MedWatch Form FDA 3500A: Mandatory Reporting of Adverse Reactions Related to Human Cells, Tissues, and Cellular and Tissue-Based Products (HCT/Ps). US Food and Drug Administration. http://www.fda.gov/BiologicsBlood Vaccines/GuidanceComplianceRegulatoryInformation/Guidances/Tissue/ucm074000.htm. Accessed September 26, 2014.

182. MedWatch: The FDA Safety Information and Adverse Event Reporting Program. US Food and Drug Administration. http://www.fda.gov/Safety/MedWatch/default.htm. Accessed September 26, 2014.

Acknowledgements

LEAD AUTHOR
Sharon A. Van Wicklin, MSN, RN, CNOR, CRNFA, CPSN, PLNC
Perioperative Nursing Specialist
AORN Nursing Department
Denver, CO

CONTRIBUTING AUTHORS
Scott A. Brubaker, CTBS
Chief Policy Officer
American Association of Tissue Banks
McLean, VA

Ramona Conner, MSN, RN, CNOR
Manager, Standards and Guidelines
AORN Nursing Department
Denver, CO

The authors and AORN thank Marie A. Bashaw, DNP, RN, NEA-BC, CNOR, Clinical Assistant Professor, Wright State University College of Nursing and Health, Dayton, OH; Patricia Graybill-D'Ercole, MSN, RN, CNOR, CHL, CRCST, Clinical Specialist, Integra Life Science, York, PA; and Deborah Farina Mulloy, PhD, RN, Associate Chief Nurse, Quality and Center for Nursing Excellence, Brigham and Women's Hospital, Boston, MA, for their assistance in developing this guideline.

PUBLICATION HISTORY
Originally published in November 2014 in *Perioperative Standards and Recommended Practices* online.

Minor editing revisions made in November 2014 for publication in *Guidelines for Perioperative Practice*, 2015 edition.

GUIDELINE FOR A SAFE ENVIRONMENT OF CARE, PART 1

The following Guideline for a Safe Environment of Care, Part 1 has been approved by the AORN Recommended Practices Advisory Board. It was presented as proposed recommendations for comments by members and others. The guideline is effective December 15, 2012. The recommendations in this guideline are intended to be achievable and represent what is believed to be an optimal level of practice. Policies and procedures will reflect variations in practice settings and/or clinical situations that determine the degree to which the guideline can be implemented. AORN recognizes the various settings in which perioperative nurses practice; therefore, this guideline is adaptable to various practice settings. These practice settings include traditional operating rooms (ORs), ambulatory surgery centers, physicians' offices, cardiac catheterization laboratories, endoscopy suites, radiology departments, and all other areas where operative and other invasive procedures may be performed.

Purpose

This document provides guidance for providing a safe environment of care related to patients and perioperative personnel and the equipment used in the perioperative environment. They include information on

- musculoskeletal injury,
- fire safety,
- electrical equipment,
- clinical and alert alarms,
- blanket- and solution-warming cabinets,
- medical gas cylinders,
- waste anesthesia gases,
- latex,
- chemicals including methyl methacrylate bone cement, and
- hazardous waste.

The potential for injuries related to exposure to bloodborne pathogens, radiation, surgical smoke, and chemotherapeutic agents are outside the scope of this document. Patient injuries related to incorrect tubing connections and requirements for heating, ventilation, and air conditioning also are outside the scope of this document. The recommendations for these topics are addressed in other AORN guidelines.

Evidence Review

A medical librarian conducted a systematic literature search of the databases MEDLINE®, CINAHL®, Scopus®, and Cochrane Database of Systematic Reviews for meta-analyses, randomized and nonrandomized trials and studies, systematic and nonsystematic reviews, and opinion documents and letters. Search terms included *operating room, ambulatory surgery center, perioperative nursing, nursing, nurses, surgical procedures, anesthesia, electrosurgery, diathermy, ventilation, smoke, surgical smoke, security measures, violence, occupational accidents, occupational diseases, musculoskeletal diseases, lifting, transportation of patients, patient positioning, human engineering, ergonomics, latex hypersensitivity, security measures, violence, security risk, fire blanket, fire safety, fires, smoke plume, clinical alarms, anesthetics, gas scavengers, compressed gas, compressed medical gas, methyl methacrylate, occupational exposure, hazardous waste, hazardous substances, waste products, hazardous upon disposal, protective clothing, tubing misconnection, spontaneous abortion, miscarriage,* and *abnormality*.

The search was limited to articles published in English and between the years 2005 and 2011; the librarian also established continuing alerts on the environment of care topics and contacted a federal agency for guidance. The lead author and medical librarian also identified relevant guidelines from government agencies and standards-setting bodies and consulted equipment specifications. In addition, the lead author identified and requested other guidelines and professional literature as deemed appropriate.

Articles identified by the search were provided to the project team for evaluation. The team consisted of the lead author, three members of the Recommended Practices Advisory Board, one member of the Research Committee, and one doctorally prepared evidence appraiser. The lead author divided the search results into topics and assigned members of the team to review and critically appraise each article using the Johns Hopkins Evidence-Based Practice Model and the Research or Non-Research Evidence Appraisal Tools as appropriate. The literature was independently evaluated and appraised according to the strength and quality of the evidence. Each article was then assigned an appraisal score as agreed upon by consensus of the team. The appraisal score is noted in brackets after each reference, as applicable.

The collective evidence supporting each intervention within a specific recommendation was summarized and used to rate the strength of the evidence using the AORN Evidence Rating Model. Factors considered in review of the collective evidence were the quality of research, quantity of similar studies on a given topic, and consistency of results supporting a recommendation. The evidence rating is noted in brackets after each intervention.

Editor's note: MEDLINE is a registered trademark of the US National Library of Medicine's Medical Literature Analysis and Retrieval System, Bethesda, MD. CINAHL,

ENVIRONMENT OF CARE, PART 1

Cumulative Index to Nursing and Allied Health Literature, is a registered trademark of EBSCO Industries, Birmingham, AL. Scopus is a registered trademark of Elsevier B.V., Amsterdam, Netherlands.

Recommendation I

Precautions should be taken to mitigate the risk of occupational injuries that may result in death, days lost from work, work restrictions, medical treatment beyond first aid, and loss of consciousness.[1]

Occupational injuries include injuries that result in breaking of the skin and musculoskeletal injuries from slips, trips, falls, or ergonomic stressors.[2,3] Musculoskeletal injuries involve the muscles, nerves, tendons, ligaments, joints, cartilage, and spinal discs. Contributing factors, including duration, frequency, and magnitude, determine the effect of each ergonomic stressor. Examples of ergonomic stressors encountered in the perioperative environment include

- forceful tasks (eg, pushing a stretcher and patient up a ramp),
- repetitive motions (eg, passing instruments, opening suture packets, typing),
- awkward postures (eg, holding retractors during a surgical procedure, lifting or holding patient extremities),
- static postures (eg, standing for long periods of time in one position),
- moving or lifting patients and equipment (eg, lifting without assistance),
- carrying heavy instruments and equipment, and
- overexertion (eg, protecting a combative patient emerging from anesthesia).[1,4,5]

Perioperative nurses expressed more complaints regarding neck and shoulder injuries than non-specialized and intensive care nurses in a descriptive study involving 3,169 employees in eight university hospitals in the Netherlands.[6] In another descriptive study of direct patient caregivers (n = 5,991 nurses, n = 1,543 aides), aides had a higher rate of injury than nurses. The back was the most common body part injured that resulted in days away from work. Sharps injury was the most frequent injury that did not require time away from work. The OR had the highest number of injuries that did not require time away from work, and perioperative nurses had the second highest rate of injuries that resulted in days away from work.[1]

A study of musculoskeletal injuries in a tertiary medical center revealed that nurse's aides had a higher rate of injury than nurses, and the stressors for injury were equally distributed between lifting, pushing, and pulling equipment; patient handling; and slips, trips, and falls.[7] A descriptive study of endoscopy nurses showed that about 50% of the sample (N = 38) experienced upper extremity injuries.[8] In a descriptive study, researchers determined that patient transfers, clean-up duties, basic patient care, and bed making all resulted in the nurse assuming a stressful trunk posture, which can lead to back injury.[5]

The advent of laparoscopic surgery has created ergonomic stressors in addition to those usually encountered during open surgery.[9] These stressors are created by the need to view a monitor and the need to maintain a static posture related to holding a camera.[10,11] The instruments may not be configured appropriately for the user or the patient, which can lead to stress on the user's arms and neck.[12]

A 2010 report from the Bureau of Labor Statistics indicated that musculoskeletal disorders accounted for 29% of all workplace injuries that led to time away from work. Back injuries were the most frequent claim overall, and shoulder injuries were the most severe injury for all occupations. Among registered nurses, 55.1% reported back injuries and 13.2% reported shoulder injuries. Although back injuries were the most frequently reported, abdominal injuries and leg injuries resulted in the greatest number of days away from work, at 19 days and 13 days, respectively. The rates for nursing assistants were higher than those for registered nurses.[13]

Perioperative team members are prone to pain and fatigue from the need to maintain static postures during surgical procedures.[4] A cross-sectional study in Greece of 350 nursing personnel revealed that 51% experienced lower back pain and 23% experienced knee pain. Personnel who perceived that their jobs demanded high physical exertion or that they had moderate to bad general health had a higher odds ratio of experiencing low back or knee pain.[14]

A survey of 425 German surgeons indicated that they perceive that OR design, equipment (eg, lights, tables, monitors), cables and tubes, instrument design, and working posture all contribute to ergonomic stressors in the OR.[15]

I.a. Risk-reduction strategies (ie, administrative, engineering, behavioral controls) for injury prevention should be identified, developed, and implemented. *[2: Moderate Evidence]*

Education on techniques to improve posture and ergonomics has been shown to decrease the incidence of occupational injuries overall.[16] In an endoscopy suite with 120 employees, various strategies that were implemented reduced the number of reported injuries (eg, trips over cords, head traumas, crushing injuries to the hand).[3] In another study of endoscopy suites, strategies such as combining cables into one bundle, covering cables and tubes on the floors, and using electrical plugs anchored in the ceiling were shown to reduce the incidence of team members tripping over exposed wires and tubes.[2]

After changing to a zero-transfer system, one facility reported a 100% decrease in staff member injuries related to patient transfers, which was sustained for two years.[17] The zero-transfer system involved using a chair with wheels that, when in position, became the OR bed. A pre- and post-intervention study of 766 injury cases in six facilities showed that a combination of administrative and engineering controls significantly reduced personnel injuries and disabilities related to patient handling.[18] A qualitative study of 126 patient-caregiver encounters revealed that the complexity of care, patient treatment goals, the amount of time to complete the task, knowledge of patient moving techniques, and equipment issues all influence the nurse's decision on the best way to move a patient.[19] A descriptive, exploratory study in a facility with 950 nurses investigated nurses' satisfaction with the use of mechanical lift equipment, the frequency of use, and the efficacy of employing a hands-on bedside mechanical lift equipment facilitator in increasing the use of lift equipment. The study revealed a decrease in lost work days and in the cost of worker's compensation claims after the interventions were employed.[20]

I.a.1. Administrative controls for an ergonomically healthy perioperative environment should include
- developing a culture of ergonomic safety,
- developing and implementing a policy for manual patient handling,
- using patient care ergonomic assessment protocols,
- educating personnel in the use of patient handling devices and strategies to prevent musculoskeletal injury,[16]
- using ergonomic workstations,
- having adequate personnel present during patient handling and other situations resulting in ergonomic stress, and
- having ergonomic clinical advisors or resources available.[20]

A comparative study involving 16 nurses revealed that education on safe patient handling techniques improves compliance.[21] A report from a 958-bed hospital in Florida showed a 62% reduction in injuries related to patient handling during a six-year period after the creation of a lift team.[22] Similar injury reductions were noted in an Australian study after a no-lift policy was implemented in the entire state of Victoria.[23]

I.a.2. Engineering controls for an ergonomically healthy perioperative environment should include
- having appropriate assistive patient handling equipment available[22,23];
- limiting the weight of instrument trays to 25 lb total weight[24];
- adapting workstations, tools, and equipment for ergonomic safety; and
- providing adequate lighting.[25]

I.a.3. Behavioral controls for an ergonomically healthy perioperative environment include
- wearing nonskid footwear;
- eliminating clutter, including removing wires or tubes from the floor;
- covering equipment cables across the floor;
- keeping cabinet and room doors closed;
- placing monitors straight in front of personnel and slightly lower than eye level[10];
- cleaning up spills or debris as soon as possible;
- using anti-fatigue mats;
- using lift teams and assistive devices to transfer or lift patients; and
- cleaning furniture wheels frequently.

A retrospective study of medical records, employee records, and interviews of personnel who worked in endoscopy rooms showed a decrease in injuries from collisions when spills were cleaned up as soon as possible, booties were not worn over shoes, and monitors were placed at eye level and were replaced with lighter weight models.[3] Another study revealed a reduction in injuries when cords or tubing lying on the floor were removed or were bundled and covered.[2]

I.b. The physical environment should provide
- hydraulic or electric booms mounted to the ceiling or wall when structurally feasible;
- adequate room lighting;
- adequate storage; and
- floor surfaces that allow for easy movement of patient handling equipment.[26]

[2: Moderate Evidence]

Using hydraulic or electric ceiling-suspended equipment decreases the risk of injuries to perioperative team members.[10,27] Low lighting levels have been shown to increase the risk of tripping.[2,9] A review of accident reports revealed an injury resulting from tripping over an improperly stored wheelchair.[3]

I.c. Perioperative personnel should follow the algorithms outlined in the AORN "Guidance statement: safe patient handling and movement in the perioperative setting"[27] and organizational policies and procedures while completing activities such as
- performing a lateral patient transfer from a stretcher to the OR bed;
- positioning or repositioning the patient on the OR bed;
- lifting and holding the patient's head or extremities for prepping;
- standing for a prolonged period;
- retracting tissue;
- lifting and carrying supplies or equipment; and
- pushing, pulling, or moving equipment on wheels.[27]

[2: Moderate Evidence]

The AORN guidance statement provides evidence-based directions for decreasing ergonomic stressors that, if they are not recognized, can cause personnel injury.[28-34]

ENVIRONMENT OF CARE, PART 1

Recommendation II

Potential hazards associated with fire safety in the practice setting should be identified, and safe practices for communication, prevention, suppression, and evacuation should be established and followed.

Fire is a risk to both patients and personnel in the OR because all three elements of the fire triangle (Figure 1) that are necessary for a fire—fuel, oxidizer, ignition source—typically are present.[35,36] Surgical fires are estimated to occur in the United States about 550 to 650 times a year.[36,37] The ECRI Institute states that surgical fires occur most frequently on the patient (70%), and 29% occur in the patient. Forty-four percent of fires occurring on the patient involve the head, neck, and upper chest, and 26% occur elsewhere. Twenty-one percent of fires are located in the airway, and 8% occur at other locations in the body.[36] The majority of fatal fires are airway fires.[37] Fires have been reported to occur during different types of surgical procedures (eg, coronary bypass graft, otolaryngology procedures).[38-40] One explosion was reportedly caused by cutting the wires from the battery pack of a battery-operated lavage system.[41]

II.a. A written fire prevention and management plan should be developed by a multidisciplinary group composed of key stakeholders within the organization such as
- perioperative RNs,
- perioperative unlicensed assistive personnel,
- anesthesia professionals,
- physicians,
- a local fire department representative,
- risk management personnel,
- the safety officer, and
- facilities/engineering personnel.[35]

[2: Moderate Evidence]

II.a.1. The fire prevention and management plan should include
- perioperative team members' responsibilities, including communication;
- methods of prevention;
- processes to safely manage different fire scenarios;
- alarm activation procedures;
- methods to extinguish a fire;
- the preferred routes and levels of evacuation;
- a description of the facility's fire risk assessment tool (Figure 2); and
- the required content for and frequency of fire safety education, including frequency of and procedures for fire drills.[35]

II.b. A fire risk assessment should be completed and communicated to the entire perioperative team before beginning a surgical procedure. [2: Moderate Evidence]

Fire prevention experts and professional associations support the importance of completing the risk assessment.[35,42] In one case report that involved a fire caused by the electrosurgical electrode igniting a sponge during open heart surgery, a lack of communication may have contributed to the fire. In this situation, there was a delay in communicating to the surgeon a decrease in the tidal volumes that was caused by a ruptured bleb. The rupture caused oxygen to leak into the patient's chest cavity and created an oxygen-enriched environment.[39]

II.b.1. The fire risk assessment should identify
- fuels that are present,
- ignition sources that are present,
- the potential for the presence of an oxygen-enriched environment,
- the specific type of fire extinguisher that is required based on the fuel and involvement of electrical current, and
- additional preventive measures that are required as determined by the location of the fire and fuel sources.

II.c. Ignition sources (eg, active electrosurgical electrodes, lasers, electrocautery devices, fiber-optic light cords) should be used according to manufacturers' instructions for use and AORN guidelines.[9,43,44] [2: Moderate Evidence]

Manufacturers' written instructions for use and labels include fire safety information, such as the laser resistance of the endotracheal tube and methods of disposal for equipment (eg, battery packs).[37,41,45] Electrosurgical units provide the ignition source, especially when they are used in the presence of oxidizers, flammable solutions, or volatile or combustible chemicals or liquids.[36,44] Lasers provide the ignition source

FIGURE 1. AORN FIRE TRIANGLE

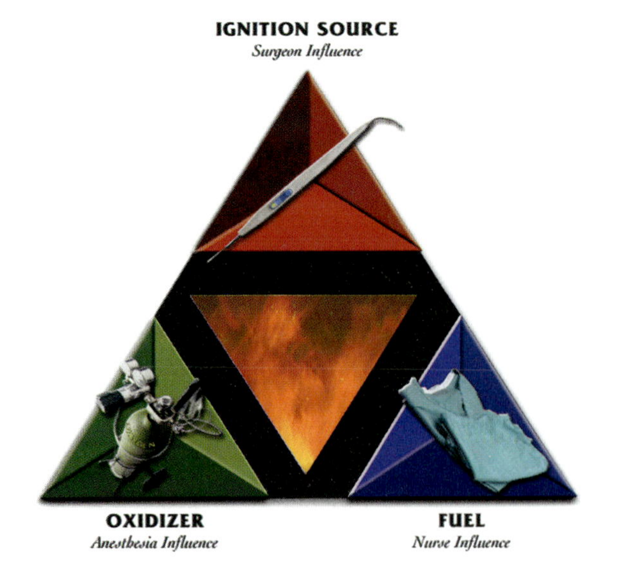

IGNITION SOURCE
Surgeon Influence

OXIDIZER
Anesthesia Influence

FUEL
Nurse Influence

The AORN Fire Triangle illustrates the three elements necessary for a fire and the members of the perioperative team who frequently influence the element.

when they are used in the presence of oxidizers, flammable solutions, or volatile or combustible chemicals or liquids.[36,37,43] Fiber-optic light cables may provide an ignition source if they are disconnected from the working element and are allowed to remain in contact with drapes, sponges, or other fuel sources.[9,46]

II.c.1. Saline should be used to cool devices that create heat during use (eg, drills, burrs, saw blades).[36]

II.c.2. Defibrillator paddles and pads should be an appropriate size for the patient and applied using only manufacturer-recommended lubricants.

Using paddles that are the correct size and with manufacturer-recommended lubricants decreases both sparking and the amount of energy required for defibrillation.[36]

II.d. Fuels (eg, alcohol-based skin antiseptic agents, collodion, drapes, gowns, endotracheal tubes) should be managed to prevent contact with ignition sources. *[2: Moderate Evidence]*

Preventing contact between fuels and ignition sources breaks the fire triangle, thereby preventing fire.[47] Many potential fuels that will not burn in ambient air will burn in an oxygen-enriched environment, which may be present in the OR.[36,37,42]

II.d.1. The flammable or combustible rating of a skin antiseptic agent should be determined by reviewing the applicable material safety data sheet (MSDS) or safety data sheet (SDS).

Prep solutions can be rated as "flammable" or "combustible" on the MSDS or SDS. A combustible solution will burn but requires a higher temperature to cause ignition. A rating of "flammable" indicates a solution that has a flash point of less than 100° F (37.8° C). A solution with a rating of "combustible" has a flash point of greater than 100° F (37.8° C).[48]

II.d.2. Flammable skin antiseptic agents should be prevented from pooling or soaking into linens or the patient's hair by
- using reusable or disposable sterile towels to absorb drips and excess solution during application,
- removing materials that are saturated with the skin antiseptic agent before draping the patient, and
- wicking excess solution with a sterile towel to help dry the surgical prep area completely.[36,37,42]

II.d.3. Adequate time should be provided to allow flammable skin antiseptic agents to dry completely and to allow any fumes to dissipate before applying surgical drapes or using a potential ignition source.[35,42]

FIGURE 2. AORN FIRE RISK ASSESSMENT TOOL

Fire Risk Assessment Tool

A. Is an alcohol-based skin antiseptic or other flammable solution being used preoperatively?
  ❏ Yes
  ❏ No

B. Is the operative or other invasive procedure being performed above the xiphoid process or in the oropharynx?
  ❏ Yes
  ❏ No

C. Is open oxygen or nitrous oxide being administered?
  ❏ Yes
  ❏ No

D. Is an electrosurgical unit, laser, or fiber-optic light being used?
  ❏ Yes
  ❏ No

E. Are there other possible contributors (eg, defibrillators, drills, saws, burrs)?
  ❏ Yes
  ❏ No

The AORN Fire Risk Assessment Tool illustrates components that should be included in an assessment tool.

Allowing adequate time for skin antiseptic agents to dry before applying drapes helps prevent the accumulation of volatile fumes beneath the drapes.[47] The volatile fumes are flammable and may ignite without a connection between the ignition source and the actual surgical antiseptic agent.[36,37]

II.d.4. For surgical procedures that involve the head or neck, a water-soluble gel should be used to cover the patient's facial hair, and any eye lubricants that are used should be water based.

The patient's hair is a fuel source, and covering facial hair with water-soluble gel decreases the risk of combustion because it raises the temperature that is required for ignition.[36]

II.d.5. Local and state fire regulations should be followed regarding the storage of flammable liquids (eg, alcohol-based skin antiseptic solutions, hand sanitizer, alcohol, acetone, collodion) and the location of dispensers.[42,49-51]

II.e. Oxidizers (eg, oxygen, nitrous oxide) should be used with caution near any ignition or fuel sources. *[2: Moderate Evidence]*

An oxygen-enriched environment is when the oxygen concentration is greater than 21% by volume.[35] In an oxygen-enriched environment, the temperature and energy required for fuels to ignite is lower than that of ambient or medical air. Nitrous oxide is considered an oxidizer and requires the same precautions that are used with oxygen.[36,37,42,49]

II.e.1. The anesthesia circuit should be free of leaks.

Leaks in the anesthesia circuit can increase the oxygen concentration under the drapes, creating an oxygen-enriched environment that increases the risk of fire.[35,37,52] The anesthesia circuit includes the endotracheal tube, the seal between the tube and the patient's airway, the bag reservoir, and the tubing that leads from the anesthesia machine to the endotracheal tube.

II.e.2. Accumulated anesthetic gas should be evacuated using a metal suction cannula before an ignition source is used in or near an oxygen-enriched environment.

The suction will assist with removing excess oxidizing agents to create an atmosphere that is closer to ambient air.[36,37] A metal suction cannula will not ignite.[37]

II.e.3. The lowest possible concentration of oxygen that provides adequate patient oxygen saturation should be used for a patient who requires supplemental oxygen.[35-37,52,53]

II.e.4. A laryngeal mask airway or an endotracheal tube should be used when the patient requires supplementary oxygen greater than 30% unless using the tube is contraindicated by the procedure (eg, the patient is required to respond verbally during the procedure).

Use of a laryngeal mask airway or an endotracheal tube decreases the risk of fire by decreasing the oxygen concentration under the drapes and in the patient's upper airway.[35-37,54]

II.e.5. Drapes should be placed over the patient's head in a manner that allows the oxygen to flow freely and prevents accumulation under the drapes.[36,37,47,52]

II.e.6. When using a warming blanket with an attached head drape, the following precautions should be used:
- cut a hole in the drape around the endotracheal tube;
- place the drape over the patient's head in a manner that allows the oxygen to flow freely and prevents accumulation under the drapes;
- lift and reposition the patient's head frequently, if possible; and
- keep the warmer blower on while the drape is in place.

These precautions have been shown to decrease the oxygen concentration under the drapes, which assists in preventing an oxygen-enriched environment.[52]

II.e.7. A second delivery system that administers 5 L/minute to 10 L/minute of medical air should be used when supplemental oxygen is administered under the drapes.

A second delivery system, which consists of a flow meter that is connected to a medical air source and tubing that delivers air beneath the drapes, assists with flushing oxygen from under the drapes. Mixing oxygen with nonflammable gases, such as medical air, reduces the risk of fire by preventing an oxygen-enriched environment.[36,37]

II.e.8. When performing surgical procedures on anatomical structures that present special fire hazards (eg, bowel, trachea), additional precautions should be taken (eg, using a scalpel rather than an electrosurgical active electrode to create the incision).

Hydrogen and methane, which are flammable gases, may be present in the bowel and ignite when they are exposed to an ignition source, such as an active electrosurgical electrode.[36,47,55] An oxygen-enriched environment may be present within the trachea because of the presence of anesthesia gases.[37,55]

II.f. The risk of airway fires should be minimized during surgical procedures involving the airway by placing wet radiopaque sponges in the back of the throat and inflating endotracheal tube cuffs with tinted solutions. *[2: Moderate Evidence]*

Wet radiopaque sponges placed in the back of the throat help decrease or prevent oxygen leaks.[35,40] Inflating endotracheal tube cuffs with tinted solutions improves visibility in the event of a cuff rupture.[35-37]

II.g. Communication, suppression, and evacuation procedures should be followed in the event of a fire. *[2: Moderate Evidence]*

Following established procedures assists in protecting patients and perioperative personnel from injury or may decrease the severity of sustained injuries.[56]

II.g.1. Perioperative team members should be alerted to the presence of a fire by the person who discovers the fire.

Alerting the team allows team members to carry out their responsibilities and decreases the risks of injury to the patient and personnel.[36]

II.g.2. Water or normal saline or a safe method for smothering should be used to extinguish a fire, if it can be accomplished safely.

Extinguishing a fire as soon as possible decreases the risk of injury to the patient and personnel.[36,37]

II.g.3. In the event of an airway fire, the endotracheal tube should be removed and normal saline should be poured into the airway. These steps should occur in collaboration with the anesthesia care professional.

Removing the endotracheal tube removes the source of the fuel, and normal saline cools burned tissue.[35,37,56,57]

II.g.4. In the event of a non-airway fire, the fuel source should be removed from the patient and the fire extinguished. Simultaneously, the anesthesia care professional should discontinue administration of airway gases.[36,56,57]

II.g.5. After the fuel source has been removed from the patient, ventilation should be reestablished, the patient assessed, and the findings reported to the physician.[56,57]

II.g.6. After safely extinguishing the fire, perioperative team members should follow required procedures for reporting and should save all items that were involved in the fire.

Saving all items that are involved in the fire is necessary to provide evidence for an investigation. This investigation may be accomplished by the quality or risk management department personnel but also may involve the local fire department.[36,37]

II.g.7. The OR should be evacuated according to the facility fire plan if perioperative team members are unable to extinguish a fire.

Evacuation protects the patient and perioperative team members from injury from the by-products of fire or the fire itself.[36]

II.h. Equipment that emits unanticipated smoke, whether in use or not, should be disconnected from the electrical current source. The equipment and all of the accessories in use should be moved to a safe area, if this can be done safely. *[2: Moderate Evidence]*

Smoke suggests the presence of fire, and equipment may be an ignition source for nearby items. Disconnecting the piece of equipment from the electrical current source may remove the ignition source and thereby extinguish the fire. Moving the equipment out of the OR decreases the risk to the patient and perioperative team members in that room.[36] An overheated ventilator circuit has been reported to be the cause of two different fires.[58]

II.h.1. The room should be immediately evacuated if the equipment cannot be removed safely.[36]

II.i. Fire extinguishers should be located within 30 to 75 feet from the center of the OR, or as required by the local authority with jurisdiction, depending on the fuel source and extinguisher.[59] *[2: Moderate Evidence]*

II.i.1. Fire extinguishers should be selected according to standards established by the National Fire Protection Association (NFPA) and the local authority with jurisdiction. Factors that help determine the appropriate type of fire extinguisher include
- types of fuel that are present,
- potential fire size,
- hazards that are present and may create adverse chemical reactions with the extinguishing agent,
- electrical equipment that is present,
- ease of use,
- physical abilities of potential users, and
- maintenance requirements.[59]

The NFPA recommends either a water mist or carbon dioxide extinguisher be used in the OR. Water mist extinguishers are rated Class 2A:C.[59] Carbon dioxide extinguishers are rated Class B and Class C, but also may be used for Class A fires.[59]

II.i.2. Fire extinguishing equipment and supplies should be regularly inspected, tested, and maintained.[59]

II.i.3. Fire extinguishers should not be used as a first line of defense in a fire.

Extinguishing a fire using noncombustible and nonflammable solutions from the back table or a smothering technique can be faster than obtaining a fire extinguisher.[36]

II.j. All personnel should be able to identify medical gas control valves, including the areas that they control, and have the ability to shut down medical gases in the event of a fire. *[2: Moderate Evidence]*

Removing the oxidizer by turning off the medical gas supply assists with breaking the fire triangle.[36,42] A medical gas control valve may control more than one OR.

II.k. Equipment (eg, case carts, stretchers, supply carts, patient beds) should not be stored in locations that block access to pull alarms, medical gas control valves, or electrical panels.[49] *[2: Moderate Evidence]*

II.l. Fire blankets should not be used in an OR.

Fire blankets may trap fire next to or under the patient and cause more harm. Fire blankets are made of wool and can burn in an oxygen-enriched environment.[36,60] During the application of the fire blanket, instruments may be dislodged, causing injury to the patient. Usage can

ENVIRONMENT OF CARE, PART 1

lead to wound contamination or spread the fire.[36,56] [2: Moderate Evidence]

II.m. Evacuation routes should be established for the perioperative environment, be developed in collaboration with local authorities, and be guided by NFPA regulations.[49] [2: Moderate Evidence]

II.m.1. Personnel and emergency responders should be educated about how to implement the evacuation plan.[42,49]

II.m.2. Evacuation routes should be clearly displayed in multiple locations throughout the health care facility.[49]

II.m.3. The evacuation destination should be the closest safe location where patient care can be continued.[36]

II.n. All personnel should receive education and competency verification on
- the elements of the fire triangle;
- use of the perioperative fire risk assessment;
- fire extinguisher locations;
- use of fire extinguishers and other firefighting equipment;
- evacuation routes for each room;
- medical gas panel locations and operation, including how to turn them off in an emergency;
- the location of shut off controls for ventilation and electrical systems;
- the location of fire alarm pull stations;
- procedures for turning off the ventilation and electrical systems;
- how and when to activate the fire safety and evacuation plan;
- how and when to contact the local fire department; and
- the roles and responsibilities of each team member in various fire scenarios.[36,37,49,56]

[2: Moderate Evidence]

The need for education is identified in a report of a fire simulation in an obstetric OR that revealed personnel did now know the locations of the fire extinguishers or fire safe zones.[61]

II.n.1. Fire drills should occur periodically as required by the local authority with jurisdiction.

The NFPA 101 recommends that fire drills occur at least quarterly on each shift.[49] The NFPA 99 recommends fire drills to include evacuation annually or as determined by the relevant building code.[42] The local authority with jurisdiction may not have adopted the most current NFPA guidelines and therefore may be following the earlier edition.

Recommendation III

Precautions should be taken to mitigate the risk of injury associated with the use of electrical equipment.

Injuries to patients, personnel, or visitors may occur from medical equipment that has frayed cords, from damaged outlets, or from extension cords.[42] In 2011 the Joint Commission received 39 reports of medical equipment–related events, and the ECRI Institute received reports of events related to ceiling-mounted booms that created the potential for or resulted in injuries.[62,63]

III.a. All electrical equipment, including ceiling- and wall-mounted equipment (eg, booms, monitors), and all loaned equipment should be inspected for damage periodically and before each use. Inspection should include checking power cords for fraying and examining strain relief and plugs for damage. [2: Moderate Evidence]

Damaged electrical equipment and power cords can cause unsafe conditions. Power cords are frequently subject to damage from daily use.[42] Fires related to improper cleaning or malfunctions of booms and other equipment has been reported.[62,64]

III.b. Equipment, including the electrical cord, that is found to be in disrepair should be removed immediately from service. [2: Moderate Evidence]

Using equipment that is in a state of disrepair can create unsafe conditions.[42]

III.c. Device cords should be secured and have the appropriate characteristics for the intended use, including adequate length. [2: Moderate Evidence]

Cords that do not lie flat create the risk of tripping or accidental unplugging of the equipment.[2,3] An inappropriate cord may cause damage to the machine if it does not meet the necessary electrical characteristics (eg, grounding resistance, power cord ampacity, correct polarization).[42]

III.c.1. Device cords should not be changed unless the replacement cord meets the electrical characteristics of the original.

Changing the device cord may nullify the device warranty. The cord may cause damage to the equipment if the electrical characteristics do not match the characteristics of the original cord.[42]

III.c.2. Cords should be secured in a safe manner with an "electrically safe device"[42] that is disposable and able to be cleaned.

Safely securing cords helps prevent trips and falls.[2,3] Using an electrically safe device to secure cords decreases the potential for an electrical shock.[42] Using a device that is disposable or that can be cleaned decreases the risk of transmitting an infection to the patient by contact with the contaminated device.[65,66]

III.c.3. An extension cord should be used only if it has the correct electrical characteristics.

Incorrect electrical characteristics can cause damage to the equipment and overheating of the cord.[42]

III.c.4. Multiple outlet connections should be mounted to a movable equipment assembly (eg, cart, table, pedestal, boom), provided that the cord and the connection have the capacity to allow the total number of amps used to pass through the cord without creating unsafe conditions. The total number of amps should be calculated by adding the amps required by each piece of equipment together.

The use of a multiple outlet connection allows for multiple pieces of equipment to be plugged in to one connection. This connection has only one cord on the floor instead of one cord for each piece of equipment.[42]

III.d. All electrical equipment charger adaptor cords should be labeled with the name of the piece of equipment to which they belong. *[3: Limited Evidence]*

Equipment has been reported to overheat and malfunction when incorrect charger adaptor cords are used.[67]

Recommendation IV

Precautions should be taken to mitigate hazards associated with non-functioning clinical and alert alarms or with personnel failing to hear or failing to act on alarms.

A clinical alarm (eg, cardiac monitor, ventilator, anesthesia machine) is patient specific and used for the purpose of alerting staff members to a patient emergency. An alert alarm (eg, medical gas systems, blood bank refrigerators, fire alarms, code blue alarms, ethylene oxide level alarms, water treatment alarms) is connected to a system and alerts personnel to system failures that would affect multiple patients. Alarms can be auditory, visual, or a combination of both.[68] Patients have experienced injuries and near-misses because of alarms being turned off or being inaudible.[69-71]

IV.a. Clinical and alert alarms should be tested on initial setup.[72] *[2: Moderate Evidence]*

IV.b. Clinical and alert alarms should be tested according to organizational policy and procedures. *[2: Moderate Evidence]*

Periodic testing assists with maintaining a working system.[69,71]

IV.c. An inventory of clinical and alert alarms should be conducted periodically as a collaborative effort between clinical engineering and perioperative personnel. *[2: Moderate Evidence]*

Clinical engineering and perioperative personnel provide a broad spectrum of information for the team.[69,71] Completing an assessment assists with identifying the pieces of equipment that have alarms, maintaining an accurate alarm inventory, and tracking testing. This information also may assist with setting optimal alarm limits.[71]

IV.c.1. The alarm inventory should include all devices with alarms, including
- blood bank refrigerators,
- medication refrigerators,
- security systems,
- electrosurgical units (ESUs),
- pneumatic tourniquets,
- patient monitoring devices (eg, cardiac monitors, oximeters),
- carbon dioxide (CO_2) insufflators,
- anesthesia equipment,
- sequential compression devices, and
- infusion pumps.

IV.d. Clinical and alert alarms should be sufficiently loud to allow them to be heard above competing noise, and competing noise should be reduced so that alarms can be heard. *[2: Moderate Evidence]*

Competing noise makes it difficult to hear and differentiate between alarms.[69,71] The OR is a very noisy atmosphere with competing noise from alarms on anesthesia monitors and other equipment (eg, tourniquets) and operating alerts, such as the alert on the ESU.[73] A study that evaluated the amount of competing noise in the OR revealed that in 25 consecutive elective cardiac surgery procedures, an anesthesia alarm sounded an average of every 1.2 minutes.[70] AORN recommends that noise-reduction interventions be incorporated into action plans intended to decrease distractions.[74]

IV.e. Changes in alarm default parameters (eg, volume, high or low limits) should be communicated verbally and visually during changes of personnel, including using a clearly distinguishable visual cue, such as posting a sign, to indicate the change in the default. *[2: Moderate Evidence]*

Communicating changes to alarm settings notifies the oncoming personnel that the default settings have been changed and prepares them to respond appropriately.[75]

Recommendation V

Precautions should be taken to avoid thermal injuries related to warming solutions, blankets, and patient linens in blanket- and solution-warming cabinets.

The danger of burns from heated blankets, solutions, or linens is increased in the perioperative setting because patients are unconscious or sedated and cannot feel an increase in temperature or communicate discomfort. Even when solutions and blankets do not feel warm to the touch, heat continues to build up in these items and can be transferred to the patient.[76] Injuries to the patient can result from irrigation solution being warmed to high temperatures. In one report, a patient experienced full thickness skin burns and joint damage from irrigation solutions that were warmed in a cabinet in which the temperature ranged from 100.4° F (38° C) on the top shelf to 118.4° F (48° C) on the bottom shelf.[77]

V.a. Solutions, blankets, and patient linens should be stored in separate warming cabinets or in cabinets with separate compartments that have independent temperature controls. [3: Limited Evidence]

Using separate warming cabinets allows for better temperature control compared to dual compartment or single compartment cabinets. Separate compartments with separate controls allow for each compartment to be set to an individual temperature and for accurate regulation of both cabinets.[76,78] Fluids should not be warmed to the same temperature as blankets because fluids attain a higher temperature and retain that temperature longer, presenting a greater risk of thermal injury.[76]

V.a.1. Warming cabinets should be labeled to identify items that may be placed within the cabinet and the maximum permissible temperature setting. If the cabinet has separate compartments, each compartment should be labeled.[76]

V.b. Warming cabinet temperatures should be set, maintained, monitored, and documented according to organizational policy. [2: Moderate Evidence]

Monitoring and documenting the temperature of warming cabinets is necessary to verify that temperature settings are maintained within specified limits.[76] A malfunctioning cabinet can cause temperature variation.[77]

V.b.1. Temperatures should be documented on a temperature log or recorded with an electronic recording system.

V.b.2. A specific team member should be assigned to set, maintain, monitor, and document the temperature of the warming cabinets.[76]

V.b.3. Precautions should be taken when a warming cabinet malfunctions, including
- removing the cabinet from service,
- labeling the cabinet as out of order,
- removing all blankets and solutions from the warmer,
- not using blankets if they are overheated until the temperatures are within the acceptable range,
- following fluid manufacturers' written instructions to determine usability of solutions, and
- reporting the malfunction to the clinical engineering department for maintenance.

V.b.4. Warming cabinet contents should be rotated on a first-in, first-out basis.

V.c. The number of warming cabinets should be sufficient to support the anticipated need for warmed items. [2: Moderate Evidence]

Three blankets may be required per patient to decrease the amount of heat loss. Blankets may take eight to 12 hours to reach the set temperature.[76] Perioperative staff members have been reported to use unsafe means to warm blankets, such as in autoclaves or microwaves.[79] When the supply of warm blankets is not sufficient, staff members may increase the temperature of the warmer, which can cause overheating of the blankets and potentially lead to burns. The use of methods such as forced-air warming devices may decrease the number of warming cabinets required.[76,80]

V.d. Warming cabinets should be located close to the point of use. [2: Moderate Evidence]

One single-site quality improvement project that measured blanket temperatures showed that if a blanket is warmed to 110° F (43.3° C), its temperature drops to 82° F (27.8° C) within five minutes, and if a blanket is warmed to 150° F (65.6° C), its temperature drops to 83° F (28.3° C) within five minutes.[79]

V.e. Warming cabinet or compartment temperatures used for blankets and other patient linens should not exceed 130° F (54.4° C). [2: Moderate Evidence]

In one limited quality improvement project, blankets were warmed to 150° F (65.6° C) without harmful effects to the subjects, who were alert and not under the effects of any anesthetic agents.[79] However, this recommendation is based on stronger evidence that shows temperatures greater than 130° F (54.4° C) increase the potential for burns.[76,78]

V.f. Solution manufacturers' instructions for use should be followed regarding the maximum temperature and length of time solutions should remain in the warming cabinet or compartment and for usability after removal. [3: Limited Evidence]

Solution manufacturers' recommendations for maximum temperature setting, time limit that solutions may remain in the warming device, and for solution use after removal vary. Manufacturers' settings may be determined by the stability of the container and the solution.[76]

V.f.1. When solutions are placed in warming cabinets, they should be labeled with the date of insertion or date of removal.

Labeling helps determine when the solution has reached its maximum shelf life and prevents overheating related to being left in the warmer too long.

V.f.2. The temperature of solutions on the sterile field should be remeasured before administration.

ENVIRONMENT OF CARE, PART 1

Burns have been associated with the administration of overheated solutions.[9,76,77,80]

V.g. Solutions intended for IV administration should only be warmed using technology designed for this purpose. *[3: Limited Evidence]*

Warming IV solutions in warming cabinets can overheat the solution from inconsistencies in temperature within the warming cabinet and variances in the temperature of the cabinet.[76,78]

V.h. Skin antiseptic agents should not be warmed, unless otherwise directed by the manufacturer's instructions for use.[81] *[2: Moderate Evidence]*

Recommendation VI

Precautions should be taken to mitigate risks associated with handling, storage, and use of compressed medical gas cylinders and liquid oxygen containers.

The US Food and Drug Administration (FDA) has received reports of patient deaths and injuries related to hook-up errors in medical gas systems.[82]

VI.a. Storage conditions for medical gases should be determined by the volume stored in a location, the need for immediate use, and regulatory requirements.[42] *[2: Moderate Evidence]*

The NFPA and regulatory agencies have determined and enforce the various medical gas storage condition requirements.[42]

VI.a.1. An adequate emergency supply of oxygen should be stored at the facility to provide an uninterrupted supply for one day.[42] *Amb*

VI.a.2. Medical gases must be stored in a secure area with controlled access and separately from industrial gases.

The FDA considers compressed medical gases to be drugs for dispensing by prescription only.[42,83,84]

VI.a.3. The combined volume of medical gas cylinders not considered to be for immediate patient use should not exceed 3,000 ft^3 per smoke compartment.

Cylinders on patient gurneys are considered in use or for immediate patient use. Cylinders and carts directly associated with a specific patient are considered "in use." Cylinders and carts not directly associated with a specific patient for 30 minutes or more are considered not in use or in storage.[42]

VI.a.4. Medical gas cylinders that are not intended for immediate use should be stored indoors and
- in a room with a minimum one-hour fire resistance rating,
- in a room that has negative pressure and eight air exchanges per hour,[26]
- in a holder or storage rack with a chain-like securing device, and
- away from heat sources.

Securing cylinders with a chain-like device or in racks prevents the cylinders from falling over. Cylinders and carts directly associated with a specific patient are considered "in use." Cylinders and carts not directly associated with a specific patient for 30 minutes or more are considered not in use or in storage.[42]

VI.a.5. Medical gas cylinders should not be stored in an egress hallway.[42]

VI.a.6. Empty medical gas cylinders should be marked and segregated from full cylinders.

Segregating empty cylinders from full ones minimizes the risk of connecting to an empty cylinder and delaying administration of vital gases.[42]

VI.b. Medical gas cylinders should be transported and secured in a carrier that is designed to prevent the cylinders from tipping or being dropped or damaged. *[2: Moderate Evidence]*

Transporting a cylinder without using an appropriate carrier increases the potential of damage to the cylinder and causing sudden release of the compressed gas, which can cause propulsion of the cylinder and subsequent injury.[42]

VI.c. Medical gas cylinders used during patient transport should be secured to the transport cart or bed in holders designed for this purpose and not placed on top of the bed or cart next to the patient. *[2: Moderate Evidence]*

Holders minimize the risk of the cylinder falling, which can cause propulsion of the cylinder and subsequent injury. Many transport carts are available with built-in holders.[42]

VI.d. Before use, gas cylinders should be checked for the appropriate label, pin-index safety system connector, and color coding. *[2: Moderate Evidence]*

The color of the cylinder, written labels, and a unique pin-index safety system connector are used to clearly identify the medical gas contained within medical gas cylinders.[42]

The pin-index safety system connector for different medical gases prevents connecting the wrong gas to the delivery system.[85] The Compressed Gas Association has approved standardized colors for identification of different medical gases (eg, green indicates oxygen).[42,86] Serious injuries and deaths have resulted from the use of an incorrectly identified medical gas.[82]

VI.e. Fittings on medical gas cylinders and hoses should not be altered under any circumstances.[42] *[2: Moderate Evidence]*

249

Serious injuries and deaths have resulted from altering the pin-index safety system, thereby permitting delivery of an incorrect gas into the medical gas administration system.[82,87]

VI.e.1. If the fitting does not easily connect, the label on the gas cylinder or hose should be rechecked to verify that it is correct.[42,87]

VI.e.2. If the label is correct, the cylinder should be returned to the distributor for examination.[42]

VI.e.3. If the label is incorrect, the cylinder should be replaced with a correctly labeled gas cylinder.[42]

VI.f. Only approved regulators or other flow control devices should be used.[42,87] *[2: Moderate Evidence]*

VI.f.1. The regulator, gasket, and washers should be inspected before use.[87]

VI.f.2. The regulator should be tightened with a T-handle until it is firmly in place.

VI.g. Precautions should be followed when using medical gas cylinder valves. *[2: Moderate Evidence]*

Improper use of medical gas cylinder valves can result in contamination of the gas and leakage of the contents into the environment.[42]

VI.g.1. When a cylinder valve is opened, a small amount of gas should be released before attaching the regulator.

Opening the valve removes any dust that may have accumulated.[42,87]

VI.g.2. The valve should be opened slowly to determine whether there is a leak, and the valve should be closed quickly if a leak is found.

VI.g.3. Compressed medical gas tank valves should be opened fully during use.[42]

VI.g.4. The valves on medical gas cylinders should be closed properly to avoid leaking during storage. *Amb*

VI.h. Liquid oxygen containers must be handled, filled, stored, and transported according to state and federal regulations and manufactures' written instructions and labeling.[42] *[2: Moderate Evidence]*

VI.h.1. Liquid oxygen containers should be stored
- in a cool, dry place outside of the building or
- inside the building, as long as the containers are secured to prevent them from tipping over, they do not interfere with foot traffic, they are not exposed to open flames or high-temperature devices, and they are not subject to damage from falling devices.[42]

Recommendation VII

Precautions should be taken to mitigate hazards related to waste anesthesia gases.

All anesthesia machines have the potential to leak, which increases the level of waste anesthesia gases in the ambient air.[88] A study of 15,317 live births between 1990 and 2000 to 9,433 mothers who were exposed to waste anesthesia gases consisting of halothane, isoflurane, or sevoflurane revealed a potential exposure-response relationship between gas exposure and the development of congenital anomalies in the children, although the study did not establish a causal link. Results suggest the anomalies may correlate with the type of waste anesthesia gas to which the mother was exposed.[89]

A report of two cases from 2008 suggests a potential relationship between personnel exposure to high nitrous oxide concentrations and persistent cognitive deficits.[90] A study in Poland involving 55 female nurses and 29 male anesthesiologists showed a link between the levels of waste nitrous oxide and DNA damage. If the concentration of nitrous oxide exceeded the occupational exposure level of 180 mg/m^3, the genetic injury was aggravated.[91] A British study revealed a link between lower vitamin B12 metabolism and levels of nitrous oxide greater than the occupational exposure level, but no link existed if the level was less than the occupational exposure level.[92]

A correlation between levels of waste anesthesia gases and DNA damage was revealed in a study involving 30 OR personnel compared to 30 non-OR personnel. There also was a correlation between DNA damage and an increased oxidative stress index and total oxidative status.[93] In a study of 50 OR personnel in Croatia, where a scavenging system was in use at the facility, researchers found DNA damage.[94] Similar results were found from a study in India that involved a group of 90 OR personnel.[95] A descriptive study in Turkey revealed that a group of anesthesiologists who were exposed to higher than acceptable levels of waste anesthesia gases experienced higher levels of sister chromatid exchanges (ie, DNA mutation) compared to internists who did not work in the OR, and the levels dropped after a two-month absence from the OR. These ORs did not have scavenging systems or low-leakage anesthesia machines, and no preventative maintenance had been performed.[96]

A literature review revealed that the effects of waste anesthesia gases are controversial and the acceptable occupational levels vary by country.[97] A report by the National Institute for Occupational Safety and Health (NIOSH) showed inconsistencies in the literature regarding the effects of waste anesthesia gases, confirmed the means of exposure, and provided guidance for reducing exposures.[98]

VII.a. The health care organization should establish a waste anesthesia gas management program to be in compliance with the NIOSH recommendations. *[2: Moderate Evidence]*

ENVIRONMENT OF CARE, PART 1

The NIOSH standard for nitrous oxide exposure levels is no more than 25 parts per million (ppm) during an eight-hour period and no more than 2 ppm of any halogenated anesthetic agent in one continuous hour.[99]

VII.a.1. Anesthesia circuits should be inspected before each use to verify the absence of leaks.[72]

One study showed various types of leaks were present during anesthesia administration, including within the circuitry and from inadequate control by the anesthesia professional during administration.[100] Higher levels of waste anesthesia gases related to the use of uncuffed endotracheal tubes and during induction with a mask were reported in a review of the literature.[101] A study comparing four different administration techniques revealed that variance in the level of waste anesthesia gases was related to the administration technique.[102]

VII.a.2. Air sampling for the most frequently used anesthesia gases should be conducted every six months to evaluate occupational exposure and the effectiveness of control measures.[88,99]

VII.b. A scavenging system must be used to remove waste anesthesia gases.[88,99] *[1: Regulatory Requirement]*

A Polish study that involved 35 ORs in 10 hospitals showed that the combination of a scavenging system and air exchanges of more than 12 per hour was required to maintain a level of nitrous oxide below the acceptable occupational exposure limit. Use of ventilation systems with up to 15 air exchanges per hour were not adequate alone to keep the nitrous oxide level below the acceptable occupational exposure limit.[103]

VII.b.1. Scavenging systems should be tested for leaks at installation and daily, and testing compliance documentation should be maintained.[72,99]

VII.b.2. Scavenging systems must be vented to an area where waste anesthesia gases will not be reintroduced into the intake air vents or into the recirculating system.[26,88]

VII.c. Ventilation systems in rooms where anesthesia gases are administered should have an air exchange rate of at least 15 exchanges per hour.[26] *[2: Moderate Evidence]*

A descriptive study revealed less waste anesthesia gases in the ambient air when an air exchange rate of at least 15 exchanges per hour was maintained.[100]

VII.d. Anesthesia delivery systems located throughout the facility must be in proper working order and maintained on a regularly scheduled basis, consistent with the manufacturer's written instructions and organizational policy and procedures.[88,99] *[1: Regulatory Requirement]*

A report summarizing the results of one facility's 24 anesthesia machine testing revealed differing high- and low-level leaks at the time of testing. One group of machines had leaks primarily at the absorbent canister bases. The remainder of the machines had leaks in other locations.[104] It is required by OSHA and recommended by NIOSH that a program for routine inspection and maintenance of all anesthesia machines be in place.[88,99]

Recommendation VIII

A protocol to establish a natural rubber latex–safe environment should be developed and implemented.

In a review of the literature, natural rubber latex was identified as a common cause of anaphylaxis during surgical and interventional procedures.[105-107] An observational study performed at two facilities in Wisconsin determined that health care providers are exposed to latex antigens from airborne sources, and the use of powder-free latex gloves reduces the risk of sensitization.[108]

Health care personnel and patients are at a high risk of developing a latex sensitivity from exposure to latex.[109] There are several routes of exposure to natural rubber latex, including

- direct external contact (eg, gloves, natural rubber latex face masks, blood pressure cuff tubing);
- airborne sources that can affect the mucous membranes of the eyes, nose, trachea, bronchi and bronchioles, and oropharynx;
- particles that are swallowed after entering the nasopharynx or oropharynx;
- direct contact of the mucous membranes with indwelling natural rubber latex devices such as catheters;
- internal patient exposure from health care provider use of natural rubber latex gloves during surgical procedures; and
- internally placed natural rubber latex devices, such as wound drains.[105]

The reactions to latex can include urticaria; blisters; rash; dry, cracked, or irritated skin; bronchospasm; and anaphylactic shock.[105] The quality of life for those allergic to latex is improved by avoiding latex.[110] The symptoms of a reaction may resolve quickly after the source of the latex protein has been removed, but the immunoglobulin E (IgE)—a class of antibody that indicates continued sensitivity—remains in the body for at least five years.[111]

VIII.a. Latex-free products, as determined by their labels, should be purchased, if available. *[4: Benefits Balanced with Harms]*

In 1997, the FDA required that all medical devices containing latex be labeled as such and carry a warning that latex can cause allergic reactions.[112]

ENVIRONMENT OF CARE, PART 1

VIII.a.1. A list of supplies for which there are no latex-free alternatives should be maintained.

The American Latex Allergy Association maintains an electronic listing of products that contain latex and alternatives that do not.[113]

VIII.b. All patients should be assessed preoperatively for risk factors for latex sensitivity. *[1: Strong Evidence]*

Early recognition of risk factors for sensitivity can prevent the progression of anaphylaxis. Anaphylaxis to latex usually presents 30 to 60 minutes after induction of anesthesia. Latex sensitization reportedly occurs in as many as 12% of health care workers, in 75% of patients with spina bifida, and in patients with a history of multiple surgical procedures.[109]

VIII.b.1. The preoperative assessment should include risk factors for latex sensitivity, including
- a history of long-term bladder care[114];
- a history of spina bifida and genitourinary abnormalities in children[109,114];
- a history of multiple surgical procedures[109,114];
- occupational exposure to latex, such as work in health care[109];
- food allergies (eg, banana, kiwi, avocado, chestnut, raw potato)[105,114]; and
- a history of symptoms of
  - contact dermatitis (ie, type IV sensitivity), especially of the hands,
  - contact urticaria, or
  - hay fever, rhinitis, or asthma.[114]

In a study of children with latex allergies, the researchers concluded that the greater the total number of risk factors, the greater the seriousness of the allergy.[114] The presence of contact dermatitis may permit greater amounts of latex to penetrate the skin.[105]

VIII.b.2. The perioperative RN should document and communicate patient latex sensitivity or allergy information to the perioperative team.

VIII.c. Latex precautions should be implemented for patients with latex sensitivity or allergy. *[2: Moderate Evidence]*

A seven-year study involving patients with latex allergies demonstrated the effectiveness of establishing a latex-safe management program, as evidenced by known allergic patients having no allergic reactions.[114]

VIII.c.1. Personnel should remove latex gloves, wash their hands, and don latex-safe gloves before entering the room of a patient with a known or suspected latex sensitivity or allergy.

Natural rubber latex proteins on gloves bind to the glove powder (eg, cornstarch powder) and release allergens into the air when gloves are removed.[108,109]

VIII.c.2. Patients with a sensitivity or allergy to latex should be identified by a wristband or bracelet, as well as a label on the patient's bed and a label or electronic flag on the patient's health record.[105,109]

These interventions provide multiple visual cues for health care team members and promote patient safety.

VIII.c.3. The following steps should be followed during care of a patient with a latex sensitivity who requires surgery or another invasive procedure in a non–latex-safe environment:
- remove all latex-containing products from the room the evening before the procedure, except those that are sealed or contained;
- do not use latex products during terminal cleaning of the room the evening before the procedure;
- schedule an elective surgery as the first procedure of the day;
- restrict traffic and equipment in the OR before and during the procedure; and
- when no latex-safe alternative is available, cover latex-containing equipment that comes into direct contact with the patient with stockinette.

Removing latex-containing products from the room the evening before the procedure and using non-latex products during terminal cleaning is thought to help reduce the release of latex particles.[115] Scheduling elective procedures as the first of the day provides time for room air to be completely exchanged after terminal cleaning. Covering latex-containing equipment with stockinette provides a barrier between the equipment and the skin.[116]

VIII.c.4. Signs indicating "latex allergy" should be posted on all doors leading into the OR where the procedure will be performed before the start of the procedure.[116]

VIII.c.5. Postoperatively, the patient should be transferred to a latex-safe care area.[106]

VIII.c.6. Latex sensitivity should be included in all hand-off communications during the transfer of patient care.[106]

VIII.c.7. Rubber stoppers should not be removed from medication vials when withdrawing the medication. The stopper should only be punctured once.

In a review of the literature, no evidence was found to support the removal of medication vial stoppers. Removing the stopper does not reduce contamination of the contents with latex protein because the medication already may contain latex absorbed from the stopper during transport and storage. Not all stoppers contain latex, and the amount of latex in each stopper varies. Requirements for labeling medication vials regarding the latex content of the stopper have not been established.[107]

Multiple punctures of the stopper increase the opportunity for introducing latex proteins into the contents.[107]

VIII.d. Perioperative personnel should wear low-protein, powder-free, natural rubber latex gloves or latex-free gloves. *[1: Strong Evidence]*

Health care personnel are susceptible to developing latex allergies when they are exposed to latex gloves and glove powder.[110] A study that involved 325 health care workers in Kenya showed 16% had an allergy to latex gloves; wearing gloves for more than one hour per day and more years of service increased the risk factors for latex allergy. This study also showed, with statistically marginal significance, that working in an environment where others are wearing latex gloves increases the risk of latex allergy.[117]

Use of low-protein, powder-free natural rubber latex gloves or latex-free gloves can minimize latex exposure and the risk of reactions in both health care workers and patients.[108-110,117,118] A systematic review of the literature showed that using low-protein, powder-free, natural rubber latex gloves or latex-free gloves significantly reduces natural rubber latex aeroallergens in the environment, as well as sensitivity and asthma in health care workers.[118]

Quality-of-life scores improved in health care workers with latex allergies after latex products were removed from the workplace. Participants were asked to complete a questionnaire that addressed quality-of-life scores related to skin, eye, and respiratory symptoms that they experienced as a result of exposure to latex in the workplace.[110]

A study in two hospitals involving 805 health care workers showed that the amount of latex in the air duct systems decreased with the introduction of powder-free gloves. This study also identified a reduction in the latex sensitization of seven of the 28 previously sensitized employees.[108]

Recommendation IX

Precautions must be taken to mitigate the risks associated with the use of chemicals in the perioperative setting (eg, methyl methacrylate, glutaraldehyde, formalin, ethylene oxide).[119,120]

Improper handling of chemicals can result in injury to health care workers and patients. Injuries may result from exposure to any portion of the body, including the integumentary or respiratory systems.[121,122] A study of 12 physicians and eight nurses in 10 states revealed the presence of a variety of chemicals (eg, mercury, tricloscan, perfluorminated compounds [PFCs]) in the participants' blood or urine; however, the levels were consistent with general population studies conducted by the US Centers for Disease Control and Prevention National Report on Biomonitoring.[123]

IX.a. Health care organizations must follow the most stringent federal, state, or local regulations for chemical handling and disposal. *[1: Regulatory Requirement]*

State and local requirements may be more stringent than federal regulations.[119,124,125] The most stringent regulations take precedence over less-restrictive regulations.

IX.b. For every potentially hazardous chemical, MSDSs or SDSs must be readily accessible to employees within the practice setting.[119] *[1: Regulatory Requirement]*

The Occupational Safety and Health Administration (OSHA) has changed the title of the "material safety data sheet" to "safety data sheet" and changed the requirements for what information manufacturers must provide on the sheets. The updated requirements now align with international requirements. The updated SDSs include information on hazard identification, recommendations for precautions or special handling, signs and symptoms of toxic exposure, and first aid treatments for exposure, as well as provide more information, including pictograms and signal words (eg, danger, warning).[119]

IX.c. A chemical hazard risk assessment for all chemicals within the unit or facility must be performed annually using the MSDS or SDS and the manufacturer's instructions for use for each chemical. The assessment should include
- the concentration of each ingredient;
- the means of exposure (eg, respiratory, skin, eye, inhalation);
- handling precautions;
- first aid measures if an exposure occurs;
- spill management procedures;
- storage requirements;
- appropriate disposal methods;
- required personal protective equipment (PPE) for handling and spill management;
- whether a chemical that has less risk of causing and injury can be used[121]; and
- whether a chemical that is present is no longer being used and therefore should be disposed of.

[1: Regulatory Requirement]

The risk assessment helps determine the precautions to take and provides information for developing an action plan in the event of spills or exposures.[119]

IX.d. All chemicals must be handled according to their respective MSDS or SDS and the manufacturer's instructions for use,[119] including

ENVIRONMENT OF CARE, PART 1

- disinfectants and sterilants (eg, glutaraldehyde, ortho-phthalaldehyde, ethylene oxide, hydrogen peroxide, peracetic acid),[24,126]
- tissue preservatives (ie, formalin),[127] and
- antiseptic agents (eg, hand hygiene products, surgical prep solutions).[42,81,128]

[1: Regulatory Requirement]

IX.e. An emergency spill plan should be developed for all chemicals listed in the chemical hazard risk assessment if required by regulation. [1: Regulatory Requirement]

Some chemicals may not require an emergency spill plan, or the requirement may be based on the volume of the chemical spilled (eg, formaldehyde, glutaraldehyde).[125]

IX.f. Chemicals must be stored according to
- MSDS or SDS information;
- manufacturer instructions for use;
- flammability and combustibility;
- patient and perioperative personnel safety requirements; and
- local, state, and federal regulations.[129]

[1: Regulatory Requirement]

IX.g. Personal protective equipment must be provided, as applicable, for employees who must handle chemicals in the workplace. [1: Regulatory Requirement]

Defined as any clothing or other equipment that protects a person from exposure to chemicals, PPE may include gloves, aprons, chemical splash goggles, and impervious clothing.[129] Scrubs and lab coats worn by health care workers are not considered PPE because they are not impervious.

IX.h. A respiratory protection plan applicable to each chemical listed in the chemical hazard risk assessment must be developed. [1: Regulatory Requirement]

Respiratory protection includes local exhaust ventilation (eg, hoods) or general ventilation above a designated number of air changes per hour. Respirators are required as a portion of the respiratory protection plan for certain chemicals and if the appropriate ventilation cannot be provided.[130]

IX.i. Eyewash stations, either plumbed or self contained, must be provided where chemicals that are hazardous to the eyes are located.[131] [1: Regulatory Requirement]

IX.i.1. Plumbed eyewash stations should deliver warm water (ie, 60° F to 100° F [15.6° C to 37.8° C]) at a rate of 1.5 L/minute.[132]

IX.i.2. Plumbed eyewash stations should be flushed weekly.

Weekly flushing removes stagnant water, which may contain microbial contamination, from the system.[132]

IX.i.3. Eyewash stations should be located so that travel time is no greater than 10 seconds from the location of chemical use or storage, or should be immediately available if the chemical is caustic or is a strong acid.[132]

IX.j. Health care organizations must provide education to employees about the hazardous chemicals in the workplace.[119] [1: Regulatory Requirement]

IX.k. Safe practices should be established for the use of methyl methacrylate bone cement. [1: Regulatory Requirement]

Bone cement is a combination of methyl methacrylate monomer, which is a liquid, and beads of polymethyl methacrylate or a polymethyl methacrylate-based polymer.[133] The liquid portion of methyl methacrylate can be absorbed through the skin and respiratory tract and by ingestion and may cause irritation to the area exposed.[134,135] The permissible exposure limit that OSHA set for methyl methacrylate is 100 ppm or a time-weighted average of 410 mg/m^3.[134,135]

One study revealed that morbidity among orthopedic surgeons was higher than general surgeons related to esophageal and myeloproliferative malignancies, but a direct link to methyl methacrylate was not determined.[122] Methyl methacrylate has not been proven to be carcinogenic.[136]

IX.k.1. Eye protection must be worn when mixing and inserting methyl methacrylate bone cement.[134]

Methyl methacrylate fumes may irritate the eyes.[135,137]

IX.k.2. Mixed cement should not come in contact with gloves until it has reached the dough stage. A second pair of gloves, made of the material recommended in the methyl methacrylate manufacturer's instructions, should be worn and then be discarded after contact with the cement.

Methyl methacrylate can penetrate many plastic and latex compounds and can be absorbed through the skin, leading to contact dermatitis.[135,137]

IX.k.3. A closed mixing system or mixing gun should be used for mixing methyl methacrylate.

Closed mixing systems and mixing guns help reduce chemical handling. Closed mixing systems with or without a vacuum release less methyl methacrylate vapor into the breathing zone of the surgical team compared with open mixing systems.[136]

IX.k.4. Direct contact with methyl methacrylate monomer should be avoided.

The liquid monomer is a mild skin irritant and may induce skin sensitization.[133]

IX.k.5. Discarded bone cement should not be left in contact with the patient's skin.

During the curing process, the cement releases heat and has been shown to cause patient burns during total hip arthroplasty.[138]

IX.k.6. When methyl methacrylate liquid is spilled,
- the spill area should be ventilated until the odor has dissipated,
- all sources of ignition should be removed,
- appropriate PPE should be worn during cleanup as required by the MSDS or SDS or the manufacturer's instructions for use,
- the spill area should be isolated,
- the liquid should be covered with an activated charcoal absorbent, and
- the waste product should be disposed of in a hazardous waste container.[134]

IX.k.7. Methyl methacrylate monomer is hazardous waste and must be disposed of according to state, local, and federal requirements.[139]

IX.l. Safe handling practices for glutaraldehyde should be developed as required by federal, state, and local regulation and as described in the AORN "Guideline for high-level disinfection."[124,126] *[2: Moderate Evidence]]*

Exposure to glutaraldehyde for greater than one hour continuously has been shown to increase the risk of a spontaneous abortion, according to a study that involved 6,707 live births and 775 spontaneous abortions.[140]

IX.l.1. Alternatives for glutaraldehyde should be considered if any are listed in the manufacturer's instructions for use for the device being high-level disinfected.

Several alternative methods of high-level disinfection or sterilization that are less toxic to humans and the environment than glutaraldehyde are available.[124,126]

IX.m. Safe handling practices must be developed for handling formalin.[127] *[1: Regulatory Requirement]*

Formaldehyde, the active ingredient in formalin, is a known carcinogen and may cause other acute and chronic health conditions, including sensitization leading to asthma and contact dermatitis.[127]

IX.m.1. Locations where formalin is used should
- be free of ignition sources,
- have posted signs warning of formaldehyde use, and
- have ventilation systems with adequate capacity to maintain levels below the permissible exposure limits (ie, eight-hour total weighted average of 0.75 ppm; 15-minute, short-term exposure limit of 2.0 ppm).[127]

Formalin is a combustible liquid. The permissible exposure limits are set by OSHA and individual states.[127,141]

IX.m.2. Formaldehyde should not be stored in the OR unless the ventilation system is adequate to keep the levels within the recommended exposure limits.

IX.m.3. Personnel handling formaldehyde must wear proper PPE based on the potential for exposure, including gloves, impervious clothes, aprons, chemical splash goggles, and respiratory protection.

Latex gloves provide no protection against formaldehyde. Butyl and nitrile gloves provide eight hours of protection, and polyethylene gloves provide four hours of protection. Providing respiratory protection (eg, respirators, ventilation hoods) is required if the levels of formalin in the area are greater than 100 ppm.[141]

IX.m.4. Medical surveillance must be provided if workers are exposed to levels of formaldehyde above the permissible exposure limits.[142]

IX.m.5. Health care organizations must monitor levels of formaldehyde
- when the agent is introduced into the space where it will be stored or used;
- if there is a change in processes or practices involving formaldehyde;
- periodically after introduction,
- after a change in processes or practices unless permission has been granted by the regulatory agency with jurisdiction to stop monitoring after two consecutive measurements that were taken at least seven days apart showed the levels were below the recognized safe limits; and
- when an employee reports symptoms of respiratory or dermal exposure.[127,142]

IX.n. Safe handling precautions for ethylene oxide must be developed as required by federal, state, and local regulations and as described in the AORN "Guideline for sterilization."[24,124,129] *[1: Regulatory Requirement]*

Recommendation X

Precautions should be taken to avoid hazards associated with handling waste.

The types of precautions taken when handling wastes are based on the US Environmental Protection Agency (EPA) classifications (eg, hazardous, non-hazardous). Hazardous waste is further classified by the EPA as listed waste, characteristic waste, universal waste, and mixed waste. Medical waste is considered non-hazardous waste and disposal may or may not be regulated.[143]

X.a. The most stringent of federal, state, or local laws that govern the disposal of hazardous and non-hazardous waste must be followed.[143] *[1: Regulatory Requirement]*

ENVIRONMENT OF CARE, PART 1

Legal requirements vary by state and local jurisdiction. The most stringent requirement supersedes others.

X.a.1. The appropriate regulatory body should be consulted for the applicable definition of medical waste (ie, regulated, non-regulated), which may include specific requirements (eg, volume of body fluids, type of waste exposed to human body fluids) to classify the item as a regulated medical waste.[143]

X.b. Waste that is classified as hazardous must be placed in hazardous waste containers at the point of use.[143] *[1: Regulatory Requirement]*
This action alerts handlers to take precautions during disposal.

X.b.1. The waste container must be labeled with the type of waste it contains (eg, red bags indicate regulated medical waste, yellow bags indicate hazardous waste such as waste contaminated by chemotherapy agents).[143]

X.b.2. The waste container must protect the personnel handling the container against exposure to the contents (eg, a container used to dispose of sharps must be puncture-resistant, the container for hazardous liquids must be fracture-resistant, the lid of the waste container must seal).[143]

X.b.3. Batteries that contain cadmium, lead, or silver must be disposed of as hazardous waste.[139]

X.b.4. Any product that contains mercury must be disposed of as a hazardous waste.[139]

X.b.5. Flammable liquids (eg, alcohol, benzoin, collodion, formalin, methyl methacrylate monomer, silver nitrate) are considered characteristic wastes and must be contained and placed into a hazardous waste receptacle for disposal.[143]
These chemicals pose fire and environmental hazards if they are discarded into the regular waste stream.

X.c. Medications should be disposed of in accordance with guidelines from the state or local regulatory body with jurisdiction and the AORN "Guideline for medication safety,"[144] and in consultation with the health care organization's pharmacist. *[1: Regulatory Requirement]*
Regulations that cover medication disposal vary between states and locality. The category of waste, which dictates the method of disposal, may vary based on the volume of waste and other conditions.[143]

Recommendation XI

Perioperative personnel should receive initial and ongoing education and complete competency verification activities for establishing and maintaining a safe environment of care.[50,51]

Initial and ongoing education of perioperative personnel on establishing and maintaining a safe environment of care facilitates the development of knowledge, skills, and attitudes that affect safe patient care.

Periodic educational programs provide the opportunity to reinforce the knowledge of potential environmental hazards to patients and personnel, and to introduce new information on equipment or practice changes.

Competency verification measures individual performance and provides a mechanism for documentation. Competency assessment verifies that perioperative personnel have an understanding of potential environmental hazards to patients and personnel.

XI.a. Perioperative team members should receive education and complete competency verification activities that address specialized knowledge and skills related to providing a safe environment of care. Education and competency verification activities should review topics related to maintaining a safe environment of care, including
- the available ergonomic equipment and safe lifting and moving practices;
- the safe use of medical equipment in the perioperative environment;
- appropriate responses to and the meanings of clinical and alert alarms[69,71];
- the safe use of blanket- and solution-warming cabinets[76];
- fire prevention, suppression, and risk assessment;
- the safe use and handling of medical and anesthetic gases;
- precautions for handling and storage of all chemicals listed in the chemical hazard risk assessment[119];
- latex precautions and procedures for handling latex-related reactions;
- hazardous and medical waste disposal; and
- an introduction to and review of organizational policies and procedures.

[1: Regulatory Requirement]
Specialized knowledge includes empirical knowledge (eg, technical understanding), practical knowledge (eg, clinical experience), and aesthetic knowledge (eg, patient advocacy). Ongoing development of knowledge and skills and documentation of personnel participation is a regulatory and accreditation requirement for both hospitals and ambulatory settings.[145-151]

XI.a.1. Simulation demonstrations, such as fire and other emergency drills, should be used to educate perioperative personnel when applicable.

ENVIRONMENT OF CARE, PART 1

Simulation has been reported to assist with identifying strengths and weaknesses in systems.[61]

XI.b. Employers must provide education and competency verification for perioperative personnel who work with chemicals and other potentially hazardous agents in the workplace.[119,120] Education should include safe handling practices, a description of potential hazards, exposure prevention practices, and spill management procedures. *[1: Regulatory Requirement]*

Recommendation XII

Documentation reflecting activities related to providing a safe environment of care should be recorded in a manner consistent with the health care organization's policies and procedures.

Documentation demonstrates compliance with regulatory and accrediting agency requirements and identifies trends and quality improvement opportunities. Highly reliable data collection is not only necessary to chronicle patient responses to nursing interventions, but also to demonstrate the health care organization's progress toward quality care outcomes.[152]

XII.a. Documentation related to providing a safe environment of care should include
- the date and the name of the person who performs inspection, testing, and maintenance of equipment and alarms;
- the date and the name of the person who performs inspection, testing, and maintenance of eyewash stations;
- results of blanket- and solution-warming cabinet temperature monitoring[76];
- the date and name of the person who performs testing of anesthesia systems and waste gas scavenging systems[42,139];
- the date and the name of the person who performs inspection, testing, and maintenance of fire extinguishing equipment[153];
- employee injuries; and
- patient and visitor injuries.

[1: Regulatory Requirement]

Effective management and collection of health care information that accurately reflects the patient's care and treatment, as well as measures taken to ensure employee, patient, and visitor safety, are regulatory and accreditation requirements for both hospitals and ambulatory settings.[50,51,154-158]

XII.b. Records should be maintained for a time period specified by the health care organization and in compliance with local, state, and federal regulations.[119] *[1: Regulatory Requirement]*

Recommendation XIII

Policies and procedures for the provision of a safe environment of care should be developed, reviewed periodically, revised as necessary, and readily available in the practice setting.

Policies and procedures assist in the development of patient safety, quality assessment, and performance improvement activities. Policies and procedures establish authority, responsibility, and accountability within the organization. Policies and procedures also serve as operational guidelines that are used to minimize patient risk for injury or complications, to standardize practice, to direct perioperative personnel, and to establish continuous performance improvement programs.

XIII.a. Policies and procedures should be consistent across disciplines, be supported by administrative leaders, and reflect the rules and recommendations of regulatory and accreditation bodies.[119,120] Policies and procedures related to maintaining a safe environment of care should describe or define the requirements for
- safe patient handling and movement in the perioperative setting[27];
- processes to effectively manage medical equipment, including selection, purchase, inspection, maintenance, and removal from service in the event of a malfunction;
- the use of extension cords;
- the monitoring and recording of warming cabinet temperatures;
- inspection, testing, and maintenance of fire extinguishing equipment and supplies[42];
- who is responsible for and has the authority to turn off medical gas valves;
- the monitoring of nitrous oxide levels and the levels of other inhalation anesthetics;
- the maintenance of anesthesia delivery systems, including scheduling and testing criteria;
- alert and clinical alarm testing and criteria for setting alarm limits[68,69,75];
- who is permitted to change alarm limits, including default limits[68,69,71,75];
- chemical storage[125]; and
- effective management of patients and health care personnel who are at risk for natural rubber latex sensitivity or allergy.

[1: Regulatory Requirement]

Establishing policies and procedures that guide and support patient care, treatment, and services is a regulatory and accreditation requirement for both hospitals and ambulatory settings.[50,51,159-161]

Recommendation XIV

Perioperative personnel should participate in a variety of quality assurance and performance improvement activities that are consistent with the health care organization's plan to improve understanding of and compliance with the principles and processes of maintaining a safe environment of care.

Quality assurance and performance improvement programs assist in evaluating the quality of patient care, the presence of environmental safety hazards, and the formulation of plans for taking corrective actions.

ENVIRONMENT OF CARE, PART 1

These programs provide data that may be used to determine whether an individual organization is within benchmark goals and meets regulatory requirements, and if not, to identify areas that may require corrective actions.

XIV.a. A quality management plan should be developed by a multidisciplinary team that includes representatives from all disciplines of the perioperative team and should include guidance for

- collecting and analyzing information about adverse outcomes associated with the environment of care (eg, latex allergy) as a part of the organization-wide performance improvement program that addresses adverse events and near misses;
- monitoring actual and potential risks in each care area on a regular basis (eg, at least monthly environment of care rounds) and by a team that includes clinicians, administrators, and support personnel;
- monitoring and reporting incidents of equipment malfunction that lead to patient harm, as outlined in the Safe Medical Devices Act of 1990[162];
- monitoring and reporting incidents of alarm malfunction and events related to the inability of the team members to respond to alarms[68,69,71];
- conducting scheduled "walk around" safety rounds to test clinical and alert alarms and to observe staff member responses to the alarms;
- monitoring compliance with requirements for safe handling of chemicals and hazardous wastes in the workplace;
- developing processes to regularly inspect, test, and maintain fire extinguishing equipment and supplies;
- critiquing fire drill performance by a team that includes representatives from all disciplines of the perioperative department to identify deficiencies and opportunities for improvement; and
- reporting work-related health problems, such as using the E-OSHA 300 log.[163]

[1: Regulatory Requirement]

Collecting data to monitor and improve safety, patient care, treatment, and services is a regulatory and accreditation requirement for both hospitals and ambulatory settings.[50,51,155,164,165]

XIV.a.1. Personnel in the perioperative setting should
- identify safety hazards,
- take appropriate corrective actions, and
- report hazards according to organizational policy.

Glossary

Alert alarm: An alarm connected to a system such as medical gas systems, blood bank refrigerators, and fire alarms.

Characteristic wastes: Wastes that do not meet any of the criteria to be considered a listed waste, but exhibit ignitability, corrosivity, reactivity, or toxicity.

Combustible: A substance that can burn, but requires a flash point that is higher than a flammable substance and is at or above 100° F.

Compressed medical gas: A liquefied or vaporized gas alone, or in combination with other gases, which is defined as a drug by the US Food and Drug Administration (eg, oxygen, nitrogen, nitric acid, nitrous oxide, carbon dioxide, helium, medical air).

Flammable: A substance that can burn, but requires a flash point, which is less than a combustable substance, and less than 100° F.

Flash point: The temperature of a liquid at which sufficient vapor is given off forming a mixture with the air that will ignite when exposed to an ignition source.

Industrial gases: Gases that are not filtered to remove oils from the compressor and other contaminants.

References

1. Boden LI, Sembajwe G, Tveito TH, et al. Occupational injuries among nurses and aides in a hospital setting. *Am J Ind Med.* 2012;55(2):117-126. doi:10.1002/ajim.21018; 10.1002/ajim.21018. [IIIA]
2. Cappell MS. Injury to endoscopic personnel from tripping over exposed cords, wires, and tubing in the endoscopy suite: a preventable cause of potentially severe workplace injury. *Dig Dis Sci.* 2010;55(4):947-951. doi:10.1007/s10620-009-0923-0. [VB]
3. Cappell MS. Accidental occupational injuries to endoscopy personnel in a high-volume endoscopy suite during the last decade: mechanisms, workplace hazards, and proposed remediation. *Dig Dis Sci.* 2011;56(2):479-487. doi:10.1007/s10620-010-1498-5. [VB]
4. Esser AC, Koshy JG, Randle HW. Ergonomics in office-based surgery: a survey-guided observational study. *Dermatol Surg.* 2007;33(11):1304-1313. doi:10.1111/j.1524-4725.2007.33281.x. [IIIB]
5. Freitag S, Ellegast R, Dulon M, Nienhaus A. Quantitative measurement of stressful trunk postures in nursing professions. *Ann Occup Hyg.* 2007;51(4):385-395. doi:10.1093/annhyg/mem018. [IIIC]
6. Bos E, Krol B, van der Star L, Groothoff J. Risk factors and musculoskeletal complaints in non-specialized nurses, IC nurses, operation room nurses, and X-ray technologists. *Int Arch Occup Environ Health.* 2007;80(3):198-206. doi:10.1007/s00420-006-0121-8. [IIIC]
7. Pompeii LA, Lipscomb HJ, Dement JM. Surveillance of musculoskeletal injuries and disorders in a diverse cohort of workers at a tertiary care medical center. *Am J Ind Med.* 2008;51(5):344-356. doi:10.1002/ajim.20572. [IVB]
8. Drysdale SA. The incidence of upper extremity injuries in endoscopy nurses. *Gastroenterol Nurs.* 2007;30(3):187-192. [IIIB]
9. Guideline for minimally invasive surgery. *Guidelines for Perioperative Practice.* Denver, CO: AORN, Inc; 2015:525-552. [IVB]

10. van Det MJ, Meijerink WJ, Hoff C, Totte ER, Pierie JP. Optimal ergonomics for laparoscopic surgery in minimally invasive surgery suites: a review and guidelines. *Surg Endosc*. 2009;23(6):1279-1285. doi:10.1007/s00464-008-0148-x. [VB]

11. Lee G, Lee T, Dexter D, et al. Ergonomic risk associated with assisting in minimally invasive surgery. *Surg Endosc*. 2009;23(1):182-188. doi:10.1007/s00464-008-0141-4. [VC]

12. Matern U. Ergonomic deficiencies in the operating room: examples from minimally invasive surgery. *Work*. 2009;33(2):165-168. doi:10.3233/WOR-2009-0862. [VB]

13. Nonfatal occupational injuries and illnesses requiring days away from work, 2010 [news release]. Washington, DC: US Department of Labor Bureau of Labor Statistics; November 9, 2011. http://www.bls.gov/news.release/pdf/osh2.pdf. Accessed September 27, 2012.

14. Alexopoulos EC, Tanagra D, Detorakis I, et al. Knee and low back complaints in professional hospital nurses: occurrence, chronicity, care seeking and absenteeism. *Work*. 2011;38(4):329-335. doi:10.3233/WOR-2011-1136. [IIIA]

15. Matern U, Koneczny S. Safety, hazards and ergonomics in the operating room. *Surg Endosc*. 2007;21(11):1965-1969. doi:10.1007/s00464-007-9396-4. [IIIB]

16. Reddy PP, Reddy TP, Roig-Francoli J, et al. The impact of the alexander technique on improving posture and surgical ergonomics during minimally invasive surgery: pilot study. *J Urol*. 2011;186(4 Suppl):1658-1662. doi:10.1016/j.juro.2011.04.013. [IC]

17. Timmons L. Creating a no-lift, no-transfer environment in the OR. *AORN J*. 2009;89(4):733-736. doi:10.1016/j.aorn.2008.12.025. [VB]

18. Black TR, Shah SM, Busch AJ, Metcalfe J, Lim HJ. Effect of transfer, lifting, and repositioning (TLR) injury prevention program on musculoskeletal injury among direct care workers. *J Occup Environ Hyg*. 2011;8(4):226-235. doi:10.1080/15459624.2011.564110. [IIIB]

19. de Ruiter HP, Liaschenko J. To lift or not to lift: patient-handling practices. *AAOHN J*. 2011;59(8):337-343. doi:10.3928/08910162-20110718-02; 10.3928/08910162-20110718-02. [IIIB]

20. Meeks-Sjostrom D, Lopuszynski SA, Bairan A. The wisdom of retaining experienced nurses at the bedside: a pilot study examining a minimal lift program and its impact on reducing patient movement related injuries of bedside nurses. *Medsurg Nurs*. 2010;19(4):233-236. [IIC]

21. Resnick ML, Sanchez R. Reducing patient handling injuries through contextual training. *J Emerg Nurs*. 2009;35(6):504-508. doi:10.1016/j.jen.2008.10.017. [IIIC]

22. Kutash M, Short M, Shea J, Martinez M. The lift team's importance to a successful safe patient handling program. *J Nurs Adm*. 2009;39(4):170-175. doi:10.1097/NNA.0b013e31819c9cfd. [VA]

23. Martin PJ, Harvey JT, Culvenor JF, Payne WR. Effect of a nurse back injury prevention intervention on the rate of injury compensation claims. *J Safety Res*. 2009;40(1):13-19. doi:10.1016/j.jsr.2008.10.013. [VC]

24. Guideline for sterilization In: *Guidelines for Perioperative Practice*. Denver, CO: AORN, Inc; 2015:665-692. [IVA]

25. Illuminating Engineering Society of North America. *Lighting for Hospitals and Health Care Facilities*. New York, NY: Illuminating Engineering Society of North America; 2006. [IVC]

26. Facility Guidelines Institute. *Guidelines for Design and Construction of Health Care Facilities*. Washington, DC: American Society for Healthcare Engineering (ASHE) of the American Hospital Association; 2010. [IVC]

27. AORN guidance statement: safe patient handling and movement in the perioperative setting. In: *Perioperative Standards and Recommended Practices*. Denver, CO: AORN, Inc; 2012:689-710. [IVB]

28. Waters T, Lloyd JD, Hernandez E, Nelson A. AORN ergonomic tool 7: pushing, pulling, and moving equipment on wheels. *AORN J*. 2011;94(3):254-260. doi:10.1016/j.aorn.2010.09.035. [VA]

29. Waters T, Baptiste A, Short M, Plante-Mallon L, Nelson A. AORN ergonomic tool 6: lifting and carrying supplies and equipment in the perioperative setting. *AORN J*. 2011;94(2):173-179. doi:10.1016/j.aorn.2010.09.033. [VA]

30. Spera P, Lloyd JD, Hernandez E, et al. AORN ergonomic tool 5: tissue retraction in the perioperative setting. *AORN J*. 2011;94(1):54-58. doi:10.1016/j.aorn.2010.08.031. [VA]

31. Hughes NL, Nelson A, Matz MW, Lloyd J. AORN ergonomic tool 4: solutions for prolonged standing in perioperative settings. *AORN J*. 2011;93(6):767-774. doi:10.1016/j.aorn.2010.08.029. [VA]

32. Waters T, Spera P, Petersen C, Nelson A, Hernandez E, Applegarth S. AORN ergonomic tool 3: lifting and holding the patient's legs, arms, and head while prepping. *AORN J*. 2011;93(5):589-592. doi:10.1016/j.aorn.2010.08.028. [VA]

33. Waters T, Short M, Lloyd J, et al. AORN ergonomic tool 2: positioning and repositioning the supine patient on the OR bed. *AORN J*. 2011;93(4):445-449. doi:10.1016/j.aorn.2010.08.027. [VA]

34. Waters T, Baptiste A, Short M, Plante-Mallon L, Nelson A. AORN ergonomic tool 1: lateral transfer of a patient from a stretcher to an OR bed. *AORN J*. 2011;93(3):334-339. doi:10.1016/j.aorn.2010.08.025. [VA]

35. American Society of Anesthesiologists Task Force on Operating Room Fires; Caplan RA, Barker SJ, Connis RT, et al. Practice advisory for the prevention and management of operating room fires. *Anesthesiology*. 2008;108(5): 786-801. doi:10.1097/01.anes.0000299343.87119.a9. [IVB]

36. ECRI. New clinical guide to surgical fire prevention. *Health Devices*. 2009;38(10):314-332. [IVC]

37. ECRI. Fighting airway fires. *Healthcare Risk Control*. 2010;4(Surgery and Anesthesia 10):1-11. [VC]

38. Friedrich M, Tirilomis T, Schmitto JD, et al. Intrathoracic fire during preparation of the left internal thoracic artery for coronary artery bypass grafting. *J Cardiothorac Surg*. 2010;5:10. doi:10.1186/1749-8090-5-10. [VA]

39. Moskowitz M. Fire in the operating room during open heart surgery: a case report. *AANA J*. 2009;77(4):261-264. [VA]

40. Richter GT, Willging JP. Suction cautery and electrosurgical risks in otolaryngology. *Int J Pediatr Otorhinolaryngol*. 2008;72(7):1013-1021. doi:10.1016/j.ijporl.2008.03.006. [IIIA]

41. Mirsaidi N. Cutting a battery pack cable can start a fire. Nursing. 2008;38(8):13-14. doi:10.1097/01.NURSE.0000327465.69676.1c. [IIIA]

42. Bielen RP, Lathrop JK. *Health Care Facilities Code Handbook*. 9th ed. Quincy, MA: National Fire Protection Association; 2012. [IVB]

43. Guideline for laser safety. In: *Guidelines for Perioperative Practice*. Denver, CO: AORN, Inc; 2015:139-152. [IVB]

44. Guideline for electrosurgery. In: *Guidelines for Perioperative Practice*. Denver, CO: AORN, Inc; 2015:121-138. [IVB]

45. Guidleine for product selection. In: *Guidelines for Perioperative Practice*. Denver, CO: AORN, Inc; 2015:179-186. [IVB]

46. ECRI. Reducing the risk of burns from surgical light sources. *Risk Management Reporter*. 2009;28(6):15-17. [VB]

47. Rinder CS. Fire safety in the operating room. *Curr Opin Anaesthesiol*. 2008;21(6):790-795. doi:10.1097/ACO.0b013e328318693a. [VC]

48. NFPA 30: *Flammable and Combustible Liquids Code*. Quincy, MA: National Fire Protection Association; 2012. [IVB]

49. *NFPA 101: Life Safety Code*. Quincy, MA: National Fire Protection Association; 2012. [IVB]

50. Ambulatory Surgical Services, 42 CFR §416 (2011).

51. Conditions of Participation for Hospitals, 42 CFR §482 (2010).

52. Chapp K, Lange L. Warming blanket head drapes and trapped anesthetic gases: understanding the fire risk. *AORN J*. 2011;93(6):749-760. doi:10.1016/j.aorn.2010.08.030. [IIIA]

53. Roy S, Smith LP. What does it take to start an oropharyngeal fire? Oxygen requirements to start fires in the operating room. *Int J Pediatr Otorhinolaryngol*. 2011;75(2):227-230. doi:10.1016/j.ijporl.2010.11.005. [VA]

54. Militana CJ, Ditkoff MK, Mattucci KF. Use of the laryngeal mask airway in preventing airway fires during adenoidectomies in children: a study of 25 patients. *Ear Nose Throat J*. 2007;86(10):621-623. [IIIB]

55. Nishiyama K, Komori M, Kodaka M, Tomizawa Y. Crisis in the operating room: fires, explosions and electrical accidents. *J Artif Organs*. 2010;13(3):129-133. doi:10.1007/s10047-010-0513-0. [VC]

56. Yardley IE, Donaldson LJ. Surgical fires, a clear and present danger. *Surgeon*. 2010;8(2):87-92. doi:10.1016/j.surge.2010.01.005. [VB]

57. Watson DS. Surgical fires: 100% preventable, still a problem. *AORN J*. 2009;90(4):589-593. doi:10.1016/j.aorn.2009.09.012. [VB]

58. Laudanski K, Schwab WK, Bakuzonis CW, Paulus DA. Thermal damage of the humidified ventilator circuit in the operating room: an analysis of plausible causes. *Anesth Analg*. 2010;111(6):1433-1436. doi:10.1213/ANE.0b013e3181ee8092. [VA]

59. National Fire Protection Association Technical Committee on Portable Fire Extinguishers. NFPA 10: Standard for Portable Fire Extinguishers. Quincy, MA: National Fire Protection Association; 2010. [IVB]

60. Water-Jel fire blankets [product sheet]. Carlstadt, NJ: Water-Jel; #FB 1110-0.

61. Berendzen JA, van Nes JB, Howard BC, Zite NB. Fire in labor and delivery: simulation case scenario. *Simul Healthc*. 2011;6(1):55-61. doi:10.1097/SIH.0b013e318201351b. [VA]

62. ECRI. Hazard report: prevent surgical boom fires with routine maintenance. *Health Devices*. 2008;January:24-26. [VC]

63. Sentinel event statistics data—event type by year (1995-2011). The Joint Commission. http://www.jointcommission.org/sentinel_event.aspx. Accessed June 21, 2012. [VB]

64. Kuczkowski KM. Anesthesia machine as a cause of intraoperative "code red" in the labor and delivery suite. *Arch Gynecol Obstet*. 2008;278(5):477-478. doi:10.1007/s00404-008-0610-y. [VC]

65. US Department of Health and Human Services Centers for Disease Control and Prevention. Guidelines for environmental infection control in health-care facilities. http://www.cdc.gov/ncidod/dhqp/pdf/guidelines/Enviro_guide_03.pdf ed. Accessed September 27, 2012. [IVA]

66. Guideline for environmental cleaning. *Guidelines for Perioperative Practice*. Denver, CO: AORN, Inc; 2015:9-30. [IVB]

67. Hargrove M, Aherne T. Possible fire hazard caused by mismatching electrical chargers with the incorrect device within the operating room. *J Extra Corpor Technol*. 2007;39(3):199-200. [VC]

68. Phillips J. Clinical alarms: complexity and common sense. *Crit Care Nurs Clin North Am*. 2006;18(2):145-156. [VB]

69. Clinical Alarms Task Force. Impact of clinical alarms on patient safety: a report from the American College of Clinical Engineering Healthcare Technology Foundation. *J Clin Eng*. 2007;32(1):22-33. [VB]

70. Schmid F, Goepfert MS, Kuhnt D, et al. The wolf is crying in the operating room: patient monitor and anesthesia workstation alarming patterns during cardiac surgery. *Anesth Analg*. 2011;112(1):78-83. doi:10.1213/ANE.0b013e3181fcc504. [IIIB]

71. *A Siren Call to Act: Priority Issues from the Medical Device Alarms Summit*. Arlington, VA: Association for the Advancement of Medical Instrumentation; 2011. [VC]

72. 2008 recommendations for pre-anesthesia checkout procedures. American Society of Anesthesiologists. http://asatest.asahq.org/clinical/fda.htm. Accessed October 9, 2012. [IVB]

73. Hagenouw RR. Should we be alarmed by our alarms? *Curr Opin Anaesthesiol*. 2007;20(6):590-594. doi:10.1097/ACO.0b013e3282f10dff. [VC]

74. Position statement on noise in the perioperative practice setting. AORN, Inc. http://www.aorn.org/WorkArea/DownloadAsset.aspx?id=21925. Accessed September 27, 2012. [IVB]

75. Brown JC, Anglin-Regal P. Patient safety focus. Clinical alarm management: a team effort. *Biomed Instrum Technol*. 2008;42(2):142-144. [VA]

76. Warming cabinets. *Oper Room Risk Manag*. 2010;2(Surgery 7). [VC]

77. Huang S, Gateley D, Moss AL. Accidental burn injury during knee arthroscopy. *Arthroscopy*. 2007;23(12):1363.e1–1363.e3. doi:10.1016/j.arthro.2006.08.015. [VB]

78. Limiting temperature settings on blanket and solution warming cabinets can prevent patient burns. *Health Devices*. 2005;34(5):168-171. [VC]

79. Bujdoso PJ. Blanket warming: comfort and safety. *AORN J*. 2009;89(4):717-722. [VB]

80. Guideline for the prevention of unplanned perioperative hypothermia. In: *Guidelines for Perioperative Practice*. Denver, CO: AORN, Inc; 2015:479-490. [IVB]

81. Guideline for preoperative patient skin antisepsis. In: *Guidelines for Perioperative Practice*. Denver, CO: AORN, Inc; 2015:43-66. [IVB]

82. *Guidance for Hospitals, Nursing Homes, and Other Health Care Facilities*. FDA Public Health Advisory. Rockvill, MD: US Food and Drug Administration Center for Drug Evaluation and Research; 2001. http://www.fda.gov/downloads/Drugs/GuidanceComplianceRegulatoryInformation/Guidances/ucm070285.pdf. Accessed October 9, 2012.

83. US Department of Health and Human Services Food and Drug Administration. Medical gas containers and closures; current good manufacturing practice requirements. *Fed Regist*. 2006;71(68):18039-18053.

84. Compressed Medical Gases Guideline. Revised February 1989. Food and Drug Administration Center for Drug Evaluation and Research. http://www.fda.gov/Drugs/

GuidanceComplianceRegulatoryInformation/Guidances/ucm124716.htm. Accessed October 9, 2012.

85. ISO 407:2004. Small medical gas cylinders—Pin-index yoke-type valve connections. ISO. http://www.iso.org/iso/catalogue_detail.htm?csnumber=40148. Accessed October 9, 2012. [IVB]

86. Compressed Gas Association. *Standard Color Marking of Compressed Gas Cylinders Intended for Medical Use*. 4th ed. Chantilly, VA: Compressed Gas Association; 2004. [IVB]

87. ECRI. Compressed gases. *Healthcare Risk Control*. 2007;3(Environmental Issues 17.1). [VB]

88. Anesthetic gases: guidelines for workplace exposures. US Department of Labor Occupational Safety & Health Administration. http://osha.gov/dts/osta/anestheticgases/index.html. Published July 20, 1999. Revised May 18, 2000. Accessed October 9, 2012.

89. Teschke K, Abanto Z, Arbour L, et al. Exposure to anesthetic gases and congenital anomalies in offspring of female registered nurses. *Am J Ind Med*. 2011;54(2):118-127. doi:10.1002/ajim.20875; 10.1002/ajim.20875. [IIIB]

90. Dreyfus E, Tramoni E, Lehucher-Michel MP. Persistent cognitive functioning deficits in operating rooms: two cases. *Int Arch Occup Environ Health*. 2008;82(1):125-130. doi:10.1007/s00420-008-0302-8. [VC]

91. Wronska-Nofer T, Palus J, Krajewski W, et al. DNA damage induced by nitrous oxide: study in medical personnel of operating rooms. *Mutat Res*. 2009;666(1-2):39-43. doi:10.1016/j.mrfmmm.2009.03.012. [IIIB]

92. Krajewski W, Kucharska M, Pilacik B, et al. Impaired vitamin B12 metabolic status in healthcare workers occupationally exposed to nitrous oxide. *Br J Anaesth*. 2007;99(6):812-818. doi:10.1093/bja/aem280. [IIIB]

93. Baysal Z, Cengiz M, Ozgonul A, Cakir M, Celik H, Kocyigit A. Oxidative status and DNA damage in operating room personnel. *Clin Biochem*. 2009;42(3):189-193. doi:10.1016/j.clinbiochem.2008.09.103. [IIIB]

94. Rozgaj R, Kasuba V, Brozovic G, Jazbec A. Genotoxic effects of anaesthetics in operating theatre personnel evaluated by the comet assay and micronucleus test. *Int J Hyg Environ Health*. 2009;212(1):11-17. doi:10.1016/j.ijheh.2007.09.001. [IIIB]

95. Chandrasekhar M, Rekhadevi PV, Sailaja N, et al. Evaluation of genetic damage in operating room personnel exposed to anaesthetic gases. *Mutagenesis*. 2006;21(4):249-254. doi:10.1093/mutage/gel029. [IIIB]

96. Eroglu A, Celep F, Erciyes N. A comparison of sister chromatid exchanges in lymphocytes of anesthesiologists to nonanesthesiologists in the same hospital. *Anesth Analg*. 2006;102(5):1573-1577. doi:10.1213/01.ane.0000204298.42159.0e. [IIIB]

97. Oliveira CR. Occupational exposure to anesthetic gases residue. *Rev Bras Anestesiol*. 2009;59(1):110-124. [VC]

98. *Waste Anesthetic Gases: Occupational Hazards in Hospitals* [DHHS (NIOSH) Publication No. 2007-151]. Atlanta, GA: National Institute for Occupational Safety and Health; 2007. [IVB]

99. NIOSH Criteria Documents: Criteria for a Recommended Standard: Occupational Exposure to Waste Anesthetic Gases and Vapors. Atlanta, GA: National Institute for Occupational Safety and Health; 1977:194. http://www.cdc.gov/niosh/docs/1970/77-140.html. Accessed October 9, 2012. [IVB]

100. Sartini M, Ottria G, Dallera M, Spagnolo AM, Cristina ML. Nitrous oxide pollution in operating theatres in relation to the type of leakage and the number of efficacious air exchanges per hour. *J Prev Med Hyg*. 2006;47(4):155-159. [IIIB]

101. Irwin MG, Trinh T, Yao CL. Occupational exposure to anaesthetic gases: a role for TIVA. *Expert Opin Drug Saf*. 2009;8(4):473-483. doi:10.1517/14740330903003778. [VA]

102. Barberio JC, Bolt JD, Austin PN, Craig WJ. Pollution of ambient air by volatile anesthetics: a comparison of 4 anesthetic management techniques. *AANA J*. 2006;74(2):121-125. [IVA]

103. Krajewski W, Kucharska M, Wesolowski W, Stetkiewicz J, Wronska-Nofer T. Occupational exposure to nitrous oxide—the role of scavenging and ventilation systems in reducing the exposure level in operating rooms. *Int J Hyg Environ Health*. 2007;210(2):133-138. doi:10.1016/j.ijheh.2006.07.004. [VB]

104. Smith FD. Management of exposure to waste anesthetic gases. *AORN J*. 2010;91(4):482-494. [VA]

105. Pollart SM, Warniment C, Mori T. Latex allergy. *Am Fam Physician*. 2009;80(12):1413-1418. [VB]

106. Mertes PM, Lambert M, Gueant-Rodriguez RM, et al. Perioperative anaphylaxis. *Immunol Allergy Clin North Am*. 2009;29(3):429-451. doi:10.1016/j.iac.2009.04.004. [VB]

107. Heitz JW, Bader SO. An evidence-based approach to medication preparation for the surgical patient at risk for latex allergy: is it time to stop being stopper poppers? *J Clin Anesth*. 2010;22(6):477-483. doi:10.1016/j.jclinane.2009.12.006. [VC]

108. Kelly KJ, Wang ML, Klancnik M, Petsonk EL. Prevention of IgE sensitization to latex in health vare workers after reduction of antigen exposures. *J Occup Environ Med*. 2011;53(8):934-940. doi:10.1097/JOM.0b013e31822589dc. [IIIC]

109. Lieberman P, Nicklas RA, Oppenheimer J, Kemp SF, Lang DM, eds. The diagnosis and management of anaphylaxis practice parameter: 2010 update [published correction appears in *J Allergy Clin Immunol*. 2010;126(6):1104]. *J Allergy Clin Immunol*. 2010;126(3):477-480.e42. doi:10.1016/j.jaci.2005.01.010. [IVA]

110. Power S, Gallagher J, Meaney S. Quality of life in health care workers with latex allergy. *Occup Med (Lond)*. 2010;60(1):62-65. doi:10.1093/occmed/kqp156. [IIIC]

111. Smith AM, Amin HS, Biagini RE, et al. Percutaneous reactivity to natural rubber latex proteins persists in health-care workers following avoidance of natural rubber latex. *Clin Exp Allergy*. 2007;37(9):1349-1356. doi:10.1111/j.1365-2222.2007.02787.x. [IIIC]

112. Natural rubber-containing medical devices; user labeling. Final rule. *Fed Regist*. 1997;62(189):51021-51030.

113. Online resource manual section 1: latex-free product lists—consumer, dental, hospital. American Latex Allergy Association. http://www.latexallergyresources.org/latex-free-products. Accessed October 9, 2012. [IVC]

114. Gentili A, Lima M, Ricci G, et al. Perioperative treatment of latex-allergic children. *J Patient Saf*. 2007;3(3):166-172. [IIIB]

115. Bernardini R, Catania P, Caffarelli C, et al. Perioperative latex allergy. *Int J Immunopathol Pharmacol*. 2011;24(3 Suppl):S55-S60. [VB]

116. AANA latex protocol. American Latex Allergy Association. http://www.latexallergyresources.org/articles/aana-latex-protocol. Accessed October 9, 2012. [IVC]

117. Amarasekera M, Rathnamalala N, Samaraweera S, Jinadasa M. Prevalence of latex allergy among healthcare workers. *Int J Occup Med Environ Health*. 2010;23(4):391-396. doi:10.2478/v10001-010-0040-5. [IIIB]

118. LaMontagne AD, Radi S, Elder DS, Abramson MJ, Sim M. Primary prevention of latex related sensitisation and occupational asthma: a systematic review. *Occup Environ Med.* 2006;63(5):359-364. doi:10.1136/oem.2005.025221. [IIIB]

119. Hazard Communication: Toxic and Hazardous Substances, 29 CFR §1910.1200 (2012). http://www.osha.gov/pls/oshaweb/owadisp.show_document?p_table=STANDARDS&p_id=10099. Accessed October 9, 2012.

120. Occupational Safety and Health Standards, Toxic and Hazardous Substances, Definition of "Trade Secret" (Mandatory), 29 CFR §1910.1200E (2012). http://www.osha.gov/pls/oshaweb/owadisp.show_document?p_table=STANDARDS&p_id=10104. Accessed October 9, 2012.

121. Gunson TH, Smith HR, Vinciullo C. Assessment and management of chemical exposure in the Mohs laboratory. *Dermatol Surg.* 2011;37(1):1-9. doi:10.1111/j.1524-4725.2010.01807.x; 10.1111/j.1524-4725.2010.01807.x. [VC]

122. Diaz JH. Proportionate cancer mortality in methyl methacrylate-exposed orthopedic surgeons compared to general surgeons. *J Med Toxicol.* 2011;7(2):125-132. doi:10.1007/s13181-011-0134-x. [IIIC]

123. Wilding BC, Curtis K, Welker-Hood K. *Hazardous Chemicals in Health Care: A Snapshot of Chemicals in Doctors and Nurses.* Washington, DC: Physicians for Social Responsibility. http://www.psr.org/assets/pdfs/hazardous-chemicals-in-health-care.pdf. Accessed October 9, 2012. [IIIA]

124. ECRI. Ethylene oxide, formaldehyde, and glutaraldehyde. *Healthcare Risk Control.* 2011;3(Environmental Issues 6). [VC]

125. Occupational Safety and Health Standards, Hazardous Materials, Hazardous Waste Operations and Emergency Response, 29 CFR §1910.120 (2012). http://www.osha.gov/pls/oshaweb/owadisp.show_document?p_table=standards&p_id=9765. Accessed October 9, 2012.

126. Guideline for high-level disinfection. In: *Guidelines for Perioperative Practice.* Denver, CO: AORN, Inc; 2015:601-614. [IVB]

127. Occupational Safety and Health Standards, Toxic and Hazardous Substances, Formaldehyde, 29 CFR §1910.1048 (2012). http://www.osha.gov/pls/oshaweb/owadisp.show_document?p_table=STANDARDS&p_id=10075. Accessed October 9, 2012.

128. Guideline for hand hygiene. In: *Guidelines for Perioperative Practice.* Denver, CO: AORN, Inc; 2015:31-42. [IVB]

129. Occupational Safety and Health Standards, Personal Protective Equipment, General Requirements, 29 CFR §1910.132 (2011). http://www.osha.gov/pls/oshaweb/owadisp.show_document?p_table=STANDARDS&p_id=9777. Accessed October 9, 2012.

130. Occupational Safety and Health Standards, Personal Protective Equipment, Respiratory Protection. 29 CFR §1910.134 (2011). http://www.osha.gov/pls/oshaweb/owadisp.show_document?p_table=STANDARDS&p_id=12716. Accessed October 9, 2012.

131. Occupational Safety and Health Standards, Medical and First Aid, Medical Services and First Aid. 29 CFR §1910.151 (1998). http://www.osha.gov/pls/oshaweb/owadisp.show_document?p_table=STANDARDS&p_id=9806. Accessed October 9, 2012.

132. *ANSI/ISEA Z358.1-2009: American National Standard for Emergency Eyewash and Shower Equipment.* New York, NY: American National Standards Institute; 2009. [IVC]

133. Leggat PA, Smith DR, Kedjarune U. Surgical applications of methyl methacrylate: a review of toxicity. *Arch Environ Occup Health.* 2009;64(3):207-212. doi:10.1080/19338240903241291. [IVC]

134. International Chemical Safety Cards: Methyl methacrylate. International Programme on Chemical Safety. http://www.cdc.gov/niosh/ipcsneng/neng0300.html. Accessed October 9, 2012.

135. Chemical sampling information: methyl methacrylate. Occupational Safety and Health Administration. http://www.osha.gov/dts/chemicalsampling/data/CH_254400.html. Updated April 27, 2007. Accessed October 9, 2012.

136. Ungers LJ, Vendrely TG, Barnes CL. Control of methyl methacrylate during the preparation of orthopedic bone cements. *J Occup Environ Hyg.* 2007;4(4):272-280. doi:10.1080/15459620701223843. [IIIB]

137. Medical devices; reclassification of polymethylmethacrylate (PMMA) bone cement. Final rule. *Fed Regist.* 2002;67(137):46852-46855.

138. Burston B, Yates P, Bannister G. Cement burn of the skin during hip replacement. *Ann R Coll Surg Engl.* 2007;89(2):151-152. doi:10.1308/003588407X168262. [VC]

139. Protection of Environment, Chapter 1: Environmental Protection Agency, Subchapter I: Solid Wastes. 40 CFR §260, 266 (2011).

140. Lawson CC, Rocheleau CM, Whelan EA, et al. Occupational exposures among nurses and risk of spontaneous abortion. *Am J Obstet Gynecol.* 2012;206(4):327.e1–327.e8. doi:10.1016/j.ajog.2011.12.030. [IIIB]

141. Occupational Safety and Health Standards, Toxic and Hazardous Substances, Substance Technical Guidelines for Formalin, 29 CFR §1910.1048A (2006). http://www.osha.gov/pls/oshaweb/owadisp.show_document?p_table=STANDARDS&p_id=10076. Accessed October 9, 2012.

142. Occupational Safety and Health Standards, Toxic and Hazardous Substances, Sampling Strategy and Analytical Methods for Formaldehyde, 29 CFR §1910.1048B. http://www.osha.gov/pls/oshaweb/owadisp.show_document?p_table=STANDARDS&p_id=10077. Accessed October 9, 2012.

143. Wastes. Environmental Protection Agency. http://www.epa.gov/epawaste/index.htm. Accessed October 9, 2012.

144. Guideline for medication safety. In: *Guidelines for Perioperative Practice.* Denver, CO: AORN, Inc; 2015:291-329. [IVB]

145. Centers for Medicare & Medicaid Services. *State Operations Manual Appendix A—Survey Protocol, Regulations and Interpretive Guidelines for Hospitals.* Rev. 78; 2011.

146. Centers for Medicare & Medicaid Services. *State Operations Manual Appendix L: Guidance for Surveyors: Ambulatory Surgical Centers.* Rev. 76; 2011.

147. HR.01.05.03: Staff participate in ongoing education and training. In: *Comprehensive Accreditation Manual: CAMH for Hospitals.* Oakbrook Terrace, IL: The Joint Commission; 2012.

148. HR.01.05.03: Staff participate in ongoing education and training. In: *Comprehensive Accreditation Manual for Ambulatory Care.* Oakbrook Terrace, IL: Joint Commission; 2012.

149. Quality management and improvement. In: 2012 *Accreditation Handbook for Ambulatory Health Care.* Skokie, IL: Accreditation Association for Ambulatory Health Care; 2012:34-39.

150. Personnel. Personnel records. In: *Procedural Standards and Checklist for Accreditation Ambulatory*

Facilities. Version 1. Gurnee, IL: American Association for Accreditation of Ambulatory Facilities; 2008:51-52.

151. Knowledge, skill & CME training. In: *Procedural Standards and Checklist for Accreditation Ambulatory Facilities*. Version 1. Gurnee, IL: American Association for Accreditation of Ambulatory Facilities; 2008:53.

152. Guideline for perioperative health care information management. In: *Guidelines for Perioperative Practice*. Denver, CO: AORN, Inc; 2015:491-512. [IVB]

153. *NFPA 99 : Health Care Facilities Code*. 2012 ed. Quincy, MA: National Fire Protection Association; 2011. [IVB]

154. RC.01.01.01: The hospital maintains complete and accurate medical records for each individual patient. In: *Hospital Accreditation Standards 2012*. Oakbrook Terrace, IL: Joint Commission on Resources; 2012.

155. PI.03.01.01: The hospital improves performance on an ongoing basis. In: *Hospital Accreditation Standards 2012*. Oakbrook Terrace, IL: Joint Commission on Resources; 2012.

156. Medical records. *Procedure room records*. In: *Procedural Standards and Checklist for Accreditation Ambulatory Facilities*. Version 1. Gurnee, IL: American Association for Accreditation of Ambulatory Facilities; 2008:42-43.

157. Medical records. General. In: *Procedural Standards and Checklist for Accreditation Ambulatory Facilities*. Version 1. Gurnee, IL: American Association for Accreditation of Ambulatory Facilities; 2008:39-40.

158. Clinical records and health information. In: *2012 Accreditation Handbook for Ambulatory Health Care*. Skokie, IL: Accreditation Association for Ambulatory Health Care; 2012:40-42.

159. LD.04.01.07: The hospital has policies and procedures that guide and support patient care, treatment, and services. In: *Hospital Accreditation Standards 2012*. Oakbrook Terrace, IL: Joint Commission on Resources; 2012.

160. LD.04.01.07: The organization has policies and procedures that guide and support patient care, treatment, or services. In: *Standards for Ambulatory Care 2012: Standards, Elements of Performance Scoring Accreditation Polices*. Oakbrook Terrace, IL: The Joint Commission; 2012.

161. Governance. In: *2012 Accreditation Handbook for Ambulatory Health Care*. Skokie, IL: Accreditation Association for Ambulatory Health Care; 2012:20-27.

162. Safe Medical Devices Act of 1990 and the Medical Device Amendments of 1992. HHS Publication FDA 93-4243. Washington, DC: US Dept. of Health and Human Services, Public Health Service/Food and Drug Administration, Center for Devices and Radiological Health; 1993.

163. Randall SB, Pories WJ, Pearson A, Drake DJ. Expanded occupational safety and health administration 300 log as metric for bariatric patient-handling staff injuries. *Surg Obes Relat Dis*. 2009;5(4):463-468. doi:10.1016/j.soard.2009.01.002. [IIIA]

164. PI.03.01.01: The organization improves performance. In: *Standards for Ambulatory Care 2012: Standards, Elements of Performance Scoring Accreditation Polices*. Oakbrook Terrace, IL: The Joint Commission; 2012.

165. Quality assessment/quality improvement. Quality improvement. In: *Procedural Standards and Checklist for Accreditation Ambulatory Facilities*. Version 1. Gurnee, IL: American Association for Accreditation of Ambulatory Facilities; 2008:44.

ENVIRONMENT OF CARE, PART 1

Acknowledgments

LEAD AUTHOR
Byron Burlingame, MS, BSN, RN, CNOR
Perioperative Nursing Specialist
AORN Nursing Department
Denver, Colorado

CONTRIBUTING AUTHOR
Ramona Conner, MSN, RN, CNOR
Manager, Standards and Guidelines
AORN Nursing Department
Denver, Colorado

The authors and AORN thank Antonia B. Hughes, MA, BSN, RN, CNOR, Perioperative Education Specialist, Baltimore Washington Medical Center, Glen Burnie, Maryland; Elizabeth A. P. Vane, MSN, RN, CNOR, Chief, Perioperative Nursing Services, Walter Reed National Military Medical Center, Bethesda, Maryland; Rebecca M. Patton, MSN, RN, CNOR, FAAN, Atkinson Scholar in Perioperative Nursing, Case Western Reserve University, Lakewood, Ohio; and Rev Donna S Nussman, PhD, RN, Surgical Health Care Consultant, and Adjunct Professor, College of Mechanical Engineering/BioEngineering Department, University of North Carolina – Charlotte, for their assistance in developing this guideline.

PUBLICATION HISTORY

Originally published February 1988, *AORN Journal*, as "Recommended practices for safe care through identification of potential hazards in the surgical environment." Revised March 1992.

Revised November 1995; published March 1996, *AORN Journal*. Reformatted July 2000.

Revised; published March 2003, *AORN Journal*.

Revised 2007; published in *Perioperative Standards and Recommended Practices*, 2008 edition, as "Recommended practices for a safe environment of care."

Revised November 2009 for online publication in *Perioperative Standards and Recommended Practices*.

Minor editing revisions made in November 2010 for publication in *Perioperative Standards and Recommended Practices*, 2011 edition.

Revised and reformatted December 2012 for online publication in *Perioperative Standards and Recommended Practices*.

Evidence ratings revised 2013 to conform to the AORN Evidence Rating Model.

Minor editing revisions made in November 2014 for publication in *Guidelines for Perioperative Practice*, 2015 edition.

AMBULATORY SUPPLEMENT: SAFE ENVIRONMENT OF CARE, PART 1

Recommendation VI

Precautions should be taken to mitigate risks associated with handling, storage, and use of compressed medical gas cylinders and liquid oxygen containers.

VI.a.1. An adequate emergency supply of oxygen should be stored at the facility to provide an uninterrupted supply for one day.[A1]

> *Amb* Oxygen delivery may only be available on certain days, and emergency supplies may be unavailable.

> *Amb* An alarm system should indicate oxygen reserve status and one-day supply.[A2-A4]

> *Amb* Oxygen supply levels should be verified daily when the facility is open for business.[A2,A3]

> *Amb* Surgical procedures should not be started until a sufficient oxygen supply is confirmed.

VI.g.4. The valves on medical gas cylinders should be closed properly to avoid leaking during storage.

> *Amb* Gas cylinder valves and oxygen delivery unit valves (eg, anesthesia machines, flow meters) should be checked at the close of business to confirm they are in the off position.
>
> A cylinder valve or delivery unit valve left open overnight or over the weekend may deplete the facility's entire oxygen supply.

Recommendation XIII

Policies and procedures for the provision of a safe environment of care should be developed, reviewed periodically, revised as necessary, and readily available in the practice setting.

Amb Policies and procedures should include
- the minimum oxygen supply level to be maintained,[A4]
- oxygen storage capabilities,[A4]
- the oxygen procurement process,[A4]
- the amount of time needed for routine and emergency oxygen delivery,[A3,A4]
- processes for verifying the daily oxygen supply,[A2,A3] and
- processes for checking gas cylinder valves and oxygen delivery unit valves (eg, anesthesia machines, flow meters) at the close of business to confirm they are in the off position.

References

A1. Bielen RP, Lathrop JK. *Health Care Facilities Code Handbook*. 9th ed. Quincy, MA: National Fire Protection Association; 2012. [IVB]

A2. EC.02.05.09: The organization inspects, tests, and maintains medical gas and vacuum systems. In: *Comprehensive Accreditation Manual for Ambulatory Care*. Oakbrook Terrace, IL: Joint Commission; 2013.

A3. Anesthesia services. In: 2013 *Accreditation Handbook for Ambulatory Health Care*. Skokie, IL: Accreditation Association for Ambulatory Health Care; 2013:47.

A4. *NFPA 99: Health Care Facilities Code*. 2012 ed. Quincy, MA: National Fire Protection Association; 2011. [IVB]

GUIDELINE FOR A SAFE ENVIRONMENT OF CARE, PART 2

The Guideline for a Safe Environment of Care, Part 2 has been approved by the AORN Guidelines Advisory Board. It was presented as a proposed guideline for comments by members and others. The guideline is effective May 15, 2014. The recommendations in the guideline are intended to be achievable and represent what is believed to be an optimal level of practice. Policies and procedures will reflect variations in practice settings and/or clinical situations that determine the degree to which the guideline can be implemented. AORN recognizes the many diverse settings in which perioperative nurses practice; therefore, this guideline is adaptable to all areas where operative and other invasive procedures may be performed.

Purpose

The physical design and environment of the perioperative suite should support safe patient care, workplace safety, and security. This document provides guidance for the design of the building structure; movement of patients, personnel, supplies, and equipment through the suite; safety during construction; environmental controls (eg, heating, ventilation, air conditioning [HVAC]); maintenance of structural surfaces; power failure response planning; security; and control of noise and distractions. Disaster response and recovery are outside the scope of this document.

Evidence Review

A medical librarian conducted a systematic review of the MEDLINE®, CINAHL®, and Scopus® databases and the Cochrane Database of Systematic Reviews for meta-analyses, randomized and nonrandomized trials and studies, and systematic and nonsystematic reviews. Search terms included *restricted area, semi-restricted area, nonrestricted area, transition zone, traffic patterns, traffic, foot traffic, traffic flow, door swings, hospital design and construction, hospital construction, facility design and construction, Aspergillus, aspergillosis, spores, mycoses, fungi, dust, debris, operating rooms, operating theatres, operating suites, surgicenters, ambulatory surgery centers, hospitals, air microbiology, filtration, indoor air pollution, infection control, surgical site infection, surgical wound infection, Health Insurance Portability and Accountability Act, HIPAA, privacy, confidentiality, controlled environment, heating, ventilation, air conditioning, HVAC, equipment contamination, cardboard, ventilation, heating, laminar flow, laminar airflow, Staphylococcus, enterococcus, enterococci, Staphylococcaceae, microbial colony count, security measures, violence, ultraviolet disinfection, ultraviolet rays, ultraviolet, disinfection, terminal cleaning,* *company representatives, industry representatives, sales representatives, equipment manufacturers, humidity, temperature, health personnel, surgical attire, clothing, clothes, textiles, fabric, lighting, illumination, electricity,* and *electric power supplies*.

Articles specific to animals and the topics of refuse disposal, waste management, sanitary engineering, waste products, and the food industry were excluded. In addition, the librarian reviewed the search results related to laminar airflow and removed from them articles that were not relevant to infection or the environment. The lead author and the medical librarian identified and obtained relevant guidelines from government agencies, other professional organizations, and standards-setting bodies.

The initial search was conducted in February 2011; an April 2012 follow-up search included additional topics. In both cases, search results were limited to literature published in the five years prior to the date of the search. The lead author also consulted the results of a 2013 literature search on distractions in the perioperative environment for recent studies on this topic. The librarian established continuing alerts on the topics included in this guideline and provided relevant results to the lead author.

Editor's note: *MEDLINE is a registered trademark of the US National Library of Medicine's Medical Literature Analysis and Retrieval System, Bethesda, MD. CINAHL, Cumulative Index to Nursing and Allied Health Literature, is a registered trademark of EBSCO Industries, Birmingham, AL. Scopus is a registered trademark of Elsevier B.V., Amsterdam, Netherlands.*

Recommendation I

The health care organization should establish a multidisciplinary team that is responsible for the oversight of any surgical suite construction or renovation project.

A multidisciplinary team can provide expertise on functional design, the functional needs of the users, infection prevention, sustainability, and regulatory requirements.[1-3]

I.a. The multidisciplinary team should consist of
- representatives of the health care organization, including perioperative nurses and an infection preventionist[1,2];
- representatives from all affected disciplines;
- external representatives including the design team (eg, architects, interior designers, engineers); and

- representatives of equipment manufacturers whose equipment requires provisions for structural support, space, and utilities.
  [2: Moderate Evidence]

  Representatives of the health care organization possess the clinical expertise necessary to identify the functional needs of the users and assess the design for possible constraints (eg, infection prevention, functional workflow).[1,3] Representatives of equipment manufacturers can provide critical equipment installation specifications to the design team at the time of planning and design. This information is needed to help avoid costly adjustments to the plan after construction has begun.

I.a.1. A perioperative registered nurse (RN) should provide input into the selection of equipment, proposed flow of people and equipment, and space utilization during the planning stages of the project.

Perioperative RNs possess the clinical expertise to provide input on these topics and to advocate for patient safety.[4]

I.b. The multidisciplinary team should participate in all phases of the project including planning, design, construction, and commissioning.[5-7]
[2: Moderate Evidence]

Involvement of the multidisciplinary team in the process helps hold all parties responsible for taking the necessary precautions to prevent or decrease the risk to patients.[3]

I.b.1. The multidisciplinary team should create a functional plan to include
- intended use of the space,
- projected volume of procedures,
- utility requirements,
- environmental requirements,
- security requirements,
- communication requirements,
- location of support areas,
- storage requirements, and
- traffic patterns.

The functional plan defines the requirements for the space and provides the framework upon which designers will create the design for the project.[7]

I.b.2. The multidisciplinary team should obtain and be familiar with federal, state, and local regulatory requirements and applicable construction guidelines (eg, Occupational Safety and Health Administration [OSHA], Centers for Medicare & Medicaid Services, National Fire Protection Association [NFPA], Facility Guidelines Institute, American Society for Healthcare Engineering).[6-11]

I.c. The multidisciplinary team should perform an initial and ongoing risk assessment beginning early in the planning phase, continuing throughout the project, and ending at commissioning.
[2: Moderate Evidence]

The assessment identifies potential risks to patients and personnel that could be caused by the construction and the need for precautions to prevent the spread of infection to patients after the building project is completed.[1-3]

I.c.1. The risk assessment should identify factors that support a safe design and create the criteria for the selection of finishes, surfaces, and HVAC systems.

I.c.2. The assessment should identify the risks created during construction that affect patient care and workplace safety, including
- infection prevention,
- air quality,
- utilities,
- noise,
- vibration, and
- security.[3,7]

Recommendation II

The multidisciplinary team should use evidence-based design concepts in the planning and design of the surgical suite.

Evidence-based design can be cost-effective and may positively affect the safety, quality, and efficiency of perioperative patient care. In an analysis of the business case for evidence-based design, Henriksen et al determined that the upfront capital costs related to using evidence-based design would be paid for in two to three years. The hypothetical facility used in this analysis was a 300-bed hospital with an original construction cost of $240 million. The upfront capital costs for the evidence-based design improvements was $12 million. Using the cost data available, the authors determined that the evidence-based design improvements could save the facility $7 million annually by decreasing the cost of operations and increasing revenues.[13]

II.a. During the surgical suite planning and design phase, a simulated room or suite setup should be used. [2: Moderate Evidence]

Simulation has been shown to assist in determining factors that affect the performance of tasks in an area.[14] Birnbach et al conducted a quantitative study to determine whether simulation could predict possible errors in design. The indicator measured in this study, which involved 52 physicians and residents, was hand hygiene completion. The variable that was manipulated was the location of the hand hygiene dispenser.[15]

The hand hygiene solution dispenser was placed in the designer's chosen location for group 1 (n = 26). In this group, 11.5% (n = 3) of the participants performed hand hygiene using the dispenser. For group 2 (n = 26), the dispenser was placed in clear view of the physicians as they observed patients. In this group, 53.8% (n = 14) used the dispenser. Based on these data, the researchers concluded that simulation is effective and can be an inexpensive way to quantitatively evaluate proposed design solutions to patient safety hazards.[15]

II.a.1. The perioperative RN should verify that the components required (eg, surgical table, anesthesia machine, suction canister, back table) in an operating room (OR) are present in the simulated OR.

II.b. Traffic patterns should be designed to facilitate movement of patients, personnel, equipment, and supplies into, through, and out of defined areas within the surgical suite. *[2: Moderate Evidence]*

The surgical suite design should include three designated areas that are defined by the activities performed in each area (Table 1):

- **Unrestricted area:** An area of the building that is not defined as semi-restricted or restricted. This area includes a central control point for designated personnel to monitor the entrance of patients, personnel, and materials into the semi-restricted areas. This area may include locker rooms, break rooms, offices, waiting rooms, the preoperative admission area, Phase I and Phase II postanesthesia care units (PACUs), and access to procedure rooms (eg, endoscopy rooms, laser treatment rooms). Street clothes are permitted in this area. Public access to the area may be limited based on the facility's policy and procedures.
- **Semi-restricted area:** The peripheral support areas of the surgical suite. The area may include storage areas for equipment and clean and sterile supplies; work areas for processing instruments; sterilization processing room(s); scrub sink areas; corridors leading from the unrestricted area to the restricted area of the surgical suite; and the entrances to locker rooms, the preoperative admission area, the PACU, and sterile processing. This area is entered directly from the unrestricted area past a nurses' station or from other areas. Semi-restricted areas have specific HVAC design requirements associated with the intended use of the space (See Recommendation IV).[7] Personnel in the semi-restricted area should wear surgical attire and cover all head and facial hair.[16] Access to the semi-restricted area should be limited to authorized personnel and patients accompanied by authorized personnel.
- **Restricted area:** A designated space contained within the semi-restricted area and accessible only through a semi-restricted area. The restricted area includes the operating and other rooms in which operative or other invasive procedures are performed. Restricted areas have specific HVAC design requirements associated with the intended use of the space (See Recommendation IV).[7] Personnel in the restricted area should wear surgical attire and cover head and facial hair. Masks should be worn when the wearer is in the presence of open sterile supplies or of persons who are completing or have completed a surgical hand scrub.[16,17] Only authorized personnel and patients accompanied by authorized personnel should be admitted to this area.

The HVAC, surgical attire, and traffic pattern requirements of the surgical suite are designed to be more stringent as one moves from unrestricted to restricted areas.[2] The progression of restrictions is intended to provide the cleanest environment in the restricted area.

II.b.1. The designated areas should be separated by
- signage indicating the attire required for entering the area and who may access the area;
- doors separating the restricted area from the semi-restricted area; and
- doors, signage, or a line of demarcation to identify the separation between the unrestricted and semi-restricted areas.

Signs provide a visual cue that alerts persons to the restrictions required for entry into each area. The doors provide a physical barrier to assist in maintaining control of the HVAC.

II.c. When a hybrid OR is to be included in the construction or renovation project, the hybrid room should
- be sized to accommodate the equipment to be used based on the manufacturers' specifications;
- have radiation protection based on the type and amount of protection required for the type of system used;
- include the size and location of the radiation system control room; and
- have, at a minimum, the same traffic restrictions and ventilation system requirements as an OR.

[2: Moderate Evidence]

Meeting these recommendations will help provide a safe environment for patients and for personnel working in these areas, help avoid unnecessary construction expenses and late change orders, and help ascertain that the room will accommodate the equipment.[7]

II.d. Laminar airflow may be used in the restricted area. *[2: Moderate Evidence]*

The results of studies involving laminar airflow conflict; some support and some refute the benefits of laminar airflow in the OR.[18-29] This is an unresolved issue and additional research is needed. The studies define and measure laminar flow differently or do not provide a definition of laminar flow, making comparison and analysis difficult.

ENVIRONMENT OF CARE, PART 2

Table 1: Unit/Area Designation of Restriction	
Unit/area	Level of restriction
Postanesthesia care unit	Unrestricted or semi-restricted
Endoscopy suite	Unrestricted
Pain clinic/procedure room	Unrestricted
Locker room/administrative office/waiting room	Unrestricted
Sterile processing area	Semi-restricted
Equipment and sterile supply storage	Semi-restricted
Sterile processing decontamination area	Semi-restricted
Operating room	Restricted
Invasive procedure room	Restricted
Preoperative/postoperative patient care area	Unrestricted

A review of the literature by Howard and Hanssen concluded that vertical laminar airflow is more effective than horizontal airflow.[22] The authors pointed out that when horizontal laminar airflow is used, persons passing or standing between the unit and the patient can disrupt the airflow. The authors recommended that the patient and all instruments be within the clean air zone during use of a vertical laminar system.[22]

One limited study by Hall suggests that vertical laminar airflow may be affected by the design of the surgical light. In this study, a large dome type light either blocked or altered the airflow.[28]

Researchers conducting an Austrian study of 80 orthopedic surgical procedures that compared no laminar airflow to use of laminar flow systems of 19.83 m² and 4.56 m² found that the 19.83 m² system provided a significant reduction in the number of viable microorganisms on the instrument table and an insignificant reduction on the other locations measured (ie, at the patient's head, the instrument table, the right side of the patient at about waist level, the left side of the patient's head but away from the table).[20]

A retrospective study conducted by Hooper et al in 2011 included 51,485 total hip arthroplasties and 36,826 total knee replacements. The researchers defined laminar flow as 300 air changes per hour (ACH) and conventional airflow rate as 30 ACH. They concluded that the rate of prosthetic revisions for early deep infections was not reduced by using laminar flow and protective suits with hoods and self-contained exhaust systems when compared with procedures performed with a conventional air change rate and without protective suits.[25]

A comparative study conducted in the United Kingdom between the years 2000 and 2004 involved 435 patients who required re-operation after an Austin-Moore hemiarthroplasty. The researchers did not provide a definition of laminar airflow. They determined that the rate of re-operation for all indications in the non-laminar airflow theater group was four times greater than in the laminar airflow group. Based on these findings, they recommended the use of laminar airflow.[24]

In a quasi-experimental study of 140 patients having total hip or total knee replacements (n = 70 in the control group, n = 70 in the experimental group for whom laminar air flow was used), Knobben et al cultured used instruments, unused instruments, and bone removed from each patient. Laminar airflow was defined as an airflow of 8,100 m³/hour; air inflow speed was 20 cm/second, resulting in the total number of air changes in the entire OR of 60 ACH. The standard airflow was 2,700 m³/hour with an air inflow speed of 10 cm/second and 22 ACH. The researchers concluded that use of laminar airflow reduced the occurrence of prolonged wound discharge and superficial surgical site infection (SSI) and, when compared to standard airflow, laminar airflow was shown to decrease intraoperative bacterial contamination.[26]

Friberg and Friberg compared an upward displacement (ie, a thermal convection system) with 17 ACH to a vertical downward flow system with 16 ACH, with bacterial air and surface counts as the measure of performance. Use of the vertical delivery system resulted in lower bacterial counts than use of the thermal convection system. The researchers also found that vertical, horizontal, and exponential laminar airflow systems all performed equally well.[27]

In a quasi-experimental study comparing bacterial contamination of wood (n = 10), plastic (n = 10), and stainless steel (n = 10) tiles placed within and outside the laminar flow area, Da Costa et al found no less contamination of the tiles placed outside the laminar flow than those placed within the laminar flow area. Based on the results of this study, the researchers suggested that placing instruments and implants outside the laminar flow area is a safe practice.[21]

Hirsch et al tested four ventilation systems (ie, window-based ventilation, supported air nozzle canopy, low-turbulence displacement airflow, and low-turbulence displacement airflow with flow stabilizer) for intraoperative contamination using a descriptive study technique. The study included 277 procedures performed in six ORs in five German hospitals. The researchers found that use of the window-based ventilation system resulted in the highest intraoperative contamination and use of the low-turbulence displacement airflow with flow stabilizer system resulted in the lowest intraoperative contamination. The low-turbulence displacement airflow with flow stabilizer system is equivalent to the vertical laminar airflow system used in the United States.[29]

A retrospective study involving 63 surgical departments in 55 German hospitals (N = 99,230 surgical procedures) showed higher SSI rates with use of laminar airflow in the OR when compared with turbulent clean air for hip prosthesis; for knee prosthesis and abdominal surgery (ie, appendectomy, cholecystectomy, colon surgery, herniorrhaphy) no significant differences were found. The researchers performed active SSI surveillance using the methods and definitions of the US National Nosocomial Infection Surveillance system. They suggested that the results may not be generalizable because of factors that were not controlled in the study.[19]

A survey of orthopedic program administrators in 256 hospitals in which 8,288 total knee replacements were performed in 2000 found no significant difference in the rate of deep infection after total knee replacement. The survey asked whether the facility used or did not use laminar airflow or body exhaust suits. The overall 90-day cumulative incidence of deep infection requiring subsequent surgery was used for measurement. Twenty-eight of the 8,288 procedures required subsequent surgery (0.34%) because of the presence of an infection.[23]

II.d.1. If the multidisciplinary team chooses to consider the use of laminar airflow, a risk/benefit/cost analysis should be performed during the planning phase. Analysis should include the direction of the airflow (eg, from ceiling to floor, lateral).

II.e. A ventilation setback strategy may be used for periods when the OR is unoccupied. *[2: Moderate Evidence]*

A ventilation setback strategy provides a cost savings by allowing the amount of air supplied to an OR to be reduced when the room is not in use. The cost savings occurs because the amount of energy used in heating or cooling the air is decreased.[30]

II.e.1. An HVAC system setback that reduces the number of ACH may be used if
- the temperature and humidity settings are maintained within the design parameters as stated in Recommendation IV and
- the positive-pressure relationship of the OR to the adjacent area is maintained.[7,30]

II.e.2. A risk/benefit/cost analysis should be performed during the planning phase to determine whether use of such a system is acceptable. The analysis of ventilation system setback should include
- actual or projected usage;
- the needs, preferences, and perceptions of the system's users;
- local climate;
- facility type (eg, hospital, ambulatory surgery center);
- applicable local building code requirements;
- existing ventilation system design;
- cost of system maintenance;
- energy savings; and
- necessary components of the system (eg, occupancy sensor, manual control, timed control, combined control).[30]

II.f. Ultraviolet (UV) light for air purification may be used in the restricted area. If the multidisciplinary team chooses to consider the use of UV light, a risk/benefit/cost analysis should be performed during the planning phase. *[2: Moderate Evidence]*

There are a number of published studies regarding UV light use for infection prevention. The study designs are varied and not all relate directly to the OR, but the results may be generalizable to the OR.[31-39]

In a study that was performed in a patient room to compare the effects of UV light on methicillin-resistant *Staphylococcus aureus* (MRSA), vancomycin-resistant enterococcus (VRE) and *Clostridium difficile*, Nerandzic and Donskey concluded that UV-C light kills all three of the organisms. A 3-log reduction in *Clostridium difficile* was achieved after an exposure to 20,000-microwatt seconds/cm^2 for 45 minutes. If the *Clostridium difficile* was first exposed to a germination solution, the 3-log reduction occurred in 10 minutes. There was a 3-log reduction in the MRSA and VRE counts with both of the exposure conditions. In this study, the UV light was administered by an automated room decontamination device.[32]

In a single facility comparative study published in 2007, Ritter et al reviewed the records of 5,980 patients undergoing total joint surgery performed by a single surgeon between 1986 and 2005. The study compared the infection rate when laminar flow was used (n = 1,071) to the infection rate when a downward pointing UV light was used (n = 4,909). The infection rate was 1.77% when laminar flow was used and 0.57% when UV light was used. The researchers concluded that when proper safety precautions were taken, use of downward-pointing UV lights appeared to be an effective method of reducing the infection rate in total joint replacement surgeries.[33]

In a report by the National Institute of Occupational Safety and Health (NIOSH), the use of upper room UV lights was found to be beneficial when there were 6 ACH. The air changes in this study were not the same as the recommended changes for the OR (ie, 15 to 25 ACH); therefore, the effect of UV lights in the OR may not match the results in this study.[37] The air exchanges are significant because UV germicidal irradiation is effective at a low air change rate, but its efficacy diminishes as the rate increases. The decrease in efficacy occurs because the kill rate is dependent on the length of exposure of the microbe to the UV light. The high air change rate in an OR decreases the exposure time; therefore, the efficacy is significantly decreased.[35] Similar results were found in other studies and in literature reviews.[35,36,38,39]

A review of the literature published in 2010 concluded that direct down-pointing UV lights should not be used in the OR because of the risk of injury to personnel and the decreased efficacy related to the rate of ACH. This review also suggests that UV light could be used as an adjunct to other infection prevention measures.[35]

II.f.1. The risk/benefit/cost analysis should include
- the design of the light system to be used (eg, within the duct work, upper room, downward pointing, portable),[31]
- the safety measures required (eg, protective clothing, eye wear), and
- room down time and other use restrictions.

Ultraviolet light exposure may cause harmful effects to the eyes and the skin.[34,35] The required safety measures, including wearing protective clothing and keeping the room vacant, are dependent on the type of system used.[35]

II.g. An environmental impact assessment of construction materials and design features should be performed during the planning phase. *[2: Moderate Evidence]*

If amounts of volatile chemicals are high, "sick building syndrome" may result, which may cause personnel and patients to experience headaches, dizziness, nausea, dry cough, nasal dryness, watery or itchy eyes, skin rashes, and difficulty concentrating.[40]

The literature frequently describes efforts to produce a low environmental impact as *green design*, *green building*, and *sustainable design*, which are synonyms and encompass all aspects of building design.[41] Green design features may include a high-efficiency HVAC system, surfaces and finishes that use low volatile organic compounds, natural lighting, and reclamation or recycling of materials disposed of during construction.[1,42] The financial effects of green design may be short or long term and positive or negative.[41,42]

II.g.1. The environmental impact assessment should include the projected water and energy consumption; the biodegradability and environmental toxicity of the building materials; and the ability to recycle, reuse, or renew building materials.

II.h. The perioperative environment should be planned with electrical safeguards in place as described in *NFPA 70: National Electrical Code*[43]; *Guidelines for Design and Construction of Hospitals and Outpatient Facilities*[7]; and local, state, and national regulations.[10] *[2: Moderate Evidence]*

Electrical hazards in the OR may lead to fires, burns, and electrical shocks. These conditions result from electric current flowing through inappropriate pathways (eg, through the patient's or perioperative team member's body to ground).[44]

II.i. The OR lighting system should be planned and designed to provide
○ light for monitoring the patient, illumination of the surgical field, and performance of other patient care tasks;
○ dimmable lighting;
○ low operating and maintenance cost; and
○ surgical field lighting that
  - causes minimal interference with air circulation,
  - has the required ceiling support system,
  - causes minimal interference with other ceiling-mounted equipment,
  - provides the ability to focus and control the spot size,
  - generates minimal heat,
  - requires minimal time and effort for lamp replacement,
  - provides the desired color and temperature,
  - limits the amount of shadow produced,
  - is easy to clean,
  - requires a low amount of energy for movement and focusing, and
  - provides the ability to control settings at the sterile field.

[2: Moderate Evidence]

Lighting in the OR that is comfortable, safe, and provides optimal visibility and color recognition should provide a satisfactory visual environment and meet the requirements of the OR personnel.[45] The shape and size of the surgical lights have been shown to affect the airflow patterns during use of laminar airflow.[28] Surgical lights may produce high amounts of radiant heat that may cause damage to exposed tissues and discomfort to the surgical team.[46] The color of light produced can change the color and appearance of the skin and other tissue.[46,47] Shadows may be produced by equipment that blocks the light.

Lights require frequent cleaning to protect against infections caused by dust.[47] An observational study of 46 hours of surgery revealed that high forces were required to move the lights, and an interruption was caused by adjustment of the lights, which at times required assistance from the RN circulator.[48] In a comparison of different surgical lights, varying levels of inclusion of these criteria (eg, amount of force required to move the lights, amount of interruption caused during adjustment) were found among the different light manufacturers.[49,50]

Incidents of patient burns from surgical lights have been reported. The reported incidents occurred when multiple light heads were aimed at one small area and operating at or near maximum power.[51]

II.j. The building design should provide functionally equivalent space for decontamination and sterilization of surgical instruments in all locations where sterilization processes are performed.[7,52,53] When instrument sterilization is to be performed within the surgical suite, a sterile processing room should have
- separate clean and decontamination spaces, which may be rooms or areas;
- decontamination and clean spaces that are separated by one of three methods:
  - a wall with a door or pass-through,
  - a partial wall or partition that is at least 4-ft high and at least the width of the counter, or
  - a distance of 4 ft between the instrument-washing sink and the area where the instruments are prepared for sterilization;
- provisions for sterilization equipment and storage of related supplies in the clean area;
- separate sinks for washing instruments and washing hands;
- decontaminating equipment (eg, automated washer, ultrasonic cleaner); and
- storage space for personal protective equipment (PPE) and cleaning supplies in the decontamination area.[7]

[2: Moderate Evidence]

The requirements for reprocessing of reusable medical devices do not vary by location. Equivalent procedures, supplies, and equipment are needed in all locations where sterilization is performed.

ENVIRONMENT OF CARE, PART 2

II.k. All surfaces (eg, floors, walls, ceilings, cabinets) should be durable, smooth, and cleanable. *[2: Moderate Evidence]*

Surfaces that are durable, smooth, and cleanable allow for ease of cleaning and assist in preventing buildup of dirt and debris in crevices.[2,7,54]

II.k.1. In the semi-restricted and restricted areas,
- surfaces should withstand cleaning chemicals;
- floors should have no seams or have sealed seams and a cove base;
- walls should be smooth with no seams or sealed seams;
- cabinets should have a smooth surface and be made of laminate, stainless steel, or glass; and
- absorbent material, such as exposed wood, should not be used.[2,7]

II.k.2. Ceilings in semi-restricted areas should be smooth and may be either monolithic or drop-in ceiling tiles.

II.k.3. Ceilings in restricted areas should be monolithic. Drop-in ceiling tiles should not be used.[7]

II.l. The surgical suite should have security controls (eg, door security systems, video surveillance, tracking systems, electronic identification access tracking systems, visitor logs).[55,56] *[2: Moderate Evidence]*

Security controls help limit unauthorized access to the semi-restricted and restricted areas of the surgical suite. Video surveillance assists with monitoring of access at all times. Tracking systems (eg, electronic identification access tracking systems, visitor logs) assist in identifying who is present in the perioperative suite.

II.l.1. Security measures should be selected based on a risk assessment and may include the use of devices (eg, alarm systems, video surveillance, shatter-proof glass, metal detectors, locked doors).

Recommendation III

During renovation and construction in the close vicinity of an occupied health care facility, measures for preventing environmental contamination should be established, maintained, and monitored by perioperative team members and the infection preventionist in accordance with applicable state regulations and the ongoing risk assessment.

Multiple studies have been published that demonstrate contamination of the internal environment by infectious agents present in the external environment during renovation and construction.[57-60]

Pini et al measured *Aspergillus* levels in two units of a facility during construction. The levels were greater in the corridor connected to the construction area in comparison with the restricted access rooms.

ENVIRONMENT OF CARE, PART 2

The researchers recommended ongoing surveillance of the levels of *Aspergillus* during construction.[57]

III.a. Infection prevention measures should include
- barriers applicable to the type of construction occurring;
- maintenance of barrier integrity;
- surgical attire for construction workers;
- special construction-related traffic pathways, entrances, and exits;
- negative pressure and use of high-efficiency particulate air (HEPA) filters on the construction side of the barrier;
- regular maintenance of the air-handling system; and
- other infection control prevention and surveillance measures (eg, particulate counts).

[2: Moderate Evidence]

A prospective air and surface sampling study examined the amount of *Aspergillus* in air samples and on surfaces in a facility during construction outside the building. The measurements were completed in three units with high populations of immunocompromised patients. The researchers found no increase in the amount of *Aspergillus* when protective measures, described as use of HEPA filtration systems, wet brooming, and wetting down of the outside construction site, were taken and the importance of environmental cleaning was reinforced.[61]

A limited study conducted during two separate renovation projects requiring exterior demolition at a hospital in Japan compared the effectiveness of adhesive tape with the effectiveness of an adhesive poly film applied to the window frames as a weather stripping for the purpose of creating an additional dust barrier. The amount of dust in the air was measured before construction and during construction. The results revealed that the adhesive tape was more effective than the poly film, but both controlled the amount of dust in the air.[58]

An outbreak of *Bacillus* species in a neonatal care unit was linked to contamination resulting from excavation during construction. After precautions were taken, including replacing air filters, cleaning surfaces in the unit, emphasizing hand hygiene, and relocating the loading dock for linen and supply delivery, the rate of patient infection decreased to zero.[59]

A review of the literature published in 2006 revealed that more than 500 reported cases of surgical infections were caused by airborne *Aspergillus*. This review included patients having surgery in various specialities but did not specify whether the infections occurred during construction. In the majority of the cases, it was presumed that the source of the *Aspergillus* causing the infection was the air in the OR. The authors recommended routine maintenance of the air-handling system.[60]

Infection prevention during construction and renovation is a complex issue dependent on multiple variables specific to the setting.

III.a.1. High-efficiency particulate air filters should be used to filter the incoming air during construction occurring outside of the building.

III.a.2. Construction workers should don surgical attire if they are required to enter the semi-restricted area.[16]

III.a.3. Barriers (eg, solid fiberboard or sheetrock walls, sealed plastic walls) should be placed between the construction site and the perioperative environment and maintained at all times.

III.a.4. Traffic plans for construction personnel and movement of supplies, equipment, and debris should be developed, communicated, and implemented.

Traffic plans assist surgical team members in moving from place to place without contaminating their surgical attire and in moving supplies and equipment by a route that minimizes contamination from the construction site. The traffic plans also help prevent exposure of construction workers to soiled or potentially infectious materials.

III.a.5. Perioperative RNs should participate in the construction process by
- verifying the presence and integrity of barriers and infection prevention measures,
- participating in construction meetings,
- monitoring the progress of the project by visual inspection,
- communicating to the perioperative team the progress of the project and information that will affect the daily functions of the surgical suite (eg, presence of new barriers, additional cleaning required, noise and vibration that will be caused by the construction), and
- collaborating with perioperative team members to resolve unanticipated problems as they arise.

Recommendation IV

The health care organization should create and implement a systematic process for monitoring HVAC performance parameters and a mechanism for resolving variances.

Heating, ventilation, and air conditioning systems control room air quality, temperature, humidity, and air pressure of the room in comparison to the surrounding areas. The HVAC system is intended to reduce the amount of environmental contaminates (eg, microbial-laden skin squames, dust, lint) in the surgical suite. The restricted areas are intended to be the cleanest; therefore, the HVAC requirements for the restricted areas are the most stringent. The HVAC system reduces the amount of environmental contamination by carrying airborne contaminates away from the sterile field and removing these contaminants through the return duct vents located at the periphery of the room.[62,63]

IV.a. Designated perioperative team members in collaboration with a multidisciplinary team should perform a risk assessment of the surgical suite if a variance in the parameters of the HVAC system occurs. *[5: No Evidence]*

The literature search did not reveal any evidence of clinical significance related to the degree of variance in the HVAC system design parameters. Additional research is needed.

The effect of the HVAC system parameters falling out of range is variable. A small variance for a short period of time may not be of clinical concern, whereas a large variance for a longer period may have clinical significance.

IV.a.1. The multidisciplinary team should include
- a perioperative nurse,
- an infection preventionist,
- a surgeon,
- a facility plant engineer or designated person,
- sterile processing department personnel, and
- facility and perioperative managers.

IV.a.2. Based on the risk assessment, corrective measures may include
- rescheduling or redirecting procedures to areas of the surgical suite where the HVAC system is functioning within parameters,
- delaying elective procedures,
- limiting surgical procedures to emergency procedures only,
- closing the affected OR(s), or
- taking no action.

IV.a.3. Based on the risk assessment, measures that should be taken to restore the surgical suite to full functionality after the HVAC system variance has been corrected may include
- terminal cleaning when there is evidence of contamination on surfaces[54];
- reprocessing or discarding any supplies with packaging that may have been compromised[53]; and
- inventorying discarded, damaged supplies for insurance claim purposes and to obtain replacements.

IV.b. Personnel who identify an unintentional variance in the predetermined HVAC system parameters should report the variance according to the health care organization's policy and procedures. *[5: No Evidence]*

Rapid communication between affected and responsible personnel can help facilitate resolution of the variance.

IV.c. The minimum number of ACH including the percentage of outdoor air should be maintained within the HVAC design parameters at the rate that was applicable at the time of design or of the most recent renovation of the HVAC system (Table 2). *[2: Moderate Evidence]*

Filtered air minimizes the recirculation of indoor contaminants within the perioperative area. In a comparative study conducted in a Turkish hospital OR, researchers compared the number of live airborne microorganisms in the air in one OR in which the HEPA filters were turned on and one OR in which the HEPA filters were turned off during a weekend. The OR in which the HEPA filters were turned off experienced a rise in the air microbial load. The airborne microorganism load in the OR in which the HEPA filter was operating was 222.44 colony-forming units (cfu)/m^3; the airborne microorganism load in the OR in which the HEPA filter was not operating was 536.66 cfu/m^3. The researchers concluded that operational HEPA filtration systems reduce the air microbial load.[64]

Hirsch et al compared four ventilation systems to determine the system with the greatest efficiency at preventing bacterial emission into the sterile field. The study included 277 surgical procedures performed in 60 ORs located in five German hospitals. The ventilation systems tested included window-based, supported air nozzle canopy, low-turbulence displacement airflow, and low-turbulence displacement airflow with flow stabilizer. The low-turbulence displacement airflow with flow stabilizer system was found to be the most efficient in preventing bacterial emission into the sterile field. The low-turbulence displacement airflow with flow stabilizer system described in this document is similar to the system used in the United States.[29]

In a comparative study conducted in Poland, researchers assessed the level of occupational exposure to nitrous oxide using different ventilation and scavenging systems. Thirty-five ORs in 10 hospitals were equipped with different ventilation systems with active or passive scavenging systems. The ventilation systems included natural ventilation with supplementary fresh air provided by a pressure ventilation system at 6 ACH, pressure and exhaust systems equipped with ventilation units supplying fresh air to maintain the ACH rate at about 10 ACH to 15 ACH, and laminar flow air-conditioning systems that maintain the ACH at a rate of 15 or higher. The researchers concluded that at least 12 ACH in addition to use of a scavenging system reduces the levels of waste anesthesia gases below the Polish occupational exposure levels of 180 mg/m^3.[65]

A study conducted in Taiwan compared the air particulate level in two ORs with two different

ENVIRONMENT OF CARE, PART 2

Table 2: HVAC Design Parameters[1,2]

Functional area	Minimum outdoor air changes per hour	Minimum total air changes per hour*	Humidity	Temperature	Settings for airflow patterns (pressure)
Operating room	4	20	20% to 60%	68° F to 75° F (200 C to 240 C)	positive
Soiled workroom/decontamination room	2	6	NR	72° F to 78° F (22° C to 26° C)	negative
Sterilizer equipment access	NR	10	NR	72° F to 78° F (22° C to 26° C)	negative
Preparation and packaging/clean workroom	2	4	Maximum 60%	72° F to 78° F (22° C to 26° C)	positive
Clean/sterile storage	2	4	Maximum 60%	72° F to 78° F (22° C to 26° C)	positive
Restroom/housekeeping	NR	10	NR	NR	negative
Postanesthesia care unit	2	6	20% to 60%	70° F to 75° F (21° C to 24° C)	NR
Procedure room	3	15	20% to 60%	70° F to 75° F (21° C to 24° C)	positive
Gastrointestinal endoscopy procedure room	2	6	20% to 60%	68° F to 73° F (20° C to 23° C)	NR
Gastrointestinal endoscope cleaning room	2	10	NR	NR	negative
Semi-restricted corridor	NR	NR	NR	NR	NR

NR = No recommendation
* Total air changes per hour is the sum of the outdoor air changes plus the recirculated air changes.

Reference
1. Facility Guidelines Institute, US Department of Health and Human Services, American Society for Healthcare Engineering. Guidelines for Design and Construction of Hospitals and Outpatient Facilities. Chicago, IL: American Society for Healthcare Engineering of the American Hospital Association; 2014.
2. Centers for Medicare & Medicaid Services. State Operations Manual Appendix A—Survey Protocol, Regulations and Interpretive Guidelines for Hospitals. Rev. 78; 2011.

rates of air changes. One OR had an air change rate of 23 ACH and the other OR had a rate of 15 ACH. The comparison revealed that the OR with 23 ACH had lower levels of particulate matter in the air. The researchers concluded that a higher air change rate may reduce microbial contamination in the OR.[66]

Perdelli et al measured airborne microbial concentrations in various environments including ORs in 10 hospitals in Saudi Arabia. They found that the fungal concentration was lower inside the building compared to the outside environment. The fungal concentration levels were the lowest in the ORs that were equipped with HEPA filters (efficiency = 99.97%), had at least 15 ACH, and had positive pressure.[67]

IV.c.1. The ACH in a restricted area should be maintained at 20 total changes per hour, with a minimum of five air changes of outdoor air per hour or at the rate that was applicable at the time of design or of the most recent renovation of the HVAC system.[7]

IV.c.2. The ACH in a semi-restricted area are related to the function performed in that area:
- clean/sterile storage—4 total and 2 outdoor air changes
- soiled workroom/decontamination room—6 total and 2 outdoor air changes
- sterilizer equipment access—10 total and no recommendation for outdoor air changes[7]

IV.c.3. The ACH in an unrestricted area are related to the function performed in that area:
- postanesthesia care unit—6 total and 2 outdoor air changes
- procedure room—15 total and 3 outdoor air changes
- gastrointestinal endoscopy procedure room—6 total and 2 outdoor air changes[7]

IV.d. The incoming air should be sequentially filtered through two filters. The first filter should be rated as 7 MERV (ie, minimum efficiency reporting value) and the second should be rated as 14 MERV.[7] *[2: Moderate Evidence]*

In a comparative study in a French hospital under construction, Fournel et al evaluated the benefits of a filtration system by measuring the amount of *Aspergillus* found inside the facility before and during construction. The study found the levels of *Aspergillus* inside did not increase during construction outside, even though there was a rise in the amount of *Aspergillus* outside. The researchers attributed the results to the use of filtration systems in the building. The filtration systems were either HEPA filters or a mobile air treatment decontamination unit. The decontamination unit used a novel technology based on nonthermal-plasma reactors instead of mechanically filtering the air.[61]

In a study comparing two different hematology departments, one with and one without HEPA filters, Crimi et al found that incoming air filtered with HEPA filters had a lower amount of microbic and *Aspergillus* contamination at the air output grille, in the middle of the room, and at the air intake grille.[68] In another study, researchers found lower airborne particulate counts in the OR when the air was filtered using two filters with efficiency ratings of 30% and 90%.[69]

A study in Taiwan compared two ORs, one with HEPA filtration and 23 ACH and one with no HEPA filtration and 15 ACH. The researchers found the room with HEPA filtration and 23 ACH had significantly reduced levels of particulate matter in the air.[66]

A comparative study measured airborne microbial concentrations in various departments including the OR in 10 hospitals equipped with air conditioning. The researchers found the fungal concentration inside the building was lower than that in the outside environment. The levels were the lowest in the ORs that were equipped with HEPA filters (99.97% efficiency) and had at least 15 ACH and positive pressure. The other areas of the buildings had a lower percentage of filtration and number of air changes. The authors concluded that air-handling systems are effective in reducing fungal concentrations.[67]

The outside air requires filtration continuously because airborne fungi are present at all times, but the level of the fungi can vary with the season. A descriptive study in Egypt investigated the effect of air pollutants and environmental parameters on the survivability of airborne fungi. The researchers found that the amount of airborne fungi and the species of fungi in outdoor air varied among seasons of the year. The two largest predictors of the amount and species of fungus were temperature and relative humidity. The fungi count was the lowest in the summer and highest in the autumn. The researchers concluded that environmental parameters were the most significant indicator of fungal survival.[70]

IV.e. Relative humidity should be maintained within the HVAC design parameters. *[2: Moderate Evidence]*

The effect of relative humidity on bacterial, fungal, and viral growth is inconclusive. Additional research is required to determine optimal relative humidity levels for control of environmental contamination.

In a descriptive study, Panagopoulou et al examined air and surface fungal levels in four units in a Greek tertiary care hospital during a 12-month period. Two of the units were in building A and two were in building B. In building A, each room had a separate air conditioning unit; building B had a central air conditioning unit. The researchers determined that the fungal levels were higher during the months when the temperature and humidity levels were higher, independent of the method of air conditioning. They also determined that the air conditioning system in building B was more effective.[71]

The authors of a literature review on the effects of humidity on bacterial survival found that various levels of humidity created differing responses in different strains of bacteria. The responses included structural changes and death. The bacterial survival rates are dependent on the species. A generalization of a link between humidity and bacterial survival cannot be made.[72]

In a laboratory setting, Thompson et al found that aerosolized *Staphylococcus epidermidis*, used as a surrogate for *Staphylococcus aureus*, survived at relative humidity levels of < 20%, 40% to 60%, 70% to 80%, and > 90%. The researchers concluded that the *Staphylococcus epidermidis* was not affected by the level of relative humidity.[73]

In a literature review of 120 articles, Memarzadeh found no conclusive evidence to support a maximum or minimum relative humidity level to decrease the survival rate of viruses and the ability of viruses to cause diseases.[74]

ENVIRONMENT OF CARE, PART 2

IV.e.1. The relative humidity in a restricted area should be maintained within a range of 20% to 60%.[7]

IV.e.2. The humidity in a semi-restricted area is related to the function performed in that area:
- clean/sterile storage—maximum 60%
- soiled workroom/decontamination room—no recommendations
- sterilizer equipment access—no recommendations
- semi-restricted corridor—no recommendations[7]

IV.e.3. The humidity in an unrestricted area is related to the function performed in that area:
- PACU—20% to 60%
- gastrointestinal endoscopy procedure room—20% to 60%
- procedure room—20% to 60%[7]

IV.f. The temperature should be maintained within the limits recommended for each area (ie, unrestricted, semi-restricted, restricted). The temperature of the room may be intentionally adjusted based on the individual needs of the patient. *[2: Moderate Evidence]*

No research studies linking variations in temperature to SSIs were found in the literature search. However, literature reviews by Tang[72] and Memarzadeh[74] discuss the effect of temperatures on bacterial and viral survival rates. Neither review is directly related to the OR, nor is either review generalizable to the OR because they recommend temperatures that are beyond the OR comfort zone.

The review by Tang details factors affecting the survival of airborne bacteria in hospitals. This review suggests that temperatures above 75° F (24° C) decrease bacterial survival rates by varying amounts for gram-negative, gram-positive, and intracellular bacteria.[72] The review by Memarzadeh, which includes 120 research studies, indicated that temperatures greater than 60° C (140° F) for longer than 60 minutes will inactivate viruses, and the level of inactivation is dependent on the presence of organic materials.[74]

The only literature regarding room temperature ranges for the surgical suite found in the literature search were guidelines developed by the American Society for Healthcare Engineering, which are the accepted professional guidelines for HVAC systems in the United States.[7]

IV.f.1. The temperature range in a restricted area should be 68° F to 75° F (20° C to 24° C) but the range may be intentionally adjusted for a limited time based on the individual needs of the patient.[7]

Individual patients, such as pediatric surgical patients or patients undergoing procedures that require intentional hypothermia, may require that room temperature be adjusted outside of the recommended range.

IV.f.2. The temperature in a semi-restricted area should be dependent on the use of the area:
- clean/sterile storage—72° F to 78° F (22° C to 26° C)
- soiled workroom/decontamination room—72° F to 78° F (22° C to 26° C)
- sterilizer equipment access—no recommendations
- semi-restricted corridor—no recommendations[7]

IV.f.3. The temperature of an unrestricted area should be between 70° F and 75° F (21° C and 24° C).[7]

IV.g. The airflow direction (ie, pressure relationship of one area to adjacent areas) should be maintained within the HVAC design parameters. *[2: Moderate Evidence]*

The direction of the airflow from one room to the adjacent area is designed and engineered to minimize the flow of contaminates from clean to less-clean areas.[75] Disruptions in the airflow patterns within the OR can redirect contaminants onto the sterile field.[62,76]

IV.g.1. The restricted area should have a positive pressure relationship to the adjacent areas.[7]

IV.g.2. The pressure relationship of the semi-restricted area to the adjacent area should be based on the use of the area:
- clean/sterile storage—positive
- soiled workroom/decontamination room—negative
- sterilizer equipment access—negative
- semi-restricted corridor—no recommendations[7]

IV.g.3. Equipment and supplies should be located away from return ducts.

An unobstructed airflow out of the room is required to maintain the correct pressure within the area.

IV.h. Free-standing fans, portable HEPA filtering devices, humidifiers, air conditioners, and dehumidifiers should not be used in restricted areas or sterile processing areas. *[2: Moderate Evidence]*

A retrospective study of 180 patients undergoing total knee arthroplasties revealed that 5.6% (n = 10) of the patients developed a superficial infection and 3.9% (n = 7) developed a deep infection. The procedures were performed in an OR with a nonstandard air conditioner installed above a door, which produced a horizontal airflow. An instrument-washing sink was located on the intake side of the air conditioner. After the sink and the air conditioner were removed, a repeat study was completed two years later. In the repeat study, the infection rate fell to 2.2% or one in 45 patients. The investigators concluded that removing the sink and the wall air conditioner resulted in a decrease in SSIs.[77]

Free-standing fans can disrupt airflow patterns, resulting in contamination of the sterile field. A pilot study compared the airflow patterns created by two free-standing HEPA filters and a portable anteroom system with HEPA filtration. The researchers examined a single OR and used smoke plumes to indicate airflow direction. The airflow pattern during use of the free-standing HEPA filter systems moved upward into the breathing zones of the personnel and over the patient. The portable anteroom system maintained the downward airflow pattern. This study also found the noise level was increased with the use of the portable units compared to the portable anteroom system. The authors concluded that use of free-standing HEPA filters in an OR should be avoided and that the portable anteroom system with HEPA filtration was effective in removing airborne infectious agents, which may enhance patient safety.[76]

IV.h.1. For patients who require airborne precautions when no airborne infection isolation room is available, a portable, industrial grade HEPA filter should be used to supplement air cleaning.[78]

IV.i. Preventive maintenance, including regular inspection and changing of filters, should be performed on HVAC systems. *[2: Moderate Evidence]*

A properly functioning HVAC system minimizes the risk of contamination to the sterile field and is an essential component in SSI prevention.[2]

The authors of a study conducted in a Polish hospital concluded that the air filtering system requires regular maintenance, including filter changes, based on the amount of *Aspergillus* in the air samples. The filter should be changed according to the manufacturer's instructions for use because as the air filter ages, its effectiveness decreases.[79]

An investigation of an outbreak of postoperative shoulder arthritis (ie, four cases within one month) caused by *Propionibacterium acnes* infection revealed that the HVAC system was not functioning properly. After repair of the system and increased environmental cleaning, no additional cases were reported.[80]

IV.i.1. Health care personnel in consultation with the HVAC design engineer and plant operations personnel should determine the frequency of filter changes and establish a mechanism for maintaining the system.

IV.j. Doors to the operating or invasive procedure room should be kept closed except during the entry and exit of patients and personnel. *[2: Moderate Evidence]*

Several studies have demonstrated the effects of OR door openings. The studies all support keeping the doors closed during the surgical procedure except when opening is required for a procedure-related reason.[81-86]

A quasi experimental cohort study conducted in a Dutch hospital involved 284 colorectal procedures performed between June 2009 and October 2011. The researchers measured the relationship between personnel compliance with a bundle of interventions and the rate of SSI. The bundle consisted of four interventions including removal of razors previously used for hair removal during preoperative skin preparation, an explicit and uniform protocol for perioperative antibiotic prophylaxis, preoperative application of a warming blanket, and recommendations to reduce the number of OR door openings.

The researchers concluded that a significant relationship existed between the development of an SSI and the higher number of door openings. The primary reasons for door openings were noted to be for non-procedure–related conversation, obtaining equipment required for the procedure, and providing breaks for staff members. A decrease in the number of door openings and a corresponding SSI rate decrease were noted after implementation and enforcement of procedures such as providing breaks at different times and having all necessary equipment in the OR before the beginning of the procedure. The researchers stated that a limitation of the study was not including confounding factors for the door opening, such as complications occurring during surgery.[81]

When the doors are left open, the HVAC system is unable to maintain critical environmental control parameters.[2] Leaving the door open can disrupt pressurization. The ventilation system in the OR is designed to administer air pressure that is greater than the pressure in the semi-restricted area. The ventilation system is also designed to facilitate 20 total room ACH.[7]

In a descriptive study completed in three parallel ORs during 30 orthopedic trauma surgeries, door openings were shown to increase the CFUs present in the air. The characteristics of the ORs in this study included positive pressure in relation to the hallway, one doorway, and an upward air displacement system. The researchers also examined the reasons for the door openings, which included consultation between two experts, obtaining supplies or instruments, relief of personnel, required entrance of personnel while the wound was open, logistic reasons, social visits, and no detectable reason. The researchers concluded

ENVIRONMENT OF CARE, PART 2

that the traffic flow in the OR should be reduced because increased traffic flow has a negative effect on the OR environment.[82]

A descriptive study of the number of door openings during total joint arthroplasties found that the door to the OR was opened 0.69 times per minute. The three most frequent reasons for opening the door were to obtain supplies, to exchange information, and unknown purposes. The door was opened by the RN circulator 26% of the time, by other members of the nursing team 19% of the time, and by the equipment representative 20.3% of the time. The researchers concluded that strategies such as storage of instruments and supplies in the OR will decrease the number of door openings.[83]

In response to an unexplained increase in SSIs, Lynch et al conducted a comprehensive review of infection prevention practices. The review recorded the number of OR door openings, who opened the doors, and the reasons for door openings. The researchers found that during 28 procedures, the door was opened 3,071 times. Door openings varied across specialities and were most often related to requests for information. They also determined that the duration for the OR door to be open was 20 seconds and when multiplied by the number of openings per surgical procedure, the door was open for seven to 20 minutes per hour. The authors suggested that to decrease the number of SSIs, the number of OR door openings should be decreased.[85]

In a descriptive study of 46 consecutive surgical procedures, Young and O'Regan noted an increased potential for the development of an SSI related to the number of door openings during the procedure. There were five infections in 46 procedures; the mean frequency of door openings was 94 times during the procedures that resulted in an infection and 76.4 times during those that did not result in an infection.[84]

A study conducted during 23 surgeries performed in three different ORs evaluated the relationship between biological and dust contamination. Scaltriti et al found that the number of dust particles in the air of the OR decreased as the number of door openings increased, but the presence of bacteria increased as the frequency of door opening increased. The researchers suggested that behaviors such as frequently opening the door may affect the air quality in the OR.[86]

IV.j.1. The health care organization should have a quality monitoring process to monitor rates of and reasons for OR door openings that occur while sterile supplies are open.
A quality improvement initiative in a pediatric hospital revealed that observation alone did not decrease the number of door openings. This study also revealed that the door was opened frequently for communication, and the number of door openings increased with the length of the procedure and the number of people in the room. The authors recommended that a quality plan include measures that describe the reason for OR door openings.[87]

IV.j.2. Measures to reduce the number of door openings may include
- preplanning so that turbulence from opening the door is minimized during the procedure or when sterile supplies are opened,[85,87]
- keeping the surgeons' preference cards current,[87]
- confirming that all instruments and supplies are present before the incision is made,
- posting a sign on the door to restrict traffic while a procedure is in progress,[87]
- using means of communication that do not involve opening the door during procedures,[85,87]
- installing locks on OR doors that can be opened from the inside only,
- analyzing the stage of the procedure before relieving for breaks,[85,87]
- analyzing the culture in the perioperative environment, and
- providing education about the effects of opening the doors.[82]

Recommendation V

The integrity of structural surfaces (eg, doors, floors, walls, ceilings, cabinets) should be maintained, and surfaces should be repaired when damaged.

Surfaces can be damaged through use. Damaged surfaces can lead to an inability to clean and could create a fall or other injury hazard.[2,54]

V.a. Personnel should report damage to floors, walls, ceilings, cabinets, and other structural surfaces according to the health care organization's policy. *[5: No Evidence]*
Damaged structural surfaces may create a reservoir for the collection of dirt and debris that cannot be removed during cleaning. Damage to floor surfaces may create a trip or fall hazard.

V.a.1. Repair priorities should be based on a risk assessment.

Recommendation VI

The health care organization emergency preparedness plan should include procedures for power failure.

There have been multiple reports of power failures in ORs.[88-90]

VI.a. The power failure plan should include procedures for a failure during which the emergency generator works and a failure during which the emergency generator does not work. *[2: Moderate Evidence]*

Advanced preparation will assist in emergency response to an electrical power failure.[89] Generators are designed to operate until there is no fuel; however, generator failure has been reported.[91,92] Reports of organizational experiences and expert opinions recommend various steps to be taken before an electrical outage to assist in preventing negative outcomes.[88-93]

VI.a.1. The power failure plan should identify which essential equipment should be connected to the outlets powered by the emergency generator.[90]

VI.a.2. The power failure plan should identify alternate power sources, including
- working flashlights in every OR and on every anesthesia machine,
- manual monitoring equipment (eg, blood pressure cuff, stethoscope),
- long extension cords,
- battery-operated communication devices, and
- paper documentation forms/records.

VI.a.3. Personnel should be aware of
- the locations of alternate sources of lighting, power, and supplies for use when the normal power is interrupted and
- which life-sustaining medical equipment has battery backup.[43]

Battery power can assist in keeping the equipment operating in case of a power failure involving the main electrical circuit.[90,91]

VI.a.4. Perioperative personnel should confirm batteries are
- labeled with their expiration date,
- checked monthly for expiration, and
- replaced as needed.[94]

VI.b. The power failure plan should include personnel education, including
○ what equipment can operate on battery power[90,93] and
○ the location and availability of
  - charged transport monitors,
  - manual monitoring devices (eg, manual blood pressure cuff, stethoscope),
  - flashlights,
  - the power failure emergency procedures manual,
  - back-up resources for documentation and for supplies that are secured in devices that require power to open,
  - long extension cords, and
  - nonelectrical powered communication devices.[90,91,93]

[2: Moderate Evidence]

VI.c. The power failure plan should include procedures for restoring an OR to service after loss of power, including the required assessment and interventions to perform based on the assessment. *[2: Moderate Evidence]*

The assessment is completed to determine whether there is damage and the extent of damage to equipment, supplies, and the facility.[92]

VI.c.1. Designated perioperative RNs should perform an assessment of the surgical suite in collaboration with a multidisciplinary team that includes
- an infection preventionist,
- a facility plant manager,
- sterile processing personnel, and
- biomedical personnel.

VI.c.2. The assessment should include
- environmental cleanliness (eg, condensation on surfaces including walls and flooring, dirt, debris),
- integrity of sterile supplies (eg, presence of condensation on package surfaces, signs of water damage),
- functionality of the power supply (eg, fully restored, emergency generator in use), and
- availability of water (eg, water pressure, water quality, steam supply).

VI.c.3. Interventions should be completed by the designated perioperative team members to restore the surgical suite to full functionality, based on the results of the assessment (Table 3).

Recommendation VII

The facility-wide security plan should include provisions for security of the surgical suite.

Security measures provide for the safety of patients, personnel, and visitors; prevention of drug diversion and theft; and protection of patient information.[16,95-97] Including the surgical suite in the facility-wide plan takes into consideration the unique security risks created by the presence of high-value equipment, supplies, and pharmaceuticals and the variable hours when the suite may be unoccupied.[98]

Preliminary data released by the US Bureau of Labor Statistics in 2012 shows that in the previous year, there were 11 fatal injuries in which the victim was a nurse.[99]

VII.a. A multidisciplinary team should develop the security plan in consultation with security personnel or law enforcement representatives. *[2: Moderate Evidence]*

Security personnel and law enforcement representatives have expertise in identifying security risks and in prevention and mitigation tactics.[98]

VII.a.1. The security plan should be reviewed and updated based on security breaches that have occurred, potential or actual changes

279

ENVIRONMENT OF CARE, PART 2

Table 3: Assessments and Interventions After a Power Failure[1-3]

Assessment	Intervention
Environmental cleanliness	• Perform terminal cleaning.
Integrity of sterile supplies	• Reprocess or discard any sterile items suspected of damage. • Inventory and record discarded, damaged supplies for insurance claim purposes and to obtain replacements. • Contact manufacturers of sterile supplies to obtain the method of determining package integrity.
Functionality of power supply	• Delay elective procedures until the power supply is restored. • Complete surgeries already in progress. • Redirect procedures to areas of the surgical suite where the power supply is functioning.
Availability of water	• Perform a quality check on steam sterilizers and automated cleaning equipment before returning them to service. • Collaborate with engineering department personnel to determine whether water is safe to use.

Reference

1. Mangram AJ, Horan TC, Pearson ML, Silver LC, Jarvis WR. Guideline for prevention of surgical site infection, 1999. Hospital Infection Control Practices Advisory Committee. Infect Control Hosp Epidemiol. 1999;20(4):250-278.
2. ANSI/AAMI ST79:2010 & A1:2010 & A2:2011 & A3:2012 (Consolidated Text) Comprehensive Guide to Steam Sterilization and Sterility Assurance in Health Care Facilities. Arlington, VA: AAMI; 2012.
3. Mitchell L, Anderle D, Nastally K, Sarver T, Hafner-Burton T, Owens S. Lessons learned from Hurricane Ike. AORN J. 2009;89(6):1073-1078.

related to construction, and changes in technology.[56,96]

VII.a.2. The security plan should include the prevention of workplace violence and address
- mandatory education,
- tracking and analysis of incidents and potential risk,
- a response plan,
- follow-up care for personnel, and
- the process for event reporting.[55,56]

Workplace violence is defined by the Federal Bureau of Investigation as violent acts
- directed at anyone within the workplace and committed by criminals not connected to the workplace,
- directed at employees and committed by those who have a direct connection to the workplace (eg, customers, clients, students),
- directed at employees and committed by present or former employees, or
- directed at employees or customers and committed by a person with whom they have had a personal relationship.[55]

Workplace violence is defined by the US Bureau of Labor as "violent acts directed towards a person at work or on duty (eg, physical assaults, threats of assault, harassment, intimidation, or bullying)."[100] In private industry in 2011, 11,760 persons were intentionally injured by another person. None of these injuries resulted in death but the recovery required the injured party to take days off from work.[100]

Incidents of violence against health care workers have been reported including fatal and nonfatal attacks. Between 1997 and 2006, 113 incidents of assault, rape, or homicide were reported to The Joint Commission.[96]

In 2007, 291 nurses in a German hospital participated in a retrospective cross-sectional survey. Seventy-two percent of the nurses reported having experienced verbal violence from a patient or visitor and 42% reported having experienced physical violence from a patient or visitor in the previous 12 months. The violence sometimes resulted in physically injury (23%) and in one or more days of sick leave (14%).[56,101]

A security risk assessment and an analysis of incidents can help identify the actual or potential risk of workplace violence.[55]

VII.a.3. The security plan should include methods for protecting the patient's health information and personal identifiable information, such as during broadcast surgery or use of social media and photography.

The Health Insurance Portability and Accountability Act requires facilities to keep patient's protected health information and personal identifiable information confidential.[94,102] Protected health information includes the information shared during surgery broadcast using any technology.[103]

It has been reported that social media has been used to share confidential information, which may be considered a breach of the confidentiality regulations.[104] One descriptive study on social media involving 88 residents and 127 faculty members at a school of medicine found that 64% and 22% respectively had a Facebook® profile. Fifty percent of the Facebook pages were public; 31% of the public pages were found to have work-related postings, and patient-specific information was shared in 14% of those with work-related postings. The researchers concluded that individuals have personal responsibility for managing their usage of social media. Health care organizations should have guidelines to guard against professional truancy and violation of patient confidentiality.[104]

In a report summarizing malpractice, battery, and invasion-of-privacy cases, Segal and Sacopulos noted that monetary awards have been received by patients whose photographs have been used for purposes other than those intended or whose photograph was taken without the patient's consent. They concluded that the facility should have plans in place and have the necessary forms completed to limit liability when photographs of patients are taken.[105]

A survey of 205 patients undergoing plastic surgery measured patients' perceptions of the correct use of their photographs. Ninety-eight percent of the patients felt their photographs could be used by their treating physicians but other uses had varying lesser percentages of acceptance (eg, by other physicians [74%], for student teaching [82%], for patient education [88%]). The authors concluded that photography is acceptable to most patients and appropriate consents should be obtained to maximize the patient's acceptance of use.[106]

A case involving a breach of confidentiality was reported related to sharing of confidential patient information on the telephone. In this case, the nurse called the patient's home and spoke with a person whom she knew to be the patient's mother and not the patient. The patient had left specific instructions that the home telephone number was not to be used. The jury awarded the patient $365,000. The legal commentary reminds nurses to be aware of the significance of patient confidentiality and their role in it.[107]

VII.b. Identification badges should be worn by all persons entering the perioperative suite. The identification should be worn on the upper body and be visible. *[2: Moderate Evidence]*

Identification badges support security measures and help identify persons authorized to access the surgical suite.[16]

VII.b.1. Individuals with limited or temporary access to the perioperative environment (eg, students, law enforcement agents, parents of pediatric patients, health care industry representatives) should be identified as visitors and should wear temporary identification badges.[108,109]

Recommendation VIII

Noise and distractions that are not related to patient care should be minimized.

Noise and distractions are created by conversation, clinical and alert alarms, HVAC systems, telephones and other communication devices, and tools related to the provision of surgical procedures (eg, instruments, powered instruments, electrosurgical units, smoke evacuators). Some noise is unavoidable in the perioperative environment but certain noises can be controlled.[110-112]

In one investigation, NIOSH measured noise levels in 18 ORs and found that the noise levels were the highest in the orthopedic and neurosurgery rooms. The levels were higher the closer the person was to the source of the sound (eg, higher for the people in the sterile field compared to the RN circulator). The authors concluded that noise protection was not required because the noise levels were below the NIOSH recommended criterion level of 85 decibels A-Scale (dBA). The NIOSH criterion level describes level of noise exposure that can be safely tolerated during an eight-hour shift without ear protection. There were peak levels that exceeded the threshold level of 90 dBA but that lasted for only short periods of time. The researchers also concluded that the levels were high enough to potentially cause interference with understanding of the spoken word.[113]

In a comparative study involving 10 participants performing robotic-assisted suture tying and mesh alignment, Siu et al concluded that music with high rhythmicity (eg, hip-hop, Jamaican music) had a beneficial effect on performance of both tasks, and music played in the surgical environment may improve surgical education and increase the efficiency of the acquisition of surgical skills. The study compared performance when classical, jazz, hip-hop, or Jamaican music was played. The best performance was noted when Jamaican music was played and when the person performing the task liked the music being played. The study did not consider volume as a variable.[114]

In a review of the literature, Joseph and Ulrich found that noise can induce stress and increase work pressure, annoyance, fatigue, emotional exhaustion and burnout, and communication difficulties. The authors found conflicting articles regarding the effect of noise on performance of health care personnel. Based on the studies reviewed, the authors concluded that it took more effort to maintain a high level of performance when loud noise was present. They also conclude that an increased level of noise frequently required raising the volume of the voice to enable accurate comprehension.[115]

In an observational study performed during 10 surgical procedures, Christian et al recorded 11 events that had the potential to compromise patient safety (eg, counting errors, the RN circulator needing to leave the room). They identified communication and information flow problems, work flow, and competing tasks as possible sources of the events.[116]

A total of 9,830 patients were involved in a prospective study assessing underlying errors that contribute to surgical complications. The study was performed during a 12-month period in an academic department of surgery. The tool used was a survey completed by surgeons. Of the 9,830 patients, 322 experienced a complication (eg, prolonged hospitalization, temporary disability, permanent disability, death) related to an error (eg, incomplete understanding of problem, carelessness/inattention to detail, judgment error, error of omission, technique error). The researchers concluded that errors contributed more than 50% to the complications. Two percent of the 322 errors were attributed to communication errors.[117]

In another study, 62 perioperative professionals (ie, physicians, nurses, nurse anesthetists) completed the Disruptions in Surgery Index. The participants perceived that the disruptions had a greater effect on others than on themselves. The number of disruptions was reported to be the highest for the nurses and the least for the surgeons. The issues considered to be disruptions included individuals' personality and skills, the OR environment, communication, coordination/situational awareness, patient-related disruptions, team cohesion, and the organizational culture.[118]

In a 2010 survey of 439 perfusionists, 55.6% of the respondents admitted to using a cell phone while performing cardiopulmonary bypass.[119]

VIII.a. Non-procedure–related conversation and activities should be prohibited during critical phases of the surgical procedure.[120] [2: Moderate Evidence]

The effects of interruptions and distractions are well documented in the literature.[121-126] In an observational study, interruptions and distractions diverting the attention of the operator from the task at hand caused 44% of errors in simulated procedures being performed by 18 medical students who had varying amounts of education. The authors concluded that distractions and interruptions in the OR could cause surgical residents to commit operative errors.[121]

In a controlled laboratory study, 12 medical interns performing a task related to laparoscopic surgery experienced a significant decline in performance and an increased level of irritation when distracted by music, conversation, and non-optimal handling of the laparoscope. The researchers concluded that the social and technological sources of irritation should be evaluated with a goal of increasing safety for patients.[122]

In a controlled study involving 96 undergraduate university students, Altmann and Trafton found that after an interruption, it took an average of 3.8 seconds for the students to collect their thoughts and return to the activity. The test group partially completed activity A, which was followed by an interruption, and then the time to return to activity A was measured. The control group completed activity A without interruption and then the time to begin activity B was measured at only 1.9 seconds.[123]

Interruptions were shown to increase error rates in a study involving 300 undergraduate university students performing tasks of various lengths with varying types of interruptions. The researchers found the longer the interruption, the greater the error rate.[124]

An observational study in a hospital setting examined the causes of work interruptions during medication administration. The study involved 59 hours and two minutes of medication administration time. The researchers found the work interruptions were caused primarily by nurse colleagues.[125]

In an observational study that examined distractions and interruptions in anesthesia care, Campbell et al noted 424 distracting events, 22% of which had a negative effect. The study involved 30 surgeries lasting a total of 31 hours and two minutes. The researchers suggested that to decrease the potential for committing errors, the anesthesia professional should ignore inappropriate intrusions or conversations, ask personnel who have entered the OR for non-procedure–related reasons to return later, prepare all supplies well in advance, and not participate in irrelevant conversation.[126]

VIII.b. Noise and distraction created by the following sources should be minimized:
- portable communication devices (eg, beepers, cell phones, personal digital assistants, computers),
- fixed communication devices (eg, overhead pages and announcements, telephones, computers),
- electronic music devices (eg, radios, CD players, digital audio players),
- the environment (eg, HVAC system, pneumatic tube systems),
- medical equipment and devices (eg, radiology equipment, waste management system, smoke evacuator, powered surgical instruments, monitors, clinical and alert alarms, metal instruments),
- electronic activities (eg, e-mail, texting, social media [eg, Facebook, YouTube®, Twitter®, LinkedIn®], Internet, games), and
- behavioral activities (eg, nonessential and extraneous conversations, personnel movement in and out of the room).

[2: Moderate Evidence]

The sources of noise and distractions are well documented in the literature, and minimizing various sources is supported by professional organizations.[111-113,127-141] The American College of Surgeons and the American Association of Nurse Anesthetists both support the creation of a policy that limits the use of mobile communication devices in the OR.[140,141]

In an evaluation of noise pollution in ORs in nine hospitals during 43 surgeries, Tsiou et al found that noise pollution came from many sources including the building, machinery, tools, and people. Based on these findings, they recommended a multidisciplinary approach to solving the noise pollution problem.[131]

In a prospective study including 50 trauma procedures, the average noise level was 85 dB with a range of 40 dB to 130 dB. The researchers also noted an average of 60.8 interruptions and distractions per procedure (range, 5 to 192). The distractions and interruptions were caused by team members entering and leaving the room, equipment alarms, parallel conversations, and telephones or pagers. The main effect of distractions and interruptions was disruption in the continuous flow of surgical activities.[112]

A study involving 15 physicians using simulated OR noise and music showed that when music was added to the noise and a task was being performed, the level of auditory processing was decreased. Auditory processing was measured by the surgeon's ability to understand and repeats words using a revised version of the Speech in Noise Test.[137]

The amount of noise generated by pneumatic power tools during orthopedic procedures includes saws at 95 dBA, drills at 90 dBA, K-wire drivers at 85 dBA, and hammers at 65 dBA.[135] These are short-term exposures, and this level of noise is not consistent for the eight-hour shift required in the NIOSH recommended limits of 85 dBA of noise exposure for an eight-hour shift without ear protection.[113]

The results of a cohort observational study involving 11 nurses showed that higher average sound levels were related to higher self-reported levels of stress and annoyance.[133]

Juang et al studied noise created in the hospital unit and outside the unit at three hospitals in Taiwan. The study, which involved 573 patients and personnel, found noise was created by multiple factors including doors opening and closing, people talking, alarms, and equipment. The effects of the noise on the participants' emotion and physiology varied depending on gender, age, religion, work experience, and other factors.[138]

In a review of the literature on occupational exposure to noise, Oliviera and Arenas concluded that noise pollution in ORs can cause a breakdown in communications.[111] They reported that to enable good communication, the spoken voice needs to be 10 dB higher than the surrounding noise.[111]

In a pilot study involving 35 patients undergoing open abdominal procedures, a connection was found between sound levels and the development of SSIs. The authors speculated this may be caused by decreased concentration or a stressful environment.[132]

Nurses in the ORs in three different facilities identified that speech comprehension difficulties were related to the amount of noise in the OR. This difficulty led to more vocal effort being required to achieve speech comprehension.[139] The procedures performed during this study involved various specialties. Similar results were found in a nine-hospital study in which background noise and average noise were measured during surgical procedures performed in different subspecialties. In this study, Stringer et al found noise levels to be higher than those recommended by the World Health Organization for locations in a hospital where patient care occurs.[139] This study and one by Kracht et al[129] found the orthopedic ORs had the highest levels of noise, and other specialities were less noisy. The comparative specialities varied in these studies.[129,139]

A review of the literature conducted in 2010 revealed that the primary effect of noise on personnel was impaired communication.[128]

Arora et al investigated the frequency of stress being produced by distractions and interruptions and the severity of that stress. The study participants were the personnel involved in 55 elective procedures in the United Kingdom. The participants rated distractions and interruptions as frequent cause of stress but rated these least severe on the severity scale. The example of distractions and interruptions stated in the article was telephone calls that led to conveying and replying to nonurgent messages.[127]

In a study of 78 endo-urological procedures, a distraction occurred every 1.8 minutes. Equipment problems and relevant and irrelevant conversations were rated as the most frequent and most distracting events.[130]

In a study in which 10 participants performed robot-assisted suturing and were simultaneously multitasking, the time to secondary task completion was longer and the speed of the primary task was slower compared with a control group.[134]

One case was reported in which a person texting an order was interrupted by a personal text. The interruption resulted in the order not being completed, and the patient received an overdose of anticoagulation medication.[135]

VIII.b.1. Portable communication devices (eg, pagers, smart phones, cell phones, wireless communication systems, hand held two-way radio transceivers [eg, walkie-talkies]) should be

ENVIRONMENT OF CARE, PART 2

- placed on vibrate or silent mode,
- off unless directly needed for job performance, or
- left at a common location outside of the OR.

VIII.b.2. Fixed communication devices (eg, overhead paging systems, intercoms, telephones) should be used
- only for essential communications,
- at the lowest volume possible, and
- for essential communication instead of opening the door and entering the OR.

The use of fixed communication devices is preferred to opening the door because opening the door causes a greater distraction and affects the airflow within the surgical suite.[83]

VIII.b.3. The volume level of electronic music devices (eg, radios, digital audio players, CD players) should be low enough to allow communication among team members.

VIII.b.4. Alarms and verbal communications should be audible above competing environmental noise.

The level of environmental noise (eg, HVAC system, pneumatic tube systems, radiology equipment, suction, smoke evacuator, drills monitors, alarms) may compete with critical communications.

VIII.b.5. The health care organization should establish a policy and procedure for the use of mobile communication devices that includes
- use of personal devices,
- use of facility-owned devices,
- locations or prohibited locations for use, allowable information that may be conveyed by the mobile device (eg, patient-related information only, photography),
- level of encryption and security controls, and
- device cleaning.

VIII.b.6. The health care organization should establish a policy and procedure for distraction control that includes
- portable communication devices (eg, pagers, cell phones, personal digital assistants, computers),
- fixed communication devices (eg, overhead pages and announcements, telephones, computers),
- electronic music devices (eg, radios, CD players, digital audio players),
- the environment (eg, HVAC system, pneumatic tube systems),
- medical equipment and devices (eg, radiology equipment, waste management system, smoke evacuator, powered surgical instruments, monitors, clinical and alert alarms, metal instruments),
- use of electronic activities (eg, e-mail, texting, social media [eg, Facebook, YouTube, Twitter, LinkedIn], Internet, games), and
- personal conduct (eg, essential and extraneous conversations, personnel movement in and out of the room).

VIII.c. The level of noise generated by a piece of equipment or instrument should be a part of the evaluation criteria for purchasing decisions. *[2: Moderate Evidence]*

A health hazard evaluation report conducted by NIOSH at a large teaching facility demonstrated that different amounts of noise are generated by different type of instruments that perform the same function (eg, a modified design produced less noise than the standard design).[113]

VIII.d. Before use, the user should verify that the mobile communication device is
- approved for sharing patient-related information,
- approved for photography,
- equipped with the required level of encryption and security controls, and
- approved for use within the surgical suite.

[3: Limited Evidence]

The advantages of mobile communication technology include easy access to clinical data and patient information, ease of bedside documentation, automated reminders, and ease of access to the device. Devices may be easily lost and personal information contained on the device may be stolen.[135,142]

Cases have been reported in which electro-mechanical interference was caused by cell phone use (ie, the use of a cell phone changed the operation of a medical device).[142]

Editor's note: *Facebook is a registered trademark of Facebook, Inc, Menlo Park, CA. YouTube is registered trademark of Google, Inc, Mountain View, CA. Twitter is a registered trademark of Twitter, Inc, San Francisco, CA. LinkedIn is a registered trademark of LinkedIn Corp, Mountain View, CA.*

Glossary

Commissioning: A quality process used to achieve, validate, and document that facilities and component infrastructure systems are planned, constructed, installed, tested, and are capable of being operated and maintained in conformity with the design intent or performance expectations.

Cove base: Molding or trim used to create a curved right-angle transition from the wall to the floor.

Displacement airflow system: An airflow system in which the air entry point is located low on the wall, the air exit point is located near the ceiling, and the filtered air is introduced at a low velocity.

Distraction: An event that causes a diversion of attention during performance of a task or diverts the person's concentration from the task.

Evidence-based design: A process used by architects, interior designers, and facility managers in the planning, design, and construction of health care facilities. Individuals using evidence-based design make decisions based on the best information available from research, project evaluations and evidence gathered from client operations. An evidence-based design should result in improvements to an organization's outcomes, economic performance, productivity, and customer satisfaction.

Interruption: An unplanned or unexpected event causing discontinuation of a task.

Laminar air delivery system: An air delivery system that delivers particle-free air that moves over the sterile field at a uniform velocity of 0.3 to 0.5 micrometers/second. Laminar airflow is recirculated air that is filtered through a HEPA filter. Laminar air flow can be either vertical or horizontal. Synonym: *ultra clean air.*

Monolithic: A surface constructed to be free of fissures, cracks, and crevices.

Noise: Any sound that interferes with normal hearing and is undesired.

Overhead air delivery system: An airflow system in which the air entry point is located in the ceiling, the air exit point is located low on the wall, and the filtered air is introduced at various velocities.

Procedure room: A room designated for the performance of procedures that do not require a restricted environment but may require the use of sterile instruments or supplies.

References

1. Bartley JM, Olmsted RN, Haas J. Current views of health care design and construction: practical implications for safer, cleaner environments. *Am J Infect Control.* 2010;38(5 Suppl 1):S1-12. [VB]
2. Allo MD, Tedesco M. Operating room management: operative suite considerations, infection control. *Surg Clin North Am.* 2005;85(6):1291-1297, xii. [VC]
3. Lee L. Clean construction. Infection control during building and renovation projects. *Health Facil Manage.* 2010;23(4):36-38. [VB]
4. Guideline for product selection. In: *Guidelines for Perioperative Practice.* Denver, CO: AORN, Inc; 2015:179-186. [IVA]
5. Chang CC, Athan E, Morrissey CO, Slavin MA. Preventing invasive fungal infection during hospital building works. *Intern Med J.* 2008;38(6b):538-541. [VC]
6. American Society of Heating Refrigerating and Air-Conditioning Engineers. Room design. In: *HVAC Design Manual for Hospitals and Clinics.* 2nd ed. Atlanta, GA: ASHRAE; 2013:151-202. [IVB]
7. Facility Guidelines Institute, US Department of Health and Human Services, American Society for Healthcare Engineering. *Guidelines for Design and Construction of Hospitals and Outpatient Facilities.* Chicago, IL: American Society for Healthcare Engineering of the American Hospital Association; 2014.[IVB]
8. National Fire Protection Association. *NFPA 101: Life Safety Code.* Quincy, MA: National Fire Protection Association; 2012. [IVB]
9. National Fire Protection Association. *NFPA 99: Health Care Facilities Code.* 2012 ed. Quincy, MA: National Fire Protection Association; 2011. [IVB]
10. 42 CFR 482.41—Condition of participation: Physical environment. http://www.gpo.gov/fdsys/granule/CFR-2011-title42-vol5/CFR-2011-title42-vol5-sec482-41/content-detail.html. Accessed April 7, 2014.
11. 42 CFR 416.44—Condition for coverage: Environment. http://www.gpo.gov/fdsys/granule/CFR-2012-title42-vol3/CFR-2012-title42-vol3-sec416-44/content-detail.html. Accessed April 7, 2014.
12. Haiduven D. Nosocomial aspergillosis and building construction. *Med Mycol.* 2009;47(Suppl 1):S210-S216. [VB]
13. Henriksen K, Isaacson S, Sadler BL, Zimring CM. The role of the physical environment in crossing the quality chasm. *Jt Comm J Qual Patient Saf.* 2007;33(11 Suppl):68-80. [VA]
14. Lin F, Lawley M, Spry C, McCarthy K, Coyle-Rogers PG, Yih Y. Using simulation to design a central sterilization department. *AORN J.* 2008;88(4):555-567. [IIIC]
15. Birnbach DJ, Nevo I, Scheinman SR, Fitzpatrick M, Shekhter I, Lombard JL. Patient safety begins with proper planning: a quantitative method to improve hospital design. *Qual Saf Health Care.* 2010;19(5):462-465. [IIB]
16. Guideline for surgical attire. In: *Guidelines for Perioperative Practice.* Denver, CO: AORN; 2015:97-120. [IVB]
17. Guideline for hand hygiene. In: *Guidelines for Perioperative Practice.* Denver, CO: AORN; 2015:31-42. [IVB]
18. Mangram AJ, Horan TC, Pearson ML, Silver LC, Jarvis WR. Guideline for prevention of surgical site infection, 1999. Hospital Infection Control Practices Advisory Committee. *Infect Control Hosp Epidemiol.* 1999;20(4):250-278. [IVA]
19. Brandt C, Hott U, Sohr D, Daschner F, Gastmeier P, Ruden H. Operating room ventilation with laminar airflow shows no protective effect on the surgical site infection rate in orthopedic and abdominal surgery. *Ann Surg.* 2008;248(5):695-700. [IIIA]
20. Diab-Elschahawi M, Berger J, Blacky A, et al. Impact of different-sized laminar air flow versus no laminar air flow on bacterial counts in the operating room during orthopedic surgery. *Am J Infect Control.* 2011;39(7):e25-e29. [IIIB]
21. Da Costa AR, Kothari A, Bannister GC, Blom AW. Investigating bacterial growth in surgical theatres: establishing the effect of laminar airflow on bacterial growth on plastic, metal and wood surfaces. *Ann R Coll Surg Engl.* 2008;90(5):417-419. [IIC]
22. Howard JL, Hanssen AD. Principles of a clean operating room environment. *J Arthroplasty.* 2007;22(7 Suppl 3):6-11. [VC]
23. Miner AL, Losina E, Katz JN, Fossel AH, Platt R. Deep infection after total knee replacement: impact of laminar airflow systems and body exhaust suits in the modern operating room. *Infect Control Hosp Epidemiol.* 2007;28(2):222-226. [IIIB]
24. Kakwani RG, Yohannan D, Wahab KH. The effect of laminar air-flow on the results of Austin-Moore hemiarthroplasty. *Injury.* 2007;38(7):820-823. [IIIB]
25. Hooper GJ, Rothwell AG, Frampton C, Wyatt MC. Does the use of laminar flow and space suits reduce early deep infection after total hip and knee replacement?: the ten-year results of the New Zealand Joint Registry. *J Bone Joint Surg Br.* 2011;93(1):85-90. [IIIA]
26. Knobben BA, van Horn JR, van der Mei HC, Busscher HJ. Evaluation of measures to decrease intra-operative bacterial contamination in orthopaedic implant surgery. *J Hosp Infect.* 2006;62(2):174-180. [IIB]
27. Friberg B, Friberg S. Aerobiology in the operating room and its implications for working standards. *Proc Inst Mech Eng H.* 2005;219(2):153-160. [IIIB]

28. Hall G. Air flow disruption must be minimised. *Health Estate.* 2005;59(3):53-55. [VC]

29. Hirsch T, Hubert H, Fischer S, et al. Bacterial burden in the operating room: impact of airflow systems. *Am J Infect Control.* 2012;40(7):e228-e232. [IIIB]

30. *Operating Room HVAC Setback Strategies.* Chicago, IL: American Society for Healthcare Engineering; 2011. [VB]

31. Chan DWT, Law KC, Kwan CHS, Chiu WY. Application of an air purification system to control air-borne bacterial contamination in a University clinic. *Transactions Hong Kong Institution of Engineers.* 2005;12(1):17-21. [IIIB]

32. Nerandzic MM, Donskey CJ. Triggering germination represents a novel strategy to enhance killing of *Clostridium difficile* spores. *PLoS One.* 2010;5(8):e12285. [IIB]

33. Ritter MA, Olberding EM, Malinzak RA. Ultraviolet lighting during orthopaedic surgery and the rate of infection. *J Bone Joint Surg Am.* 2007;89(9):1935-1940. [IIIA]

34. ACGIH. *Ultraviolet Radiation: TLV Physical Agents. Documentation.* 7th ed. Cincinnati, OH: American Conference of Industrial Hygienists; 2010. [IVB]

35. Memarzadeh F, Olmsted RN, Bartley JM. Applications of ultraviolet germicidal irradiation disinfection in health care facilities: effective adjunct, but not stand-alone technology. *Am J Infect Control.* 2010;38(5 Suppl 1):S13-S24. [VA]

36. Escombe AR, Moore DA, Gilman RH, et al. Upper-room ultraviolet light and negative air ionization to prevent tuberculosis transmission. *PLoS Med.* 2009;6(3):e43. [IA]

37. National Institute for Occupational Safety and Health Centers for Disease Control and Prevention. *Environmental Control for Tuberculosis: Basic Upper-Room Ultraviolet Germicidal Irradiation Guidelines for Healthcare Settings.* DHHS (NIOSH) Publication Number 2009-105. Atlanta, GA: National Institute for Occupational Safety and Health. Centers for Disease Control and Prevention; 2009. [IVB]

38. Rutala WA, Gergen MF, Weber DJ. Room decontamination with UV radiation. *Infect Control Hosp Epidemiol.* 2010;31(10):1025-1029. [IIB]

39. McDevitt JJ, Milton DK, Rudnick SN, First MW. Inactivation of poxviruses by upper-room UVC light in a simulated hospital room environment. *PLoS One.* 2008;3(9):e3186. [IIB]

40. Stichler JF. Enhancing safety with facility design. *J Nurs Adm.* 2007;37(7-8):319-323. [VB]

41. Guenther R, Hall AG. Healthy buildings: impact on nurses and nursing practice. *Online J Issues Nurs.* 2007;12(2):2. [VB]

42. Stichler JF. Code green: a new design imperative for healthcare facilities. *J Nurs Adm.* 2009;39(2):51-54. [VC]

43. *NFPA 70: National Electrical Code.* Quincy, MA: National Fire Protection Association; 2011. [IVB]

44. Barker SJ, Doyle DJ. Electrical safety in the operating room: dry versus wet. *Anesth Analg.* 2010;110(6):1517-1518. [VB]

45. Illuminating Engineering Society of North America. *Lighting for Hospitals and Health Care Facilities.* New York, NY: Illuminating Engineering Society of North America; 2006. [IVB]

46. Cockram A. Correct lighting of hospital buildings. 1976. *Health Estate.* 2007;61(4):21-23. [VC]

47. Verrinder J. Use of right lighting levels essential. *Health Estate.* 2007;61(6):31-32. [VC]

48. Knulst AJ, Mooijweer R, Jansen FW, Stassen LP, Dankelman J. Indicating shortcomings in surgical lighting systems. *Minim Invasive Ther Allied Technol.* 2011;20(5):267-275. [VC]

49. Baillie J. Stars of the theatre show true colours. *Health Estate.* 2012;66(1):31-40. [VC]

50. Surgical lights. An illuminating look at the LED marketplace. *Health Devices.* 2010;39(11):390-402. [VB]

51. ECRI Institute. Hazard report. Overlap of surgical lighthead beams may present burn risk. *Health Devices.* 2009;38(10):341-342. [IVC]

52. *ANSI/AAMI ST79:2010 & A1:2010 & A2:2011 & A3:2012 (Consolidated Text) Comprehensive Guide to Steam Sterilization and Sterility Assurance in Health Care Facilities.* Arlington, VA: AAMI; 2012. [IVB]

53. Guideline for sterilization. In: *Guidelines for Perioperative Practice.* Denver, CO: AORN; 2015:665-692. [IVA]

54. Guideline for environmental cleaning. In: *Guidelines for Perioperative Practice.* Denver, CO: AORN; 2015:9-30. [IVA]

55. Warren B. Workplace violence in hospitals: safe havens no more. *J Healthc Prot Manage.* 2011;27(2):9-17. [VC]

56. Guidelines for preventing workplace violence for health care & social service workers. OSHA 3148-01R 2004. Occupational Safety & Health Administration. http://www.osha.gov/Publications/OSHA3148/osha3148.html. Accessed April 7, 2014. [IVA]

57. Pini G, Faggi E, Donato R, Sacco C, Fanci R. Invasive pulmonary aspergillosis in neutropenic patients and the influence of hospital renovation. *Mycoses.* 2008;51(2):117-122. [IIIC]

58. Yahara K, Miura M, Masunaga K, et al. Comparison of two control measures of weatherstripping in reducing blowing dust during hospital renovations. *J Infect Chemother.* 2010;16(6):431-435. [IIIC]

59. Campbell JR, Hulten K, Baker CJ. Cluster of Bacillus species bacteremia cases in neonates during a hospital construction project. *Infect Control Hosp Epidemiol.* 2011;32(10):1035-1038. [VA]

60. Pasqualotto AC, Denning DW. Post-operative aspergillosis. *Clin Microbiol Infect.* 2006;12(11):1060-1076. [VA]

61. Fournel I, Sautour M, Lafon I, et al. Airborne Aspergillus contamination during hospital construction works: efficacy of protective measures. *Am J Infect Control.* 2010;38(3):189-194. [IIIB]

62. American Society of Heating Refrigerating and Air-Conditioning Engineers. Infection control. In: *HVAC Design Manual for Hospitals and Clinics.* 2nd ed. Atlanta, GA: ASHRAE; 2013:19-34. [IVB]

63. Eames I, Tang JW, Li Y, Wilson P. Airborne transmission of disease in hospitals. *J R Soc Interface.* 2009;6(Suppl 6):S697-S702. [VB]

64. Aydin Cakir N, Ucar FB, Haliki Uztan A, Corbaci C, Akpinar O. Determination and comparison of microbial loads in atmospheres of two hospitals in Izmir, Turkey. *Ann Agric Environ Med.* 2013;20(1):106-110. [IIIC]

65. Krajewski W, Kucharska M, Wesolowski W, Stetkiewicz J, Wronska-Nofer T. Occupational exposure to nitrous oxide—the role of scavenging and ventilation systems in reducing the exposure level in operating rooms. *Int J Hyg Environ Health.* 2007;210(2):133-138. [IIIB]

66. Wan GH, Chung FF, Tang CS. Long-term surveillance of air quality in medical center operating rooms. *Am J Infect Control.* 2011;39(4):302-308. [IIIB]

67. Perdelli F, Cristina ML, Sartini M, et al. Fungal contamination in hospital environments. *Infect Control Hosp Epidemiol.* 2006;27(1):44-47. [IIA]

68. Crimi P, Valgiusti M, Macrina G, et al. Evaluation of microbial contamination of air in two haematology departments equipped with ventilation systems with different filtration devices. *J Prev Med Hyg.* 2009;50(1):33-36. [IIIC]

69. Stocks GW, Self SD, Thompson B, Adame XA, O'Connor DP. Predicting bacterial populations based on airborne particulates: a study performed in nonlaminar flow operating rooms during joint arthroplasty surgery. *Am J Infect Control.* 2010;38(3):199-204. [IIIB]

70. Abdel Hameed AA, Khoder MI, Ibrahim YH, Saeed Y, Osman ME, Ghanem S. Study on some factors affecting survivability of airborne fungi. *Sci Total Environ.* 2012;414:696-700. [IIIC]

71. Panagopoulou P, Filioti J, Farmaki E, Maloukou A, Roilides E. Filamentous fungi in a tertiary care hospital: environmental surveillance and susceptibility to antifungal drugs. *Infect Control Hosp Epidemiol.* 2007;28(1):60-67. [IIIB]

72. Tang JW. The effect of environmental parameters on the survival of airborne infectious agents. *J R Soc Interface.* 2009;6(Suppl 6):S737-S746. [VB]

73. Thompson KA, Bennett AM, Walker JT. Aerosol survival of *Staphylococcus epidermidis*. *J Hosp Infect.* 2011;78(3):216-220. [IIIB]

74. Memarzadeh F. Literature review of the effect of temperature and humidity on viruses. *ASHRAE Transactions.* 2012;118(1):1046-1060. [VB]

75. American Society of Heating Refrigerating and Air-Conditioning Engineers. Overview of health care HVAC. In: *HVAC Design Manual for Hospitals and Clinics.* Atlanta, GA: American Society of Heating, Refrigerating and Air-Conditioning Engineers, Inc; 2003:33-45. [IVB]

76. Olmsted RN. Pilot study of directional airflow and containment of airborne particles in the size of *Mycobacterium tuberculosis* in an operating room. *Am J Infect Control.* 2008;36(4):260-267. [IIB]

77. Babkin Y, Raveh D, Lifschitz M, et al. Incidence and risk factors for surgical infection after total knee replacement. *Scand J Infect Dis.* 2007;39(10):890-895. [IIIB]

78. Guideline for prevention of transmissible infections. In: *Guidelines for Perioperative Practice.* Denver, CO: AORN, Inc; 2015:419-451. [IVA]

79. Gniadek A, Macura AB. Air-conditioning vs presence of pathogenic fungi in hospital operating theatre environment. *Wiad Parazytol.* 2011;57(2):103-106. [IIIB]

80. Berthelot P, Carricajo A, Aubert G, Akhavan H, Gazielly D, Lucht F. Outbreak of postoperative shoulder arthritis due to *Propionibacterium acnes* infection in nondebilitated patients. *Infect Control Hosp Epidemiol.* 2006;27(9):987-990. [VB]

81. Crolla RM, van der Laan L, Veen EJ, Hendriks Y, van Schendel C, Kluytmans J. Reduction of surgical site infections after implementation of a bundle of care. *PLoS One.* 2012;7(9):e44599. [IIB]

82. Andersson AE, Bergh I, Karlsson J, Eriksson BI, Nilsson K. Traffic flow in the operating room: an explorative and descriptive study on air quality during orthopedic trauma implant surgery. *Am J Infect Control.* 2012;40(8):750-755. [IIIB]

83. Panahi P, Stroh M, Casper DS, Parvizi J, Austin MS. Operating room traffic is a major concern during total joint arthroplasty. *Clin Orthop Relat Res.* 2012;470(10):2690-2694. [VC]

84. Young RS, O'Regan DJ. Cardiac surgical theatre traffic: time for traffic calming measures? *Interact Cardiovasc Thorac Surg.* 2010;10(4):526-529. [IIIC]

85. Lynch RJ, Englesbe MJ, Sturm L, et al. Measurement of foot traffic in the operating room: implications for infection control. *Am J Med Qual.* 2009;24(1):45-52. [VB]

86. Scaltriti S, Cencetti S, Rovesti S, Marchesi I, Bargellini A, Borella P. Risk factors for particulate and microbial contamination of air in operating theatres. *J Hosp Infect.* 2007;66(4):320-326. [IIIB]

87. Parikh SN, Grice SS, Schnell BM, Salisbury SR. Operating room traffic: is there any role of monitoring it? *J Pediatr Orthop.* 2010;30(6):617-623. [VB]

88. Riley RH. Power failure to a tertiary hospital's operating suite. *Anaesth Intensive Care.* 2010;38(4):785. [VB]

89. Yasny J, Soffer R. A case of a power failure in the operating room. *Anesth Prog.* 2005;52(2):65-69. [VB]

90. Carpenter T, Robinson ST. Case reports: response to a partial power failure in the operating room. *Anesth Analg.* 2010;110(6):1644-1646. [VA]

91. Preventing adverse events caused by emergency electrical power system failures. *Sentinel Event Alert.* Septemper 6, 2006;37. The Joint Commission. http://www.jointcommission.org/assets/1/18/SEA_37.PDF. Accessed April 7, 2014. [IVA]

92. Mitchell L, Anderle D, Nastally K, Sarver T, Hafner-Burton T, Owens S. Lessons learned from Hurricane Ike. *AORN J.* 2009;89(6):1073-1078. [VB]

93. Eichhorn JH, Hessel EA 2nd. Electrical power failure in the operating room: a neglected topic in anesthesia safety. *Anesth Analg.* 2010;110(6):1519-1521. [VB]

94. Routine maintenance and operational testing. In: *NFPA 110: Standard for Emergency and Standby Power Systems.* Quincy, MA: National Fire Protection Association; 2013:110-19–110-21. [IVB]

95. 45 CFR Parts 160, 162, 164: General administrative requirements, Administrative requirements, Security and privacy. http://www.gpo.gov/fdsys/search/pagedetails.action?collectionCode=CFR&searchPath=Title+45%2FSubtitle+A%2FSubchapter+C&granuleId=&packageId=CFR-2007-title45-vol1&oldPath=Title+45%2FSubtitle+A%2FSubchapter+A%2FPart+2&fromPageDetails=true&collapse=true&ycord=2372. Accessed April 7, 2014.

96. The Joint Commission. Protecting your health care workers from violence in the workplace. *Joint Commission: The Source.* 2006;4(4):1-2, 10. [VB]

97. Centers for Medicare & Medicaid Services (CMS) DHHS. Medicare and Medicaid programs; hospital conditions of participation: patients' rights. Final rule. *Fed Regist.* 2006;71(236):71378-71428. http://www.cms.gov/CFCsAndCoPs/downloads/finalpatientrightsrule.pdf. Accessed April 7, 2014.

98. Potter AN. Developing a strategic security plan. *J Healthc Prot Manage.* 2011;27(2):59-65. [VC]

99. United States Census of Fatal Occupational Injuries, 2011. Bureau of Labor Statistics. http://www.bls.gov/iif/oshcfoi1.htm. Accessed April 7, 2014. [IIIA]

100. Injuries, illnesses, and fatalities: frequently asked questions (FAQs). US Bureau of Labor Statistics. http://www.bls.gov/iif/oshfaq1.htm#q05. Accessed April 7, 2014. [VA]

101. Hahn S, Muller M, Needham I, Dassen T, Kok G, Halfens RJ. Factors associated with patient and visitor violence experienced by nurses in general hospitals in Switzerland: a cross-sectional survey. *J Clin Nurs.* 2010;19(23-24):3535-3546. [IIIB]

102. Department of Health and Human Services. HIPAA administrative simplification: standard unique health identifier for health care providers; final rule. *Fed Regist.* 2004;69(15):3434-3469. http://frwebgate.access.gpo.gov/cgi-bin/getpage.cgi?dbname=2004_register&position=all&page=3434. Accessed April 7, 2014.

103. Williams JB, Mathews R, D'Amico TA. "Reality surgery"—a research ethics perspective on the live broadcast of surgical procedures. *J Surg Educ.* 2011;68(1):58-61. [VB]

104. Landman MP, Shelton J, Kauffmann RM, Dattilo JB. Guidelines for maintaining a professional compass in the era of social networking. *J Surg Educ.* 2010;67(6):381-386. [IIIC]

105. Segal J, Sacopulos MJ. Photography consent and related legal issues. *Facial Plast Surg Clin North Am.* 2010;18(2):237-244. [VA]

106. Lau CK, Schumacher HH, Irwin MS. Patients' perception of medical photography. *J Plast Reconstr Aesthet Surg.* 2010;63(6):e507-e511. [IIIB]

107. How aware of patient confidentiality are you? *Nurs Law Regan Rep.* 2007;48(7):2. [VB]

108. AORN position statement on the role of the health care industry representative in the perioperative/invasive procedure setting. 2006. AORN, Inc. http://www.aorn.org/Clinical_Practice/Position_Statements/Position_Statements.aspx. Accessed April 7, 2014. [VC]

109. Health care industry representatives in the operating room. *Clin Privil White Pap.* 2005;(1010):1-12. [IVB]

110. Healey AN, Sevdalis N, Vincent CA. Measuring intra-operative interference from distraction and interruption observed in the operating theatre. *Ergonomics.* 2006;49(5-6):589-604. [IIIB]

111. Oliveira CR, Arenas GW. Occupational exposure to noise pollution in anesthesiology. *Rev Bras Anestesiol.* 2012;62(2):253-261. [VB]

112. Pereira BM, Pereira AM, Correia Cdos S, Marttos AC Jr, Fiorelli RK, Fraga GP. Interruptions and distractions in the trauma operating room: understanding the threat of human error. *Rev Col Bras Cir.* 2011;38(5):292-298. [IIIB]

113. Chen L, Brueck SE. Health hazard evaluation report: evaluation of potential noise exposures in hospital operating rooms, Morgantown, WV [NIOSH HETA No. 2008-0231-3105]. Cincinnati, OH: US Department of Health and Human Services, Centers for Disease Control and Prevention, National Institute for Occupational Safety and Health; 2010. [IIIB]

114. Siu KC, Suh IH, Mukherjee M, Oleynikov D, Stergiou N. The effect of music on robot-assisted laparoscopic surgical performance. *Surg Innov.* 2010;17(4):306-311. [IIIC]

115. Joseph A, Ulrich R. *Sound Control for Improved Outcomes in Healthcare Settings*. Concord, CA: Center for Health Design; 2007. [VA]

116. Christian CK, Gustafson ML, Roth EM, et al. A prospective study of patient safety in the operating room. *Surgery.* 2006;139(2):159-173. [IIIB]

117. Fabri PJ, Zayas-Castro JL. Human error, not communication and systems, underlies surgical complications. *Surgery.* 2008;144(4):557-563. [IIIC]

118. Sevdalis N, Forrest D, Undre S, Darzi A, Vincent C. Annoyances, disruptions, and interruptions in surgery: the Disruptions in Surgery Index (DiSI). *World J Surg.* 2008;32(8):1643-1650. [IIIB]

119. Smith T, Darling E, Searles B. 2010 Survey on cell phone use while performing cardiopulmonary bypass. *Perfusion.* 2011;26(5):375-380. [IIIB]

120. AORN position statement on noise in the perioperative practice setting. 2009. AORN, Inc. http://www.aorn.org/Clinical_Practice/Position_Statements/Position_Statements.aspx. Accessed April 7, 2014. [VA]

121. Feuerbacher RL, Funk KH, Spight DH, Diggs BS, Hunter JG. Realistic Distractions and interruptions that impair simulated surgical performance by novice surgeons. *Arch Surg.* 2012;147(11):1026-1030. [IIIC]

122. Pluyter JR, Buzink SN, Rutkowski AF, Jakimowicz JJ. Do absorption and realistic distraction influence performance of component task surgical procedure? *Surg Endosc.* 2010;24(4):902-907. [IIB]

123. Altmann EM, Trafton JG. Task interruption: resumption lag and the role of cues. In: *Proceedings of the 26th Annual Conference of the Cognitive Science Society*. Austin, TX: Cognitive Science Society; 2004. [IA]

124. Altmann EM, Trafton JG, Hambrick DZ. Momentary interruptions can derail the train of thought. *J Exp Psychol Gen.* 2014;143(1):215-226. [IIA]

125. Biron AD, Lavoie-Tremblay M, Loiselle CG. Characteristics of work interruptions during medication administration. *J Nurs Scholarsh.* 2009;41(4):330-336. [IIIB]

126. Campbell G, Arfanis K, Smith AF. Distraction and interruption in anaesthetic practice. *Br J Anaesth.* 2012;109(5):707-715. [IIIB]

127. Arora S, Hull L, Sevdalis N, et al. Factors compromising safety in surgery: stressful events in the operating room. *Am J Surg.* 2010;199(1):60-65. [IIIB]

128. Hasfeldt D, Laerkner E, Birkelund R. Noise in the operating room—what do we know? A review of the literature. *J Perianesth Nurs.* 2010;25(6):380-386. [VA]

129. Kracht JM, Busch-Vishniac IJ, West JE. Noise in the operating rooms of Johns Hopkins Hospital. *J Acoust Soc Am.* 2007;121(5 Pt1):2673-2680. [IIIB]

130. Persoon MC, Broos HJ, Witjes JA, Hendrikx AJ, Scherpbier AJ. The effect of distractions in the operating room during endourological procedures. *Surg Endosc.* 2011;25(2):437-443. [IIIB]

131. Tsiou C, Efthymiatos G, Katostaras T. Noise in the operating rooms of Greek hospitals. *J Acoust Soc Am.* 2008;123(2):757-765. [IIIA]

132. Kurmann A, Peter M, Tschan F, Muhlemann K, Candinas D, Beldi G. Adverse effect of noise in the operating theatre on surgical-site infection. *Br J Surg.* 2011;98(7):1021-1025. [IIIC]

133. Morrison WE, Haas EC, Shaffner DH, Garrett ES, Fackler JC. Noise, stress, and annoyance in a pediatric intensive care unit. *Crit Care Med.* 2003;31(1):113-119. [IIIC]

134. Suh IH, Chien JH, Mukherjee M, Park SH, Oleynikov D, Siu KC. The negative effect of distraction on performance of robot-assisted surgical skills in medical students and residents. *Int J Med Robot.* 2010;6(4):377-381. [IIIC]

135. Halamka J. Order interrupted by text: multitasking mishap. *AHRQ Web M&M* [serial online]. http://webmm.ahrq.gov/case.aspx?caseID=257. Published December 2011. Accessed April 7, 2014. [VB]

136. Siverdeen Z, Ali A, Lakdawala AS, McKay C. Exposure to noise in orthopaedic theatres—do we need protection? *Int J Clin Pract.* 2008;62(11):1720-1722. [IIIB]

137. Way TJ, Long A, Weihing J, et al. Effect of noise on auditory processing in the operating room. *J Am Coll Surg.* 2013;216(5):933-938. [IIIC]

138. Juang DF, Lee CH, Yang T, Chang MC. Noise pollution and its effects on medical care workers and patients in hospitals. *Int J Environ Sci Tech.* 2010;7(4):705-716. [IIIB]

139. Stringer B, Haines TA, Oudyk JD. Noisiness in operating theatres: nurses' perceptions and potential difficulty communicating. *J Perioper Pract.* 2008;18(9):384-391. [IIIA]

140. American College of Surgeons Committee on Perioperative Care. Statement on use of cell phones in the operating room. *Bull Am Coll Surg.* 2008;93(9):33-34. [IVB]

141. Position statement number 2.18: mobile device use. *AANA J.* 2013;81(1):12. [IVB]

142. Judgment call. *Health Devices.* 2012;41(10):314-329. [VC]

ENVIRONMENT OF CARE, PART 2

Acknowledgements

LEAD AUTHOR
Byron Burlingame, MS, BSN, RN, CNOR
Perioperative Nursing Specialist
AORN Nursing Department
Denver, Colorado

CONTRIBUTING AUTHOR
Ramona Conner, MSN, RN, CNOR
Manager, Standards and Guidelines
AORN Nursing Department
Denver, Colorado

The authors and AORN thank Antonia B. Hughes, MA, BSN, RN, CNOR, Perioperative Education Specialist, Baltimore Washington Medical Center, Edgewater, MD; Sandy Albright, MSHM, BSN, RN, CNOR, Nurse Consultant, Synergy Health North America, Tampa, FL; Janice Neil, PhD, RN, Associate Professor and Chair, Department of Undergraduate Nursing Science, College of Nursing, East Carolina University, Greenville, NC; Rodney W. Hicks, PhD, RN, FNP-BC, FAANP, Professor, Western University of Health Sciences, Pomona, CA: Bill Rostenberg, FAIA, FACHA, ACHE, EDAC, Principal and Director of Research, Anshen + Allen Architects, San Francisco, CA, for their assistance in developing this guideline.

PUBLICATION HISTORY
Originally published in May 2014 in *Perioperative Standards and Recommended Practices* online.

Minor editing revisions made in November 2014 for publication in *Guidelines for Perioperative Practice*, 2015 edition.

ENVIRONMENT OF CARE, PART 2

GUIDELINE FOR MEDICATION SAFETY

The Guideline for Medication Safety has been approved by the AORN Recommended Practices Advisory Board. It was presented as proposed recommendations for comments by members and others. The guideline is effective December 1, 2011. The recommendations in this guideline are intended to be achievable and represent what is believed to be an optimal level of practice. Policies and procedures will reflect variations in practice settings and/or clinical situations that determine the degree to which the guideline can be implemented. AORN recognizes the various settings in which perioperative nurses practice; therefore this guideline is adaptable to various practice settings. These practice settings include traditional operating rooms (ORs), ambulatory surgery centers, physicians' offices, cardiac catheterization laboratories, endoscopy suites, radiology departments, and all other areas where operative and other invasive procedures may be performed.

Purpose

This document provides guidance to perioperative RNs to develop, implement, and evaluate safe medication management practices specific to the perioperative setting. Evidence-based approaches to medication safety in perioperative settings are not well established; therefore, guidance emerges from broad knowledge of adverse events and strategies to prevent medication errors identified in other settings.[1-3] Medication errors may go undetected, but when they are reported, the sources of the errors are multidisciplinary and multifactorial. Results of medication errors can include substantial threats to patients, increased health care costs, and compromised patient confidence in the health care system.[4,5]

Awareness of medication errors increased after the 1999 Institute of Medicine report *To Err Is Human: Building a Better Health System* stated that "medication errors account for one out of 131 outpatient deaths and one out of 854 inpatient deaths."[6] Since that time, the Joint Commission's *Sentinel Event Alert* reports have indicated that medication errors resulting in death or permanent loss of function continue to occur each year.[7]

The recommendations that follow are consistent with the six phases of the medication use process, including procuring, prescribing, transcribing, dispensing, administering, and monitoring.[4] Medication errors can originate at any point in the medication use process and affect patients of all ages. Perioperative settings present additional challenges for safe medication practices. Factors affecting the medication process in the perioperative environment include, but are not limited to,

- the aseptic transfer of medications onto the sterile field,
- the presence of an intermediary who is in sterile attire to receive and transfer dispensed medications to the licensed independent practitioner who is in sterile attire (eg, surgeon),
- time-sensitive conditions, and
- sensory distractions intrinsic to the environment.

Potential risks associated with medication errors in the perioperative setting include, but are not limited to,

- inconsistent communication of current and previous medication regimens (ie, medication reconciliation);
- confusion in the medication order (eg, name, strength, dose) caused by muffled verbal orders delivered through surgical masks;
- incomplete, ambiguous, incorrect, or illegible written or spoken orders;
- inaccurate, illegible, or outdated surgical preference cards;
- medication that is removed from the original manufacturer's packaging to aseptically deliver contents onto the sterile field;
- allied heath professionals in sterile attire who receive medications onto the sterile field having limited knowledge of medications;
- inconsistent labeling of medications on and off the sterile field;
- medication dispensed to the sterile field that may be handled by multiple individuals before reaching the licensed individual administering the medication;
- medication preparations without a pharmacist in the setting to perform or oversee the preparation or provide consultation;
- high-alert medications that are available in multiple dose forms and concentrations;
- look-alike and sound-alike medications stored in close proximity;
- patient care complexity that requires rapid perioperative interventions;
- extended work hours leading to health care worker fatigue;
- care provided by multiple health care providers simultaneously;
- multiple patient hand offs between care providers; and
- misuse or failure of medical devices used to store, dispense, or administer medications.

Safe medication practices require open, honest, and clear communication throughout the medication use process and the perioperative continuum of care. The following recommendations for perioperative settings are consistent with established professional standards of care for the medication use process. In addition, these recommendations provide guidance for the comprehensive planning required for managing medication inventory across the medication use process. Perioperative administrators can use these evidence-based recommendations to facilitate policy development and provide a foundation for creating quality-improvement and process-improvement monitors. For the purposes of this document, medication includes prescription products, IV and irrigation fluids, medication patches, implanted devices that contain or deliver medication, medical gases, herbal and dietary supplements, and over-the-counter agents.

Recommendation I

A multidisciplinary team approach for medication management and the prevention of medication errors should be used throughout the phases of perioperative care.

Involving all health care professionals who participate in the medication use process assists with identifying medication error risk factors from a variety of perspectives. In many settings, the nurse may be the primary person administering medications. However, there is still a need for collaboration between all stakeholders (eg, nurse, physician, pharmacist) to address issues relating to the medication management plan and to ensure that the plan is effective.[8] In the perioperative setting, there are medication hand offs among perioperative team members, and medications may be given concurrently by the sterile team members and anesthesia professionals, which adds further justification for collaborating to prevent medication errors. Creating quality improvement teams that include stakeholders relevant to this patient safety issue was among the recommendations identified in a report from the Agency for Healthcare Research and Quality describing successful initiatives nurses can use to guide efforts to improve quality.[9]

I.a. A pharmacy and therapeutics committee or medication safety committee should be established.[5]

A committee that is focused on medication safety issues helps to ensure ongoing interaction among health care providers. The American Society of Health-System Pharmacists states that it is a minimum standard in both hospital and ambulatory settings to have a multidisciplinary team for medication-use policy development and to make decisions concerning medication use.[10,11] A multidisciplinary approach may help balance pharmaceutical cost containment and the risk of adverse drug events in patient settings.[12]

I.a.1. The medication safety committee should include key stakeholders (eg, nurses, physicians, anesthesia professionals, pharmacists, risk management personnel, purchasing personnel, administrators) who participate in the medication use process. *Amb*

I.b. A medication management plan should be developed by a multidisciplinary team to identify risk-reduction strategies for each of the six phases of the medication use process, including procuring, prescribing, transcribing, dispensing, administering, and monitoring. The medication management plan should be communicated to all members of the perioperative team and implemented consistently in all perioperative practice settings (eg, preoperative, intraoperative, day surgery, postoperative).

Developing a medication management plan that incorporates structures, processes, and professional responsibilities into each of the six phases of the medication use process allows for identification of latent and active failures. The medication error can be associated with the point of origin in the medication use process and targeted interventions can be identified.[4]

Increasing the perioperative team's awareness of the health care organization's medication management plan disseminates a broader picture of medication risk-reduction strategies and can help communicate the interdependency of the team's actions to provide safe medication practices. Promoting effective team functioning is among the five principles for creating safe systems of health care delivery reported in the Institute of Medicine report on medical errors.[6] Involving key people is among the strategies for developing a strategic plan for medication safety in the 2002 Pathways for Medication Safety report developed by the Institute for Safe Medication Practices (ISMP) in a partnership with American Hospital Association and the Health Research and Educational Trust.[13] The report indicated that involvement of informal leaders from the front line, senior administrative leaders, physicians, and managers helps garner support and enthusiasm, nurtures broad networks, and provides feedback about levels of support needed to ensure a meaningful and effective medication management plan.[13] Although there are not many quantitative research findings that document the relationship between team behaviors and outcomes in health care, research supports developing surgical teams to focus on sharing potential problems, inquiries, and briefings.[14,15]

Consistent implementation of the medication management plan across all phases of perioperative patient care establishes clarity and decreases ambiguity. Consistency between perioperative practice settings establishes the same standard of care for patients regardless of where a surgical or other invasive procedure is performed.

I.b.1. Nurses, prescribers, and pharmacists should collaborate with each other and assess the needs of patients and their designated support persons to develop a structured and

MEDICATION SAFETY

systematic approach to the medication management plan.[16,17]

A systems approach to patient-centered medication administration includes interprofessional collaboration.[8] A model strategic plan for medication safety also may include involvement from patients, people who are designated to support patients, and community leaders to promote community medication safety initiatives and medication self-management programs.[13] Multidisciplinary and patient collaboration to enhance the effectiveness of medication reconciliation was identified as a primary medication error risk-reduction strategy based on a review of eight studies focusing on prescribing and medication reconciliation.[16]

I.b.2. Pharmacists should be involved in the planning, development, and continuous evaluation of the medication management plan.

Pharmacists are trained to detect potential medication errors and to identify contraindications of medications and drug-drug interactions.[4,18,19] One of the roles of the pharmacist is to prepare and present drug product evaluation reports that consider all aspects of safety, effectiveness, and cost to the pharmacy and therapeutics committee to evaluate the need for policy development or revisions to existing medication-use policies.[10]

I.b.3. The medication management plan should promote the use of integrated technology whenever possible during the medication use process. Medication technology may include, but is not limited to,
- automated dispensing storage systems that have patient profiles and drug formularies,
- smart infusion pumps,
- electronic medical record systems that contain decision support systems,
- automated medication dosage calculations, and
- bar-coding technology.

The Institute of Medicine identified the use of well-designed technologies as a priority for health care organizations for the delivery of safe medication care.[17] Researchers who conducted a review reported evidence that information technology has been used to facilitate medication reconciliation activities including obtaining medication information, comparing medications, and clarifying discrepancies (eg, duplication, appropriateness).[20]

An interdisciplinary group of practitioners convened in 2007 to identify medication error risk-reduction strategies. The strategies identified include positioning computer monitors or a means to access drug information resources and the medical administration record in close proximity to an automated dispensing storage system or medication storage.[21] The group also identified profiled automated dispensing storage systems as a strategy that can be implemented to comply with the Joint Commission medication management accreditation requirement that specifies that a pharmacist should review all new orders before they are available for selection and administration by the nurse, respiratory therapist, or physician.[21,22]

One study showed a substantial reduction in medication errors at patient admission after implementation of a process that mapped data between a medication reconciliation system and a computerized-provider order (CPOE) entry system.[23] Another study showed a reduction in potential adverse medication events after an information technology application designed to facilitate medication reconciliation was integrated into the CPOE system.[24] Clinical decision support systems alert the perioperative team member administering the medication to possible out-of-range doses or contraindications with other medications to help identify and avert medication errors.[24-26] When fully implemented, use of bar-code technologies during medication administration provides a way for the perioperative team member who is administering the medication to confirm patient identification, dose, and product, and it allows pharmacy personnel to confirm order verification.[27,28]

I.b.4. The medication management plan should include strategies for providing immediate access (preferably electronic information resources) to current medication information resources for perioperative personnel who administer medications. Current medication information resources should be available for all new medications and acceptable concentrations that will be dispensed or accessible.

Health care organizations have the responsibility to provide easily accessible and current information resources to assist perioperative personnel who administer medications.[17] Important information includes, but is not limited to, nutrition and herbal supplement interactions (eg, calcium channel blockers and grapefruit) and medication allergies or side effects associated with other medications (eg, amoxicillin and cephalexin). Dose errors or omissions may occur in printed medication references or the information provided may not match the medication concentrations that are acceptable for use in critical care settings.[29]

MEDICATION SAFETY

Newly released medications present risk for error because nurses are less likely to be familiar with them and information often cannot be found in printed medication references.[29]

I.c. Pharmacists should be available for consultation with members of the perioperative team in all facilities, including ambulatory surgery centers and office-based surgery facilities, and at each phase of the medication use process.[30]

Errors may be more likely to occur when medication products and dosing strengths are available without pharmacist review. Collaboration between pharmacists and members of the perioperative team to determine special considerations for medications (eg, temperature ranges for medication storage, disposal of medications) or patient conditions (eg, medication reconciliation, allergies, weight-based dosing, side effect management) decreases the opportunity for medication errors.

Recommendation II

Medications, chemicals, reagents, and related supplies should be procured and stored in a manner that facilitates safe and efficient delivery to the patient.

Medication errors have been traced back to procurement, the first phase of the medication use process.[1] Risk for errors at this phase can be reduced by making proactive decisions about unit-of-use versus multidose containers, shelf life, and the general supply chain (ie, medication availability, delivery, and protection during transit from the wholesaler to the end user).[4]

II.a. The health care organization's medication management plan should incorporate considerations for procurement including, but not limited to,
- obtaining medications from manufacturers or suppliers with established quality programs; [Amb]
- developing procedures for current or potential product shortages, discontinuations, and recalls;
- implementing procedures for verifying accuracy of medications upon receipt; and
- implementing processes that promote accurate medication stocking and restocking.

Medication manufacturers and suppliers that define target product profiles relating to quality, safety, and efficacy (eg, dosage form, bioavailability, strength, stability) and identify critical quality attributes are more likely to provide timely notification of recalls or shortages.[31] An investigation of a multi-state outbreak of *Serratia marcescens* related to contaminated prefilled syringes revealed poor compliance with Food and Drug Administration (FDA) Good Manufacturing Practices and quality system regulations.[32] The same investigation also revealed that National Drug Codes are the most reliable method for identifying potentially contaminated syringes because some had gone through three distribution steps before reaching the end user and others bore the name of a subsidiary company to the original manufacturer.[32]

Errors at the procurement phase have been reported when medications that are received are not verified with what was ordered before they are stocked. The Pennsylvania Patient Safety Authority reports two circumstances involving errors in stocking 1,000 mL bags of IV solutions. One involved 1,000 mL of sterile water for injection that was mistakenly dispensed and stored on a dialysis unit instead of 0.9% saline solution. The other involved a wholesaler who mistakenly delivered 1,000 mL of sterile water for injection instead of 5% dextrose solution.[33]

II.a.1. Medications in perioperative storage areas should be rotated based on the expiration date indicated on the medication label.

Medication storage areas that are organized to avoid outdated items helps to reduce the risk of administering expired medications to patients. Medications that are stored on emergency or special procedure carts may not be used frequently and have increased risk of becoming outdated before they are used. Rotating low volume medications back through a central or regional pharmacy or through vendor agreements may save money in spite of potential restocking fees and also reduces potential environmental pharmaceutical waste.

II.a.2. Processes should be implemented when stocked medications are not available because of shortages, discontinuations, or recalls. Processes should include, but not be limited to,
- removing recalled items from storage and returning them to the appropriate location,
- procuring substitutions, and
- communicating to licensed independent practitioners and staff members who participate in medication management.

Removing and substituting medications that are recalled or discontinued for safety reasons by the manufacturer decreases the risk of administering an unsafe medication. Communication about shortages, discontinuations, or recalls decreases the risk of prescribing, dispensing, or administering a recalled or discontinued medication.[5,10]

II.a.3. Medications should be delivered and placed in storage areas (eg, automated dispensing storage systems, refrigerated areas, anesthesia carts, emergency carts), and unused medications should be returned to a specific secured return storage area according to established policy.

Inaccurate placement of medications may occur during restocking, which increases the risk of error when the next person retrieves an item from the medication storage area.[21]

II.a.4. Standardized processes should be implemented for timely replacement of used emergency medications or supplies.

Availability of fully stocked emergency and specialty carts promotes safe patient care.

II.a.5. Emergency medications for all populations served should be readily available (eg, separate emergency carts for adults and pediatric patients).

II.b. The health care organization's medication management plan should incorporate safety practices to reduce opportunities for product-related or equipment-related medication errors.

II.b.1. Health care organizations should periodically review a list of look-alike, sound-alike medications prepared by national medication safety organizations[34] and compare the list with medication inventory to determine action plans relating to procurement and storage.

The FDA name differentiation project focuses on the appearance of manufacturer's medication labels to minimize medication errors resulting from look-alike confusion. In 2001, the FDA sent 142 letters to manufacturers encouraging them to revise their medication labels by using "tall man" letters to visually differentiate product names.[35] Periodically reviewing look-alike medications increases awareness of updated data regarding tall-man lettering and other strategies for reducing errors with look-alike medications and provides the opportunity to incorporate new strategies into the procurement and storage section of the medication management plan.[36]

II.b.2. Safety practices should be implemented including, but not limited to,
- obtaining equipment with Luer connectors that are not compatible with other connectors on other devices,
- ensuring that appropriate supplies and equipment are in place to avoid creative work-arounds, and
- standardizing medication delivery equipment (eg, infusion pumps).

Multiple reports show that patient injuries have been caused by interchangeable Luer connectors that allow different equipment to be incorrectly connected because female and male Luer connections match.[37,38] Examples of reported errors include blood pressure monitors being connected to needleless IV ports and oxygen tubing being connected to needleless IV ports. Other reported errors include enteral misconnections where an enteral feeding system has been inadvertently connected to an IV line, peritoneal catheter, tracheostomy tube cuff, or medical gas tubing.[39] Small bore connectors, such as Luer locks or Luer tips, are examples of systems that do not have a design feature that prevents inadvertent connection and, therefore, carry a high risk for patient injury.[40,41] Until equipment design solutions are available from manufacturers, it is necessary to implement administrative controls to prevent tubing misconnections.[37]

II.c. Medications should be stored according to manufacturer's medication storage requirements.

Medications may have sensitive structures that require storage at specific temperature ranges to ensure stability or avoid inactivation.[31] Manufacturers are required to provide supporting stability data for products that are sensitive to external conditions that can affect the product's potency, purity, and quality.[42] Product information should include the manufacturer's directions about temperature requirements for shipping and storage. Failure to control the temperature of medication storage areas may result in decreased therapeutic levels caused by inactivation, a change in pH, a change in concentration, or spoilage.

II.c.1. Temperature-sensitive medications should be stored within the required temperature range.[10,11]

II.c.2. Medications that require refrigeration should be stored in a segregated area with restricted access.[43]

Segregating medications facilitates routine inspection to assess and document compliance with environmental requirements and any storage conditions that may have fostered medication deterioration.[10,11,43] Restricted access reduces the risk of diversion and tampering.

II.d. Health care organizations and personnel must comply with federal laws to register with the Drug Enforcement Agency and follow the agency's regulations related to security and documentation of controlled (ie, Schedule II to IV) substances.[44,45]

II.d.1. To prevent incidences of drug diversion, only authorized personnel should have access to medications, including controlled substances, and medication supplies.[43,44]

II.d.2. All medications and related supplies should be securely stored in areas with limited access, including refrigerated areas, anesthesia carts, and emergency carts.[43]

II.e. Automated dispensing storage systems should be considered as a strategy for inventory management to restrict and document access to medications.

MEDICATION SAFETY

Contributing factors in medication errors include busy, chaotic work environments.[46,47] Automated dispensing storage systems are designed to manage medication inventory.[21] Automated dispensing storage systems can be beneficial for controlling and providing automated documentation of who has accessed medications in the storage device and when the medications were restocked.[21,44,48]

II.f. Medications should be stored in a standardized manner throughout all perioperative areas.

Standardizing placement of medications in the supply area is an effective strategy for reducing medication errors.[18] In ambulatory surgery or office-based settings, the development of a drug formulary that contains a complete list of medications approved for administration in the setting can serve as a foundation for the standardized storage system.[49] Standardized medication areas throughout perioperative areas facilitates the development of a uniform unit-based drug library that can identify medication alerts and provide clinical and decision support.[21,50]

Whether the standardization approach to medication storage is a manual inventory control system or involves automated dispensing storage systems, the consistency between units within the perioperative area will provide perioperative personnel with more familiarity in the way in which medications are stored and their location in the medication storage area, emergency carts, specialty carts, or anesthesia carts to help reduce human factor errors (eg, retrieving the wrong product).

Standardization of medication storage is not a stand-alone strategy to replace risk-reduction practices at the administration end of the medication use process. In spite of standardization through automated dispensing storage systems, there have been reports of errors such as a nurse retrieving phenylephrine from an adjacent compartment when the intent was to obtain an antiemetic agent. The wrong medication was administered and caused the patient to spend additional time in the postanesthesia care unit (PACU) to manage the effects of the phenylephrine.[18]

II.f.1. Nursing and pharmacy personnel should collaborate to establish, monitor, and periodically review medications that are routinely stocked at par level in various bins or drawers in all medication storage areas (eg, automated dispensing storage systems, refrigerated areas, anesthesia carts, emergency carts).

Collaboration between nursing and pharmacy personnel may help to identify changes in storage that will reduce errors related to the wrong medication being retrieved for the procedure case cart. When perioperative RNs and surgical technologists implement the medication orders as specified on surgeon preference cards, they may identify areas of potential confusion and have recommendations for standardizing units of use and concentrations. Sharing information with pharmacists that will contribute to changes relating to procurement and storage is one way that front-line practitioners can help to ensure the safe delivery of medications to patients.[1]

II.f.2. Medications in the storage area should be organized using safety considerations including, but not limited to,
- separating medications by generic name and packaging;
- separating look-alike, sound-alike medications;
- separating high-alert medications;
- providing separate bins or dividers for all medications in storage;
- labeling storage bins, using enhanced lettering when possible, with both the medication's generic and brand names;
- positioning medication containers so that their labels are visible; and
- avoiding alphabetical storage.[35,51-57]

More than 1,400 medications (ie, 57% brand or proprietary names, 43% generic names) have been involved in look-alike, sound-alike medication errors. Almost 800 medications have been identified as a distinct pair, meaning look-alike, sound-alike errors were associated with only one other product. More than 600 medications were paired with two or more distinct medications.[46] Even though the largest percentage of look-alike, sound-alike medication errors originated in the dispensing phase of the medication use process,[46] obtaining the wrong medication from a storage area has resulted in patient injury or death.[46] Anticipating a look-alike, sound-alike medication error and adjusting the organization of the medication storage area accordingly is an effective medication error risk-reduction strategy.

II.f.3. Medications and related supplies stored on anesthesia carts should be standardized within perioperative areas and, if possible, in the community when anesthesia professionals rotate between multiple health care organizations. Medications should be organized according to order of use, frequency of use, similarity of action, severity of harm from misuse, and lack of similar appearance.[58]

The Anesthesia Patient Safety Foundation identified standardization within all anesthesia workstations in an institution as a risk-reduction strategy for medication errors related to anesthesia medication administration.[25] When anesthesia professionals rotate from one facility to another within the community, standardized anesthesia carts provide consistency and may reduce human factor errors. Studies of human error show that many errors involve deviation from routine practice. Standardization of equipment and problems with medication stock control, including delivery to and from storage, were among the unsafe acts described in a classic paper about the nature and likelihood of anesthesia errors.[59] A case report described an incident of unexplained apnea during surgery caused by a mix-up with cefazolin and vecuronium located in adjacent compartments in the anesthesia drawer.[60]

II.f.4. Medications and related supplies stored in emergency and specialty carts in perioperative areas should be standardized and be available in unit-dose, age-specific, and ready-to-use forms.

Consistency between emergency carts will facilitate efficiency in the medication use process and reduce the risk of error. Studies of human error show that many errors involve deviation from routine practice.[59]

II.g. Medications should be procured in limited varieties of concentrations and dosages and standardized in all perioperative medication storage areas.

Standardizing medication concentrations and dosing is a strategy that can be implemented to ensure that excessive amounts of medication are not available. This creates a forcing function intended to promote patient safety. Safety principles include restricting access to high concentrations of heparin (eg, 10,000 units per mL). Another example may be to have morphine routinely available in doses smaller than 10 mg/mL (eg, 2 mg or 4 mg), which would still allow for dose titration.[18]

Epinephrine in concentrations of 1:1,000 is a high-alert medication that has been reported to cause harm when it is not diluted.[61] Warning labels may help to reduce confusion when a high-alert medication requires dilution, but it may be more effective to store the vials in the pharmacy to reduce the risk of error.[61] *Amb*

Toxic dose calculations for pediatric and adult dosages can be clarified more easily when there is a standardization and limited number of medications in the storage area.[62] Drug libraries for infusion pumps serve as a resource for toxic dose calculations but cannot be established without standardizing the medications on hand.[50]

II.g.1. Concentrated electrolytes including, but not limited to, sodium chloride solutions more concentrated than 0.9%, potassium chloride, and potassium phosphate should be ordered from the pharmacy when needed rather than stored at the unit level or in ambulatory surgery centers.[63]

Mortality has been reported as a result of concentrated electrolytes being mistakenly administered too rapidly and without proper dilution.[63] A neonate died as a result of a nurse mistakenly removing a vial of concentrated (23.4%) sodium chloride from the unit medication storage area and administering the solution intravenously, instead of administering normal saline (0.9% sodium chloride) flush.[63]

II.h. Perioperative RNs should collaborate with pharmacists to procure and store single-dose vials rather than multidose vials.

Multidose vials of medication contain a preservative to help prevent bacterial growth, single-use vials do not.[64] There may be viral contamination of multidose vials because the preservative may be effective only for inhibiting bacterial growth.[65] With some multidose vials, the preservative may not become entirely effective until two hours after it has been opened, which leaves the possibility of the presence of bacterial organisms in the meantime.[66]

Nurses can provide practical insight by investigating ways to decrease the use of multidose vials.[67] The rationale for stocking multidose vials may be related to cost savings or because there is a short supply of the medication available on the market. When medications are supplied in quantities that exceed the amount typically given, health care workers may be at risk of misinterpreting the amount in the vial, or may use the vial for more than one patient in an effort to avoid waste.[66]

Primary safety concerns related to the use of multidose vials include, but are not limited to, potential
- cross contamination from one patient to another,[65]
- risk of administering too much medication,
- confusion in labeling and expiration dates with open vials, and
- issues of proper disposal of unused pharmaceuticals and inconsistent documentation of waste.[68-71]

II.h.1. Medications labeled as single-use vials that are found opened should not be used and should be discarded.

II.h.2. Opened multidose medication containers must be dated to indicate expiration within 28 days of opening and should be discarded immediately upon expiration.[30] When a product has been opened or a vial cap has been punctured or removed, the manufacturer's expiration date is no longer valid and should be replaced with a new date.

MEDICATION SAFETY

The Centers for Medicare & Medicaid Services requires that over-the-counter medications, including cough and pediatric elixirs, be disposed of within 28 days of breaking the label regardless of manufacturer's printed expiration date on the multidose container.[30]

The manufacturer's labeled expiration date represents the beyond-use date for a product that has not been opened. The effectiveness of the bacteriostatic agent used in the multidose vial is only tested by the manufacturer of the product for a period of 28 days. There is increased risk for bacterial growth the longer the seal is broken and a container is open.

II.h.3. Multidose medications used for more than one patient should not be stored in the immediate area where direct patient contact occurs and should be separated from single-dose vials in the storage area.[30]

There is an increased risk for a dosage medication error if multidose medications are stored in the same area as single-dose vials. Expiration dates on multidose medications that are opened are likely to be shorter than the single-dose vials, which increases the risk that an expired medication could be administered. Separating opened multidose vials in the storage area facilitates checking for outdated stock.

II.i. Nonmedication solutions and chemicals should not be stored in medication storage areas.

Storing bleach, formaldehyde, cleaning products, and other chemicals in areas where medications are stored may increase the risk of mistaking the solution as a medication.

II.i.1. Chemicals and reagents (eg, formalin, Lugol's solution, radiopaque dyes, glutaraldehyde) should be procured and stored with the same care and caution as medications.

Nonmedication solutions may be packaged in containers that look similar and can be confused with medications or confused with each other. One incident of acetone being mistaken for an ingestible solution has been published.[72] Other examples of confusion have occurred with hydrogen peroxide/denatured ethyl alcohol and hydrogen peroxide/ethanol. Both solutions have been reported to be mistaken for eye drops because the containers are similar in size and shape.[63]

II.i.2. Chemicals and reagents should be stored in their original containers with the original labels.

Errors resulting in patient injury have been reported as a consequence of chemicals being stored in unlabeled containers.[73]

II.i.3. Potential hazards associated with medical gases in the practice setting should be identified, and safe practices should be established. Medical gases should be stored separately from industrial gases in a secure area with controlled access.[74]

The FDA considers compressed medical gases to be prescription drugs that can only be dispensed by prescription.[75] According to FDA reports, medical gas mix-ups have resulted in at least seven deaths and 15 serious injuries.[74,76]

Recommendation III

Prescribing personnel should provide clear, unambiguous, and accurate medication orders.

Medication errors can occur at the point of prescribing.[4,18] In perioperative settings, surgeons, anesthesia professionals, and advanced practice nurses are examples of prescribers who are licensed to write orders, give verbal orders, or verify standing orders. Having three distinct prescribing processes rather than one contributes to the complexity of the prescription process in perioperative areas. Complex processes open more opportunities for errors related to increased variables and breakdowns in communication.[9,77]

III.a. Prescribers should have access to all pertinent patient data and reference material.

Medication errors have occurred because prescribers have insufficient patient data (eg, allergy information, current medications) or medication information (eg, indications for special populations, laboratory parameters).[51,78-82] Not having access to patient information has led to errors across the perioperative continuum, with a larger percentage of prescribing errors occurring in the outpatient setting.[4] Researchers of one study reported that higher rates of prescribing errors occurred with less frequently prescribed analgesics, new medications when they are first introduced to the organization, and older medications that are used in new or uncommon ways.[79]

Preference cards are not directly linked to patient data, but rather are related to systems level data (eg, type of procedure). This can increase the risk for error when patient information is not integrated into the care plan on the day of surgery.

III.b. Prescribers should incorporate the Beers criteria or other tools for identifying potentially inappropriate medication use for special populations.

The Beers criteria identify appropriate medications for adult patients who are older than 65 years of age and calls to attention medications that are inappropriate because of the heightened risk for adverse outcomes.[83] Application of the Beers criteria and other tools enables prescribers to carefully weigh the benefits against the

MEDICATION SAFETY

risks of using such medications.[83,84] Prescribing approaches that apply to younger adult patients and guidelines for patients with specific chronic disorders may not be effective or safe for frail, elderly patients.[85] Older patients, patients with multiple health conditions, and pediatric patients often are excluded from evidence-generating, randomized, controlled trials.[85-87] A study of the frequency of off-label prescribing to children showed that the majority of pediatric outpatient visits involve off-label prescribing. The researchers concluded that up-to-date tools for pediatric prescribing information should be included as a priority for medication safety.[86]

III.c. Medication orders that appear in preprinted forms, standing orders, and preference cards should be reviewed annually by perioperative team members including perioperative RNs, prescribers, and pharmacists.

Medications listed on preference cards are not considered to be standing orders unless they have been reviewed and signed by the prescriber. Annually reviewing medication orders allows prescribers and pharmacists to collaborate with other members of the perioperative team to confirm or update all forms and documents associated with perioperative care.[4,88-90]

III.c.1. Evidence of the review should be documented on the preprinted forms, standing orders, and preference cards, as should the adoption date and subsequent revision dates.

III.c.2. Standing orders should be reviewed and approved by the prescriber when they are created and whenever changes are made.

Researchers of one study reported that changes made to preference cards by perioperative nurses are not always verified and approved by the prescriber. In addition, researchers found that medication orders on preference cards were outdated or missing information, or were not what the surgeon intended to use.[91]

III.d. Verbal medication orders should be limited,[92] especially with medications identified as high risk for sound-alike errors or for having commonly confused names.[93]

Verbal orders can be misinterpreted for a number of reasons including, but not limited to, regional dialects, background noise, muffled voices behind surgical masks, and orders involving sound-alike or commonly confused medication names.[4,94,95] Verbal orders have been the source of medication errors.[4,94] In one study aimed at understanding the content and context of verbal orders, researchers reported that 80% of the verbal orders given by physicians and received by nurses included medication-related orders. Further examination revealed that 20% of the orders that matched medications listed on the ISMP's list of commonly confused medications were verbal orders involving fentanyl, furosemide, lidocaine 1% injection, midazolam, or dextrose 50% syringe. Of the medication orders that involved high-alert medications, 20% were verbal orders involving narcotic medicines, sedating agents, anticoagulants, and low-molecular-weight heparin. The risk of verbal orders may be further compounded because commonly confused medications and high-alert medications are often involved.[95]

III.d.1. When verbal orders are necessary, they should be received and carried out only by persons who are authorized to do so and consistent with federal and state law and the health care organization policy and procedures.[92]

Medication use is included in the professional licensing process. State regulations identify the scope of practice for unlicensed personnel related to participation in medication administration.

III.d.2. Perioperative RNs should confirm verbal medication orders by reading back the order to the prescriber digit by digit and spelling out the medication name, if necessary.

Verification of critical components of perioperative verbal orders, before the implementation of the order, affords an opportunity to confirm the accuracy of the verbal order.[5,77,94,96]

III.d.3. Perioperative RNs should immediately record verbal medication orders in the patient's record.

Immediate documentation of verbal orders in the patient's record increases accuracy and allows the recipient of the order to read it back to the prescriber for confirmation.

III.d.4. Prescribers should review, validate, and sign the transcribed verbal medication order on the patient's record as close as possible to the time of the medication administration.

Verifying the accuracy of the documented verbal order allows for confirmation that the intended medication order matches what is administered to the patient.[96] Verifying the verbal order as close as possible to the time the medication is administered allows timely corrective action to be taken if a medication error is discovered.

III.e. When available, prescribers should use CPOE systems.

Computerized-provider order entry systems, especially those with clinical rule-based decision support aids, have reduced opportunity for errors.[97,98] Between April and August 2008, researchers used a simulation tool to assess 62 hospitals, representing about 8% of US hospitals

MEDICATION SAFETY

with CPOE systems, and found wide variation in the type of decision support aids used to provide alerts and advice for medication orders that have a high risk of resulting in harm to patients. This study showed that the hospitals had higher scores for basic clinical decision support, and the most reliably detected adverse drug event was a drug-to-allergy contraindication. This study also showed that drug-to-diagnosis contraindications, including pregnancy, were only detected 15% of the time, leading the researchers to emphasize the importance of pharmacy and nursing review processes to intercept medication errors until advanced clinical decision support tools can be integrated into CPOE systems.[80]

Providers who use CPOE systems support pay-for-performance initiatives and quality outcomes that are clinically driven.[4] Computerized provider order entry systems allow for an electronic record of medication administration and decrease the risk for misinterpretation of medication orders from illegible handwriting or misunderstood verbal orders.[99] When studying the characteristics of verbal orders at a tertiary children's hospital, researchers found that CPOE system implementation reduced verbal orders and unsigned verbal orders.[100]

III.e.1. Computerized-provider order entry systems should be designed with prescriber input and evaluated continually for effectiveness.

The authors of one systematic review noted that continual evaluation of the CPOE system is necessary to study the interfaces of CPOE systems with the normal flow of actions in the prescribing processes and other subtle design features (eg, inconvenient logging procedures may encourage physicians to order medications at computer terminals not yet "logged out" by other physicians if the log-out time is slow).[101] Authors of another systematic review noted the substantial difference in how studies on CPOE systems are conducted in terms of setting, design, quality, and definition of the measured outcome variable and noted that electronic prescribing systems could increase the number of medication errors if the system is not designed and implemented appropriately.[102]

Recommendation IV

Safe medication order transcribing processes should be implemented.

Transcribing is the point in the medication use process that involves anything related to the act of recording or transferring an order by someone other than the prescriber for order processing.[1] When inaccuracies occur during the transcribing process, there is a risk for medication error (eg, medication given to the wrong patient) at the administering phase of the medication use process or omission errors may occur (eg, medication is not transcribed, so the patient misses the dose that was ordered).[4]

IV.a. Perioperative RNs should be alert to potential transcribing errors throughout each phase of perioperative care.

Medication errors attributed to the transcribing phase are reported to occur less frequently than other phases in the medication use process.[4] However, case studies and data analysis reports reflect errors in perioperative settings. Examples include an outpatient setting where a staff nurse incorrectly stamped the wrong patient name on a hand-written medication order, resulting in the wrong patient receiving a medication[4]; an omission error in the PACU where a patient did not receive a calcium replacement because postoperative orders were not transcribed[4]; and an error with transcription during the medication reconciliation process that resulted in an overdose of blood pressure medication being administered, resulting in the patient developing asystole while in the OR.[103]

Recommendation V

Pharmacists should be actively involved in dispensing aspects of perioperative medication use across all perioperative settings.

Dispensing is the fourth phase of the medication use process. This phase begins with a pharmacist's assessment of a medication order and continues to the point of release of the product for use by another health care professional.[1] When pharmacists identify prescribing errors at the dispensing phase of the medication use process, it reduces the risk of errors at the administration phase of the medication use process.

Regulatory agencies, accreditation, and standards-setting organizations recommend pharmacy oversight of the medication management practices.[5,30]

V.a. Pharmacists should review medication orders before administration. In perioperative settings, this review should include standing orders (eg, preference cards). *Amb*

Pharmacists are trained to detect errors, contraindications of medications, and drug-drug interactions.[4,5] When a pharmacist reviews medication orders, it increases the potential of identifying errors in prescribing early in the medication use process.[5]

V.b. The health care organization should comply with local, state, and federal regulations for pharmacy resources and ensure solutions are prepared according to national standard specified in *The United States Pharmacopeia,* Chapter <797>.[104]

The Centers for Medicare & Medicaid Services regulations specify that hospitals must have pharmaceutical services that meet the needs of patients and that all compounding, packaging, and dispensing of medications must be under the supervision of a pharmacist and performed consistently with state and federal laws.[105] The regulation does not require a pharmacist to be on site unless an ambulatory surgery center is in a state that has passed a law that requires a licensed pharmacist to provide oversight or consultation for pharmaceutical services.[30] The federal regulations for ambulatory surgery centers state that a designated licensed health care professional must be "routinely present during regular business hours."[30] *Amb*

The United States Pharmacopeia, Chapter <797>, addresses sterile parental products.[104] Sterile preparations reduce microbial contamination.[106] When perioperative nurses are mixing, diluting, or compounding medications, they bypass the dispensing function of the pharmacy oversight that is intended to ensure the correct ingredient identity, purity, strength, and sterility in addition to accurate labeling on the appropriate type of container.[106,107]

V.c. Perioperative administrators should investigate the feasibility of implementing a decentralized perioperative pharmacy located within the perioperative suite.[4]

Decentralized (eg, satellite) pharmacies provide support to perioperative staff members with mixing, diluting, and compounding medications to ensure compliance with the specific national standard that pertains to sterility of parenteral products.[25,107]

V.d. Pharmacists should provide oversight of automated dispensing storage system processes.

Automated dispensing storage systems are an extension of the pharmacy department; therefore, these systems fall under their jurisdiction.[106] The safe use of automated dispensing storage systems is dependent on cooperation between nursing and pharmacy personnel.[21] Automated dispensing storage systems are complex and have design and function variations that require specific maintenance and education. When these systems are not used appropriately, there can be a compromise in patient safety.[106]

Recommendation VI

The perioperative RN should assess the patient and review the patient's record to confirm the patient's metric weight, medication history, and current medication orders before administering medications.

Medication administration is the fifth phase of the medication use process.[1] This phase begins with nursing assessment and continues through planning and intervention. Coupling the medication use process with the nursing process allows risk-reduction strategies to be identified at each step of each process across all phases of perioperative care. Thorough nursing assessment and patient record review is the foundation for planning and implementing the nursing medication plan.[108]

VI.a. The perioperative RN should confirm that the patient's weight is documented accurately in both pounds and kilograms in the patient's record.

Many medication dosages are calculated according to a patient's weight. There is an increased risk for dosage medication error when the patient's weight is not documented or is inaccurately documented, or when the health care worker estimates the patient's weight.[109] According to the Pennsylvania Patient Safety Authority Advisory, 479 medication error events between June 2004 and November 2008 were associated with inaccurate patient weights with approximately 65% of those reported resulting in an over- or under-dose of the medication ordered.[110,111]

VI.a.1. Electronic or paper patient record forms should be designed to clearly reflect weight in both metric (eg, kilograms) and English (eg, pounds) measurements.

VI.b. The perioperative RN should collaborate with personnel in other disciplines and participate in medication reconciliation activities.

Medication reconciliation is a strategy to promote safe patient outcomes by facilitating patient-centered care, providing insight into preexisting disease processes, reducing opportunities for errors, and detecting duplicate therapies.[3,17,112-114] Medication errors related to transcribing and prescribing may be prevented through the medication reconciliation process.[81,115]

Identifying home medication bottles accurately and collaborating with pharmacists to review home medications may help to identify transcribing errors. In a case report analysis where 75 mg of metoprolol was mistakenly identified as a daily dose on the patient's list of home medications, the author identified the pharmacist as the one more likely to point out that metoprolol is only available in 25-mg or 50-mg tablets.[103] The patient received a fourfold overdose of the medication when the dose was increased from 75 mg to 100 mg. The prescriber's intent was to increase the home dose by 25 mg, but because of a transcribing error, he did not realize that the home dose was 25 mg per day as opposed to 75 mg per day.[103]

VI.b.1. The perioperative RN should actively involve the patient or authorized representative in obtaining a complete list of the patient's current medications, including dietary supplements and over-the-counter products as well as dosages and allergies to the same.[17,103,116]

Researchers from one study in an ambulatory setting found that the accuracy of

MEDICATION SAFETY

medication lists improved from 23.1% to 37.7% when perioperative staff members called patients the day before their appointments and reminded them to bring their original medication containers or an updated list of medications for their appointment.[117]

VI.b.2. When compiling information from the medication history during the preoperative assessment, the perioperative RN should collaborate with pharmacy personnel to investigate medications identified by the patient that have no corresponding disease or condition in the patient's record.

Researchers who conducted one study found that medication-condition matching may decrease unnecessary medication use in older adult populations and allow prescribers to make more educated decisions about continuing or discontinuing home medications at the time of patient discharge.[118] In another study, researchers found that it may be useful to identify patients ahead of time who have a higher risk of medication reconciliation errors so that proactive arrangements can be made for pharmacy personnel involvement during transitions in patient care (eg, medication histories upon admission, medication counseling at discharge).[114]

VI.b.3. The perioperative RN should confirm with the patient routes of administration for every product identified during the medication reconciliation process. When they are providing their medication history, patients should be reminded to include all medications they are taking, not just oral medications, injections, or those taken regularly, but also those only taken PRN.

Reports indicate patient injury has resulted from fentanyl and nitroglycerin skin patches when they are not removed before clinical interventions.[119,120] Transdermal patches may contain aluminum or other metals that can overheat during a magnetic resonance imaging (MRI) scan and cause skin burns in the immediate area of the patch.[121]

VI.b.4. Perioperative RNs should use a standardized, multidisciplinary medication reconciliation format that is readily available for review at every transition of patient information.[114,122]

A retrospective chart review revealed that the most accurate method of obtaining complete medication lists at the time of hospital admission is a combination of techniques including compiling a list of medication names and strengths from admission patient interviews as well as from a pharmacy claims database.[123]

VI.c. In the preoperative phase of care, the perioperative RN should confirm that medications and herbal supplements were taken as prescribed or discontinued on the day of surgery or the designated number of days before surgery as per physician orders.

Pharmacokinetic information is not available for most herbs and, therefore, it is not known how long it takes for most herbal products to be cleared from the body. Patients are often instructed to discontinue herbal products five to seven days before surgery.[124] Herbs that are known to affect clotting include bromelain, cayenne pepper, chamomile, cinchona bark, dong quai, fenugreek, feverfew, garlic, ginger, ginkgo, ginseng, guggul, horse chestnut, vitamin E (ie, more than 1,200 IU), and willow bark.[124] Fish oil, glucosamine, flax seed, saw palmetto, chondroitin, mild thistle, and green tea are other examples of natural products that may need to be discontinued two to three weeks before surgery, but the guidelines for discontinuation are not well defined.[125] Researchers report that aspirin may not need to be stopped before surgical or invasive procedures unless the risk of bleeding exceeds the thrombotic risk from withholding the medication.[126]

VI.d. Medication allergy and reaction information should be obtained from patients, family members, legal guardians, and/or previous medical records and should be documented clearly in the patients' records.

In a two-year period, researchers reported 35 incidents in a surgical setting involving medications that were prescribed for or administered to elective surgery patients who had a previous allergy to that medication or a related medication.[127] The Pennsylvania Patient Safety Authority identified documenting allergies and the reaction that a patient experiences to the medication upon admission to a health care facility as an important risk-reduction strategy.[128]

Recommendation VII

Across all phases of care and in all perioperative settings, the perioperative RN should develop a nursing medication plan.

The administering phase of the medication use process requires perioperative RNs to use their knowledge of pharmacology and the patient's condition to establish an individualized medication plan before obtaining or giving medications to the patient.[107,129]

VII.a. The nursing medication plan should include, but not be limited to,
- incorporating findings from the medication history and medication reconciliation process,
- verifying medication orders associated with the patient's planned surgical or other invasive procedure, and

MEDICATION SAFETY

- collaborating with other professionals to resolve discrepancies.

Interpreting and comparing the findings from the medication reconciliation with medication plans outlined for the scheduled surgical or invasive procedure allows communication and revisions to the plan early in the patient's encounter if revisions to the plan are determined to be necessary.[129] Verifying medication orders and seeking pharmacy consultation to confirm contraindications, drug-drug interactions, or specific medication information for special populations are examples of action items in the medication planning stage of the nursing process. Collaborating with other professionals to resolve discrepancies and clarify medication orders is a risk-reduction strategy for establishing an individualized medication care plan that produces maximum benefit from the medications and minimizes harm.[108,129]

VII.a.1. The perioperative RN should contact the prescriber when clarification is needed for medication orders, including medications specified on surgeon preference cards as standing or preprinted orders.

VII.a.2. The perioperative RN should collaborate with the pharmacist when it is necessary to obtain unique medications that are not in the standardized department inventory.

VII.b. The nursing medication plan should include verifying high-risk medications and toxic dosage ranges for products with a narrow therapeutic range, especially in pediatric patients, older adults, and patients who are pregnant, to decrease the risk for adverse effects.

Reports indicate a higher frequency of medication errors or more harm resulting from medication errors for pediatric patients and older adults.[4,83,130,131] Patients who are pregnant are at risk for potentially narrow therapeutic ranges and teratogenic medications.[132]

VII.b.1. Perioperative team members should not be interrupted when verifying an independent dose confirmation of high-alert medications or medications intended for pediatric use.

High-alert medications have a higher risk of causing harm when an error occurs.[13] Most medications administered to pediatric patients have a narrow therapeutic range.[130] Medication calculation errors are five times more likely to occur with pediatric patients.[4,130]

Distractions are a contributing factor in all phases of perioperative care.[4] The presence of interruptions and the frequency of interruptions have been found to be a contributing factor to medication errors,[133] with more interruptions resulting in a greater severity of error.[47] Environments that promote safe medication use are described as locations where the potential for distraction or interruption can be minimized.[134]

VII.b.2. Perioperative team members should use specific weight-based conversion charts or other technological devices for each of the major error-prone medications identified for the population at risk.

VII.b.3. When possible, pharmacists should be consulted to oversee calculations.

Recommendation VIII

The perioperative RN should implement the medication care plan by using safe medication practices to obtain, verify, prepare, and administer medications throughout all phases of perioperative care and in all perioperative settings.

Failure to follow current medication safety practices can lead to adverse effects.[4,9] Medication administration is performed at the intervention level of the nursing process. Medication administration is the point where the medication interfaces with the patient.[1] This phase is the point in the medication use process that represents the last opportunity to detect an error to avoid potential harm to the patient.

VIII.a. The perioperative RN should retrieve medications for only one patient at a time from storage bins or automated dispensing storage systems.

Retrieving medications for more than one patient at a time increases the risk for error.[135] Medication administration errors have occurred because a perioperative nurse retrieved the wrong product from an automated dispensing system.[18] If a restocking error has occurred, it is more likely to be caught if the nurse is focused on each medication required for the individual patient at the time the medication is being retrieved.

VIII.b. The perioperative RN should verify all medications retrieved against the original medication order or preference card.

The original medication order, including preprinted order forms, prescriptions, or preference cards, establishes what medication the prescriber intended to be given to the patient.

Automated dispensing storage systems have been reported to have up to a 5% misfill rate.[4] As medications are obtained, an additional visual confirmation of the order and product will help establish accuracy in administering the correct medication.

VIII.c. Perioperative personnel who administer medications should not be interrupted or distracted when preparing and administering medications.

Distractions are the second most common reason for error in the medication use process.[4] Distraction may cause a person to forget to perform a key task and thus may contribute to a chain of events that results in error.[1,130,133,136-138]

303

MEDICATION SAFETY

VIII.d. When preparing medications for administration, the perioperative RN should use safety devices (eg, infusion pumps, filtered needles, sterile transfer devices).

VIII.e. Medications should be prepared as close as possible to the time of use. *Amb*

Medications prepared ahead of time may have an increased risk for contamination and increase the risk for being administered to the wrong patient.[70] A root cause analysis revealed that having a medication available before it was needed contributed to a fatal mix-up. Because it was available early, medication for epidural pain management was administered intravenously instead of the intended antibiotic solution.[139]

VIII.e.1. Intravenous solution containers should be punctured as close as possible to time of use. Opened and unused medication vials, solution bags, bottles, syringes, and compounded sterile preparations should be discarded within one hour of opening.[104]

The Association for Professionals in Infection Control and Epidemiology (APIC) recommends that spiked IV solutions be used within one hour of being prepared.[70] According to the US Pharmacopeia, opened or needle-punctured single-dose containers are to be used within one hour if they are not opened in a protected environment that is designed for preparation of sterile medications.[104]

VIII.e.2. If a pharmacist is not available to prepare a compounded sterile preparation in the perioperative area, sterile medication preparation should include, but not be limited to, the following guidelines:
- Perioperative personnel who have adequate training and licensure should prepare sterile solutions (eg, eye blocks) for one patient at a time, using aseptic technique, and as close as possible to the time of use.
- The compounded sterile preparation should be labeled with patient identification information, the names and amounts of all ingredients, the name or initials of the person who prepared the preparation, the date of preparation, and the beyond-use date and time.[104]
- When the compounded sterile preparation is completed, it should be continuously observed if not immediately administered.[104]

The United States Pharmacopeia, Chapter <797>, states that prepared solutions require continuous supervision to decrease the risk of mix-ups with other compounded sterile preparations and contamination from contact with nonsterile surfaces or introduction of particulates.[104]

VIII.e.3. Compounded sterile preparations that are not administered within one hour after the start of preparation should be discarded according to local, state, and federal regulations and health care organization policy.[104]

VIII.e.4. Medications should not be pre-drawn up and stored on the anesthesia cart or elsewhere unless the pre-filled syringes are supplied by the manufacturer or pharmacy.

VIII.e.5. Perioperative team members should not prepare medication products in advance and then store them in clothing or pockets.[4,70]

Preparing medications in advance and storing medications in clothing or pockets increases the risk for contamination and errors. At least one medication error resulting in a life-threatening event has been reported involving an anesthesia care professional removing from their pocket and administering a paralytic agent outside of the OR.[4]

VIII.f. Unless the medication is to be administered immediately, all medications removed from the original package and transferred to a secondary container should be clearly marked and easily identifiable. At a minimum, the secondary container should be labeled with the medication and dose in accordance with the health care organization's policy.

Medications that are removed from the original package and not labeled cannot be verified before administration, increasing the risk for administering the wrong medication.

VIII.f.1. Medications that are removed from the original package and found in a secondary container without a label should be discarded.

VIII.g. The use of multidose vials should be avoided. Whenever a multidose vial is used, perioperative personnel who administer medications should use safe practices associated with multidose vials including, but not limited to, the following guidelines:
- The rubber septum on a multidose container that is used for more than one patient should be disinfected with alcohol and allowed to dry before each entry.
- Needleless entry devices should be used whenever possible to withdraw contents from multidose vials.
- A new needle or needleless device and new syringe should be used every time the multidose vial is accessed.
- Needles and syringes should not be reused for multidose containers.
- When medications are needed from more than one multidose container, separate needles and syringes should be used.

Primary concerns related to the use of multidose vials include, but are not limited to, risk of

MEDICATION SAFETY

cross contamination from one patient to another, administering too much medication, improper labeling of expiration dates on opened vials, and improper disposal and documentation of unused pharmaceuticals.[68-71]

Cross contamination has been reported in the use of multidose containers.[70] Failure to follow aseptic technique increases the risk of introducing contamination into the container.[51,65,70,71] Alcohol disinfection helps to decrease the risk of cross contamination when multidose vials are used.[70]

Using the same needle to withdraw medications from two different multidose vials may increase the risk of particulate matter from one medication or rubber septum entering the second multidose container.

VIII.h. Perioperative personnel who administer medications should implement the seven rights of safe medication practices (ie, right patient, right medication, right dose, right time, right route, right indication, right documentation) as a final check before administering the medication to the patient.[140]

The tradition of the five rights of medication safety has been expanded to seven rights to include the right indication and the right documentation. Adhering to the seven rights of safe medication practices is the professional responsibility of the licensed perioperative team member.[1,18]

Practitioners who administer medications are expected to know the right indication for a medication and understand the contraindications for the medication's use. In an appellate court ruling, a hospital was found negligent for its staff members not recognizing contraindications.[1,141] The same court ruling established "right documentation" as an expectation for medication safety.[1,18,141] Missing or incomplete documentation has been associated with medication errors during perioperative care.[4]

A report on medication error findings describes wrong patient, wrong medication product, wrong dose, wrong timing, and wrong route medication errors that have occurred during perioperative care.[4] Wrong dose errors can result from illegible handwriting and incorrect placement of decimal points.[130] Wrong dose errors include either too much (ie, excessive) or too little of the intended medication. The most serious errors that have been reported in the OR include an excessive dose (20-fold extra) of heparin administered during a plastic surgery case, leading to loss of soft tissues, and a tenfold overdose of digoxin administered to an infant, resulting in cardiac toxicity and death.[4] In the outpatient setting, 3.3% of wrong-dose errors resulted in patient harm.[4]

Wrong time errors are defined as medication administration outside of the health care organization's parameters. A reported example involved a mannitol order that was delayed 5.5 hours from the time ordered postoperatively, resulting in increased intracranial pressure.[18]

Wrong route errors are defined as the medication being administered via a route other than intended. Wrong route errors are the second most commonly reported type of harmful medication errors.[4] Tubing misconnections often contribute to wrong route errors and have serious outcomes.[18,142] Examples of wrong route errors include antimicrobial agents intended for parenteral administration (eg, IV piggyback) being connected and infused through epidural or intrathecal catheters, and epidural medication infusions being connected to IV catheters. Other wrong route errors included IV fluids connected to indwelling catheters as bladder irrigants and a harmful case in which an antimicrobial agent delivered via IV piggyback was mistakenly connected to an external ventricular drain.[18] Cases also have been reported where magnesium sulfate was infused through epidural catheters instead of the intended mixture of local anesthetic and narcotic analgesics.[143]

VIII.h.1. Perioperative personnel who administer medications should verify patient identification using at least two patient identifiers before administering medication.

VIII.h.2. Perioperative personnel who administer medications should verify all medications just before administration, giving special consideration (eg, independent double check) to high-alert medications[82,144,145] and products that have been identified as high risk because they sound-alike or look-alike.

VIII.h.3. Perioperative personnel who administer medications should verify the correct dose of the medication before administration. Medication dose verification should include, but not be limited to,
- confirming doses to be administered to vulnerable populations;
- using caution with medications that are available in multiple strengths or concentrations;
- using caution to draw up the proper dose of a medication that is packaged in a multidose container;
- using dosage conversion charts or electronic aids to calculate maximum dose limits, especially for high-alert medications;
- identifying out of range or toxic limits;
- confirming correct standard infusion pump settings; and
- recognizing special circumstances that require checks by two individuals, such as independent verification of high-alert doses and pain-controlled-analgesia

MEDICATION SAFETY

pump settings, or that require independent confirmation of calculations for weight-based medications.

VIII.h.4. Perioperative personnel who administer medications should verify the right medication administration time. Medication timing should include, but not be limited to,
- verifying the timing of antibiotic administration and
- collaborating with members of the perioperative team on what medications have been or are about to be administered.

VIII.h.5. Perioperative personnel who administer medications should administer the medication via the right route. Considerations for the right medication route should include, but not be limited to,
- labeling multiple lines, catheters, and connection ports (eg, spinal, parenteral, drains, indwelling catheters);
- confirming the potential for adverse effects related to medication administration that is not consistent with manufacturer's recommendation (eg, rapid vancomycin infusion)[146]; and
- verifying the integrity of the parenteral site.

VIII.h.6. Perioperative personnel who administer medications should have knowledge about the medication's intent for use and any contraindications. In confirming the right indication, perioperative personnel should identify considerations including, but not limited to,
- abnormal renal and hepatic function,
- off-label use for special populations (eg, pediatric use, pregnancy), and
- triggering agents for patients who are known to be susceptible to malignant hyperthermia.

VIII.h.7. Medications should be documented in the patient record as close as possible to the time they were administered.

VIII.i. Perioperative personnel who administer medications should follow the medication manufacturer's directions for use.

All medication products have an FDA-approved package insert with instructions for dosage and administration. Some medications have specific timing for administration.[146] Medication errors have been reported as a result of failure to follow manufacturer directions for administration.[4]

VIII.j. Perioperative personnel who administer medications should comply with constraints and forcing functions that have been initiated to minimize risks related to medication administration.

Constraints and forcing functions are human factors-proven interventions that reduce risk and are deployed at the sharp end of patient care.[6] Constraints are approaches that make a medication error difficult. Examples include dose limit protocols, automatic stop orders, redundant checks, and labeling all medications that are removed from their original containers. Another example of a constraint would be obtaining medication packaged in the final unit of use (ie, single-dose preparations). When there is extra product in the container, it increases the potential for the practitioner to draw up the entire amount, risking an overdose.

Forcing functions are approaches that reduce the potential for medication errors and are set around processes put into place that minimize opportunity for work-arounds. Examples include removing certain medications (eg, cytotoxic agents, concentrations of saline higher than 0.9%) from the OR. Other examples include medical gas connectors (eg, oxygen versus nitrous) that are not interchangeable and password-protected access to electronic equipment or storage devices.[75]

VIII.k. Perioperative team members should implement known safe practices when identifying conditions related to medication administration that have been associated with adverse effects (eg, multiple tubings, potential confusion with patient names, equipment risks, handling sharps).

Multiple patient injuries have been caused by incorrect tubing connections. Tubing connections errors include
- blood pressure monitors connected to needleless IV ports,
- oxygen tubing connected to needleless IV ports, and
- enteral feeding systems connected to an IV catheter, peritoneal catheter, tracheostomy tube cuff, or medical gas tubing.[37-39]

Medication errors and omissions have been reported in association with medication-related equipment and sharps.[4,147]

VIII.k.1. Perioperative personnel who administer medications should implement known safe practices that minimize the risks associated with tubing including, but not limited to,
- tracing all tubing to the point of origin and point of insertion,
- labeling all tubing and injection ports,
- avoiding use of y-port extension tubing,
- aligning tubing to avoid tangling and to facilitate easy identification, and
- avoiding use of standard Luer-lock syringes for medications intended for oral or enteric administration.

VIII.k.2. Perioperative team members should implement safety practices that minimize the risk of administering medications to the wrong

MEDICATION SAFETY

patient because of patients who have the same or similar names.

Implementing safety measures for patients who have the same or similar names is a risk-reduction strategy that has prevented a medication being administered to the wrong patient on several occasions.[148]

VIII.k.3. Perioperative team members should implement safety practices that minimize the risk from equipment including, but not limited to,
- eliminating free-flow IV tubing,
- programming non-smart IV pumps (eg, key-bounce errors),
- avoiding work-arounds associated with automated dispensing storage systems and other technologies,
- ensuring activation of all medication reconstitution devices (eg, planned IV piggybacks), and
- complying with sharps safety guidelines.

Recommendation IX

Safe medication practices should be used when transferring medications to, handling medications on, and administering medications from the sterile field.

Transferring medications to the sterile field poses increased risks for contamination of the medication, the sterile field, or both. Information is displaced and verification processes are different because the medications are removed from their original containers.

Safe practices include accurately labeling medications in their new sterile containers to provide consistency for communication when handing off medications that will be administered on the sterile field. Hand offs involving multiple personnel increase the risk for miscommunication. Enhancing communication among the perioperative team has been recognized as a strategy to reduce medication errors.[4]

IX.a. Aseptic technique should be used when transferring medications to the sterile field.

Medication vials are not designed to aseptically pour the contents into a secondary container on the sterile field. Transfer devices are designed to minimize splashing, spilling, and the need to reach over the sterile field, which could cause contamination of the sterile field.

IX.a.1. The RN circulator should obtain commercially available sterile transfer devices (eg, sterile vial spike, filter straw, plastic catheter) to prepare products for aseptic presentation to the sterile field.

IX.a.2. Stoppers should not be removed from vials for the purpose of pouring medications.

IX.a.3. The RN circulator should check the expiration date and visually inspect the medication for any indication that the medication was compromised during the storage process (eg, particulates, discoloration) before transferring the medication to the sterile field. If there is any question of compromise, the item should not be transferred to the sterile field.

Medications that have signs of being compromised may have reduced effectiveness or could be contaminated.

IX.b. The RN circulator should transfer one medication at a time to the sterile field in an environment without distraction or interruption.

Focusing on transferring one medication at a time without distraction or interruption facilitates performance of aseptic technique and accurate identification of the medication being transferred.

IX.b.1. The RN circulator should confirm dose limits previously established before he or she transfers the medication to the sterile field.

IX.b.2. The RN circulator transferring the medication to the sterile field and the perioperative team member receiving the medication should concurrently verify the medication name, strength, dosage, and expiration date.

IX.b.3. If there is no designated scrub person, the RN circulator should confirm the medication visually and verbally with the licensed independent professional performing the procedure.

IX.c. Immediately upon receipt of the medication to the sterile field, the person receiving the medication should label the medication container. The label should include, at a minimum, the medication name, strength, and concentration.[149,150]

Fatal errors directly related to unlabeled containers of medication have been reported.[4,151-156] One study suggests that scrub personnel are more likely to label medications and medication-delivery devices when preprinted labels are provided.[150]

IX.c.1. The label should be confirmed by both the RN circulator and the scrub person.

IX.c.2. Any solution or medication found on the sterile field without an identification label should be discarded.

IX.d. Verbal confirmation should be given when handing medications to the licensed independent practitioner for subsequent administration, even when only one medication is on the sterile field.

A standardized method of communication helps reduce the risk of error involving medications on the sterile field.[4]

IX.e. All medications on the sterile field should be verified with the relief person during any personnel changes (eg, shift relief, breaks).

MEDICATION SAFETY

A standardized method of communication helps to reduce the risk of error involving medications on the sterile field.[4]

IX.f. Perioperative team members should use safe injection practices (eg, one syringe and one needle) when infiltrating medications (eg, local anesthetics) to multiple areas within the same surgical site.

Using needles and syringes more than once increases the risk of infection.

IX.f.1. A syringe and needle should be used only once to administer a medication to a single patient, after which the syringe and needle should be discarded. When administering incremental doses to a single patient from the same syringe is an integral part of the procedure, the same syringe and needle may be reused, with strict adherence to aseptic technique, for the same patient as part of a single procedure. The syringe should never be left unattended and should be discarded immediately at the end of the procedure.

IX.g. Perioperative team members should retain and isolate all delivery devices and original medication containers for medications that have been delivered to the sterile field until the end of the procedure.

The practice of maintaining possession of delivery devices and medication containers until the patient leaves the OR or invasive procedure room is important in the event of a medication-related error or adverse reaction.[153] Maintaining possession of these containers may facilitate the root cause analysis of an adverse event. Isolating broken ampoules or other glass containers may reduce the risk of sharps injuries.

IX.h. Unused, opened irrigation or IV solutions should be discarded at the end of the procedure.

Irrigation and IV containers and supplies are considered single-patient use. Using surplus volume from any irrigation or IV solution containers or supplies for more than one patient increases the risk of cross contamination.

Recommendation X

Perioperative team members should monitor the patient for therapeutic effect or adverse reactions to medications.

Evaluating and documenting the patient's physical, emotional, or psychological response to medications is part of the monitoring phase of the medication use process, which is the sixth and final phase. This phase allows an opportunity to detect both therapeutic and adverse effects of products, as well as detect errors.[1,4]

X.a. Perioperative team members should observe the patient for effectiveness of medications that are administered.

Monitoring the patient for effects of medications is a core principle of pharmacotherapy and is consistent with professional standards associated with the medication use process.[108,129]

X.a.1. Perioperative personnel should document patient responses as close as possible to the time the medication was administered and the response is observed.

X.a.2. As appropriate to their roles, perioperative team members should reevaluate ineffective responses to determine whether further investigation is warranted.

Reports indicate that health care professionals may divert pain medications and the patient may receive a replacement of lesser or no strength.[44,48,157] By evaluating the effectiveness for pain management and sedation (eg, amount given and expected response), perioperative team members may be able to correlate findings from patient assessment data with inventory management documents.

X.b. Perioperative team members should observe the patient for adverse reactions to medication and should document patient responses as close as possible to the time the response is observed.

Assessing and documenting the patient's response to medication provides vital information related to dose effectiveness and the presence of a potential medication-related adverse effect. Adverse effects of medication use include allergy (eg, anaphylaxis), toxicity, oversedation, and underusage.[4,18,151-156,158]

Immediate documentation of untoward effects is a medicolegal standard and contributes to planning, intervening, and supporting continuity of care. Documentation also serves as a means for systems review to improve processes related to medication use.

X.c. Perioperative team members should implement role-appropriate processes to detect and report potential hazards and near-misses, as well as actual medication errors.

Medication errors (eg, adverse effects) may occur earlier in the medication use process but can be detected in the monitoring phase.[4]

X.c.1. In the event of unexpected patient responses, all pertinent data and all the steps of the medication use process should be reviewed to determine a plausible explanation.

Recommendation XI

In final phases of the postanesthesia care (eg, phase 2 recovery), the perioperative RN should coordinate patient education plans that are focused on discharge and aftercare instructions related to medication use.

Clearly delineated postprocedural orders provide the basis for patient safety after the patient leaves the health care organization. Adherence to aftercare instructions is an essential component to facilitate recovery and prevent complications. After discharge, patients and their designated support person(s) are often responsible for incorporating new postprocedure medications into their old medication regimens and identifying symptoms of reactions and monitoring for effectiveness.[159] Effective communication between the patient, designated support person(s), and perioperative team members enhances the patient's capacity for medication self-management after discharge.[17,160]

XI.a. The perioperative RN should review postprocedure physician medication orders, resolve any discrepancies, and plan care accordingly.

Reviewing the medication orders before the patient is discharged is a strategy to reduce medication errors or omissions after the patient leaves the health care organization.

XI.a.1. When reviewing patient medications after a surgical or other invasive procedure, the perioperative RN should understand the procedure performed and the patient's pre-existing conditions before he or she compares those considerations with the medications prescribers have initiated, resumed, or discontinued to verify medications are consistent with the therapeutic objective and relevant medical history.

XI.a.2. Perioperative RNs should clarify medication orders that are not specific including, but not limited to, "resume previous orders."

The Joint Commission discourages prescribers from resuming previous orders.[161] Improving communication between physicians who are writing discharge orders and patients' primary care physicians has been identified as a key issue for promoting effective transitions of care at discharge.[159]

XI.b. Using the medication reconciliation process, the perioperative RN should collaborate with physicians and pharmacists to develop effective medication plans for educating patients and their designated support persons at the time of discharge.

Discrepancies found through the medication reconciliation process often occur at the discharge phase of care.[162] Effective medication reconciliation is a strategy to promote safe patient outcomes by reducing opportunities for errors and detecting duplicate therapies.[112,163,164] Researchers have reported that patients whose medications are electronically reconciled have a greater understanding of medication administration and the potential adverse effects of the medications they are taking at the time of hospital discharge.[165] Some medications (eg, oral antidiabetic agent metformin) cause complications (eg, contrast-induced nephropathy) if resumed too soon after the procedure.[166,167] Researchers report that patients who have a prescription to take warfarin are more likely to discontinue the medication after an overnight hospitalization for elective surgery or an ambulatory procedure compared with the general population.[168] There is a need for active communication between patients and their prescribers about when to resume anticoagulation therapy because there is increased potential for miscommunication when the prescriber discontinuing the medication therapy is different from the prescriber expected to write the order for resuming the therapy.[168]

Patients and the people who support them may be at risk for medication errors or less effective treatment when they have limited health literacy that influences their ability to understand instructions on prescription medication labels.[169,170] Using appropriate teaching strategies based on the patient's needs (eg, learning readiness, language preference, cognitive ability) and adjusting teaching strategies based on feedback are key components of the AORN "Standards of perioperative nursing" that can be applied at the time of patient discharge.[108]

XI.b.1. The discharge medication plan should include instructions for the patient to follow up with the primary care provider to determine when to resume maintenance medications (eg, medications for blood pressure, diabetes).

XI.b.2. The discharge medication plan should include follow-up instructions regarding laboratory tests that may be needed to assess levels of medications.

XI.b.3. The discharge medication plan should specify when to discontinue medications.

XI.b.4. The discharge medication plan should include provisions for patients and their designated support persons who cannot read or when English is the second language.

XI.c. The perioperative RN should use the discharge medication plan to educate patients and their designated support persons about how to implement the plan in their aftercare setting.

Patient-centered care is facilitated by linking the procedure just performed and preexisting conditions to the medication plan. Teaching enhances compliance with the medication plan.[17,49,171]

Because medication labels and the medication package inserts are often confusing, patients and the people who support them in

MEDICATION SAFETY

aftercare need access to up-to-date information (eg, patient education fact sheets, online resources) about how to use their medications safely.[5,51]

XI.c.1. The perioperative RN should instruct patients and their designated support persons regarding medication use in the aftercare setting.[164,170] Instructions should include, but not be limited to,
- emphasizing the importance of carrying a medication list that has up-to-date information, including prescriptions, over-the-counter medications, and dietary supplements[17] and
- explaining how to schedule, administer, and use adjunct equipment and supplies.

XI.d. The perioperative RN should be familiar with state pharmacy laws regarding dispensing medications.

State pharmacy laws vary regarding dispensing medications for patient use. Pharmacists are accountable for ensuring compliance with state laws pertaining to dispensing medications for aftercare use.[10,11]

XI.d.1. Facility-based pharmacists should be available if any medications or pharmaceutical products are to be sent home with the patient from the perioperative area. Partially used solutions (eg, ear drops, eye drops) should only be sent home with the patient after being properly labeled by a pharmacist in a manner that is consistent with state pharmacy laws regarding dispensing.

XI.e. The perioperative RN should coordinate medication orders, written or electronic, with third-party providers.

The complexity of aftercare requires coordination with third-party providers (eg, pharmacy, durable medical equipment, home health agencies) to ensure appropriate medications, equipment (eg, patient-controlled analgesia pump), and supplies are available for aftercare use by patients or their designated support persons.

XI.f. The perioperative RN should perform an aftercare assessment (eg, telephone call).

Aftercare patient assessment is a safety strategy that can identify patient status, response to medications, actual adverse conditions (eg, nausea, vomiting, ineffective pain control, inability to perform activities of daily living), and knowledge and compliance with the medication plan. Additional elements (eg, infection prevention, wound care/management, patient satisfaction) also can be collected during the aftercare assessment.[160]

XI.f.1. The perioperative RN performing the aftercare patient assessment should document the findings as soon as possible and take action as appropriate.

XI.g. Perioperative RNs and pharmacists should be involved in developing suitable aftercare medication written instruction forms that take into consideration age-specific requirements (eg, large print), special populations (eg, readability and suitability, language requirements), and health literacy.[10,11,17]

Enhancing communication about medications and enabling patients to better understand their medications can be accomplished by creating a patient-friendly medication schedule tool.[116] Safety issues (eg, incorrect dispensing of eardrops instead of eyedrops; patient self administering with glaucoma eye drops instead of anti-inflammatory eye drops) have been reported with look-alike, sound-alike ophthalmic medications.[172] Patients who have limited or impaired vision may need additional care to encourage them to verify labels on medications that will be used at home after discharge. Including direct caregivers in the development of patient teaching tools enhances the effectiveness of the tools because they can supply information based on patient feedback.[116]

Recommendation XII

A comprehensive safety program should be developed to identify special care and handling of hazardous medications that are used in perioperative environments.

To be in compliance with the Occupational Safety and Health Administration (OSHA) hazard communication standard, health care organizations are required to have practice-specific assessments for hazardous medications that are used within the organization.[173,174]

XII.a. The health care organization must have a hazard communication program that identifies a continually updated list of hazardous medications that may be encountered by perioperative staff members. The list of hazardous medications must be posted to ensure worker safety.[173,174]

Hazard communication programs help inform health care workers about the risk of exposure to medications that are defined as hazardous but that have dosage formulations that are solid or intact (eg, coated tablets or capsules) and may not pose a significant risk of direct occupational exposure unless they are altered (eg, crushing tablets, making solutions from capsules outside of a ventilated cabinet).[174]

XII.a.1. A current material safety data sheet must be immediately available for all hazardous medications that are used in the workplace.[173,175]

XII.b. Hazardous medications or solutions should be stored in segregated areas with clear signage and warning labels.

MEDICATION SAFETY

Clear signage and warning labels in storage areas separate from other medications helps to reduce the risk of errors in medication administration and the risk of injury to the health care worker. Immediately available spill kits and waste containers facilitates containment of spilled hazardous substances and reduces the risk of injury to persons in the area.[176,177]

XII.b.1. Spill kits and waste containers for hazardous medications should be stored with hazardous medications or solutions in the storage area.

XII.c. Hazardous medications should be transported in sealed containers with Luer caps and no needles attached. The transport container should be
- leak proof,
- resistant to breakage, and
- labeled with warning labels to alert personnel that contents are hazardous.[174,178]

XII.d. Personnel handling hazardous medications should wear personal protective equipment (PPE) consistent with the type of exposure that can reasonably be anticipated. Personal protective equipment should include the following:
- chemical protective gowns and two pairs of gloves when handling hazardous medications in the storage area or transporting hazardous medications to the point of use,[176,178]
- face shields when there is a potential for splashing or splattering, and
- gloves.

An impervious or chemotherapy-rated gown protects perioperative team members' skin, especially on the arms and torso, from exposure to the hazardous medication when reconstituting or admixing medications.[174,178]

Face shields protect mucous membranes, skin, and eyes from injury that can be caused by some cytotoxic agents.[174]

Double-gloving and changing the outer glove after contact with hazardous medications protects perioperative team members from exposure when administering or handling open containers of chemotherapy drugs.[174]

XII.d.1. Gloves worn for chemotherapy administration should meet the American Society for Testing and Materials D 6978 standards.[179]

XII.e. Perioperative team members should follow the medication manufacturer's recommendations for cleaning and handling of instrumentation exposed to the chemotherapeutic agent, for disposal of body fluids of patients receiving chemotherapeutic agents, and for disposal of unused medication.

Some cytotoxic agents leave a residue on instruments and require specific PPE and cleaning techniques. Traces of the medication may be retained in body fluids, making special disposal considerations necessary. Hazardous medications may have different disposal requirements than other medications.

XII.f. The hazardous medication safety plan should include medical surveillance of personnel who handle cytotoxic agents.

Cytotoxic drugs have the potential to cause serious health risks to health care workers who are exposed to them.[176] These medications are often mutagenic, carcinogenic, and teratogenic and may cause local injury when they come into direct contact with skin, eyes, or mucous membranes.[180] Safe levels of exposure to these drugs have not been determined by OSHA, and no reliable system is currently available to monitor exposure levels.[175]

Recommendation XIII

Medications should be disposed of according to local, state, and federal regulations; manufacturer's instructions; and health care organization policy.

A medication may be classified as a controlled substance or a medical hazardous waste and have federal, state, or local requirements for disposal. Factors influencing the decision for how to dispose of medication waste include the ease of, access to, and cost of disposal.[181]

The Resource Conservation and Recovery Act is the federal law for management and disposal of solid and hazardous waste.[69,182] Hazardous and non-hazardous waste regulations are defined by the Environmental Protection Agency and enforced at both the federal and state levels.[183]

The FDA web site is a source for information on medications that are safe to be flushed. Restrictions on flushing pharmaceuticals and related waste can be found in the federal Clean Water Act,[184] as well as in state and local regulations. Fines and warnings of future penalties may be issued for failure to comply with restrictions for disposing of pharmaceutical waste into waterways.[69]

XIII.a. Perioperative RNs should collaborate with pharmacists to determine compliance with federal, state, or local regulations and manufacturer recommendations for disposal of hazardous medications or solutions.

In general, about 5% of pharmaceuticals are considered hazardous because they have one or more of the following characteristics: waste ignitability, corrosivity, reactivity, or toxicity.[69,182,183] Hormonal agents and hazardous medications may not be identified as hazardous waste at the federal level but may be managed as hazardous waste at the state level.[178] Because of the complexity of hazardous pharmaceutical waste disposal, pharmacy consultation may be necessary to determine compliance.[183]

XIII.a.1. Medications should be disposed of by one of the following methods:
- returning to the manufacturer,

MEDICATION SAFETY

- donating the unused portion for reuse,
- flushing down the drain,
- disposing into a landfill, or
- incinerating.[181]

XIII.a.2. Medication disposal should be performed in a manner that does not contaminate the water supply. When prescription medications are not labeled as safe for flushing, pharmacists should advise health care workers as to the appropriate method for disposal at the point of use or if the item should be returned to the pharmacy for proper disposal.[69]

XIII.b. Perioperative RNs should collaborate with pharmacy personnel to develop processes for determining the proper methods of disposal and how unused and unopened medications in the medication storage areas are to be returned to the pharmacy.

Medication storage and control are important components of the medication management system.[43] Returning medications to pharmacies increases the accuracy for accounting for unused medications. Returning unopened medications to pharmacies may increase the chances for exchanging the medications to avoid outdates and consequent waste.

XIII.c. Perioperative personnel who administer medications or handle medications within their scope of practice must follow established practices to validate controlled substance (Schedule II to IV) waste.

Licensed individuals are accountable for adhering to the Controlled Substance Act. Such adherence extends to retrieving and administering medication, and documenting the wasting of unused products.[45]

XIII.c.1. Licensed perioperative team members should participate in inventory management of controlled substances.

XIII.c.2. Licensed perioperative team members should waste unused scheduled medications in accordance with federal regulations and health care organization policy. *Amb*

Recommendation XIV

Perioperative personnel should receive initial and ongoing education and demonstrate competency in the performance of safe medication practices at least on an annual basis.

Initial and periodic education on safe medication practices provides direction for personnel in providing safe patient care. Additional periodic educational programs provide opportunities to reinforce previous learning and introduce new information on adjunct technology, its use, and potential risks. Competency validation serves as an indicator that personnel have an understanding of safe medication practices. Evolving technology interfaces associated with infusion pumps, computerized order entry, and automated dispensing systems require initial and ongoing training to achieve the benefit of equipment designed to reduce medication errors.[21,25,185]

XIV.a. An introduction to and review of policies and procedures for safe medication practices should be included in orientation and ongoing education of personnel.

Reviewing policies and procedures assists health care personnel in developing knowledge, skills, and attitudes that affect patient outcomes.

XIV.b. At a minimum, education, training, and competency validation should address the following areas:
- the medication use process;
- at-risk behaviors in perioperative settings;
- the nurse's role in medication reconciliation;
- medications associated with emergency care;
- education tools for patients and their support persons about prescribed medications;
- pharmaceutical waste; and
- new regulations, technology, and procedures relevant to safe medication practices.

XIV.b.1. Competency validation should be documented.

Documented competency validation serves as a basis for staff development, quality improvement, and performance evaluation. Documentation tools facilitate objectivity and consistency and remove subjectivity from the validation process.

XIV.c. Perioperative team members who handle medication products should demonstrate competency in the procuring process.

Product shortages occur in the procuring phase of the medication use process. Automatically substituting other medication products increases the risk for human errors.[186] When perioperative team members understand the medication purchasing process for perioperative patient care areas and participate in or serve on medication safety committees, more clinically relevant decisions can be made to reduce the risk for human errors.

XIV.c.1. Education should include product packaging considerations (eg, single-dose, multi-dose vials, inner sterile wrap), bioequivalent issues, and pharmacotherapeutic issues that potentially increase the risk for error.

XIV.c.2. Education and competency validation should include safety considerations related to medication inventory and par levels including, but not limited to,
- standardizing strength and concentration,
- identifying distinct pairs for look-alike, sound-alike medication products,
- separating look-alike medication products, and

MEDICATION SAFETY

- disseminating information about product shortages and recalls.

XIV.c.3. Education should include risk-reduction strategies for inventory management including, but not limited to,
- establishing temperature control for medications,
- rotating stock,
- processing product returns, including outdated medications, and
- securing medication inventory (ie, both scheduled and non-scheduled products).

XIV.d. Education and competency validation should include barriers to successful prescribing including, but not limited to,
  ○ determining scope of practice boundaries;
  ○ recognizing what constitutes prescribing;
  ○ receiving and processing verbal, written, or electronic orders; and
  ○ maintaining preference cards and standing order forms.

Educating perioperative team members about the parameters of the perioperative prescribing process is a strategy designed to reduce opportunities for adverse events. By establishing a broad understanding and appreciation of how their role supports accuracy in the prescribing process, perioperative team members are more likely to be accountable for ensuring the accuracy of verbal and standing orders.

XIV.e. Education should include the risks inherent to the transcribing process.

From a national perspective, approximately 22% of the reported errors occurred at the point of transcribing.[4]

XIV.f. Education and competency validation should include barriers to successful dispensing.

There are variations in dispensing processes across perioperative settings. Educating perioperative team members about safety parameters that are designed into the dispensing phase of the medication use process is a strategy intended to improve compliance with medication verification and accuracy before the medication intersects with direct patient care.

XIV.f.1. Education and competency validation should include retrieving or returning medications from automated dispensing storage systems or medication storage areas.

XIV.f.2. Education should include the pharmacist's role regarding safety parameters in the dispensing process.

In the dispensing process, pharmacists review medication orders, prepare products for perioperative use, serve as consultants to perioperative team members, and participate in inventory management with automatic dispensing systems. Some perioperative settings do not have a direct opportunity for pharmacists' participation and, therefore, have reduced support in the dispensing process. Educating perioperative team members about pharmacists' contributions at the dispensing phase will increase their awareness of safety parameters that are necessary to build into safe medication practices in perioperative settings.

XIV.g. Perioperative team members should demonstrate competency appropriate to their roles in the perioperative medication administration process.

Through education, perioperative RNs are able to exercise critical judgment in administering medications with the intent to reduce infections and adverse medication events. Licensed individuals other than RNs have multiple ways to demonstrate competency, such as medical staff appointment processes (eg, credentialing process), peer review, and quality reports. Through education, unlicensed personnel are able to demonstrate appropriate handling of medications (eg, labeling, handing off).

Medication errors occur at the administration phase and across all phases of care in perioperative settings.[4] Knowledge and performance deficits and calculation errors have been reported among the five leading causes of pediatric medication errors.[130] Effective training, education, and support are identified as key elements to the success of using computer-entry systems to reduce medication errors.[185]

XIV.g.1. Perioperative RNs should demonstrate age-specific competencies in obtaining, preparing, and administering medications.

XIV.g.2. Perioperative team members should demonstrate competency in aseptic technique when preparing, handling, and administering medications.

XIV.g.3. Perioperative team members should demonstrate competency appropriate to their roles regarding recommended safety practices for medication administration including, but not limited to,
- confirming the medication with visual and verbal validation,
- labeling medications on the sterile field,
- labeling medications when outside of their original container regardless of the perioperative setting, and
- confirming safe dosage limits and dosage calculations.

XIV.g.4. Perioperative team members should demonstrate competency appropriate to their roles related to safe injection practices including, but not limited to,
- using one needle per injection,
- using one syringe per injection, and
- complying with sharps safety measures.

MEDICATION SAFETY

XIV.g.5. Perioperative team members should demonstrate competency appropriate to their roles related to the use of medication containers, adjunct equipment, and supplies including, but not limited to,
- ampoules;
- filtered needles for use with ampoules;
- devices used to transfer medications to the sterile field;
- infusion pumps;
- volume injectors;
- IV and irrigation tubing and connectors; and
- syringes, needles, stopcocks, and sharp-safety systems.

XIV.g.6. Perioperative team members should demonstrate competency appropriate to their roles related to documenting medication administration.

XIV.g.7. Perioperative team members should be able to describe how the following conditions act as barriers to successful medications administration:
- hand off, shift relief, and breaks;
- noise;
- distractions;
- lighting;
- interruptions;
- muffled voices through masks;
- regional dialects; and
- staff member age-related sensory changes (eg, hearing, vision).

XIV.g.8. Perioperative team members should demonstrate safe handling of hazardous medications and solutions (eg, cytotoxic and chemotherapeutic agents) including, but not limited to,
- preventing exposure,
- managing spills,
- disposing of hazardous wastes, and
- handling of instruments that are exposed to chemotherapeutic agents.

Education and competency validation of the perioperative team members who work with the hazardous agents are essential to minimize exposure and promote workplace safety.[174,175]

XIV.h. Perioperative team members should demonstrate competency appropriate to their roles in monitoring patients' responses to medications including, but not limited to, recognizing
- effectiveness,
- ineffective responses, and
- adverse reactions to medications.

Education helps to support perioperative team members in exercising critical judgment in evaluating patients' physical, emotional, or psychological responses to the medication and recording such findings.[46]

XIV.h.1. Perioperative team members should demonstrate competency appropriate to their roles related to documenting patients' responses to medications.

XIV.h.2. Perioperative team members should be able to describe how the following conditions act as barriers to successful monitoring:
- shift changes,
- interruptions,
- noise,
- distractions, and
- patient transfers to other phases of perioperative care.

XIV.i. Perioperative team members should demonstrate competency in emergency medication administration and management (eg, malignant hyperthermia, cardiac arrest, respiratory depression).

XIV.i.1. Education should include mock drills for malignant hyperthermia, cardiac arrest, and other emergencies related to adverse medication responses.

Mock drills help perioperative team members develop critical thinking skills.

XIV.j. Education sessions for perioperative team members should be initiated when new regulations, technologies, and procedures related to safe medication practices become available.

Regulations regarding pharmaceutical waste and safe medication administration continue to be updated. Technologies and new procedures relating to safe medication practices continue to evolve. When perioperative team members are up to date on recent regulatory developments and new equipment or product trends, they will be better prepared to comply with regulations, identify safety issues, and take appropriate actions.

Recommendation XV

Perioperative team members, consistent with their roles, should document all activities related to the medication use process throughout all phases of perioperative patient care.

Documentation throughout the medication use process is a professional medicolegal standard. Documentation is applicable at the systems level and the patient care level. At the systems level, documentation serves as basis for monitoring compliance and measuring performance. At the patient care level, documentation facilitates continuity of patient care through clear communication and supports collaboration between health care team members.

XV.a. Perioperative team member participation in the procuring process should be documented in a retrievable manner (eg, committee minutes, logs, reports).

MEDICATION SAFETY

Documentation serves as the medicolegal standard to measure adherence with safety practices including, but not limited to,
- selecting standardized products for use;
- rotating stock;
- returning products, including outdated medications;
- securing medication inventory (ie, both scheduled and non-scheduled products);
- reversing distribution or disposing of unused medications; and
- controlling temperature for temperature-sensitive medications.

XV.b. Perioperative team members' involvement in the prescribing process should be documented in a manner that is consistent with their roles and scopes of practice.

Documentation serves as the medicolegal standard to measure adherence with prescribing processes.

XV.b.1. Medication orders, regardless of origin (eg, standing, verbal, written, electronic), should be documented and signed by the prescriber.

XV.b.2. Medication orders should be legible and reflect legible signatures of the prescriber initiating the order and the caregiver transcribing the verbal order.

It is the responsibility of the health care practitioner, in concert with the health care organization, to ensure that documentation clearly and unambiguously reflects the individualized treatment of the patient. Having all health care providers use block print and sign their names to all written and verbal orders is one risk-reduction strategy designed to improve communication among caregivers. The extra step of block-printing the name of the prescriber affords the caregiver an opportunity to contact the provider if a question, concern, or issue were to arise related to the written order. If the receiver of the order is unable to hear the order correctly or the caregiver is unable to read the written order, confusion or misinterpretation could result and lead to an adverse patient event.[4]

XV.b.3. Verbal and telephone orders should be authenticated with the prescriber's signature and date and time.

XV.b.4. Standing medication orders should contain evidence of periodic review for accuracy.

Medication errors can occur from a failure to update standing orders or to individualize patient care by assessing the standing order for appropriateness to a specific patient condition or clinical situation.[3] One study revealed that intraoperative standing orders in the form of preference cards increased the risk of potential medication errors.[91] The following were among the major concerns from the study findings:
- Surgeons were not double-checking changes made to the preference cards.
- Medications listed on the preference cards were not what the surgeon wanted or intended to use.[91]

In another study, researchers implemented preprinted physician orders for pediatric procedural sedation and reported an increase in documentation compliance (ie, legibility, completeness) and a decrease in medication ordering errors.[89]

XV.c. Perioperative team members' involvement in the transcribing process should be documented in a manner that is consistent with their roles.

Documentation serves as the medicolegal standard to measure adherence with transcribing processes.

XV.d. Perioperative team members' involvement in the dispensing process should be documented in a manner that is consistent with their roles and scopes of practice.

Documentation serves as the medicolegal standard to measure adherence with dispensing processes.

XV.d.1. Documentation should reflect a pharmacist's review of all medication orders. Automated dispensing systems and pharmacy computer systems may be used to document pharmacist validation of medication orders.[21]

XV.e. Medications administered should be documented in a manner that
- is legible and easily accessible,
- is free of unapproved abbreviations and acronyms,
- is timely,
- identifies the concentrations of the medication and solutions administered and the route of administration,
- identifies the person who administered the medication, and
- indicates total amounts administered when there are multiple injections of the same medication (eg, lidocaine) administered during a procedure.

Documentation serves as the medicolegal standard to measure adherence with administering processes. Documenting the total amount of medication administered when a medication is administered repeatedly over a course of time decreases the risk of injecting medications at toxic levels.

XV.e.1. Documentation should reflect that Schedule II through V products that were not administered to the patient were disposed of in accordance with local, state, and federal law, as well as with the health care organization's policy.

MEDICATION SAFETY

XV.f. Documentation should reflect patient responses to administered medications.

Documentation serves as the medicolegal standard to measure adherence with monitoring processes.

XV.f.1. In the presence of ineffective response or adverse events, documentation should reflect actions initiated or interventions that were implemented.

XV.g. Documentation should reflect the discharge process related to medication reconciliation and the instructions presented to patients and their designated support persons for medications.[187]

Documentation serves as the medicolegal standard to measure adherence with medication reconciliation processes and to reflect the patient's or designated support person's response to the instructions given about medications.

XV.h. Documentation should reflect the aftercare process including, but not limited to, a nursing evaluation of the patient's postprocedure progress and follow-up activities that are deemed necessary based on the aftercare phone call.

Documentation serves as the medicolegal standard to measure adherence to aftercare processes.

XV.i. Medication documentation should include correct placement of zeroes and be free of unapproved abbreviations, acronyms, symbols, and dose designations.

Confusing or easily misinterpreted abbreviations, acronyms, or symbols put caregivers at risk of making errors and compromising patient safety.[188] A misplaced decimal point, a "U" interpreted as a "0" (zero), "QOD" confused with "QID," or "AS" misinterpreted as "OS" puts patients at risk for medical errors with potentially serious results (eg, overdose, inadequate dose, omission due to laterality error, wrong medication administered, error in frequency of administration). Improving communication by reducing abbreviations, acronyms, and symbols is a significant step toward reducing the occurrence of errors related to the inability to accurately read and interpret written medical orders and transcribed verbal orders.[189]

Computer systems designed for medication documentation may increase the risk of errors when their programs include
- abbreviated medication names because of character length limitations,
- medication names listed in alphabetical order without mixed-case lettering or alternating colored lines as differentiators, or
- unclear expressions of drug dosages (eg, 40000 versus 40,000).[185]

XV.i.1. Documentation should reflect that the minimally required list of do-not-use items in the health care organization's policy has been augmented to include problem-prone, high-risk, and high-volume abbreviations, acronyms, and symbols that are unique to medications in the perioperative practice setting.

XV.i.2. Abbreviations related to laterality should not be used when documenting activities related to medications.

XV.i.3. Documentation should include leading zeroes (eg, 0.X mg rather than .X mg) and be free of trailing zeroes (eg, X mg rather than X.0 mg).

XV.i.4. Medication orders should not be numbered.

XV.j. Across all perioperative settings and all phases of the medication use process, perioperative RNs should incorporate the Perioperative Nursing Data Set (PNDS) taxonomy when documenting medications whenever possible.

The PNDS is the standardized perioperative nursing vocabulary.[190] Standardized documentation promotes nursing research.

Recommendation XVI

Policies and procedures for safe medication practices should be developed, readily available in the practice setting, and reviewed periodically, and they should address direct patient care situations as well as organizational level situations. *Amb*

Policies and procedures are the operational guidelines that can be used to minimize patient risk factors while strategically linking the health care organization's mission to its day-to-day operations. Policies and procedures establish authority, responsibility, and accountability within the organization. Policies and procedures assist perioperative team members in developing guidelines for continuous performance improvement and activities that support patient safety.

In addition to dosing errors and miscommunication, ineffective policies have been reported as one of the main categories associated with causes of error.[130] Policies are needed in perioperative settings to help clarify the increased complexities that occur at several points in the medication use process, including communications related to verbal orders, medications removed from original containers, and sensory distractions.[130] In addition, policies may help with improving inconsistent practices for communicating current and previous medication regimens (ie, medication reconciliation) and reporting drug diversion in perioperative settings.[44,130] Administrative policies that are developed with participation from a variety of perspectives are more likely to provide guidance at the point of care, including education and training and appropriate documentation, as well as to provide for workplace safety and to set the tone for a culture of safety.

XVI.a. Policies and procedures should be developed collaboratively by stakeholders who are knowledgeable and are willing to advocate for safe

MEDICATION SAFETY

practices in the various phases of the medication use process.

Involving all stakeholders in the process strengthens policies and procedures, contributes to interprofessional respect, and enhances teamwork and, therefore, compliance.

XVI.a.1. Stakeholders who are involved in policy and procedure development should be willing to advocate for culturally sensitive medication practices within the communities served including, but not limited to,
- age-specific populations,
- special populations (eg, women's services, ophthalmology, oncology), and
- ethnically diverse populations.

XVI.a.2. Stakeholders should help identify the types of resources that should be provided to the perioperative team via policies and procedures. Examples include, but are not limited to,
- up-to-date online reference materials,
- access to Drug Information Centers, and
- defined parameters for supplemental staff members (eg, agency nurse, consulting pharmacist).

XVI.a.3. Stakeholders in the medication use process should identify barriers and solutions to achieving immediate access to medication safety policies and procedures at the time needed regardless of setting.

Ready access to policies and procedures provides clarity and guidance and reduces variance across the medication use process.

XVI.b. Perioperative administrators should conduct a periodic review of the policies and procedures for the health care organization's medication use process that is specific enough to consider external changes in medication safety best practices and the regulatory landscape in which the organization must comply.

Periodic reviews identify new knowledge, new regulatory guidelines, and internal limitations or weaknesses that may exist in the medication use process, as well as determine continued relevance to setting.

XVI.c. Policies and procedures should promote safe medication practices throughout the medication use process and establish authority, responsibility, and accountability at the point of care.

Establishing authority, responsibility, and accountability for medication use at the point of care is a risk-reduction strategy that supports patient safety by facilitating development of quality assessment measures and guidelines for continuous performance improvement. The framework created through the health care organization's policies and procedures pertaining to medication-use-process activities contributes to patient safety by aligning perioperative team members' roles and responsibilities with their respective scopes of practice.

XVI.c.1. Policies and procedures for procuring medications should include, but not be limited to,
- therapeutic considerations for formulary management (eg, generation of antibiotics, addition of new products to formulary);
- packaging considerations (eg, standardization, look-alike, sound-alike, unit of use);
- security for medication inventory (ie, both scheduled and non-scheduled products);
- rotation of stock (eg, first in, first out);
- plans for medication disposal (eg, unused, outdated) and product returns; and
- standardization of all locations where medications are stored including, but not limited to,
  - anesthesia carts,
  - emergency medication carts,
  - refrigerators, freezers, or warmers,
  - automated dispensing storage systems,
  - satellite pharmacies,
  - storage areas with controlled access, and
  - storage devices associated with scheduled substances.

XVI.c.2. Policies and procedures for prescribing medications should include, but not be limited to,
- what constitutes prescribing;
- parameters regarding who can prescribe;
- the format (eg, verbal, written, electronic) for medication prescribing;
- clear medication orders (eg, no unapproved abbreviations);
- a process for creating, maintaining, and reviewing preference cards and standing order forms;
- verbal order verification (eg, read back, whiteboard);
- environmental conditions that interfere with successful prescribing (eg, noise, interruptions);[134] and
- forcing functions and constraints when appropriate.

When the health care organization has an electronic environment for prescribing medications (eg, CPOE system), the policies and procedures should be consistent with information technology policies for user verification and password security.

XVI.c.3. Policies and procedures for transcribing medications should include, but not be limited to,
- the roles and responsibilities of the person involved in transcribing;

- the health care organization's specific forms (eg, medication administration record);
- a process for verifying accurate patient identification on all forms;
- the process for documenting that the order has been transcribed; and
- how to transmit the order to the pharmacy for processing, if appropriate.

XVI.c.4. Policies and procedures for dispensing medications should include, but not be limited to,
- what constitutes dispensing;
- parameters regarding who can dispense;
- pharmacy or a comparable type of oversight for medication management processes;
- par levels of medications in storage areas, including automated dispensing storage systems;
- a process for retrieving or returning medications from automated dispensing storage systems or medication storage areas;
- a process for how medications are prepared (eg, compliance with *The United States Pharmacopeia* Chapter <797> guidelines[104]);
- forcing functions for certain medications; and
- a process for restocking medication storage areas, including automated dispensing storage systems (ie, replenishment).

XVI.c.5. Policies and procedures for administering medications should include, but not be limited to,
- what constitutes medication administering;
- parameters regarding who can administer what medications;
- forcing functions and constraints when appropriate;
- weight-based dose conversion charts into practice;
- practices that incorporate the use of at least two patient identifiers to medication order;
- competencies and verification processes for administering medications;
- use of labels when medications are removed from their original containers;
- guidelines for holding all containers until the end of the procedure;
- disposal of unused medications and containers;
- compliance with federal regulations (eg, Controlled Substances Act[45] Resource Conservation and Recovery Act[182]); and
- documentation of all medications administered, including compliance with documentation standards and do-not-use abbreviations and symbols.

XVI.c.6. Policies and procedures should define the role of perioperative team members with regard to monitoring patients' responses to medications. Considerations should include, but not be limited to,
- parameters (eg, how long, how often) for observing patients' responses to medications,
- competencies for monitoring patients' responses to medications, and
- documentation of nursing activities related to the monitoring process (eg, evaluation findings, steps taken for adverse reactions).

XVI.d. Policies and procedures should establish authority, responsibility, and accountability, consistent with scope of practice boundaries, for safe medication practices and should be standardized across all phases of perioperative patient care.

Standardizing the process for transfer of medication information with the broader process for transferring perioperative patient care information provides consistency and improves the accuracy, reliability, and quality of the information reported.[191]

XVI.d.1. Policies and procedures should define the roles of perioperative team members with regard to the medication reconciliation, discharge, and aftercare processes.

In addition to policies for the medication use process, policies for other processes that involve medications (eg, medication reconciliation, discharge, aftercare, transfer of information) provide a framework for safe patient care.[192]

XVI.d.2. Contents of the medication transfer-of-patient-information report for each phase of perioperative care should include, but not be limited to, the following:

Preoperative phase:
- medication allergies;
- medication side effects;
- vital signs (eg, temperature, pulse, respiration, blood pressure);
- pain assessment; and
- medication profile, including preoperative medications.

Intraoperative phase:
- medication allergies;
- medication side effects;
- anesthesia type and route;
- current or pending laboratory or other test results that relate to medications;
- medications administered, including dose and time; and
- administered IV and irrigation fluids.

Postoperative phase:
- anesthesia type and route;

MEDICATION SAFETY

- anesthesia professional's orders related to IV medications;
- infusion pump settings;
- surgeon's orders for medications;
- medications administered, including dose and time;
- patient responses to medications; and
- administered IV fluids and irrigation.[191]

XVI.e. Health care organizations' policies and procedures should outline processes for initial education, training, ongoing competency validation, and annual review across the medication use process.

Policies and procedures assist in the development of activities that support patient safety, quality assessment, and the establishment of guidelines for continuous performance improvement. Standardizing processes for performance expectations between perioperative settings facilitates continuity of care and reduces the risk of error when staff members rotate between areas.

XVI.e.1. The processes for training, competency validation, and annual review pertaining to the medication use process should be standardized between perioperative settings within the health care organization.

XVI.f. Health care organizations should standardize perioperative documents and develop policies and procedures that include a list of do-not-use abbreviations, acronyms, and symbols that are inappropriate for inclusion in perioperative care documentation.

Perioperative settings may have three or more forms related to timing of doses (eg, preoperative records, intraoperative records, postanesthesia records, anesthesia forms). Standardizing methods of documenting on the medication administration record and perioperative records will facilitate continuity of care.

XVI.g. Policies and procedures should promote a safe workplace as it relates to medication-related equipment and supplies.

Appropriate methods to protect health care workers from exposure to hazardous materials or bloodborne pathogens and to decrease the risk of disease transmission through sharps injuries are specified in OSHA regulations.[193] Injuries from hollow-bore needles constitute the majority of injuries and pose the highest risk of exposure to bloodborne pathogens.[194] To help prevent hollow-bore percutaneous injuries during injections and bodily fluid retrieval, health care organization policies can establish a priority throughout perioperative settings to supply safety devices such as needleless systems; sharps with engineered sharp injury protection devices; blunt cannulas to withdraw medications and fluids from vials; retractable, protective sheath or self-resheathing systems; and hinged re-cap needles to administer local anesthetics and other injectable medications.

XVI.g.1. Policies and procedures should establish multidisciplinary teams to evaluate safety devices.

Staff members who work directly with medication safety devices are key members of the team.[67]

XVI.g.2. Policies and procedures should define required training and education on the use of appropriate sharps safety devices and risk-reduction strategies for preventing sharps injuries.

XVI.h. Policies and procedures should promote a culture of safety including, but not limited to,
- establishing systems that promote recognition of conditions that are associated with adverse effects related to medication use[137,138,195-197];
- defining communication expectations and types of team training to be implemented;
- designating time out procedures to be performed before each surgical or other invasive procedure that include a review of medications, allergies, and anticipated doses;
- establishing protocols that address situations when patients have the same or similar names[198];
- offering guidance for open discussion of barriers to safe medication use[15,192,199,200];
- establishing systems that promote open reporting of medication errors[201];
- establishing mechanisms to counter staff member fatigue[202-208]; and
- requiring adequate illumination where medications are obtained, prepared, and administered.[134]

XVI.h.1. Policies and procedures should outline processes for reporting to the quality improvement committee and disclosing to patients and their designated support persons when a medication error or near-miss occurs.

XVI.i. Policies and procedures should address pharmaceutical waste.

Pharmaceutical waste disposal is a complex issue. Providing clarity and guidance about how to dispose of unused or outdated medications will facilitate compliance with waste disposal regulations.

XVI.j. Policies and procedures should address impaired workforce members and drug diversion in perioperative settings including, but not limited to,
- aligning with state licensing laws and other state regulations,
- complying with human resource department policies,
- defining channels for reporting suspected cases to appropriate authorities,

MEDICATION SAFETY

- providing approved guidance for participating in evidence collection as directed by appropriate authorities,
- listing peer-assistance programs approved for referrals,
- identifying reentry to practice programs in accordance with licensing requirements, and
- restricting access to controlled substances after reentry to practice.

Recommendation XVII

Perioperative team members should participate in a variety of quality improvement activities that are consistent with the health care organization's plan and improve safe medication use by meeting or exceeding expectations from published national patient safety initiatives. *Amb*

Health care organizations that use a variety of quality improvement activities (eg, failure modes and effects analysis [FMEA], root cause analysis, Plan-Do-Study-Act) have better patient outcomes.[9,209] All improvement processes require stakeholders to be actively engaged.

XVII.a. Perioperative team members should participate in developing prospective strategies and identifying improvements across the medication use process.

Successful procurement programs aid in formulary decisions, purchasing decisions, and inventory management. Identifying the nature of the errors that occur at the prescribing phase allows perioperative team members to design interventions and monitor effectiveness. Improving communication and documentation can improve transcribing. Errors that originate at the point of dispensing may be identified through an evaluation of the chain of custody of medications from the point of fulfilling the order through to the point of administering the medication, returning unused medications, and replenishing medication par levels. Process improvements for the administration phase often include verification strategies and systems that reduce distractions and fatigue.[4] Observation may be a useful method of evaluating assessments in the monitoring phase of the medication use process.

Computer-entry errors may occur at any phase of the medication use process. To identify effective risk-reduction strategies to reduce computer-entry errors, it is important to focus on how the perioperative team members work, what activities are organized around the use of computers, and who will be open and willing to share their perspectives. Investing in training programs is another important component of performance improvement strategies related to computer-entry or computer-related errors.[185] Training programs may include how to use computer systems effectively, how to build robust clinical decision-support databases, or how to establish full integration and connectivity with other key information systems (eg, laboratory, pharmacy).

XVII.a.1. Perioperative team members should incorporate prospective risk-reduction strategies (eg, FMEA) into the procurement process to examine areas including, but not limited to,
- identifying inventory items with sound-alike, look-alike drug names;
- identifying inventory items with similar packaging;
- restricting types of medications and concentrations based on pharmacy and therapeutics committee recommendations;
- defining processes for product shortage situations;
- defining processes for determining replacement systems when recalls or system malfunction trends are identified; and
- defining processes for reverse distribution of unopened, unused, or expired products.

XVII.a.2. Perioperative prescribers should develop proactive risk-reduction strategies for the prescribing process including, but not limited to,
- adopting electronic health records,
- avoiding verbal orders,
- using clear handwriting without abbreviations,
- standardizing forms, and
- using Beers criteria.

XVII.a.3. Perioperative team members should develop risk-reduction strategies for the transcribing process including, but not limited to,
- clearly communicating medication orders in the medication administration record or the perioperative record and
- minimizing manual order transcription.

XVII.a.4. Perioperative team members should develop risk-reduction strategies for the dispensing process including, but not limited to,
- controlling and recording access to inventory management when perioperative staff members obtain medications,
- developing a methodology for accurate replenishing of automated dispensing storage systems within an established time frame, and
- implementing processes for irrigant and solution preparation by pharmacy staff members.

XVII.a.5. Perioperative team members should develop risk-reduction strategies for the administering process including, but not limited to,
- increasing the use of technology (eg, bar coding, dose confirmation software),
- standardizing and simplifying dosing charts,

- reporting medication allergies and medication contraindications,
- verifying timing of prophylactic antibiotics, and
- ensuring timely and adequate documentation.

XVII.a.6. Perioperative team members should develop risk-reduction strategies for the monitoring process including, but not limited to,
- auditing for documentation of the effects of medications and
- selecting appropriate equipment for use in the medication use process (eg, smart infusion pumps, adjunct equipment).

XVII.a.7. When making financial investments for performance-improvement strategies related to computer-entry or computer-related errors, considerations should include
- training programs for health care practitioners about how to use computer systems effectively,
- robust clinical decision-support databases, and
- full integration and connectivity with other key information systems (eg, laboratory, pharmacy).[185]

Bar-code technology and computer documentation are examples of performance-improvement strategies designed to increase compliance with documentation for medication administration. One study revealed a 21.7% increase in the number of medications documented per cardiac surgery case when a bar-code medication administration system was used by anesthesia professionals.[210] Another practice report discussed findings that revealed new opportunities for wrong dose or wrong drug errors when computer systems were used depending on the configuration of how medication names and dosages were displayed on the computer screen.[185]

Training programs increase familiarity with new systems. Robust clinical decision-support databases are designed to alert users about computer-entry errors to allow correction before the error is made.

XVII.b. Perioperative team members should develop processes for monitoring the medication management system to identify risk factors associated with medication errors and to strive for compliance with safety measures.

Monitoring provides a means to identify medication errors at the time or before the time they occur. Monitoring compliance with safety measures provides a means to correct situations at the time of occurrence and collect data for use in process-improvement projects. As a system, monitoring in the medication use process allows for process improvement and compliance with regulatory standards.

XVII.b.1. The health care organization should include a variety of error-detection strategies in the monitoring process including, but not limited to,
- spontaneous reports;
- computerized triggers;
- random chart reviews, including medication audits; and
- a classification reporting system, such as one endorsed by the World Health Organization (eg, Eindhoven Classification Model).[211,212]

Using more than one strategy facilitates identification of errors and risks for errors from multiple perspectives.

XVII.b.2. Perioperative team members should observe each other at various points in the medication use process to monitor for processes that inhibit safe medication use, including safe injection practices.

Observing interactions between working conditions, equipment, and people may reveal vulnerability for medication errors and opportunities for spontaneous coaching interactions to engage staff members in identifying risks (eg, discussion with a staff member not responding to clinical alarms).

XVII.b.3. Perioperative team members should monitor aftercare processes.

XVII.b.4. Perioperative team members should monitor compliance with safe handling of chemicals, cytotoxic agents, and hazardous waste in the workplace.

XVII.b.5. When observing for potential risks where medications are stored or used, perioperative team members should address environmental conditions including, but not limited to,
- space,
- illumination,
- noise, and
- interruptions.

XVII.b.6. Perioperative team members should monitor for potential risks for medication errors related to equipment including, but not limited to,
- equipment alarms (eg, temperature, pumps),
- infusion pumps,
- tubing interconnectivity, and
- hood or ventilation requirements for compounding irrigants.

XVII.b.7. Perioperative team members should actively participate in monitoring the health care organization's medication management system.

MEDICATION SAFETY

Given that there are numerous failures in medication management systems,[6] perioperative team members bear the responsibility for actively identifying system level barriers that impede safe medication use.[17] Actively participating in the improvement process requires monitoring of the medication use process to identify patterns and trends. Armed with such information, perioperative team members can close the divide between expected care and actual care that is delivered.[213]

XVII.b.8. Perioperative team members should monitor for a blame-free culture.

A culture of safety provides an atmosphere where perioperative team members can openly discuss errors, process improvements, or system issues without fear of reprisal.

XVII.c. The quality improvement/process improvement (QI/PI) program should include a routine review and update of all performance improvement activities.

Reviewing the established QI/PI program may identify failure points contributing to medication errors and may aid in improving patient safety.

XVII.c.1. The perioperative QI/PI program should include periodic evaluation of the medication management process; for example, a routine review and update of all preprinted order sheets and facility-approved standing orders for clarity of
- medication choice,
- dose, and
- delivery method.

XVII.c.2. The PNDS should be used to establish guidelines to monitor and manage institutional improvements with regard to medication safety and to identify desired outcomes including, but not limited to,
- the patient receives appropriate prescribed medication(s) safely administered during the perioperative period,
- the patient demonstrates knowledge of medication management, and
- the patient demonstrates knowledge of pain management.[190]

XVII.c.3. Medication performance improvement indicators should include structure, process, and outcome metrics. A baseline and a target should be used for routine reviews of performance indicators including, but not limited to,
- reducing the number of preoperative antibiotics administered outside of the acceptable time frame;
- eliminating the number of medication range orders without specification;
- reducing the number of medications drawn up in unlabeled syringes;
- reducing the number of outdated medications found;
- reducing the number of clinical staff members who do not demonstrate knowledge of the proper verbal order process, including "read back";
- reducing the number of times unapproved abbreviations occur in nursing documentation; and
- reducing the number of illegible entries of medications that occur in nursing documentation.[49]

XVII.c.4. Standardized medication safety event measurements should be incorporated into performance improvement reviews. Measurements should include, but not be limited to,
- event definitions,
- event severity classification,
- event preventability criteria,
- control event capture,
- standardized recording tools, and
- rater training and ongoing inter-rater reliability evaluation.[214]

XVII.d. Quality improvement activities (eg, root cause analysis) should be used to investigate and document all actual or potential (eg, near miss) medication errors across the medication use process.

Quality improvement activities are expectations for all professionals within the health care team.[215] Documenting such activities fulfills regulatory and accreditation requirements.

XVII.e. Health care organizations should adopt a standardized approach to reporting (eg, incident report, hotline) errors and near misses related to medications and medication administration equipment.

Standardization helps to achieve consistency in reporting.

XVII.e.1. Perioperative team members should actively participate in error reporting regardless of where the error originates within the medication use process and regardless of whether patient harm results from the error.

Information from near-miss and medication error reports can be used to identify trends, develop new safety measures, and educate members of the perioperative team to increase awareness of and improve compliance with safe medication practices.

XVII.e.2. Health care organizations should participate in a national medication error reporting program.

Participation in national medication error programs (eg, ISMP National Medication Error Reporting Program) and state reporting programs will enhance the data available to identify trends for medication errors in perioperative settings. The information collected by the national medication error programs is used to educate regulatory agencies, professional organizations, front-line practitioners, consumers, and the pharmaceutical industry about preventing future adverse drug events.[1]

XVII.e.3. Health care organizations should have a process to monitor and report incidents of equipment malfunction that lead to patient harm as outlined in the Safe Medical Devices Act of 1990.[216]

XVII.e.4. Health care organizations should have a process to report serious adverse events, product quality problems, or product use errors to the ISMP and FDA through the MedWatch web site.

The data from these reports are used to maintain safety surveillance of products associated with medication administration and may be used to prompt a modification in use or design of the product to improve its safety profile and patient safety.[51]

XVII.f. Perioperative team members who serve on their organization's quality improvement committee or root cause analysis group should be included when analyzing findings from medication error reports and planning corrective interventions.

XVII.f.1. When a medication error or near-miss occurs, perioperative administrators should collaborate with the health care organization's quality improvement committee members regarding disclosure of medication errors to patients and their designated support persons.

Glossary

Compounding: The process of combining two or more different medications. Compounding does not include mixing, reconstituting, or similar acts that are performed in accordance with the directions contained on approved labeling that is provided by the product's manufacturer or other manufacturer directions consistent with that labeling.

Multidose vial: Defined by the Safe Injection Practices Coalition (SIPC) as a bottle of injectable medication that contains more than one dose of medication and has a label to indicate approval by the US Food and Drug Administration for use on more than one person.

Par level: Minimum inventory level that has been identified to match the volume typically used within a specified time frame to promote rotation of stock and avoid outdates.

References

1. Wanzer LJ, Hicks RW, Goeckner B, Cole L. A focused review: perioperative safe medication use. *Perioper Nurs Clin.* 2008;3(4):305-316. doi:10.1016/j.cpen.2008.08.001.
2. Wanzer LJ, Hicks RW. Medication safety within the perioperative environment. *Annu Rev Nurs Res.* 2006;24:127-155.
3. Beyea S. Safe medication practices in perioperative settings. *Perioper Nurs Clin.* 2006;1(3):283-288.
4. Hicks RW, Becker SC, Cousins DD. *MEDMARX Data Report: A Chartbook of Medication Error Findings from the Perioperative Settings from 1998-2005.* Rockville, MD: US Center for the Advancement of Patient Safety; 2006.
5. ASHP guidelines on preventing medication errors in hospitals. In: *Best Practices for Hospital & Health-System Pharmacy: Position & Guidance Documents of ASHP.* Bethesda, MD: American Society of Health-System Pharmacists; 2009:178-186.
6. Kohn LT, Corrigan JM, Donaldson MS, eds. *To Err Is Human: Building a Safer Health System.* Washington, DC: National Academy Press; 1999. http://www.nap.edu/openbook.php?record_id=9728. Accessed September 27, 2011.
7. Sentinel event data: event type by year, 1995-third quarter 2010. The Joint Commission. http://www.jointcommission.org/se_data_event_type_by_year_/. Accessed September 9, 2011.
8. Macdonald M. Patient safety: examining the adequacy of the 5 rights of medication administration. *Clin Nurse Spec.* 2010;24(4):196-201. doi:10.1097/NUR.0b013e3181e3605f.
9. Hughes RG. Tools and strategies for quality improvement and patient safety. In: Hughes RG, Smith JD, Jones RA, eds. *Patient Safety and Quality: An Evidence-Based Handbook for Nurses; volume 3.* Rockville, MD: Agency for Healthcare Research and Quality; 2008:22-43.
10. ASHP guidelines: minimum standard for pharmaceutical services in ambulatory care. In: *Best Practices for Hospital & Health-System Pharmacy: Position & Guidance Documents of ASHP.* Bethesda, MD: American Society of Health-System Pharmacists; 2009:392-400.
11. ASHP guidelines: minimum standard for pharmacies in hospitals. In: *Best Practices for Hospital & Health-System Pharmacy: Position & Guidance Documents of ASHP.* Bethesda, MD: American Society of Health-System Pharmacists; 2009:401-406.
12. ASHP guidelines on medication cost management strategies for hospitals and health systems. In: *Best Practices for Hospital & Health-System Pharmacy: Position & Guidance Documents of ASHP.* Bethesda, MD: American Society of Health-System Pharmacists; 2009:314-328.
13. American Hospital Association, Health Research & Educational Trust, Institute for Safe Medication Practices. *Pathways for Medication Safety: Leading a Strategic Planning Effort.* Chicago, IL: Health Research and Educational Trust; 2002.
14. Mazzocco K, Petitti DB, Fong KT, et al. Surgical team behaviors and patient outcomes. *Am J Surg.* 2009;197(5):678-685. doi:10.1016/j.amjsurg.2008.03.002.
15. Neily J, Mills PD, Young-Xu Y, et al. Association between implementation of a medical team training program and surgical mortality. *JAMA.* 2010;304(15):1693-1700. doi:10.1001/jama.2010.1506.
16. Brady AM, Malone AM, Fleming S. A literature review of the individual and systems factors that contribute to medication errors in nursing practice. *J Nurs Manag.* 2009;17(6):679-697. doi:10.1111/j.1365-2834.2009.00995.x.
17. Institute of Medicine. *Preventing Medication Errors: The Quality Chasm Series.* Washington, DC: The

18. Hicks RW, Becker SC, Windle PE, Krenzischek DA. Medication errors in the PACU. *J Perianesth Nurs.* 2007;22(6):413-419. doi:10.1016/j.jopan.2007.08.002.

19. ASHP statement on standards-based pharmacy practice in hospitals and health system. In: *Best Practices for Hospital & Health-System Pharmacy: Position & Guidance Documents of ASHP.* Bethesda, MD: American Society of Health-System Pharmacists; 2009:312-313.

20. Bassi J, Lau F, Bardal S. Use of information technology in medication reconciliation: a scoping review. *Ann Pharmacother.* 2010;44(5):885-897. doi:10.1345/aph.1M699.

21. *Guidance on the Interdisciplinary Safe Use of Automated Dispensing Cabinets.* Horsham, PA: Institute for Safe Medication Practices; 2008. http://www.ismp.org/tools/guidelines/ADC_Guidelines_Final.pdf. Accessed September 27, 2011.

22. Medication management. In: *Comprehensive Accreditation Manual for Hospitals.* E-dition v3.6.0.0. Oakbrook Terrace, IL: Joint Commission Resources; 2011.

23. Agrawal A, Wu WY. National patient safety goals. Reducing medication errors and improving systems reliability using an electronic medication reconciliation system. *Joint Comm J Qual Patient Saf.* 2009;35(2):106-114.

24. Schnipper JL, Hamann C, Ndumele CD, et al. Effect of an electronic medication reconciliation application and process redesign on potential adverse drug events: a cluster-randomized trial. *Arch Intern Med.* 2009;169(8):771-780. doi:10.1001/archinternmed.2009.51.

25. Eichhorn JH. APSF hosts medication safety conference: consensus group defines challenges and opportunities for improved practice. *APSF Newsletter.* 2010;25(1):1, 3-8.

26. Medication safety. *Healthcare Risk Control.* 2011;4(Pharmacy and Medications 1):1-32.

27. Poon EG, Keohane CA, Yoon CS, et al. Effect of barcode technology on the safety of medication administration. *N Engl J Med.* 2010;362(18):1698-1707. doi:10.1056/NEJMsa0907115.

28. Cochran GL, Jones KJ, Brockman J, Skinner A, Hicks RW. USP medical safety forum. Errors prevented by and associated with bar-code medication administration systems. *Joint Comm J Qual Patient Saf.* 2007;33(5):293-301.

29. Paparella S. Drug information resources: essential but may be error prone. *J Emerg Nurs.* 2010;36(3):250-252. doi:10.1016/j.jen.2010.01.012.

30. Appendix L: Guidance for surveyors: Ambulatory surgical centers [Rev. 56, 12-30-09]. In: *State Operations Manual.* Washington, DC: Centers for Medicare & Medicaid Services; 2009

31. *Guidance for Industry: Q8(R2) Pharmaceutical Development.* Rev. 2. Washington, DC: Food and Drug Administration; 2009.

32. Blossom D, Noble-Wang J, Su J, et al. Multistate outbreak of *Serratia marcescens* bloodstream infections caused by contamination of prefilled heparin and isotonic sodium chloride solution syringes. *Arch Intern Med.* 2009;169(18):1705-1711. doi:10.1001/archinternmed.2009.290.

33. Sterile water should not be given "freely." *Pa Patient Saf Advis.* 2008;5(2):53-56.

34. *ISMP's List of Confused Drug Names.* Horsham, PA: Institute for Safe Medication Practices; 2009.

35. FDA Name Differentiation Project. http://www.fda.gov/Drugs/DrugSafety/MedicationErrors/ucm164587.htm. Updated June 18, 2009. Accessed September 27, 2011.

36. Kelly WN, Grissinger M, Shaw Phillips M. Look-alike drug name errors: is enhanced lettering the answer? *Patient Saf Qual Healthc.* 2010;July/August:22-26.

37. Preventing misconnections of lines and cables. *Health Devices.* 2006;35(3):81-95.

38. Beyea SC, Simmons D, Hicks RW. Caution: tubing misconnections can be deadly. *AORN J.* 2007;85(3):633-635.

39. Guenter P, Hicks RW, Simmons D, et al. Enteral feeding misconnections: a consortium position statement. *Jt Comm J Qual Patient Saf.* 2008;34(5):285-292, 245.

40. Simmons D, Graves K. Tubing misconnections—a systems failure with human factors: lessons for nursing practice. *Urol Nurs.* 2008;28(6):460-464.

41. Simmons D, Phillips MS, Grissinger M, Becker SC; USP Safe Medication Use Expert Committee. Error-avoidance recommendations for tubing misconnections when using Luer-tip connectors: a statement by the USP Safe Medication Use Expert Committee. *Jt Comm J Qual Patient Saf.* 2008;34(5):293-6, 245.

42. *Guideline for Industry: Quality of Biotechnological Products: Stability Testing of Biotechnological/Biological Products.* Food and Drug Administration; 1996.

43. ASHP technical assistance bulletin on hospital drug distribution and control. *Am J Hosp Pharm.* 1980;37:1097-1103.

44. Drug diversion in healthcare: risks and prevention. *Risk Management Reporter.* 2007;26(5):1, 3-10.

45. Controlled Substance Act, 21 USC §801-971 (2006).

46. Hicks RW, Becker SC, Cousins DD, eds. *MEDMARX Data Report: A Report on the Relationship of Drug Names and Medication Errors in Response to the Institute of Medicine's Call for Action.* Rockville, MD: Center for the Advancement of Patient Safety, US Pharmacopeia; 2008.

47. Westbrook JI, Woods A, Rob MI, Dunsmuir WT, Day RO. Association of interruptions with an increased risk and severity of medication administration errors. *Arch Intern Med.* 2010;170(8):683-690. doi:10.1001/archinternmed.2010.65.

48. Bryson EO, Silverstein JH. Addiction and substance abuse in anesthesiology. *Anesthesiology.* 2008;109(5):905-917. doi:10.1097/ALN.0b013e3181895bc1.

49. Burden N. A comprehensive medication management program in the ambulatory surgery setting. *J Perianesth Nurs.* 2007;22(1):40-46. doi:10.1016/j.jopan.2006.12.002.

50. *Infusing Patients Safely: Priority Issues From the AAMI/FDA Infusion Device Summit.* Arlington, VA: Association for the Advancement of Medical Instrumentation; 2010. http://www.aami.org/infusionsummit/AAMI_FDA_Summit_Report.pdf. Accessed September 28, 2011.

51. *FDA's Safe Use Initiative: Collaborating to Reduce Preventable Harm from Medications.* Silver Spring, MD: Food and Drug Administration; 2009. http://www.fda.gov/downloads/Drugs/DrugSafety/UCM188961.pdf. Accessed September 30, 2011.

52. Labeling Issuance, 21 CFR §211.125 (2010). http://edocket.access.gpo.gov/cfr_2005/aprqtr/pdf/21cfr211.130.pdf. Accessed September 30, 2011.

53. Garnerin P, Perneger T, Chopard P, et al. Drug selection errors in relation to medication labels: a simulation study. *Anaesthesia.* 2007;62(11):1090-1094. doi:10.1111/j.1365-2044.2007.05198.x.

54. Santell JP, Cousins DD. Medication errors related to product names. *Jt Comm J Qual Patient Saf.* 2005;31(11):649-654.

55. McCoy LK. Look-alike, sound-alike drugs review: include look-alike packaging as an additional safety check. *Jt Comm J Qual Patient Saf.* 2005;31(1):47-53.

56. Gabriele S. The role of typography in differentiating look-alike/sound-alike drug names. *Healthc Q.* 2006;9 Spec No:88-95.

57. High-alert medications. *Healthc Risk Control.* 2004;4(Pharmacy and Medications 1.4):1-7.

58. Shultz J, Davies JM, Caird J, Chisholm S, Ruggles K, Puls R. Standardizing anesthesia medication drawers using human factors and quality assurance methods. *Can J Anaesth.* 2010;57(5):490-499. doi:10.1007/s12630-010-9274-8.

59. Reason J. Safety in the operating theatre—part 2: human error and organisational failure. *Qual Saf Health Care.* 2005;14(1):56-60.

60. Girard NJ. Unexplained apnea during surgery. *AORN J.* 2008;87(6):1288, 1216.

61. Paparella S. Fatal confusion with epinephrine: 1:1,000 is not 1:10,000. *J Emerg Nurs.* 2005;31(1):86-88. doi:10.1016/j.jen.2004.09.016.

62. Bullock J, Jordan D, Gawlinski A, Henneman EA. Standardizing IV infusion medication concentrations to reduce variability in medication errors. *Crit Care Nurs Clin North Am.* 2006;18(4):515-521. doi:10.1016/j.ccell.2006.08.008.

63. Smetzer JL, Cohen MR. Preventing drug administration errors. In: Cohen MR, ed. *Medication Errors.* 2nd ed. Washington, DC: American Pharmacists Association; 2007:235-274.

64. Paparella S. The risks associated with the use of multidose vials. *J Emerg Nurs.* 2006;32(5):428-430. doi:10.1016/j.jen.2006.05.016.

65. Perz JF, Thompson ND, Schaefer MK, Patel PR. US outbreak investigations highlight the need for safe injection practices and basic infection control. *Clin Liver Dis.* 2010;14(1):137-151. doi:10.1016/j.cld.2009.11.004.

66. Pugliese G, Gosnell C, Bartley JM, Robinson S. Injection practices among clinicians in United States health care settings. *Am J Infect Control.* 2010;38(10):789-798. doi:10.1016/j.ajic.2010.09.003.

67. Recommended practices for product selection in perioperative practice settings. In: *Perioperative Standards and Recommended Practices.* Denver, CO: AORN, Inc; 2011: 191-200.

68. Dangers associated with shared multidose vials. *Pa Patient Saf Advis.* 2008;5(2):68.

69. Pharmaceutical waste disposal practices get legal evil eye. *Environ Care Lead.* 2010;15(3):1, 5-6.

70. Dolan SA, Felizardo G, Barnes S, et al. APIC position paper: safe injection, infusion, and medication vial practices in health care. *Am J Infect Control.* 2010;38(3):167-172. doi:10.1016/j.ajic.2010.01.001.

71. Vonberg R, Gastmeier P. Hospital-acquired infections related to contaminated substances. *J Hosp Infect.* 2007;65(1):15-23.

72. Kushakovskyy V. Acetone on the labour ward: an accident waiting to happen. *Int J Obstet Anesth.* 2008;17(3):285-286. doi:10.1016/j.ijoa.2008.02.002.

73. Smędra-Kaźmirska A, Żydek L, Barzdo M, Machała W, Berent J. Accidental intravenous injection of formalin. *Anaesthesiol Intensive Ther.* 2009;XLI(3):133-135.

74. Feigal DW Jr, Woodock J. FDA public health advisory: potential for injury from medical gas misconnections of cryogenic vessels [medical device safety: alerts and notices]. Silver Spring, MD: US Food and Drug Administration; July 20, 2001. http://www.fda.gov/MedicalDevices/Safety/AlertsandNotices/PublicHealthNotifications/ucm062189.htm. Accessed September 28, 2011.

75. Center for Drug Evaluation and Research, Food and Drug Administration. Compressed medical gases guideline. http://www.fda.gov/Drugs/GuidanceComplianceRegulatoryInformation/Guidances/ucm124716.htm. Updated February 1989. Accessed September 28, 2011.

76. Medical gas errors. *Practitioners' Reporting News.* June 19, 2001.

77. Greenberg CC, Regenbogen SE, Studdert DM, et al. Patterns of communication breakdowns resulting in injury to surgical patients. *J Am Coll Surg.* 2007;204(4):533-540. doi:10.1016/j.jamcollsurg.2007.01.010.

78. Engum SA, Breckler FD. An evaluation of medication errors—the pediatric surgical service experience. *J Pediatr Surg.* 2008;43(2):348-352. doi:10.1016/j.jpedsurg.2007.10.042.

79. Smith HS, Lesar TS. Analgesic prescribing errors and associated medication characteristics. *J Pain.* 2011;12(1):29-40. doi:10.1016/j.jpain.2010.04.007.

80. Metzger J, Welebob E, Bates DW, Lipsitz S, Classen DC. Mixed results in the safety performance of computerized physician order entry. *Health Aff (Millwood).* 2010;29(4):655-663.

81. Picone DM, Titler MG, Dochterman J, et al. Predictors of medication errors among elderly hospitalized patients. *Am J Med Qual.* 2008;23(2):115-127. doi:10.1177/1062860607313143.

82. Grissinger MC, Hicks RW, Keroack MA, Marella WM, Vaida AJ. Harmful medication errors involving unfractionated and low-molecular-weight heparin in three patient safety reporting programs. *Jt Comm J Qual Patient Saf.* 2010;36(5):195-202.

83. Fick DM, Cooper JW, Wade WE, Waller JL, Maclean JR, Beers MH. Updating the Beers criteria for potentially inappropriate medication use in older adults: results of a US consensus panel of experts. *Arch Intern Med.* 2003;163(22):2716-2724. doi:10.1001/archinte.163.22.2716.

84. Stefanacci RG, Cavallaro E, Beers MH, Fick DM. Developing explicit positive Beers criteria for preferred central nervous system medications in older adults. *Consult Pharm.* 2009;24(8):601-610.

85. Kaur S, Mitchell G, Vitetta L, Roberts MS. Interventions that can reduce inappropriate prescribing in the elderly: a systematic review. *Drugs Aging.* 2009;26(12):1013-1028. doi:10.2165/11318890-000000000-00000;10.2165/11318890-000000000-00000.

86. Bazzano ATF, Mangione-Smith R, Schonlau M, Suttorp MJ, Brook RH. Off-label prescribing to children in the United States outpatient setting. *Acad Pediatr.* 2009;9(2):81-88.

87. Woo T. Pharmacology of cough and cold medicines. *J Pediatr Health Care.* 2008;22(2):73-82. doi:10.1016/j.pedhc.2007.12.007.

88. Hamilton T. "Standing orders" in hospitals—revisions to S&C memoranda [memorandum]. Baltimore, MD: Department of Health & Human Services; 2008. Ref: S&C-09-10.

89. Broussard M, Bass PF III, Arnold CL, McLarty JW, Bocchini JA Jr. Preprinted order sets as a safety intervention in pediatric sedation. *J Pediatr.* 2009;154(6):865-868. doi:10.1016/j.jpeds.2008.12.022.

90. Straube BM. Letter to David T. Tayloe Jr. [written communication]. Baltimore, MD: Department of Health & Human Services; 2010. http://practice.aap.org/public/Straube%20Letter%20to%20Tayloe.PDF. Accessed September 30, 2011.

91. Dawson A, Orsini MJ, Cooper MR, Wollenburg K. Medication safety—reliability of preference cards. *AORN J.* 2005;82(3):399-414.

92. Medicare and Medicaid programs; hospital conditions of participation: requirements for history and physical examinations; authentication of verbal orders; securing medications; and postanesthesia evaluations. Final rule. *Fed Regist.* 2006;71(227):68671-68695. http://edocket.access.gpo.gov/2006/pdf/E6-19957.pdf. Accessed September 30, 2011.

93. Recommendations to reduce medication errors associated with verbal medication orders and prescriptions. National Coordinating Council for Medication Error Reporting and Prevention. http://www.nccmerp.org/council/council2001-02-20.html. Published February 20, 2001. Updated February 24, 2006. Accessed September 28, 2011.

94. Lambert BL, Dickey LW, Fisher WM, et al. Listen carefully: the risk of error in spoken medication orders. *Soc Sci Med.* 2010;70(10):1599-1608. doi:10.1016/j.socscimed.2010.01.042.

95. Wakefield DS, Brokel J, Ward MM, et al. An exploratory study measuring verbal order content and context. *Qual Saf Health Care.* 2009;18(3):169-173.

96. Wakefield DS, Wakefield BJ. Are verbal orders a threat to patient safety? *Postgrad Med J.* 2009;85(1007):460-463. doi:10.1136/qshc.2009.034041.

97. Kaushal R, Goldmann DA, Keohane CA, et al. Medication errors in paediatric outpatients. *Qual Saf Health Care.* 2010;19(6):e30. doi:10.1136/qshc.2008.031179.

98. Bates DW, Leape LL, Cullen DJ, et al. Effect of computerized physician order entry and a team intervention on prevention of serious medication errors. *JAMA.* 1998;280(15):1311-1316.

99. Computerized provider order-entry systems. *Healthcare Risk Control.* 2002;suppl A(Pharmacy and Medications 6):1-21.

100. Kaplan JM, Ancheta R, Jacobs BR. Inpatient verbal orders and the impact of computerized provider order entry. *J Pediatr.* 2006;149(4):461-467.

101. Khajouei R, Jaspers MW. The impact of CPOE medication systems' design aspects on usability, workflow and medication orders: a systematic review. *Methods Inf Med.* 2010;49(1):3-19. doi:10.3414/ME0630.

102. Ammenwerth E, Schnell-Inderst P, Machan C, Siebert U. The effect of electronic prescribing on medication errors and adverse drug events: a systematic review. *J Am Med Inform Assoc.* 2008;15(5):585-600. doi:10.1197/jamia.M2667.

103. Weber RJ. Medication reconciliation pitfalls. *AHRQ WebM&M* [serial online]. February 2010. http://www.webmm.ahrq.gov/case.aspx?caseID=213. Accessed September 28, 2011.

104. United States Pharmacopeia Convention. Committee of Revision. Pharmaceutical compounding—sterile preparations. In: *The United States Pharmacopeia.* 27th ed. Rockville, MD: United States Pharmacopeial Convention, Inc; 2009:318-354.

105. Centers for Medicare & Medicaid Services, US Department of Health and Human Services. Condition of Participation: Pharmaceutical Services. 42 CFR §482.25 (2009). http://edocket.access.gpo.gov/cfr_2010/octqtr/pdf/42cfr482.25.pdf. Revised November 27, 2006. Accessed September 12, 2011.

106. ASHP guidelines on quality assurance for pharmacy-prepared sterile products. In: *Best Practices for Hospital & Health-System Pharmacy: Position & Guidance Documents of ASHP.* Bethesda, MD: American Society of Health-System Pharmacists; 2009:71-89.

107. Hicks RW, Wanzer L, Goeckner B. Perioperative pharmacology: a framework for perioperative medication safety. *AORN J.* 2011;93(1):136-145. doi:10.1016/j.aorn.2010.08.020.

108. Standards of perioperative nursing. In: *Perioperative Standards and Recommended Practices.* Denver, CO: AORN, Inc; 2011:3-20.

109. Hicks RW, Becker SC, Cousins DD. Harmful medication errors in children: a 5-year analysis of data from the USP's MEDMARX program. *J Pediatr Nurs.* 2006;21(4):290-298. doi:10.1016/j.pedn.2006.02.002.

110. Annual Report 2009. Pennsylvania Patient Safety Authority. April 28, 2010. http://patientsafetyauthority.org/PatientSafetyAuthority/Documents/Annual_Report_2009.pdf. Accessed September 12, 2011.

111. Medication errors: significance of accurate patient weights. *Pa Patient Saf Advis.* 2009;6(1):10-15.

112. Murphy EM, Oxencis CJ, Klauck JA, Meyer DA, Zimmerman JM. Medication reconciliation at an academic medical center: implementation of a comprehensive program from admission to discharge. *Am J Health Syst Pharm.* 2009;66(23):2126-2131. doi:10.2146/ajhp080552.

113. Schwarz M, Wyskiel R. Medication reconciliation: developing and implementing a program. *Crit Care Nurs Clin North Am.* 2006;18(4):503-507. doi:10.1016/j.ccell.2006.09.003.

114. Pippins JR, Gandhi TK, Hamann C, et al. Classifying and predicting errors of inpatient medication reconciliation. *J Gen Intern Med.* 2008;23(9):1414-1422. doi:10.1007/s11606-008-0687-9.

115. Boockvar KS, Carlson LaCorte H, Giambanco V, Fridman B, Siu A. Medication reconciliation for reducing drug-discrepancy adverse events. *Am J Geriatr Pharmacother.* 2006;4(3):236-243. doi:10.1016/j.amjopharm.2006.09.003.

116. Fredericks JE, Bunting RF Jr. Implementation of a patient-friendly medication schedule to improve patient safety within a healthcare system. *J Healthc Risk Manag.* 2010;29(4):22-27. doi:10.1002/jhrm.20030.

117. Nassaralla CL, Naessens JM, Hunt VL, et al. Medication reconciliation in ambulatory care: attempts at improvement. *Qual Saf Health Care.* 2009;18(5):402-407. doi:10.1136/qshc.2007.024513.

118. Gizzi LA, Slain D, Hare JT, Sager R, Briggs F III, Palmer CH. Assessment of a safety enhancement to the hospital medication reconciliation process for elderly patients. *Am J Geriatr Pharmacother.* 2010;8(2):127-135. doi:10.1016/j.amjopharm.2010.03.004.

119. Frolich MA, Giannotti A, Modell JH. Opioid overdose in a patient using a fentanyl patch during treatment with a warming blanket. *Anesth Analg.* 2001;93(3):647-648.

120. Wrenn K. The hazards of defibrillation through nitroglycerin patches. *Ann Emerg Med.* 1990;19(11):1327-1328.

121. Public health advisory: risk of burns during MRI scans from transdermal drug patches with metallic backings. US Food and Drug Administration. http://www.fda.gov/Drugs/DrugSafety/PostmarketDrugSafetyInformationforPatientsandProviders/DrugSafetyInformationforHeathcareProfessionals/PublicHealthAdvisories/ucm111313.htm. Published March 5, 2009. Updated June 23, 2010. Accessed September 30, 2011.

122. Sullivan C, Gleason KM, Rooney D, Groszek JM, Barnard C. Medication reconciliation in the acute care setting: opportunity and challenge for nursing. *J Nurs Care Qual.* 2005;20(2):95-98.

123. Warholak TL, McCulloch M, Baumgart A, Smith M, Fink W, Fritz W. An exploratory comparison of medication lists at hospital admission with

administrative database records. *J Manag Care Pharm.* 2009;15(9):751-758.

124. Kuhn MA. Herbal remedies: drug-herb interactions. *Crit Care Nurse.* 2002;22(2):22-35.

125. King AR, Russett FS, Generali JA, Grauer DW. Evaluation and implications of natural product use in preoperative patients: a retrospective review. *BMC Complement Altern Med.* 2009;9:38. doi:10.1186/1472-6882-9-38.

126. O'Riordan JM, Margey RJ, Blake G, O'Connell PR. Antiplatelet agents in the perioperative period. *Arch Surg.* 2009;144(1):69-76. doi:10.1001/archsurg.144.1.69.

127. Farooq M, Kirke C, Foley K. Documentation of drug allergy on drug chart in patients presenting for surgery. *Ir J Med Sci.* 2008;177(3):243-245. doi:10.1007/s11845-008-0166-7.

128. Medication errors associated with documented allergies. *Pa Patient Saf Advis.* 2008;5(3):75-80.

129. Lehne RA. Application of pharmacology in nursing practice. In: *Pharmacology for Nursing Care.* 7th ed. St Louis, MO: Saunders/Elsevier; 2010:5-14.

130. Payne CH, Smith CR, Newkirk LE, Hicks RW. Pediatric medication errors in the postanesthesia care unit: analysis of MEDMARX data. *AORN J.* 2007;85(4):731-744. doi:10.1016/S0001-2092(07)60147-1.

131. Chuo J, Hicks RW. Computer-related medication errors in neonatal intensive care units. *Clin Perinatol.* 2008;35(1):119-139. doi:10.1016/j.clp.2007.11.005.

132. Kfuri TA, Morlock L, Hicks RW, Shore AD. Medication errors in obstetrics. *Clin Perinatol.* 2008;35(1):101-117. doi:10.1016/j.clp.2007.11.015.

133. Ozkan S, Kocaman G, Ozturk C, Seren S. Frequency of pediatric medication administration errors and contributing factors. *J Nurs Care Qual.* 2011;26(2):136-143. doi:10.1097/NCQ.0b013e3182031006.

134. <1066> Physical environments that promote safe medication use. *USP Revision Bull.* October 2010:1-6.

135. ISMP Guidelines for Standard Order Sets. Institute for Safe Medication Practices. http://www.ismp.org/tools/guidelines/StandardOrderSets.pdf. Published 2010. Accessed September 28, 2011.

136. Hicks RW, Sikirica V, Nelson W, Schein JR, Cousins DD. Medication errors involving patient-controlled analgesia. *Am J Health Syst Pharm.* 2008;65(5):429-440. doi:10.2146/ajhp070194.

137. Biron AD, Loiselle CG, Lavoie-Tremblay M. Work interruptions and their contribution to medication administration errors: an evidence review. *Worldviews Evid Based Nurs.* 2009;6(2):70-86. doi:10.1111/j.1741-6787.2009.00151.x.

138. Biron AD, Lavoie-Tremblay M, Loiselle CG. Characteristics of work interruptions during medication administration. *J Nurs Scholarsh.* 2009;41(4):330-336. doi:10.1111/j.1547-5069.2009.01300.x.

139. Smetzer J, Baker C, Byrne FD, Cohen MR. Shaping systems for better behavioral choices: lessons learned from a fatal medication error. *Jt Comm J Qual Patient Saf.* 2010;36(4):152-163.

140. Best practices for safe medication administration. *AORN J.* 2006;84(Suppl 1):S45-S56.

141. *Schroeder v. Northwest Community Hospital,* NE 2d, 2006 WL 3615559 (Ill App, December 12, 2006).

142. Hicks RW, Becker SC, Jackson DG. Understanding medication errors: discussion of a case involving a urinary catheter implicated in a wrong route error. *Urol Nurs.* 2008;28(6):454-459.

143. Goodman EJ, Haas AJ, Kantor GS. Inadvertent administration of magnesium sulfate through the epidural catheter: report and analysis of a drug error. *Int J Obstet Anesth.* 2006;15(1):63-67. doi:10.1016/j.ijoa.2005.06.009.

144. Otoya M. Heparin safety in the neonatal intensive care unit: are we learning from mistakes of others? *Newborn Infant Nurs Rev.* 2009;9(1):53-61. doi:10.1053/j.nainr.2008.12.007.

145. Medication errors with the dosing of insulin: problems across the continuum. *Pa Patient Saf Advis.* 2010;7(1):9-17.

146. Vancomycin [package insert]. Lake Forest, IL: Akorn-Strides, LLC; July 2009.

147. AORN guidance statement: Sharps injury prevention in the perioperative setting. In: *Perioperative Standards and Recommended Practices.* Denver, CO: AORN, Inc; 2011:639-644.

148. Lee ACW, Leung M, So KT. Managing patients with identical names in the same ward. *Int J Health Care Qual Assur.* 2005;18(1):15-23.

149. Seitz IA, Tojo D, Schechter LS. Anatomy of a medication error: inadvertent subcutaneous injection of neosynephrine during nasal surgery. *Plast Reconstr Surg.* 2010;125(3):113e-114e. doi:10.1097/PRS.0b013e3181cb68f9.

150. Jennings J, Foster J. Medication safety: just a label away. *AORN J.* 2007;86(4):618-625. doi:10.1016/j.aorn.2007.04.003.

151. Haas D. In memory of Ben. *Risk Management Reports.* 1998;12.

152. Cohen MR, Smetzer JL. Unlabeled containers lead to patient's death. *Jt Comm J Qual Patient Saf.* 2005;31(7):414-417.

153. Case update: epinephrine death in Florida. *ISMP Medication Safety Alert!.* December 4, 1996.

154. Hass D. Moving beyond blame to create an environment that rewards reporting. In: Youngberg BJ, Hatlie MJ, eds. *Patient Safety Handbook.* Sudbury, MA: Jones and Bartlett Publishers; 2004:415-421.

155. Loud wake-up call: Unlabeled containers lead to patient's death. *ISMP Medication Safety Alert!.* December 2, 2004.

156. Fatal outcome after inadvertent injection of topical EPINEPHrine. *ISMP Medication Safety Alert!.* March 26, 2009.

157. McCormick CG, Henningfield JE, Haddox JD, et al. Case histories in pharmaceutical risk management. *Drug Alcohol Depend.* 2009;105(Suppl 1):S42-S55. doi:10.1016/j.drugalcdep.2009.08.003.

158. Devlin JW, Mallow-Corbett S, Riker RR. Adverse drug events associated with the use of analgesics, sedatives, and antipsychotics in the intensive care unit. *Crit Care Med.* 2010;38(Suppl 6):S231-S243. doi:10.1097/CCM.0b013e3181de125a.

159. Kripalani S, Jackson AT, Schnipper JL, Coleman EA. Promoting effective transitions of care at hospital discharge: a review of key issues for hospitalists. *J Hosp Med.* 2007;2(5):314-323. doi:10.1002/jhm.228.

160. Zavala S, Shaffer C. Do patients understand discharge instructions? *J Emerg Nurs.* In press. doi:10.1016/j.jen.2009.11.008.

161. Joint Commission. MM.04.01.01: Medication orders are clear and accurate. In: *Comprehensive Accreditation Manual for Hospitals.* E-edition v3.6.0.0. Oakbrook Terrace, IL: Joint Commission Resources; 2011.

162. Varkey P, Cunningham J, O'Meara J, Bonacci R, Desai N, Sheeler R. Multidisciplinary approach to inpatient medication reconciliation in an academic setting. *Am J Health Syst Pharm.* 2007;64(8):850-854. doi:10.2146/ajhp060314.

163. Unroe KT, Pfeiffenberger T, Riegelhaupt S, Jastrzembski J, Lokhnygina Y, Colon-Emeric C. Inpatient medication reconciliation at admission and discharge: A retrospective cohort study of age and other risk factors for medication discrepancies. *Am J Geriatr Pharmacother.* 2010;8(2):115-126. doi:10.1016/j.amjopharm.2010.04.002.

164. Davis TC, Federman AD, Bass PF 3rd, et al. Improving patient understanding of prescription drug label instructions. *J Gen Intern Med.* 2009;24(1):57-62. doi:10.1007/s11606-008-0833-4.

165. Kramer JS, Hopkins PJ, Rosendale JC, et al. Implementation of an electronic system for medication reconciliation. *Am J Health Syst Pharm.* 2007;64(4):404-422. doi:10.2146/ajhp060506.

166. Schweiger MJ, Chambers CE, Davidson CJ, et al. Prevention of contrast induced nephropathy: recommendations for the high risk patient undergoing cardiovascular procedures. *Catheter Cardiovasc Interv.* 2007;69(1):135-140. doi:10.1002/ccd.20964.

167. Glucophage, Glucophage XR [package insert]. Princeton, NJ: Bristol-Myers Squibb Company; January 2009.

168. Bell CM, Bajcar J, Bierman AS, Li P, Mamdani MM, Urbach DR. Potentially unintended discontinuation of long-term medication use after elective surgical procedures. *Arch Intern Med.* 2006;166(22):2525-2531. doi:10.1001/archinte.166.22.2525.

169. Persell SD, Osborn CY, Richard R, Skripkauskas S, Wolf MS. Limited health literacy is a barrier to medication reconciliation in ambulatory care. *J Gen Intern Med.* 2007;22(11):1523-1526. doi:10.1007/s11606-007-0334-x.

170. Wolf MS, Davis TC, Bass PF, et al. Improving prescription drug warnings to promote patient comprehension. *Arch Intern Med.* 2010;170(1):50-56. doi:10.1001/archinternmed.2009.454.

171. National Patient Safety Agency. *Safety in Doses: Improving the Use of Medicines in the NHS.* London, England: National Health Service; 2009. http://www.nrls.npsa.nhs.uk/resources/?entryid45=61625. Accessed September 29, 2011.

172. Betz R. Letter to Margaret Hamburg [written communication]. Arlington, VA: American Association of Eye and Ear Centers of Excellence. January 11, 2010.

173. Hazard Communication, 29 CFR §1910.1200 (2010). http://www.osha.gov/pls/oshaweb/owadisp.show_document?p_table=standards&p_id=10099. Accessed September 29, 2011.

174. National Institute for Occupational Safety and Health. *Preventing Occupational Exposure to Antineoplastic and Other Hazardous Drugs in Health Care Settings.* Cincinnati, OH: US Department of Health and Human Services; 2004. NIOSH Alert; publication No. 2004-165.

175. Occupational Safety and Health Administration. Controlling occupational exposure to hazardous drugs. In: *OSHA Technical Manual.* Washington, DC: US Department of Labor; 1999. http://www.osha.gov/dts/osta/otm/otm_vi/otm_vi_2.html. Accessed September 29, 2011.

176. Huber C. The safe handling of hazardous drugs. *Am J Nurs.* 2010;110(10):61-63. doi:10.1097/01.NAJ.0000389679.57273.c1.

177. Hazardous spills: the safe handling of hazardous drugs. *Pa Patient Saf Advis.* 2008;5(3):96-99.

178. ASHP guidelines on handling hazardous drugs. In: *Best Practices for Hospital & Health-System Pharmacy: Position & Guidance Documents of ASHP.* Bethesda, MD: American Society of Health-System Pharmacists; 2009:49-68.

179. *ASTM D6978-05 Standard Practice for Assessment of Resistance of Medical Gloves to Permeation by Chemotherapy Drugs.* West Conshohocken, PA: ASTM International; 2005.

180. Lehne RA. Anticancer drugs I: cytotoxic agents. In: *Pharmacology for Nursing Care.* 7th ed. St Louis, MO: Saunders/Elsevier; 2010: 1181-1196.

181. *Unused Pharmaceuticals in the Health Care Industry: Interim Report.* Washington, DC: Environmental Protection Agency; 2008. http://water.epa.gov/scitech/swguidance/ppcp/upload/2010_1_11_ppcp_hcioutreach.pdf. Accessed September 29, 2011.

182. Solid Waste Disposal Act (Resource Conservation and Recovery Act): as amended through P.L. 107–377, 42 USC §6901–6992k (2002). http://epw.senate.gov/rcra.pdf. Accessed September 29, 2011.

183. Managing pharmaceutical waste. *Healthcare Hazard Control.* 2005;(Waste Management 7):1-9.

184. Federal Water Pollution Control Act (Clean Water Act): as amended through P.L. 107–303, November 27, 2002, 33 USC §1251-1387 (2002). http://epw.senate.gov/water.pdf. Accessed September 29, 2011.

185. Santell JP, Kowiatek JG, Weber RJ, Hicks RW, Sirio CA. Medication errors resulting from computer entry by nonprescribers. *Am J Health Syst Pharm.* 2009;66(9):843-853. doi:10.2146/ajhp080208.

186. Hicks RW, Becker SC. An overview of intravenous-related medication administration errors as reported to MEDMARX, a national medication error-reporting program. *J Infus Nurs.* 2006;29(1):20-27.

187. Lafata JE, Simpkins J, Kaatz S, et al. What do medical records tell us about potentially harmful co-prescribing? *Jt Comm J Qual Patient Saf.* 2007;33(7):395-400.

188. Brunetti L, Santell JP, Hicks RW. The impact of abbreviations on patient safety. *Jt Comm J Qual Patient Saf.* 2007;33(9):576-583.

189. Medical abbreviations. *Healthcare Risk Control.* 2010;2(Medical Records 2):1-9.

190. Petersen C. *Perioperative Nursing Data Set.* 3rd ed. Denver, CO: AORN, Inc;2011.

191. Recommended practices for transfer of patient care information. In: *Perioperative Standards and Recommended Practices.* Denver, CO: AORN, Inc; 2011: 381-387.

192. Paparella S. Choosing the right strategy for medication error prevention—part II. *J Emerg Nurs.* 2008;34(3):238-240. doi:10.1016/j.jen.2008.01.011.

193. Bloodborne Pathogens, 29 CFR §1910.1030 (2010). http://www.osha.gov/pls/oshaweb/owadisp.show_document?p_table=standards&p_id=10051. Accessed September 29, 2011.

194. *Preventing Needlestick Injuries in Health Care Settings* [Publication No. 2000 108]. Morgantown, WV: National Institute for Occupational Safety and Health; 1999.

195. Smith DS, Haig K. Reduction of adverse drug events and medication errors in a community hospital setting. *Nurs Clin North Am.* 2005;40(1):25-32. doi:10.1016/j.cnur.2004.09.014.

196. Dennison RD. Creating an organizational culture for medication safety. *Nurs Clin North Am.* 2005;40(1):1-23. doi:10.1016/j.cnur.2004.10.001.

197. Elganzouri ES, Standish CA, Androwich I. Medication administration time study (MATS): nursing staff performance of medication administration. *J Nurs Adm.* 2009;39(5):204-210. doi:10.1097/NNA.0b013e3181a23d6d.

198. Gray JE, Suresh G, Ursprung R, et al. Patient misidentification in the neonatal intensive care unit: quantification of risk. *Pediatrics.* 2006;117(1):e43-e47.

199. Koppel R, Wetterneck T, Telles JL, Karsh BT. Workarounds to barcode medication administration systems: their occurrences, causes, and threats to patient safety. *J Am Med Inform Assoc.* 2008;15(4):408-423. doi:10.1197/jamia.M2616.

200. Chang YK, Mark BA. Antecedents of severe and nonsevere medication errors. *J Nurs Scholarsh.* 2009;41(1):70-78. doi:10.1111/j.1547-5069.2009.01253.x.

201. Potylycki MJ, Kimmel SR, Ritter M, et al. Nonpunitive medication error reporting: 3-year findings from one hospital's primum non nocere initiative. *J Nurs Adm.* 2006;36(7-8):370-376.

202. Parshuram CS, To T, Seto W, Trope A, Koren G, Laupacis A. Systematic evaluation of errors occurring during the preparation of intravenous medication. *CMAJ.* 2008;178(1):42-48. doi:10.1503/cmaj.061743.

203. Wright MC, Phillips-Bute B, Mark JB, et al. Time of day effects on the incidence of anesthetic adverse events. *Qual Saf Health Care.* 2006;15(4):258-263. doi:10.1136/qshc.2005.017566.

204. Seki Y, Yamazaki Y. Effects of working conditions on intravenous medication errors in a Japanese hospital. *J Nurs Manag.* 2006;14(2):128-139. doi:10.1111/j.1365-2934.2006.00597.x.

205. Warren A, Tart RC. Fatigue and charting errors: the benefit of a reduced call schedule. *AORN J.* 2008;88(1):88-95. doi:10.1016/j.aorn.2008.03.016.

206. Rogers AE, Dean GE, Hwang WT, Scott LD. Role of registered nurses in error prevention, discovery and correction. *Qual Saf Health Care.* 2008;17(2):117-121. doi:10.1136/qshc.2007.022699.

207. Lockley SW, Barger LK, Ayas NT, et al. Effects of health care provider work hours and sleep deprivation on safety and performance. *Jt Comm J Qual Patient Saf.* 2007;33(Suppl 11):7-18.

208. Garrett C. The effect of nurse staffing patterns on medical errors and nurse burnout. *AORN J.* 2008;87(6):1191-1204. doi:10.1016/j.aorn.2008.01.022.

209. Schillie SF. Quality improvement in healthcare. *Perspectives in Prevention from the American College of Preventive Medicine: MedscapeCME Public Health & Prevention.* Published September 12, 2007. Accessed September 29, 2011.

210. Nolen AL, Rodes WD 2nd. Bar-code medication administration system for anesthetics: effects on documentation and billing. *Am J Health Syst Pharm.* 2008;65(7):655-659. doi:10.2146/ajhp070167.

211. Meyer-Massetti C, Cheng CM, Schwappach DL, et al. Systematic review of medication safety assessment methods. *Am J Health Syst Pharm.* 2011;68(3):227-240. doi:10.2146/ajhp100019.

212. Simmons D. Sedation and patient safety. *Crit Care Nurs Clin North Am.* 2005;17(3):279-285. doi:10.1016/j.ccell.2005.04.009.

213. Nyssen AS, Aunac S, Faymonville ME, Lutte I. Reporting systems in healthcare from a case-by-case experience to a general framework: an example in anaesthesia. *Eur J Anaesthesiol.* 2004;21(10):757-765.

214. Snyder RA, Fields W. A model for medication safety event detection. *Int J Qual Health Care.* 2010;22(3):179-186. doi:10.1093/intqhc/mzq014.

215. Moss J. Reducing errors during patient-controlled analgesia therapy through failure mode and effects analysis. *Jt Comm J Qual Patient Saf.* 2010;36(8):359-364.

216. Safe Medical Devices Act of 1990, Pub L No. 101-629, HR 3095. http://thomas.loc.gov/cgi-bin/bdquery/z?d101:H.R.3095:. Accessed October 3, 2011.

Acknowledgments

Lead Author
Bonnie Denholm, MS, BSN, RN, CNOR
Perioperative Nursing Specialist
AORN, Inc
Denver, Colorado

Contributing Authors
Rodney W. Hicks, PhD, ARNP, RN, FAANP, FAAN
Professor
Western University of Health Science
Pomona, California

Linda J. Wanzer, DNP(C), MSN, RN, CNOR, COL (Ret)
Director
Perioperative Clinical Nurse Specialist Program
Assistant Professor of Nursing
Uniformed Services University of the Health Sciences,
Graduate School of Nursing
Bethesda, Maryland

Publication History
Originally published December 2011 online in *Perioperative Standards and Recommended Practices.*

Reformatted September 2012 for publication in *Perioperative Standards and Recommended Practices*, 2013 edition.

Minor editing revisions made in November 2014 for publication in *Guidelines for Perioperative Practice,* 2015 edition.

AMBULATORY SUPPLEMENT: MEDICATION SAFETY

Recommendation I

A multidisciplinary team approach for medication management and the prevention of medication errors should be used throughout the phases of perioperative care.

I.a.1. The medication safety committee should include key stakeholders (eg, nurses, physicians, anesthesia professionals, pharmacists, risk management personnel, purchasing personnel, administrators) who participate in the medication use process.

Amb If an on-site pharmacist is not available, the organization should contract with a pharmacist to provide consultative services.

Amb The contracted pharmacist should be a member of the organization's committee that has oversight responsibility for medication safety.[A1]

Recommendation II

Medications, chemicals, reagents, and related supplies should be procured and stored in a manner that facilitates safe and efficient delivery to the patient.

II.a. The health care organization's medication management plan should incorporate considerations for procurement including, but not limited to,
- obtaining medications from manufacturers or suppliers with established quality programs.

   Amb Assessment criteria should be used to select a compounding pharmacy (Table 1).[A2]

II.g. Medications should be procured in limited varieties of concentrations and dosages and standardized in all perioperative medication storage areas.

Epinephrine in concentrations of 1:1,000 is a high-alert medication that has been reported to cause harm when it is not diluted.[A3] Warning labels may help to reduce confusion when a high-alert medication requires dilution, but it may be more effective to store the vials in the pharmacy to reduce the risk of error.[A3]

Amb High-alert medication vials that require dilution should be secured from unauthorized access if there is no pharmacy.

Amb Prescription pads should be secured, not pre-signed and/or postdated.[A4]

Recommendation V

Pharmacists should be actively involved in dispensing aspects of perioperative medication use across all perioperative settings.

V.a. Pharmacists should review medication orders before administration. In perioperative settings, this review should include standing orders (eg, preference cards).

Amb Centers for Medicare & Medicaid Services (CMS)-certified facilities must meet CMS requirements for pharmaceutical services.[A5]

---

§416.48 Condition for Coverage: Pharmaceutical Services

The [Ambulatory surgery center] ASC must provide drugs and biologicals in a safe and effective manner, in accordance with accepted professional practice, and under the direction of an individual designated responsible for pharmaceutical services.

§416.48 Condition for Coverage: Pharmaceutical Services. In: Centers for Medicare & Medicaid Services. *State Operations Manual Appendix L—Guidance for Surveyors: Ambulatory Surgical Centers.* Rev. 89; 2013.

Interpretive Guidelines: §416.48

The ASC must designate a specific licensed healthcare professional to provide direction to the ASC's pharmaceutical service. That individual must be routinely present when the ASC is open for business, but continuous presence is not required, particularly when the ASC is open for longer periods of time to accommodate the recovery of patients for up to 24 hours. Ideally the ASC should have available a pharmacist who provides oversight or consultation on the ASC's pharmaceutical services, but this is not required by the regulation, unless the ASC is performing activities which under State law may only be performed by a licensed pharmacist.

Interpretive Guidelines: §416.48. In: Centers for Medicare & Medicaid Services. *State Operations Manual Appendix L—Guidance for Surveyors: Ambulatory Surgical Centers.* Rev. 89; 2013.

V.b. The health care organization should comply with local, state, and federal regulations for pharmacy resources and ensure solutions are prepared according to national standard specified in *The United States Pharmacopeia*, Chapter <797>.[A6]

The [CMS] regulation does not require a pharmacist to be on site unless an ambulatory

AMBULATORY SUPPLEMENT: MEDICATION SAFETY

Table 1. Compounding Pharmacy Assessment Criteria

Licenses-Permits

- Is the pharmacy licensed and in good-standing with the state board of pharmacy?
- Has the pharmacy ever been disciplined for any infractions related to its compounding services?
- If the pharmacy is in a different state than the purchasing institution, is the pharmacy licensed to dispense/distribute/provide medications in this state as well?
- What is the license number?
- Is the permit in good standing?
- Will the pharmacy become licensed?
- Has the pharmacy ever been disciplined for any infractions related to its compounding services in those states in which it currently or formerly had a license/permit?
- If the pharmacy is in a different state than the purchasing institution, is the pharmacist-in-charge or another full-time pharmacist licensed in the state as well?
  - What is the license number(s)?
- If not, will the pharmacy agree to have one of its staff pharmacists become licensed?
- Has the pharmacist ever been disciplined for any infractions related to his/her compounding services?
- Has the pharmacy demonstrated it meets national quality standards by earning accreditation by the Pharmacy Compounding Accreditation Board (PCAB)? Current accreditation can be verified at http://www.pcab.org
- Is the pharmacy accredited by any other accrediting bodies? If so, which ones?
- Are the pharmacist(s) and/or pharmacy staff members of the International Academy of Compounding Pharmacists (IACP)?
- Of the American Society of Health-System Pharmacists?

Compounding Services Provided

- What types of dosage forms does the pharmacy prepare (eg, injectables, capsules, troches, oral liquids, suppositories, topicals, ophthalmics, inhalations)?
- How long has the pharmacy compounded these various dosage forms?
- Does the pharmacy provide sterile compounding services?
- If so, what level of complexity?

Internal Controls and Quality Assurance

- Does the pharmacy have written and active standard operating procedures (SOPs) in place for all compounding activities?
- Does the pharmacy obtain its pharmaceutical ingredients from a US Food and Drug Administration- and Drug Enforcement Agency-registered pharmaceutical ingredients supplier?
- How is that documented?
- Are SOPs in place to demonstrate verification of supplier registration status?
- Does the pharmacy obtain certificates of analysis (CoA) for all formula ingredients from its suppliers?
- Are those available for verification?
- Does the pharmacy have an SOP in place in case of a recall?
- Has the pharmacy had a recall in the last 24 months?
- Does the pharmacy have an SOP on how a customer can report problems to the pharmacy?
- Has the pharmacy staff been trained and evaluated in proper aseptic technique, gowning, and cleanroom procedures?
- What SOPs exist that show performance compliance with those procedures?
- Does the pharmacy compound sterile preparations?
- What level of sterile compounding is performed by the pharmacy using the commonly named "low-risk, medium-risk, and/or high-risk" categories?
- Does the pharmacy comply with current *US Pharmacopeia (USP)* <797> standards for sterile compounding?
- How is that compliance documented through SOPs?
- Does the pharmacy compound nonsterile preparations?
- Are the preparations simple, medium, and/or complex?
- Does the pharmacy comply with the current *USP* <795> standards for nonsterile compounding?
- How is that compliance documented through SOPs?

continued on next page.

AMBULATORY SUPPLEMENT: MEDICATION SAFETY

TABLE 1 CONTINUED. COMPOUNDING PHARMACY ASSESSMENT CRITERIA

Testing and Verification

- Does the pharmacy use published information or stability studies to establish the preparations' beyond-use dating?
- What sources are used?

- Does the pharmacy have in place quality-assurance and continuous quality-improvement programs?
- Give an example.

- Does the pharmacy staff participate in ongoing training and continuing education that is specific to compounding pharmacy practice?

- Does the pharmacy have its compounded preparations regularly tested for potency to ensure the concentration on the container is what is stated on the label?
- Which laboratories does the pharmacy use for potency assessments?
- How frequently are batches tested for potency?
- What SOPs are in place governing the frequency of testing?

- Do the pharmacy's preparations meet the +/- 10% of stated concentration that is required from USP?
- How is that documented?

- Will the pharmacy provide written documentation of all testing results to the purchasing institution?

- Has the air quality in the pharmacy's designated compounding areas been independently tested and/or certified?
- Please provide details.

- Does the pharmacy perform or contract with an analytical laboratory to perform sterility testing according to *USP* <71> Sterility Tests and *USP* <85> Bacterial Endotoxin (Pyrogen) Tests?
- Which laboratories does the pharmacy use for sterility assessments?
- How frequently are batches tested for sterility?
- What SOPs are in place governing the frequency of testing?

- How are the compounded preparations delivered or shipped?
- Does the pharmacy assure proper storage conditions are maintained through delivery?

- What is the turn-around time for delivery once the order has been placed?

- What information is on the labeling of the preparation?
- How does the labeling look?
- Does the pharmacy color code labels?

- How are the preparations packaged?
  - Unit-dose or multiple-dose?
  - Tamper-evident?
  - Protected from light?
  - Overwrapped?

- Does the pharmacy accept site visits?
- How can a site visit be arranged?

Compounding Pharmacy Assessment Questionnaire (CPAQTM). Adapted with permission of the International Academy of Compounding Pharmacists 2012.

surgery center is in a state that has passed a law that requires a licensed pharmacist to provide oversight or consultation for pharmaceutical services.[A1] The federal regulations for ambulatory surgery centers state that a designated licensed health care professional must be "routinely present during regular business hours."[A1]

Amb "Records and security are maintained to ensure the control and safe dispensing of drugs, including samples, in compliance with federal and state laws."[A4(p58)]

Recommendation VIII

The perioperative RN should implement the medication care plan by using safe medication practices to obtain, verify, prepare, and administer medications throughout all phases of perioperative care and in all perioperative settings.

VIII.e. Medications should be prepared as close as possible to the time of use.

Amb Regardless of time pressures for surgical procedures of short duration, medication preparation, including IV solutions, should be done as close as possible to the time of administration.

Recommendation XIII

Medications should be disposed of according to local, state, and federal regulations; manufacturer's instructions; and health care organization policy.

A medication may be classified as a controlled substance or a medical hazardous waste and have federal, state, or local requirements for disposal. Factors influencing the decision for how to dispose of medication waste include the ease of, access to, and cost of disposal.[A7]

AMBULATORY SUPPLEMENT: MEDICATION SAFETY

XIII.c. Perioperative personnel who administer medications or handle medications within their scope of practice must follow established practices to validate controlled substance ([Drug Enforcement Agency regulations] Schedule II to IV) waste.

Licensed individuals are accountable for adhering to the Controlled Substance Act. Such adherence extends to retrieving and administering medication, and documenting the wasting of unused products.[A8]

XIII.c.1. Licensed perioperative team members should participate in inventory management of controlled substances.

XIII.c.2. Licensed perioperative team members should waste unused scheduled medications in accordance with federal regulations and health care organization policy.

 Facilities accredited by the CMS must meet the conditions for coverage requirements for pharmaceutical services.[A5]

> **Interpretive Guidelines: §416.48(a)**
>
> Is the ASC's system is capable of readily identifying loss or diversion of all controlled substances in such a manner as to minimize the time frame between the actual losses or diversion to the time of detection and determination of the extent of loss or diversion?
>
> §416.48(a) Standard: Administration of Drugs. Interpretive Guidelines: §416.48(a). In: Centers for Medicare & Medicaid Services. *State Operations Manual Appendix L—Guidance for Surveyors: Ambulatory Surgical Centers.* Rev. 89; 2013.

Recommendation XVI

Policies and procedures for safe medication practices should be developed, readily available in the practice setting, and reviewed periodically, and they should address direct patient care situations as well as organizational level situations.

 Facilities certified by the CMS must have a medication administration policy and procedure.[A5]

> **Interpretive Guidelines: §416.48(a)**
>
> The ASC must have policies and procedures designed to promote medication administration consistent with acceptable standards of practice. The policies and procedures should address issues including, but not limited to:
> - A physician or other qualified member of the medical staff acting within their scope of practice must issue an order for all drugs or biologicals administered in the ASC. The administration of the drugs or biologicals must be by, or under the supervision of, nursing or other personnel in accordance with applicable laws, standards of practice and the ASC's policies.
> - Following the manufacturer's label, including storing drugs and biologicals as directed; disposing of expired medications in a timely manner; using single-dose vials of medication for one ASC patient only; etc.
> - Avoiding preparation of medications too far in advance of their use. For example, while it may appear efficient to pre-draw the evening before all medications that will be used for surgeries scheduled the following day, this practice may, depending on the particular drug or biological, promote loss of integrity, stability or security of the medication.
> - Any pre-filled syringes must be initialed by the person who draws it, dated and timed to indicate when they were drawn, and labeled as to both content and expiration date.
> - Employing standard infection control practices when using injectable medications.
>
> §416.48(a) Standard: Administration of Drugs. Interpretive Guidelines: §416.48(a). In: Centers for Medicare & Medicaid Services. *State Operations Manual Appendix L—Guidance for Surveyors: Ambulatory Surgical Centers.* Rev. 89; 2013.

Recommendation XVII

Perioperative team members should participate in a variety of quality improvement activities that are consistent with the health care organization's plan and improve safe medication use by meeting or exceeding expectations from published national patient safety initiatives.

 Facilities certified by the CMS must have a plan for quality assessment and performance improvement.[A5]

> **§416.43 Condition for Coverage: Quality Assessment and Performance Improvement**
>
> The ASC must develop, implement and maintain an ongoing, data-driven quality assessment and performance improvement (QAPI) program.
>
> §416.43 Condition for Coverage: Quality Assessment and Performance Improvement. In: Centers for Medicare & Medicaid Services. *State Operations Manual Appendix L—Guidance for Surveyors: Ambulatory Surgical Centers.* Rev. 89; 2013.

> **Interpretive Guidelines: §416.43**
>
> - Ongoing – ie, the program is a continuing one, not just a one-time effort. Evidence of this would include, but is not limited to, things like collection by the ASC of quality data at regular intervals; analysis of the updated data at regular intervals; and updated records of actions taken to

AMBULATORY SUPPLEMENT: MEDICATION SAFETY

address quality problems identified in the analyses, as well as new data collection to determine if the corrective actions were effective.
- *Data-driven – ie, the program must identify in a systematic manner what data it will collect to measure various aspects of quality of care; the frequency of data collection; how the data will be collected and analyzed; and evidence that the program uses the data collected to assess quality and stimulate performance improvement.*

Interpretive Guidelines: §416.43. In: Centers for Medicare & Medicaid Services. *State Operations Manual Appendix L—Guidance for Surveyors: Ambulatory Surgical Centers.* Rev. 89; 2013.

§416.43(a) Standard: Program Scope

1) *The program must include, but not be limited to, an ongoing program that demonstrates measurable improvement in patient health outcomes, and improves patient safety by using quality indicators or performance measures associated with improved health outcomes and by the identification and reduction of medical errors.*
2) *The ASC must measure, analyze, and track quality indicators, adverse patient events, infection control and other aspects of performance that includes care and services furnished in the ASC.*

§416.43(a) Standard: Program Scope. In: Centers for Medicare & Medicaid Services. *State Operations Manual Appendix L—Guidance for Surveyors: Ambulatory Surgical Centers.* Rev. 89; 2013.

§416.43(c) Standard: Program Activities

1) *The ASC must set priorities for its performance improvement activities that –*
   (i) *Focus on high risk, high volume, and problem-prone areas.*
   (ii) *Consider incidence, prevalence and severity of problems in those areas.*
   (iii) *Affect health outcomes, patient safety and quality of care.*

§416.43(c) Standard: Program Activities. In: Centers for Medicare & Medicaid Services. *State Operations Manual Appendix L—Guidance for Surveyors: Ambulatory Surgical Centers.* Rev. 89; 2013.

References

A1. Centers for Medicare & Medicaid Services. *State Operations Manual Appendix L—Guidance for Surveyors: Ambulatory Surgical Centers.* Rev. 89; 2013. http://www.cms.gov/Regulations-and-Guidance/Guidance/Manuals/downloads/som107ap_l_ambulatory.pdf. Accessed October 20, 2013.

A2. Compounding Pharmacy Assessment Questionnaire (CPAQTM). International Academy of Compounding Pharmacists. http://www.iacprx.org/associations/13421/files/CPAQ%20REV%20with%20updated%20member%20number%20October%202012.pdf. Accessed October 20, 2013.

A3. Paparella S. Fatal confusion with epinephrine: 1:1,000 is not 1:10,000. *J Emerg Nurs.* 2005;31(1):86-88. doi:10.1016/j.jen.2004.09.016.

A4. Pharmaceutical services. In: *2013 Accreditation Handbook for Ambulatory Health Care.* Skokie, IL: Accreditation Association for Ambulatory Health Care; 2013:58-59.

A5. §416.48 Condition for Coverage: Pharmaceutical Services and Interpretive Guidelines. In: Centers for Medicare & Medicaid Services. *State Operations Manual Appendix L—Guidance for Surveyors: Ambulatory Surgical Centers.* Rev. 89; 2013. http://www.cms.gov/Regulations-and-Guidance/Guidance/Manuals/downloads/som107ap_l_ambulatory.pdf. Accessed October 20, 2013.

A6. United States Pharmacopeia Convention. Committee of Revision. Pharmaceutical compounding—sterile preparations. In: *The United States Pharmacopeia.* 27th ed. Rockville, MD: United States Pharmacopeial Convention, Inc; 2009:318-354.

A7. *Unused Pharmaceuticals in the Health Care Industry: Interim Report.* Washington, DC: Environmental Protection Agency; 2008. http://water.epa.gov/scitech/swguidance/ppcp/upload/2010_1_11_ppcp_hcioutreach.pdf. Accessed October 20, 2013.

A8. Controlled Substance Act, 21 USC §801–971 (2006).

GUIDELINE FOR REDUCING RADIOLOGICAL EXPOSURE

The Guideline for Reducing Radiological Exposure was developed by the AORN Recommended Practices Committee and was approved by the AORN Board of Directors. It was presented as proposed recommended practices for comments by members and others. The guideline is effective January 1, 2007. The recommendations in the guideline are intended to be achievable and represent what is believed to be an optimal level of practice. Policies and procedures will reflect variations in practice settings and/or clinical situations that determine the degree to which the guideline can be implemented. AORN recognizes the numerous types of settings in which perioperative nurses practice; therefore, this guideline is adaptable to various practice settings. These practice settings include traditional operating rooms, ambulatory surgery centers, physicians' offices, cardiac catheterization suites, endoscopy suites, radiology and interventional radiology departments, and all other areas where operative and other invasive procedures may be performed.

Purpose

Radiological procedures are an invaluable medical diagnostic and treatment tool and, if proper safety procedures are followed, create only minimal risks to both the patient and medical personnel. Ionizing radiation is useful for diagnostic, interventional, and therapeutic procedures. Ionizing radiation can damage living tissues and may produce long-term effects. Patients and personnel should be protected from unsafe levels of radiation that are not medically indicated because of the potential hazardous effects of ionizing radiation exposure on tissue over time. Evidence has demonstrated that ionizing radiation also can harm a developing embryo. The greatest risk is the development of cancer. Health care workers who do not protect themselves from scatter radiation are especially at risk when performing interventional procedures because of significantly increased exposure time and close proximity during the procedure.

Prevention of radiation injury requires the application of principles of physics and radiological safety standards. Policies addressing education, credentialing, and radiological safety and maintenance must be in accordance with national regulatory standards and manufacturers' documented instructions.[1]

The overall goal of a radiation safety program should be to keep the risks from ionizing radiation as low as reasonably achievable.[2] Time, distance, and shielding should be employed to keep radiation exposure within safe levels. The National Council on Radiation Protection and Measurements has established guidelines for total dose radiation limits for radiation workers. In 1995, the Conference of Radiation Control Program Directors, a nonregulatory organization, published recommendations for state regulatory agencies.[3] Each state develops and implements regulations governing safe use of radiation-producing equipment and radioactive materials. Using safety measures of limiting exposure time and using protective shields (eg, thyroid shields, lead aprons, protective eyeglasses) is addressed.[4] Radiology departments use both diagnostic and interventional techniques in a wide variety of invasive applications and are included in this recommended practice. Interventional radiology nurses assist with procedures that include, but are not limited to, intravascular repairs such as

- inserting stents;
- placing shunts;
- performing embolization procedures;
- performing genitourinary procedures (eg, percutaneous nephrostomy tube placement, stone obliteration, balloon dilatation);
- draining abscesses; and
- performing laparoscopic tumor biopsies.

A primary responsibility of the interventional radiology nurse is to protect personnel and patients from high doses of radiation used during these procedures.[4]

Low dose-rate and high dose-rate brachytherapy both use ionizing radiation and are included in this guideline. Brachytherapy is the use of radioactive isotopes to treat malignancies and benign conditions. The radioactive source is inserted close to the treatment site or tumor. This therapy is used to treat tumors of the head, neck, breast, cervix, prostate, and endometrium, and to treat obstructive esophageal and bronchial lesions. Delivering high dose-rate brachytherapy, including that which is used during cardiovascular revascularization procedures, requires limiting radiation exposure to the patient and personnel. Personnel should have a thorough understanding of the physical effects of radiation and the regulatory guidelines established to ensure patient and personnel safety.[5]

Lasers, which are recognized to be nonionizing radiation, are not within the scope of this guideline. This document provides guidance for developing institutional policies and procedures that can be used collaboratively by personnel in the radiology and surgical services departments and by the facility radiation safety officer.

The primary nursing diagnosis applicable in this guideline is the risk for impaired skin integrity from the effects of gamma radiation. To ensure optimal outcomes, the perioperative nurse should assess the patient at the end of the procedure to ensure that the patient's skin remains smooth, intact, and free from unexpected redness, blistering, or tenderness.[6] Each of the following recommendations is a nursing intervention intended to protect the patient and staff members and ensure optimal outcomes.

REDUCING RADIOLOGICAL EXPOSURE

Recommendation I

The patient's exposure to radiation should be minimized.

1. The patient's exposure to radiation should be limited to situations in which it is medically indicated and to the anatomical structures being treated. Fluoroscopy delivers some of the largest doses of radiation to patients.[7] Serious skin injuries to patients undergoing certain fluoroscopic procedures have been reported. The greatest dose of radiation to the patient occurs on the patient's skin, where the beam enters the body. The decision to use fluoroscopy during medical or surgical procedures should be approached with caution, weighing the benefits afforded by the technology against the need to keep radiation exposure limited.[7]

2. The perioperative registered nurse should review the patient record for relevant history involving radiation exposure and record study parameters such as fluoroscopy time and area irradiated. He or she also should advise the treating physician of any pertinent information that would be important in reducing patient risk.

3. The perioperative registered nurse should assess the patient for any previous procedure involving radioactive material (ie, nuclear medicine, radiation oncology). It may be necessary to delay the procedure if there is significant radioactive material remaining in the patient. The physician responsible for the radiation treatment or diagnostic procedure should be consulted to determine exposure levels.

4. All reasonable means of reconciling an incorrect sponge, needle, or instrument count should be attempted before using a radiological examination to locate a sponge, sharp, or instrument that may be missing. Certain procedures, because of the complexity of the number of instruments used, may necessitate a postoperative x-ray as stated in the "Recommended practices for sponge, sharp, and instrument counts."[8] Controlling the amount of total fluoroscopic beam "on" time for these procedures through judicious control of the exposure time may help ensure that radiation exposure is as low as reasonably achievable.[4]

Recommendation II

The patient should be protected from unnecessary radiation exposure.

1. Care should be taken to keep extraneous body parts out of the radiation beam to prevent injury. Reports have shown that arms and breast tissue have been injured as a result of increased unintended radiation.[6] Parts of the patient's body not included in the intended radiation field that are located on the x-ray tube side can accumulate dose rapidly.[4] Implementing protective measures (eg, protective lead shielding) helps to prevent injury from radiation sources.[1] Lead shielding should be placed between the patient and the source of radiation.[9] Shielding placed on the wrong side (ie, away from the source) can actually increase the dose to the patient. Lead shielding should not be in the beam in fluoroscopic procedures (eg, hand surgery).

2. Lead shielding should be used, when possible, to protect the thyroid during x-ray studies of the upper extremities, trunk, and head. Thyroid and lymphoid tissues are shown to be sensitive to radiation exposure.[9]

3. Lead shielding should be used, when possible, to protect the patient's ovaries or testes (ie, gonads) during x-ray studies, including those performed on the hips and upper legs.

4. Female patients of childbearing age should be questioned about the possibility of pregnancy.
   - If the possibility of pregnancy exists, the surgeon should be notified to determine the advisability of continuing or postponing the procedure.
   - Lead shielding should be used to protect the fetus when other areas of a pregnant woman's body are x-rayed. The fetus is highly sensitive to ionizing radiation. Scatter radiation may expose the fetus to low-level radiation. Radiation to the abdomen and pelvis in women who are pregnant or may be pregnant poses an increased risk to the fetus and may result in childhood cancers.[10,11] Proper safety measures minimize the actual risk. The perioperative nurse should assess the history of all premenopausal women to ensure that they are aware of radiation exposure risks during pregnancy.[6]

Recommendation III

Occupational exposure to radiation should be minimized.

Guidelines for radiation safety are based on the principles of time, distance, and shielding. When exposed to radiation at a constant rate, the total dose equivalent received depends on the length of time exposed. If the distance from the point source of radiation is doubled, the exposure is quartered.[1] Radiation that scatters as the x-ray beam passes through the patient is the main source of radiation exposure. Passage through materials reduces the amount of radiation. State and government regulations that stipulate the dose limits for occupational exposure are described in the glossary.

1. Warning signs should be posted to alert personnel to potential radiation hazards at entrances to ORs and procedure rooms where radiological equipment is in use, as required by state regulations. State regulations provide requirements for posting warning signs at entrances to rooms where radiation is a potential hazard. These

REDUCING RADIOLOGICAL EXPOSURE

requirements apply equally to all areas where radiological equipment is used. Applicable state regulations should be followed.

2. Personnel should limit the amount of time spent in close proximity to the radiation source when exposure to radiation is possible.[12] Minimizing beam "on" time during fluoroscopic procedures by using the last-image hold feature may decrease the dose of radiation to the patient and personnel.[4,7]

3. The radiation equipment operator should notify personnel present in the treatment room before activating the equipment.[12]

4. During intracoronary brachytherapy, close contact with the patient should be limited to less than five minutes whenever possible. An authorized user, medical physicist, or radiation safety officer should be present before the therapy is initiated to ensure staff member safety. Designated safe areas should be determined before initiating treatment to allow staff members to distance themselves from exposure to increased radiation levels.[13]

5. Personnel should be aware of scatter radiation that is emitted from the patient in all directions in both radiological and fluoroscopic procedures.[13] Scatter radiation is a significant hazard to personnel, especially in fluoroscopic procedures. Variability exists as to the total amount of radiation that is emitted due to the intensity of the radiation primary beam, the size of the beam area, and the patient's dimensions. Larger patients may require greater radiation beam intensity in order to produce greater image quality, which may result in greater radiation scatter.[12]

6. During fluoroscopic procedures, personnel should keep the patient as close as possible to the image intensifier side of the fluoroscopic unit and away from the tube side of the unit. Keeping the patient close to the image intensifier side lowers the dose required to produce an image, decreases the amount of radiation scatter, and decreases the amount of radiation emitted to the personnel assisting with the procedure. Doubling the distance from the source of emitting radiation reduces the intensity of the radiation by a factor of four.[12]

7. To reduce exposure, personnel involved in fluoroscopic procedures should stand on the image intensifier side of the fluoroscopic unit whenever possible.[14] Using fluoroscopy in lateral views tends to produce greater radiation scatter from the patient. Personnel standing on the same side as the image intensifier experience a decrease in radiation intensity.[3,12]

8. Personnel assisting with radiological procedures should not hold the patient manually for a study because of the risk of exposure by the direct beam.[12] Slings, traction devices, and sandbags should be used to maintain patient position during radiation exposure. Cassette holders should be used to position films. If manual holding cannot be avoided, the individual should be protected from the primary x-ray beam. A 0.5 mm lead-equivalent shield or apron should be worn.

9. Whenever possible, shielding should be employed to provide attenuation of the radiation being delivered to the personnel potentially exposed.[14] Types of shielding available to personnel may include, but are not limited to,
   * walls, windows, control booths, and doors;
   * mobile rigid shields on wheels for transport to various areas;
   * ceiling-suspended transparent barriers;
   * flexible aprons (eg, wraparound, open backs), vests, skirts, thyroid shields, and gloves; and
   * leaded safety eyeglasses with side shields.

10. Personnel who may have to stand with their backs to the radiation beam should wear wraparound aprons to decrease the risk of exposure. It is important to note, however, that wraparound aprons may not provide the same level of protection to both sides of the staff member because the front of the apron usually is double in thickness.[3] Personnel should turn toward the radiation beam when possible to minimize the dose of radiation during a procedure and maximize safety. Lightweight aprons that meet the thickness requirements should be considered for comfort and user compliance.

11. Shielding of the upper legs of personnel near the radiation beam (eg, oblique imaging with the x-ray tube in close proximity to the lower body of the operator) should be initiated to protect the long bones and bone marrow from increased doses of radiation. Aprons should be as long and as wide as needed to provide protection.[12]

12. Shielding of the upper chest and neck of personnel nearest the x-ray tube (eg, oblique imaging with the x-ray tube in close proximity to the upper chest of the operator) may reduce radiation risk. Thyroid shields should be worn to protect the thyroid whenever the likelihood of the procedure (eg, orthopedic spinal fixation procedures) places the operator at higher risk because of increased exposure.[15] Females should protect their breasts from radiation exposure and aprons should cover the area completely.[3]

13. Some individuals who will be farther away from the x-ray beam may choose to wear aprons with less protection because they are lighter and cause less muscle strain. If aprons with different levels of protection are stored in the same area, the aprons that have less protection should be easily identified to avoid confusion as to the level of safety afforded to the personnel who are wearing them. State regulations should be followed concerning the minimum thickness required for aprons in the facility.[3]

14. Shielding the lens of the eye by using leaded face shields or leaded eyeglasses with wraparound side shields should be used to reduce scatter radiation to the operator when it is anticipated that increased fluoroscopic time may be necessary. Repeated exposure of the eyes over time can produce ulceration of the cornea and cataracts.[16] Leaded eyewear is recommended for personnel who are likely to receive levels of radiation measured by collar badge readings above 15,000 millirem roentgen equivalent unit (mrem) per year annually. Side eye shields also may be beneficial for personnel who perform procedures during which it is necessary to turn away from the radiation beam.[12]

15. Personnel participating in fluoroscopic procedures during which they are less than 24 inches (ie, 70 cm) away from the x-ray beam may consider routinely wearing a thyroid shield and leaded eyeglasses especially during procedures where increased time/dose to the patient are performed.[17]

16. In general, no part of the operator's body should be in the direct x-ray beam. If the operator's hand will be in the direct beam, radiation attenuation gloves should be considered. These gloves afford some protection and may be of benefit in reducing the amount of radiation exposure during a procedure. Most radiation attenuation gloves provide only 33% to 35% safety attenuation.[15] Outside the direct beam, protective gloves are very cumbersome and the inconvenience may outweigh any protective advantage. Even if protective gloves are worn, hands still should be kept out of the x-ray beam as much as possible. Remote handling devices (eg, forceps) should be used whenever possible to minimize the need for the operator's hand to be exposed to radiation.[12]

17. Occupational exposure should be minimized during sentinel node biopsy. Sentinel node biopsy is useful in demonstrating evidence of micrometastatic disease. A gamma-emitting radiocolloid (ie, technetium-99m) can be injected into the patient's tissue to find the sentinel node.[18] The use of time, distance, and shielding should be employed during these procedures to limit personnel exposure to the radioactive isotope. The risk of radiation exposure in these procedures is minimal. Sentinel nodes demonstrating radioactivity should be labeled as radioactive before transporting the specimens from the OR.

18. Personnel with known or suspected pregnancy should declare this condition to the radiation safety officer or other appropriate facility channels. State regulations vary regarding pregnant personnel and radiation safety. State guidelines are based upon the US Nuclear Regulatory Commission (NRC) guidelines regarding confidentiality in the pregnant worker. Disclosure of the pregnancy, even if it is obvious, is not required. A written, voluntary, official declaration that includes the estimated date of conception may be used to base the total dose limit to the pregnant person.[3] The NRC guidelines include the following:
    - Occupational dose to the embryo or fetus of an occupationally exposed staff member who has declared her pregnancy must not exceed 0.5 rem during the entire gestational period.
    - Dose should be uniform over time and not all at once (ie, at one point in the gestational period).
    - Deep-dose equivalent of the declared pregnant worker must be used as the dose to the embryo or fetus. The dosimeter should be worn at the waist under the apron shield.[3] Radiation must pass through several layers of tissue before reaching the fetus; therefore, this dosimeter reading does not reflect the amount of radiation reaching the fetus. Leaded shielding will attenuate 95% to 98% of the radiation.

19. State regulations regarding the monitoring of radiation in pregnant workers may monitor radiation differently as evidenced by the number of dosimeters worn, the area(s) the dosimeters are placed on the body, and whether the dosimeters are placed under or over shielding during the procedure.[3]

20. Maternity aprons may be worn to decrease the amount of radiation to the embryo or fetus. Although there is double thickness in the area where most pregnant workers need the protection, caution should be used by the pregnant worker when turning away from the x-ray beam. Most aprons do not shield the back of the pregnant worker.[3] These aprons are heavier and may be more difficult to wear, placing extra strain on the shoulders of the pregnant worker. Organizations may decide to purchase these aprons for pregnant workers and should mark the aprons to make the aprons easy to identify and ensure that they will be available for those who choose to wear them.

Recommendation IV

Shielding devices should be handled carefully, visually examined before use, and x-rayed at least annually to detect and prevent damage that could diminish their effectiveness.

1. Newly purchased leaded protective devices should be tested for attenuation and for shielding properties to check for cracks and holes in shipping before use. Subsequently, all leaded protective devices should be checked for defects and wear at least annually and whenever damage is suspected.[3] The frequency of testing is dependent upon the type of device used and the care that the device receives as it is used because excessive misuse can increase the risk of cracks and damage.[19,20]

REDUCING RADIOLOGICAL EXPOSURE

2. Leaded aprons and thyroid shields should be stored flat or hung vertically and should not be folded. Leaded aprons and shields are susceptible to cracking, which can reduce the apron's effectiveness as a shielding barrier.

3. Testing documentation of all leaded protective devices should be maintained in the radiology department or in the facility safety office. Areas that purchase new aprons should notify the department where the testing is performed so records are kept up-to-date and accurate. All aprons should be labeled or numbered so that each apron can be tracked if necessary.

4. Protective devices should be cleaned with an EPA-registered hospital disinfectant after every use.

Recommendation V

Individuals should be protected from exposure to patients who have received diagnostic or therapeutic radionuclides that may pose a radiation risk.

1. Facilities that use therapeutic radionuclides should employ a radiation safety officer. This individual should determine specific organizational policies and procedures. The primary function of the radiation safety officer is supervision of the daily operation of the radiation safety program to ensure that individuals are protected from radiation. The radiation safety officer should determine which individuals are in frequent proximity to radiation, which should wear monitoring devices, and how occupational exposure is monitored and recorded. *Amb*

2. Personnel should use the principles of time, distance, and shielding when caring for patients who have received therapeutic radionuclides. Radionuclide materials are absorbed by the body and safety precautions are required depending on the absorption and excretion of the radionuclide.[3] Patients who have received radionuclides emit radiation until the nuclide has decayed or has been eliminated.[20] Body fluids and tissue removed from patients who have undergone recent diagnostic nuclear medicine studies should be handled according to radiation safety procedures and standard precautions and should be labeled radioactive. These procedures should be based on government regulations and recommendations.

3. Contamination-control measures should be applied to the use of unsealed radioactive materials.[1] When transferring patients who received therapeutic radionuclides in the OR, perioperative personnel should notify personnel receiving the patients of the radiation source and anatomical location before patient transfer. All radiation precautions should be observed during transfer of the patient from one area or unit to another. The radiation safety officer should establish policies concerning how patients are transferred after receiving therapeutic radionuclides to minimize exposure to staff members. Advance communication allows personnel time to protect themselves, the patient's visitors and family members, and other patients from unnecessary exposure to radiation.[5]

4. Preparation of sealed radionuclides, such as prostatic seeds, may require sterilization before use. Manufacturers' written instructions should be followed for sterilization. Sealed radionuclides requiring sterilization should be packaged and sterilized according to the "Recommended practices for sterilization in perioperative practice settings."[21] Prevacuum sterilization cycles should not be used because the vacuum may displace the seeds and potentially cause a radiation hazard to personnel.[22] Flash sterilization of the seeds should be avoided. Implantable medical devices should not be flash sterilized because of possible patient complications and because it is difficult to ensure aseptic delivery and personnel safety. Varying sterilization times have been cited in the literature. Health care facilities may wish to purchase pre-sterilized seeds or needles to minimize the risk to personnel who have to prepare these devices for use.[23]

5. Manufacturers' written instructions for preparation of eye plaques should be followed. Eye plaques are a form of brachytherapy used for treatment of choroidal melanoma.[24] Radionuclide seeds are placed in silicone tubes and secured to gold discs sutured next to the tumor. Gold is used to decrease the amount of scatter radiation to the adjacent retina, choroid, and optic nerve. The same guidelines should be used as for other types of radioactive seeds. The radiation safety officer or a designee should ensure containment of the seeds.

6. The radiation safety officer or a designee should ensure compliance with NRC regulations when prostatic radionuclides are sterilized and used in the OR. This person should control and maintain strict surveillance of the radionuclides that are in controlled or unrestricted areas and that are not in storage.[25]

7. If radionuclide seeds such as prostate seeds are processed for use in a central processing department, the seeds must remain in constant surveillance during the entire processing period and delivery to the OR.[25] Central processing supervisors should consult the radiation safety officer for questions concerning dose limits and surveillance in central processing. Dosimeter monitoring and specific training may be required to ensure that dose limits fall within the established guidelines. Staff members who sterilize prostatic seeds should receive training from the radiation safety officer that includes techniques for
    * handling radioactive nuclides;

REDUCING RADIOLOGICAL EXPOSURE

- minimizing exposure to radiation (ie, as low as reasonably achievable);
- controlling and providing security for the material (ie, constant surveillance); and
- emergency response to spills of radioactive material.[23]

Recommendation VI

Radiation monitors or dosimeters should be worn by personnel who are in frequent proximity to radiation as determined by the radiation safety officer.

1. Individuals must comply with state regulations concerning placement of the monitors worn. Personnel who routinely are involved in fluoroscopic procedures should wear at least one radiation monitor approved by the National Voluntary Laboratory Accreditation Program.[26] When single monitoring devices are used, they should be worn on the same area of the body by all health care personnel. Radiation monitoring devices are the principal mechanism for monitoring radiation exposure of the personnel on a day-to-day basis and, therefore, should be used consistently by health care personnel working with radiation.[14]

2. State regulations for radiation monitoring must be followed. When two monitoring devices are used, one usually is worn at the neckline outside the leaded apron and the other inside the leaded apron. The monitor worn under the apron measures whole-body levels, while the one at the neckline measures head, neck, and lens of the eye exposure.[26] The radiation safety officer may require that the monitors be worn at other sites depending on the dose information desired. Personnel monitoring is required for individuals who have a reasonable probability of exceeding 10% of the occupational dose equivalent limit of 0.05 Sievert (Sv) (ie, 5 rem) per year.[27] Practitioners who perform interventional vascular, biliary tract, or genitourinary tract procedures should wear a finger monitor in the same location for every procedure.[26]

3. Radiation monitors or radiation dosimeters should be worn at the waist for all pregnant personnel and read monthly, not quarterly.[1]

4. Radiation monitoring devices or dosimeters should be removed and stored at the facility at the end of every workday. Radiation monitoring devices should not be removed and taken home because the device will collect ionizing radiation from other sources (eg, sun, soil, airport scanners). Documentation of the readings of the dosimeters should be kept in the facility's safety office.

Recommendation VII

Therapeutic radiation sources should be handled minimally to minimize exposure. Protective measures are implemented to prevent injury.[2,6]

1. Radioactive materials always should be used under direct supervision of the radiation safety officer or an authorized user. Radioactive materials should be kept in a protective container. The container reduces, but does not eliminate, exposure to radiation. Radioactive sources should never be left unattended when not in use.[1] Transport containers should remain under the direct supervision of the radiation safety officer or authorized user, or locked in a safe storage area.[13] Radioactive waste should never be placed in a nonradioactive waste container.

2. Radioactive sealed sources (eg, capsules, seeds, needles) should be handled with forceps, tongs, or tube racks. Forceps are used to increase the distance between the health care worker and the radiation source. Health care workers should never handle a sealed source with hands or fingers. Radiation protective gloves and aprons do not provide adequate shielding of therapeutic radionuclides; their inconvenience precludes their use for therapy. Examination gloves do not provide radiation shielding. They serve to control contamination if the radionuclide is a liquid or an unsealed source.[1]

3. Radioactive spills must be contained and disposed of in accordance with state and federal regulations. The source should be contained and completely removed, and the area cleaned thoroughly to remove any residual contamination. The area should be tested to verify that all radioactive material has been removed. Supplies used for cleanup should be discarded as radioactive waste. Perioperative registered nurses who work in this environment must receive training from the radiation safety officer or designee annually.[1]

4. An appropriate label (ie, radioactive waste label) must be placed on all radioactive waste. Such labels should include at least
   - radioisotope name,
   - activity,
   - date of disposal, and
   - radiation personnel's/authorized user's full name and contact information.[1]

Recommendation VIII

Measures taken to protect patients during the procedure from the risks of direct and indirect radiation exposure should be documented on the perioperative nursing record.

1. Perioperative nursing documentation should include the type of patient protection and the area(s) protected. Documentation of nursing interventions promotes continuity of patient care, improves communication among health care team

REDUCING RADIOLOGICAL EXPOSURE

members, and serves as a medical legal record of patient care.[28] Documentation of the protective measures used is necessary to track outcomes and ensure safety of the patient and staff members.

2. Documentation should include the perioperative nurse's patient skin assessment, including signs and symptoms of injury to the skin and tissue as evidenced by
   - redness,
   - abrasions,
   - bruising,
   - blistering, or
   - edema.[2]

3. The Perioperative Nursing Data Set (PNDS), the uniform perioperative nursing vocabulary, should be used to document patient care and to develop policies and procedures related to radiological safety. The expected outcome of primary importance to this recommended practice is "The patient is free from signs and symptoms of radiation injury." This outcome falls within the domain of Safety. The associated nursing diagnosis is "Risk of impaired skin integrity." The associated interventions that may lead to the desired outcome may be "Assesses history of previous radiation exposure"; "Verifies operative procedure, surgical site, and laterality"; and "Implements protective measures to prevent injury due to radiation sources."[6]

Recommendation IX

Policies and procedures regarding radiation exposure should be written, reviewed periodically, and readily available within the practice setting.

1. Policies and procedures should be developed collaboratively and approved by perioperative personnel, the radiation safety officer, or the director of the radiology department in cooperation with safety committee members or the radiation safety expert in accordance with government regulations. Polices and procedures should be reviewed by a medical radiation physicist. Collaboration should ensure compliance with current radiation safety policies and contribute to quality patient care.[1]

2. Polices and procedures should include, but are not limited to,
   - establishing authority, responsibility, and accountability for radiation safety;
   - identifying measures for protecting patients and personnel from unnecessary exposure to ionizing radiation;
   - developing procedures for handling and disposing of body fluids and tissue that may be radioactive;
   - ensuring that appropriate personnel wear radiation monitoring devices; and
   - scheduling radiographic testing of leaded protective devices.

3. Policies and procedures should be established in conjunction with the radiation safety officer for radiation safety training and competency in special handling techniques for personnel in the central processing department if sterilization of radiation seeds is performed there.

Recommendation X

Personnel should receive initial education, training, and competency validation and at least annual updates on new regulations and procedures.

1. All authorized users and radiation workers should complete initial training to include
   - radiation safety (eg, risk, hazards, spill containment);
   - biological effects of radiation;
   - regulatory requirements; and
   - environmental workplace techniques and procedures.

2. Documentation of training should include the above components and be maintained by the radiation safety officer.[1] Personnel who have not been involved in radiation procedures during the preceding two-year period should complete a refresher education and training program.

3. The radiation safety officer should provide annual competency validation, to include
   - a refresher course and testing for radiation safety and
   - a review of new regulations or procedures.

4. Educational programs should be developed to enhance knowledge that minimizes patient, personnel, and public risk of unnecessary exposure.

Recommendation XI

Only personnel who have received specific state-approved radiological training may be permitted to operate radiographic equipment.[26]

1. State-specific regulations must be followed regarding who may operate radiographic equipment. Legislation has been issued in various states restricting the use of this equipment to specific personnel who have demonstrated successful completion of formal education and training.

2. Operators of miniature mobile fluoroscopy units must adhere to the same state and federal regulations as all other radiological sources. The manufacturer's safety recommendations for the use of the device should be used when writing policies and procedures for the facility.

Glossary

Absorbed dose: The energy imparted to matter by ionizing radiation per unit mass of irradiated material at the place of interest. The special units of absorbed

REDUCING RADIOLOGICAL EXPOSURE

dose are the radiation absorbed dose (rad) (ie, 0.01 joule per kilogram) and gray (gy) (ie, one joule per kilogram), which is equal to 100 rads). The units for biological effective dose are the rem and sievert (sv).

Attenuation: The process by which a beam of radiation is reduced in intensity when passing through some material.

Authorized user: A physician or someone who has received special training or is credentialed to use radioactive materials and understands radiation physics, radiobiology, radiation safety, and radiation management.

Beam: A unidirectional flow of particle or electromagnetic radiation.

Conference of Radiation Control Program Directors (CRCPD): A nonregulatory organization that is a 501(c)(3) nonprofit, nongovernmental, professional organization dedicated to radiation protection.

Deep dose equivalent: The dose equivalent at a tissue depth of 1 cm; applies to the external whole body exposure.

Distance: The physical space between a source of radiation and its target (or the distance away from a source of radiation). The greater the distance an individual or target is from the source of radiation, the less the amount of radiation exposure. The inverse-square law applies—at a 4-ft distance from the source, the exposure received is approximately one quarter of that received at a 2-ft distance. Likewise, at a 6-ft distance the radiation is one ninth that received at a 2-ft distance.

Dosimeter: A device that is used to determine the external radiation dose that a person has received.

Equipment operator: A person with demonstrated qualifications and competency to operate a fluoroscopic system while exposing a patient to radiation. According to the American College of Radiology technical standard, only a physician is qualified to hold this title. Registered and/or licensed radiologic technologists or radiation therapists may perform fluoroscopic procedures if they are monitored by a supervising physician who is readily available.

Exposure: A measure of the total quantity of radiation reaching a specific point measured in the air. The unit of measure is based on the amount of ionization produced in air by a specified amount of x-ray energy. Radiation exposure is controlled in three ways—time, distance, and shielding.

External dose: That portion of the dose equivalent received from radiation sources outside the body.

Fluoroscopy: Observation of the internal features of an object by means of the fluorescence produced on a screen by x-rays transmitted through the object.

Gamma radiation: The emission of electromagnetic energy from the nucleus of an atom.

Gonad: Ovary or testis.

Gonad shield: A leaded device used to reduce x-ray exposure to the reproductive organs.

High radiation area: An area in which radiation levels could result in an individual receiving a dose equivalent in excess of 100 mrem per hour.

Internal dose: That portion of the dose equivalent received from radioactive material taken into the body.

Ionizing radiation: Electromagnetic radiation (eg, x-rays, gamma rays) that yields ions as it passes through an absorbing material (eg, air, tissue). The ions produce chemical reactions that are responsible for the biological expression of radiation (eg, cancer).

Leaded apron: A leaded-rubber material worn to protect personnel from scatter radiation.

Occupational dose: Annual exposure limits that took effect in 1994.[11]

- Total effective dose equivalent (TEDE) to radiation workers—5 rem.
- Dose equivalent to the eye—15 rem.
- Shallow dose equivalent to the skin, extremities—50 rem.
- TEDE to any other individual organ—50 rem.
- TEDE to an embryo or fetus of declared pregnant woman—0.5 rem.
- Minors—10% of worker limit.
- Members of the public—0.1 rem.

Quantify amount: A millirem is one one-thousandth of a rem.

Rad: Radiation absorbed dose.

Radioactivity: The property, possessed by certain nuclides, of spontaneously emitting particles of gamma radiation or of emitting radiation after orbital electron capture or spontaneous fission.

Radionuclide: A radioactive atom used in nuclear medicine that shows radioactive disintegration and emits alpha and beta particles or gamma rays. Some radionuclides are used for diagnostic studies to trace the function and structure of most organs. Those emitting beta particles are used primarily for treating malignant tumors.

Rem: A special unit of dose equivalent. The dose equivalent in rems is numerically equal to the absorbed dose in rads multiplied by the quality factor, which for most medical radiation is one.

Scatter radiation: Radiation is scattered when an x-ray beam strikes a patient's body, as it passes through the patient's body, and as it strikes surrounding structures (eg, walls, OR furniture).

Sealed and unsealed sources: Many radioactive pharmaceuticals come in the form of liquids or capsules and are administered orally. These are classified as unsealed sources. Some radioactive materials are sealed in small containment vessels, such as seeds, for implanting into tumors. These are classified as sealed sources.

Shallow dose equivalent: The dose equivalent at a tissue depth of 0.007 cm averaged over an area of 1 cm.[1]

Shielding: Radiation interacts with any type of material, and the amount of radiation is reduced during passage through materials. A thin layer of lead can absorb most scattered diagnostic x-rays. Gamma radiation from medically useful radionuclides is substantially attenuated by 1 to 2 inches of lead.

Time factor: The less time a person is exposed to radiation, the less radiation one absorbs. Remaining close to a source of radiation for 15 minutes, an individual receives one-half the radiation dose received if the exposure time was 30 minutes.

Total effective dose equivalent: The sum of deep-dose equivalent (ie, external exposures) and the committed effective dose equivalent (ie, internal exposures).

US Nuclear Regulatory Commission (NRC): A government group that regulates use of nuclear materials and assists with formulation of regulations that protect workers, the public, and the environment. The NRC also regulates nuclear materials that are used in science, medicine, and industry. The NRC issues licenses to those who operate power plants or use nuclear materials and conducts inspections to make sure these facilities are following established regulations.

X-ray intensifier: The radiation detector that produces the image in fluoroscopy.

X-ray tube: The radiation sources for x-ray and fluoroscopic machine.

References

1. "Radiation safety manual," (August 1999) Centers for Disease Control and Prevention Radiation Safety Committee, http://www.cdc.gov/od/ohs/manual/radman.htm (accessed 23 May 2004).
2. "Radiation safety guide, chapter 11: Permissible exposure levels (dose limits)," (May 14, 2004) National Institute of Environmental Health Sciences, http://www.niehs.nih.gov/odhsb/radhyg/radguide/sectxi.htm (accessed 12 Dec 2006).
3. L Brateman, "The AAPM/RSNA physics tutorial for residents: Radiation safety considerations for diagnostic radiology personnel," (May 11, 1999) RadioGraphics, http://radiographics.rsnajnls.org/cgi/content/full/19/4/1037 (accessed 1 Sept 2006).
4. L Strangio, "Interventional uroradiologic procedures," *AORN Journal* 66 (August 1997) 286-294.
5. "ACR practice guideline for the performance of low-dose-rate brachytherapy," (Jan 1, 2001) American College of Radiology, http://www.acr.org/s_acr/bin.asp?CID=0&DID=12243&DOC=FILE.PDF (accessed 30 Aug 2006).
6. S C Beyea, ed, *Perioperative Nursing Data Set: The Perioperative Nursing Vocabulary,* second ed (Denver: AORN, Inc, 2002) 100-101.
7. T G Norris, "Radiation safety in fluoroscopy," *Radiologic Technology* 73 no 6 (July-August, 2002) 511-533.
8. "Recommended practices for sponge, sharp, and instrument counts," in *Standards, Recommended Practices, and Guidelines* (Denver: AORN, Inc. 2006) 459-468.
9. L K Otto, S Davidson, "Radiation exposure of certified registered nurse anesthetists during ureteroscopic procedures using fluoroscopy," *Journal of the American Association of Nurse Anesthetists* 67 (February 1999) 53-58.
10. D Gilmour, "Risks for the new or expectant mother," *British Journal of Perioperative Nursing* 10 (June 2000) 306-310.
11. US Nuclear Regulatory Commission, Office of Nuclear Regulatory Research, *Instruction Concerning Prenatal Radiation Exposure,* Regulatory Guide 8.13, Revision 3 (June 1999) 8.13.11– 8.13.12.
12. S M Fishman et al, "Radiation safety in pain medicine," *Regional Anesthesia and Pain Medicine* 27 (May/June 2002) 296-305.
13. B G Bass, "How to maximize safety and minimize radiation exposure for cath lab personnel," *Cardiovascular Disease Management/COR Healthcare Resources* 7 (March 2001) 5-7.
14. J Newman, "Radiation protection for radiologic technologists," *Radiologic Technology* 71 no 3 (2000) 273-286.
15. Y R Rampersaud, K T Foley, A C Shen, et al "Radiation exposure to the spine surgeon during fluoroscopically assisted pedicle screw insertion," *Spine* 25 no 20 (2000) 2637-2645.
16. E Brailsford, P L Williams, "Evidence based practice: An experimental study to determine how different working practice affects eye radiation dose during cardiac catheterization," *Radiography* 7 no 1 (2000) 21-30.
17. C T Mehlman, T G DiPasquale, "Radiation exposure to the orthopaedic surgical team during fluoroscopy: How far away is far enough?" *Journal of Orthopaedic Trauma* 11 no 6 (1997) 392-398.
18. "Practice guideline for breast conservation therapy in the management of invasive breast carcinoma," (January 1, 2002) American College of Radiology, http://www.acr.org/s_acr/bin.asp?CID=0&DID=12238&DOC=FILE.PDF (accessed 30 Aug 30, 2006).
19. "Testing of lead aprons for QA," Pulse Medical, Inc, http://www.rci-pulsemed.com (accessed 30 Aug 2006).
20. "Recommended guidelines for controlling noninfectious health hazards in hospitals," Standard 5.2.3.6, in *Guidelines for Protecting the Safety and Health of Health Care Workers,* National Institute for Occupational Safety and Health, http://www.cdc.gov/niosh/hcwold5d.html (accessed 30 Aug 2006).
21. "Recommended practices for sterilization in the perioperative practice setting," in *Standards, Recommended Practices, and Guidelines* (Denver: AORN, Inc, 2006) 629-643.
22. Y Yu et al, "Permanent prostate seed implant brachytherapy: Report of the American Association of Physicists in Medicine task group No. 64," *Medical Physics* 26 (October 1999) 2054-2076.
23. T Lembcke, "Sterile loading of radioactive materials into needles," in *Trans-Rectal Ultrasound-Guided Trans-Perineal Implants of the Prostate Using ^{125}I and ^{103}P and $HDR(^{192}Ir)$,* Oconee Regional Cancer Center, http://www.oconeecancercenter.com/prostate/prosbk10.htm (accessed 30 Aug 2006).
24. J I Hui, T G Murray, "Radioactive plaque therapy," *International Ophthalmology Clinics* 46 no 1 (Winter 2006) 51-68.
25. "What are safe and legal options for radioactive source security during sterilization?" answer to question #212 submitted to "Ask the experts," Health Physics Society, http://www.hps.org/publicinformation/ate/q212.html (accessed 30 August 2006).
26. "ACR technical standard for management of the use of radiation in fluoroscopic procedures," (Jan 1, 2003) *Management of Fluoroscopic Procedures,* American College of Radiology, http://www.acr.org/s_acr/bin.asp?CID=0&DID=12244&DOC=FILE.PDF (accessed 30 Aug 2006).
27. E C Lipsitz et al, "Does the endovascular repair of aortoiliac aneurysms pose a radiation safety hazard to vascular surgeons?" *Journal of Vascular Surgery* 32 (October 2000) 704-710.
28. "Recommended practices for documentation of perioperative nursing care," in *Standards, Recommended Practices, and Guidelines* (Denver: AORN, Inc, 2006) 477-479.

REDUCING RADIOLOGICAL EXPOSURE

PUBLICATION HISTORY

Originally published October 1989, *AORN Journal*. Published as proposed recommended practices September 1993.

Revised and reformatted; published January 2001, *AORN Journal*.

Revised 2006; published in *Standards, Recommended Practices, and Guidelines*, 2007 edition.

Minor editing revisions made to omit PNDS codes; reformatted September 2012 for publication in *Perioperative Standards and Recommended Practices*, 2013 edition.

Minor editing revisions made in November 2014 for publication in *Guidelines for Perioperative Practice*, 2015 edition.

AMBULATORY SUPPLEMENT: REDUCING RADIOLOGICAL EXPOSURE

Ambulatory surgery centers (ASCs) that seek reimbursement from Medicare must comply with the hospital conditions of participation for radiological services.[A1]

> §416.49(b) Standard: Radiologic Services, Specific Conditions for Coverage
>
> *(1) The ASC must have procedures for obtaining radiological services from a Medicare approved facility to meet the needs of patients.*
> *(2) Radiologic services must meet the hospital conditions of participation for radiologic services specified in 482.26.*
>
> §416.49(b) Standard: Radiologic Services. In: Centers for Medicare & Medicaid Services. *State Operations Manual Appendix L—Guidance for Surveyors: Ambulatory Surgical Centers.* Rev. 89; 2013.
>
> §482.26 Condition of Participation: Radiologic Services
>
> *The hospital must maintain, or have available, diagnostic radiologic services. If the therapeutic services are also provided, they, as well as the diagnostic services, must meet professionally approved standards for safety and personnel qualifications.*
>
> §482.26 Condition of Participation: Radiologic Services. In: Centers for Medicare & Medicaid Services. *State Operations Manual Appendix A—Survey Protocol, Regulations and Interpretive Guidelines for Hospitals.* Rev. 89; 2013.

Recommendation V

Individuals should be protected from exposure to patients who have received diagnostic or therapeutic radionuclides that may pose a radiation risk.

1. Facilities that use therapeutic radionuclides should employ a radiation safety officer. This individual should determine specific organizational policies and procedures. The primary function of the radiation officer is supervision of the daily operation of the radiation safety program to ensure that individuals are protected from radiation. The radiation safety officer should determine which individuals are in frequent proximity to radiation, which should wear monitoring devices, and how occupational exposure is monitored and recorded.

   Patients receiving brachytherapy should receive specific discharge instructions for limiting radiation exposure to others upon discharge from the ambulatory facility.[A2]

REFERENCES

A1. §416.49(b) Standard: Radiologic Services. In: Centers for Medicare & Medicaid Services. *State Operations Manual Appendix L—Guidance for Surveyors: Ambulatory Surgical Centers.* Rev. 89; 2013. http://www.cms.gov/Regulations-and-Guidance/Guidance/Manuals/downloads/som107ap_l_ambulatory.pdf. Accessed October 20, 2013.

A2. National Council on Radiation Protection & Measurements. Patient-release criteria. In: *Management of Radionuclide Therapy Patients* [NCRP Report No. 155]. Bethesda, MD: NCRP Publications; 2007:141-160.

AMBULATORY SUPPLEMENT: REDUCING RADIOLOGICAL EXPOSURE

GUIDELINE FOR PREVENTION OF RETAINED SURGICAL ITEMS

The Guideline for Prevention of Retained Surgical Items was developed by the AORN Recommended Practices Committee and was approved by the AORN Board of Directors. It was presented as proposed recommendations for comments by members and others. The guideline is effective July 15, 2010. The recommendations in the guideline are intended to be achievable and represent what is believed to be an optimal level of practice. Policies and procedures will reflect variations in practice settings and/or clinical situations that determine the degree to which the guideline can be implemented. AORN recognizes the various settings in which perioperative nurses practice; therefore, this guideline is adaptable to various practice settings. These practice settings include traditional operating rooms (ORs), ambulatory surgery centers, physicians' offices, cardiac catheterization laboratories, endoscopy suites, radiology departments, and all other areas where operative and other invasive procedures may be performed.

Purpose

This document provides guidance to perioperative registered nurses (RNs) in preventing retained surgical items (RSIs) in patients undergoing surgical and other invasive procedures. Avoiding injuries from the care that is intended to help patients was identified by the Institute of Medicine as one of six goals to achieve a better health care system.[1] Counts for soft goods (eg, radiopaque sponges, radiopaque towels); sharps; and instruments are performed to account for all items used on the surgical field and to lessen the potential for injury to the patient as a result of an RSI. Health care organizations are responsible for employing standardized, transparent, verifiable, reliable practices to account for all surgical items used during a procedure to lessen the potential for patient harm as a result of retention. There is a potential for inaccurate counts with both current variable manual counting practices and the use of adjunct technology.[2-7] Therefore, behavioral change and an understanding of risk reduction strategies unique to each setting should be employed when adopting system(s) to account for all surgical items. A reliable system to account for all surgical items includes, but is not limited to, complete and accurate counting, radiological confirmation, and the use of adjunct technology, to promote optimal perioperative patient outcomes.

Current law does not prescribe what methodologies should be used, who should use them, or even that they need to be used. It does, however, require that surgical items not intended to remain in the patient be removed. The doctrine of *res ipsa loquitur* (ie, "the thing speaks for itself") is most applicable in RSI incidents. Therefore, the time and effort in legal tort cases is spent assigning blame or fault for the act because it is not always necessary to prove negligence. The "captain of the ship" doctrine is no longer assumed to be true, and members of the entire surgical team can be held liable in litigation for RSIs.[8-10]

Retained surgical items are considered a preventable occurrence. Many states require public reporting when these events occur. Federal and state agencies, accrediting bodies, third-party payers, and professional associations consider an RSI a sentinel event or "never event." Health care organizations and providers will not be reimbursed for additional care provided as a result of "never events."[8,11-15]

The incidence of RSIs is well-documented in the literature dating as early as the 1800s.[2,3,5-7,16-18] There is immense variability, however, in the occurrence rates and identified risks. In a study of retained foreign items, 52% were radiopaque sponges and 43% were instruments.[7] The RSIs in this study were associated with multiple major procedures being performed at the same time. Another study reported count discrepancies in 29 procedures (ie, 45% for radiopaque sponges, 34% for instruments, 21% for needles).[5] The study suggests that emergency procedures and unexpected changes in procedures correlated to an increased risk of RSIs. Closed claim studies conducted between 1985 and 2001 demonstrated that roughly 69% of reported cases of RSIs involved radiopaque sponges.[2]

Although the majority of retained radiopaque sponges are found in the abdomen and pelvis, there are reports in the literature discussing retained radiopaque sponges in the vagina, thorax, spinal canal, face, brain, and extremities.[2,6,8] The risk exists for RSIs even in the smallest of incisions.[3] A general strategy for preventing RSIs is to account for all items opened or used in a procedure at the end of the procedure because the potential risk for retention cannot always be predicted.

Common strategies in the literature that have been used to mitigate the incidence of RSIs include development of standardized procedures combined with manual counting; enhanced communication; multidisciplinary teamwork; radiological verification; and use of adjuncts (eg, count bags, technology to supplement manual sponge count procedures). Health care organizations are responsible for drafting policies and procedures applicable to their practice setting. It is imperative to value teamwork and hold all perioperative personnel accountable for the adoption, implementation, and review of their designated procedures and practices.

RETAINED SURGICAL ITEMS

Recommendation I

A consistent multidisciplinary approach for preventing RSIs should be used during all surgical and invasive procedures.

Retained surgical items are preventable events that can be reduced by implementing multidisciplinary system and team interventions.[12,19,20] Retained surgical items may result in morbidity and mortality for the patient and prove to be costly to health care organizations.[3,13,14,21]

Establishing a system that accounts for all surgical items opened and used during a procedure constitutes a primary and proactive injury-prevention strategy. Performing surgical item counts is one RSI-prevention strategy. Accounting systems that involve counting and detection are, at a minimum, team-based activities composed of input from multiple team members. The practices employed should be standardized, transparent, verifiable, and reliable. All items need to be accounted for at the end of a procedure so that all team members can be sure that a surgical item is not left in the patient.[22]

I.a. All perioperative team members should be responsible for the prevention of RSIs.

I.a.1. Any individual who observes an item dropped from the surgical field should immediately inform the RN circulator and other members of the perioperative team.[3]

I.a.2. Any perioperative team member (eg, anesthesia care provider, float RN) who assists the surgical team by opening sterile items such as extra sutures or radiopaque sponges onto the sterile field should
- count the items with the scrub person;
- add the counted items to the count documentation (ie, count sheet, whiteboard); and
- promptly inform the RN circulator about what was added.[3,23]

Other team members may be asked to open supplies while the RN circulator is occupied with other patient care activities. Opening extra supplies without properly adding them to the count sheet or whiteboard may lead to a discrepancy at the end of the procedure.

I.a.3. A count may be initiated by any member of the perioperative team involved in the counting process.

I.a.4. Unnecessary activity and distractions should be curtailed during the counting process to allow the scrub person and RN circulator to focus on counting tasks.

An environment that is filled with noise and distractions is likely to result in ineffective communication.[19,24-26] Distractions during counting can lead to incorrect counts.[4,27,28] Distractions may include excessive noise (eg, radio, equipment, pagers, telephones); multi-tasking (eg, patient care, charting, retrieving supplies, adding surgical items to the field); and interruptions or breaks in attention (eg, conversations not related to patient care).[24,29,30] It is unlikely that all activities can be eliminated during the counting process; however, communication can be enhanced with reliable team-based practices that withstand the interruptions and conflicting activities that are part of the surgical environment.

I.a.5. Counts and events that would require a count (eg, relief of scrub person or RN circulator) should not be performed during critical portions of the procedure.

I.b. The RN circulator should actively participate in safety measures to prevent RSIs during all phases of a procedure and observe the sterile field to assist in the reduction of RSIs.

Accurately accounting for items used during a surgical procedure is a primary responsibility of the RN circulator and the perioperative team members.[31] The RN circulator plays a leading role in implementing measures to account for surgical items.

I.b.1. The RN circulator should facilitate the count process by initiating the count, performing count procedures in concert with the perioperative team, documenting count reconciliation activities, and reporting any count discrepancy. (See Recommendation VI.)

I.c. The scrub person and the RN circulator should perform standardized procedures when accounting for all surgical items opened or used during a procedure as required by the health care organization's policy.

Reason's study of human error has shown that errors involve some kind of deviation from routine practice.[32] Deliberate, consistent application and adherence to standardized procedures are necessary to prevent the retention of surgical items.[2-4,7,28,33-36]

I.c.1. The scrub person should maintain an organized sterile field with minimal variation between scrub persons.

Maintaining an organized sterile field facilitates accounting for all objects during and after the operative procedure. Standardized sterile setups established by the health care organization's policy reduce variation and may lessen risk of error.

I.c.2. Sharps should be confined and contained in specified areas of the sterile field or within a sharps containment device.

I.c.3. The scrub person should maintain awareness of the location of soft goods (eg, radiopaque sponges, towels, textiles); miscellaneous

RETAINED SURGICAL ITEMS

items; and instruments on the sterile field during the course of the procedure. It is the scrub person's responsibility to

- know the character and configuration of soft goods, instruments, and devices that are used by the surgeons and first assistants;
- verify the integrity and completeness of soft goods when they are counted;
- ensure that the RN circulator sees surgical items being counted;
- confirm that instruments or devices that are returned from the operative site are intact; and
- speak up when a discrepancy exists.

A standardized, transparent, verifiable, reliable process of accounting for soft goods, sharps, needles, instruments, and small items may decrease the incidence of RSIs. Although there is a greater incidence of RSIs for soft goods, the risk also exists for retained instruments and device fragments.[3,5,7,37]

I.d. Surgeons should engage in safe practices that support prevention of RSIs.

The American College of Surgeons recognizes patient safety as "the highest priority and strongly urges individual hospitals and healthcare organizations to take all reasonable measures to prevent the retention of foreign bodies in the surgical wound."[36] It is the responsibility of all perioperative team members to engage in safe practices for the prevention of RSIs.

I.d.1. The surgeon(s) and surgical first assistant(s) should maintain awareness of all soft goods, instruments, and sharps used in the surgical wound during the course of the procedure. The surgeon does not perform the count but should facilitate the count process by
- using only radiopaque surgical items in the wound;
- communicating placement of surgical items in the wound to the perioperative team for notation (eg, whiteboard);
- acknowledging awareness of the start of the count process;
- removing unneeded soft goods and instrumentation from the surgical field at the initiation of the count process;
- performing a methodical wound exploration when closing counts are initiated;
- accounting for and communicating about surgical items in the surgical field; and
- notifying the scrub person and RN circulator about surgical items returned to the surgical field after the count.

I.e. Anesthesia care providers should maintain situational awareness and engage in safe practices that support the prevention of RSIs.

Situational awareness is the process of recognizing a threat and taking steps to avoid the threat.

I.e.1. Anesthesia care providers should plan anesthetic milestone actions so that these actions do not pressure the perioperative team to perform insufficient accounting practices.[3]

Completion of the proper counting procedures is the responsibility of the entire perioperative team.

I.e.2. Anesthesia care providers should not use counted items.

I.e.3. Anesthesia care providers should verify that throat packs, bite blocks, and other similar devices are removed from the oropharynx and communicate to the perioperative team when these items are inserted and removed.

I.f. Complete and detailed communication between OR personnel and radiologic technologists and radiologists should occur when requesting radiological support to prevent RSIs. (See Recommendation VI.)

These activities focus the radiologist's view and aid in the best chance of being able to see the surgical items on the radiograph. Radiological imaging along with other perioperative activities may mitigate the risk of RSIs.[38]

Recommendation II

Radiopaque surgical soft goods (eg, sponges, towels, textiles) opened onto the sterile field should be accounted for during all procedures for which soft goods are used.

Accurately accounting for radiopaque sponges throughout a surgical procedure should be a priority and requires a multidisciplinary effort.[22,39-41]

Reports in surgical literature document that gossypiboma (ie, the unintentional retention of soft goods) can occur after a wide variety of surgical procedures.[2,37,42,43] Clinical presentation of gossypiboma is either acute or delayed. Acute presentations generally follow a septic course with abscess and/or granuloma formation. Delayed presentations may occur months or years after the original surgical intervention, with adhesion formation and encapsulation.[3,4,36,37,41,44-46]

II.a. Initial counts of radiopaque soft goods should be performed and recorded for all surgical procedures.

Performing and recording initial counts establishes a baseline for subsequent counts on all procedures. Deliberate, consistent application and adherence to standardized procedures are necessary to prevent the retention of surgical items.[2-4,7,28,33-36]

RETAINED SURGICAL ITEMS

II.b. Counts of soft goods should be performed
- before the procedure to establish a baseline and identify manufacturing packaging errors (ie, initial count);
- when new items are added to the field;
- before closure of a cavity within a cavity (eg, uterus);
- when wound closure begins;
- at skin closure at the end of the procedure or at the end of the procedure when counted items are no longer in use (ie, final count); and
- at the time of permanent relief of either the scrub person or the RN circulator, although direct visualization of all items may not be possible.

Deliberate, consistent application and adherence to standardized procedures are necessary to prevent RSIs.[2-4,7,28,33-36] A standardized count procedure assists in achieving accuracy, efficiency, and continuity among perioperative team members. Studies of human error have shown that many errors involve some kind of deviation from routine practice.[32]

II.c. Radiopaque sponges should be completely separated, viewed concurrently by two individuals, one of whom should be an RN circulator, and counted audibly.

Concurrent verification of counts by two individuals may lessen the risk of inaccurate counts. Separating radiopaque sponges during the initial baseline count helps to determine whether a sponge has been added to or removed from a sterilized package and that a radiopaque marker or identifying tag is present on each surgical sponge.

II.c.1. Packages containing an incorrect number of radiopaque sponges or a manufacturing defect should be removed from the field, bagged, labeled, isolated from the rest of the radiopaque sponges in the OR, and excluded from the count. Packages containing an incorrect number of radiopaque sponges may be removed from the room before the patient's entry.

The initial sponge count is performed to determine that all packages of radiopaque sponges contain the correct number and the appropriate radiopaque marker or identification bar code, tag, or chip. Incorrect numbers of items or product defects within a package do occur.

Isolating the entire package containing an incorrect number of sponges may help reduce the potential for error in subsequent counts. Packages containing an incorrect number of radiopaque sponges may be removed from the room before the patient's entry to decrease confusion and the likelihood of error.

II.c.2. If the surgical sponge package is banded, the band should be broken and discarded before counting.

Leaving the package band in place may prevent the ability of each individual to see the sponges and allow one or more sponges to be undetected.

II.d. Additional radiopaque sponges added to the field should be counted at that time and recorded as part of the count documentation.

Counting and recording radiopaque sponges as they are added to the field is required to account for all items at the conclusion of the procedure.

II.e. Sponges should be left in their original configuration and should not be cut or altered in any way.

Altering a sponge by cutting or removing radiopaque portions invalidates counts and increases the risk of a portion being retained in the wound.

II.f. Soft goods counts should be conducted in the same sequence each time as defined by the health care organization. The counting sequence should be in a logical progression (eg, large to small item size, proximal to distal from the wound).

A standardized count procedure (ie, following the same sequence) assists in achieving accuracy, efficiency, and continuity among perioperative team members.[7,36] Studies of human error have shown that many errors involve some kind of deviation from routine practice.[32]

II.g. All soft goods used in the surgical wound should be radiopaque and easily differentiated from non-radiopaque soft goods (eg, sponges, towels).

Radiopaque indicators facilitate locating by radiograph an item presumed lost or left in the surgical field when a count discrepancy occurs.

Retained surgical towels have resulted in patient injury.[3,20,47,48] Surgical towels found in the abdomen and chest have been reported, as have instances of surgical towels found at autopsy or as a retained item after root cause analysis or focused case review.[49,50] When placed in a body cavity, an unmarked towel not included in the count may not be detected and increases the possibility of an RSI.

II.g.1. Non-radiopaque sponges used for skin preps that have a similar appearance to counted radiopaque sponges should be isolated before beginning the procedure to avoid possible confusion with the counted radiopaque sponges.

II.g.2. Radiopaque sponges should not be used as postoperative wound dressings.

The use of radiopaque sponges as surface dressings may invalidate subsequent counts

RETAINED SURGICAL ITEMS

if the patient is returned to the OR. The use of surgical sponges as surface dressings may appear as foreign items on postoperative radiographs and suggest a retained item.[51,52]

II.g.3. Non-radiopaque gauze dressing materials should be withheld from the field until the final count is conducted.

Separating dressing materials from the actual counted radiopaque sponges may help prevent intermingling with the sponges used in the procedure.

II.g.4. Dressing sponges included in custom packs should remain sealed and isolated on the field until the final count is resolved.

II.h. The final count should not be considered complete until all sponges used in closing the wound are removed from the wound and returned to the scrub person.

Sponges used in closing the wound could be left in the wound.

II.i. All counted radiopaque sponges should remain within the OR or procedure room during the procedure.

Confining all counted radiopaque sponges to the OR may help eliminate the possibility of a count discrepancy and aid in the disposal of all the radiopaque sponges to prevent carryover to subsequent procedures.

II.i.1. Pocketed sponge bags or similar systems should be used on all procedures where a soft goods count is performed.

Using a pocketed bag or other system for separating used radiopaque sponges facilitates the ability to see sponges for counting. Separating radiopaque sponges after use minimizes errors caused by sponges sticking together.

Draping used surgical sponges over the sides of the kick bucket is discouraged because it may be difficult for all team members to see each individual sponge. Wet, used sponges may drip blood and other potentially infectious fluids on the floor.

II.i.2. If a sponge is passed or dropped from the sterile field, the RN circulator should retrieve it using standard precautions, show it to the scrub person, isolate it from the field, and include it in the final count.

II.i.3. Linen and waste containers should not be removed from the OR or procedure room until all counts are completed and reconciled and the patient has been transferred out of the room.

II.i.4. Radiopaque surgical sponges should be disposed of and removed from the OR or procedure room at the end of the procedure after the patient has left the room.

Removing soft goods from the room at the end of the procedure may prevent potential count discrepancies between patients.

II.j. When soft goods are used as therapeutic packing (eg, intracavity, oral) and the patient leaves the OR with this packing in place, a standardized procedure should be defined and implemented to communicate the location of packing and the plan for eventual removal of the items.

II.j.1. When soft goods are intentionally used as therapeutic packing and the patient leaves the OR with this packing in place, the number and types of items placed should be documented in the medical record
- as reconciled and confirmed by the surgeon when this information is known with certainty, or
- as incorrect if the number and type of sponges used for therapeutic packing is not known with certainty.

II.j.2. The number and types of soft goods used for therapeutic packing should be included and communicated as part of the transfer of patient care information.[53]

II.j.3. When the patient is returned to the OR for a subsequent procedure or to remove therapeutic packing,
- the number and type of radiopaque soft goods removed should be documented in the medical record,
- the radiopaque sponges removed should be isolated and not included in the counts for the removal procedure,
- the surgeon and the surgical team should perform a methodical wound examination and consider taking an intraoperative radiograph, and
- the count on the removal procedure should be noted as reconciled if all radiopaque soft goods have been accounted for.

Additional safety measures may help to ensure that no soft goods remain in the patient when the number and type of radiopaque soft goods used for therapeutic packing is not known.

II.j.4. The surgeon should inform the patient of any soft good(s) purposely left in the wound at the end of the procedure and the plan for removing the item.[54]

Recommendation III

Sharps and other miscellaneous items that are opened onto the sterile field should be accounted for during all procedures for which sharps and miscellaneous item are used.

Needles may account for up to 50% of identified RSIs.[55] Miscellaneous items may be non-radiopaque

RETAINED SURGICAL ITEMS

and unintentionally retained in the surgical wound. Accurately accounting for sharps and other miscellaneous items during a surgical procedure is a primary responsibility of the RN circulator and the perioperative team members.

III.a. Initial sharps (eg, scalpels, needles) counts should be performed and recorded for all surgical procedures.

Performing and recording initial counts establishes a baseline for subsequent counts on all procedures. Deliberate, consistent application and adherence to standardized procedures is necessary to prevent the retention of surgical items.[2-4,7,28,33-36]

III.a.1. Standardized practices, manual counting procedures, and containment devices for sharps and needles should be employed to prevent needle miscounts, needle loss, and needlestick injuries.

Counting sharps and miscellaneous items is important to prevent item retention and reduce the risk of injuries to health care personnel and patients.[56] Operating room, sterile processing, housekeeping, laundry, and morgue personnel are at an increased risk for needlestick injury resulting in undue exposure to transmissible infections.[33,57] There are multiple reported cases of needlestick-associated injuries to health care personnel.[58-60] A standardized count procedure (ie, following the same sequence) assists in achieving accuracy, efficiency, and continuity among perioperative team members. Studies of human error have shown that many errors involve some kind of deviation from routine practice.[32]

III.a.2. All suture needles, regardless of size, should be counted for all surgical procedures.

Even small needles left in the patient may cause injury. Needles less than 10 mm, however, may be difficult to see radiographically when retention is suspected.[3,5,60] One study showed that radiologists inconsistently see small needles on intraoperative imaging studies.[55]

III.b. Counts of sharps and miscellaneous items should be performed
- before the procedure to establish a baseline and identify manufacturing packaging errors (ie, initial count);
- when new items are added to the field;
- before closure of a cavity within a cavity (eg, uterus);
- when wound closure begins;
- at skin closure at the end of the procedure or at the end of the procedure when counted items are no longer in use (ie, final count); and
- at the time of permanent relief of either the scrub person or the RN circulator, although the ability to directly see all items may not be possible.

III.b.1. Miscellaneous items that should be accounted for include, but are not limited to,
- defogger solution bottle, bottle cap, and associated accessories (eg, wipe, sponge);
- electrosurgery active electrode blades;
- electrosurgery scratch pads;
- endostaple reload cartridges;
- laparotomy sponge rings;
- Raney clips;
- trocar sealing caps;
- umbilical and hernia tapes;
- vascular inserts;
- vessel clip bars; and
- vessel loops.

III.c. Sharps and miscellaneous items should be counted audibly and viewed concurrently by two individuals, one of whom should be an RN circulator.

Concurrent verification of counts by two individuals may lessen the risk for count discrepancies.

III.d. Additional sharps and miscellaneous items added to the field should be counted when they are added and recorded as part of the count documentation.

Counting and recording sharps and miscellaneous items as they are added to the field may reduce the risk of error and may prevent an inaccurate count at the conclusion of the procedure.

III.e. Suture needles should be counted when the package is opened, verified by the scrub person, and recorded.

Viewing each needle will help ensure an accurate needle count.

III.e.1. Empty suture packages should not be used to rectify a discrepancy in a closing needle count.

The actual number of needles may not be the same as the number of empty packages.

III.f. The scrub person should account for and confine all sharps on the sterile field until the final count is reconciled.

Unconfined sharps remaining on the sterile field may be unintentionally introduced into the incision, dropped on the floor, or penetrate barriers. Confinement and containment of sharps may minimize the risk of needlestick injury to personnel as well as RSIs.

III.f.1. Used sharps on the sterile field should be kept in a puncture-resistant container.

Collecting used needles in a puncture-resistant container helps ensure their containment on the sterile field and assists in counting at the conclusion of the procedure.

RETAINED SURGICAL ITEMS

III.g. Sharps counts should be conducted in the same sequence each time as defined by the health care organization. The counting sequence should be in a logical progression (eg, sterile field to table to off the field).

A standardized count procedure (ie, following the same sequence) assists in achieving accuracy, efficiency, and continuity among perioperative team members. Studies of human error have shown that many errors involve some kind of deviation from routine practice.[32]

III.h. The scrub person should assess the condition of sharps or other items and verify that they are intact when returned from the operative site.

Breakage or separation of parts can occur during open and minimally invasive surgical procedures. Verifying that all broken parts are present or accounted for helps prevent RSIs within the patient.[61,62]

III.h.1. If a broken or separated item is returned from the operative site, the scrub person should immediately notify the perioperative team.

III.i. The final count should not be considered complete until all the sharps used in closing the wound are removed from the wound and returned to the scrub person.

Suture needles and other sharp items used in closing the wound could be left in the wound.

III.j. All counted sharps should remain within the OR or procedure room during the procedure.

Confining all sharps to the OR or procedure room helps minimize the possibility of a count discrepancy.

III.j.1. If a sharp is passed or dropped from the sterile field, the RN circulator should retrieve it using standardized precautions, show it to the scrub person, isolate it from the field, and include it in the final count.

III.j.2. Linen or waste containers should not be removed from the OR or procedure room until all counts are completed and reconciled and the patient has been transferred out of the room.

Recommendation IV

Instruments should be accounted for on all procedures in which the likelihood exists that an instrument could be retained.

Instrument counts protect the patient by reducing the likelihood that an instrument will be retained in the patient, including during minimally invasive procedures (eg, laparoscopy, thoracoscopy). Instrument counts are a proactive injury-prevention strategy. Retention of surgical instruments accounts for approximately one-third of retained item case reports.[5] Case studies demonstrate that many types and sizes of retained instruments have been found, ranging from small serrafine clamps to moderately sized hemostats (ie, 6 to 10 inches) to 13-inch-long retractors.[3,4]

IV.a. Counts of instruments should be performed
- before the procedure to establish a baseline (ie, initial count);
- when new instruments are added to the field;
- at wound closure or at the end of the procedure when counted items are no longer in use (ie, final count); and
- at the time of permanent relief of either the scrub person or the RN circulator, although the ability to directly see all items may not be possible.

Deliberate, consistent application and adherence to standardized procedures are necessary to prevent RSIs (eg, surgical instruments).[2-4,7,28,33-36]

IV.a.1. Instruments should be counted when sets are assembled for sterilization.

A count of the instruments at assembly of the instrument set provides a basic inventory reference for the instrument set but is not considered the initial count before the surgical procedure. A count performed outside of the OR that is considered an initial count increases the number of variables that can contribute to a count discrepancy and unnecessarily extends responsibility to personnel not involved in direct patient care.

IV.b. The health care organization's policy should clearly define circumstances in which the instrument count may be waived.

Procedures in which accurate instrument counts may not be achievable or practical include, but are not limited to,
- complex procedures involving large numbers of instruments (eg, anterior-posterior spinal procedures)[6];
- trauma[2,45,63];
- procedures that require complex instruments with numerous small parts; and
- procedures where the width and depth of the incision is too small to retain an instrument.

IV.c. Instruments should be counted audibly and viewed concurrently by two individuals, one of whom should be the RN circulator.

Concurrent verification of counts by two individuals assists in ensuring accurate counts.

IV.d. Individual pieces of assembled instruments (eg, suction tips, wing nuts, blades, sheaths) should be accounted for separately and documented on the count sheet.

Counting individual pieces of assembled instruments before and after a procedure reduces the risk of leaving a piece behind if the instrument becomes disassembled for any reason. Removable instrument parts can be purposefully removed or become loose and fall into the wound or onto or off of the sterile field.[61]

RETAINED SURGICAL ITEMS

IV.e. Additional instruments should be counted and recorded as part of the count documentation when they are added to the sterile field.

Counting and recording instruments as they are added to the sterile field may prevent an inaccurate count at the conclusion of the procedure.

IV.f. Members of the surgical team should account for instruments in their entirety that may have broken or become separated within the confines of the surgical site.

Breakage or separation of parts can occur during open or minimally invasive surgical procedures. Verifying that the instrument is intact or that all broken parts are present and accounted for helps prevent RSIs within the patient.[61,62]

IV.g. Instrument counts should be conducted in the same sequence each time as defined by the health care organization. The counting sequence should be in a logical progression (eg, large to small item size, proximal to distal from the wound).

A standardized count procedure (ie, following the same sequence) assists in achieving accuracy, efficiency, and continuity among perioperative team members. Studies of human error have shown that many errors involve some kind of deviation from routine practice.[32]

IV.h. The final instrument count should not be considered complete until those instruments used in closing the wound (eg, malleable retractors, needle holders, scissors) are removed from the wound and returned to the scrub person.

Incidents of retained surgical instruments used in closing the wound have been reported.[64,65]

IV.i. All counted instruments should remain within the OR or procedure room during the procedure until all counts are completed and resolved.

Confining all counted instruments to the room helps eliminate the possibility of a count discrepancy.

IV.i.1. Counted items either passed off or dropped from the sterile field should be retrieved by the RN circulator, isolated, and included in the final count.

IV.j. All instruments should be accounted for and removed from the room during end-of-procedure cleanup.

Accounting for all instruments facilitates inventory control, as well as patient and personnel safety. Removing all instruments from the room helps prevent potential count discrepancies during subsequent procedures.

IV.k. Preprinted count sheets should be used to record the counted instruments.

Preprinted count sheets provide organization and efficiency, which are key to preventing retained surgical instruments.

IV.k.1. The circulating nurse should record only the number of instruments opened for the procedure.

IV.l. Instrument sets should be standardized with the minimum number and variety of instruments needed for the procedure.

Reducing the number and types of instruments and streamlining standardized sets improves ease and efficiency of counting.

IV.l.1. Instruments that are not routinely used on procedures should be removed from sets.

Specialty instruments, if needed, can be opened and added to the count at the time of the procedure.

Recommendation V

Measures should be taken to identify and reduce the risks associated with unretrieved device fragments.

Each year, the US Food and Drug Administration (FDA) Center for Devices and Radiological Health receives nearly 1,000 adverse event reports related to unretrieved device fragments. Serious adverse events have been associated with unretrieved device fragments. The FDA defines an unretrieved device fragment as "a fragment of a medical device that has separated unintentionally and remains in the patient after a procedure."[66]

V.a. In the event that an unretrieved device fragment is left in the surgical wound (eg, broken instrument tip), the surgeon should inform the patient of the nature of the item and the risks associated with leaving it in the wound.

Health care professionals are encouraged to maintain public confidence by communicating with patients regarding their treatment and outcomes. Organizations are held accountable for informing patients of their rights when they enter the health care system.[54]

V.a.1. Information provided to the patient should include, but is not limited to,
- material composition of the fragment (if known);
- size of the fragment (if known);
- location of the fragment;
- potential mechanisms for injury (eg, migration, infection);
- procedures or treatments that should be avoided, such as magnetic resonance imaging (MRI) examinations in the case of ferrous metallic fragments, which may help reduce the possibility of a serious injury from the fragment; and
- risks and benefits of retrieving the fragment as opposed to leaving it in the wound.

RETAINED SURGICAL ITEMS

Recommendation VI

Standardized measures for investigation and reconciliation of count discrepancies should be taken during the closing count and before the end of surgery. When a discrepancy in the count(s) is identified, the surgical team should carry out steps to locate the missing item.[27,67]

Rapid intervention when an incorrect count is identified may reduce procedural time. Assessing the surgical site before closure decreases the time a patient remains under anesthesia and the risk of extended surgical time if the wound has to be reopened.[5] Early identification of RSIs decreases the likelihood that a surgical wound would need to be reopened and reduces or eliminates the need for radiographs to detect an RSI.[8]

VI.a. The RN circulator should inform and receive verbal acknowledgment from the surgeon and surgical team as soon as a discrepancy in a surgical count is identified.[5,68]

The RN circulator has a responsibility and ethical obligation to speak up promptly when a discrepancy is identified. Clear and timely communication reinforces a safe patient culture.[3,31,69] A count discrepancy is a potential RSI incident.[70]

VI.a.1. The RN circulator should visually inspect the area surrounding the surgical field, including the floor, kick buckets, and linen and trash receptacles in an effort to locate the missing surgical item.

VI.a.2. The scrub person should assist with visual inspection of the area surrounding the sterile field when there is a count discrepancy.

VI.b. When a discrepancy in the count is identified, the surgeon(s) should
- suspend closure of the wound if the patient's condition permits,
- perform a methodical wound examination by actively looking for the missing item,
- cooperate in the attainment of radiographs or other modalities as indicated to find the missing item, and
- remain in the OR until the item is found or it is determined with certainty not to be in the patient.[3,4]

VI.c. If a missing item is not recovered, intraoperative imaging should be performed to rule out a retained item before final closure of the wound if the patient's condition permits. If the patient's condition is unstable, a radiograph should be taken as soon as possible in the next phase of care.[3,60]

Obtaining a radiograph when all other efforts have failed and before the patient's wound is closed allows the surgical team to remove a potential RSI before the wound is closed completely. In some jurisdictions, this also will prevent the necessity of reporting an RSI.

VI.c.1. In situations when accurate counting of surgical items is not possible, intraoperative imaging should be performed before the patient is transferred from the OR.[3,17,27,34]

VI.c.2. If intraoperative imaging is not available, the health care organization should have a policy and procedure describing the actions and communication required between referring and receiving organizations. `Amb`

VI.c.3. A radiograph to locate a possible retained item may be waived under certain circumstances as defined in the health care organization's policy and procedure.

There are situations when it may be medically appropriate for the surgeon to determine it is not in the individual patient's best interest to perform an intraoperative radiograph to locate a potential RSI.

VI.c.4. Complete and detailed communication between OR personnel and radiologic technologists and radiologists should occur when requesting radiological support to prevent RSIs. The OR radiology request should include standardized information about the missing surgical item, including, but not limited to,
- the room where the procedure is being performed or the patient is located,
- the type of radiograph and views needed,
- a description of the missing surgical item,
- the operation performed, and
- the surgical site.[21,38]

These activities focus the radiologist's attention and aid in his or her ability to see the surgical items on the radiograph. Radiological imaging along with other perioperative activities may mitigate the risk of RSIs.[38]

VI.c.5. The radiologic technologist should be called promptly and respond expeditiously when an incorrect count occurs in the OR.[21]

VI.c.6. Intraoperative imaging should provide coverage of the surgical site and should include any views deemed necessary by the surgeon or radiologist to exclude the potential for RSIs. Radiological views should be obtained using recommended techniques and quality films or digital images to capture the full extent of the wound.

Progressive radiological techniques are recommended for successful identification of RSIs, including, but not limited to, multiple images, which may be necessary for full coverage. Images may include
- initial portable anterior and posterior (A&P) views followed by an oblique view if the A&P is negative;
- fluoroscopy, which may be used as an alternative technique if the RSI cannot be

- excluded with the intraoperative study; and
- unenhanced computerized tomography (CT), which should be considered if previous techniques are negative and a high suspicion remains for an RSI.[38]

VI.c.7. The radiologist should be consulted for guidance on the most appropriate available radiographic equipment to use to maximize the opportunity to identify a missing surgical item.[3,38]

Although some literature suggests that a radiograph taken in a radiology suite may be of better quality than a portable film taken in an OR, this would preclude finding a potential RSI before the wound is closed and the patient is taken out of the OR.[3,35,71] There is no evidence to support the use of a portable radiograph versus an image intensifier (ie, fluoroscopy). Portable radiographs have limitations, such as lower tube power; reduced ability to determine the character (eg, needle size and type) of an RSI; and limited placement options for film cassettes.[71]

VI.c.8. Intraoperative imaging for RSIs should be read by a radiologist and the results communicated directly to the surgeon in a timely manner.[3,38] Interpretation of intraoperative films should be communicated by direct report to the OR with read-back verbal confirmation between the radiologist and the surgeon.[21,38]

VI.c.9. Health care organizations should define needle size limit criteria where radiographs will effectively assist in identifying retained needles.

There is no definitive evidence to indicate how effective radiographs are in detecting small suture needles. Recent studies have demonstrated that needles 10 mm and smaller may not be consistently visible on a radiograph.[3,59,72,73] There is conflicting evidence regarding the visibility of 10-mm to 13-mm needles on radiographs.[3,19,20,35,55,60,72,73]

VI.c.10. The surgeon should inform the patient of the possibility of a retained needle as a result of an unresolved needle count and counsel the patient on the possible risks.

Recommendation VII

Perioperative staff members may consider the use of adjunct technologies to supplement manual count procedures.

Soft goods, such as radiopaque sponges and towels, represent the majority of RSIs. Paradoxically, studies suggest that the final count was documented as correct in 62% to 88% of RSI cases.[2,8,22,70,74] Manual counts can result in errors, especially during emergencies and unexpected surgical events. Intraoperative radiographs also are not always effective in identifying RSIs. In one study, 67% of intraoperative radiographs were read as negative when an RSI actually was present.[17]

Technologies have recently become available that are designed to supplement manual counting of soft goods, primarily radiopaque sponges, in an attempt to reduce RSIs.[20,75,76] Early identification of a retained sponge reduces the likelihood of delaying patient care; requiring additional measures, such as intraoperative radiographs to locate and retrieve the retained sponge; having to reopen the wound; or returning the patient to surgery for removal of the retained item at a later date. Use of this technology may allow timely detection of retained sponges even when a manual sponge count does not reveal a missing sponge. These technologies can be classified as count, detect, or count and detect.[20,70,75,77-81] In the future, adjunct technologies for accounting of needles and instruments may become available as well.

VII.a. A mechanism for evaluating and selecting existing and emerging adjunct technology products should be implemented.[82]

Patient safety is a primary concern of perioperative personnel. Safety concerns are the impetus for perioperative personnel as they participate in evaluating and selecting medical devices and products for use in practice settings.

VII.a.1. Perioperative RNs, physicians, and other health care providers involved in the use of products and medical devices for prevention of RSIs should be part of a multidisciplinary product evaluation and selection committee when the health care organization is evaluating the purchase of adjunct technology.[82]

VII.a.2. Perioperative personnel should evaluate existing and emerging adjunct technology to determine the application that may be most suitable in their setting.

Several adjunct technology products are currently available, and the technology is rapidly evolving.[44,75-77,79]

VII.a.3. Technology product standardization and value analysis processes should reflect functional and reliable products that are safe, cost-effective, environmentally friendly, and that promote quality patient care.[77,81,83]

VII.b. Adjunct technology may be used, where available, as an extra measure of safety to verify count accuracy throughout the reconciliation process.

The literature suggests that a combination of standardized procedures with manual counting; enhanced communication; multidisciplinary teamwork; radiological verification; and the use of adjuncts (eg, count bags, technology to supplement manual sponge count procedures) may decrease the incidence of RSIs.[2-4,7,17,19,44,48]

VII.b.1. Perioperative personnel should be aware of and competent in the proper use and application of adjunct technologies if used within the health care organization.[77]

Technological systems are dependent on proper usage and technique.

Recommendation VIII

Personnel should receive initial and ongoing education and demonstrate competency in the performance of standardized measures to prevent RSIs.

Initial and periodic education on practices for the prevention of RSIs provides direction for personnel in providing safe patient care. Additional periodic educational programs provide opportunities to reinforce previous learning and introduce new information on adjunct technology, its use, and potential risks. Competency validation serves as an indicator that personnel have an understanding of safe practices for the prevention of RSIs; the risks of injury (eg, needlesticks) to the patient and to health care personnel; and corrective actions that should be implemented when a process failure occurs.

VIII.a. An introduction and review of policies and procedures for prevention of RSIs should be included in orientation and ongoing education of personnel.

Reviewing policies and procedures assists health care personnel in developing knowledge, skills, and attitudes that affect patient outcomes.

VIII.b. Perioperative personnel should be knowledgeable about all accounting procedures, equipment, and technology used in the health care organization.

Rapid advances in clinical evidence and technology require continuous learning and skills updates to maintain competency.

VIII.b.1. Perioperative personnel should receive education and demonstrate competency in, but not limited to, the following:
- the performance of manual count procedures (eg, soft goods, instruments, sharps, miscellaneous items);
- the use of adjunct technology, following manufacturers' written instructions, if available;
- the roles, responsibilities, and accountability of each perioperative team member;
- measures for reconciliation of count discrepancies; and
- reporting of known or suspected RSIs.

Instruction and return demonstration in proper manual counting procedures and adjunct technology usage minimizes the risk of error. Competencies based on manufacturers' instructions provide personnel with information regarding the proper use of adjunct technologies. Incorrect use can result in RSIs and serious patient injury. Equipment instruction manuals assist in developing operational, safety, and maintenance guidelines and serve as a reference for safe, appropriate use.

Recommendation IX

Measures taken for the prevention of RSIs should be documented in the patient's medical record.

Documentation of all nursing activities performed is legally and professionally important for clear communication and collaboration between health care team members and for continuity of patient care.[84]

IX.a. Sponge, sharp, and instrument counts should be documented on the patient's intraoperative record by the RN circulator.[84]

IX.b. Documentation of measures taken for the prevention of RSIs should include, but not be limited to,
- types of counts (eg, radiopaque sponges, sharps, instruments, miscellaneous items);
- number of counts;
- names and titles of personnel performing the counts;
- results of surgical item counts;
- surgeon notification of count results;
- any adjunct technology that was used and any associated records;
- an explanation for any waived counts;
- number and location of any instruments intentionally remaining with the patient or radiopaque sponges intentionally retained as therapeutic packing;
- unretrieved device fragments left in the wound, including
  - material composition,
  - size,
  - location (if known), and
  - manufacturer;
- actions taken if count discrepancies occur, including all measures taken to recover the missing item or device fragment and any communication regarding the outcome;
- rationale if counts are not performed or completed as prescribed by policy; and
- the outcome of actions taken.

Documentation of nursing activities related to the patient's perioperative care provides an account of the nursing care administered and provides a mechanism for comparing actual versus expected outcomes.[84] Such documentation is considered sound professional practice and demonstrates that all reasonable efforts were made to protect the patient's safety.[1] Extreme patient emergencies and certain individual patient considerations may necessitate waived counts to preserve a patient's life or limb. Documenting the rationale for waived counts and for variation in standard practice provides a record of the occurrence and an alert to subsequent caregivers that the patient may be at an increased risk for an RSI.

Recommendation X

Policies and procedures for the prevention of RSIs and unretrieved device fragments should be developed, reviewed periodically, revised as necessary, and readily available in the practice setting.

Policies and procedures establish authority, responsibility, and accountability. Policies and procedures assist in the development of patient safety, quality assessment, and quality improvement (QI) activities.[1] They also serve as operational guidelines that are used to minimize patient risk factors, standardize practice, direct staff members, and establish guidelines for continuous performance improvement activities. Best practices are subject to change with the emergence of new evidence and the advent of new technologies; therefore, periodic review and revision of the health care organization's policy is needed.

X.a. A multidisciplinary team should establish a policy and procedure for prevention of RSIs.[2,3,36,85] These policies and procedures should include, but not be limited to,
- items to be counted;
- directions for performing counts (eg, sequence, item grouping);
- waived count procedures in which baseline and/or subsequent counts may be exempt;
- alternative or additional safety measures for special circumstances;
- use of adjunct technology;
- measures necessary to reduce the risk of unretrieved device fragments including, but not limited to,
  - use of the medical device in accordance with its labeled indications and the manufacturer's instructions for use, especially during insertion and removal,
  - inspection of the medical device before use for damage during shipment or storage, as well as any out-of-box defects that could increase the likelihood of fragmentation during a procedure,
  - inspection of the medical device immediately after removal from the patient for any signs of breakage or fragmentation, and
  - retention of any damaged medical device to assist with the manufacturer's analysis of the event;
- the multidisciplinary team actions and procedures for count discrepancy reconciliation;
- when radiographic screening should be used in accounting for surgical items;
- documentation and reporting procedures for removal of RSIs; and
- competency validation.

All perioperative team members should be committed to and involved in establishing meaningful policies and procedures related to the prevention of RSIs. Detailed, clear, and concise policies provide consistent, standardized direction for the team. In situations with increased risk for RSIs, radiographic screening has been identified as an excellent method for improving early identification.[3,6,45]

X.a.1. Polices and procedures should meet the requirements of regulatory and accrediting agencies.

X.a.2. A policy and procedure for reporting product packaging defects to manufacturers should be established.

X.a.3. Policies and procedures related to the use of adjunct technology should be based on the manufacturer's written instructions for use.

X.a.4. If intraoperative imaging is not available, the health care organization should have a policy and procedure describing actions necessary and communication required between referring and receiving organizations. *Amb*

X.b. Based on risk analysis, the health care organization should establish policies that define when additional measures for prevention of RSIs must be performed or when they may be waived (eg, trauma, cystoscopy, ophthalmology).

Even in the smallest of incisions, the risk exists for RSIs.[3] The size of a pediatric patient may dictate a correspondingly small incision that would make retention of an instrument in the surgical wound unlikely; however, RSIs can occur in the smallest of incisions.[3] Careful consideration should be given when establishing a policy for waived counts for the pediatric patient because it is difficult to determine whether there is no risk of an RSI.

Some situations that have been identified as potentially contributing to the risk for RSI include,
- the emergent nature of a procedure[8,63];
- an unexpected change in the procedure[2];
- patient obesity[2,7,8,44,45];
- multiple surgical teams;
- shift changes[7];
- pressure to increase throughput (ie, reduce operating time)[44]; and
- staff member inexperience.[86]

X.c. Policies and procedures should include RSI prevention measures for organ procurement procedures.

Counted items that are sent with the donated organ(s) increase the risk for RSIs for the organ recipient. Counted sharps and instruments that are retained in the donor may contribute to inventory loss or injury to other health care workers. Counted items left in the OR or procedure room may increase the risk of inaccuracy in subsequent procedure counts or create sharps injury hazards for personnel.[87]

Recommendation XI

A quality assurance/performance improvement process should be in place to evaluate the incidence and risks of RSIs and to improve patient safety.

Quality and performance improvement functions may ensure that organizations design processes well and systematically monitor, analyze, and improve outcomes.[3,12,88-90] Continuous QI opportunities arise from documented and structured quality processes and measures that can define and resolve problems.

XI.a. A multiphase, multidisciplinary process improvement program should be implemented, including, but not limited to,
- an ongoing risk assessment and review (eg, failure mode effect analysis);
- policy design and review;
- a review of published evidence, internal data collection, and data analysis; and
- plans for the ongoing monitoring and analysis of processes, near misses, and adverse events related to the prevention of RSIs.

A comprehensive QI program may identify opportunities for minimizing the risk of RSI events.

XI.b. A critical investigation should be conducted regarding any adverse event or near miss related to RSIs.[1]

Error and near miss reporting are the first steps to addressing error reduction.[89,91] The distraction-prone environment of the perioperative practice setting makes it more likely that errors can be made during routine tasks, including surgical counts.[3,6] Errors can be divided into two categories: those at the human interface in a complex system (ie, active), and those representing a failed system design (ie, latent). There are a number of analysis methods (eg, root cause analysis, appreciative inquiry) available to health care organizations that may be used to conduct a critical investigation of adverse events.[7,12,90,92]

XI.b.1. Multidisciplinary teams should be involved in the review process and address any changes in policy that can improve patient safety.[1]

XI.c. Reporting mechanisms for adverse events and near misses related to RSIs should be established.

Many states require public reporting when these events occur. Federal and state agencies, accrediting bodies, third-party payers, and professional associations consider RSIs a sentinel event or "never event," which should be reported and investigated.[12-14,93-100]

XI.c.1. Events that necessitate reopening a wound to retrieve an RSI should be reported in compliance with health care organizational policy, as well as local, state, and federal regulatory agencies.

XI.d. Health care organizations should value learning and respond to errors with a focus on process improvement rather than individual blame.[69]

Systematic performance measures (ie, indicators) and/or priority areas are identified as opportunities for improvement based on the functions and processes of the perioperative episode.[51,89-91,101] Each perioperative team member has an ethical obligation to perform his or her role and responsibilities with appropriate competence and the highest level of personal integrity.[31]

XI.d.1. Errors should be evaluated in such a manner that contributing factors are first reviewed and then accountability is determined in relation to actions.

Continuous QI opportunities arise from documented and structured quality processes and measures that can define and resolve problems.

XI.d.2. Personnel should identify and respond to opportunities for improvement.

To evaluate the quality of patient care and formulate plans for corrective action, it is necessary to maintain a system of evaluation.

Glossary

Baseline: "A set of critical observations or data used for comparison or a control." (Source: Association for the Advancement of Medical Instrumentation. *Comprehensive Guide to Steam Sterilization and Sterility Assurance in Health Care Facilities; ANSI/AAMI ST79:2006*. Arlington, VA: Association for the Advancement of Medical Instrumentation; 2006:54-111.)

Gossypiboma: Surgical sponge or towel unintentionally retained in the body following surgery. Synonym: Textiloma.

Instruments: Surgical tools or devices designed to perform a specific function, such as cutting, dissecting, grasping, holding, retracting, or suturing.

Minimally invasive surgery: Surgical procedures performed through one or more small incisions using endoscopic instruments, radiographic and magnetic resonance imaging, computer-assisted devices, robotics, and other emerging technologies.

Miscellaneous items: In relation to items on the sterile field that require counting, this may include vessel clip bars, vessel loops, umbilical and hernia tapes, vascular inserts, electrosurgery scratch pads, trocar sealing caps, and any other small items that have the potential for being retained in a surgical wound.

RETAINED SURGICAL ITEMS

Near miss: An occurrence that could have resulted in an accident, injury, or illness but did not by chance, skillful management, or timely intervention. "Any process variation that did not affect the outcome (for the patient or personnel), but for which a recurrence carries a significant chance of a serious adverse outcome. Such a near miss falls within the scope of the definition of a sentinel event, but those outside the scope of sentinel events that are subject to review by the Joint Commission under its Sentinel Event Policy." (Source: Glossary. In: *Hospital Accreditation Standards*. Oak Brook Terrace, IL: Joint Commission on Accreditation of Healthcare Organizations; 2002:331, 345, 351, 354, 360.)

Radio frequency identification (RFID): A system that transmits the identity (in the form of a unique serial number) of an object wirelessly using radio waves.

Root cause analysis: A retrospective approach to error analysis that focuses on failures of system design as related to common root causes of adverse events. "A process for identifying the basic or causal factors that underlie variation in performance, including the occurrence or a sentinel event. A root cause analysis focuses primarily on systems and processes, not individual performance. It progresses from special causes in clinical processes to common causes in organizational processes and identifies potential improvements in processes or systems that would tend to decrease the likelihood of such events in the future, or determines, after analysis that no such improvement opportunities exist." (Source: Sentinel events. In: *Hospital Accreditation Standards*. Oak Brook Terrace, IL: Joint Commission on Accreditation of Healthcare Organizations; 2002:51-52.)

Sentinel event: "An unexpected occurrence involving death or serious physical or psychological injury, or the risk thereof. Serious injury specifically includes loss of limb or function. The phrase 'or the risk thereof' includes any process variation for which a recurrence would carry a significant chance of a serious adverse outcome. Such events are called 'sentinel' because they signal the need for immediate investigation and response." (Source: Official accreditation policies and procedures. In: *Hospital Accreditation Standards*. Oak Brook Terrace, IL: Joint Commission on Accreditation of Healthcare Organizations; 2002:48-49.)

Sharps: Items with edges or points capable of cutting or puncturing through other items. In the context of surgery, items include, but are not limited to, suture needles, scalpel blades, hypodermic needles, electrosurgical needles and blades, instruments with sharp edges or points, and safety pins.

Sponges: Soft goods (eg, gauze pads, cottonoids, peanuts, dissectors, tonsil/laparotomy sponges) used to absorb fluids, protect tissues, or apply pressure or traction.

Waived count: Surgical procedures in which accurate accounting for sponges, instruments, and miscellaneous items is determined to be unachievable or in situations in which the time required to perform the count may present an unacceptable delay in patient care (eg, trauma procedures, anterior-posterior spinal procedures).

References

1. Institute of Medicine Committee on Quality of Health Care in America. *Crossing the Quality Chasm: A New Health System for the 21st Century*. Washington, DC: National Academy Press; 2001.
2. Gawande AA, Studdert DM, Orav EJ, Brennan TA, Zinner MJ. Risk factors for retained instruments and sponges after surgery. *N Engl J Med*. 2003;348(3):229-235.
3. Gibbs VC, Coakley FD, Reines HD. Preventable errors in the operating room: retained foreign bodies after surgery—part I. *Curr Probl Surg*. 2007;44(5):281-337.
4. Gibbs VC. Patient safety practices in the operating room: correct-site surgery and nothing left behind. *Surg Clin North Am*. 2005;85(6):1307-1319.
5. Greenberg CC, Regenbogen SE, Lipsitz SR, Diaz-Flores R, Gawande AA. The frequency and significance of discrepancies in the surgical count. *Ann Surg*. 2008;248(2):337-341.
6. Egorova NN, Moskowitz A, Gelijns A, et al. Managing the prevention of retained surgical instruments: what is the value of counting? *Ann Surg*. 2008;247(1):13-18.
7. Lincourt AE, Harrell A, Cristiano J, Sechrist C, Kercher K, Heniford BT. Retained foreign bodies after surgery. *J Surg Res*. 2007;138(2):170-174.
8. ECRI. Sponge, sharp, and instrument counts. *Healthcare Risk Control*. 2003;4(Surgery and Anesthesia 5):1-7.
9. Murphy EK. "Captain of the ship" doctrine continues to take on water. *AORN J*. 2001;74(4):525-528.
10. Surgical nurses: sponge count is strictly nurses' responsibility, court rules. *Legal Eagle Eye Newsl Nurs Prof*. 2000;8(9):2.
11. Focus on five. Preventing retained foreign objects: improving safety after surgery. *Joint Comm Perspect Patient Saf*. 2006;6(3):11.
12. Sentinel event policy and procedures. The Joint Commission. http://www.jointcommission.org/SentinelEvents/PolicyandProcedures/. Updated July 2007. Accessed July 1, 2010.
13. Centers for Medicare & Medicaid Services (CMS) HHS. Medicare program: changes to the hospital outpatient prospective payment system and CY 2008 payment rates, the ambulatory surgical center payment system and CY 2008 payment rates, the hospital inpatient prospective payment system and FY 2008 payment rates; and payments for graduate medical education for affiliated teaching hospitals in certain emergency situations Medicare and Medicaid programs: hospital conditions of participation; necessary provider designations of critical access hospitals. Interim and final rule with comment period. *Fed Regist*. 2007;72(227):66579-67226.
14. Centers for Medicare & Medicaid Services (CMS) HHS. Medicare program; proposed changes to the hospital inpatient prospective payment systems and fiscal year 2009 rates; proposed changes to disclosure of physician ownership in hospitals and physician self-referral rules; proposed collection of information regarding financial relationships between hospitals and physicians; proposed rule. *Fed Regist*. 2008;73(84):23527-23938.
15. Rosenthal MB. Nonpayment for performance? Medicare's new reimbursement rule. *N Engl J Med*. 2007;357(16):1573-1575.
16. Wilson C. Foreign bodies left in the abdomen after laparotomy. *Trans Am Gynecol Soc*. 1884;9:109-112.
17. Cima RR, Kollengode A, Garnatz J, Storsveen A, Weisbrod C, Deschamps C. Incidence and characteristics of potential and actual retained foreign object events in surgical patients. *J Am Coll Surg*. 2008;207(1):80-87.

18. Bani-Hani KE, Gharaibeh KA, Yaghan RJ. Retained surgical sponges (gossypiboma). *Asian J Surg.* 2005;28(2):109-115.

19. Joint Commission Resources Inc. Preventing retention of foreign bodies after surgery. In: *Safety in the Operating Room.* Oakbrook Terrace, IL: Joint Commission on Accreditation of Healthcare Organizations; 2006:105-110.

20. Beyond the count: preventing retention of foreign objects. *Pa Patient Saf Advis.* 2009;6(2):39-45.

21. Retained surgical instruments and other items. NoThing Left Behind®. http://www.nothingleftbehind.org/Instruments.html. Accessed July 1, 2010.

22. Cima RR, Kollengode A, Storsveen AS, et al. A multidisciplinary team approach to retained foreign objects. *Jt Comm J Qual Patient Saf.* 2009;35(3):123-132.

23. *Implementation Manual Surgical Safety Checklist.* 1st ed. Geneva, Switzerland: World Health Organization; 2008. http://www.who.int/patientsafety/safesurgery/tools_resources/SSSL_Manual_finalJun08.pdf. Accessed July 6, 2010.

24. Sevdalis N, Healey AN, Vincent CA. Distracting communications in the operating theatre. *J Eval Clin Pract.* 2007;13(3):390-394.

25. Kracht JM, Busch-Vishniac IJ, West JE. Noise in the operating rooms of Johns Hopkins Hospital. *J Acoust Soc Am.* 2007;121(5 Pt1):2673-2680.

26. Joint Commission Resources Inc. Improving communication and avoiding distractions. In: *Safety in the Operating Room.* Oakbrook Terrace, IL: Joint Commission on Accreditation of Healthcare Organizations; 2006:3-19.

27. Jackson S, Brady S. Counting difficulties: retained instruments, sponges, and needles. *AORN J.* 2008;87(2):315-321.

28. Best practices for preventing a retained foreign body. *AORN J.* 2006;84(Suppl 1):S30-S36, S58-S60.

29. Healey AN, Primus CP, Koutantji M. Quantifying distraction and interruption in urological surgery. *Qual Saf Health Care.* 2007;16(2):135-139.

30. Healey AN, Sevdalis N, Vincent CA. Measuring intra-operative interference from distraction and interruption observed in the operating theatre. *Ergonomics.* 2006;49(5-6):589-604.

31. Standards of perioperative nursing. In: *Perioperative Standards and Recommended Practices.* Denver, CO: AORN, Inc; 2010:9-62.

32. Reason J. Safety in the operating theatre—part 2: human error and organisational failure. *Qual Saf Health Care.* 2005;14(1):56-60.

33. Brown J, Feather D. Surgical equipment and materials left in patients. *Br J Perioper Nurs.* 2005;15(6):259-262.

34. Porteous J. Surgical counts can be risky business! *Can Oper Room Nurs J.* 2004;22(4):6-8.

35. VHA Directive 2006-030. *Prevention of Retained Surgical Items* [corrected copy]. Washington, DC: Department of Veterans Affairs; May 17, 2006.

36. Statement on the prevention of retained foreign bodies after surgery. American College of Surgeons. http://www.facs.org/fellows_info/statements/st-51.html. Accessed July 1, 2010.

37. Kernagis LY, Siegelman ES, Torigian DA. Case 145: retained sponge. *Radiology.* 2009;251(2):608-611.

38. Whang G, Mogel GT, Tsai J, Palmer SL. Left behind: unintentionally retained surgically placed foreign bodies and how to reduce their incidence—pictorial review. *AJR Am J Roentgenol.* 2009;193(6 Suppl):S79-S89.

39. Catalano K. Knowledge is power: averting safety-compromising events in the OR. *AORN J.* 2008;88(6):987-995.

40. Murphy EK. Protecting patients from potential injuries [OR Nursing Law]. *AORN J.* 2004;79(5):1013-1016.

41. Kim CK, Park BK, Ha H. Gossypiboma in abdomen and pelvis: MRI findings in four patients. *AJR Am J Roentgenol.* 2007;189(4):814-817.

42. Tammelleo AD. Gauze pad left in pt. during reversal of tubal ligation surgery. *Nurs Law Regan Rep.* 2004;45(7):4.

43. Is M, Karatas A, Akgul M, Yildirim U, Gezen F. A retained surgical sponge (gossypiboma) mimicking a paraspinal abscess. *Br J Neurosurg.* 2007;21(3):307-308.

44. Berkowitz S, Marshall H, Charles A. Retained intra-abdominal surgical instruments: time to use nascent technology? *Am Surg.* 2007;73(11):1083-1085.

45. Teixeira PG, Inaba K, Salim A, et al. Retained foreign bodies after emergent trauma surgery: incidence after 2526 cavitary explorations. *Am Surg.* 2007;73(10):1031-1034.

46. Tandon A, Bhargava SK, Gupta A, Bhatt S. Spontaneous transmural migration of retained surgical textile into both small and large bowel: a rare cause of intestinal obstruction. *Br J Radiol.* 2009;82(976):e72-e75.

47. Whang G, Mogel GT, Tsai J, Palmer SL. Left behind: unintentionally retained surgically placed foreign bodies and how to reduce their incidence—self-assessment module. *AJR Am J Roentgenol.* 2009;193(6 Suppl):S90-S93.

48. Camazine B. The persistent problem of the retained foreign body. *Contemp Surg.* 2005;8:398-400.

49. Wells J. Hospitals must disclose doctor errors. Oversight panel seeks to cut preventable patient injuries. *San Francisco Chronicle.* December 24, 2000;A:1.

50. Hartlaub P. S.F. settles suit over a painful pair of surgeries. Towel, tubing left inside woman. *San Francisco Chronicle.* June 28, 2001;A:13.

51. Retained surgical sponges. New York State Department of Health - NYPORTS. *NYPORTS News & Alert.* Department of Health, Issue 11. September 2002. http://www.health.state.ny.us/nysdoh/hospital/nyports/annual_report/2000-2001/news_and_alerts.htm. Accessed July 1, 2010.

52. Gencosmanoglu R, Inceoglu R. An unusual cause of small bowel obstruction: gossypiboma—case report. *BMC Surg.* 2003;3:6.

53. Recommended practices for transfer of patient care information. In: *Perioperative Standards and Recommended Practices.* Denver, CO: AORN, Inc; 2010:371-378.

54. Rights and Responsibilities of the Individual: RI.01.01.03: The hospital respects the patient's right to receive information in a manner he or she understand. In: *2010 Comprehensive Accreditation Manual for Hospitals.* Oak Brook, IL: Joint Commission Resources; 2010.

55. Use of x-rays for incorrect needle counts. *Pa Patient Saf Advis.* 2004;1(2):5-6.

56. Dagi TF, Berguer R, Moore S, Reines HD. Preventable errors in the operating room—part 2: retained foreign objects, sharps injuries, and wrong site surgery. *Curr Probl Surg.* 2007;44(6):352-381.

57. Perry J, Parker G, Jagger J. EPINet report: 2001 percutaneous injury rates. *Adv Expo Prev.* 2003;6(3):32-36.

58. Jagger J, Berguer R, Phillips EK, Parker G, Gomaa AE. Increase in sharps injuries in surgical settings versus non-surgical settings after passage of national needlestick legislation. *J Am Coll Surg.* 2010;210(4):496-502.

59. Berguer R, Heller PJ. Preventing sharps injuries in the operating room. *J Am Coll Surg.* 2004;199(3):462-467.

60. Ponrartana S, Coakley FV, Yeh BM, et al. Accuracy of plain abdominal radiographs in the detection of retained surgical needles in the peritoneal cavity. *Ann Surg.* 2008;247(1):8-12.

61. Thomas EJ, Moore FA. The missing suction tip [Case & Commentary]. *Morbidity & Mortality Rounds on the Web.* Surgery/Anesthesia. November 2003. http://www.webmm.ahrq.gov/case.aspx?caseID=37. Accessed July 1, 2010.

62. Milankov M, Savic D, Miljkovic N. Broken blade in the knee: a complication of arthroscopic meniscectomy. *Arthroscopy.* 2002;18(1):E4.

63. Murdock D. Trauma: when there's no time to count. *AORN J.* 2008;87(2):322-328.

64. Retained surgical retractor. Closed claim studies—general surgery. Texas Medical Liability Trust. http://www.tmlt.org/newscenter/closedclaims/generalsurgery.html?x=1. Accessed July 1, 2010.

65. Abdomen: retained retractor bolt on plain film. Lieberman's Classics Collections in Radiology. http://eradiology.bidmc.harvard.edu/Classics/item.aspx?section=Patient+Safety+-+Retained+Surgical+Devices&labelpk=9e5a943e-3b2e-415e-82d8-e364853cf0a8&pk=ec2ea0b8-4c64-4c71-b2af-f00f047c673f. Accessed July 1, 2010.

66. Public health notification: unretrieved device fragments. US Food and Drug Administration. http://www.fda.gov/cdrh/safety/011508-udf.html. Accessed July 1, 2010.

67. Beyea SC. Counting instruments and sponges. *AORN J.* 2003;78(2):290, 293-294.

68. Eskreis-Nelson T. Nursing case law update. Medical errors and the need for nurses' continuing education. *J Nurs Law.* 2000;7(3):49-59.

69. AORN guidance statement: creating a patient safety culture. In: *Perioperative Standards and Recommended Practices.* Denver, CO: AORN, Inc; 2010:523-528.

70. Greenberg CC, Diaz-Flores R, Lipsitz SR, et al. Barcoding surgical sponges to improve safety: a randomized controlled trial. *Ann Surg.* 2008;247(4):612-616.

71. *Health Care Protocol: Prevention of Unintentionally Retained Foreign Objects During Vaginal Deliveries.* 2nd ed. Bloomington, MN: Institute for Clinical Systems Improvement; 2008.

72. Barrow CJ. Use of x-ray in the presence of an incorrect needle count. *AORN J.* 2001;74(1):80-81.

73. Macilquham MD, Riley RG, Grossberg P. Identifying lost surgical needles using radiographic techniques. *AORN J.* 2003;78(1):73-78.

74. Pelter MM, Stephens KE, Loranger D. An evaluation of a numbered surgical sponge product. *AORN J.* 2007;85(5):931-936.

75. Rogers A, Jones E, Oleynikov D. Radio frequency identification (RFID) applied to surgical sponges. *Surg Endosc.* 2007;21(7):1235-1237.

76. Regenbogen SE, Greenberg CC, Resch SC, et al. Prevention of retained surgical sponges: a decision-analytic model predicting relative cost-effectiveness. *Surgery.* 2009;145(5):527-535.

77. ECRI. Radio-frequency surgical sponge detection: a new way to lower the odds of leaving sponges (and similar items) in patients. *Health Devices.* 2008;37(7):193-203.

78. Fabian CE. Electronic tagging of surgical sponges to prevent their accidental retention. *Surgery.* 2005;137(3):298-301.

79. Macario A, Morris D, Morris S. Initial clinical evaluation of a handheld device for detecting retained surgical gauze sponges using radiofrequency identification technology. *Arch Surg.* 2006;141(7):659-662.

80. Shojania KG, Duncan BW, McDonald KM, Wachter RM, eds. *Making Health Care Safer: A Critical Analysis of Patient Safety Practices. Evidence Report/Technology Assessment* Number 43. Rockville, MD: Agency for Healthcare Research and Quality; 2001.

81. RF surgical sponge detection: lowering the odds of retention. *ORRM Newsletter.* 2009;18(2).

82. Recommended practices for product selection in the perioperative practice setting. In: *Perioperative Standards and Recommended Practices.* Denver, CO: AORN, Inc; 2010:189-192.

83. Van der Togt R, Van Lieshout EJ, Hensbroek R, Beinat E, Binnekade JM, Bakker PJ. Electromagnetic interference from radio frequency identification inducing potentially hazardous incidents in critical care medical equipment. *JAMA.* 2008;299(24):2884-2890.

84. Recommended practices for documentation of perioperative nursing care. In: *Perioperative Standards and Recommended Practices.* Denver, CO: AORN, Inc; 2010:289-292.

85. Perioperative nursing: sponge inside patient, nurses faulted, but consequences disputed. *Legal Eagle Eye Newsl Nurs Prof.* 2004;12(7):8.

86. Riley R, Manias E, Polglase A. Governing the surgical count through communication interactions: implications for patient safety. *Qual Saf Health Care.* 2006;15(5):369-374.

87. Burton JL. Health and safety at necropsy. *J Clin Pathol.* 2003;56(4):254-260.

88. Berryman R. Why count instruments and sponges in the operating room? Stories from home and abroad. *ACORN.* 2004;17(4):20, 22-4.

89. Dunn D. Incident reports—their purpose and scope. *AORN J.* 2003;78(1):45-66.

90. Root cause analysis. United States Department of Veterans Affairs. http://www.patientsafety.gov/rca.html. Accessed July 1, 2010.

91. Liang BA. The adverse event of unaddressed medical error: identifying and filling the holes in the health-care and legal systems. *J Law Med Ethics.* 2001;29(3-4):346-368.

92. Shendell-Falik N, Feinson M, Mohr BJ. Enhancing patient safety: improving the patient hand-off process through appreciative inquiry. *J Nurs Adm.* 2007;37(2):95-104.

93. Incorporating selected national quality forum and never events into Medicares list of hospital-acquired conditions [fact sheet]. Baltimore, MD: Centers for Medicare & Medicaid Services; April 14, 2008. http://www.cms.hhs.gov/apps/media/press/factsheet.asp?Counter=3043&intNumPerPage=10&checkDate=&checkKey=&srchType=1&numDays=3500&srchOpt=0&srchData=&keywordType=All&chkNewsType=6&intPage=&showAll=&pYear=&year=&desc=false&cboOrder=date. Accessed July 1, 2010.

94. Department of Health and Human Services, Office of the Inspector General. *Adverse Events in Hospitals: State Reporting Systems.* Washington, DC: HHS; 2008.

95. Hospital medical error reporting rule. 410 Indiana Administrative Code 15-1.4-2 (2009).

96. *Clinical Definitions Manual.* Version 4. Albany, NY: New York Patient Occurrence and Tracking System; 2005.

97. *Patient Safety Act.* New Jersey PL 2004 c. 9 26:2H-12.23-12.25.

98. California Health and Safety Code. Section 1275-1289.5.

99. Facility requirements to report, analyze, and correct. Minnesota statutes 144.7065 (2009).

100. *National Integrated Accreditation for Healthcare Organizations (NIAHO) Interpretive Guidelines and*

Surveyor Guidance. Revision 8.0. Cincinnati, OH: DNV Healthcare Inc; 2009.

  101. Sentinel event statistics. The Joint Commission. http://www.jointcommission.org/SentinelEvents/Statistics/. Accessed July 1, 2010.

Acknowledgments

LEAD AUTHORS

Sheila Mitchell, MS, BSN, RN, CNOR
Perioperative Nursing Specialist
AORN Center for Nursing Practice
Denver, Colorado

Judith L. Goldberg, MSN, RN, CNOR
Clinical Director, Sterile Processing Department
The William W. Backus Hospital
Norwich, Connecticut

CONTRIBUTING AUTHORS

Maria C. Arcilla, BSN, RN, CNOR
Education Coordinator
Texas Childrens Hospital
Houston, Texas

David L. Feldman, MD, MBA, CPE, FACS
Vice President, Perioperative Services
Maimonides Medical Center
Brooklyn, New York

PUBLICATION HISTORY

Originally published May 1976, *AORN Journal,* as "Standards for sponge, needle, and instrument procedures." Format revision March 1978, July 1982.

Revised March 1984, March 1990.

Revised November 1995; published October 1996, *AORN Journal.*

Revised; published December 1999, *AORN Journal.* Reformatted July 2000.

Revised November 2005; published as "Recommended practices for sponge, sharp, and instrument counts" in *Standards, Recommended Practices, and Guidelines,* 2006 edition. Reprinted February 2006, *AORN Journal.*

Revised July 2010 for online publication in *Perioperative Standards and Recommended Practices.*

Reformatted September 2012 for publication in *Perioperative Standards and Recommended Practices,* 2013 edition.

Minor editing revisions made in November 2014 for publication in *Guidelines for Perioperative Practice,* 2015 edition.

AMBULATORY SUPPLEMENT: RETAINED SURGICAL ITEMS

Recommendation VI

Standardized measures for investigation and reconciliation of count discrepancies should be taken during the closing count and before the end of surgery. When a discrepancy in the count(s) is identified, the surgical team should carry out steps to locate the missing item.

VI.c.2. If intraoperative imaging is not available, the health care organization should have a policy and procedure describing the actions and communication required between referring and receiving organizations.

> [Amb] The ambulatory surgery facility should have a policy and procedure describing actions to take when on-site radiology services are not available to perform a radiograph and interpret the result.
>
> [Amb] A surgeon with perioperative radiologic privileges may consider the use of fluoroscopy to locate the retained item.[A1]
>
> [Amb] Fluoroscopy may be used and a preliminary reading obtained by a surgeon with privileges to interpret radiographic studies.[A1]

Recommendation X

Policies and procedures for the prevention of RSIs [retained surgical items] and unretrieved device fragments should be developed, reviewed periodically, revised as necessary, and readily available in the practice setting.

X.a. A multidisciplinary team should establish a policy and procedure for prevention of RSIs.[A2-A5]

X.a.4. If intraoperative imaging is not available, the health care organization should have a policy and procedure describing actions necessary and communication required between referring and receiving organizations.

> [Amb] Policies and procedures should include circumstances in which the patient should be transferred to the post-anesthesia care unit and a subsequent receiving facility for further radiologic imaging.

References

A1. §482.26(b)(4). In: Centers for Medicare & Medicaid Services. *State Operations Manual Appendix A—Survey Protocol, Regulations and Interpretive Guidelines for Hospitals.* Rev. 89; 2013. http://www.cms.gov/Regulations-and-Guidance/Guidance/Manuals/downloads/som107ap_a_hospitals.pdf. Accessed October 20, 2013.

A2. Gawande AA, Studdert DM, Orav EJ, Brennan TA, Zinner MJ. Risk factors for retained instruments and sponges after surgery. *N Engl J Med.* 2003; 348(3):229-235.

A3. Gibbs VC, Coakley FD, Reines HD. Preventable errors in the operating room: retained foreign bodies after surgery—part I. *Curr Probl Surg.* 2007; 44(5):281-337.

A4. Statement on the prevention of retained foreign bodies after surgery. American College of Surgeons. http://www.facs.org/fellows_info/statements/st-51.html. Accessed November 7, 2013.

A5. Perioperative nursing: sponge inside patient, nurses faulted, but consequences disputed. *Legal Eagle Eye Newsl Nurs Prof.* 2004;12(7):8.

GUIDELINE FOR SHARPS SAFETY

The following Guideline for Sharps Safety has been approved by the AORN Recommended Practices Advisory Board. It was presented as proposed recommendations for comments by members and others. The guideline is effective June 15, 2013. The recommendations in the guideline are intended to be achievable and represent what is believed to be an optimal level of practice. Policies and procedures will reflect variations in practice settings and/or clinical situations that determine the degree to which the guideline can be implemented. AORN recognizes the various settings in which perioperative nurses practice; therefore, this guideline is adaptable to various practice settings. These practice settings include traditional operating rooms (ORs), ambulatory surgery centers, physicians' offices, cardiac catheterization laboratories, endoscopy suites, radiology departments, and all other areas where operative and other invasive procedures may be performed.

Purpose

This document provides guidance to perioperative registered nurses (RNs) in identifying potential sharps hazards and developing and implementing best practices to prevent sharps injuries and reduce bloodborne pathogen exposure to perioperative patients and personnel.

Health care workers are at risk for percutaneous injury, exposure to bloodborne pathogens, and occupational transmission of disease.[1] Annually, an estimated 384,325 hospital health care workers sustain a percutaneous injury.[2] When non-hospital health care workers are included, the number increases to more than 500,000.[3] Percutaneous injuries are associated primarily with occupational transmission of hepatitis B virus (HBV), hepatitis C virus (HCV), and HIV, but also may be implicated in the transmission of other pathogens.[1,3-17] A 2006 review of pathogens transmitted in published cases since 1966 showed transmission of 60 pathogens or species, which included 26 viruses, 18 bacteria or *Rickettsia*, 13 parasites, and three yeasts.[18]

The occupational risk of HBV transmission is dependent on the level of exposure to blood and the type of hepatitis B antigens.[19] Since the widespread adoption of HBV immunizations, the number of HBV infections in health care workers has declined significantly.[19-23] The reported number of HBV-infected providers in 1983 was 10,000 compared to approximately 100 in 2009.[20,21] The rate of anti-HCV seroconversion after an occupational exposure to HCV positive blood ranges from 0% to 7% with an average rate of 1.8%.[13,19,21,24,25] Although the risk of occupational transmission of HIV depends on the type and severity of the exposure,[19,26-28] the average risk is 0.3%.[12,19,26,28,29]

Percutaneous injuries carry risks not only to perioperative personnel but to patients as well.[20,21,25,30-33] If a health care worker infected with a bloodborne pathogen experiences a percutaneous injury and the object that caused the injury reconnects with the patient or the health care worker's glove perforation is undetected, the patient is at risk for infection.[34] There have been 132 documented cases of health care provider to patient transmission of HBV, HCV, or HIV worldwide.[17,20,31,35-37]

The bloodborne pathogens standard 29 CFR 1910.1030 became effective March 6, 1992.[38] The standard includes definitions, an exposure control plan, engineering and work practice controls (eg, personal protective equipment [PPE]), vaccinations, post-exposure follow-up, employee training, and record keeping.[38] The purpose of the bloodborne pathogen standard is to limit health care worker exposure to HBV, HCV, HIV, and other potentially infectious materials in the workplace through the implementation of engineering and work practice controls.[39]

The Needlestick Safety and Prevention Act was signed into law on November 6, 2000.[40] The act directs the Occupational Safety and Health Administration (OSHA) to revise the bloodborne pathogens standard. The revisions included adding engineering control definitions; including requirements for technology changes that eliminate or reduce bloodborne pathogen exposure in exposure control plans; including input from frontline, non-managerial employees in the identification, evaluation, and selection of safety-engineered devices and work practice controls; annually documenting the evaluation in the exposure control plan; including employee input in the exposure control plan; and maintaining a sharps injury log.[40-42]

Sharps injury prevention is a concern for all members of the perioperative team. Many perioperative professional associations have developed sharps safety position and guidance statements. AORN adopted its "Position statement on workplace safety" in 2003, identifying bloodborne pathogen exposures from percutaneous injuries as a risk in the perioperative environment.[43] The "AORN guidance statement: Sharps injury prevention in the perioperative setting," published in 2005, assisted perioperative nurses in developing sharps injury prevention programs and provided strategies to overcome compliance obstacles. Risk-reduction strategies included double gloving, using the neutral or hands-free zone, and using safety-engineered devices.[44]

The Association of Surgical Technologists (AST) adopted its "Guideline statement for the implementation of the neutral zone in the perioperative environment" in 2006.[45] The AST "Recommended standards of practice for sharps safety and use of the neutral zone" were developed the same year to provide support for and reinforce sharps safety and the use of a neutral zone.[46]

The American Academy of Orthopaedic Surgeons issued a statement on preventing the transmission of bloodborne pathogens in 2001.[32] Prevention strategies included employers establishing a prevention and treatment-of-exposure plan, providing PPE, and promoting double gloving and the use of a neutral zone.[32]

The American College of Surgeons (ACS) developed and approved its statement on sharps safety [ST-58] in 2007. The ACS recommends the universal adoption of double gloving, using blunt suture needles to close the fascia and muscle, using hands-free techniques, and using sharps injury prevention devices.[47]

The Council on Surgical & Perioperative Safety (CSPS)—a member organization composed of AORN, the American Association of Nurse Anesthetists, the American Association of Surgical Physician Assistants, the ACS, the American Society of Anesthesiologists, the American Society of PeriAnesthesia Nurses, and the AST—endorsed sharps safety measures to prevent injury during perioperative care. Sharps safety measures should include double gloving, using blunt suture needles for closing facia and muscle, and using a neutral zone when appropriate to avoid hand-to-hand passage of sharps. The CSPS sharps statement was adopted in 2007 and modified in 2009.[48]

In November 2010, a consensus statement and call to action was drafted by members of the steering committee at the 10th Anniversary of the Needlestick Safety and Prevention Act: Mapping Progress, Charting a Future Path conference, sponsored by the International Healthcare Worker Safety Center at the University of Virginia. The consensus statement was released in 2012 and endorsed by 20 organizations. It lists improving sharps safety in surgical settings as the number-one priority to reduce percutaneous injuries.[49]

In a joint safety communication, the US Food and Drug Administration (FDA), the National Institute for Occupational Safety and Health (NIOSH), and OSHA encourage health care professionals in surgical settings to use blunt-tip suture needles for suturing muscle and fascia when it is clinically appropriate.[50] Blunt-tip suture needles reduce the risk of needlestick injury and the risk of bloodborne pathogen transmission.[50]

Understanding the etiology of percutaneous injuries in the perioperative setting is paramount to developing a sharps injury prevention program. The perioperative setting is a high-risk environment for exposure to bloodborne pathogens from percutaneous injuries.[51] The International Healthcare Worker Safety Center at the University of Virginia compared percutaneous injury surveillance data of 87 participating hospitals before and after the passage of the Needlestick Safety and Prevention Act of 2000. The analysis showed a 6.5% increase in injuries in the surgical setting compared to a 31.6% decrease in nonsurgical settings.[36,51] There were 7,186 sharps injuries to surgical personnel reported between 1993 and 2006.[51] When surgeons and surgical residents sustained a sharps injury, they were the original user of the device in 81.9% and 67.3% of the injuries, respectively. Nurses and surgical technologists were injured by devices used by others in 77.2% and 85.1% of the injuries, respectively. The majority of injuries occur to surgeons and surgical residents during use, while the sharps injuries to nurses and surgical technologists occur during passing, disassembling, and disposal.[51] The perioperative environment is unique in health care.[51] Perioperative personnel are at a distinct risk of percutaneous injury because of the presence of large quantities of blood and other potentially infectious body fluids, prolonged exposure to open surgical sites, frequent handling of sharp instruments, and the requirement for coordination between team members while passing sharp surgical instruments.[51,52]

An economic analysis of a retrospective survey estimated the effect of an occupational exposure from a needlestick injury. Associated costs included post-exposure health services, post-exposure testing, post-exposure prophylaxis, missed work days, and loss of productivity. Based on the findings, researchers projected the national economic burden per year at $65 million.[53] A convenience sample of health care facilities provided information on the cost of managing an occupational exposure, including reporting time, follow-up, salaries, and laboratory testing of the source individual and exposed health care worker. Overall costs ranged from $71 to $4,838 per exposure.[54] An analysis of the estimated costs of needlestick injuries and subsequent infections for hospital and non-hospital-based health care workers for testing, prophylaxis, and long-term infection suggests a range of $100.7 million to $405.9 million annually based on 2004 statistics.[55] The emotional burden of an occupationally acquired infection to the health care worker and his or her family members and the time spent waiting and wondering cannot be measured.[56]

Sharps safety is a priority in the perioperative environment and includes considerations for standard precautions, health care worker vaccination, post-exposure protocols and follow-up treatment, and treatment for health care workers infected with a bloodborne pathogen. These topics are addressed in other AORN guidelines, and although they are mentioned briefly where applicable (eg, standard precautions), broader discussions of these topics are outside the scope of this document.

Evidence Review

A medical librarian conducted a systematic review of MEDLINE®, CINAHL®, Scopus®, and the Cochrane Database of Systematic Reviews for meta-analyses, randomized and nonrandomized trials and studies, systematic and nonsystematic reviews, guidelines, case reports, and opinion documents and letters. Search terms included *needlestick injuries, sharps injuries, blood-borne pathogens, occupational accidents, occupational injuries, medical staff, nurses, perioperative nursing, operating room nursing, perioperative nurses, operating room nurses, operating rooms, surgical procedures, surgical instruments, safety devices, sutures, scalpels, sharps, scalpel injuries, needlesticks, needle sticks, safety scalpels, safety-engineered sharps, blunt-tip needles, hands-free passing, neutral zone, double gloving,* and *double-gloving.*

The lead author and medical librarian identified and obtained relevant guidelines from government agencies, other professional organizations, and standards-setting bodies. The lead author assessed additional professional literature, including some that initially appeared in other articles provided to the author.

The initial search was conducted in 2011 and was limited to articles published in English from 1992, when OSHA's Bloodborne Pathogens Final Standard was established. The librarian established continuing alerts on sharps safety-related topics and provided relevant results to the lead author. The lead author and medical librarian also identified relevant guidelines from accreditation organizations, government agencies, and standards-setting bodies. In addition, the lead author requested other articles identified through literature appraisal and other outside sources.

Articles identified by the search were provided to the project team for evaluation. The team consisted of the lead author, three members of the Recommended Practices Advisory Board, two members of the Research Committee, and a doctorally prepared evidence appraiser. The lead author divided the search results into topics and assigned members of the team to review and critically appraise each article using the Johns Hopkins Evidence-Based Practice Model and the Research or Non-Research Evidence Appraisal Tools as appropriate. The literature was independently evaluated and appraised according to the strength and quality of the evidence. Each article was then assigned an appraisal score as agreed upon by consensus of the team. The appraisal score is noted in brackets after each reference, as applicable. The collective evidence supporting each intervention within a specific recommendation was summarized and used to rate the strength of the evidence using the AORN Evidence Rating Model. Factors considered in review of the collective evidence were the quality of research, quantity of similar studies on a given topic, and consistency of results supporting a recommendation. The evidence rating is noted in brackets after each intervention.

Editor's note: *MEDLINE is a registered trademark of the US National Library of Medicine's Medical Literature Analysis and Retrieval System, Bethesda, MD. CINAHL, Cumulative Index to Nursing and Allied Health Literature, is a registered trademark of EBSCO Industries, Birmingham, AL. Scopus is a registered trademark of Elsevier B.V., Amsterdam, Netherlands.*

Recommendation I

Health care facilities must establish a written bloodborne pathogens exposure control plan.[38]

Bloodborne pathogens are pathogenic microorganisms that are present in human blood and can cause disease (eg, HBV, HCV, HIV).[28] Federal and state regulations and organizational standards that mandate bloodborne pathogen guidelines are intended to reduce health care provider exposure and to minimize the risk of infection.[38,57] The bloodborne pathogens standard 29 CFR 1910.1030 includes a requirement for an exposure control plan.[38]

I.a. The exposure control plan must be reviewed and updated at least annually and whenever new or modified tasks or procedures are implemented.[38] *[1: Regulatory Requirement]*

I.a.1. The review and update should include changes in technology that reduce or eliminate bloodborne pathogen exposure[38] and should document the annual trial and implementation of effective, commercially available, safer medical devices that are designed to eliminate or minimize bloodborne pathogen exposure.[38]

I.a.2. The employer must ask for input from nonmanagerial employees responsible for direct patient care who may potentially be exposed to injuries from contaminated sharps to identify, evaluate, and select effective engineering and work practice controls. The employer must document the process in the exposure control plan.[38]

I.b. The employer must prepare an exposure determination of any employee with the potential for exposure to bloodborne pathogens.[38] *[1: Regulatory Requirement]*

I.b.1. The exposure determination must include a list of all job classifications that place any employee in that classification at risk for bloodborne pathogen exposure.[38]

I.b.2. The exposure determination must be based on the level of risk when the employee is wearing no PPE.[38]

I.c. As part of the written bloodborne pathogens exposure control plan, the organization's plan to reduce sharps injuries should include
- a profile of how sharps injuries occur,
- the occupational group sustaining the most injuries,
- the location (ie, department, work area) where the injuries occur,
- the sharps devices involved in the injuries,
- the procedures (eg, recapping needles) that most commonly contribute to sharps injuries, and
- the sharps injury reduction devices that have been implemented.[4]

[1:Strong Evidence]

Monitoring sharps injury data allows results to be compared to a predetermined level of quality. Reviewing the findings provides information to identify problems and trends, which can be used to improve practice.[4,13]

SHARPS SAFETY

I.d. The priority of risk-reduction strategies should be determined and should be based on the greatest risk of bloodborne pathogen exposure, frequency of injury, and problem-prone areas with frequent sharps injuries.[4] [1: Strong Evidence]

Analysis of sharps injury logs or other sharps surveillance programs aids in identifying the types of injuries, types of devices, frequency of injuries, and work areas where exposure has occurred.[58]

I.d.1. Sharps hazard control methods should be based on a hierarchy of controls to include
- elimination of the hazard,
- engineering controls,
- work practice controls,
- administrative controls, and
- PPE.[13,24,59,60]

Elimination of the hazard includes removing the sharp object from use (eg, using electrosurgery instead of a scalpel for the incision). Engineering controls include using a safety-engineered device (eg, safety scalpel). Work practice controls include using a neutral or safe zone for passing sharp instruments and devices and wearing proper PPE, including double gloving.[24,59,60] Administrative controls include developing policies and procedures, incorporating sharps safety prevention into a new or existing committee structure, implementing an exposure control plan, and providing education and training.

I.e. The health care organization must establish a process for selecting and evaluating sharps safety devices as part of the written bloodborne pathogens exposure control plan.[24,38] [1: Regulatory Requirement]

I.e.1. A multidisciplinary committee that includes frontline workers should develop, implement, and evaluate a plan to reduce sharps injuries in the perioperative setting and to evaluate sharps safety devices.[24,61] The multidisciplinary team may include representatives from clinical staff, materials management, infection prevention and control, risk management, administration, occupational health, sterile processing, environmental cleaning services, and waste management, depending on the device being evaluated.[61]

I.e.2. Priorities should be identified and should be based on the mechanism of sharps injuries, frequency of injuries, procedure-specific risks, relative risk of disease transmission, and the devices involved in sharps injuries.[24,61] Highest priority should be given to the device that will have the greatest effect on reducing sharps injuries.[24,61]

I.e.3. Device selection factors should include patient and worker safety, efficiency, user acceptability, and overall performance.[24] Safety features should be simple, reliable, clear, and easily understood.[61]

Safety device design may be passive, active, or integrated, or a safety device may be an accessory.[62] A passive safety device requires no worker action for the safety feature to function. An active safety device requires the worker to take an action to initiate the safety feature.[62] A multicenter study of different types of safety-engineered devices showed that passive devices are associated with fewer sharps injuries.[62] An integrated safety design is an integral part of the device. An accessory safety device is an external feature to the device that is affixed either temporarily or permanently.[61]

I.e.4. Product evaluation should be accomplished by a representative group of frontline users of the safety device who have been educated and trained in the correct use of the device. The length of the evaluation period should be established, and a survey tool that includes the criteria and measures for the evaluation should be used.[24,61]

Factors that may influence product evaluation outcomes include the end user's experience with the safety device and the current device in use, the end user's previous experience in product evaluations, the product evaluation team members' attitudes and involvement, and the end user's peer opinions, as well as time intervals between distribution of the product and the survey, self-selection biases,[61] and the availability of the current product during the evaluation period.

I.e.5. The survey form should be easy to complete and score (eg, a Likert-type scale), limited to a single page, contain established performance criteria, have space for comments, and collect product user information (eg, name, title).[61]

I.e.6. Final product selection should be based on data analysis of the completed product evaluation forms.[61,63]

I.e.7. Final product selection should not be based on cost alone.[63] Cost analysis should include the cost of the sharps safety product, the potential cost savings of reducing or eliminating sharps injuries, and the cost of educating and training personnel.[61]

I.e.8. After the introduction of a new safety device, an assessment should be performed to evaluate acceptance, correct usage, usage rate, device performance, and the effect on the rate of sharps injuries.[24]

I.e.9. Safety-engineered devices must be evaluated annually.[38] Current devices should be evaluated for efficacy in reducing or preventing sharps injuries.[64] If current devices are not preventing sharps injuries, new devices should be evaluated.[42]

I.e.10. The safety-engineered device product evaluation process must be documented as part of the exposure control plan.[38,42]

I.f. The exposure control plan must be accessible to all employees.[38] [1: Regulatory Requirement]

Recommendation II

Perioperative personnel must use sharps with safety-engineered devices (ie, engineering controls).[38]

The Needlestick Safety and Prevention Act of 2000 mandates that employers provide safety-engineered devices in the health care setting to prevent sharps injuries.[40] According to OSHA, engineering controls are safety-engineered devices that isolate or remove the risk of a bloodborne pathogen exposure.[38] Safety-engineered devices include sharps with engineered sharps injury protection (SESIP) and needleless systems. A SESIP is a sharp with a built-in safety feature or mechanism that reduces the risk of a bloodborne pathogen exposure, such as safety or sheathed scalpels, blunt suture needles, and safety syringes and needles.

Sharps injuries increase the risk of bloodborne pathogen exposure in the OR. A review of 17 studies that evaluated safety-engineered device implementation and percutaneous injury rates showed a substantial decrease in percutaneous injuries after implementation of safety-engineered devices in all of the studies. The range of percutaneous injury reduction was 22% to 100%.[65] Researchers conducting a multisite survey compared the injury rates of different safety-engineered devices. During the time frame of the study, 22 million safety-engineered devices were purchased and evaluated with the conclusion that passive (ie, automatic) safety-engineered devices are the most effective in preventing percutaneous injuries.[62]

In a quasi-experimental trial with before-and-after intervention evaluations, researchers reported a 93% reduction in relative risk when safety devices were used. The researchers concluded that the proper use of safety-engineered devices is an effective measure to prevent percutaneous injuries.[66]

Researchers conducted a controlled, retrospective, interventional study of safety-engineered device implementation. Percutaneous injuries resulting from a safety-engineered device (ie, an intravenous catheter stylet with a retractable protection shield) were compared to sharp suture needle injuries in the control group. There was a statistically significant decrease in percutaneous injuries from intravenous catheter styli during the 18-month study period. Percutaneous injury rates from sharp suture needles increased from 5.3 to 10.7 per 1,000 health care workers during the same 18-month period.[67]

Researchers using the Massachusetts Sharps Injury Surveillance System examined trends in sharps injury rates by occupation, hospital size, and device. Seventy-six hospitals reported 16,158 sharps injuries to the surveillance system. During the five-year surveillance period, the overall annual sharps injury rate declined by 22%. Injury rates decreased when sharps with engineered sharps injury protection devices were available and used.[68]

The International Healthcare Worker Safety Center at the University of Virginia analyzed 16,871 sharp object injuries using data collected through the EPI-Net™ system. The data analysis found that 94% of the reported injuries were caused by a conventional device and only 6% were caused by a safety-engineered device.[58]

Researchers conducting a retrospective review of 161 injuries found that an estimated 65% of the injuries could have been prevented by using a device with safety-engineered features.[69] A prospective study of 952 health care worker occupational needlestick injuries estimated that 52% could have been prevented by use of a safety-engineered device.[70]

II.a. Blunt suture needles should be used unless clinically contraindicated (eg, scarred or thick fascia).[14,47,48,50,71-74] [1: Strong Evidence]

Blunt suture needles may prevent percutaneous injuries. Sharp suture needles account for 51% to 77% of the percutaneous injuries to surgical personnel.[52,75,76] Blunt suture needles decrease the occurrence of glove perforations, percutaneous injuries, and exposure risks to blood and body fluids by reducing the number of needlestick injuries.[52,71,72,76-82] A Cochrane review of 10 randomized controlled trials evaluated blunt versus sharp needles for preventing percutaneous exposure incidents in surgical staff members. Using blunt needles versus sharp suture needles reduced glove perforation risk by 54% as well as reduced the risk of infectious disease transmission.[71]

In a randomized controlled trial that compared blunt tapered and sharp needles in closing abdominal fascia in 200 general surgery patients undergoing laparotomy, the glove perforation rate for blunt suture needles was 12% compared to 28% for sharp needles. The researchers concluded that use of blunt tapered suture needles reduce the incidence of glove perforations.[72]

In a 15-month surveillance study of occupational blood exposures in the ORs of six hospitals, researchers reported 197 suture needle injuries; 59% of the injuries were attributable to suture needles used to suture muscle or fascia. Use of blunt suture needles as a prevention strategy could reduce percutaneous injuries in the OR by 30%.[52]

A randomized controlled study compared wound morbidity after cesarean deliveries using blunt suture needles and sharp suture needles.

SHARPS SAFETY

The researchers concluded that blunt-tip suture needles do not increase wound morbidity.[83]

The use of blunt suture needles is supported by OSHA, the FDA, NIOSH, and the ACS when clinically indicated.[47,50] Additionally, OSHA has identified blunt suture needles as an acceptable engineering control.[73]

II.a.1. Blunt suture needles should be used for perineal laceration and episiotomy repair.[84-86]

In a survey of obstetricians regarding the use of blunt suture needles for episiotomy and laceration repair, 95% of respondents reported that blunt suture needles were an excellent to good alternative to sharp suture needles. There were no needlestick injuries or glove perforations reported during the time frame of the study.[84]

A randomized, controlled trial compared the number of glove perforations when using blunt-tip needles to sharp needles for suturing perineal tears and episiotomies. Researchers reported that the rate of glove punctures with blunt-tip needles was 8.6% and the rate with sharp needles was 16.5%.[85]

A randomized, prospective trial compared the rate of surgical glove perforations when blunt and sharp suture needles were used to repair obstetrical lacerations. There were five glove perforations in the sharp suture needle group and four glove perforations in the blunt suture group. The difference between the two groups was not statistically significant.[87]

II.b. Safety scalpel devices should be used when clinically feasible.[88] *[1: Regulatory Requirement]*

Scalpel injuries are the second most common injury in the perioperative setting, comprising 17% of injuries.[51,89] Scalpel injuries pose a risk of injury to the skin and underlying tissue and a bloodborne pathogen exposure risk.[4] Scalpel injuries occur to the surgeon or assistant, the original user of the device, as well as to the nurses and surgical technologists when scalpels are passed or blades are removed.[51]

II.b.1. There are several types of safety scalpel devices that may be used in the perioperative setting, each of which has an associated reduced risk of injury.
- Single-use scalpel handles and blades that do not require disassembly (ie, removal of the blade) are associated with 68% fewer percutaneous injuries.[90]
- Retracting scalpel blades withdraw the blade into the handle when they are passed between perioperative team members and when not in use.[91,92] When they are used consistently and correctly, there is the potential to prevent 65% of scalpel injuries.[90]
- Shielded or sheathed scalpel blades allow the blade to be covered by the shield or sheath when passed between perioperative team members and when not in use.[91] When used consistently and correctly, there is the potential to prevent 65% of scalpel injuries.[90]
- Rounded tip scalpel blades[4] may be effective in reducing scalpel injuries. No studies were found in the literature review regarding effectiveness of rounded tip scalpel blades in reducing scalpel injuries.
- Scalpel blade removal devices permit the safe removal of the blade at the conclusion of the procedure.[91] In a retrospective study of a metropolitan hospital's sharps injuries database, chart review, and hypothetical modeling of the data, researchers concluded that 44.5% of scalpel injuries could be prevented by using a combination of hands-free techniques and a scalpel blade removal device.[91]

II.c. Alternative wound closure devices should be used when clinically indicated.[93,94] *[2: Moderate Evidence]*

Alternative skin closure devices reduce the use of sharp suture needles and the incidence of percutaneous injuries.[52,94,95] A systematic review of 14 randomized, controlled trials evaluated the tissue effects on surgical wound healing when tissue adhesives were used for skin closure. Researchers found no significant difference between sutures and adhesives in regard to infection, patient and user satisfaction, and cost. Sutures were better than adhesives for minimizing wound dehiscence in 10 trials, and were significantly faster to use. Adhesive tapes were faster to use than adhesives.[95]

Researchers conducting a single-center, prospective study that compared arthroscopy portal wound closure methods found comparable wound healing with adhesive wound closure strips and nylon suture. Eliminating the suture reduces the possibility of a percutaneous injury.[94] A randomized controlled animal study compared a fascial closure device to traditional suture closure. The researchers evaluated the amount of time needed to close the fascia, accuracy of placement, and abdominal bursting pressures. Fascial closure time was reduced by 24% with the closure device, and both methods had comparable closure integrity. Fascial closure devices may reduce percutaneous injuries by reducing the use of sutures to close the fascial layer.[96]

II.c.1. Alternative closure methods may include
- fascial closure devices,[92,96]
- tissue staplers,[92]
- tissue adhesives,[92] and
- adhesive skin closure strips.

SHARPS SAFETY

II.d. Perioperative team members should use syringes, needles, and IV catheters that incorporate safety-engineered features. *[1: Regulatory Requirement]*

Appropriate methods to protect health care workers from exposure to bloodborne pathogens and to decrease the risk of disease transmission through sharps injuries are specified in OSHA regulations.[38]

Researchers prospectively monitored needlestick injuries for two years after the introduction of safety-engineered devices (ie, retractable syringes, needle-free IV systems) and compared injury rate to pre-intervention needlestick injury data at a large teaching hospital. All needlestick injuries decreased by 49%. Needlestick injuries related to IV line access decreased 81%. Hollow-bore needlestick injuries were reduced by 57%.[97]

A prospective surveillance study of 76 acute care hospitals examined sharps injuries over time, occupation, hospital size, and device. The sharps injury rates decreased steadily and significantly for hypodermic needles and syringes when safety-engineered devices were available and used. The rate of sharps injury decreased 3.5% per year.[68]

A three-year controlled retrospective interventional study analyzed injury data of health care workers with the potential to be exposed to bloodborne pathogens. Use of an IV catheter with a safety-engineered feature was implemented. Injuries from IV catheters decreased significantly from 2.3 to 2.5 percutaneous injuries per 1,000 health care workers during the pre-intervention period to 0.2 to 1.9 percutaneous injuries per 1,000 health care workers during the post-intervention period.[67]

II.d.1. Safety-engineered syringes and needles that may be used in the perioperative setting include
- a syringe or needle with a sliding sheath that covers the needle after use,
- a hinged needle guard that is attached to the hub of the needle and manually folds over the needle,
- a sliding shield needle guard that moves forward to cover the needle after use, and
- a syringe with a needle that retracts inside the syringe after use.[4]

II.d.2. Needleless systems should be used for
- the collection or withdrawal of bodily fluids after the initial access is established,
- the administration of medications or fluids, and
- any other procedure involving the potential for occupational exposure to bloodborne pathogens because of percutaneous injuries from contaminated sharps.[38]

Needleless systems protect against bloodborne pathogen exposure by eliminating the use of needles. A review of 17 studies evaluated the effect of safety-engineered device implementation on the rate of percutaneous injuries. Researchers evaluated needleless systems in eight of the 17 studies and reported a 22% to 100% reduction in overall percutaneous injuries.[65] In another review of 11 studies, authors concluded that the use of a needleless IV system and surgical assist devices led to a significant reduction in glove perforations.[98]

One study of needlestick injuries at an 800-bed university hospital in Australia indicated that introducing safety-engineered devices (ie, retractable syringes, needle-free IV systems, safety winged butterfly needles) reduced hollow-bore needlestick injuries by 49%.[97] The investigators also noted a 57% reduction in high-risk injuries after introducing retractable syringes and a virtual elimination of needlestick injuries related to accessing IV lines.[97]

II.d.3. A blunt cannula should be used to withdraw medication and fluid from a vial.[99]

Recommendation III

Perioperative personnel must use work practice controls when handling scalpels, hypodermic needles, suture needles, bone fragments, K-wires, burrs, saw blades, drill bits, trocars, razors, bone cutters, towel clips, scissors, electrosurgical tips, skin hooks, retractors, and other sharp devices.[38,100,101]

Work practice controls, as required by OSHA, reduce the likelihood of exposure by changing the method of performing a task to minimize the risk of exposure to blood or other potentially infectious materials.[38,42,101]

III.a. Sharps should be confined and contained in specified areas of the sterile field or within a sharps containment device.[102] *[2: Moderate Evidence]*

III.a.1. The scrub person should account for and confine all sharps on the sterile field until the patient is transferred out of the room.[102]

Unconfined sharps that remain on the sterile field may be unintentionally introduced into the incision, may be dropped on the floor, or may penetrate barriers. Confinement and containment of sharps may minimize the risk of injury to personnel as well as reduce the risk of retained surgical items.

III.a.2. Used sharps on the sterile field should be kept in a puncture-resistant container.

Collecting used sharps (eg, needles, blades) in a puncture-resistant container helps ensure their containment on the sterile field.

III.a.3. When a needle disposal container on the sterile field is full, an additional, new container should be used. Sharps are included in the count and should not be removed from the OR until the final count reconciliation is completed and the patient has been taken from the room.[102]

III.a.4. Needle containers should be securely closed before disposal.

III.b. Surgical team members should use a neutral zone or hands-free technique for passing sharp instruments, blades, and needles.[12,14,46-48,92,103-107]
[1: Strong Evidence]

Analysis of percutaneous injury surveillance data from 87 hospitals in the United States during a 13-year period showed that most sharps injuries occur when suture needles or sharps are passed between perioperative team members.[51] Changes in surgical practice to minimize manual manipulation of sharps (ie, neutral zone or no-touch techniques) can have a major effect on these injuries. Creation of a neutral zone (ie, where instruments are put down and picked up rather than passed hand to hand) may decrease injuries from sharp instruments.[4] In a 2007 standards interpretation letter, OSHA recommends the use of the neutral zone.[108]

The use of a no-touch technique (ie, no two people touch a sharp at the same time) was described in 1988 as a means to minimize the risk of a sharps injury and exposure to HIV.[109] The author advocated the use of a magnetic pad as the neutral zone and for scrubbed team members to provide verbal warnings of sharps in use.

A pre-intervention and post-intervention study investigated whether preventative practice changes (ie, reducing the use of sharp instruments, using a neutral zone, using a no-touch technique) during orthopedic procedures would decrease the risk of blood exposure for the surgical technologist, first assistant, surgeon, and patient. Researchers defined the no-touch technique as using an instrument instead of manually manipulating any sharp (eg, suture needle, scalpel blade). Before the introduction of preventative practice changes, the researchers studied sharps injuries and glove perforations for 347 procedures and 1,068 staff members using traditional working methods that included hand-to-hand passing of sharp instruments. During the pre-intervention phase, there were 24 incidents (ie, 13 injuries, 11 glove perforations) during 6.8% of procedures. After introducing preventative practice changes, researchers studied sharps injuries and glove perforations for 383 orthopedic procedures and 1,058 staff members using the no-touch and neutral zone techniques. During the post-intervention phase, there were 10 incidents (ie, six injuries, four glove perforations) during 2.7% of procedures.[103]

In a pre-intervention and post-intervention study, researchers used a hands-free technique training video as the intervention to increase the use of the hands-free technique and reduce bloodborne pathogen exposures. They found that use of the video and technique were effective in reducing injuries, glove tears, and contaminations.[107]

In a prospective study of 3,765 procedures performed in inpatient and outpatient settings, RN circulators recorded the use of the hands-free technique during each procedure. The rates of incidents (ie, percutaneous injuries, glove tears, contaminations) were compared in procedures during which the technique was and was not used. The effectiveness of the hands-free technique in decreasing percutaneous injuries was evaluated, and researchers found that it was more effective in surgeries with blood loss greater than 100 mL.[110]

In a study evaluating behavioral treatment that combined goal setting, task clarification, and feedback as a means to increase the use of the hands-free technique, researchers found the combined treatment increased use of the hands-free technique from 32% to 64% in the inpatient setting and from 31% to 70% in the outpatient setting. Sharps injuries declined from 10.3 per quarter to six per quarter.[111]

A self-administered questionnaire surveyed the use of the hands-free technique among 158 perioperative nurses in seven different facilities. Data analysis showed a significant association between hands-free technique education and the perceived need for using it. Researchers concluded that increasing education on the hands-free technique could increase its use.[104]

A 1997 randomized, prospective study of the use of a neutral zone during cesarean births showed no statistically significant difference in the number of glove perforations between the control and intervention groups. Based on their findings, the researchers concluded that while there are no proven benefits, there are few adverse effects of using a passing tray.[112]

III.b.1. Use of a neutral zone should include
- identifying the neutral zone in the preoperative briefing[45,46,106,109];
- using a basin, instrument mat, magnetic pad, or designated area on the Mayo stand as the neutral zone[45,46,103,106,109,113,114];
- giving verbal notification when a sharp is in the neutral zone[45,46,109,114];
- placing one sharp at a time in the neutral zone[45,46];
- orienting the sharp for easy retrieval by the surgeon[45,46];
- handling of a sharp item by only one team member at a time[106,109]; and
- placing sharp items in the neutral zone after use.[106]

III.b.2. A modified neutral zone (eg, a limited hands-free passing technique) should be used during procedures that require the use of a microscope. The scrub person should place the sharp in the surgeon's hand. The surgeon should return the sharp to the designated neutral zone.

Low lighting, microscope magnification, and a narrow field of vision contribute to sharps injury risks during microscopic procedures.[115] A retrospective review of reported sharps injuries during ophthalmic procedures in a six-year period showed that most of the sharps injuries occurred while the device was being used or passed between health care workers in the OR.[115] A modified neutral zone (eg, limited hands-free passing technique) may reduce sharps injuries.[115]

III.c. A no-touch technique should be used when handling sharps.[32,103,109,116] *[2: Moderate Evidence]*

The no-touch technique minimizes manual handling of sharp devices and instruments, reducing the risk of injury to perioperative team members.[103,109]

III.c.1. Suture needles should not be manipulated with gloved hands.[12,103]

Suture needle injuries occur when loading the needle holder or repositioning the needle.

III.c.2. When suture is being loaded on a needle holder, the suture packet should be used to position the suture needle in the needle holder without touching the needle.

III.c.3. A blunt instrument (eg, forceps) should be used to manipulate and guide the suture needle through tissue to avoid finger contact with the suture needle or the tissue being sutured.[103,109,117]

The most common site of percutaneous injuries in the perioperative setting is to the non-dominant hand during suturing. In a randomized clinical trial, the rate of glove perforations of the non-dominant hand occurred in 88% of the procedures for the surgeon and in 78% of the procedures for assistants.[72] The researchers found that the use of a blunt instrument-assisted technique reduced the need for finger contact with the suture needle or the tissue being sutured.

III.c.4. The perioperative team member performing suturing should use a forceps to turn the suture needle 90 degrees toward the box lock of the needle holder before returning the loaded needle holder to the Mayo stand if a hands-free zone is not being used.[103,117,118]

Turning the loaded needle may reduce the risk of sharps injury during instrument passing.[118]

III.c.5. An instrument should be used to pick up sharp items (eg, scalpel blades, suture needles) that have fallen off the sterile field.

III.d. Sharp instruments (eg, retractors, towel clips) should be used only when clinically necessary.[52,114] Sharp devices should be used only when there is no safer alternative available.[52] *[2: Moderate Evidence]*

A study about the feasibility of performing specific general surgery procedures without sharp instruments (eg, scalpels, sutures) was evaluated. Researchers identified 91 procedures preoperatively as appropriate non-sharp procedures. A total of 86.8% of the procedures were completed without the use of sharp instrumentation, eliminating the risks of sharps injury to perioperative personnel.[93]

III.e. Safe scalpel handling methods should be used when clinically feasible. *[2: Moderate Evidence]*

Scalpel injuries are the second most common injury in the perioperative setting, comprising 17% of the injuries.[51,89] Scalpel injuries pose a risk of injury to the skin and underlying tissue and a risk of bloodborne pathogen exposure.[4]

Scalpel injuries occur to the surgeon or assistant, the original user of the device, as well as to the nurses and surgical technologists when scalpels are passed or blades are removed.[51]

III.e.1. An instrument should be used for loading a scalpel blade on a knife handle when a safety-engineered device is not available.[103]

III.e.2. A scalpel blade remover or instrument should be used to remove the blade when a safety-engineered device is not available.[103,119]

III.f. Alternative cutting devices (eg, electrosurgery, diathermy, electrosurgical plasma; adapted electrosurgical tips) should be used when clinically indicated. *[1: Strong Evidence]*

A systematic review and meta-analysis compared cutting diathermy (ie, electrosurgery) to the use of a scalpel for skin incisions. The researchers concluded that skin incisions using electrosurgical instruments were quicker, associated with less blood loss, and resulted in no difference in wound rate complications or pain.[120]

III.f.1. A hand piece that uses electrosurgical plasma induced with pulsed radio-frequency energy to cut tissue may be used as an alternative to scalpels.[121]

A hand piece that uses electrosurgical plasma induced with pulsed radio-frequency energy may reduce the risk of sharps injuries by decreasing the use of sharp instruments.[121]

SHARPS SAFETY

- III.f.2. Specially adapted electrosurgical tips for cutting with power mode may be used as an alternative to scalpels.

- III.g. Perioperative team members should use additional sharps safety practices, including
  - maintaining situational awareness of all sharps on the sterile field[14,114];
  - communicating the location of sharps on the sterile field with other members of the perioperative team during the procedure and at times of personnel change;
  - removing suture needles from the suture before tying (eg, cutting, control release);
  - retracting tissue with instruments (eg, retractors) rather than hands;
  - handling (eg, applying, passing, using, removing) saw blades, sharp K-wires, burrs, and other sharp devices with caution[114]; and
  - covering with a protective cap or cutting the exposed ends of sharp pins or K-wires after they have passed through the patient's skin.[32]

  [2: Moderate Evidence]

  A multi-center surveillance study identified patterns of blood exposure and exposure-prevention strategies. Researchers reported 386 percutaneous exposure events during a 15-month period in six OR suites. Manual tissue retraction accounted for 3.4% of the injuries.[52]

- III.h. Perioperative team members should use safe practices when injecting medications or withdrawing bodily fluids.[99] [1: Regulatory Requirement]

  Safe injection practices protect health care workers from exposure to bloodborne pathogens and decrease the risk of disease transmission through sharps injuries. These practices are specified in OSHA regulations.[38]

  - III.h.1. Needles should not be recapped. When a safe needle device is not available and recapping is required, a one-handed scooping recapping technique must be used.[38,122]

    Two-handed recapping of hypodermic needles is associated with an increased incidence of injuries.[4] A study comparing the incidence of sharps injuries in medical students before and after a demonstration of the scooping recapping technique and a lecture on the dangers of sharps injuries showed a reduction in the incidence of sharps injuries from 17.4% to 2.8%.[123]

  - III.h.2. Contaminated needles and other contaminated sharps must not be bent, recapped, or removed unless there is no alternative or the action is required because of a specific medical or dental procedure.[38]

  - III.h.3. Needleless entry devices should be used whenever possible to withdraw contents from multidose vials.[99]

- III.i. Perioperative team members should practice ampule safety to minimize percutaneous injury during or after opening of an ampule.[124] [2: Moderate Evidence]

  Safety measures may include
  - using a reusable or disposable ampule breaker that covers the neck of the ampule during the breaking process or
  - wrapping a sterile gauze pad around the ampule neck before breaking the top.[125]

  Opening a glass ampule may produce glass fragments and a jagged or sharp edge. The Centers for Disease Control and Prevention (CDC) estimated that glass devices account for 2% of percutaneous injuries among all health care personnel.[4] A cross-sectional survey of 864 nurses at a large teaching hospital showed that 29% of the injuries were related to use of ampules or vials.[126] A randomly completed survey of all anesthetists at the Bristol Royal Infirmary after an anesthetic session indicated there was a 6% incidence of hand laceration after opening a glass ampule.[127] In one study, researchers used a questionnaire-based methodology to investigate the prevalence and cause of needlestick injuries in a cross-section of 274 nursing students. The results demonstrated an injury rate of 36% when opening an ampule.[128] A multi-center study determined the incidence and causes of anesthesia professionals' hazards by data analysis. Broken glass ampules were the causative factor in 54.2% of the incidents.[129]

Recommendation IV

Perioperative personnel must use PPE.

The use of PPE is required by OSHA where there is a risk of occupational exposure to blood, body fluids, or other potentially infectious materials after engineering and work practice controls are implemented. Personal protective barriers are required when it can be reasonably anticipated that a health care worker will be exposed to bloodborne pathogens or other potentially infectious materials.[42] The use of PPE (eg, gloves) protects health care worker's skin from coming into contact with blood, body fluids, and other potentially infectious materials.[38,130]

- IV.a. Health care personnel should use standard precautions when caring for all patients in the perioperative setting.[131] [1: Strong Evidence]

  Standard precautions are the foundation for preventing transmission of infectious diseases. Standard precautions apply to all patients across all health care settings (eg, hospitals, ambulatory surgery centers, free-standing specialty care sites, interventional sites).[130,132] Standard precautions include practices for hand hygiene, PPE, patient resuscitation, environmental control, respiratory hygiene/cough etiquette, sharps safety, and textiles and laundry.[130]

IV.b. Scrubbed team members should wear two pairs of surgical gloves, one over the other, during surgical and other invasive procedures that have the potential for exposure to blood, body fluids, or other potentially infectious materials.[12,32,46-48,131,133-135] *[1: Strong Evidence]*

Wearing two pairs of gloves reduces the risk of glove perforation and percutaneous injury. A systematic review of 31 randomized controlled trials of gloving practices demonstrated that double gloving minimizes the risk of exposure to blood during invasive procedures by providing a protective barrier.[136] The studies compared single gloves to double gloves; double gloves to indicator gloves; double gloves to double latex gloves plus a glove liner; double gloves to latex inner gloves with knitted outer gloves; double gloves to latex inner gloves with steel-weave outer gloves; and double gloves to triple gloves.[136] Double gloving (eg, two pairs of gloves, indicator glove with over glove) is more effective than single gloving in reducing glove perforations.[82,136-143]

Double gloving minimizes bloodborne pathogen exposure.[137,144-147] Studies have demonstrated that double gloving reduces contact with blood by a factor of 5.8 to 10.[144,148] When two pairs of gloves are worn (ie, double gloving), in most instances only the outer glove is perforated when punctured by a sharp device. In addition, research demonstrates that when two pairs of gloves are worn and a puncture occurs, the volume of blood on a solid sharp device (eg, suture needle) is reduced by as much as 95%. There is evidence that double gloving can reduce the risk of exposure to blood and body fluids by as much as 87% if the outer glove is punctured.[76,133,149]

A prospective cohort study compared the frequency of glove perforations in single and double gloves by testing 1,000 pairs of gloves after the end of pelvic surgery procedures. Of the single glove sets, 11% had a perforation, and 2% of the double glove sets had a perforation in the inner and outer gloves.[145]

A prospective study investigated the efficacy of double gloving by comparing the frequency of glove perforations from 100 consecutive major and 100 consecutive minor orthopedic procedures. All surgical team members wore double gloves. Researchers examined the gloves for perforations after the procedures. The overall perforation rate was 15.8%. Major procedures had a 21.6% perforation rate while minor procedures had a 3.6% perforation rate. The outer glove perforation rate was 22.7% while the inner glove perforation rate was 3.7%; inner gloves were perforated only in major procedures. The majority of outer glove perforations (72.7%) were not detected by the surgical team members. The most common site of perforation occurred on the dominant thumb. Based on these results, the authors recommended routine double gloving during orthopedic procedures given the integrity of the inner gloves.[150]

A prospective, randomized, controlled trial calculated the rate of barrier breaches when personnel were single and double gloved in 99 procedures. Single gloves were breached at a rate of 35% per procedure and 21% per individual.[151] Only one breach was immediately detected by the wearer. The breach rate in the outer glove of personnel who wore double gloves was similar to those wearing single gloves, but none of the inner gloves were breached, which reduced the risk of bloodborne pathogen exposure.[151]

IV.b.1. When double gloves are worn, perforation indicator systems should be used.[81,152]

A perforation indicator system uses a colored pair of gloves worn beneath a standard pair of gloves. When glove perforation occurs, moisture from the surgical field seeps through the perforation between the layers of gloves, revealing the underlying color and signaling a perforation.[60,81,151,153] Perforations are detected more frequently and reliably with a perforation indicator glove system.[133,136,149,151,153-155]

A double-blind, randomized study evaluated the ability of participants to locate a 30-micron sized hole in various glove configurations (ie, single gloves, double gloves, double gloves using a glove perforation indicator system) during simulated surgery. While wearing the indicator system, participants detected 84% of the perforations with the latex indicator system and 56% of the perforations with the synthetic indicator system.[155]

IV.b.2. When indicated by a clinical need for high tactile sensitivity, a single pair of gloves may be worn.

IV.c. Perioperative personnel should monitor gloves for punctures. *[1: Strong Evidence]*

Careful inspection of glove integrity throughout the procedure may prevent unnoticed glove perforation. Undetected glove perforation during operative or other invasive procedures may present an increased risk for bloodborne pathogen transmission to perioperative team members related to prolonged exposure to blood, body fluids, or other potentially infectious materials.

Intact gloves provide a barrier that reduces the passage of microorganisms from surgical team members' hands to the operative field. Intact gloves also provide a barrier that prevents bloodborne pathogen exposure to the wearer. Glove failures can be caused by punctures, tears by sharp devices, or spontaneous failures. The ASTM Standard Specification for Rubber Surgical Gloves allows for a 1.5% glove hole failure rate.[152,156] A comparison study of single and double gloving analyzed the frequency of glove perforations during surgery. The rate of perforations during surgical procedures that lasted fewer than two hours was 4.21%; the rate of perforations during procedures that were longer than two hours was 11.69%.[149] Researchers calculated the increased perforation risk per additional 10 minutes of operating time to be 1.115 times.[140,149] When single gloves were worn, the detection rate of a perforation was 36.84%. When a double glove puncture indication system was worn, the detection rate for a perforation was 86.52%.[149]

A prospective study assessed glove perforation rates in 130 consecutive orthopedic procedures. A total of 1,452 gloves from all surgical team members were tested. The overall perforation rate was 3.58%. Perforations went unnoticed 61.5% of the time. Single glove perforations occurred at a rate of 10.87% compared to 3.34% when two pairs of gloves were used. When double gloves were used, the inner glove was perforated at a rate of 0.36%.[139]

A study of glove perforations when team members double gloved during hip and knee arthroplasty showed a perforation rate of 18.4% to the outer glove and 8.4% to the inner glove. The most frequent site of perforation was the second finger of the nondominant hand.[157] A prospective study of four brands of latex-free gloves used during arthroplasty showed a higher perforation rate and poorer handling properties than latex gloves.[158] A randomized controlled study of personnel scrubbed on primary cemented total hip replacement surgeries evaluated the incidence of glove perforation and contamination when outer gloves were changed at specific intervals. In the study group, outer gloves were changed every 20 minutes, prior to cementation, and when a visible puncture was detected. In the control group, outer gloves were changed prior to cementation and when a visible puncture was detected. There was a statistically significant lower rate of perforations for surgeons and scrub persons in the study group compared with surgeons and scrub persons in the control group. There also was a statistically significant lower rate of glove contamination in the study group compared to the control group. The researchers found that regular glove changes during a procedure can reduce the incidence of perforation and contamination.[159]

Researchers in a cross sectional study investigated the incidence and recognition of glove perforations during gynecological procedures. Perforations occurred in 24.4% of the procedures and were detected 37.5% of the time by the gynecologist.[160] A randomized study of single and double gloving analyzed glove punctures during major gynecological surgery. When the staff physician and resident were single gloved, the rate of perforation was 22.1%. The perforation rate was 2.7% when the staff physician and resident were double gloved.[134]

Glove microperforations were studied by testing 180 pairs of gloves with both the water load test and electrical conductance following use in endoscopic, laparoscopic, and open urology procedures. The glove defect rate was 29% in all urologic procedures. The rate of glove perforations was 15% in endoscopy procedures, 25% in laparoscopic procedures, and 30.6% in open urologic procedures. The investigators concluded that double gloving in urologic procedures protects the patient from cross contamination and protects the surgical team from occupational exposure.[161]

A prospective, randomized study compared glove perforations between perioperative nurses who were single and double gloved. Perforations were detected in 8.9% of nurses wearing single gloves and 11.3% in the outer glove of nurses wearing double gloves. No inner gloves were perforated. The average time for a perforation to occur was 69.8 minutes after the beginning of surgery. The researchers concluded that double gloving was effective in preventing exposure to bloodborne pathogens.[141]

IV.c.1. Gloves should be changed when a suspected or actual perforation occurs or a visible defect is noted.[60]

Surgical gloves develop microperforations depending on the length of time the gloves are worn. Perforations allow bacteria to pass from the surgical site through the glove.[162]

IV.d. Virus-inhibiting protective gloves may be worn. [2: Moderate Evidence]

Virus-inhibiting gloves reduce the amount of virus transmitted when a glove is perforated.[163-165] An automatic apparatus was used to study the influence of the puncture and type of glove on the volume of blood transferred during a simulated percutaneous injury with a hollow bore needle. The researchers found an 81% reduction in virus transmission with virus-inhibiting gloves compared to single or double latex glove systems.[164] A study of virus transmission showed a 15-fold or greater reduction in virus transmission with virus-inhibiting gloves compared to standard gloves of the same thickness.[165] The researchers concluded that virus-inhibiting gloves could provide increased protection against HIV and HCV exposures.[165]

A prospective clinical study evaluated the tolerance, ergonomics, and glove barrier value of virus-inhibiting gloves. The researchers examined 834 gloves from 100 procedures and concluded that the virus-inhibiting gloves afforded mechanical protection against punctures and may be recommended in high-risk surgical procedures.[163] In another study, researchers randomly assigned study volunteers into one of three groups: single gloves, double gloves, and antimicrobial gloves. The researchers found a significant reduction in microbial passage with antimicrobial gloves.[166]

Recommendation V

Sharp devices must be contained and disposed of safely.

Containing sharps in an appropriate container can reduce sharps injuries. Causes of container-related injuries include a sharp protruding from disposal container; a sharp piercing the side of a disposal container; a sharp left on or near the disposal container; a sharp left on the floor, table, or other inappropriate place; and a sharp protruding from a trash bag or inappropriate disposal container.[167]

The OSHA bloodborne pathogens standard requires the safe disposal of contaminated sharps devices to minimize the risk of bloodborne pathogen transmission.[38,168] Analysis of data reported to a national surveillance system compared percutaneous injuries from sharps device disposal from two time periods, before and after the regulatory-driven improvements in sharps disposal practices. Between 1992 and 1994, 36.8% of percutaneous injuries were attributed to disposal of sharps devices. Between 2006 and 2007, 19.3% of percutaneous injuries were attributed to disposal of sharps devices.[168] The 53% decline in container-related injuries is attributable to widespread use of point-of-use, puncture-resistant sharps containers.[168,169]

V.a. Selection criteria for sharps containers should include functionality, accessibility, accommodation, and visibility.[169] [2: Moderate Evidence]

Sharps disposal injuries have been attributed to inappropriate sharps containment practices by the user, inadequate sharps disposal container design, inappropriate sharps container placement, and over-filling of sharps disposal containers.[169]

V.a.1. Functional selection criteria for a sharps disposal container should include that the container
- is durable (ie, resistant to punctures and chemical or liquid leaks),
- has a mechanism for closing that minimizes exposure to contents and hand injuries during handling and that is resistant to being opened manually,
- is stable (ie, is not prone to tipping), and
- is of a size and shape to accommodate the type of sharps that require disposal.[169]

V.a.2. Accessibility criteria for a sharps disposal container should include that
- the container is placed in close proximity to the point of use,
- there is an obstacle-free pathway between the point of use and the container, and
- the container is reachable by personnel of varied heights.[169]

V.a.3. Accommodation criteria for a sharps disposal container should include that the container requires minimal training to use and provides ease of storage, assembly, and operation.[169]

V.a.4. Visibility criteria for a sharps disposal container should include that the container
- is easily recognizable (eg, has a hazard warning label or container color),
- is visible to the user,
- has a visible fill level, and
- is placed under sufficient illumination.[169]

V.b. All sharps must be handled and disposed of safely.[38] [1: Regulatory Requirement]

Safe handling of contaminated sharps protects the original user and environmental services, laundry, sterile processing, and waste disposal personnel. One waste disposal company reported 40 sharps injuries occurring at a rate of one per 29,000 labor hours. Causes of the injuries were improperly closed or overfilled sharps containers and incorrect disposal of sharps into plastic garbage bags.[170]

V.b.1. Disposable sharps contaminated with blood or other potentially infectious materials should be disposed of in a closeable, puncture-resistant container that is leak-proof on its sides and bottom and is labeled or color-coded.[38]

V.b.2. Sharps disposal receptacles should be
- appropriately sized with a fill line that is readily visible,
- located close to the point of use,
- maintained upright when in use, and
- routinely replaced and not overfilled.[38]

V.b.3. Container devices with enhanced engineering (eg, counterbalanced tray, one-hand sharp deposit, hand entry restriction, tamper proof locks) should be used.

Researchers conducting a nonrandomized intervention and cohort study from 2006 to 2008 evaluated sharps injury rates during use of an enhanced engineered sharps container compared to during use of an existing sharps container. The enhanced engineering controls included a large horizontal aperture, counterbalanced tray, one-hand sharp deposit, and hand entry restriction. The study device was associated with a 30% reduction in after-procedure sharps injuries; a 57% reduction in disposal-related sharps injuries; and an 81% reduction in container-associated sharps injury. The control group had no significant reductions in sharps injuries.[167]

V.c. Sharps/needle counter devices should be used to contain and isolate sharps on the sterile back table. Sharps/needle counter devices should be
○ puncture resistant,

SHARPS SAFETY

- labeled or color-coded in accordance with the bloodborne pathogens standard, and
- leak proof on the sides and bottom.[38]

[1: Regulatory Requirement]

Sharps/needle counter devices protect scrubbed personnel during procedures by segregating sharps in one location until disposal at the end of the procedure.

V.d. Contaminated, reusable sharps (eg, skin hooks, trocars) should be segregated from non-sharp instruments after use for transport to the decontamination area in a puncture-resistant container that is labeled as biohazardous. *[1: Regulatory Requirement]*

Segregating sharp instruments minimizes the risk of injury to personnel handling the instruments during decontamination. Processes that require employees to place their hands into basins of sharp instruments are prohibited by OSHA because of the risk of percutaneous exposure to bloodborne pathogens.[38]

Recommendation VI

The perioperative RN should demonstrate personal and professional responsibility in preventing sharps injuries and preventing the transmission of bloodborne pathogens.

It is the perioperative RN's responsibility to evaluate his or her practice in context with current professional practice standards, rules, and regulations.[171]

VI.a. The perioperative RN should observe local, state, and federal regulations (eg, OSHA regulations).[171] *[1: Regulatory Requirement]*

It is the perioperative RN's responsibility to practice nursing in accordance with the standards and guidelines of regulatory bodies.[38,171]

VI.b. The perioperative RN and other surgical team members should comply with methods of protection (eg, PPE, HBV immunization) against disease transmission.[13,20,22,23,131] *[1: Strong Evidence]*

Occupational exposure to bloodborne pathogens is a risk for all health care workers.[14] There is potential increased risk in the OR because of the nature of the work, amount of blood exposure, and use of sharp devices.[14,51] There have been 132 documented cases of health care provider to patient transmission of HBV, HCV, or HIV worldwide.[17,31,35,36] Protective barriers contribute to the prevention of occupational and patient exposure.[14]

Since the widespread adoption of HBV immunizations, the number of HBV infections in health care workers has declined significantly.[19-23] The reported number of HBV-infected providers in 1983 was 10,000 compared to approximately 100 in 2009.[20,21]

VI.b.1. Perioperative personnel should be immunized against the hepatitis B virus.[20,131]

Hepatitis B is highly contagious and can be transmitted via percutaneous exposure (eg, needlestick injury) or mucosal exposure to infected blood or body fluids. The risk of acquiring HBV infection from occupational exposure depends on the frequency of percutaneous and mucosal exposure to blood or body fluids that contain the virus. Risks to health care providers from sharps injuries and blood and body fluid exposure have been reduced as a result of widespread HBV immunization.[131] Although rare, health care personnel who have HBV or HCV have transmitted these infections to patients.[17,31,35,36] The HBV vaccine, given in three intramuscular injections, induces a protective antibody response in 90% of healthy recipients.[13] Since 1991, OSHA requires employers of persons at risk for occupational exposure to provide the hepatitis B vaccine at no cost to the employee.[38]

VI.b.2. Perioperative personnel should report sharps injuries immediately.

Reporting facilitates prophylaxis against bloodborne pathogen exposure. Post-exposure prophylactic medication reduces the risk of acquiring HIV, immunoglobulin and vaccination reduces the risk of HBV infection, and surveillance for HCV detects an acquired infection and facilitates prompt treatment.[172]

Researchers examined blood exposure, percutaneous injury, and reporting in a stratified random sample of 5,123 physicians, nurses, and medical technologists. Under-reporting of percutaneous injuries varied by occupation but, overall, 32% did not report an exposure.[173] A questionnaire surveying perioperative personnel showed that 90.4% knew how to report a sharps injury, but 32.4% admitted to not reporting a percutaneous injury.[172] Reasons for not reporting an injury included not considering the patient to be high risk, finding the reporting process to be too difficult, and not having enough time.[172,174,175]

VI.c. Perioperative team members should use devices with safety features that are provided by the employer.[38] *[1: Regulatory Requirement]*

Safety devices are only effective when used (see Recommendation II).

VI.c.1. Perioperative personnel should actively participate in the safety conversion process and help others adapt to the change.

Recommendation VII

Personnel should receive initial and ongoing education and competency verification on their understanding of the principles of and performance of the processes for sharps safety.[176]

Health care organizations are responsible for providing initial and ongoing education and evaluating the competency of perioperative team members in the use of sharps safety devices and the performance of sharps safety measures.

Initial and ongoing education on sharps safety practices facilitates the development of knowledge, skills, and attitudes that affect safe patient care and workplace safety with regard to the prevention of percutaneous injuries.[13,66,82,177-180] Ongoing development of knowledge and skills and documentation of personnel participation is a regulatory and accreditation requirement for both hospitals and ambulatory settings.[181-184]

Periodic education programs provide the opportunity to reinforce the principles of sharps safety as well as explain safety-engineered devices and potential hazards to patients and personnel. Periodic education programs also provide the opportunity to introduce information on technology changes and new applications.[59]

Competency assessment measures individual performance, provides a mechanism for documentation, and verifies that perioperative personnel have an understanding of sharps safety and facility policies. Every nurse is responsible for being personally accountable for maintaining competency validation.[185]

There are no universally accepted or mandated ways to perform or validate competency, and strategies to accomplish this differ among states. The goal of competency strategies is to reassure the public that nurses have the knowledge, skills, and judgment to provide safe and effective care.[186]

VII.a. Perioperative personnel should receive education that addresses sharps safety practices upon orientation to the perioperative setting. Continuing education should be provided when new equipment or processes are introduced. *[2: Moderate Evidence]*

Sharps injuries may be minimized and safety improved with regularly scheduled education, training, and competency demonstrations.[177,187-189]

Residents, students, and personnel with less experience are at an increased risk for percutaneous injuries.[75,175,190-192] A survey of surgeons-in-training at 17 medical centers showed that 83% had a needlestick injury during training. By the end of their five-year training period, 99% had sustained an injury.[75] A retrospective review of the occupational health records of surgical trainees showed that senior and chief residents had a lower exposure rate than junior residents.[193]

VII.a.1. The perioperative RN should participate in education about bloodborne pathogens and follow recommended infection prevention practices.[38,131]

VII.a.2. Perioperative team members should practice using safety devices.

Practice before use will establish familiarity and experience with the device before use in clinical practice.

VII.b. Health care personnel who are occupationally exposed to blood or other potentially infectious materials must receive training before assignment to tasks during which occupational exposure may occur, at least annually thereafter, and when changes to procedures or tasks affect occupational exposure.[36,38] *[1: Regulatory Requirement]*

Employers are responsible for providing training on bloodborne exposure guidelines at no cost to the employee during working hours. Employers are also responsible for ensuring employees participate in the training program and for offering materials in appropriate languages and at appropriate literacy levels.[38]

Providing the basis for the prevention of bloodborne pathogen exposure may instill an understanding of the processes that need to be followed and thereby prevent disease transmission. Education and training efforts are equally important in promoting awareness of hazards and acceptance of safe work practices and material-handling procedures in the workplace.[59,194] Educating employees on safe work practices (eg, using PPE) can help protect staff members, their family members, and the community from disease transmission.

VII.b.1. Education and competency assessment related to sharps safety and injury prevention should include a review of
- exposure control plans,
- safety-engineered devices,
- blunt suture needle use,
- neutral or safe zone concepts,
- no-touch technique,
- double gloving, and
- sharps disposal.

VII.b.2. Sharps safety should be included in the organization's annual bloodborne pathogens training program.[38,131]

Recommendation VIII

Documentation should reflect activities related to sharps safety.[38]

Documentation related to sharps safety is applicable at the systems level. Documentation serves as a basis for monitoring compliance, measuring performance, maintaining employee records, and logging exposure incidents.

VIII.a. Employers must maintain training records for three years. The records must include
- training dates,
- the content or a summary of the training,
- the names and qualifications of the trainer(s), and
- the names and job titles of the trainees.[38]

[1: Regulatory Requirement]

SHARPS SAFETY

VIII.b. Health care facilities must have a documented exposure control plan.[38] *[1: Regulatory Requirement]*

VIII.b.1. As part of the health care facility's written exposure control plan, all incidents of occupational exposure to blood or other potentially infectious materials must be documented.[38,195] Documentation must include
- the employee's name and identification;
- the employee's hepatitis B vaccination status, including vaccination dates, and other relevant medical information for both individuals;
- results of all related examinations, medical tests, and post-exposure evaluation and follow-up procedures;
- a licensed health care professional's written evaluation of the risk of transmission; and
- a copy of the information provided to the employee.[38]

Additional documentation should include
- the route of exposure;
- the circumstances associated with the exposure; and
- the source individual's serological status, if known.

Documenting each exposure incident provides a record of the incident, what follow-through was taken, and the current status of the incident.

VIII.b.2. Input from non-managerial health care workers should be solicited and documented in the exposure control plan with regard to identifying, evaluating, and selecting safety-engineered sharp devices.[38]

VIII.b.3. The employer should document in the exposure control plan that safety-engineered sharps devices and needleless systems have been evaluated and implemented.[38]

VIII.c. Employers must maintain a sharps injury log to document all percutaneous injuries from contaminated sharps and must maintain the log in such a way that an injured employee's identification remains confidential.[38] At a minimum, a sharps injury log must include
- the type and brand of device involved in the incident,
- the department or work area where the exposure incident occurred, and
- an explanation of how the incident occurred.

[1: Regulatory Requirement]

VIII.c.1. Documentation related to exposure incidents must be maintained for the employee's duration of employment plus 30 years.[38]

Recommendation IX

Policies and procedures for sharps safety processes and practices should be developed, reviewed periodically, revised as necessary, and readily available in the practice setting.

Policies and procedures assist in the development of patient and workplace safety, quality assessment, and performance improvement activities. Policies and procedures establish authority, responsibility, and accountability within the facility. Policies and procedures also serve as operational guidelines that are used to minimize patient and health care worker risks, to standardize practice, and to direct perioperative personnel.

IX.a. Policies and procedures should be developed to guide, support, and monitor adherence to sharps safety and injury prevention practices, including the use of systems that should be used to collect, analyze, and communicate information related to sharps safety.[130] *[1: Strong Evidence]*

Definitive policies and procedures as part of an overall administrative strategy can demonstrate a commitment to preventing sharps injuries by incorporating sharps safety into the organizational objectives for patient and occupational safety.

IX.b. Policies and procedures should be developed and implemented for
- double gloving,
- neutral (hands-free) zone,
- safety-engineered devices (eg, blunt suture needles, scalpels, safety syringes and needles),[196]
- post-exposure protocols,[19,131] and
- safety-engineered device selection and evaluation.[38]

[1: Regulatory Requirement]

IX.c. Policies and procedures designed to minimize or eliminate health care personnel exposure to blood and other potentially infectious materials must be developed and implemented.[38] *[1: Regulatory Requirement]*

A written bloodborne pathogens exposure plan that is consistent with federal, state, and local rules and regulations and that governs occupational exposure to bloodborne pathogens, is reviewed periodically, and is readily available in the practice setting promotes safety with medical devices and blood and body fluids.[38]

IX.d. Policies should be developed in accordance with federal and state guidelines and should be consistent with existing impaired-provider and disability guidelines to define work restrictions for health care personnel who have a transmissible bloodborne infection (eg, HIV, HBV, HCV).[197] The policies should define work restrictions based on whether the employee

- has a viral burden above the recommended threshold for the relevant virus;
- has a medical condition or conditions that result in an inability to perform assigned tasks;
- has experienced documented untoward events (eg, having transmitted HBV, HCV, or HIV);
- refuses or is unable to follow recommended guidelines to prevent transmission of infectious diseases; or
- is unable to perform regular duties, assuming that reasonable accommodation has been offered for the disability.[22]

[1: Strong Evidence]

IX.e. Policies and procedures should include processes for initial education, training, ongoing competency validation, and annual review for issues related to sharps injury prevention.[183,184]
[1: Regulatory Requirement]

Policies and procedures assist in the development of activities that support patient safety, quality assessment, and the establishment of guidelines for continuous performance improvement. Standardizing processes for performance expectations between perioperative settings facilitates continuity of care and reduces the risk of error when personnel rotate among areas.

Recommendation X

Perioperative team members should participate in a variety of quality improvement activities to monitor and improve the prevention of sharps injuries.

Quality assurance and performance improvement programs assist in evaluating worker safety and formulating plans for corrective actions. These programs provide data that may be used to determine whether an individual organization is within benchmark goals and, if not, identify areas that may require corrective actions. These programs may also provide ongoing feedback regarding whether problems are improving, stabilizing, or worsening.

X.a. Quality indicators should be developed to measure improvement in sharps injury prevention. Quality indicators for measuring sharps safety in the perioperative setting should include rates of percutaneous injuries and near misses.
[1: Strong Evidence]

Quality indicators are measurable and demonstrate that facilities are using specific interventions to provide safe patient care.[198] According to the Agency for Healthcare Research and Quality (AHRQ), "An adequate quality indicator must have sound clinical or empirical rationale for its use. It should measure an important aspect of quality that is subject to provider or health care system control."[198(p3)] The AHRQ quality indicators are one response to the need for multidimensional, accessible quality measures that can be used to gauge performance in health care. The quality indicators are evidence based and can be used to identify variations in the quality of care provided on both an inpatient and outpatient basis.

X.b. Process monitoring should be a part of every perioperative setting as part of an overall sharps injury prevention program. Process monitoring should include
- sharps injury data,[4]
- double gloving compliance,
- standard and transmissible infection precaution compliance,
- safety-engineered device compliance, and
- neutral zone implementation.

[1: Strong Evidence]

Monitoring sharps injury data allows results to be compared to a predetermined level of quality. Reviewing the findings provides information to identify problems and trends, which can be used to improve practice.[4,13]

X.b.1. Perioperative personnel should report all percutaneous injuries according to organizational policy.

Injury reports provide data that can be used to identify problems and trends, and thus used used to improve safety. Health care workers in the perioperative setting under-report percutaneous injuries.[4,30,174] A questionnaire study asked surgeons how often they reported a sharps injury. Only 25.8% reported all of their injuries, 22.5% reported some of their injuries, and 51.7% reported none of their injuries.[199] In a retrospective survey of surgeons' needlestick injuries, only 9% reported the injury.[200]

X.b.2. Sharps injury logs should be reviewed to identify trends in types and frequency of injuries.

X.b.3. The organization should perform periodic audits for compliance with policies and use of safety-engineered devices, work practice controls, and barrier protection methods.

X.b.4. Processes and systems should be evaluated after any sharps injury by using a quality improvement tool (eg, process map, flow chart, fishbone or cause-and-effect diagram, affinity diagram, root cause analysis).[4]

X.c. The health care organization must conduct a yearly product evaluation and selection of safety-engineered devices.[38] *[1: Regulatory Requirement]*

X.d. Perioperative nurses should contribute to creating a culture of safety.

Health care organizations that support and promote safety may have a reduction in occupational exposures to bloodborne pathogens.[13,126,177,201-206]

SHARPS SAFETY

A culture of safety is created through
- management initiatives that improve patient and health care personnel safety,[201,207,208]
- health care personnel participation in safety planning,[4,201,209]
- the availability of appropriate PPE and safety devices for identified tasks,[4]
- the influence of group norms regarding appropriate safety practices,[207] and
- the facility's socialization process for newly hired personnel.[4]

[2: Moderate Evidence]

Glossary

Bloodborne pathogens: Pathogenic microorganisms that are present in human blood and can cause disease in humans. These pathogens include, but are not limited to, hepatitis B virus (HBV), hepatitis C virus (HCV), and human immunodeficiency virus (HIV) as defined by OSHA bloodborne pathogens standard 1910.1030.

Engineering controls: Safety-engineered devices designed to prevent or reduce the incidence of worker injury and the risk of bloodborne pathogen exposure to the worker.

Hands-free technique: Work practice that restricts members of the perioperative team at the sterile field from touching the same sharp instrument at the same time. Synonym, neutral zone.

Neutral zone: A safe work-practice control technique used to ensure that the surgeon and scrubbed person do not touch the same sharp instrument at the same time. This technique is accomplished by establishing a designated neutral zone on the sterile field and placing sharp items within the zone for transfer of the item between scrubbed personnel. Synonym: Hands-free technique.

No-touch technique: Technique that minimizes manual handling of sharp devices and instruments.

Perforation indicator system: A double gloving system comprising a colored pair of surgical gloves worn beneath a standard pair of surgical gloves. When a glove perforation occurs, moisture from the surgical field seeps through the perforation between the layers of gloves, allowing the site of perforation to be more easily seen.

Personal protective equipment (PPE): Specialized equipment or clothing for eyes, face, head, body, and extremities; protective clothing; respiratory devices; and protective shields and barriers designed to protect the worker from injury or exposure to a patient's blood, tissue, or body fluids. Used by health care workers and others whenever necessary to protect themselves from the hazards of processes or environments, chemical hazards, or mechanical irritants encountered in a manner capable of causing injury or impairment in the function of any part of the body through absorption, inhalation, or physical contact.

Potentially infectious material: Blood; all body fluids, secretions, and excretions (except sweat), regardless of whether they contain visible blood; nonintact skin; mucous membranes; and airborne, droplet, and contact-transmitted epidemiologically important pathogens.

Sharps with engineered sharps injury protection (SESIP): A sharp with a built-in safety feature or mechanism intended to reduce the risk of sharps injury.

Sharps: Items with edges or points capable of cutting or puncturing through other items. In the context of surgery, items include, but are not limited to, suture needles, scalpel blades, hypodermic needles, electrosurgical needles and blades, instruments with sharp edges or points, and safety pins.

Standard precautions: The primary strategy for successful infection control and reduction of worker exposure. Precautions used for care of all patients regardless of their diagnosis or presumed infectious status.

Work practice controls: Measures taken to reduce the likelihood of exposure by changing the method of performing a task to minimize the risk of exposure to blood or other potentially infectious materials.

References

1. Pruss-Ustun A, Rapiti E, Hutin Y. Estimation of the global burden of disease attributable to contaminated sharps injuries among health-care workers. *Am J Ind Med.* 2005;48(6):482-490. [IVC]

2. Panlilio AL, Orelien JG, Srivastava PU, et al. Estimate of the annual number of percutaneous injuries among hospital-based healthcare workers in the United States, 1997-1998. *Infect Control Hosp Epidemiol.* 2004;25(7):556-562. [VB]

3. Weiss ES, Makary MA, Wang T, et al. Prevalence of blood-borne pathogens in an urban, university-based general surgical practice. *Ann Surg.* 2005;241(5):803-807;discussion 807-809. [VA]

4. *Workbook for Designing, Implementing, and Evaluating a Sharps Injury Prevention Program.* Centers for Disease Control and Prevention. http://www.cdc.gov/sharpssafety/pdf/sharpsworkbook_2008.pdf Accessed April 4, 2013. [IVA]

5. Vigler M, Mulett H, Hausman MR. Chronic Mycobacterium infection of first dorsal web space after accidental Bacilli Calmette-Guerin injection in a health worker: case report. *J Hand Surg Am* Vol. 2008;33(9):1621-1624. [VB]

6. Apisarnthanarak A, Mundy LM. Cytomegalovirus mononucleosis after percutaneous injury in a Thai medical student. *Am J Infect Control.* 2008;36(3):228-229. [VB]

7. Tarantola AP, Rachline AC, Konto C, et al. Occupational malaria following needlestick injury. *Emerg Infect Dis.* 2004;10(10):1878-1880. [VB]

8. Douglas MW, Walters JL, Currie BJ. Occupational infection with herpes simplex virus type 1 after a needlestick injury. *Med J Aust.* 2002;176(5):240. [VB]

9. Cone LA, Curry N, Wuestoff MA, O'Connell SJ, Feller JF. Septic synovitis and arthritis due to Corynebacterium striatum following an accidental scalpel injury. *Clin Infect Dis.* 1998;27(6):1532-1533. [VB]

10. Alweis RL, DiRosario K, Conidi G, Kain KC, Olans R, Tully JL. Serial nosocomial transmission of Plasmodium falciparum malaria from patient to nurse to patient. *Infect Control Hosp Epidemiol.* 2004;25(1):55-59. [VB]

11. Shibuya A, Takeuchi A, Sakurai K, Saigenji K. Hepatitis G virus infection from needle-stick injuries in hospital employees. *J Hosp Infect.* 1998;40(4):287-290. [IIIB]

12. Hidalgo JA, MacArthur RD, Crane LR. An overview of HIV infection and AIDS: etiology, pathogenesis, diagnosis, epidemiology, and occupational exposure. *Semin Thorac Cardiovasc Surg.* 2000;12(2):130-139. [VB]

13. MacCannell T, Laramie AK, Gomaa A, Perz JF. Occupational exposure of health care personnel to hepatitis B and hepatitis C: prevention and surveillance strategies. *Clin Liver Dis.* 2010;14(1):23-36, vii. [VA]

14. Fry DE. Occupational risks of blood exposure in the operating room. *Am Surg.* 2007;73(7):637-646. [VB]

15. Do AN, Ciesielski CA, Metler RP, Hammett TA, Li J, Fleming PL. Occupationally acquired human immunodeficiency virus (HIV) infection: national case surveillance data during 20 years of the HIV epidemic in the United States. *Infect Control Hosp Epidemiol.* 2003;24(2):86-96. [VA]

16. Tomkins S, Ncube F. Occupationally acquired HIV: international reports to December 2002. *Euro Surveill.* 2005;10(3):E050310.2. [VC]

17. Henderson DK. Managing occupational risks for hepatitis C transmission in the health care setting. *Clin Microbiol Rev.* 2003;16(3):546-568. [VA]

18. Tarantola A, Abiteboul D, Rachline A. Infection risks following accidental exposure to blood or body fluids in health care workers: a review of pathogens transmitted in published cases. *Am J Infect Control.* 2006;34(6):367-375. [VA]

19. US Public Health Service. Updated US Public Health Service guidelines for the management of occupational exposures to HBV, HCV, and HIV and recommendations for postexposure prophylaxis. *MMWR Recomm Rep.* 2001;50(RR-11):1-52. [IVA]

20. Centers for Disease Control and Prevention (CDC). Updated CDC recommendations for the management of hepatitis B virus-infected health-care providers and students. *MMWR Recomm Rep.* 2012;61(RR-3):1-12. [IVA]

21. Williams IT, Perz JF, Bell BP. Viral hepatitis transmission in ambulatory health care settings. *Clin Infect Dis.* 2004;38(11):1592-1598. [VA]

22. Advisory Committee on Immunization Practices, Centers for Disease Control and Prevention (CDC). Immunization of health-care personnel: recommendations of the Advisory Committee on Immunization Practices (ACIP). *MMWR Recomm Rep.* 2011;60(RR-7):1-45. [IVA]

23. *Combating the Silent Epidemic of Viral Hepatitis: Action Plan for the Prevention, Care & Treatment of Viral Hepatitis.* 2011. US Department of Health & Human Services. http://www.hhs.gov/ash/initiatives/hepatitis/actionplan_viralhepatitis2011.pdf. Accessed April 4, 2013. [IVA]

24. *NIOSH Alert: Preventing Needlestick Injuries in Health Care Settings.* NIOSH publication no. 2000-108. November 1999. National Institute for Occupational Safety and Health. http://www.cdc.gov/niosh/docs/2000-108/pdfs/2000-108.pdf. Accessed April 4, 2013. [IVB]

25. Mills PR, Thorburn D, McCruden EAB. Occupationally acquired hepatitis C infection. *Rev Med Microbiol.* 2000;11(1):15-22. [VA]

26. Panlilio AL, Cardo DM, Grohskopf LA, Heneine W, Ross CS; US Public Health Service. Updated US Public Health Service guidelines for the management of occupational exposures to HIV and recommendations for postexposure prophylaxis. *MMWR Recomm Rep.* 2005;54(RR-9):1-17. [IVA]

27. Young TN, Arens FJ, Kennedy GE, Laurie JW, Rutherford GW. Antiretroviral post-exposure prophylaxis (PEP) for occupational HIV exposure. *Cochrane Database Syst Rev.* 2007;(1):CD002835 [IA]

28. Cardo DM, Culver DH, Ciesielski CA, et al. A case-control study of HIV seroconversion in health care workers after percutaneous exposure. Centers for Disease Control and Prevention Needlestick Surveillance Group. *N Engl J Med.* 1997;337(21):1485-1490. [IIIB]

29. Regez RM, Kleipool AE, Speekenbrink RG, Frissen PH. The risk of needle stick accidents during surgical procedures: HIV-1 viral load in blood and bone marrow. *Int J STD AIDS.* 2005;16(10):671-672. [IVB]

30. Jagger J, Balon M. Suture needle and scalpel blade injuries: frequent but underreported. *Adv Expo Prev.* 1995;1(3):1-6. [VA]

31. Mallolas J, Gatell JM, Bruguera M. Transmission of HIV-1 from an obstetrician to a patient during a caesarean section [1]. *AIDS.* 2006;20(13):1785. [VB]

32. Information statement: Preventing the transmission of bloodborne pathogens. February 2001. Revised June 2008. Reviewed June 2012. American Academy of Orthopaedic Surgeons. http://www.aaos.org/about/papers/advistmt/1018.asp. Accessed April 4, 2013. [IVB]

33. Ross RS, Viazov S, Roggendorf M. Risk of hepatitis C transmission from infected medical staff to patients: model-based calculations for surgical settings. *Arch Intern Med.* 2000;160(15):2313-2316. [IIIB]

34. Folin AC, Nordstrom GM. Accidental blood contact during orthopedic surgical procedures. *Infect Control Hosp Epidemiol.* 1997;18(4):244-246. [VA]

35. Perry JL, Pearson RD, Jagger J. Infected health care workers and patient safety: a double standard. *Am J Infect Control.* 2006;34(5):313-319. [VB]

36. Jagger J, Perry J, Gomaa A, Phillips EK. The impact of US policies to protect healthcare workers from bloodborne pathogens: the critical role of safety-engineered devices. *J Infect Public Health.* 2008;1(2):62-71. [VA]

37. Fry DE. Hepatitis: risks for the surgeon. *Am Surg.* 2000;66(2):178-183. [VB]

38. 29 CFR 1910.1030. Occupational exposure. Bloodborne pathogens. 2009. http://www.gpo.gov/fdsys/pkg/CFR-2011-title29-vol6/pdf/CFR-2011-title29-vol6-sec1910-1030.pdf. Accessed April 4, 2013.

39. OSHA's bloodborne pathogens standard [risk analysis]. *Healthcare Risk Control.* 2008;4(Infection Control 13.1):1-20. [VA]

40. Needlestick Safety and Prevention Act of 2000. PL 106.430. http://www.gpo.gov/fdsys/pkg/PLAW-106publ430/html/PLAW-106publ430.htm. Accessed April 4, 2013.

41. Enforcement procedures for the occupational exposure to bloodborne pathogens. CPL 02-02-069. 2001. http://www.osha.gov/pls/oshaweb/owadisp.show_document?p_table=directives&p_id=2570. Accessed April 4, 2013.

42. Occupational exposure to bloodborne pathogens; needlestick and other sharps injuries; final rule. Occupational Safety and Health Administration (OSHA), Department of Labor. Final rule; request for comment on the Information Collection (Paperwork) Requirements. *Fed Regist.* 2001;66(12):5318-5325.

43. AORN position statement: workplace safety. AORN, Inc. http://www.aorn.org/uploadedFiles/Main_Navigation/Clinical_Practice/ToolKits/PosStat%20Workplace%20Safety.pdf. Accessed April 5, 2013. [IVB]

44. AORN guidance statement: sharps injury prevention in the perioperative setting. In: *Perioperative Standards and Recommended Practices.* Denver, CO: AORN; 2012:711-716. [IVB]

45. Guideline statement for the implementation of the neutral zone in the perioperative environment. 2006. Association of Surgical Technologists. http://www.ast.org/

pdf/Standards_of_Practice/Guideline_Neutral_Zone.pdf. Accessed April 5, 2013. [IVC]

46. Recommended standards of practice for sharps safety and use of the neutral zone. 2006. Association of Surgical Technologists. http://www.ast.org/pdf/Standards_of_Practice/RSOP_Sharps_Safety_Neutral_Zone.pdf. Accessed April 5, 2013. [IVC]

47. Statement on sharps safety. American College of Surgeons. http://www.facs.org/fellows_info/statements/st-58.html. Accessed April 5, 2013. [IVB]

48. Sharps Safety #5: The CSPS endorses sharps safety measures to prevent injury during perioperative care. Sharps safety measures should include double-gloving, blunt suture needles for fascial closure, and the neutral zone when appropriate to avoid hand to hand passage of sharps. (Adopted 7.15.07, Modified 2.5.09). Council on Surgical & Perioperative Safety. http://cspsteam.org/sharpssafety/sharpssafety.html. Accessed April 5, 2013. [IVA]

49. Moving the sharps safety agenda forward in the United States: concensus statement and call to action. International Healthcare Worker Safety Center at the University of Virginia. http://www.healthsystem.virginia.edu/pub/epinet/ConsensusStatementOnSharpsInjuryPrevention.pdf. Accessed April 5, 2013. [IVA]

50. FDA, NIOSH & OSHA joint safety communication: blunt-tip surgical suture needles reduce needlestick injuries and the risk of subsequent bloodborne pathogen transmission to surgical personnel. US Food and Drug Administration. http://www.fda.gov/downloads/MedicalDevices/Safety/AlertsandNotices/UCM306035.pdf. Accessed April 5, 2013. [IVA]

51. Jagger J, Berguer R, Phillips EK, Parker G, Gomaa AE. Increase in sharps injuries in surgical settings versus nonsurgical settings after passage of national needlestick legislation. *J Am Coll Surg*. 2010;210(4):496-502. [VA]

52. Jagger J, Bentley M, Tereskerz P. A study of patterns and prevention of blood exposures in OR personnel. *AORN J*. 1998;67(5):979-987. [IIIA]

53. Lee WC, Nicklasson L, Cobden D, Chen E, Conway D, Pashos CL. Short-term economic impact associated with occupational needlestick injuries among acute care nurses. *Curr Med Res Opin*. 2005;21(12):1915-1922. [IIIA]

54. O'Malley EM, Scott RD 2nd, Gayle J, et al. Costs of management of occupational exposures to blood and body fluids. *Infect Control Hosp Epidemiol*. 2007;28(7):774-782. [VB]

55. Leigh JP, Gillen M, Franks P, et al. Costs of needlestick injuries and subsequent hepatitis and HIV infection. *Curr Med Res Opin*. 2007;23(9):2093-2105. [VA]

56. Lee JM, Botteman MF, Xanthakos N, Nicklasson L. Needlestick injuries in the United States. Epidemiologic, economic, and quality of life issues. *AAOHN J*. 2005;53(3):117-133. [IIIB]

57. APIC position paper: prevention of device-mediated bloodborne infections to health care workers. Association for Professionals in Infection Control and Epidemiology, Inc. *Am J Infect Control*. 1998;26(6):578-580. [IVB]

58. Jagger J, Perry J. Using needlestick data to target safety device implementation. *Clin Occup Environ Med*. 2002;2(3):557-573. [VA]

59. Adams D. Needlestick and sharps injuries: practice update. *Nurs Stand*. 2012;26(37):49-57; quiz 58. [VA]

60. Rabussay DP, Korniewicz DM. Improving glove barrier effectiveness. *AORN J*. 1997;66(6):1043-1046. [IVB]

61. Chiarello LA. Selection of needlestick prevention devices: a conceptual framework for approaching product evaluation. *Am J Infect Control*. 1995;23(6):386-395. [VB]

62. Tosini W, Ciotti C, Goyer F, et al. Needlestick injury rates according to different types of safety-engineered devices: results of a French multicenter study. *Infect Control Hosp Epidemiol*. 2010;31(4):402-407. [IIIB]

63. Safer medical devices must be selected based on employee feedback and device effectiveness, not Group Purchasing Organizations. November 21, 2002. Occupational Safety and Health Administration. http://www.osha.gov/pls/oshaweb/owadisp.show_document?p_table=INTERPRETATIONS. Accessed April 5, 2013.

64. Employer's responsibility to re-evaluate engineering controls, i.e., safer needle devices, at least annually. January 20, 2004. Occupational Safety and Health Administration. http://www.osha.gov/pls/oshaweb/owadisp.show_document?p_table=INTERPRETATIONS&p_id=24780. Accessed April 5, 2013.

65. Tuma S, Sepkowitz KA. Efficacy of safety-engineered device implementation in the prevention of percutaneous injuries: a review of published studies. *Clin Infect Dis*. 2006;42(8):1159-1170. [IVA]

66. Valls V, Lozano MS, Yanez R, et al. Use of safety devices and the prevention of percutaneous injuries among healthcare workers. *Infect Control Hosp Epidemiol*. 2007;28(12):1352-1360. [IIA]

67. Azar-Cavanagh M, Burdt P, Green-McKenzie J. Effect of the introduction of an engineered sharps injury prevention device on the percutaneous injury rate in healthcare workers. *Infect Control Hosp Epidemiol*. 2007;28(2):165-170. [IIA]

68. Laramie AK, Pun VC, Fang SC, Kriebel D, Davis L. Sharps Injuries among employees of acute care hospitals in Massachusetts, 2002-2007. *Infect Control Hosp Epidemiol*. 2011;32(6):538-544. [IIIB]

69. Waclawski ER. Evaluation of potential reduction in blood and body fluid exposures by use of alternative instruments. *Occup Med (Lond)*. 2004;54(8):567-569. [VA]

70. Cullen BL, Genasi F, Symington I, et al. Potential for reported needlestick injury prevention among healthcare workers through safety device usage and improvement of guideline adherence: expert panel assessment. *J Hosp Infect*. 2006;63(4):445-451. [IIIB]

71. Parantainen A, Verbeek JH, Lavoie MC, Pahwa M. Blunt versus sharp suture needles for preventing percutaneous exposure incidents in surgical staff. *Cochrane Database Syst Rev*. 2011;11:CD009170. [IA]

72. Nordkam RA, Bluyssen SJ, van Goor H. Randomized clinical trial comparing blunt tapered and standard needles in closing abdominal fascia. *World J Surg*. 2005;29(4):441-445. [IA]

73. Use of blunt-tip suture needles to decrease percutaneous injuries to surgical personnel. DHHS (NIOSH) Publication No. 2008–101. 2008. http://www.cdc.gov/niosh/docs/2008-101/pdfs/2008-101.pdf. Accessed April 5, 2013. [IVA]

74. Miller SS, Sabharwal A. Subcuticular skin closure using a "blunt" needle. *Ann R Coll Surg Engl*. 1994;76(4):281. [IIIC]

75. Makary MA, Al-Attar A, Holzmueller CG, et al. Needlestick injuries among surgeons in training. *N Engl J Med*. 2007;356(26):2693-2699. [IIIA]

76. Berguer R, Heller PJ. Preventing sharps injuries in the operating room. *J Am Coll Surg*. 2004;199(3):462-467. [VA]

77. Sullivan S, Williamson B, Wilson LK, Korte JE, Soper D. Blunt needles for the reduction of needlestick injuries during cesarean delivery: a randomized controlled trial. *Obstet Gynecol*. 2009;114(2 Pt 1):211-216. [IA]

78. Centers for Disease Control and Prevention (CDC). Evaluation of blunt suture needles in preventing percutaneous injuries among health-care workers

during gynecologic surgical procedures—New York City, March 1993-June 1994. *MMWR Morb Mortal Wkly Rep.* 1997;46(2):25-29. [IIIB]

79. Hartley JE, Ahmed S, Milkins R, Naylor G, Monson JR, Lee PW. Randomized trial of blunt-tipped versus cutting needles to reduce glove puncture during mass closure of the abdomen. *Br J Surg.* 1996;83(8):1156-1157. [IB]

80. Mingoli A, Sapienza P, Sgarzini G, et al. Influence of blunt needles on surgical glove perforation and safety for the surgeon. *Am J Surg.* 1996;172(5):512-516. [IB]

81. Edlich RF, Wind TC, Hill LG, Thacker JG, McGregor W. Reducing accidental injuries during surgery. *J Long Term Eff Med Implants.* 2003;13(1):1-10. [IB]

82. Yang L, Mullan B. Reducing needle stick injuries in healthcare occupations: an integrative review of the literature. *ISRN Nurs.* 2011;2011:315432. doi:10.5402/2011/315432. [VA]

83. Stafford MK, Pitman MC, Nanthakumaran N, Smith JR. Blunt-tipped versus sharp-tipped needles: wound morbidity. *J Obstet Gynaecol.* 1998;18(1):18-19. [IB]

84. Mornar SJ, Perlow JH. Blunt suture needle use in laceration and episiotomy repair at vaginal delivery. *Am J Obstet Gynecol.* 2008;198(5):e14-e15. [IIIB]

85. Ablett JC, Whitten M, Smith JR. Do blunt tipped needles reduce the risk of glove puncture and needlestick injury in the suture of episiotomy and perineal repair? *J Obstet Gynaecol.* 1998;18(5):478-479. [IA]

86. Catanzarite V, Byrd K, McNamara M, Bombard A. Preventing needlestick injuries in obstetrics and gynecology: how can we improve the use of blunt tip needles in practice? *Obstet Gynecol.* 2007;110(6):1399-1403. [IIIB]

87. Wilson LK, Sullivan S, Goodnight W, Chang EY, Soper D. The use of blunt needles does not reduce glove perforations during obstetrical laceration repair. *Am J Obstet Gynecol.* 2008;199(6):641.e1-641.e3. [IA]

88. Limiting factors for implementing the use of engineering controls, i.e., safety scalpels, under the Bloodborne Pathogens standard. September 1, 2004. Occupational Safety and Health Administration. http://www.osha.gov/pls/oshaweb/owadisp.show_document?p_table=INTERPRETATIONS&p_id=25090. Accessed April 5, 2013.

89. Jagger J, Berguer R, Phillips EK, Parker G, Gomaa AE. Increase in sharps injuries in surgical settings versus nonsurgical settings after passage of national needlestick legislation. *AORN J.* 2011;93(3):322-330. [VA]

90. Perry J, Parker G, Jagger J. Scalpel blades: reducing injury risk. *Adv Expo Prev.* 2003;6(4):37-40. [VA]

91. Fuentes H, Collier J, Sinnott M, Whitby M. Scalpel safety: modeling the effectiveness of different safety devices' ability to reduce scalpel blade injuries. *Intern J Risk Safety Med.* 2008;20(1-2):83-89. [IIIC]

92. Dagi TF, Berguer R, Moore S, Reines HD. Preventable errors in the operating room—part 2: retained foreign objects, sharps injuries, and wrong site surgery. *Curr Probl Surg.* 2007;44(6):352-381. [VA]

93. Makary MA, Pronovost PJ, Weiss ES, et al. Sharpless surgery: a prospective study of the feasibility of performing operations using non-sharp techniques in an urban, university-based surgical practice. *World J Surg.* 2006;30(7):1224-1229. [IIIB]

94. Bhattacharyya M, Bradley H. Intraoperative handling and wound healing of arthroscopic portal wounds: a clinical study comparing nylon suture with wound closure strips. *J Perioper Pract.* 2008;18(5):194-196. [IB]

95. Coulthard P, Esposito M, Worthington HV, van der Elst M, van Waes OJ, Darcey J. Tissue adhesives for closure of surgical incisions. *Cochrane Database Syst Rev.* 2010;(5)(5):CD004287. [IA]

96. Williams CP, Rosen MJ, Jin J, McGee MF, Schomisch SJ, Ponsky J. Objective analysis of the accuracy and efficacy of a novel fascial closure device. *Surg Innov.* 2008;15(4):307-311. [IA]

97. Whitby M, McLaws ML, Slater K. Needlestick injuries in a major teaching hospital: the worthwhile effect of hospital-wide replacement of conventional hollow-bore needles. *Am J Infect Control.* 2008;36(3):180-186. [IIA]

98. Rogers B, Goodno L. Evaluation of interventions to prevent needlestick injuries in health care occupations. *Am J Prev Med.* 2000;18(4 Suppl):90-98. [IA]

99. Guideline for medication safety. In: *Guidelines for Perioperative Practice.* Denver, CO: AORN, Inc; 2015:291-329. [IVB]

100. Perry J, Parker G, Jagger JJ. EPINet report: 2003 percutaneous injury rates. *Adv Expo Prev.* 2005;7(4):42-45. [VA]

101. Perry J, Parker G, Jagger J. EPINet report: 2007 percutaneous injury rates. 2009. University of Virginia Health System. http://www.healthsystem.virginia.edu/pub/epinet/epinet-2007-rates.pdf. Accessed April 5, 2013. [VA]

102. Guideline for prevention of retained surgical items. In: *Guidelines for Perioperative Practice.* Denver, CO: AORN, Inc; 2015:347-363. [IVB]

103. Folin A, Nyberg B, Nordstrom G. Reducing blood exposures during orthopedic surgical procedures. *AORN J.* 2000;71(3):573-576. [IIB]

104. Jeong IS, Park S. Use of hands-free technique among operating room nurses in the Republic of Korea. *Am J Infect Control.* 2009;37(2):131-135. [IIIB]

105. Stringer B, Haines AT, Goldsmith CH, Berguer R, Blythe J. Is use of the hands-free technique during surgery, a safe work practice, associated with safety climate? *Am J Infect Control.* 2009;37(9):766-772. [IIIA]

106. Stringer B, Haines T. The hands-free technique: an effective and easily implemented work practice. *Perioper Nurs Clin.* 2010;5(1):45-58. [VC]

107. Stringer B, Haines T, Goldsmith CH, et al. Hands-free technique in the operating room: reduction in body fluid exposure and the value of a training video. *Public Health Rep.* 2009;124(Suppl 1):169-179. [IIB]

108. The use of safety-engineered devices and work practice controls in operating rooms; hospital responsibility to protect independent practitioners under BBP standard. January 18, 2007. Occupational Safety and Health Administration. http://www.osha.gov/pls/oshaweb/owadisp.show_document?p_table=INTERPRETATIONS&p_id=25620. Accessed April 5, 2013.

109. Bessinger CD Jr. Preventing transmission of human immunodeficiency virus during operations. *Surg Gynecol Obstet.* 1988;167(4):287-289. [VA]

110. Stringer B, Infante-Rivard C, Hanley JA. Effectiveness of the hands-free technique in reducing operating theatre injuries. *Occup Environ Med.* 2002;59(10):703-707. [IIIB]

111. Cunningham TR, Austin J. Using goal setting, task clarification, and feedback to increase the use of the hands-free technique by hospital operating room staff. *J Appl Behav Anal.* 2007;40(4):673-677. [IIA]

112. Eggleston MK Jr, Wax JR, Philput C, Eggleston MH, Weiss MI. Use of surgical pass trays to reduce intraoperative glove perforations. *J Matern Fetal Med.* 1997;6(4):245-247. [IC]

113. Stringer B, Haines T, Goldsmith CH, Blythe J, Harris KA. Perioperative use of the hands-free technique: a semistructured interview study. *AORN J.* 2006;84(2):233-248. [IIIB]

114. Lopez RA, Rayan GM, Monlux R. Hand injuries during hand surgery: a survey of intraoperative sharp injuries

of the hand among hand surgeons. *J Hand Surg Eur Vol.* 2008;33(5):661-666. [IIIA]

115. Ghauri AJ, Amissah-Arthur KN, Rashid A, Mushtaq B, Nessim M, Elsherbiny S. Sharps injuries in ophthalmic practice. *Eye.* 2011;25(4):443-448. [IIIB]

116. Raahave D, Bremmelgaard A. New operative technique to reduce surgeons' risk of HIV infection. *J Hosp Infect.* 1991;18(Suppl A):177-183. [VB]

117. Wallace CG, Browning GG. A novel technique to reduce curved needlestick injuries. *Ann R Coll Surg Engl.* 2004;86(2):128. [VB]

118. Kunishige J, Wanitphakdeedecha R, Nguyen TH, Chen TM. Surgical pearl: a simple means of disarming the "locked and loaded" needle. *Int J Dermatol.* 2008;47(8):848-849. [VC]

119. Sinnott Michael, Shaban Ramon. "Scalpel Safety," not "Safety Scalpel": A New Paradigm in Staff Safety. *Perioper Nurs Clin.* 2010;5(1):59-67. [VA]

120. Ly J, Mittal A, Windsor J. Systematic review and meta-analysis of cutting diathermy versus scalpel for skin incision. *Br J Surg.* 2012;99(5):613-620. [IA]

121. Vose JG, McAdara-Berkowitz J. Reducing scalpel injuries in the operating room. *AORN J.* 2009;90(6):867-872. [VB]

122. Hutin Y, Hauri A, Chiarello L, et al. Best infection control practices for intradermal, subcutaneous, and intramuscular needle injections. *Bull World Health Organ.* 2003;81(7):491-500. [IVA]

123. Froom P, Kristal-Boneh E, Melamed S, Shalom A, Ribak J. Prevention of needle-stick injury by the scooping-resheathing method. *Am J Ind Med.* 1998;34(1):15-19. [IIIB]

124. Carraretto AR, Curi EF, de Almeida CE, Abatti RE. Glass ampoules: risks and benefits. *Rev Bras Anestesiol.* 2011;61(4):513-521. [VB]

125. Section VI: Chapter 2: Controlling occupational exposure to hazardous drugs. In: *OSHA Technical Manual.* 1999. Occupational Health & Safety Administration. http://www.osha.gov/dts/osta/otm/otm_vi/otm_vi_2.html. Accessed April 5, 2013.

126. Smith DR, Muto T, Sairenchi T, et al. Hospital safety climate, psychosocial risk factors and needlestick injuries in Japan. *Ind Health.* 2010;48(1):85-95. [IIIA]

127. Parker MR. The use of protective gloves, the incidence of ampoule injury and the prevalence of hand laceration amongst anaesthetic personnel. *Anaesthesia.* 1995;50(8):726-729. [IIIB]

128. Smith DR, Leggat PA. Needlestick and sharps injuries among nursing students. *J Adv Nurs.* 2005;51(5):449-455. [IIIB]

129. Pulnitiporn A, Chau-in W, Klanarong S, Thienthong S, Inphum P. The Thai Anesthesia Incidents Study (THAI Study) of anesthesia personnel hazard. *J Med Assoc Thai.* 2005;88(Suppl 7):S141-S144. [IIIB]

130. Siegel JD, Rhinehart E, Jackson M, Chiarello L; Health Care Infection Control Practices Advisory Committee. 2007 Guideline for isolation precautions: preventing transmission of infectious agents in health care settings. *Am J Infect Control.* 2007;35(10 Suppl 2):S65-S164. [IVA]

131. Guideline for prevention of transmissible infections. In: *Guidelines for Perioperative Practice.* Denver, CO: AORN, Inc; 2015:419-451. [IVA]

132. Cicconi L, Claypool M, Stevens W. Prevention of transmissible infections in the perioperative setting. *AORN J.* 2010;92(5):519-527. [VB]

133. Aarnio P, Laine T. Glove perforation rate in vascular surgery—a comparison between single and double gloving. *Vasa.* 2001;30(2):122-124. [IA]

134. Plucknett B, Kaminski PF, Podczaski ES, Sorosky JI, Pees RC. Punctured surgical gloves in major gynecologic surgery: does surgical experience of the operator make a difference? *J Gynecol Surg.* 1992;8(2):77-80. [IIIC]

135. Guideline for sterile technique. In: *Guidelines for Perioperative Practice.* Denver, CO: AORN, Inc; 2015:67-96. [IVA]

136. Tanner J, Parkinson H. Double gloving to reduce surgical cross-infection. *Cochrane Database Syst Rev.* 2009;3:CD003087. [IA]

137. Kinlin LM, Mittleman MA, Harris AD, Rubin MA, Fisman DN. Use of gloves and reduction of risk of injury caused by needles or sharp medical devices in healthcare workers: results from a case-crossover study. *Infect Control Hosp Epidemiol.* 2010;31(9):908-917. [IIIB]

138. Wittmann A, Kralj N, Kover J, Gasthaus K, Lerch H, Hofmann F. Comparison of 4 different types of surgical gloves used for preventing blood contact. *Infect Control Hosp Epidemiol.* 2010;31(5):498-502. [IIA]

139. Chan KY, Singh VA, Oun BH, To BH. The rate of glove perforations in orthopaedic procedures: single versus double gloving. A prospective study. *Med J Malaysia.* 2006;61(Suppl B):3-7. [IIIB]

140. Tanner J. Surgical gloves: perforation and protection. *J Perioper Pract.* 2006;16(3):148-152. [VB]

141. Guo YP, Wong PM, Li Y, Or PP. Is double-gloving really protective? A comparison between the glove perforation rate among perioperative nurses with single and double gloves during surgery. *Am J Surg.* 2012;204(2):210-215. [IIA]

142. Thomas S, Agarwal M, Mehta G. Intraoperative glove perforation—single versus double gloving in protection against skin contamination. *Postgrad Med J.* 2001;77(909):458-460. [IB]

143. Mansouri M, Tidley M, Sanati KA, Roberts C. Comparison of blood transmission through latex and nitrile glove materials. *Occup Med.* 2010;60(3):205-210. [IB]

144. Wittmann A, Kralj N, Kover J, Gasthaus K, Hofmann F. Study of blood contact in simulated surgical needlestick injuries with single or double latex gloving. *Infect Control Hosp Epidemiol.* 2009;30(1):53-56. [IIA]

145. Lancaster C, Duff P. Single versus double-gloving for obstetric and gynecologic procedures. *Am J Obstet Gynecol.* 2007;196(5):e36-e37. http://www.ajog.org/article/S0002-9378(06)01185-9/fulltext. Accessed April 5, 2013. [VA]

146. Lefebvre DR, Strande LF, Hewitt CW. An enzyme-mediated assay to quantify inoculation volume delivered by suture needlestick injury: two gloves are better than one. *J Am Coll Surg.* 2008;206(1):113-122. [IA]

147. Chapman S, Duff P. Frequency of glove perforations and subsequent blood contact in association with selected obstetric surgical procedures. *Am J Obstet Gynecol.* 1993;168(5):1354-1357. [IIIB]

148. Bennett NT, Howard RJ. Quantity of blood inoculated in a needlestick injury from suture needles. *J Am Coll Surg.* 1994;178(2):107-110. [IB]

149. Laine T, Aarnio P. How often does glove perforation occur in surgery? Comparison between single gloves and a double-gloving system. *Am J Surg.* 2001;181(6):564-566. [IA]

150. Ersozlu S, Sahin O, Ozgur AF, Akkaya T, Tuncay C. Glove punctures in major and minor orthopaedic surgery with double gloving. *Acta Orthop Belg.* 2007;73(6):760-764. [IIIB]

151. Caillot JL, Paparel P, Arnal E, Schreiber V, Voiglio EJ. Anticipated detection of imminent surgeon-patient barrier breaches. A prospective randomized controlled trial using an indicator underglove system. *World J Surg.* 2006;30(1):134-138. [IB]

152. Edlich RF, Long WB 3rd, Gubler K, et al. Reducing accidental injuries during surgery. *J Environ Pathol Toxicol Oncol.* 2010;29(4):317-326. [VB]

153. Edlich RF, Wind TC, Heather CL, Thacker JG. Reliability and performance of innovative surgical double-glove hole puncture indication systems. *J Long Term Eff Med Implants*. 2003;13(2):69-83. [IB]

154. Edlich RF, Wind TC, Hill LG, Thacker JG. Resistance of double-glove hole puncture indication systems to surgical needle puncture. *J Long Term Eff Med Implants*. 2003;13(2):85-90. [IB]

155. Florman S, Burgdorf M, Finigan K, Slakey D, Hewitt R, Nichols RL. Efficacy of double gloving with an intrinsic indicator system. *Surg Infect (Larchmt)*. 2005;6(4):385-395. [IIB]

156. ASTM D3577-09e1: Standard specification for rubber surgical gloves. 2009. [IVB]

157. Demircay E, Unay K, Bilgili MG, Alataca G. Glove perforation in hip and knee arthroplasty. *J Orthop Sci*. 2010;15(6):790-794. [IIIA]

158. Thomas S, Aldlyami E, Gupta S, Reed MR, Muller SD, Partington PF. Unsuitability and high perforation rate of latex-free gloves in arthroplasty: a cause for concern. *Arch Orthop Trauma Surg*. 2011;131(4):455-458. [IIIB]

159. Al-Maiyah M, Bajwa A, Mackenney P, et al. Glove perforation and contamination in primary total hip arthroplasty. *J Bone Joint Surg Br*. 2005;87(4):556-559. [IA]

160. Faisal-Cury A, Rossi Menezes P, Kahhale S, Zugaib M. A study of the incidence and recognition of surgical glove perforation during obstetric and gynecological procedures. *Arch Gynecol Obstet*. 2004;270(4):263-264. [IIIB]

161. Feng T, Yohannan J, Gupta A, Hyndman ME, Allaf M. Microperforations of surgical gloves in urology: minimally invasive versus open surgeries. *Can J Urol*. 2011;18(2):5615-5618. [IIIB]

162. Harnoss JC, Partecke LI, Heidecke CD, Hubner NO, Kramer A, Assadian O. Concentration of bacteria passing through puncture holes in surgical gloves. *Am J Infect Control*. 2010;38(2):154-158. [IIA]

163. Caillot JL, Voiglio EJ. First clinical study of a new virus-inhibiting surgical glove. *Swiss Med Wkly*. 2008;138(1-2):18-22. [IIIA]

164. Krikorian R, Lozach-Perlant A, Ferrier-Rembert A, et al. Standardization of needlestick injury and evaluation of a novel virus-inhibiting protective glove. *J Hosp Infect*. 2007;66(4):339-345. [IIB]

165. Bricout F, Moraillon A, Sonntag P, Hoerner P, Blackwelder W, Plotkin S. Virus-inhibiting surgical glove to reduce the risk of infection by enveloped viruses. *J Med Virol*. 2003;69(4):538-545. [IB]

166. Daeschlein G, Kramer A, Arnold A, Ladwig A, Seabrook GR, Edmiston CE Jr. Evaluation of an innovative antimicrobial surgical glove technology to reduce the risk of microbial passage following intraoperative perforation. *Am J Infect Control*. 2011;39(2):98-103. [IIB]

167. Grimmond T, Bylund S, Anglea C, et al. Sharps injury reduction using a sharps container with enhanced engineering: a 28 hospital nonrandomized intervention and cohort study. *Am J Infect Control*. 2010;38(10):799-805. [IIB]

168. Perry J, Jagger J, Parker G, Phillips EK, Gomaa A. Disposal of sharps medical waste in the United States: impact of recommendations and regulations, 1987-2007. *Am J Infect Control*. 2011;40(4):354-358.

169. Selecting, evaluating, and using sharps disposal containers. NIOSH publication no. 97-111. 1998. National Institute for Occupational Safety and Health. http://www.cdc.gov/niosh/pdfs/97-111.pdf. Accessed April 5, 2013. [IVB]

170. Blenkharn JI, Odd C. Sharps injuries in healthcare waste handlers. *Ann Occup Hyg*. 2008;52(4):281-286. [IIIC]

171. Standards of perioperative nursing. In: *Perioperative Standards and Recommended Practices*. Denver, CO: AORN, Inc; 2012:2-20. [IVB]

172. Cutter J, Jordan S. Uptake of guidelines to avoid and report exposure to blood and body fluids. *J Adv Nurs*. 2004;46(4):441-452. [IIIB]

173. Doebbeling BN, Vaughn TE, McCoy KD, et al. Percutaneous injury, blood exposure, and adherence to standard precautions: are hospital-based health care providers still at risk? *Clin Infect Dis*. 2003;37(8):1006-1013. [IIIB]

174. Kennedy R, Kelly S, Gonsalves S, Mc Cann PA. Barriers to the reporting and management of needlestick injuries among surgeons. *Ir J Med Sci*. 2009;178(3):297-299. [IIIB]

175. Kessler CS, McGuinn M, Spec A, Christensen J, Baragi R, Hershow RC. Underreporting of blood and body fluid exposures among health care students and trainees in the acute care setting: a 2007 survey. *Am J Infect Control*. 2011;39(2):129-134. [IIIB]

176. Kak N, Burkhalter B, Cooper M-A. *Measuring the Competence of Healthcare Providers*. Operations Research Issue Paper 2(1). Bethesda, MD: Quality Assurance Project for the US Agency for International Development; 2001. http://www.hciproject.org/sites/default/files/Measuring%20the%20Competence%20of%20HC%20Providers_QAP_2001.pdf. Accessed April 5, 2013. [VA]

177. Vaughn TE, McCoy KD, Beekmann SE, Woolson RE, Torner JC, Doebbeling BN. Factors promoting consistent adherence to safe needle precautions among hospital workers. *Infect Control Hosp Epidemiol*. 2004;25(7):548-555. [IIA]

178. Holodnick CL, Barkauskas V. Reducing percutaneous injuries in the OR by educational methods. *AORN J*. 2000;72(3):461-476. [VB]

179. Brusaferro S, Calligaris L, Farneti F, Gubian F, Londero C, Baldo V. Educational programmes and sharps injuries in health care workers. *Occup Med (Oxford)*. 2009;59(7):512-514. [IIB]

180. Bakaeen F, Awad S, Albo D, et al. Epidemiology of exposure to blood borne pathogens on a surgical service. *Am J Surg*. 2006;192(5):e18-e21. [VA]

181. HR.01.05.03: Staff participate in ongoing education and training. In: *Comprehensive Accreditation Manual for Ambulatory Care*. Oakbrook Terrace, IL: The Joint Commission; 2012.

182. HR.01.05.03: Staff participate in ongoing education and training. In: *Comprehensive Accreditation Manual: CAMH for Hospitals*. Oakbrook Terrace, IL: The Joint Commission; 2012.

183. State Operations Manual. Appendix A: Survey protocol, regulations and interpretive guidelines for hospitals. Rev 78;2011. Centers for Medicare & Medicaid Services. http://www.cms.gov/Regulations-and-Guidance/Guidance/Manuals/downloads/som107ap_a_hospitals.pdf. Accessed April 5, 2013.

184. State Operations Manual. Appendix L: Guidance for surveyors: ambulatory surgical centers. Rev 76;2011. Centers for Medicare & Medicaid Services. http://www.cms.gov/Regulations-and-Guidance/Guidance/Manuals/downloads/som107ap_l_ambulatory.pdf. Accessed April 5, 2013.

185. Sportsman S. Competency education and validation in the United States: what should nurses know? *Nurs Forum*. 2010;45(3):140-149. [VA]

186. Jordan C, Thomas MB, Evans ML, Green A. Public policy on competency: how will nursing address this complex issue? *J Contin Educ Nurs*. 2008;39(2):86-91. [VA]

187. Yang YH, Liou SH, Chen CJ, et al. The effectiveness of a training program on reducing needlestick injuries/

sharp object injuries among soon graduate vocational nursing school students in southern Taiwan. *J Occup Health.* 2007;49(5):424-429. [IIIB]

188. Ling ML, Wee M, Chan YH. Sharps and needlestick injuries: the impact of hepatitis B vaccination as an intervention measure. *Ann Acad Med Singap.* 2000;29(1):86-89. [IIB]

189. Elliott SK, Keeton A, Holt A. Medical students' knowledge of sharps injuries. *J Hosp Infect.* 2005;60(4):374-377. [IIIB]

190. Hambridge K. Needlestick and sharps injuries in the nursing student population. *Nurs Stand.* 2011;25(27):38-45. [VB]

191. Blackwell L, Bolding J, Cheely E, et al. Nursing students' experiences with needlestick injuries. *J Undergrad Nurs Scholarsh.* 2007;9(1). http://www.juns.nursing.arizona.edu/articles/Fall%202007/Nursing%20Students'%20Experiences%20with%20Needlestick%20Injuries.pdf. Accessed April 5, 2013. [IIIB]

192. Salzer HJ, Hoenigl M, Kessler HH, et al. Lack of risk-awareness and reporting behavior towards HIV infection through needlestick injury among European medical students. *Int J Hyg Environ Health.* 2011;214(5):407-410. [IIIB]

193. Brasel KJ, Mol C, Kolker A, Weigelt JA. Needlesticks and surgical residents: who is most at risk? *J Surg Educ.* 2007;64(6):395-398. [VB]

194. Protecting workers' families: a research agenda. Report of the Workers' Family Protection Task Force. DHHS (NIOSH) Publication No. 2002–113. 2002. National Institute for Occupational Safety and Health. http://www.cdc.gov/niosh/docs/2002-113/pdfs/2002-113.pdf. Accessed April 5, 2013. [VA]

195. 29 CFR 1904.8. Recording criteria for needlestick and sharps injuries. 2010. US Government Printing Office. http://www.gpo.gov/fdsys/granule/CFR-2010-title29-vol5/CFR-2010-title29-vol5-sec1904-8/content-detail.html. Accessed April 5, 2013.

196. Self-assessment questionnaire: bloodborne pathogens policies and procedures. *Operating Room Risk Management.* 2010;1-28. [VB]

197. Hubbard A. The rights of healthcare professionals with blood-borne illnesses under the Americans with Disabilities Act. *Clin Occup Environ Med.* 2002;2(3):593-608. [VA]

198. Farquhar M, Hughes R, Hughes RF. AHRQ quality indicators. In: Hughes RF, ed. *Patient Safety and Quality: An Evidence-based Handbook for Nurses.* Rockville MD: Agency for Healthcare Research and Quality; 2008:41-67. http://www.ahrq.gov/qual/nurseshdbk/. Accessed April 5, 2013. [IA]

199. Kerr HL, Stewart N, Pace A, Elsayed S. Sharps injury reporting amongst surgeons. *Ann R Coll Surg Engl.* 2009;91(5):430-432. [VB]

200. Thomas WJ, Murray JR. The incidence and reporting rates of needle-stick injury amongst UK surgeons. *Ann R Coll Surg Engl.* 2009;91(1):12-17. [VB]

201. Hooper J, Charney W. Creation of a safety culture: reducing workplace injuries in a rural hospital setting. *AAOHN J.* 2005;53(9):394-398. [IIIB]

202. McIntosh KR, Rever-Moriyama SD. Using a systems approach in developing a survey to assess the contributing factors to needlestick injuries. *Proc Hum Fact Ergon Soc Annu Meet.* 1997;41(2):782-786. [IIIB]

203. McIntosh KR. Taking the blame off of health care workers: using a systems approach to determine the contributing factors to needlestick injuries. *Proc Hum Fact Ergon Soc Annu Meet.* 1998;42(14):1033-1037. [IIIB]

204. Taylor JA, Dominici F, Agnew J, Gerwin D, Morlock L, Miller MR. Do nurse and patient injuries share common antecedents? An analysis of associations with safety climate and working conditions. *BMJ Qual Saf.* 2012;21(2):101-111. [IIIB]

205. Blouin AS, McDonagh KJ. Framework for patient safety, part 1: culture as an imperative. *J Nurs Adm.* 2011;41(10):397-400. [IVB]

206. Mark BA, Hughes LC, Belyea M, et al. Does safety climate moderate the influence of staffing adequacy and work conditions on nurse injuries? *J Saf Res.* 2007;38(4):431-446. [IIIA]

207. Gershon RR, Karkashian CD, Grosch JW, et al. Hospital safety climate and its relationship with safe work practices and workplace exposure incidents. *Am J Infect Control.* 2000;28(3):211-221. [IIIB]

208. Hunt J, Murphy C. Measurement of nursing staff occupational exposures in the operating suite following introduction of a prevention programme. *Aust Infect Control.* 2004;9(2):57. [IIB]

209. Blouin AS, McDonagh KJ. A framework for patient safety, part 2: resilience, the next frontier. *J Nurs Adm.* 2011;41(11):450-452. [VA]

Acknowledgements

Lead Author
Mary J. Ogg, MSN, RN, CNOR
Perioperative Nursing Specialist
AORN Nursing Department
Denver, Colorado

Contributing Author
Ramona Conner, MSN, RN, CNOR
Manager, Standards and Guidelines
AORN Nursing Department
Denver, Colorado

The authors and AORN thank George D. Allen, PhD, MS, RN, CNOR, CIC, Director, Infection Control, Downstate Medical Center, and Clinical Assistant Professor, SUNY College of Health Related Professions, Brooklyn, NY; Amy L. Halverson, MD, American College of Surgeons; Rodney W. Hicks, PhD, ARNP, RN, FAANP, FAAN, Professor, Western University of Health Science, Pomona, CA; Elayne Kornblatt Phillips, PhD-BSN, MPH, RN, International Healthcare Worker Safety Center, University of Virginia, Charlottesville; Rev Donna S. Nussman, PhD, RN, Surgical Health Care Consultant, and Adjunct Professor, College of Mechanical Engineering/BioEngineering Department, University of North Carolina - Charlotte; and Lisa Spruce, DNP, RN, ACNS, ACNP, ANP, CNOR, Director of Evidence-based Nursing Practice, AORN, Inc, Denver, CO, for their assistance in developing this guideline.

Publication History

Originally published June 2013 online in *Perioperative Standards and Recommended Practices.*

Evidence ratings revised 2013 to conform to the AORN Evidence Rating Model.

Minor editing revisions made in November 2014 for publication in *Guidelines for Perioperative Practice,* 2015 edition.

GUIDELINE FOR SPECIMEN MANAGEMENT

The Guideline for Specimen Management has been approved by the AORN Guidelines Advisory Board. It was presented as a proposed guideline for comments by members and others. The guideline is effective May 15, 2014. The recommendations in the guideline are intended to be achievable and represent what is believed to be an optimal level of practice. Policies and procedures will reflect variations in practice settings and/or clinical situations that determine the degree to which the guideline can be implemented. AORN recognizes the many diverse settings in which perioperative nurses practice; therefore, this guideline is adaptable to all areas where operative and other invasive procedures may be performed.

Purpose

This document provides guidance for management of surgical specimens in the perioperative practice setting, including guidance for the handling of body parts being reattached to the patient, forensic and radioactive specimens, and explanted medical devices and orthopedic hardware. Surgical techniques for resection of specimens is outside the scope of this guideline. This document does not address clinical laboratory specimens obtained for diagnostic or other screening procedures performed on blood, body fluids, or other potentially infectious materials. The reader should refer to 42 CFR 493, Laboratory Requirements, for guidance in this area.[1]

Specimen management is a multifaceted, multidisciplinary process that includes

- needs assessment,
- site identification,
- collection and handling,
- transfer from the sterile field,
- containment,
- specimen identification and labeling,
- preservation,
- transport,
- disposition of the specimen, and
- documentation.

Accurate specimen management requires effective multidisciplinary communication, minimized distractions, and awareness of the potential opportunities for error. An error is an unintended act of omission (ie, failing to perform an action) or commission (ie, performing an action that results in harm).[2] Errors in specimen management leading to inaccurate or incomplete diagnosis, the need for additional procedures, and physical and psychological injury have been reported.[3-5]

In a survey commissioned by the Association of Directors of Anatomic and Surgical Pathology to assess perceptions and definitions of errors in surgical pathology and to examine and measure the frequency of errors among its members, researchers randomly surveyed pathologists in 40 academic pathology laboratories in the United States and one in Canada (N = 41). When asked to indicate where most errors in surgical pathology occurred, 53% of respondents indicated the preanalytical phase (ie, before the specimen reaches the pathology laboratory for analysis and processing), 38% indicated the analytical phase (ie, within the pathology laboratory while the specimen is being analyzed and processed), and 6% indicated the postanalytical phase (ie, after the specimen has been analyzed and processed in the pathology laboratory).[6]

Examples of errors that may occur during the preanalytical phase include incorrect

- pathology request,
- order entry,
- patient identification,
- specimen identification,
- specimen (or no specimen) in the container,
- collection or handling methods,
- container or preservative, and
- transport methods or destination.

Examples of errors that may occur during the analytical phase include

- equipment malfunction,
- specimen mix-ups, and
- undetected failure in quality control.

Examples of errors that may occur during the postanalytical phase include

- confirmation of erroneous data,
- failure or delay in pathology reporting or addressing the pathology report,
- excessive turnaround time, and
- improper data entry and manual transcription.

Errors that may have occurred during the preanalytical phase are often detected during the analytical phase because the histology visualized under the microscope does not correspond to the biopsy site specified in the accompanying documentation or clinical history.[7] There are many points in the analytical phase during which an error can occur. Errors occurring during the analytical phase have the potential to cause great patient harm because the results of the examination by the pathologist may be critical for effective patient care.[7]

Errors in specimen management may be classified as

- near misses (ie, the error has the potential to harm the patient, but does not, either by chance or because the error was detected before harm resulted),[7,8]
- adverse events (ie, the error causes the patient either inconvenience or harm),[7] or
- sentinel events (ie, the error results in significant harm to the patient).[8]

SPECIMEN MANAGEMENT

Specimen management errors may be attributed to human factors (eg, poor communication, fatigue, inadequate education or competency verification), the environment, equipment failure, or inadequate policies and procedures.[7] The causes of specimen management errors may be determined through a process of root cause analysis in which knowledgeable individuals and other persons involved in the event make a critical analysis and a determination as to the factor(s) that contributed to the error.[7]

Most errors in specimen management are a result of human errors caused by slips, lapses, and mistakes.[7]

- Slips are unintended actions[9] (eg, placing an incorrect label on a specimen container).
- Lapses are omissions of intended actions[9] (eg, omitting the last letter of a patient's name and writing "Smith" rather than "Smithe").
- Mistakes are errors of conscious thought[9] (eg, choosing to disregard known policies and procedures).

Most errors in specimen management are classified as slips and lapses. Errors caused by slips and lapses are the result of automatic actions and are therefore difficult to prevent.[7] These type of errors are often not noticed at the time they occur.[7] The result of the error may not become apparent until hours or days after it has occurred.[7]

The true frequency of errors in specimen management is difficult to quantify. Most estimates are based on studies conducted in single institutions. Estimates based on multi-institutional studies suggest that the number of errors in specimen management varies widely among institutions and is likely associated with specimen identification practices unique to the institution.[7]

Reducing errors in specimen management requires a careful examination of the preanalytical, analytical, and postanalytical phases for system flaws that may contribute to errors and be responsive to analysis and correction. The simple application of redundancy to various portions of the specimen management cycle (ie, double-checking steps of the process that may be subject to slips and lapses) has the potential to significantly reduce errors.[7,10]

Evidence Review

A medical librarian conducted a systematic search of the databases MEDLINE, CINAHL, and the Cochrane Database of Systematic Reviews for meta-analyses, systematic reviews, randomized controlled and non-randomized trials and studies, case reports, reviews, and guidelines. Scopus was also consulted, although not searched systematically. Search terms included *specimen handling, surgical specimen, specimen type, fresh specimen, fresh tissue, anticoagulants, explant, bone screws, bone plates, bone nails, calculi, gallstones, urinary calculi, kidney stones, renal calculi, surgical pathology, clinical pathology, cell biology, cytology, stone analysis, gross examination, gross evaluation, fixatives, additives, tissue preservatives, preservative, saline solution, paraffin, formaldehyde, formalin, cryoultramicrotomy, freezing, time factors, transportation, chain of custody, container, transfer, handling, mishandling, delivery, storage, organizational policy, documentation, clinical information, name, patient information, patient identification systems, labels, labeling, mislabeling, suture tags, tissue markers, medical errors, diagnostic errors, equipment contamination, specimen contamination, safety precautions, occupational health, occupational accidents, radioactive, radioactivity, forensic, wounds, gunshot, forensic pathology, law enforcement, religion, cross-cultural comparison, cultural diversity, funeral rites, radiologic health, occupational accidents, occupational health, perioperative nursing, nurse's role, intraoperative care, intraoperative period, perioperative care, surgical procedures,* and *operating rooms.*

The search was originally limited to literature published in English between January 2007 and October 2012. The medical librarian conducted the first database search on October 11, 2012. Older articles were included when there were no articles within this time period. Additional articles not identified in the original search were obtained after a review of the reference lists of the articles obtained originally. In addition, between October 2012 and January 2014, the results of alerts established at the time of the initial searches were considered. During the development of the document, the lead author requested supplementary searches and requested additional articles that either did not fit the original search criteria or were discovered during the evidence appraisal process. Finally, the lead author and the medical librarian identified relevant guidelines from government agencies and standards-setting bodies.

More than 374 articles or documents were reviewed in preparation for writing this guideline. Approximately 120 were ultimately selected for inclusion as suitable references. Articles were rejected primarily because they addressed surgical techniques for specimen resection or procedures for processing of specimens in the pathology laboratory.

As relevant research and other evidence was located, it was independently evaluated and critically appraised according to the strength and quality of the evidence using the AORN Evidence Appraisal Tools (Research and Non-Research) by the lead author and an independent reviewer. The reviewers participated in conference calls to discuss their individual appraisal scores and to establish consensus. Each article or study was assigned an appraisal score as agreed upon by the reviewers. The appraisal scores are noted in brackets at the end of each citation in the references list at the end of the document.

After the evidence was reviewed and appraised, the collective evidence supporting each intervention within a specific recommendation was rated using the AORN Evidence Rating Model. Ratings include Strong Evidence, Regulatory Requirement, Moderate Evidence, Limited Evidence, Benefits Balanced With Harms, and No Evidence. Factors considered when applying the AORN Evidence Rating Model to the collective body of evidence included the quality of research, quantity of similar studies on a given topic, consistency of results

SPECIMEN MANAGEMENT

supporting a recommendation, and whether the potential benefits of following the recommendation outweigh the harms. The evidence rating is noted in brackets following each intervention.

Editor's note: MEDLINE is a registered trademark of the US National Library of Medicine's Medical Literature Analysis and Retrieval System, Bethesda, MD. CINAHL, Cumulative Index to Nursing and Allied Health Literature, is a registered trademark of EBSCO Industries, Birmingham, AL. Scopus is a registered trademark of Elsevier B.V., Amsterdam, Netherlands.

Recommendation I

The perioperative registered nurse (RN) should incorporate specimen management needs when developing the plan of care.

Early assessment of specimen management needs may help improve processes and decrease or prevent errors related to specimen management.

I.a. Assessment of specimen management needs should begin when the need for obtaining a specimen is identified and should include
- personnel to be notified (eg, pathologist for frozen section),
- requirements for specimen collection and handling (eg, keeping the specimen moist until transfer from the sterile field),
- method of transfer (eg, using sterile technique),
- requirements for containment (eg, size of the container),
- method of preservation, (eg, type of solution),
- transport needs (eg, availability of personnel),
- disposition of the specimen (eg, disposal, returned to the patient), and
- documentation (eg, noting the location of suture tags).

[5: No Evidence]

Conducting an assessment that begins when the need for obtaining a specimen is identified may help to improve efficiency and ensure identified needs are met.

Evidence addressing the need for assessment of specimen management needs was not identified during the evidence review for this guideline. Further research is warranted.

I.a.1. When on-site pathology, laboratory, or courier services are not available and the need for these services is identified, services may be contracted with a third party.

I.b. The cultural and personal preferences of the patient should be assessed preoperatively to determine special needs for collecting, handling, or disposing of specimens. *[2: Moderate Evidence]*

Specimen management may be influenced by a patient's beliefs about his or her body that are derived from both cultural and religious contexts.[11] For example, a Vietnamese patient may be extremely fearful of operative or other invasive procedures involving blood loss.[12] The patient may refuse to have blood drawn, believing that any body tissue or fluid removed cannot be replaced and that the body suffers the loss of the removed tissue or fluid in this life and in the afterlife.[12]

According to Jewish law, blood and limbs are considered part of the human being, and therefore, should be buried.[13] Limbs that are amputated require burial in the patient's future gravesite.[13] If the amputated limb is donated for medical research, burial is required when the limb is no longer in use.[13] Muslim patients also may request that amputated limbs be made available for burial.[14]

In a qualitative study conducted to explore the cultural attitudes of 94 Hmong Americans about placental specimen disposition, Helsel and Mochel found there was a strong persistence in the traditional belief that placentas should be buried at home. The Hmong believe that after death, the spirit returns to the place the placenta is buried. The placenta is necessary for the soul to be able to rejoin ancestors in the spirit world. Hmong patients were reluctant to ask health care providers for permission to take placentas home for burial. The researchers suggested that health care providers develop an awareness of cultural practices and the reluctance of some patients to verbalize their wishes.[15]

Incorporating an approach to specimen management that acknowledges the value of cultural beliefs and encourages increasing cultural knowledge and expertise may improve the quality of perioperative nursing care related to specimen management.[11]

I.b.1. Policies and procedures should be developed to address patient requests for nontraditional specimen management.

The patient's cultural or personal preferences may require that specimens be handled in a nontraditional manner.

Baergen et al conducted a nonexperimental study to review the practices and experiences of perinatal and placental pathologists surrounding placental release, to discuss the reasons for release, and to determine problems that have been encountered. They found that requests for release of the placenta to patients had increased; however, no statistical data were provided as to the number of increased requests. The most common reason for this request was to bury the placenta. No adverse consequences or legal ramifications related to placental release were reported by any of the survey respondents. The researchers recommended that health care organizations create a multidisciplinary team that includes personnel from obstetrics, infection control, pathology, and administration to develop a policy

SPECIMEN MANAGEMENT

to follow when requests for placental release are received.[16]

I.c. Specimen management should be assessed and planned among surgical team members during the preoperative briefing before operative or other invasive procedures. *[2: Moderate Evidence]*

Management of specimens is a multidisciplinary process. Collaborative preprocedure assessment and planning may improve efficiency and communication among team members and may help to reduce or eliminate potential errors[17] in specimen management.

Recommendation II

The perioperative RN should complete a preoperative assessment that confirms the site identification of specimens to be collected.

Site identification may be necessary to confirm the location of tissue, foreign objects, or body substances to be removed from the patient and sent for pathology examination or study. Accurate preoperative identification of the site from which specimens are to be collected may help prevent wrong site surgery.

Implementing error prevention strategies for the identification and verification of the correct site of specimens to be collected may reduce the risk for error.[18]

II.a. Photographs of dermatologic lesions that will be excised or biopsied during the surgical procedure, if available, should be labeled with the patient's identification and displayed in the procedure room. *[2: Moderate Evidence]*

Photographs help to identify and verify the location of dermatologic lesions to be removed and reduce the risk of wrong site dermatological surgery.[19-22]

In an online survey of 722 members of the American College of Mohs Surgery conducted to quantify the problem of biopsy site identification on the day of surgery, Nemeth and Lawrence found that accurate biopsy site identification is a problem encountered by Mohs surgeons. The majority (89%) responded that a high-quality photograph would provide the most useful information for accurate identification of the biopsy site.[19]

McGinness and Goldstein conducted a nonexperimental study of 271 surgical sites to determine the value of preoperative biopsy site photography. Patients with preoperative biopsy-site photography of cutaneous malignancies and their physicians were asked to identify the surgical sites on the day of the procedure. The patients were not given any help in locating the lesion. The physicians were then asked to identify the lesion using only a diagram of the location of the biopsy site. The patients incorrectly identified 45 of 271 surgical sites (16.6%). The physicians incorrectly identified 16 of 271 surgical sites (5.9%). Twelve of the 271 surgical sites were incorrectly identified by both the patient and the physician (4.4%). When the patients and physicians used the preoperative biopsy site photographs, they correctly identified all sites. The results of this study support the use of preoperative photography to help reduce the incidence of wrong site surgery for removal of cutaneous lesions.[20]

In another prospective, nonexperimental study of 329 patients representing 333 skin cancers primarily located on the head and neck, Rossy and Lawrence evaluated the difficulty associated with surgical site identification. Preoperatively, patients were asked to identify and confirm the surgical site. Thirty patients (9.1%) were unable to do so. There was a statistically significant difference in the percentage of patients able to identify lesions located in an area that was visible to them versus those patients with lesions in an area not easily seen. The results of this study demonstrate the need for accurate documentation and prebiopsy site photography of skin cancers, especially those that are not visible to the patient, as a means to reduce the possibility of wrong site surgery.[21]

In an observational study of 34 biopsy sites conducted in a university-based dermatological surgery clinic, Ke et al compared the reliability of patient and blinded dermatologist surgical site identification with identification based on biopsy site photography. On the day of the procedure, the patient was asked to identify the biopsy site. The physician was then given the general body location (eg, ear, cheek) and asked to identify the site. The photograph of the biopsy site taken during the patient's previous visit to the clinic was then reviewed to verify the surgical site. The patients and the dermatologist incorrectly identified four biopsy sites (11.8%). The patients alone incorrectly identified an additional six biopsy sites, for a total of 10 sites (29.4%) incorrectly identified by patients. The results of this study support the need for preoperative biopsy site photography to prevent wrong site surgery during removal of cutaneous skin malignancies.[22]

II.a.1. The preoperative photographs should accurately depict the biopsy site, physical features, and anatomical landmarks of the area.[19,20]

- The photograph should be in focus and taken from a distance that allows for accurate identification of the biopsy site.[20]
- Additional photographs taken from a greater distance may be helpful for identification of anatomic landmarks.[20]
- Photographs including anatomic landmarks such as the lip, ear, nose, or eyebrow, or a ruler or other measuring device showing the distance to the anatomical

landmarks may be helpful for identification of the biopsy site.[20]
- Circling the biopsy site with a surgical marker before taking the photograph may help to distinguish the biopsy site from other cutaneous lesions in the biopsy site area.[20]
- Photographs taken close up may be helpful for identification of nearby cutaneous lesions or skin surface changes in the biopsy site area.[20]

Recommendation III

Specimens should be collected and handled in a manner that protects and preserves the integrity of the specimen.

Specimen collection refers to the act or process of obtaining a biopsy or resecting a specimen. Specimen handling involves holding, securing, moving, or manipulating a specimen.

Incorrect collection and handling may compromise specimens and lead to inaccurate or incomplete diagnosis or the need for additional procedures or unnecessary surgeries.

III.a. Specimens of breast tissue to be examined for cancer should be collected and handled in a manner that preserves the molecular and genetic signatures of the specimen. *[2: Moderate Evidence]*

Mishandling of specimens may compromise the accuracy of the pathology data and result in the loss of valuable histological information.

Tissue sent for pathology examination for cancer also may be used for molecular assays of nucleic acids or proteins.[23] Cancer therapy may involve limited and individualized selection and use of a drug or biologic when the targeted tumor is expressing a biological marker.[24] Current methods of tissue handling and specimen preparation are not standardized, and this lack of standardization may result in variability of the quality of the samples and the biomarkers that can be recovered from the tissue.[23,25,26]

The time required for arterial ligation and specimen removal (ie, warm ischemic time) can vary depending on the complexity of the surgical procedure. As the sample is excised, the reduction or elimination of blood flow causes progressive tissue ischemia, hypoxia, and tissue degradation.[23,25,26] Likewise, the period of time between the removal of the specimen and its placement into fixative (ie, cold ischemic time) can vary.[25,26]

During these ischemic periods, nucleic acid and protein changes occur that can negatively affect accurate histological and biomolecular evaluation of the sample;[23-26] however, these changes cease when the fixation process begins.[25,26] Keeping both the warm and cold ischemic times as short as possible and verifying that the biomarker levels are attributable to the underlying tumor and not to artifacts related to delays in fixation may help to prevent false results (positive or negative). Individualized therapy may eliminate the use of an agent that may be costly and provide little benefit to the patient.[24] False results may lead to therapeutic consequences with the potential to harm the patient and affect outcomes, as well as the inability to elicit accurate molecular and genetic signatures that are valuable for targeted treatment.[23-26]

Levels of human epidermal growth factor receptor 2 (HER2) are increased in a percentage of breast cancers.[27] In 2007, an expert panel commissioned by the American Society of Clinical Oncology (ASCO) and the College of American Pathologists (CAP) performed a systematic review of the literature to develop recommendations for improving the accuracy of HER2 testing and its usefulness as a predictive marker for therapeutic decision making for patients with breast cancer.[27,28] In 2012, an Update Committee was convened to review literature published since 2006 and to revise and update the guidelines as necessary.[29] Current recommendations of the ASCO/CAP panel include

- establishing HER2 status for all primary, recurrent, and metastatic breast cancers;
- keeping the time to specimen fixation as short as possible (ie, less than one hour); and
- recording the time to fixation for each sample.[27-29]

Estrogen receptor status in breast cancer is an important predictive biomarker for determining breast cancer prognosis after treatment with endocrine therapy.[30] In 2008, an ad hoc committee of expert pathologists, laboratory scientists, and technical experts developed consensus recommendations for standardized procedures for estrogen receptor testing in breast cancer by immunohistochemistry for the purpose of reducing what was believed to be an unacceptably high rate of false positives.[30] The committee recommended

- sectioning and placing breast resection specimens in an adequate volume of fixative (ie, one part tissue to 20 parts fixative) within a maximum time of one hour;
- processing and fixing breast core biopsies in the same manner as resected specimens;
- placing needle core biopsies immediately into fixative and recording the time of fixative placement;
- recording both the time of specimen removal and the time of placement into fixative when specimen x-rays are required;
- keeping specimens being examined for calcifications moist on saline-soaked gauze to prevent drying of the specimen before placement in fixative;
- using only 10% phosphate-buffered formalin as the fixative for breast tissue specimens to

allow for more accurate correlation of data on estrogen receptor status; and
- recording the time between removal of the specimen and placement into fixative, as well as the length of fixation time.[30]

In 2010, the ASCO/CAP panel supported the 2008 consensus recommendations of the ad hoc committee and also recommended that estrogen and progesterone receptor status be determined on all invasive breast cancers and breast cancer reoccurrences.[28] Additional studies with larger numbers of patients are needed to fully determine the effects of extended cold ischemia time on breast samples.

Nkoy et al conducted a retrospective study to test the variability in estrogen and progesterone negativity among hospitals using a single laboratory and to examine the association between prolonged specimen conditions and estrogen and progesterone receptor negativity. They studied the records of 5,077 women with breast cancers who had undergone breast surgery and estrogen- and progesterone-receptor testing between 1997 and 2003 at seven different hospitals within a single health care system. The results showed that estrogen- and progesterone-receptor negativity varied greatly among the different hospitals even when a single laboratory was used, and the negativity levels were significantly associated with prolonged specimen handling. The researchers concluded that estrogen- and progesterone-receptor expressions can be altered by prolonged exposure to room temperature before fixation, the length of the fixation, and the type of fixation.[31]

In a study conducted by Khoury et al to determine the effects of progressive delay to formalin fixation on breast cancer biomarkers, 10 palpable breast cancers were resected. Each specimen was divided into eight portions and fixed in formalin at consecutive intervals of zero, 10, and 30 minutes, and one, two, four, and eight hours. One section was placed in saline and stored at 39.2° F (4° C) as a control. The results showed that estrogen receptors began to decline at two hours and progesterone receptors at one hour. Compromise to interpretation of HER2 began at one hour and became statistically significant at two hours. The researchers recommended that specimens be placed in fixative within one hour of resection.[32]

Some researchers have argued that cold ischemia time longer than one hour may not detrimentally effect HER2 levels. In a study conducted to assess the effect of prolonged ischemic time, a modified radical mastectomy specimen with a 10-cm grade 3 invasive ductal carcinoma was processed immediately after resection. More than 80% of the specimen was removed and stored at 39.2° F (4° C) without any fixative. The unfixed specimen was cut into 97 equal samples and placed into 20 mL of one of six different preservative solutions (ie, 10% formalin, 15% formalin, Pen-Fix®, Bouin solution, Sakura® molecular fixative, zinc formalin) for zero, one, two, three, four, five, six, seven, eight, nine, 10, 11, 12, 24, 48, 72, or 168 hours. Immunohistochemical studies and fluorescence in situ hybridization were performed. The researchers found that HER2 results remained accurate beyond the ASCO/CAP recommended one hour to fixation time.[33]

In a study conducted between August 2008 and August 2009 to address the effect of cold ischemia time on HER2 levels, Portier et al identified and collected breast resection specimens from 92 patients for which the time the specimen was handed off the sterile field and the time the sample was placed in fixative had been recorded. The samples were divided into four groups representing cold ischemic times:
- < 1 hour (n = 45),
- 1 to 2 hours (n = 27),
- > 2 to 3 hours (n = 6), and
- > 3 hours (n = 6).

Each group of samples was then evaluated using two different US Food and Drug Administration (FDA)-approved methods and an immunohistochemistry assay. The researchers found that cold ischemia time up to three hours had no detrimental effect on the HER2 levels.[34]

III.a.1. The time from excision to fixation of breast cancer specimens should be less than one hour.[27-29]

Long delays between excision and fixation of the specimen may result in a decreased ability to detect breast biomarkers in samples.[30] The current ASCO/CAP recommendations include keeping the time to fixation less than one hour.[27-29]

In a study to determine the difficulty of achieving the recommended one-hour time for breast biopsies and excised breast samples to be placed in fixative, researchers implemented a rapid tissue acquisition program in which the collection time, laboratory receipt time, and fixation start time were recorded for each sample. Results showed that meeting the one-hour time was achievable but required a commitment of personnel and resources to meet this goal.[25,26]

III.a.2. Excised breast specimens should be kept moist until transfer from the sterile field and should not be placed on dry, absorbent surfaces or materials.

Air exposure can lead to desiccation of tissue.[35] Keeping specimens moist helps to prevent drying of the specimen before placement in fixative.[30] Dry, absorbent surfaces or materials may adhere to the tissue, which may result in the loss of portions of the resection margins.[35]

III.a.3. The time of excision of breast cancer specimens and the time of fixation should be recorded.

The ASCO/CAP recommendations include recording the time of removal of tissue from the patient and the time of fixation for each sample.[28] Accurate recording of times can be helpful for verification that the testing was performed during a period of time when the biomarkers were stable.[23,26]

III.b. Amputated digits to be reimplanted should be collected and handled in a manner to protect and preserve the integrity of the specimen and the potential for replantation survival. *[2: Moderate Evidence]*

Cooling of recently amputated digits may help to preserve tissue and increase the chance of replantation survival.[36-38]

In a retrospective study of 211 patients who underwent replantation surgery following complete fingertip amputation between August 1990 and March 2006, Li et al evaluated 17 independent variables to determine primary causes of unsuccessful replantation. A total of 172 patients (81.5%) had a successful replantation. The researchers found the primary factors associated with failed replantation were mechanism of injury, high platelet count, postoperative smoking, incorrect preservation of the amputated part, and the use of vein grafting. The amputated fingertips were preserved either dry at room temperature, dry at cool temperature (35.6° F to 42.8° F [2° C to 6° C]), or immersed in a preservative fluid (ie, saline or ethanol). Immersion of the digit in fluid had a higher rate of failure (43%) compared with dry storage at room temperature (20%) or dry storage at a cooler temperature (12%). The difference in survival rates of digits stored in saline versus ethanol was not calculated; however, this study demonstrated that cooling the amputated digit improved survival by 88%.[36]

Partlin et al conducted a prospective study during May and June of 2006 to compare the efficacy of six different cooling methods for preserving amputated digits for replantation, using chicken feet as surrogate tissue because of the similarity in tissue structure to a human digit. The chicken feet were trimmed to approximate a human finger and wrapped in two layers of room-temperature, sterile, saline-soaked gauze. A digital thermometer probe was inserted into each of the six surrogate tissue samples. Three samples were placed into lidded plastic specimen containers and three samples were placed into sealable plastic specimen bags. The samples were contained in a manner that allowed viewing of the temperature probe display. The temperature of each sample was measured and the contained, and bagged samples were then placed into

- a second plastic specimen bag containing 300 mg of ice cubes and 200 mL of tap water,
- a plastic kidney bowl containing 300 mg of ice cubes and 200 mL of tap water, or
- a lidded plastic denture cup containing 80 mg of ice cubes and 60 mL of tap water.

The tissue temperature was measured at the time of placement of the specimen and then measured again when the ice was completely melted. Each of the six methods was tested 12 times, resulting in 72 sets of measurements. The results showed that all methods tested achieved the target temperature of 39.2° F ± 3.6° F (4° C ± 2° C); however, the most effective method for maintaining the surrogate tissue at the target temperature for the longest duration of time was wrapping the tissue in saline-soaked gauze, placing it in a lidded specimen container, and placing the container into a sealed specimen bag of ice and water.[37]

III.b.1. Care of the amputated digit specimen should include the following:
- Preoperatively,
  - dressing the wound with sterile saline-moistened gauze[38];
  - gently wrapping the amputated digit in saline-moistened gauze and placing it into an impervious lidded or sealable container[38] (eg, specimen container, sealable plastic bag)[37];
  - placing the sealed container in a bag of ice water, keeping warm ischemic time to a minimum[37,38]; and
  - replacing the ice and water mixture approximately every four hours or sooner as needed to maintain a target temperature of 39.2° F ± 3.6° F (4° C ± 2° C).[37]
- Intraoperatively,
  - filling a sterile irrigation basin with ice[38];
  - covering the basin with a sterile plastic adhesive drape to provide a barrier[38];
  - placing a moist, sterile towel on top of the plastic barrier to the unsterile ice[38]; and
  - prepping the amputated digit and placing it on the moist towel for preliminary debridement and dissection.[38]
- Postoperatively,
  - checking the temperature of the replanted digit every hour by taping a temperature probe to the pulp of the replanted digit,
  - notifying the surgeon if the temperature drops more than 3.6° F (2° C) from the previous reading,[38] and
  - monitoring the replanted digit for engorgement.[38]

SPECIMEN MANAGEMENT

III.b.2. Education and competency verification activities related to best practices for management of amputated digits for replantation should be provided for perioperative or other health care personnel who may be involved in collecting or handling amputated digit specimens or caring for patients undergoing replantation procedures.

In a descriptive telephone survey of 50 respondents in 18 emergency departments in Wales conducted in September 2007 to ascertain perceptions of how amputated digits should be packaged and transported for reimplantation, only nine (18%) of the respondents described the recommended process correctly and sequentially. The results of this study are limited by the small sample size; however, the results indicated the need for education on best practices for correctly managing amputated digits for reimplantation.[39]

III.c. Amputated limbs to be reimplanted should be collected and handled in a manner to protect and preserve the integrity of the specimen and increase the potential for replantation survival. *[2: Moderate Evidence]*

Functional recovery of the replanted limb is dependent on reduced ischemia time and rapid revascularization.[40] Cooling of the amputated limb is beneficial for maintaining optimal muscle viability.[40]

III.c.1. Preoperative management of the amputated limb specimen should include
- handling the limb as gently as possible to avoid crushing or contaminating tissue[40];
- retaining any fragments of tissue to provide tissue for skin, nerve, or bone grafting[40];
- wrapping the limb in sterile gauze moistened with saline, then wrapping the limb again in plastic and placing it in an insulating chest containing crushed ice and water;
- preventing direct contact of the limb with ice to minimize cell damage that may hinder replantation; and
- cannulating the most proximal artery of the cooled limb with an 18-gauge cannula, infusing 1 L of tissue perfusion fluid (eg, ViaSpan) at a temperature of 50° F (10° C) and 120 cm hydrostatic pressure,[40] and leaving the infusion running continuously to help ensure a complete washout of stagnant blood from the amputated limb.[40]

III.d. Forensic specimens should be collected and handled in a manner that preserves and protects the condition of the evidence and verifies that the evidence has been in secure possession at all times. *[2: Moderate Evidence]*

Items such as bullets and bloodstained clothing may be potential evidence in a criminal investigation.[41-43] Evidence that is not correctly collected and handled may be inadmissible as evidence during a criminal investigation.[41-43] As patient advocates, perioperative nurses are responsible for identifying, collecting, preserving, and securing evidence and verifying that potential evidence of a crime is not compromised[41,42] while also protecting the patient's right to privacy and confidentiality of health care information.[43,44]

Guidelines for forensic specimen management from other professional organizations were not identified in the evidence review for this guideline.

III.d.1. When collecting, preserving, and securing potential evidence, perioperative personnel should
- don personal protective equipment (eg, gloves, eye protection)[42];
- handle all potential evidence with gloved hands[41,43];
- place each item in a separate paper bag or envelope to avoid cross contamination[41-43];
- avoid the use of plastic bags because they may trap moisture and facilitate the growth of mold, which could destroy evidence[41,43];
- keep evidence from each wound separate if there are two or more wounds[42];
- secure all of the patient's clothes and belongings, including footwear, as evidence, regardless of the condition[43];
- cut along the seams or around bullet or stab wound holes when removing clothing from the patient[41-43];
- contain and document physical evidence, such as pills or other items found in clothing[43];
- exercise caution because needles or other sharp objects may be present in pockets[43];
- handle clothing as little as possible and avoid shaking clothing to prevent important forensic evidence such as hair, fibers, blood, or DNA from being lost[41,43];
- collect and secure the transfer sheet from the preoperative stretcher to capture evidence that may have fallen from the patient's clothing onto the sheet[43];
- collect, preserve, and secure fabric or other debris removed from the wound or around the wound edges[43];
- not handle bullets with metal instruments that may scratch the bullet surface[41,43] and use instruments with rubber shods if possible[41,43];
- be aware that bullets may have sharp edges that may tear surgical gloves[43];
- handle bullets, bullet fragments, knives, or other projectiles or penetrating devices as little as possible and not wipe them[41-43];

SPECIMEN MANAGEMENT

- not handle knives or penetrating devices in the same manner as the perpetrator would have handled them, if possible[43];
- rinse bullets, bullet fragments, knives, or other projectiles or penetrating devices that have been removed surgically in water to prevent destruction of microscopic markings[41,43];
- place rinsed bullets, bullet fragments, knives, or other projectiles or penetrating devices in a nonmetal container and sealed evidence envelope and submit bullets according to local and state law enforcement regulations[41];
- for patient care, remove plastic bags that have been placed over the hands of the patient to prevent removal of gunshot residue and use cotton swabs to recover gunpowder residue[42];
- place collected body fluids (eg urine, gastric contents) into dry containers[42];
- place collected tissue (eg, bone) into a dry container and preserve it according to the facility or health care organization's policy and procedure[42];
- place the evidence directly into a designated and sealed envelope or paper bag labeled with the patient's identification, collection date and time, and name of the collector[41]; and
- submit all evidence collected according to local and state law enforcement regulations. The sealed evidence should be given directly to the responsible law enforcement officer.[41,43] If the law enforcement officer is not immediately available, personnel should follow the facility's or health care organization's policies and procedure for securing sealed evidence.

III.d.2. Documentation to establish the chain of custody and identification of persons in possession of the evidence (ie, tissue specimens, personal clothing, other personal items) should be completed from the point of evidence removal to the point of evidence examination according to facility or health care organization policies and procedures and local, state, and federal regulations.[41] Perioperative RNs should
- document informational evidence (eg, patient statements, appearance, behavior, bodily marks, blood stains, unusual odors) in detail[42,43];
- if possible, use photographs to document wounds (eg, bruises, abrasions, lacerations) and other potential evidence[41];
- if possible and applicable, take photographs before the skin prep because the prep solution may remove evidence such as bloodstains or bloody fingerprints[43];
- if possible, include a ruler or other item (eg, coin) in the photograph to indicate scale[41];
- label each photograph with patient information and place it in a sealed evidence envelope.[41]

III.d.3. Perioperative personnel should receive initial and ongoing education and complete competency verification activities on identifying, collecting, and securing evidence, and maintaining the chain of custody.[41]

Initial and ongoing education of perioperative personnel will help to develop the necessary knowledge and skills for correctly identifying, collecting, and securing evidence and maintaining the chain of custody.

Competency verification activities measure individual performance, provide a mechanism for documentation, and may verify that perioperative personnel have an understanding of the processes for correctly identifying, collecting, and securing evidence and maintaining the chain of custody.

III.d.4. Policies and procedures for identifying, collecting, and securing evidence and maintaining the chain of custody should be developed, reviewed periodically, revised as necessary, and readily available in the practice setting.[42]

Policies and procedures establish authority, responsibility, and accountability within the organization. Policies and procedures also serve as operational guidelines that are used to standardize practice, direct perioperative personnel, and establish continuous performance improvement programs. Policies and procedures should address
- criminal cases requiring investigation;
- personnel responsibilities;
- evidence collection protocols;
- documentation requirements;
- chain of custody protocols; and
- care of victims, suspected perpetrators, and family members or designated support persons.[42]

III.e. Radioactive specimens must be collected and handled according to facility or health care organization policies and procedures and local, state, and federal regulations.[45,46] *[1: Regulatory Requirement]*

Occupational doses of radiation must be maintained as low as is reasonably achievable (ALARA).[45,46] Developing policies and procedures for maintaining occupational doses of radiation ALARA is a regulatory requirement.[45]

The maximum occupational radiation exposure limit for radiation workers is 5,000 millirem (mrem) per year or 50,000 mrem per year for skin or extremities.[45] The exposure limit for women who are pregnant or for nonradiation personnel (eg, pathology personnel) is 500 mrem per year, provided that the facility or health care organization has policies and procedures in place to maintain the dose ALARA.[45]

Although radiation exposure from procedures such as radioactive seed localization and sentinel node biopsy is low, policies and procedures for specimen and seed handling are required to prevent unnecessary exposure of personnel.[47,48] The seed(s) may be removed from the tissue specimen in surgery, or the tissue specimen containing the seed may be sent to the pathology laboratory for removal of the seed and analysis of the tissue.[49] The CAP recommends having separate policies for tissues obtained during sentinel lymph node biopsy and procedures involving radiation implant devices that may have higher radiation levels.[50]

In a study by Miner et al conducted at a military medical center, researchers obtained 318 lymph nodes during 57 sentinel lymph node procedures (37 breast cancer, 20 melanoma) and determined the amount of radiation in each node at 24 and 72 hours. Specimens with readings consistent with background radiation were considered nonradioactive. The radiation dose to the hands of the surgical team members was evaluated by placing sterilized thermoluminescent dosimeter chips in the glove of the left ring finger of both the primary surgeon and first assistant.[51]

All specimens were found to be radioactive at the first reading. The radioactivity of the breast specimens was higher than the radioactivity of the melanoma specimens. All specimens were nonradioactive at the second reading. There was no radioactivity in any of the waste materials produced by the procedures. There was no significant difference noted in the radiation levels obtained from the surgeon or the first assistant or between the levels obtained during breast or melanoma procedures. The mean radiation dose to the surgeon's hand was found to be 9.6 ± 3.6 mrem of radiation per surgery. The researchers theorized that exposure to the rest of the surgeon's body would be considerably less because the surgeon's body is farther away from the surgical site than the surgeon's hands. They concluded that a surgeon could perform more than 5,000 procedures each year without approaching the regulatory exposure limits.[51]

To quantify the occupational radiation exposure of personnel performing or assisting with sentinel lymph node biopsy procedures at a university medical center, Law et al measured whole-body and finger radiation doses of surgical and pathology personnel using high-sensitivity thermoluminescent dosimeters and then compared the results with the annual dose limits recommended by the International Commission of Radiological Protection. Results showed the surgeons' left index fingers received the highest doses. The researchers suggested that this was because the surgeons' left hands were in close contact with the injection site during the radio-guided search for the lymph node basins. All other doses were measured to be less than the daily background radiation level in the institution.[52]

In a study to explore the perception of personnel that the level of radiation in sentinel node procedures was higher than in the past, Renshaw et al reviewed records of radiation levels of 2,902 specimens from sentinel node procedures performed between 2003 and 2009. Results showed that the percentage of specimens with greater than background radiation (ie, ≥ 0.2 mrem/hour) rose from 6.3% in 2003 to 34.8% in 2009. Specimens with more than 10 mrem/hour rose from 0.0% to 9.3%. The researchers theorized that the higher levels were likely a result of higher doses of radiopharmaceuticals being administered to patients, but they also considered that the higher levels could be a result of specimens being transported more rapidly to the pathology laboratory. The researchers recommended measuring radiation levels of sentinel node and primary resection specimens upon receipt in the pathology laboratory.[53]

To evaluate radiation exposure levels of the hands and whole body and establish safe work practices for personnel involved in melanoma and breast sentinel lymph node biopsy procedures, Coventry et al measured cumulative data collected from personnel dosimeters worn during melanoma and breast sentinel lymph node biopsy procedures. Results showed the extremity dose to the surgeon was measurably higher for breast cancer procedures than for melanoma procedures, despite a longer average exposure time for melanoma procedures. The researchers theorized that this was likely caused by the shorter distance of the sentinel nodes from the primary tumor in breast cancer procedures, which increased the surgeon's working time close to the injection site. However, the data showed the whole-body dose to the surgeon was negligible for either procedure.[54]

Likewise, the whole-body doses to the radiologist, pathologist, and transport personnel were negligible. The radiation dose to the perioperative RN was not measured. The researchers theorized that the dose would also be negligible for the perioperative RN because a distance of 3.3 ft to 6.6 ft (1 m to 2 m) from the surgical site is generally maintained. In addition, exposure is reduced by using forceps or other instruments to transfer radioactive specimens into specimen containers.[54]

SPECIMEN MANAGEMENT

The researchers concluded that radiation doses for all personnel were low, but good radiation handling practices should be implemented and followed to ensure that exposure is ALARA. Results of this study also confirmed the finding of Miner et al[51] that a surgeon would have to perform thousands of sentinel node biopsy procedures each year to exceed the regulatory exposure limit.[54]

III.e.1. Policies and procedures for radioactive seed localization procedures where the seed is resected with the specimen must align with 10 CFR 35.1000, Medical Use of Byproduct Material[46]; guidance documents provided by the US Nuclear Regulatory Commission (NRC)[49]; and local and state regulations.

The use of radioactive seed localization is considered an "other medical use of byproduct material" by the NRC.[46] The NRC oversees the use of radioactive materials in clinical practice and has provided guidance documents for the performance of radioactive seed localization procedures, including the safe handling of radioactive seeds.[49]

III.e.2. Policies and procedures for managing radioactive specimens should be developed by a multidisciplinary team including representatives from the pathology laboratory; a radiation safety officer; personnel from radiology, perioperative services, and risk management; and other involved perioperative team members (eg, a scrub person).

Specimen management is a multidisciplinary process. Including the radiation safety officer and representative personnel from all involved areas will help to facilitate the development of safe and effective policies and procedures.

III.e.3. Facility or health care organization policies and procedures should define when personal shielding and exposure monitoring is required.

Personnel radiation exposure monitoring devices and shielding may not be needed for the surgical team if low levels of radioactivity have been found and exposure time is limited.[45,51]

III.e.4. Personnel performing or participating in radioactive seed localization or sentinel lymph node biopsy procedures should use standard precautions.[47,48,50]

The radiopharmaceuticals used for sentinel lymph node procedures become bound to the tissue and therefore do not produce high levels of radiation.[48] For this reason, only standard precautions are required, and these precautions will also prevent any uptake of radiation by those handling the specimens.[48]

III.e.5. Forceps or other instruments should be used to place radioactive specimens that have been removed from the patient into sealed containers.[48]

III.e.6. When a radioactive seed is retrieved, the seed should be immediately placed in a sealed specimen container and labeled with patient and specimen identifiers,[47,55] the date and time the specimen was collected, and the name of the isotope (eg, ^{99m}technetium-sulfur colloid [^{99m}Tc]).[48] The container of radioactive material must be labeled, "Caution— Radioactive Material" if the container holds more than 1.0 millicuries (mCi) of ^{99m}Tc.[45] The container need not be labeled if it holds less than 1.0 mCi of ^{99m}Tc[56] or specimens are attended by individuals taking the necessary precautions (ie, standard precautions) to prevent exposure, only authorized personnel have access to the specimen containers, and the containers are accompanied with written documentation that identifies the contents.[56]

Labeling requirements are dependent on the amount of radioactive material in the specimen.[56] Doses of 0.4 mCi to 1.0 mCi of ^{99m}Tc are typically used in sentinel lymphadenectomy for melanoma or breast cancer.[50] If the facility or health care organization policies and procedures specify that only authorized personnel are permitted to handle specimens, warning labels that identify radioactive material are not required.[56]

III.e.7. The presence of a radioactive seed should be documented on the pathology requisition slip and also communicated verbally to pathology personnel at the time of specimen delivery.[47,55]

III.e.8. Specimens containing radioactive material should be promptly transported to the pathology laboratory in sealed, labeled containers.[50] Specimens should not be left unattended or in unsecured areas.[50]

III.e.9. Radioactive specimens containing more than 1 mCi of iodine-125 or 100 mCi of palladium-103 that are transferred to an outside pathology laboratory must be transferred to an NRC or Agreement State-licensed laboratory authorized to receive radioactive contaminated tissue or seed.[57]
- Specimens must be packaged and prepared in accordance with 10 CFR 71.5, Transportation of Licensed Material, or an equivalent Agreement State regulation for shipping.[58]
- Specimens may also require "Caution— Radioactive Material" labeling when
  - specimens are not attended by individuals taking the necessary precautions (ie, standard precautions) to prevent exposure[56] and

- unauthorized personnel may have access to the specimen containers.[56]

III.e.10. When the operative or other invasive procedure is completed, all instruments (eg, forceps, scissors) that had contact with the radioactive specimen should be processed using standard precautions.[48]

III.e.11. The seed should be transported to facility or health care organization nuclear medicine or radiation safety personnel for disposal.[47,55]

Nuclear medicine or radiation safety personnel should
- examine the seed before disposal to verify that radiation is at background radiation levels[48] and
- remove any "Caution—Radioactive Materials" labels that have been attached to the container before disposal.[45]

III.e.12. Radiation safety education addressing routine radiation monitoring and emergency procedures (eg, broken or leaking seed) must be provided at least annually to personnel involved in radiation seed localization procedures.[46,49]

Annual safety instruction on routine monitoring and emergency procedures for personnel involved in radiation seed localization procedures is a regulatory requirement.[46,49]

III.f. Explanted medical devices should be collected and handled according to the facility's or health care organization's policies and procedures; manufacturers' instructions; and local, state, and federal regulations. *[1: Regulatory Requirement]*

Hospitals and other health care facilities that implant medical devices are considered final distributors (ie, any person or entity that distributes a tracked device to the patient, including licensed practitioners, retail pharmacies, hospitals, and other facilities).[59] Final distributors are subject to medical device tracking requirements and are responsible for providing information to the manufacturer about explanted devices.[60]

Medical device tracking is required if the FDA issues an order to the manufacturer and the device meets one of the following criteria:
- the failure of the device (ie, failure to perform or function as intended) would likely have serious adverse health consequences (ie, significant events that are life-threatening or involve permanent or long-term injury or illness);
- the device is intended to be implanted in the human body (ie, placed into a surgically or naturally formed human body cavity to continuously assist, restore, or replace the function of an organ system or structure) for more than one year; or
- the device is a life-sustaining or life-supporting device (ie, essential to the restoration or continuation of a bodily function) used outside of the device user facility (ie, intended for use outside a hospital, nursing home, ambulatory surgery facility, or diagnostic or outpatient treatment facility).[59]

III.f.1. Explanted medical devices that are subject to medical device tracking regulation must be reported to the manufacturer.[61] Information that must be provided to the manufacturer includes the
- date the device was explanted;
- name, mailing address, and telephone number of the explanting physician; and
- date of the patient's death or the date the device was returned to the manufacturer, permanently retired from use, or otherwise disposed of permanently.[61]

The FDA has issued orders to manufacturers that require tracking of the following of implantable devices:
- temporomandibular joint prosthesis
- glenoid fossa prosthesis
- mandibular condyle prosthesis
- implantable pacemaker pulse generator
- cardiovascular permanent implantable pacemaker electrode
- replacement heart valve (mechanical only)
- automatic implantable cardioverter/defibrillator
- implanted cerebellar stimulator
- implanted diaphragmatic/phrenic nerve stimulator
- implantable infusion pumps
- abdominal aortic aneurysm stent grafts
- silicone gel-filled breast implants
- cultured epidermal autografts
- thoracic aortic aneurysm stent grafts
- transcatheter pulmonary valve prosthesis[60]

III.f.2. Manufacturers' instructions for packaging and shipping should be followed when the explanted device is returned to the manufacturer. If the manufacturer of the explanted device cannot be determined, facility personnel must attempt to locate the manufacturer and report the explant.[60] If facility personnel are unable to locate the manufacturer, a record of the explantation and an attempt to locate the manufacturer must be maintained in the facility's implant tracking records.[60]

III.f.3. Deaths related to an implanted medical device must be reported to both the FDA and the manufacturer.[61,62] Serious injury related to an implanted medical device must be reported to the device manufacturer.[61,62] If the medical device manufacturer cannot be identified, the injury should be reported to the FDA.[61,62]

Implanted medical device malfunctions are not required to be reported; however,

SPECIMEN MANAGEMENT

III.f.4. the facility or health care organization may use the voluntary MedWatch program[63] to advise the FDA of potential problems with an implanted medical device.[61,62]

III.f.4. Explanted orthopedic hardware (eg, plates, screws) to be returned to the manufacturer should be collected, handled, packaged, and shipped according to the manufacturers' instructions.

III.f.5. Explanted orthopedic hardware to be returned to the patient should be collected, handled, decontaminated, labeled, packaged, and documented according to the facility or health care organization policies and procedures.[64]
- Before returning the explanted hardware to the patient, facility or health care organization personnel should verify that the explanted hardware has not been recalled and does not need to be returned to the manufacturer.[64]
- Return of the explanted hardware should be documented in the patient's health record, including the
  ○ patient's request for return of the explanted hardware and
  ○ personnel returning the explanted hardware to the patient.[64]

III.f.6. Explanted orthopedic hardware may be excluded from submission to the pathologist for examination, provided there is an alternative policy in place for documentation of surgical removal.[65]

In a study conducted between September 2, 2004, and December 16, 2005, to evaluate the cost and effectiveness of sending explanted internal fixation hardware to the pathologist for examination, Davidovitch et al prospectively followed and analyzed 46 consecutive patients who underwent elective hardware removal after internal fixation. In all cases, it was determined that the residual pain at the fracture site was completely hardware-related and not a result of fracture disunion or infection. The researchers reviewed pathology reports for all patients. All reports had the same basic structure and content. The only information that could be discerned from the report was that the hardware had been removed from a specific location.[66]

Pathology examination of explanted hardware is costly and provides no benefit to the patient or physician. In lieu of pathologic examination, the researchers recommended a single radiographic view of the explanted hardware and documentation in the postoperative report to verify removal of the hardware.[66]

III.f.7. Explanted orthopedic hardware that is not submitted to the pathologist, returned to the manufacturer, or returned to the patient should be disposed of according to the facility or health care organization policies and procedures.

III.f.8. Policies and procedures related to collecting and handling of explanted medical devices should be developed by a multidisciplinary team including personnel from administration, risk management, pathology, infection prevention, materials management, sterile processing, and perioperative services. Policies and procedures should be in compliance with local, state, and federal regulations and should address collection and handling of explanted
- medical devices subject to medical device tracking;
- medical devices related deaths or serious injuries;[62] and
- devices to be returned to the patient.

Recommendation IV

Specimens should be transferred from the sterile field in a manner that maintains the integrity of the specimen.

Specimen transfer refers to the process of moving a specimen from the sterile field to a containment device.

Specimens that are incorrectly transferred from the sterile field may be compromised, which may lead to inaccurate or incomplete diagnostic information resulting in the need for additional procedures.

IV.a. Specimens should be passed off the sterile field as soon as possible. *[5: No Evidence]*

Passing the specimen off the sterile field as soon as possible reduces the potential for the integrity of the specimen to be compromised or for the specimen to be misplaced or lost.

Evidence addressing the need for passing the specimen off the sterile field as soon as possible was not identified during the evidence review for this guideline.

IV.b. Specimens kept on the sterile field before transfer should be sequestered, identified, and monitored. *[5: No Evidence]*

Sequestering, identifying, and monitoring specimens kept on the sterile field reduces the possibility for the specimen to be compromised or lost.

Evidence addressing the need for sequestering, identifying, and monitoring specimens kept on the sterile field was not identified during the evidence review for this guideline.

IV.c. Specimens should be kept moist until transfer from the sterile field and should not be placed on dry, absorbent surfaces or materials. *[2: Moderate Evidence]*

SPECIMEN MANAGEMENT

Air exposure can lead to desiccation of tissue.[35] Keeping specimens moist helps to prevent drying of the specimen before placement in fixative.[29] Dry, absorbent surfaces or materials may adhere to the tissue, which may result in the loss of portions of the resection margins.[35]

IV.d. Patient and specimen identification should be verified before transfer from the sterile field. Specimens transferred from the sterile field should be verbally identified by the surgeon and verified by the perioperative RN using a "write down, read back" technique.[67] *[2: Moderate Evidence]*

Verifying identification of the specimen during the transfer process minimizes opportunities for error and helps prevent misidentification of the specimen.

IV.e. Specimens should be transferred from the sterile field by personnel using standard precautions. *[1: Strong Evidence]*

Standard precautions represent the minimum infection prevention strategy to be applied during all patient care activities (regardless of suspected or confirmed infection status of the patient) in any setting in which health care is delivered.[68] Implementing standard precautions when specimens are transferred from the sterile field helps prevent exposure of personnel to blood, body fluids, or other potentially infectious materials.[68]

IV.f. Specimens should be transferred from the sterile field by personnel using sterile technique. *[5: No Evidence]*

Using sterile technique when specimens are transferred from the sterile field helps to prevent microbial contamination of the specimen.

Evidence addressing the need for transferring specimens from the sterile field using sterile technique was not identified during the evidence review for this guideline.

IV.g. The cellular structure of the specimen should be maintained during the transfer process by not crushing, twisting, or otherwise damaging the integrity of the tissue. *[5: No Evidence]*

Maintaining the cellular structure of the specimen reduces the potential for inaccurate or incomplete diagnostic information.

Evidence addressing the need for maintaining the cellular structure of the specimen during transfer from the sterile field was not identified during the evidence review for this guideline.

Recommendation V

Containment of the specimen should be completed in a manner that protects and secures the specimen and prevents exposure of health care personnel to blood, body fluids, or other potentially infectious materials.

Specimen containment involves securing the specimen by placing it in an item used for storage and transport. Containing the specimen in a manner that protects and secures the specimen may help to prevent damage to or loss of the specimen. Containing the specimen in a manner that prevents exposure of health care personnel to blood, body fluids, or other infectious materials is a regulatory requirement.[69]

V.a. Containers and collection devices needed for specimen management during the procedure should be determined and obtained before the procedure. *[5: No Evidence]*

Determining and obtaining specimen containers before the procedure may help to improve process efficiency and prevent damage to or loss of the specimen.

Evidence addressing the need for determining and obtaining containers and collection devices necessary for specimen management before the procedure was not identified during the evidence review for this guideline.

V.b. Containers must be leak proof and puncture resistant.[69] *[1: Regulatory Requirement]*

Using specimen containers that are leak proof and puncture resistant is a regulatory requirement.[69]

V.b.1. Containers should be of the correct size and type and should be large enough to fully secure the specimen and preservative fluids.

Verifying that specimen containers are of the correct size and type to fully secure the specimen and preservative fluids used may help prevent damage to the specimen. This can also prevent leakage and help protect perioperative personnel or others handling the container or its contents from unnecessary exposure to blood, body fluids, or other infectious materials.

V.b.2. The container or collection device should be large enough to allow the preservative solution, if used, to contact all surfaces of the specimen.

V.b.3. Specimen collection containers may be sterile or clean, depending on collection requirements.

V.c. The specimen should be contained and labeled immediately after transfer from the sterile field. *[2: Moderate Evidence]*

Containing specimens immediately after transfer from the sterile field may prevent damage to or loss of the specimen.

In a study to evaluate the incidence and cause of tissue biopsy loss, Sandbank et al tracked the biopsy specimens taken by a single plastic surgeon at an outpatient clinic between October 2001 and April 2005. A total of 4,400 tissue biopsy specimens were submitted, and a total of five specimens were reported as lost during the study period. Two of the specimens were located. After formal review of the remaining three lost specimens, the researchers determined that one specimen had been lost in the pathology laboratory during processing, and two specimens had been lost because they had not been inserted into the specimen container. The researchers recommended inserting the specimen into the container immediately after excision and verifying that the specimen is in the container at the end of the procedure.[70]

Recommendation VI

Specimens containers should be labeled to communicate patient, specimen, preservative,[71] and biohazard[69] information.

Specimen identification and labeling is the process of affixing to a container information that establishes or indicates the specifications or characteristics of the enclosed sample.

Misidentification of a specimen, its margins, or other information (eg, location of suture tags) could result in errors or delay in diagnosis or treatment or the need for additional procedures.

Labeling to communicate chemical preservative and biohazard information is a regulatory requirement.[69,71] Failure to communicate preservative and biohazard information could result in exposure or injury to personnel handling the contained specimen.

Evidence related to specimen identification and labeling identified during the evidence review for this guideline. revealed a number of studies and quality improvement initiatives conducted for the purpose of reducing errors in specimen identification[72-78]; however, there are variances in terminology,[77,78] quality indicators,[72,75,76] and organizational practices,[7] and there is no clear solution for eliminating errors.[7,72,77]

Makary et al conducted a prospective cohort study designed to measure the incidence and type of specimen identification errors occurring in the surgical patient population during the preanalytical phase. The study included all surgical patients (ie, outpatient and inpatient) for whom a pathology specimen was sent between October 2004 and April 2005. The researchers analyzed a total of 21,351 specimens for identification errors (ie, any discrepancy between information on the specimen requisition form and the accompanying labeled specimen received in the pathology laboratory). There were a total of 91 specimen identification errors, including

- specimen not labeled (n = 18),
- empty specimen container (n = 16),
- incorrect laterality (n = 16),
- incorrect tissue site (n = 14),
- incorrect patient (n = 11),
- no patient name (n = 9), and
- no tissue site (n = 7).[72]

Identification errors occurred in 4.3 per 1,000 surgical specimens. This translates to approximately 182 mislabeled specimens per year. These events occurred in 53 patients from outpatient clinics and 38 patients from hospital operating rooms (ORs). The most common identification errors occurred in biopsy procedures (n = 54), followed by excisional procedures (n = 24), and resection procedures (n = 3). The most common mislabeled specimens included breast tissue (n = 11), skin (n = 10), and colon (n = 8). The researchers concluded that surgical specimen identification errors are common and present an important safety risk for patients. Strategies to reduce the rate of errors should therefore be a research priority.[72]

Quillen and Murphy conducted a study of 49,955 specimens obtained between January 1, 2004, and September 30, 2005, in a university hospital, to determine the number of specimen mislabeling events, specifically major mislabeling events, and to design and implement a corrective plan of action for reducing specimen mislabeling. They recorded and classified all mislabeling events into two categories:

- minor mislabeling: truncated name or medical record number, misspelled name, missing information (eg, date, signature) or
- major mislabeling: unlabeled specimen, mismatched information on specimen and requisition, wrong blood in the tube.[73]

The overall incidence of specimen mislabeling events during the 21-month study period was 0.5% (n = 243 of 49,955). Of the mislabeling events, 47% (n = 114) were defined as major events. The researchers noted that the highest proportion of mislabeling events came from the emergency department. Weekly feedback was provided to address the mislabeling events, and within one year, the number of mislabeling events in the emergency department was reduced from 47% (n = 23 of 49) to 14% (n = 4 of 29). The researchers concluded that collecting and reviewing data on mislabeled specimens and providing timely feedback can change practice and reduce specimen mislabeling.[73]

In early 2005, the CAP conducted a survey of 120 institutions to determine the

- frequency of identification errors detected before and after verification of results,
- frequency of adverse events caused by specimen misidentification, and
- factors associated with low error rates and detection of errors.

Participants tracked data on identification errors related to all types of anatomic (ie, examining and processing of surgical specimens) and clinical (ie, laboratory testing) errors related to all inpatients and outpatients for five weeks. The term *specimen identification error* was considered to represent any result reported for the wrong specimen (or one that would have been reported for the wrong specimen without some intervention).[74]

The researchers reviewed information from a total of 6,705 identification errors. The majority (85.5%) were detected before verification, with the remaining portion (14.5%) detected after results were released. More than 50% of the identification errors resulted from specimen labeling errors, with 22% resulting from registration or order entry errors. Approximately one in 18 identification errors resulted in an adverse event, with more than 70% of adverse events resulting in patient inconvenience rather than a change in treatment or outcome. The researchers concluded that identification errors are common, but most are detected before results are released, and only a fraction are associated with adverse patient events.[74]

In April 2003, a multidisciplinary team from a state-wide children's hospital and clinics system performed an intense scrutiny of specimen labeling methods to identify areas in the current processes that might lead to potential errors. The labeling process was critically observed, recorded, and reviewed during interviews with involved personnel. The preanalytical phase was identified as the primary focus area because it was revealed that nearly two-thirds of the labeling errors occurred during this phase.[75]

The team decided to have laboratory personnel reject all specimens that were not correctly labeled. Personnel submitting the specimen could challenge the rejection by following a procedure that involved a discussion with the ordering clinician, the health care worker who collected and labeled the specimen, and the pathologist. The discussion could result in labeling or relabeling of the specimen in question. The rejection and discussion process resulted in a 75% decrease in the number of mislabeled or unlabeled specimens received in the pathology laboratory.[75]

In a study conducted during the fall of 2009 to quantify the rates of mislabeled cases, specimens, blocks, and slides; identify the sources of error; and review the ways specimen labeling errors are discovered, Nakhleh et al prospectively reviewed voluntarily submitted surgical pathology data from 136 participating institutions for eight weeks or until 30 errors (ie, mislabeled cases, specimens, blocks, slides) were identified. Study participants used the following definitions for defining mislabeling errors:
- mislabeled case: wrong patient or case number applied to the entire case
- mislabeled specimen: wrong specimen labeling (eg, right versus left)
- mislabeled block: histological block labeled with the wrong patient or case number
- mislabeled slide: histological slide labeled with the wrong patient or case number

Information collected on each labeling error included the
- work location where the defect occurred,
- item that was mislabeled,
- number of items affected,
- point of detection, and
- consequences of the mislabeling error.[76]

The rates of mislabeled cases, specimens, blocks, and slides were also tested for association with institutional demographics and practice variables. Results from a total of 1,811 mislabeling occurrences showed the overall mislabeling rates to be 27.1% of cases, 19.8% of specimens, 25.5% of blocks, and 27.7% of slides. Mislabeling of specimens most often occurred during the preanalytical or analytical phases. In most cases, the errors were detected during the steps immediately following the error. Errors were corrected before the pathology report was issued 96.7% of the time, with a corrected report necessary for only 3.2% of errors. Study participants estimated that patient care was affected for 1.3% of error occurrences.

The researchers pointed out that the results of this study failed to show a detectable benefit associated with the use of technology (eg, bar codes) or the use of processes designed to promote continuous improvement and reduce wasted resources. They concluded that there is a need for quality checks throughout the system to reduce errors in specimen labeling.[76]

Bixenstine et al convened an expert panel to develop and pilot test a tool of standardized measures and definitions to evaluate the quality of surgical specimen identification during the preanalytical phase. The panel included physicians, nurses, students, and administrators with expertise in pathology or quality improvement. The preanalytical phase was chosen because specimen identification processes in this phase are completely preventable. A literature review was conducted to identify published surgical specimen identification defects.[77]

Group consensus was achieved on a set of surgical specimen identification quality measures and also on procedures for collecting and measuring data. Quality measures included the following container and requisition defects:
- Container defects included
  - no specimen in the container or requisition received without a container,
  - no identifying label or misplaced label,
  - no patient name or incorrect patient name,
  - no numeric patient identifier or incorrect numeric patient identifier,
  - no specimen type or source or incorrect specimen type or source, and
  - no specimen laterality or incorrect specimen laterality.
- Requisition defects included
  - no requisition or a blank requisition received with the specimen container,
  - no date and time or incorrect date and time,
  - no patient name or incorrect patient name,
  - no numeric patient identifier or incorrect numeric patient identifier,
  - no specimen type or source or incorrect specimen type or source, and
  - no specimen laterality or incorrect specimen laterality.[77]

A total of 69 diverse hospitals in Michigan and one in Iowa submitted prospectively collected data during a three-month period in 2009. The results showed an average specimen identification defect rate of nearly 3%. During the three-month study period, the identified specimen identification defects involved 1,780 patients. The overall container defect rate was about 1%, with the most common container defects being omitted or incorrect specimen source or type. The overall requisition defect rate was more than 2%, with the most common requisition defect being omitted or incorrect date and time. The consequences of these defects represent a significant risk to patient safety.[77]

The researchers contended that without standardized definitions, quality measures, and methodology, it is difficult to accurately estimate and compare the incidence of defects and to identify the most common defects in specimen identification. Additional research is needed to determine whether these measures can be used to reduce the frequency of surgical specimen identification errors and improve patient safety.[77]

In a systematic study of amended pathology reports from 2001 to 2004 conducted by a university health system to determine the types of errors and the effectiveness of efforts to improve surgical pathology processes, researchers classified amended pathology reports by four root causes:

- misidentifications (ie, wrong patient, tissue, laterality, or anatomic location),
- specimen defects (ie, lost, inadequate size or volume, missing or discrepant critical measurements),
- misinterpretations (ie, diagnosis not justified by available evidence [eg, false positives]), and
- report defects (ie, transmission of erroneous information not related to misidentification, specimen defects, or misinterpretations).

Three specific interventions designed to promote continuous improvement and reduce wasted resources were applied and assessed between 2005 and 2008, including

- clinician education to reduce identification defects,
- redesign of specimen processing to reduce specimen defects, and
- double review of breast and prostate specimens before sign-out to decrease interpretation defects.[78]

During the four-year period, misidentification defects decreased from 16% to 9%; specimen defects remained variable, ranging from 2% to 11%; misinterpretations decreased from 18% to 3%; and report defects increased from 64% to 83%. The researchers concluded that misidentification, specimen defects, and misinterpretations were relatively resistant to the applied educational interventions. This finding also underscores the multiple places misidentification errors can occur during the preanalytical and analytical phases and supports the need to double check the processes that occur in these phases.[78]

Specimen defect rates remained variable because the redesign of specimen processing only reduced specimen defects during the analytical phase. The applied interventions markedly decreased specimen misinterpretations. This finding suggests that double review of specimens by pathologists to resolve discrepancies during the analytical phase may be a valuable practice. The increase in report defects demonstrates the effectiveness of capturing data when amended reports are monitored for specific root causes and also demonstrates the need to apply consistent and specific terminology.[78]

VI.a. Patient identification should be confirmed using two unique identifiers according to facility or health care organization policy at the time the specimen is removed from the patient and placed into the container. *[2: Moderate Evidence]*

Using two patient identifiers reduces the risk for misidentification. The CAP recommends two or more patient identifiers (neither of which is the patient's room number) on specimen labels.[79]

VI.b. Specimen identification should be confirmed verbally between the surgeon and the perioperative RN circulator and documented accurately, legibly, and completely using a "read back" verification of the information provided for specimen labeling. *[2: Moderate Evidence]*

Using a "write down, read back" process to confirm the communication provided for specimen labeling minimizes the risk of communication errors.[67]

In a descriptive retrospective study to develop and prioritize strategies for preventing communication breakdowns that result in surgical patient injury, Greenberg et al identified and reviewed 60 cases involving error and patient injury related to communication breakdowns. Results showed the majority of communication breakdowns were verbal (92%) and involved a single transmitter and a single receiver (64%). The most common error was failure to transmit the information followed by inaccurate communication of the information.[67]

After a qualitative assessment of the communication breakdowns, the researchers developed a set of strategic interventions to reduce communication breakdowns based on the patterns observed in the study. Strategies included identifying trigger events that require immediate communication with the physician, the standard use of read backs, and the use of structured protocols for transfer of care. The cases were reviewed a second time to determine whether the errors could have been prevented by implementing the strategies developed by the researchers. The researchers concluded that the standard use of identified triggers, read backs, and standardized protocols for transfer of care could improve communication and patient safety.[67]

VI.b.1. Specimen identification that should be confirmed and documented includes

- facility or health care organization-defined unique patient identifiers (eg, patient name and medical record number);
- originating source of the specimen including laterality, if applicable;
- type of tissue;
- clinical diagnosis, and
- additional pertinent clinical information (eg, location of suture tags).

VI.c. Specimens must be labeled to communicate chemical preservative[71] and biohazard information.[69] *[1: Regulatory Requirement]*

Labeling to communicate chemical preservative and biohazard information is a regulatory requirement.[69,71] Failure to communicate preservative and biohazard information could result in exposure or injury to personnel handling the contained specimen.

VI.d. Specimen identification labels should be securely affixed to the container, not the lid. *[2: Moderate Evidence]*

Placing the label on the container instead of the lid may help prevent loss of specimen information after the lid is removed from the container or if the lid becomes detached from the container.[79]

VI.d.1. Information on the label should include
- facility or health care organization-defined unique identifiers (eg, patient name and medical record number);
- specimen type and site including laterality, if applicable; and
- date of resection and preservation.

VI.d.2. Dark, indelible ink should be used on labels.

Using dark ink improves visibility of both handwritten and electronic labels. Using indelible ink helps prevent ink from being removed from the label.

VI.d.3. Unused printed or handwritten labels should be discarded or removed from the OR or procedure room at the end of each procedure.

Disposal or removal of unused printed or handwritten labels helps prevent the risk of an incorrect label being secured to a specimen container, pathology requisition, or other document intended for another patient.

VI.e. Specimen identification and labeling should be confirmed among surgical team members during the debriefing at the end of the operative or other invasive procedure. *[2: Moderate Evidence]*

Confirmation should include
○ visual confirmation that the specimen is in the container;
○ verification that the patient information on the label and requisition are correct and legible;
○ verification that the number and type of specimens are correct, including laterality as applicable;
○ verification that the specimens have been correctly fixed, as applicable; and
○ confirmation of other pertinent information (eg, documentation of suture tags).

Management of specimens is a multidisciplinary process. Postprocedure confirmation of the specimen identification and labeling can improve communication among team members and may help to reduce or eliminate potential errors[80] in specimen management.

VI.f. A point-of-care bar coding or radio-frequency identification (RFID) patient and specimen labeling system may be used. *[2: Moderate Evidence]*

The CAP recommends using a bar-code patient and specimen labeling system.[79] Using point-of-care bar-coding or RFID technology has the potential to significantly reduce identification errors.[7,79,81,82]

Manual entry of patient identification has an error rate of approximately one character per 300 characters entered.[7] Bar-code technology has a substitution rate of only one per 1 million characters.[7] Most bar-code systems also have a first-read rate of 95% or better, making the acquisition of patient identifying information faster and more accurate than manual methods.[7] Although bar-code technology reduces transcription errors, it does not guarantee accurate patient or specimen identification.[7] After bar codes are printed on labels, the label could be applied to the wrong specimen container, particularly when specimen containers are labeled in advance of specimen collection.[7] Using point-of-care bar-code label printers and scanners minimizes the potential for labels to be applied to the wrong container.[7]

In a quality improvement initiative conducted in December 2002 designed to reduce patient identification errors and unidentified blood glucose results for point-of-care glucose testing, manual steps involved in patient identification were automated using armbands and bar-code scanners. The process changes resulted in a gradual decrease in patient identification errors from 12.4% to 4.9%, and a reduction in the number of unidentified blood glucose results from between 400 and 500 to 274.[83]

In March 2003, the bar-code width was reduced and the wristband was placed in a protective pouch to increase ease of scanning. Data collected after the implementation of the new wristband showed a decrease in patient identification errors from 4.9% to 1.7%, and a reduction in the number of unidentified blood glucose results from 274 to 102. Additional education and nonpunitive feedback was provided to individuals with high error rates. By December 2003, patient identification errors had decreased to 0.7%, and the number of unidentified blood glucose results was reduced to 25.[83]

In a quality improvement project conducted in 2008 in the emergency department of a medical center treating more than 42,000 patients per year, the rate of mislabeled specimens (ie, two per week) was determined to be unacceptable. A multidisciplinary team was brought together to explore options, and use of a bar-coding device designed for use with bedside computers and printers was implemented in 2010. Use of the bar-coding device, in combination with dual identification of the patient, eliminated specimen labeling errors.[84]

In an integrated health care delivery system composed of three large acute care hospitals and a reference laboratory where more than 1 million point-of-care tests are performed annually, a performance improvement initiative was prompted by a number of identification errors occurring with glucose and blood gas point-of-care testing devices. Nichols et al approached the goal of reducing identification errors associated with point-of-care testing by applying two strategies. They conducted an analysis of the identification processes to determine the various ways that identification errors could occur. Data entry was determined to be the primary source of error because of the need to enter 14 digits with every test. The first strategy involved holding clinical operators accountable for mistakes in data entry. This strategy led to only partial improvements in error rates.[85]

The investigators theorized that bar coding would be the most effective means of addressing the data entry problem. Bar coding was implemented as a second strategy in November 2002. The rates of identification errors decreased significantly for both glucose and blood gas devices; however, identification errors still occurred because operators resorted to manual entry when they encountered a bar code that was difficult to scan. Errors also occurred when patients were found to have incorrect information on bar-coded wristbands. The investigators concluded that bar-coding technology significantly reduced identification errors with point-of-care testing, improved patient care, and enhanced interdisciplinary communication, but additional steps are needed to verify that patient wristbands contain accurate information.[85]

Francis et al conducted a study in a high-volume gastroenterology and colorectal surgery outpatient endoscopy unit that yields more than 30,000 specimens annually, for the purpose of eliminating the paper requisitions that accompanied tissue specimens sent for pathologic evaluation and creating a system that would automate specimen bottle tracking. The study was undertaken as an initiative to reduce specimen-labeling errors in response to a wrong site surgery that was performed as the result of a mislabeled pathology specimen. The researchers applied RFID technology to specimen bottles and initiated dual confirmation of the correct site and patient for each specimen by both the endoscopy RN and the endoscopist.

The researchers reviewed and compared the number of specimen labeling errors that occurred in the unit during January through March 2007, before the initiative, and during January through March 2008, after the initiative. Errors were categorized as
- class 1 (ie, typographical errors with no potential clinical consequences),
- class 2 (ie, minor errors unlikely to have clinical consequences), or
- class 3 (ie, significant errors with the potential to detrimentally affect patient care).[82]

During 2007, there were 646 class 1 errors (7.85%), 112 class 2 errors (1.36%), and seven class 3 errors (0.09%) for 8,229 specimens. In 2008, there were 35 class 1 errors (0.41%), 10 class 2 errors (0.12%), and two class 3 errors (0.02%) for 8,536 specimens. The researchers concluded that the dual confirmation of patient and surgical site and the initiation of an electronic requisition and RFID technology significantly reduced specimen labeling errors in every class.[82]

VI.g. Perioperative RNs responsible for specimen management should receive education and complete competency verification activities related to reducing errors in specimen identification and labeling.[10] *[2: Moderate Evidence]*

O'Neill et al conducted a retrospective study to investigate the combined effect of an educational campaign and strict enforcement of specimen labeling policy for the purpose of reducing the incidence of mislabeled and wrong blood in the tube specimens detected by blood bank personnel. The researchers calculated and compared the incidence of mislabeled and wrong blood in the tube specimens from October 1, 2001, through September 30, 2004, preceding the education and policy enforcement, and then from October 1, 2004, through September 30, 2007, after the education and policy enforcement. Results showed that following the educational campaign and strict policy enforcement, the incidence of mislabeling errors decreased by 86.4%. The incidence of wrong blood in the tube decreased by 73.5%. The researchers concluded that education and policy enforcement can lead to statistically significant decrease in the incidence of specimen mislabeling and wrong blood in the tube.[86]

VI.h. Facility or health care organization policies and procedures should provide guidance for specimen
- collection and handling,
- identification and labeling, and
- transport.[79]

[2: Moderate Evidence]

Policies and procedures provide guidance and detail responsibilities for specimen identification and labeling.[10]

In 2006, personnel at a major university hospital noted that the number of specimen identification errors was greater than desired and represented a risk to patient safety. Between 2007

SPECIMEN MANAGEMENT

and 2011, a collaborative effort between nursing and laboratory personnel was initiated to improve performance and reduce the number of errors involving inpatient, ambulatory, and surgical services areas. The improvement process began with a review of current practices to determine how the errors were occurring. The types of errors also were reviewed and categorized; they included
- unlabeled specimen,
- lack of patient identification on the request form,
- no request form,
- specimen labeled with only one patient identifier (ie, patient name), and
- specimen and request form unmatched (ie, specimen labeled with the wrong patient or request form labeled with the wrong patient).

Applied strategies for improvement included
- establishing clear expectations for specimen identification by reviewing and updating all policies and procedures related to specimen identification,
- providing education to all clinical personnel who collect specimens,
- providing individualized feedback to each employee involved in an incorrect specimen identification event, and
- addressing the process when specific types of errors occurred repeatedly.

The applied performance improvement interventions successfully reduced the number of errors from 128 per year to 30 per year (77%).[87]

Recommendation VII

Specimens should be preserved in a manner that protects the integrity of the specimen and prevents exposure of health care personnel to chemicals, blood, body fluids, or other potentially infectious materials.

Specimen preservation involves the act of protecting a specimen to preserve morphology, reduce the loss of molecular components into solution, prevent decomposition and autolysis, and prevent microbial growth.[88]

Unpreserved or incorrectly preserved specimens may be compromised and lead to inaccurate or incomplete diagnostic information or the need for additional procedures.

Containing the specimen in a manner that prevents exposure of health care personnel to chemicals, blood, body fluids, or other infectious materials is a regulatory requirement.[69,71]

A full discussion of safe practices for handling formalin or other preservative solutions or chemicals is outside of the scope of this guideline. The reader should refer to the AORN Guideline for a Safe Environment of Care: Part 1[89] for additional guidance.

VII.a. The use of preservatives or chemical additives for tissue preservation should be confirmed with the physician. *[5: No Evidence]*

Verifying the use of preservatives or chemical additives with the physician may help to prevent errors in tissue preservation.

Evidence addressing the need for confirming the use of chemical additives for preservation with the physician was not identified during the evidence review for this guideline.

VII.b. Formalin should be dispensed and stored in an area other than the OR or procedure room unless ignition sources are not used and the regulatory requirements for locations where formalin is used and stored are met. *[1: Regulatory Requirement]*

Formalin is a combustible liquid.[90] Storage and use of formalin is regulated by the Occupational Safety and Health Administration and other federal and state health regulatory agencies.[71,91]

Locations where formalin is used must have
- posted signs warning of formaldehyde use,
- eyewash stations available within the immediate area, and
- ventilation systems with adequate capacity to maintain levels below the permissible exposure limits (ie, eight-hour total weighted average of 0.75 ppm or 15-minute short-term exposure limit of 2.0 ppm).[71]

VII.b.1. Eyewash stations should be located
- so that travel time is no greater than 10 seconds from the location of chemical use or storage, or immediately next to or adjoining the area of chemical use or storage if the chemical is caustic or a strong acid and
- on the same level as the hazard, with the path of travel free of obstructions (eg, doors) that may inhibit immediate use of an eyewash station.[92]

When walking at a normal pace, the average person covers a distance of 55 feet in 10 seconds; however, a person who has experienced a chemical splash to the eyes or face may be visually impaired, in discomfort or pain, and in a state of panic. For this reason, it is prudent to consider the physical and emotional state of the person as well as the availability of assistive personnel in the immediate area when determining the location of eyewash stations.[92]

VII.c. Personnel handling formalin must wear personal protective equipment including face and eye shields, gloves, and other protective garments.[71,90,93] *[1: Regulatory Requirement]*

Formaldehyde, the active ingredient in formalin, is a potential carcinogen. It may cause acute and chronic health conditions, including sensitization leading to asthma and contact dermatitis. Formalin can be absorbed through the skin and nasal passages, splashed in the eyes, or ingested. Exposure can result in irritation, burns, or allergic reactions.[71,90,91,93]

VII.d. Specimens should be fully immersed in a ratio of fixative volume to specimen volume determined by the pathologist or receiving pathology laboratory personnel. *[2: Moderate Evidence]*

The volume of formalin required for tissue fixation is not generally agreed upon.[94] The literature is inconclusive regarding the amount of solution that should be used for specimen preservation and the suggested amounts vary.[30,88,94,95]

In a review of the literature conducted in 2007 on function and management of the pathology laboratory, common specimen types, biohazard exposure and safety, and collection of tissue for research, Bell et al recommended a volume of at least 10 times the volume of the specimen for effective fixation.[88]

In 2008, an ad hoc committee of expert pathologists, laboratory scientists, and technical experts who developed consensus recommendations for standardized procedures for estrogen-receptor testing in breast cancer recommended placing breast resection specimens in a volume of fixative that is one part tissue to 20 parts fixative.[30]

In a study published in 2010 that examined the use of under-vacuum sealing as an alternative to fixing specimens in formalin, Di Novi et al recommended a volume of fixative that is 20 times the weight of the specimen.[95]

Fixative-to-tissue volume ratios of 1:20 have been advocated because of the consideration that fixatives are poor buffers; however, this is not the case with neutral buffered formalin.[94] In addition, it has been argued that large amounts of fixative are needed to prevent dilution of the fixative, but this is primarily applicable to fixatives that do not contain water, which is not the case with neutral buffered formalin.[94]

In a study to determine the smallest amount of neutral buffered formalin to provide adequate tissue fixation, Buesa and Peshkov fixed a total of 60 tissue samples from human breast, uterus, liver, skin, and abdominal fat for eight, 24, and 48 hours at room temperature (ie, 68° F to 71.6° F [20° C to 22° C]), with neutral buffered formalin at fixative-to-tissue volume ratios of 1:1. 2:1, 5:1, and 10:1. After processing, nine pathologists from three different histopathology institutions evaluated the slides. Results showed that the fixation process is more time and temperature dependent and less related to the volume of fixative used. Preserving tissues with a fixative-to-tissue volume of 2:1 for 48 hours at room temperature was enough to ensure proper fixation and infiltration of the tissue samples, and the researchers anticipated that other tissues would show similar results. The researchers concluded that using formalin in fixative-to-tissue ratios of lower than 10:1 will improve health care worker safety while still allowing for the use of formalin as a tissue fixative solution.[94]

VII.e. Specimens and chemicals used for preservation of specimens must be disposed of according to local, state, and federal regulations.[69,71] *[1: Regulatory Requirement]*

Disposal of pathology waste and chemicals is regulated by multiple entities and jurisdictions.[69,71]

VII.f. Alternatives to formalin may be used for tissue fixation or preservation. *[2: Moderate Evidence]*

Formalin is widely used for tissue fixation; however, concerns regarding its toxicity and potential carcinogenicity in combination with the need for more effective preservation of nucleic acids have led to attempts to find a safer alternative.[95-103]

To address concerns associated with personnel exposure to formalin during fixation of surgical specimens in a university hospital, Bussolati et al purchased an under-vacuum sealing device. The under-vacuum sealing process was tested on a variety of tissue and organs (ie, colon, gallbladder, spleen, kidney) to verify histological preservation, and then the device was transferred to the hospital surgical area where it was used successfully for more than one year. The process involved placing large surgical specimens (eg, thyroid, breast, colon) into plastic bags immediately after removal from the patient and then sealing them using the under-vacuum sealing device. The sealing process takes approximately 15 seconds. The labeled specimen was then placed into a refrigerator or taken directly to the pathology laboratory. In most cases, the specimen was kept in the refrigerator for only a few hours, but in some cases specimens were kept in the refrigerator for as long as one to two days.[96]

Under-vacuum sealing decreases the autolytic processes and enhances specimen cooling because of the absence of insulating air. Under-vacuum sealing of surgical specimens results in a lightweight bag that is easier to carry than a formalin-filled plastic container. More than 2,000 specimens were processed using the under-vacuum sealing method without any problems related to morphological preservation or immunohistochemical reactivity. Although refrigeration of specimens for longer periods was not optimal, it did not in any case prevent histopathology processing and reading.[96]

Personnel found the under-vacuum sealing process to be easy and preferable to fixing specimens in formalin. One additional benefit of the under-vacuum sealing process is that because the tissues are not exposed to formalin, material can be provided for tissue banking and research. Previously, the amount of formalin used in the surgical area in this hospital was approximately 15 L per week; currently, no formalin is used.[96]

In an attempt to limit the use of formalin to the pathology laboratory where it is handled under a hood in safe environmental conditions and avoid its use in less-protected areas of the hospital, such as the surgical operating theaters, Di Novi et al proposed an alternative procedure of under-vacuum sealing specimens in plastic bags and refrigerating the sealed, labeled bags at 39.2° F (4° C) until transfer to the pathology laboratory. The under-vacuum sealing process was used successfully for more than two years in a single surgical theater and then extended to an entire teaching hospital with 1,162 beds and approximately 54,560 admissions and 40,000 histopathology examinations per year. In a study conducted between October 2008 and April 2009 to compare the feasibility of the new procedure and compliance of personnel, the researchers used surveys and interviews with all involved personnel (ie, nurses, technicians, pathologists [N = 177]) who specifically dealt with the various steps of the under-vacuum sealing process. Data analysis showed the under-vacuum sealing process to be superior in terms of both personnel satisfaction and gross anatomic preservation. No problems with histopathology preservation were encountered. The use of formalin is now confined to the pathology laboratory and its use on hospital premises is greatly reduced.[95]

In a separate study to quantify the effect of formalin on hospital workers' respiratory systems, Berton and Di Novi used data collected from the previous study and found that only 4.3% of the respondents using the under-vacuum sealing process for containing surgical specimens suffered from respiratory symptoms (eg, cough, chest pain, shortness of breath, wheezing). This figure was approximately 30 percentage points higher for respondents using formalin for fixation of surgical specimens. The researchers concluded that the effect of formalin on the short-term probability of displaying respiratory symptoms is robust and significantly positive, and the substitution of formalin fixation with the under-vacuum sealing process would markedly improve the health of personnel.[97]

In a study to compare the effect of under-vacuum sealing to the effect of cooling alone, Kristensen et al collected tissue samples from five different organs (ie, spleen, breast, kidney, liver, colon). The collected samples underwent one of four treatments:
- under-vacuum sealing and storage at room temperature (vacuum effect),
- no under-vacuum sealing and storage at 39.2° F (4° C) (cooling effect),
- under-vacuum sealing and storage at 39.2° F (4° C) (vacuum and cooling effect), or
- no under-vacuum sealing and storage at room temperature (no treatment control).[104]

The samples were tested at seven time points: one, two, four, eight, 20, 44, and 92 hours. The results showed no preserving effect of under-vacuum sealing with respect to cellular morphology, immunohistochemical reactivity, or nucleic acid integrity. Storage at cooled temperatures was found to preserve tissue to a higher degree than storage at room temperature, independent of whether the tissue was subjected to under-vacuum sealing. The researchers concluded that under-vacuum sealing is not an alternative to cooling.[104]

Al-Maaini and Bryant conducted a study in 2006 at a university college of medicine to determine the effectiveness of honey as a substitute for formalin in the histological fixation of tissue. The researchers fixed rat liver and kidney tissues at 98.6° F (37° C) and at room temperature, with and without agitation, in concentrations of honey ranging from 10% to 100% diluted with distilled water. The tissues were processed, examined, and compared with tissues fixed in 10% neutral buffered formalin. Results showed that the tissues fixed in 10% and 20% honey concentrations at room temperature with and without agitation provided comparable results to the control tissues fixed in formalin. Honey concentrations greater than 20% were less successful and resulted in slower penetration times, hardening of tissues, and difficulty in sectioning. The researchers recommended additional studies with different brands of honey and a wider range of tissues and fixation times.[98]

In a study to determine the effectiveness of pine honey for tissue fixation and to compare it to other fixatives used for histopathology, Ozkan et al obtained eight different fresh tissue samples (endometrium, breast, placenta, uterus, omentum, suprarenal, stomach, lung). Each tissue sample was divided and placed into one of three fixative solutions:
- 10% honey in distilled water,
- 10% neutral buffered formalin, or
- alcoholic formalin.[99]

All tissues were fixed for 24 hours at room temperature and then processed and examined. Results showed similar tissue histomorphology for all solutions; however, there were minor histomorphological differences among the various tissues fixed in the honey solution. The differences did not influence correct diagnostic conclusions. The researchers concluded that honey can be used as a safe alternative to formalin in histopathology.[99]

In a study that used a systematic approach to evaluate the biomolecular status of a large number of clinical tissue specimens processed using a non-formalin fixation method, Gillespie et al reviewed tissue processed with several fixatives in a major teaching university pathology laboratory to determine whether the various fixatives were sufficient to provide a clinical diagnosis. Results showed that 70% ethanol was acceptable for clinical and molecular analysis.[100]

In the second phase of the study, the researchers fixed 50 radical prostatectomy specimens in 70% ethanol and studied them during a two-year period. The researchers had no difficulty in making a clinical diagnosis in any of the samples and also determined that ethanol fixation was consistently comparable to formalin fixation. The researchers noted, however, that 70% ethanol penetrates prostate tissue at a slower rate than 10% neutral buffered formalin. The researchers concluded that specimens fixed in 70% ethanol permitted recovery of nucleic acids and proteins sufficient for molecular analysis.[100]

In a study to determine the effect of two alcohol-based fixatives on various tissues, van Essen et al fixed a wide range of fresh tissue samples in BoonFix, RCL2®, and 4% neutral buffered formalin. The tissue was stored at room temperature and processed after fixation. A blinded evaluation was conducted by two experienced pathologists. Results showed that the formalin provided significantly better staining results (84%) than RCL2 (66%) or BoonFix (60%). Omission of pepsin pretreatment was found to be important to retain morphology of immunostained tissues preserved in alcohol-based fixatives; however, alcohol-based fixatives may have advantages for molecular techniques because they cause less degradation of nucleic acids.[101]

Prento and Lyon compared the performance of six commercial fixatives (ie, HistoChoice®, Kryofix, Mirsky's Fixative™, NoTox, Omnifix II, Tissue-Tek®) with the performance of neutral buffered formalin on tissue samples of rat liver, small intestine, and kidney, to determine the
- rate of penetration,
- mode of fixation,
- extent of protein and structural immobilization,
- quality of histology and cellular structure following routine processing, and
- performance as a fixative.[103]

Results showed that only neutral buffered formalin worked equally well on all tissues tested. The researchers noted prominent histological distortion, cell shrinkage, and vacuolization when formalin substitutes or ethanol was used. The researchers concluded that none of the proposed substitutes for neutral buffered formalin was adequate for critical histology or histopathology.[103]

In a blinded study to assess histomorphology using different formalin substitute fixatives, four experienced, board-certified, surgical pathologists examined seven tissue specimens (ie, hepatocellular carcinoma, ovarian sex cord/stromal tumor, myxoid liposarcoma, uterine endometrioid adenocarcinoma, splenic follicular hyperplasia, infiltrating mammary carcinoma, cecal signet ring carcinoma) fixed with neutral buffered formalin and five proprietary formalin substitutes (ie, Glyo-Fixx™, STF-Streck®, Omnifix, HistoChoice, Histofix). In each case, the pathologists evaluated
- cellular outlines,
- cytoplasmic detail,
- nuclear detail,
- erythrocyte integrity,
- lymphocyte integrity,
- overall morphology, and
- overall staining.

The results showed that formalin fixation provided the highest morphologic quality. The researchers concluded that when discontinuing the use of formalin, pathologists should familiarize themselves with the microscopic details of the replacement fixative.[105]

Recommendation VIII

Specimens should be transported in a manner that protects the integrity of the specimen; prevents exposure of health care personnel to chemicals, blood, body fluids, or other potentially infectious materials; and maintains the confidentiality of protected patient information.[69,71]

Specimen transport refers to carrying or conveying a specimen from one location to another. Specimens that are not safely transported may be compromised, which can lead to inaccurate or incomplete diagnostic information or the need for additional procedures.

Transporting the specimen in a manner that prevents exposure of health care personnel to chemicals, blood, body fluids, or other infectious materials and ensures confidentiality of personal health information is a regulatory requirement.[69,71]

VIII.a. Clean secondary packaging or containment devices should be used to prevent contamination of personnel and the environment during transport of specimens. *[5: No Evidence]*

Containing the specimen in a manner that prevents exposure of health care personnel to chemicals, blood, body fluids, or other infectious materials is a regulatory requirement.[69,71]

VIII.a.1. Accompanying documents (eg, pathology requisition) should be protected from contamination.

VIII.b. Patient and specimen information should be verified by transport personnel at each point of exchange. *[5: No Evidence]*

Misidentification of the patient or specimen could result in errors or delay in diagnosis or treatment or the need for additional procedures.

Evidence addressing the need for transport personnel to verify patient and specimen information at each point of exchange was not identified during the evidence review for this guideline.

VIII.c. Specimens that will not be transported immediately to the pathology laboratory must be temporarily stored in a manner that maintains specimen

SPECIMEN MANAGEMENT

integrity for examination.[106] [1: Regulatory Requirement]

Maintaining optimal integrity of patient specimens and ensuring the specimen is stored properly (eg, refrigerated, kept at room temperature) is a regulatory requirement.[106]

VIII.c.1. Until transport can take place, equipment (eg, refrigerators) used for temporary storage or devices used for transport or storage should maintain specimens at the temperature established in accordance with local, state, and federal regulations by a multidisciplinary team that includes pathology laboratory representatives, facility or health care organization physicians,[65,107] and perioperative RNs.

VIII.d. Devices intended for transport of specimens must be labeled to communicate chemical[71] and biohazard information.[69] [1: Regulatory Requirement]

Labeling to communicate chemical preservative and biohazard information is a regulatory requirement.[69,71] Failure to communicate preservative and biohazard information could result in exposure or injury to personnel handling the contained specimen.

VIII.e. Specimens must be transported in a manner that helps ensure confidentiality of personal health information[44] and minimizes visibility of the specimen. [1: Regulatory Requirement]

Maintaining confidentiality of protected health information is a regulatory requirement and a standard of perioperative nursing care.[44,108,109]

Recommendation IX

Policies and procedures for disposition of specimens should be established in accordance with local, state, and federal regulations by a multidisciplinary team that includes pathology laboratory representatives, facility or health care organization physicians,[65,107] and perioperative RNs.

The pathologist's report is often the key factor in accurate clinical diagnosis and management of patient care.[107]

The CAP and the Royal College of Pathologists recommend that disposition of specimens for each facility or health care organization be determined by the pathologist in collaboration with facility representatives or health care organization physicians.[65,107] Some explanted medical devices are subject to regulatory tracking or reporting requirements.[59-62]

IX.a. Policies and procedures for disposition of specimens should
- state that a pathologist will perform an examination of the specimen when requested by the physician or licensed independent practitioner or when the pathologist determines a pathology examination is indicated;
- address the diagnostic needs of medical personnel, including the potential for discovery of significant findings in specimens that are typically exempted from pathology examination, and address the potential for medicolegal implications; and
- include an alternative procedure for documenting the removal and disposition of any specimens or devices not submitted to the pathologist for examination.[65]

[2: Moderate Evidence]

IX.a.1. A pathology report should be generated for every specimen submitted to the pathologist for examination.[65]

IX.a.2. The facility or health care organization should develop policies and procedures for
- receipt of laboratory testing or pathology reporting results,
- communication of laboratory testing or pathology reporting results to the physician, and
- verification that laboratory testing or pathology reporting results are added to the patient's health record.

IX.b. Policies and procedures should be developed to identify tissues or other specimens that require only gross identification or disposal.[65,107] [2: Moderate Evidence]

In some instances, a gross examination and documentation of the submitted specimen by the pathologist without histological examination is sufficient.[107]

The CAP recommends that each facility or health care organization develop a written policy that addresses which specimens do not need to be submitted to the pathologist and which specimens are exempted from microscopic examination.[65]

IX.b.1. Policies and procedures may be developed in accordance with CAP guidelines.[65] The CAP suggests creating two lists:
- specimens exempt from pathology examination and
- specimens to be submitted for gross examination only.[65]

IX.b.2. The following specimens may be excluded from submission to the pathologist for examination, provided there is a procedure for documenting removal and disposition:
- bone donated to the bone bank;
- bone fragments removed during corrective or reconstructive orthopedic procedures (eg, rotator cuff repair), excluding large specimens (eg, femoral heads) and knee, ankle, or elbow reconstructions;
- cataracts removed by phacoemulsification;
- dental appliances;
- fat removed by liposuction;
- foreign bodies (eg, bullets) or other medicolegal evidence given directly to law enforcement personnel;

- foreskin from circumcision of a newborn;
- intrauterine contraceptive devices without attached tissue;
- medical devices (eg, catheters, gastrostomy tubes, myringotomy tubes, stents, sutures) that have not contributed to patient illness, injury, or death;
- middle ear ossicles;
- orthopedic hardware and other radiopaque medical devices, provided there is a policy for documentation of surgical removal;
- placentas from uncomplicated pregnancies that do not meet the facility or health care organization criteria for pathology examination and appear normal at the time of delivery;
- rib segments or other tissues removed for the purpose of gaining surgical access, provided the patient does not have a history of malignancy;
- saphenous vein segments harvested for coronary artery bypass;
- skin or other normal tissue removed during a cosmetic or reconstructive procedure (eg, blepharoplasty, abdominoplasty, rhytidectomy), provided it is not contiguous with a lesion and the patient does not have a history of malignancy;
- teeth when there is no attached tissue;
- therapeutic radioactive materials; and
- normal toenails and fingernails that are incidentally removed.[65]

IX.b.3. The following specimens may be submitted for gross examination only, with exceptions at the discretion of the pathologist or physician:
- accessory digits,
- bunions and hammertoes,
- extraocular muscle from corrective surgical procedures (eg, strabismus),
- inguinal hernia sacs (with specific age requirements determined by the facility or health care organization),
- nasal bone and cartilage from rhinoplasty or septoplasty,
- prosthetic breast implants,
- tonsils and adenoids (with specific age requirements determined by the facility or health care organization),
- torn meniscus,
- umbilical hernia sacs (with specific age requirements determined by the facility or health care organization), and
- varicose veins.[65]

Recommendation X

Nursing activities related to specimen management should be documented in a manner consistent with facility or health care organization policies and procedures and regulatory and accrediting agency requirements.

Documentation of nursing activities serves as the legal record of care delivery. Documentation of nursing activities is dictated by the facility or health care organization policy and regulatory and accrediting agency requirements and is necessary to inform other health care professionals involved in the patient's care. Highly reliable data collection is not only necessary to chronicle patients' responses to nursing interventions, but also to demonstrate the facility or health care organization's progress toward quality care outcomes.[108]

X.a. Documentation related to specimen management should include
- patient identification,
- specimen identification,
- additional information pertinent to the specimen or source (eg, location of suture tags),
- pathology examination required (eg, gross only, frozen section),
- final disposition of tissue and explanted devices,
- requests for special handling (eg, return of explanted orthopedic hardware),
- date and time of specimen collection,
- physician identification and contact information, and
- perioperative RN identification.

[2: Moderate Evidence]

Perioperative documentation that accurately reflects the patient's experience is essential for the continuity of outcome-focused nursing care and for effective comparison of realized versus anticipated patient outcomes.[108]

Inaccurate, illegible, or incomplete documentation of specimen management may lead to incomplete or erroneous diagnostic information or the need for additional procedures.

Effective management and collection of health care information that accurately reflects the patient's care, treatment, and services is a regulatory and accreditation requirement for both hospitals and ambulatory settings.[110-121]

X.a.1. Specimen requisition forms and other relevant documentation should accompany the specimen, be secured to the container, and be protected from contamination.

X.b. Documentation should be completed using standardized printed tools or electronic technology. When handwriting is required, it should be legible. *[2: Moderate Evidence]*

Using a standardized printed tool assists in achieving accuracy and consistency when documenting. Studies of human error have shown that many errors involve a deviation from routine practice.[9] Common reasons for errors related to specimen management include unlabeled containers, insufficient patient identification, and incomplete or illegible information.[7] Using electronic tools minimizes errors related to handwriting.[7]

SPECIMEN MANAGEMENT

X.c. Verbal communication from the pathologist related to diagnosis or specific information about the specimen (eg, results of frozen section) should be provided directly to the physician (ie, not through a third party). *[5: No Evidence]*

Using direct verbal communication minimizes the risk of communication errors.

Evidence addressing the need for providing verbal communication related to diagnosis or specific information about the specimen directly to the physician was not identified during the evidence review for this guideline.

X.c.1. If direct verbal communication between physicians is not possible, the communication should be received by the perioperative RN and documented in the patient's health record using a "read back" verification of the information provided.

The date and time of the indirect communication should be recorded along with the signature and title of the perioperative RN receiving the communication. Using a "write down, read back" process to confirm the communication provided minimizes the risk of communication errors.[67]

Editor's note: *Pen-Fix is a registered trademark of Richard-Allen Scientific Co, Kalamazoo, MI. Sakura and Tissue-Tek are registered trademarks of Sakura Finetek, Inc, Torrance, CA. RCL2 is a registered trademark of Alphelys, Plaisir, France. HistoChoice is a registered trademark of Amresto, LLC, Solon, OH. Mirsky's Fixative is a trademark of National Diagnostics, Atlanta, GA. Glyo-Fixx is a trademark of Thermo Fisher Scientific Inc, Waltham, MA. STF-Streck is a registered trademark of Streck Laboratories, Inc, Omaha, NE.*

Glossary

Agreement State: Any state with which the Nuclear Regulatory Commission or the Atomic Energy Commission has entered into a covenant under the Atomic Energy Act of 1954.

Analytical phase: Processes for specimen analysis that occur within the pathology laboratory (eg, gross examination, microscopic examination).

Assay: A procedure for measuring the presence or amount of a drug or biochemical substance in a sample. The substance being measured is considered the target of the assay.

Autolysis: The destruction of cells or tissue of an organism by substances produced within the organism.

Background radiation: Radiation from naturally occurring sources of radioactive material and global fallout as it exists in the environment that is not subject to control.

Biomarker: A biological molecule found in blood or other body fluids that is indicative of a particular condition or disease. Biomarker levels may be used to evaluate a patient's response to treatment.

Chain of custody: A process used to maintain, secure, and document the chronological history and persons in possession of evidence in order for the evidence to be legally accepted in court.

Cold ischemic time: The period of time between removal of the specimen and placement into fixative.

Forensic evidence: Evidence for use in legal or criminal proceedings.

Gross examination: The inspection of surgical specimens by a pathologist using only visual examination to obtain diagnostic information.

Point-of-care testing: Testing conducted at or close to the location where clinical care is delivered.

Postanalytical phase: Processes that occur after the specimen has been analyzed in the pathology laboratory (eg, recording and relaying the interpretation to the clinician).

Preanalytical phase: Processes that occur before the specimen reaches the pathology laboratory for analysis (eg, transfer of information from the physician to the perioperative RN during the procedure, and subsequent labeling, containment, and transport).

Radio-frequency identification (RFID): A system that transmits the identity (in the form of a unique serial number) of an object wirelessly using radio waves.

Root cause analysis: A retrospective process for identifying basic or causal factor(s) underlying variation in performance, including the occurrence or possible occurrence of a sentinel event.

Sentinel event: An unanticipated incident involving death or serious physical or psychological injury, or the risk of serious injury or adverse outcome.

Site identification: The act or process of positively establishing or confirming the location of tissue, foreign objects, or body substances to be removed from the patient and sent for pathology examination.

Specimen: Tissue, foreign objects, or body substances removed from a patient and sent for pathology examination.

Specimen collection: The act or process of obtaining a biopsy or resecting a specimen.

Specimen containment: The act or process of securing a specimen by placing it in a container used for storage or transport.

Specimen disposition: The act of positioning or distributing tissue, foreign bodies, explanted items, or body fluids removed from a patient for pathology examination.

Specimen handling: The act or process of holding, securing, moving, or manipulating a specimen.

Specimen identification and labeling: The process of affixing information to a container that establishes or indicates the specifications or characteristics of the enclosed sample.

Specimen preservation: The act or process of protecting a specimen to maintain morphology, reduce the loss of molecular components, prevent decomposition and autolysis, and prevent microbial growth.

Specimen transfer: The process of moving a specimen from the sterile field to the containment device.

Specimen transport: The act of carrying or conveying a specimen from one location to another.

Warm ischemic time: The time required for arterial ligation and removal of a specimen.

REFERENCES

1. 42 CFR 493. Laboratory Requirements. 2013. http://www.gpo.gov/fdsys/pkg/CFR-2013-title42-vol5/pdf/CFR-2013-title42-vol5-part493.pdf. Accessed April 7, 2014.
2. Leape LL. Error in medicine. *JAMA.* 1994;272(23):1851-1857. [VA]
3. Medal of Justice Award, May 24, 2012: Molly Akers. Center for Justice & Democracy. http://centerjd.org/content/cjd-medal-justice-award-may-24-2012-molly-akers. Accessed April 7, 2014.
4. Fischer B. U of C hospitals sued for error that resulted in removal of breast. *Chicago Sun-Times.* May 11, 2005. [VC]
5. Velasco A. St Vincent's settles suits over fetal remains. *The Birmingham News.* October 24, 2009:1A-2A. [VC]
6. Cooper K. Errors and error rates in surgical pathology: an Association of Directors of Anatomic and Surgical Pathology survey. *Arch Pathol Lab Med.* 2006;130(5):607-609. [IIIC]
7. Valenstein PN, Sirota RL. Identification errors in pathology and laboratory medicine. *Clin Lab Med.* 2004;24(4):979-996, vii. [VB]
8. Smith ML, Wilkerson T, Grzybicki DM, Raab SS. The effect of a lean quality improvement implementation program on surgical pathology specimen accessioning and gross preparation error frequency. *Am J Clin Pathol.* 2012;138(3):367-373. [VB]
9. Reason J. Safety in the operating theatre—part 2: human error and organisational failure. *Qual Saf Health Care.* 2005;14(1):56-60. [VA]
10. Novis DA. Detecting and preventing the occurrence of errors in the practices of laboratory medicine and anatomic pathology: 15 years' experience with the College of American Pathologists' Q-PROBES and Q-TRACKS programs. *Clin Lab Med.* 2004;24(4):965-978. [VA]
11. Metzger LK. An existential perspective of body beliefs and health assessment. *J Religion Health.* 2006;45(1):130-146. [VB]
12. Purnell LD. Traditional Vietnamese health and healing. *Urol Nurs.* 2008;28(1):63-67. [VC]
13. Lamm M. The interment. Chabad.org. http://www.chabad.org/library/article_cdo/aid/281565/jewish/The-Interment.htm. Accessed April 7, 2014. [VB]
14. Ehman J. Religious diversity: practical points for health care providers. Penn Medicine: Pastoral Care & Education. http://www.uphs.upenn.edu/pastoral/resed/diversity_points.html. Accessed April 8, 2014. [VB]
15. Helsel DG, Mochel M. Afterbirths in the afterlife: cultural meaning of placental disposal in a Hmong American community. *J Transcult Nurs.* 2002;13(4):282-286. [IIIB]
16. Baergen R, Thaker HM, Heller DS. Placental release or disposal? Experiences of perinatal pathologists. *Pediatr Dev Pathol.* 2013;16(5):327-330. [IIIC]
17. Makary MA, Holzmueller CG, Thompson D, et al. Operating room briefings: working on the same page. *Jt Comm J Qual Patient Saf.* 2006;32(6):351-355. [VB]
18. *AORN Position Statement: Preventing Wrong-Patient, Wrong-Site, Wrong-Procedure Events.* https://www.aorn.org/PracticeResources/AORNPositionStatements/. AORN, Inc. Accessed April 8, 2014. [IVB]
19. Nemeth SA, Lawrence N. Site identification challenges in dermatologic surgery: a physician survey. *J Am Acad Dermatol.* 2012;67(2):262-268. [IIIB]
20. McGinness JL, Goldstein G. The value of preoperative biopsy-site photography for identifying cutaneous lesions. *Dermatol Surg.* 2010;36(2):194-197. [IIIB]
21. Rossy KM, Lawrence N. Difficulty with surgical site identification: what role does it play in dermatology? *J Am Acad Dermatol.* 2012;67(2):257-261. [IIIB]
22. Ke M, Moul D, Camouse M, et al. Where is it? The utility of biopsy-site photography. *Dermatol Surg.* 2010;36(2):198-202. [IIIC]
23. Hewitt SM, Lewis FA, Cao Y, et al. Tissue handling and specimen preparation in surgical pathology: issues concerning the recovery of nucleic acids from formalin-fixed, paraffin-embedded tissue. *Arch Pathol Lab Med.* 2008;132(12):1929-1935. [VB]
24. Balch CM. Reexamining our routines of handing surgical tissue in the operating room. *J Natl Cancer Inst Monogr.* 2011;2011(42):39-40. [VB]
25. Hicks DG, Kushner L, McCarthy K. Breast cancer predictive factor testing: the challenges and importance of standardizing tissue handling. *J Natl Cancer Inst Monographs.* 2011;2011(42):43-45. [VB]
26. Hicks DG, Boyce BF. The challenge and importance of standardizing pre-analytical variables in surgical pathology specimens for clinical care and translational research. *Biotechnic Histochem.* 2012;87(1):14-17. [VB]
27. Wolff AC, Hammond ME, Schwartz JN, et al. American Society of Clinical Oncology/College of American Pathologists guideline recommendations for human epidermal growth factor receptor 2 testing in breast cancer. *Arch Pathol Lab Med.* 2007;131(1):18-43. [IVB]
28. Hammond ME, Hayes DF, Dowsett M, et al. American Society of Clinical Oncology/College of American Pathologists guideline recommendations for immunohistochemical testing of estrogen and progesterone receptors in breast cancer. *J Clin Oncol.* 2010; 28(16):2784-2795. [IVB]
29. Wolff AC, Hammond ME, Hicks DG, et al. Recommendations for human epidermal growth factor receptor 2 testing in breast cancer: American Society of Clinical Oncology/College of American Pathologists clinical practice guideline update. *Arch Pathol Lab Med.* 2014;138(2):241-256. [IVB]
30. Yaziji H, Taylor CR, Goldstein NS, et al. Consensus recommendations on estrogen receptor testing in breast cancer by immunohistochemistry. *Appl Immunohistochem Mol Morphol.* 2008;16(6):513-520. [IVB]
31. Nkoy FL, Hammond ME, Rees W, et al. Variable specimen handling affects hormone receptor test results in women with breast cancer: a large multihospital retrospective study. *Arch Pathol Lab Med.* 2010;134(4):606-612. [IIIB]
32. Khoury T, Sait S, Hwang H, et al. Delay to formalin fixation effect on breast biomarkers. *Mod Pathol.* 2009;22(11):1457-1467. [IIB]
33. Moatamed NA, Nanjangud G, Pucci R, et al. Effect of ischemic time, fixation time, and fixative type on HER2/neu immunohistochemical and fluorescence in situ hybridization results in breast cancer. *Am J Clin Pathol.* 2011;136(5):754-761. [IIB]
34. Portier BP, Wang Z, Downs-Kelly E, et al. Delay to formalin fixation "cold ischemia time": effect on ERBB2 detection by in-situ hybridization and immunohistochemistry. *Mod Pathol.* 2013;26(1):1-9. [IIB]
35. Lagios MD. Pathology procedures for evaluation of the specimen with potential or documented ductal carcinoma in situ. *Semin Breast Dis.* 2000;3:42-49. [VB]
36. Li J, Guo Z, Zhu Q, et al. Fingertip replantation: determinants of survival. *Plast Reconstr Surg.* 2008;122(3):833-839. [IIIB]

37. Partlin MM, Chen J, Holdgate A. The preoperative preservation of amputated digits: an assessment of proposed methods. *J Trauma.* 2008;65(1):127-131. [IIB]

38. Allen DM, Levin LS. Digital replantation including postoperative care. *Tech Hand Up Extrem Surg.* 2002;6(4):171-177. [VA]

39. Azzopardi EA, Whitaker IS, Laing H. Perceptions of correct preoperative storage and transfer of amputated digits: a national survey of referring emergency departments. *J Plast Reconstr Aesthet Surg.* 2008;61(11):1418-1419. [IIIC]

40. Lloyd MS, Teo TC, Pickford MA, Arnstein PM. Preoperative management of the amputated limb. *Emerg Med J.* 2005;22(7):478-480. [VB]

41. Evans MM, Stagner PA, Rooms R. Maintaining the chain of custody—evidence handling in forensic cases. *AORN J.* 2003;78(4):563-569. [VA]

42. Carrigan M, Collington P, Tyndall J. Forensic perioperative nursing. Advocates for justice. *Can Oper Room Nurs J.* 2000;18(4):12-16. [VA]

43. Porteous J. Don't tip the scales! Care for patients involved in a police investigation. *Can Oper Room Nurs J.* 2005;23(3):12-16. [VA]

44. Modifications to the HIPAA privacy, security, enforcement, and breach notification rules under the Health Information Technology for Economic and Clinical Health Act and the Genetic Information Nondiscrimination Act; other modifications to the HIPAA rules. *Fed Regist.* 2013;78(17 Part 2):5566-5702. http://www.gpo.gov/fdsys/pkg/FR-2013-01-25/pdf/2013-01073.pdf. Accessed April 8, 2014.

45. 10 CFR 20. Standards for Protection Against Radiation. 2013. http://www.gpo.gov/fdsys/pkg/CFR-2013-title10-vol1/pdf/CFR-2013-title10-vol1-part20.pdf. Accessed April 8, 2014.

46. 10 CFR 35. Medical Use of Byproduct Material. 2011. http://www.gpo.gov/fdsys/pkg/CFR-2011-title10-vol1/pdf/CFR-2011-title10-vol1-part35.pdf. Accessed April 8, 2014.

47. Graham RP, Jakub JW, Brunette JJ, Reynolds C. Handling of radioactive seed localization breast specimens in the pathology laboratory. *Am J Surg Pathol.* 2012;36(11):1718-1723. [VB]

48. Michel R, Hofer C. Radiation safety precautions for sentinel lymph node procedures. *Health Phys.* 2004;86(2 Suppl):S35-S37. [VB]

49. Iodine-125 and palladium-103 low dose rate brachytherapy seeds used for localization of non-palpable lesions. US Nuclear Regulatory Commission. http://www.nrc.gov/materials/miau/med-use-toolkit/seed-localization.html. Accessed on April 8, 2014.

50. Fitzgibbons PL, LiVolsi VA. Recommendations for handling radioactive specimens obtained by sentinel lymphadenectomy. Surgical Pathology Committee of the College of American Pathologists and the Association of Directors of Anatomic and Surgical Pathology. *Am J Surg Pathol.* 2000;24(11):1549-1551. [IVB]

51. Miner TJ, Shriver CD, Flicek PR, et al. Guidelines for the safe use of radioactive materials during localization and resection of the sentinel lymph node. *Ann Surg Oncol.* 1999;6(1):75-82. [IIB]

52. Law M, Chow LW, Kwong A, Lam CK. Sentinel lymph node technique for breast cancer: radiation safety issues. *Semin Oncol.* 2004;31(3):298-303. [VB]

53. Renshaw AA, Kish R, Gould EW. Increasing radiation from sentinel node specimens in pathology over time. *Am J Clin Pathol.* 2010;134(2):299-302. [IIIB]

54. Coventry BJ, Collins PJ, Kollias J, et al. Ensuring radiation safety to staff in lymphatic tracing and sentinel lymph node biopsy surgery—some recommendations. *J Nuclear Med Rad Ther.* 2012:1-5. http://www.omicsonline.org/ensuring-radiation-safety-to-staff-in-lymphatic-tracing-and-sentinel-lymph-node-biopsy-surgery-some-recommendations-2155-9619.S2-008.php?aid=6937. Accessed April 8, 2014. [IIIC]

55. Pavlicek W, Walton HA, Karstaedt PJ, Gray RJ. Radiation safety with use of I-125 seeds for localization of nonpalpable breast lesions. *Acad Radiol.* 2006;13(7):909-915. [VB]

56. 10 CFR 20.1905. Exemptions to Labeling Requirements. 2013. http://www.gpo.gov/fdsys/pkg/CFR-2013-title10-vol1/pdf/CFR-2013-title10-vol1-part20.pdf. Accessed April 8, 2014.

57. 10 CFR 30.41. Transfer of Byproduct Material. 2013. US Nuclear Regulatory Commission. http://www.nrc.gov/reading-rm/doc-collections/cfr/part030/part030-0041.html. Accessed April 8, 2014.

58. 10 CFR 71.5 Transportation of Licensed Material. 2013. US Nuclear Regulatory Commission. http://www.nrc.gov/reading-rm/doc-collections/cfr/part071/part071-0005.html. Accessed April 8, 2014.

59. 21 CFR 821. Medical Device Tracking Requirements. 2013. US Food and Drug Administration. http://www.accessdata.fda.gov/scripts/cdrh/cfdocs/cfcfr/CFRSearch.cfm?CFRPart=821. Accessed April 8, 2014.

60. Medical device tracking; guidance for industry and FDA staff. US Food and Drug Administration. http://www.fda.gov/medicaldevices/deviceregulationandguidance/guidancedocuments/ucm071756.htm. Accessed April 8, 2014.

61. 21 CFR 803 Subpart C. User Facility Reporting Requirements. 2013. http://www.accessdata.fda.gov/scripts/cdrh/cfdocs/cfCFR/CFRSearch.cfm?CFRPart=803&showFR=1&subpartNode=21:8.0.1.1.3.3. Accessed April 8, 2014

62. Medical device reporting. US Food and Drug Administration. http://www.fda.gov/medicaldevices/safety/reportaproblem/default.htm. Accessed April 8, 2014.

63. MedWatch: The FDA Safety Information and Adverse Event Reporting Program. US Food and Drug Administration. http://www.fda.gov/Safety/MedWatch/. Accessed April 8, 2013.

64. Burlingame B. Tracking and documenting implants; Returning explants to patients. [Clinical Issues]. *AORN J.* 2012;95(2):288-296. [VA]

65. Policy on surgical specimens to be submitted to pathology for examination. Appendix M. 2007. College of American Pathologists. http://www.cap.org/apps/docs/laboratory_accreditation/build/pdf/surgical_specimens.pdf. Accessed April 8, 2014. [IVB]

66. Davidovitch RI, Temkin S, Weinstein BS, Singh JR, Egol KA. Utility of pathologic evaluation following removal of explanted orthopaedic internal fixation hardware. *Bull NYU Hosp Joint Dis.* 2010;68(1):18-21. [IIIC]

67. Greenberg CC, Regenbogen SE, Studdert DM, et al. Patterns of communication breakdowns resulting in injury to surgical patients. *J Am Coll Surg.* 2007;204(4):533-540. [IIIB]

68. Siegel JD, Rhinehart E, Jackson M, Chiarello L; the Healthcare Infection Control Practices Advisory Committee. 2007 guideline for isolation precautions: preventing transmission of infectious agents in healthcare settings. Centers for Disease Control and Prevention. http://www.cdc.gov/hicpac/pdf/isolation/isolation2007.pdf. Accessed April 8, 2014. [IVA]

69. 29 CFR 1910.1030. Hazardous Substances. Bloodborne Pathogens. 2013. Occupational Safety and

Health Administration. https://www.osha.gov/pls/oshaweb/owadisp.show_document?p_id=10051&p_table=STANDARDS. Accessed April 8, 2014. [Regulatory]

70. Sandbank S, Klein D, Westreich M, Shalom A. The loss of pathological specimens: incidence and causes. *Dermatol Surg.* 2010;36(7):1084-1086. [VB]

71. CFR 1910.1048: Hazardous substances. Formaldehyde. Occupational Safety and Health Administration. https://www.osha.gov/pls/oshaweb/owadisp.show_document?p_id=10075&p_table=STANDARDS. Accessed April 8. 2014. [Regulatory]

72. Makary MA, Epstein J, Pronovost PJ, Millman EA, Hartmann EC, Freischlag JA. Surgical specimen identification errors: a new measure of quality in surgical care. *Surgery.* 2007;141(4):450-455. [IIIA]

73. Quillen K, Murphy K. Quality improvement to decrease specimen mislabeling in transfusion medicine. *Arch Pathol Lab Med.* 2006;130(8):1196-1198. [VB]

74. College of American Pathologists; Valenstein PN, Raab SS, Walsh MK. Identification errors involving clinical laboratories: a College of American Pathologists Q-Probes study of patient and specimen identification errors at 120 institutions. *Arch Pathol Lab Med.* 2006;130(8):1106-1113. [IIIB]

75. Dock B. Improving the accuracy of specimen labeling. *Clin Lab Sci.* 2005;18(4):210-212. [VB]

76. Nakhleh RE, Idowu MO, Souers RJ, Meier FA, Bekeris LG. Mislabeling of cases, specimens, blocks, and slides: a College of American Pathologists study of 136 institutions. *Arch Pathol Lab Med.* 2011;135(8):969-974. [IIIB]

77. Bixenstine PJ, Zarbo RJ, Holzmueller CG, et al. Developing and pilot testing practical measures of preanalytic surgical specimen identification defects. *Am J Med Qual.* 2013;28(4):308-314. [IIIB]

78. Meier FA, Varney RC, Zarbo RJ. Study of amended reports to evaluate and improve surgical pathology processes. *Adv Anat Pathol.* 2011;18(5):406-413. [VB]

79. When a rose is not a rose: the problem of mislabeled specimens. Lab Med DirecTIPs. 2009. College of American Pathologists. http://www.cap.org/apps/portlets/contentViewer/show.do?printFriendly=true&contentReference=practice_management%2Fdirectips%2Fmislabeled_specimens.html. Updated February 23, 2010. Accessed April 14, 2014. [VB]

80. Makary MA, Holzmueller CG, Sexton JB, et al. Operating room debriefings. *Jt Comm J Qual Patient Saf.* 2006;32(7):407-410, 357. [VB]

81. Trask L, Tournas E. Barcode specimen collection improves patient safety. *Mlo: Medical Laboratory Observer.* 2012;44(4):42. [VB]

82. Francis DL, Prabhakar S, Sanderson SO. A quality initiative to decrease pathology specimen-labeling errors using radiofrequency identification in a high-volume endoscopy center. *Am J Gastroenterol.* 2009;104(4):972-975. [IIIB]

83. Colard D. Reduction of patient identification errors using technology. *Point of Care.* 2005;4(1):61-63. [VB]

84. Granata J. Getting a handle on specimen mislabeling. *J Emerg Nurs.* 2011;37(2):167-168. [VC]

85. Nichols JH, Bartholomew C, Brunton M, et al. Reducing medical errors through barcoding at the point of care. *Clin Leadersh Manag Rev.* 2004;18(6):328-334. [VB]

86. O'Neill E, Richardson-Weber L, McCormack G, Uhl L, Haspel RL. Strict adherence to a blood bank specimen labeling policy by all clinical laboratories significantly reduces the incidence of "wrong blood in tube." *Am J Clin Pathol.* 2009;132(2):164-168. [VB]

87. Rees S, Stevens L, Mikelsons D, Quam E, Darcy T. Reducing specimen identification errors. *J Nurs Care Qual.* 2012;27(3):253-257. [VB]

88. Bell WC, Young ES, Billings PE, Grizzle WE. The efficient operation of the surgical pathology gross room. *Biotechnic Histochem.* 2008;83(2):71-82. [VB]

89. Guideline for a safe environment of care, part 1. In: *Guidelines for Perioperative Practice.* Denver, CO: AORN; 2015:239-263. [IVA]

90. *NIOSH Pocket Guide to Chemical Hazards.* DHHS (NIOSH) Publication No. 2005-149 ed. Cincinnati, OH: National Institute for Occupational Safety and Health; 2007.

91. OSHA FactSheet: Formaldehyde. 2011. Occupational Safety and Health Administration. http://www.osha.gov/OshDoc/data_General_Facts/formaldehyde-factsheet.pdf. Accessed April 8, 2014. [Regulatory]

92. *ANSI/ISEA Z358.1-2009: American National Standard for Emergency Eyewash and Shower Equipment.* New York, NY: American National Standards Institute; 2009. [IVC]

93. Material Safety Data Sheet—Formalin 10%. 2013. American Master Tech. http://www.americanmastertech.com/PDF/SSFXBFO.PDF. Accessed April 8, 2014.

94. Buesa RJ, Peshkov MV. How much formalin is enough to fix tissues? *Ann Diagn Pathol.* 2012;16(3):202-209. [IIB]

95. Di Novi C, Minniti D, Barbaro S, Zampirolo MG, Cimino A, Bussolati G. Vacuum-based preservation of surgical specimens: an environmentally-safe step towards a formalin-free hospital. *Sci Total Environ.* 2010;408(16):3092-3095. [VB]

96. Bussolati G, Chiusa L, Cimino A, D'Armento G. Tissue transfer to pathology labs: under vacuum is the safe alternative to formalin. *Virchows Arch.* 2008;452(2):229-231. [VB]

97. Berton F, Di Novi C. Occupational hazards of hospital personnel: assessment of a safe alternative to formaldehyde. *J Occup Health.* 2012;54(1):74-78. [IB]

98. Al-Maaini R, Bryant P. The effectiveness of honey as a substitute for formalin in the histological fixation of tissue. *J Histotechnol.* 2006;29:173-176. [IIC]

99. Ozkan N, Salva E, Cakalagaoglu F, Tuzuner B. Honey as a substitute for formalin? *Biotechnic Histochem.* 2012;87(2):148-153. [IIC]

100. Gillespie JW, Best CJ, Bichsel VE, et al. Evaluation of non-formalin tissue fixation for molecular profiling studies. *Am J Pathol.* 2002;160(2):449-457. [IIB]

101. van Essen HF, Verdaasdonk MA, Elshof SM, de Weger RA, van Diest PJ. Alcohol based tissue fixation as an alternative for formaldehyde: influence on immunohistochemistry. *J Clin Pathol.* 2010;63(12):1090-1094. [IIB]

102. Buesa RJ. Histology without formalin? *Ann Diagn Pathol.* 2008;12(6):387-396. [VA]

103. Prento P, Lyon H. Commercial formalin substitutes for histopathology. *Biotechnic Histochem.* 1997;72(5):273-282. [IIB]

104. Kristensen T, Engvad B, Nielsen O, Pless T, Walter S, Bak M. Vacuum sealing and cooling as methods to preserve surgical specimens. *Appl Immunohistochem Mole Morphol.* 2011;19(5):460-469. [IIB]

105. Titford ME, Horenstein MG. Histomorphologic assessment of formalin substitute fixatives for diagnostic surgical pathology. *Arch Pathol Lab Med.* 2005;129(4):502-506. [IIB]

106. 42 CFR 493 Subpart K. Quality system for nonwaived testing. 2013. http://www.gpo.gov/fdsys/pkg/CFR-2013-title42-vol5/pdf/CFR-2013-title42-vol5-part493-subpartK.pdf. Accessed April 8, 2014.

107. *Histopathology and Cytopathology of Limited or No Clinical Value.* 2nd ed. London: Royal College of Pathologists; 2005. [IVB]

108. Guideline for perioperative health care information management. In: *Guidelines for Perioperative Practice.* Denver, CO: AORN, Inc; 2015:491-512. [IVB]

109. Standards of perioperative nursing. In: *Perioperative Standards and Recommended Practices.* Denver, CO: AORN, Inc; 2014:3-42. [IVB]

110. *State Operations Manual Appendix A: Survey Protocol, Regulations and Interpretive Guidelines for Hospitals.* Rev 84. 2013. Centers for Medicare & Medicaid Services. http://www.cms.gov/Regulations-and-Guidance/Guidance/Manuals/downloads/som107ap_l_ambulatory.pdf. Accessed April 8, 2014.

111. *State Operations Manual Appendix L: Guidance for Surveyors: Ambulatory Surgical Centers.* Rev 89. 2013. Centers for Medicare & Medicaid Services. http://www.cms.gov/Regulations-and-Guidance/Guidance/Manuals/downloads/som107ap_l_ambulatory.pdf. Accessed April 8, 2014.

112. RC.01.01.01: The hospital maintains complete and accurate medical records for each individual patient. In: *Hospital Accreditation Standards 2013.* Oakbrook Terrace, IL: Joint Commission Resources; 2013.

113. RC.02.01.03: The patient's medical record documents operative or other high-risk procedures and the use of moderate or deep sedation or anesthesia. In: *Joint Commission Comprehensive Accreditation and Certification Manual. Hospital.* e-edition release 5.1 ed. Oakbrook Terrace, IL: Joint Commission Resources; 2013.

114. RC.01.01.01: The organization maintains complete and accurate clinical records. In: *Standards for Ambulatory Care 2013: Standards, Elements of Performance Scoring Accreditation Policies.* Oakbrook Terrace, IL: The Joint Commission; 2013.

115. RC.02.01.03: The patient's clinical record documents operative or other high-risk procedures and the use of moderate or deep sedation or anesthesia. In: *Joint Commission Comprehensive Accreditation and Certification Manual. Ambulatory.* e-edition release 5.1 ed. Oakbrook Terrace, IL: Joint Commission Resources; 2013.

116. Clinical records and health information. In: *2013 Accreditation Handbook for Ambulatory Health Care.* Skokie, IL: Accreditation Association for Ambulatory Health Care; 2013:35-37.

117. Medical records: procedure room records. In: *Procedural Standards and Checklist for Accreditation of Ambulatory Surgery Facilities.* Version 3 ed. Gurnee, IL: American Association for Accreditation of Ambulatory Surgery Facilities; 2011:64-66.

118. Medical records: operating room records. In: *Regular Standards and Checklist for Accreditation of Ambulatory Surgery Facilities.* Version 13 ed. Gurnee, IL: American Association for Accreditation of Ambulatory Surgery Facilities; 2011:64-66.

119. Medical records: general. In: *Procedural Standards and Checklist for Accreditation of Ambulatory Surgery Facilities.* Version 3 ed. Gurnee, IL: American Association for Accreditation of Ambulatory Surgery Facilities; 2011:60-61.

120. Medical records: general. In: *Regular Standards and Checklist for Accreditation of Ambulatory Surgery Facilities.* Version 13 ed. Gurnee, IL: American Association for Accreditation of Ambulatory Surgery Facilities; 2011:61.

121. Medical records: pre-operative medical record. In: *Regular Standards and Checklist for Accreditation of Ambulatory Surgery Facilities.* Version 13 ed. Gurnee, IL: American Association for Accreditation of Ambulatory Surgery Facilities; 2011:62-63.

Acknowledgements

LEAD AUTHOR
Sharon A. Van Wicklin, MSN, RN, CNOR, CRNFA, CPSN, PLNC
Perioperative Nursing Specialist
AORN Nursing Department
Denver, Colorado

CONTRIBUTING AUTHOR
Ramona Conner, MSN, RN, CNOR
Manager, Standards and Guidelines
AORN Nursing Department
Denver, Colorado

The authors and AORN thank Marie A. Bashaw, DNP, RN, NEA-BC, CNOR, Clinical Assistant Professor, Wright State University College of Nursing and Health, Dayton, OH; Patricia Graybill-D'Ercole, MSN, RN, CNOR, CHL, CRCST, Clinical Specialist, Integra Life Science, York, PA; Deborah Farina Mulloy, PhD, RN, Associate Chief Nurse Quality and Center for Nursing Excellence, Brigham and Women's Hospital, Boston, MA for their assistance in developing this guideline.

PUBLICATION HISTORY

Originally approved November 2005, AORN Board of Directors. Published in *Standards, Recommended Practices, and Guidelines*, 2006 edition.

Reprinted March 2006, *AORN Journal.*

Minor editing revisions made to omit PNDS codes; reformatted September 2012 for publication in *Perioperative Standards and Recommended Practices*, 2013 edition.

Revised January 2014 for online publication in *Perioperative Standards and Recommended Practices.*

Minor editing revisions made in November 2014 for publication in *Guidelines for Perioperative Practice*, 2015 edition.

GUIDELINE FOR PREVENTION OF TRANSMISSIBLE INFECTIONS

The Guideline for Prevention of Transmissible Infections was approved by the AORN Recommended Practices Advisory Board. It was presented as proposed recommendations for comments by members and others. The guideline is effective December 15, 2012. The recommendations in the guideline are intended to be achievable and represent what is believed to be an optimal level of practice. Policies and procedures will reflect variations in practice settings and/or clinical situations that determine the degree to which the guideline can be implemented. AORN recognizes the various settings in which perioperative nurses practice; therefore, this guideline is adaptable to various practice settings. These practice settings include traditional operating rooms (ORs), ambulatory surgery centers, physicians' offices, cardiac catheterization laboratories, endoscopy suites, radiology departments, and all other areas where operative and other invasive procedures may be performed.

Purpose

The rapidly changing health care environment presents health care personnel with continual challenges in the form of newly recognized pathogens and well-known microorganisms that have become more resistant to today's therapeutic modalities. Protecting patients and health care practitioners from potentially infectious agent transmission continues to be a primary focus of perioperative registered nurses (RNs). The prevention and control of multidrug-resistant organisms (MDROs) requires that all health care organizations implement, evaluate, and adjust efforts to decrease the risk of transmission.

There are three principal elements required for an infection to occur:
- a source or reservoir,
- a susceptible host with a portal of entry to receive the infectious agent, and
- a method of transmission.[1]

This document provides guidance to perioperative RNs in implementing standard precautions and transmission-based precautions (ie, contact, droplet, airborne) to prevent infection in the perioperative practice setting. Additional guidance is provided for bloodborne pathogens; personal protective equipment (PPE); health care-associated infections and multidrug-resistant organisms (MDROs); immunization; and activities of health care workers with infections, exudative lesions, and nonintact skin. Finally, the document includes guidance for ongoing education and competency evaluation, documentation requirements, policies and procedures, and quality assurance and performance improvement processes.

Prevention of transmissible infections is a priority in the perioperative environment and includes considerations for environment of care, sharps safety and safe injection practices, hand hygiene, sterile technique, and sterilization. These topics are addressed in separate AORN guidelines and although they are mentioned briefly where applicable (eg, standard precautions), the broader discussions are outside the scope of this document.

Evidence Review

A medical librarian conducted a systematic search of the databases MEDLINE®, CINAHL®, Scopus®, and the Cochrane Database of Systematic Reviews for meta-analyses, systematic reviews, randomized controlled trials, guidelines, and additions to the *Morbidity and Mortality Weekly Report*. The report was also regularly consulted for newly added, relevant entries. Search terms included *infectious disease transmission, infectious skin diseases, soft tissue infections, blood-borne pathogens, gram-negative bacteria, gram-positive bacteria, gram-negative bacterial infections, gram-positive bacterial infections, viral hepatitis, viral meningitis, viral skin diseases, HIV infections, disease outbreaks, infectious disease transmission, needlestick injuries, occupational accidents, occupational health, occupational diseases, droplet precautions, standard precautions, isolation precautions, airborne precautions, patient isolation, microbial drug resistance, methicillin-resistant* Staphylococcus aureus, *methicillin resistance,* Staphylococcus aureus, *vancomycin resistance, vaccination, immunization, disaster planning, emergency preparedness, bioterrorism,* and *chemical terrorism.*

The search was limited to articles published in English between 1989 and 2011. The librarian established continuing alerts on the transmissible infection topics. The authors and medical librarian identified relevant guidelines from government agencies and standards-setting bodies. In addition, the authors requested articles that highlight the causes, identification, and treatment of transmissible infection, including some that were beyond the scope of this search.

Articles identified by the search were provided to the project team for evaluation. The team consisted of the lead author, three members of the Recommended Practices Advisory Board, and a doctorally prepared evidence appraiser. The lead author divided the search results into topics and assigned members of the team to review and critically appraise each article using the Johns Hopkins Evidence-Based Practice Model and the Research or Non-Research Evidence Appraisal Tools as appropriate. The literature was

TRANSMISSIBLE INFECTIONS

independently evaluated and appraised according to the strength and quality of the evidence. Each article was then assigned an appraisal score as agreed upon by consensus of the team. The appraisal score is noted in brackets after each reference, as applicable.

The collective evidence supporting each intervention within a specific recommendation was summarized and used to rate the strength of the evidence using the AORN Evidence Rating Model. Factors considered in review of the collective evidence were the quality of research, quantity of similar studies on a given topic, and consistency of results supporting a recommendation. The evidence rating is noted in brackets after each intervention.

Editor's note: *MEDLINE is a registered trademark of the US National Library of Medicine's Medical Literature Analysis and Retrieval System, Bethesda, MD. CINAHL, Cumulative Index to Nursing and Allied Health Literature, is a registered trademark of EBSCO Industries, Birmingham, AL. Scopus is a registered trademark of Elsevier B.V., Amsterdam, Netherlands.*

Recommendation I

Health care workers should use standard precautions when caring for all patients in the perioperative setting.

Standard precautions are the foundation for preventing transmission of infectious diseases. They apply to all patients and across all health care settings (eg, hospitals, ambulatory surgery centers, free-standing specialty care sites, interventional sites). Standard precautions include practices for hand hygiene, PPE, patient resuscitation, environmental control, respiratory hygiene/cough etiquette, sharps safety, and textiles and laundry.[1]

I.a. All personnel in the health care organization should follow established hand hygiene practices.[1,2] *[1: Strong Evidence]*

Hand hygiene is one of the most effective ways to prevent disease transmission and control infections in health care settings.[3]

I.b. Perioperative personnel should wear PPE whenever the possibility exists for exposure to blood or other potentially infectious materials. *[1: Strong Evidence/Regulatory Requirement]*

The use of PPE protects the health care provider's mucous membranes, airway, skin, and clothing from coming into contact with blood, body fluids, and other potentially infectious materials.[1,4] (See Recommendation VI.)

I.c. The health care provider should use a mouthpiece, resuscitation bag, or other ventilation device during resuscitation. *[1: Strong Evidence]*

Respiratory droplets are generated during cardiopulmonary resuscitation (CPR),[1] and if CPR is given to a patient with a transmissible infection, disease transfer is possible.[5-7] Mouthpieces, resuscitation bags, pocket masks with one-way valves, and other ventilation devices allow caregivers to perform CPR without exposing their nose and mouth to oral and respiratory fluids.[1]

I.d. The patient should be provided a clean, safe environment.[8-11] *[1: Strong Evidence]*

Hospital surfaces are often contaminated with health care-associated pathogens and may be responsible for cross-transmission.[12] Infections have been associated with surface contamination in hospital rooms, and the level of patient-to-patient transmission has been directly related to the level of environmental contamination.[13] In one case of an adenovirus outbreak in a military facility, during which 15 trainees were hospitalized for pneumonia, investigators recovered the infection serotype from several hospital surfaces.[14] The researchers concluded that there was a need to reinforce infection control guidelines.

Improved cleaning and disinfection of environmental surfaces can reduce the spread of numerous pathogens (eg, methicillin-resistant *Staphylococcus aureus* [MRSA], vancomycin-resistant *Enterococcus* spp [VRE], norovirus, *Clostridium difficile*, *Acinetobacter* spp).[13] Research has demonstrated that by consistently cleaning frequently touched items in the patient care environment (eg, toilet handholds, light switches, door knobs, nurse call devices, bedside rails), infections can be reduced.[10]

I.e. All people who enter the health care facility should practice respiratory hygiene and cough etiquette. *[1: Strong Evidence]*

Following an outbreak of severe acute respiratory syndrome (SARS) in 2003, the Centers for Disease Control and Prevention (CDC) expanded its guideline for infection prevention to include respiratory hygiene and cough etiquette.[1] Transmission of the virus was believed to occur because simple hygienic measures were not followed in health care facilities. Failure to use respiratory hygiene and cough etiquette may result in transmission of a respiratory tract infection.[1,15]

I.e.1. Respiratory hygiene and cough etiquette should include
- covering the mouth and nose with a tissue or a sleeve rather than the hand when coughing or sneezing;
- disposing of used tissues quickly;
- performing hand hygiene after coming into contact with respiratory secretions;
- having the person who exhibits signs of respiratory infection wear a surgical mask if he or she is able; and
- separating those who have a respiratory infection from others by more than 3 feet when possible.[1]

TRANSMISSIBLE INFECTIONS

I.e.2. Health care organizations should promote proper respiratory hygiene and cough etiquette by
- providing resources and instructions for performing hand hygiene in or near waiting areas,
- placing alcohol-based hand rub dispensers in convenient locations,
- keeping supplies for hand washing where sinks are available,
- offering surgical masks to coughing patients during periods of increased community respiratory infections (eg, as indicated by increased school absences or patients seeking care for such infections),
- encouraging patients who exhibit signs of respiratory infection to stay at least 3 feet away from others in common areas when possible, and
- posting signs at entrances and in strategic places within ambulatory and inpatient settings in all languages that are applicable to the population served and that provide instructions for proper respiratory hygiene and cough etiquette.[1]

I.e.3. Perioperative nurses should promote compliance with respiratory hygiene and cough etiquette by educating health care personnel, patients, and visitors to cover their mouth or nose with tissue or to sneeze or cough into the crook of their arm, especially during seasonal community outbreaks of viral respiratory infections (eg, influenza, adenovirus), and by providing products (eg, tissues, surgical masks, no-touch waste receptacles, hand hygiene products) as control measures for minimizing contact with respiratory secretions.[1,15]

I.f. Perioperative team members should use safe injection practices (eg, one syringe and one needle, complying with sharps safety measures).[1,16]
[1: Strong Evidence]

Using needles and syringes more than once increases the risk of infection, and unsafe medication injection practices have been implicated in outbreaks of hepatitis B and hepatitis C.[1,17-19] The CDC conducted investigations of four large outbreaks in ambulatory surgery facilities and found there is a need to reinforce safe injection practices.[19] The breaks in infection control practices were reinserting used needles into a multidose vial or solution container (eg, saline bag) and using a single needle or syringe to administer IV medication to multiple patients.

Appropriate methods to protect health care workers from exposure to hazardous materials or bloodborne pathogens and to decrease the risk of disease transmission through sharps injuries are specified in US Occupational Safety and Health Administration (OSHA) regulations.[4]

I.f.1. A syringe and needle should be used only once to administer a medication to a single patient, after which the syringe and needle should be discarded. When administering incremental doses to a single patient from the same syringe is an integral part of the procedure, the same syringe and needle may be reused, with strict adherence to aseptic technique, for the same patient as part of a single procedure. The syringe should never be left unattended and should be discarded immediately at the end of the procedure.[16]

I.f.2. Perioperative RNs should collaborate with pharmacists to procure and store single-dose vials rather than multidose vials.[16]

Reuse of multidose vials of medication is a concern as a cause of iatrogenic bloodborne pathogen infection.[18,20] Outbreaks of hepatitis B and C viruses in New York, Oklahoma, and Nebraska were attributed to unsafe injection practices that led to patient-to-patient transmission, including contamination of multidose medication vials and reuse of syringes and needles.[19]

HIV can be transmitted either parenterally or across mucous membranes. The risk of transmission from mucocutaneous exposure is estimated at 0.03%, and the risk of infection as a result of intact skin exposure is below detection.[20] Health care providers are among at-risk populations for occupational exposure to HIV, and transmission is significantly associated with procedures involving a needle placed in the source patient's blood vessel.[21]

Following fundamental infection-control principles (eg, safe injection practices, appropriate aseptic techniques) helps reduce the risk of bloodborne pathogen transmission.[18,19]

I.g. Reusable health care textiles should be changed and laundered after each patient use or when soiled. Health care textiles should be laundered in a health care-accredited laundry facility.[22]
[2: Moderate Evidence]

Health care textiles (eg, patient gowns, bed linens, privacy curtains, washcloths) may become contaminated by bacteria and fungi during wear or use, and microbes can survive on textiles for extended periods.[23,24] Contaminated textiles could contaminate the environment or health care providers' hands or clothing.[1]

Recommendation II

Contact precautions should be used when providing care to patients who are known or suspected to be infected or colonized with microorganisms that are transmitted by direct contact or indirect contact.

TRANSMISSIBLE INFECTIONS

Contact precautions are in addition to standard precautions, including PPE (eg, gloves, gowns, masks, face protection). Additional precautions include flushing mucous membranes and washing skin that is exposed to blood or other potentially infectious materials, taking special considerations for patient transport, increasing environmental cleaning, adequate cleaning and disinfection of patient care equipment and items, and coordinating with an infection preventionist.

Contact with infected patients or contaminated surfaces leads to pathogen transmission 45% of the time, according to a review of 1,022 health care-associated infection outbreaks.[25] Health care providers are at risk of spreading health care-associated infections (eg, *S aureus,* VRE) through contact, according to a study in which researchers saw positive cultures from imprints of health care providers' hands after contact with surfaces near 34 out of 64 patients.[26] Adherence to contact precautions helps prevent transmission of infectious agents, including MDROs.[1,27-29]

Clostridium difficile is known to be transmitted by contact with contaminated people or environmental surfaces,[12] and skin contamination and environmental shedding of the pathogen can persist after symptoms resolve for up to four weeks after therapy.[30] An outbreak of staphylococcal bullous impetigo during a five-month period in a maternity ward was caused by contact with an auxiliary nurse, who was an asymptomatic nasal carrier of the strain.[31] In a study of VRE transmission, researchers cultured the intact skin of 22 colonized patients and sites in the patients' rooms before and after care by 98 health care providers.[32] The health care providers touched 151 VRE-negative sites after touching a VRE-positive site. The researchers found that VRE was transferred via health care providers' hands or gloves 10.6% of the time.

Contact precautions, as part of an overall infection control program, have been shown to decrease MRSA infection and transmission[33,34] and multidrug resistant *Acinetobacter baumannii* infection.[35]

II.a. Personal protective equipment should be worn in the perioperative setting as part of contact precautions. *[1: Strong Evidence/Regulatory Requirement]*

The use of PPE protects the health care provider's mucous membranes, airway, skin, and clothing from coming into contact with blood, body fluids, and other potentially infectious materials.[1,4] (See Recommendation VI.)

II.a.1. Perioperative personnel should don PPE upon room entry and discard PPE upon exiting the room when caring for a patient who requires contact precautions.[1]

Donning a gown and gloves when treating a patient who requires contact precautions and discarding them when leaving the patient's room helps contain pathogens, especially those that can be transmitted through environmental contamination (eg, VRE, *C difficile*, norovirus).[1]

Although PPE as part of contact precautions may help contain pathogens, there is some conflicting evidence. One cluster-randomized trial in an intensive care unit setting indicated that contact precautions (ie, gloves, gowns, hand hygiene) were not significantly more effective in preventing transmission of MRSA or VRE than universal gloving.[36] In six months, there were 5,434 admissions to 10 intervention intensive care units compared with 3,705 admissions to eight control intensive care units, and the rate of colonization or infection per 1,000 patient-days at risk did not differ significantly between the intervention and control sites. However, the providers did not use contact precautions as often as required: when contact precautions were specified, gloves were used for a median of 82% of contacts, gowns for 77% of contacts, and hand hygiene after 69% of contacts.[36]

II.b. Health care providers must wash their hands and skin with soap and water or flush their mucous membranes with water immediately or as soon as possible after coming into direct contact with blood or other potentially infectious materials.[1,4] *[1: Strong Evidence/Regulatory Requirement]*

Exposure to environmental pathogens (eg, *Aspergillus* spp, *Legionella* spp) can cause illness among health care providers and adverse patient outcomes.[9] There is a risk of bloodborne disease transmission from splash injuries during endourology and other minimally invasive procedures, according to a study of 118 procedures performed by five surgeons.[37] The researchers noted that mucocutaneous and transconjunctival exposure are important portals for transmission. In a study of 25 consecutive patients who were undergoing dental surgery for impacted mandibular third molars, investigators concluded that surgeons were exposed to possible bloodborne infections by splashing in nearly 90% of the procedures.[38]

II.c. When patient transport is necessary, precautions should be taken to reduce the opportunity for transmission of microorganisms to other patients, personnel, and visitors and to reduce contamination of the environment.[1] *[1: Strong Evidence]*

II.c.1. Patient transport should be limited to essential diagnostic and therapeutic procedures that cannot be performed in the patient's room.[1]

II.c.2. When transport is necessary, appropriate barriers should be used on the patient to cover affected areas if infectious skin lesions or drainage are present. These barriers should be consistent with the route and risk of transmission.[1]

II.c.3. When a patient who requires contact precautions is transported from one area to another, the nurse should notify the receiving team members that the patient is coming and what precautions should be taken to prevent transmission.[1]

II.d. Environmental cleaning should be included as part of a program to control the transmission of MDROs.[27] *[1: Strong Evidence]*

Environmental reservoirs have been implicated in transmission of VRE and other MDROs. Thorough cleaning and disinfection practices, including of frequently touched surfaces (eg, bedrails, charts, bedside commodes, doorknobs), can help control the spread of MDROs.[27] Improved environmental cleaning can reduce the transmission of multidrug-resistant *A baumannii*, MRSA, VRE, *Acinetobacter* spp, and *C difficile*.[13,39-41]

II.d.1. Patient care areas of patients infected with *C difficile* should be cleaned with a 10% bleach solution and allowed to air dry.

Contamination of environmental surfaces contributes to the spread of *C difficile*.[42] *Clostridium difficile* is a spore that can survive for months in the environment and is not killed by standard processes for environmental cleaning.[39]

Educating housekeeping personnel on environmental cleaning practices significantly reduces the amount of contamination, according to a prospective, six-week before-and-after study.[42] When housekeeping personnel used 10% bleach solution to disinfect frequently touched surfaces (eg, bed rails, bedside tables, call buttons, telephones, toilet seats, door handles), contamination was significantly reduced, from nine rooms with positive cultures before cleaning to two rooms with positive cultures after cleaning.

II.e. All noncritical equipment (eg, commodes, IV pumps, ventilators, computers, personal electronic devices) should be cleaned and disinfected before use on another patient and should be handled in a manner to prevent health care provider or environmental contact with potentially infectious materials.[1] *[1: Strong Evidence]*

II.e.1. Dedicated noncritical equipment such as stethoscopes, blood pressure cuffs, and electronic thermometers may be used.[1,43]

II.f. Routine cleaning of environmental surfaces (eg, floors, walls) should be performed according to facility policy and more frequently when necessary.[11] *[2: Moderate Evidence]*

Surface cleaning and disinfection practices are recommended to manage outbreaks caused by *Acinetobacter* spp, *C difficile*, MRSA, norovirus, and VRE.[13] Cleaning may need to be more thorough or performed more frequently depending on the patient's level of hygiene, the degree of environmental contamination, and the type of infectious agent (eg, if the infectious reservoir is the intestinal tract).[1]

II.g. An infection preventionist should be consulted for guidance when measures are indicated to prevent the spread of highly transmissible or epidemiologically important pathogens.[1] *[1: Strong Evidence]*

II.h. Perioperative nurses should evaluate and manage any negative patient outcomes that may be caused by using contact precautions. *[1: Strong Evidence]*

Studies have shown that health care providers are half as likely to enter the rooms of or examine patients who require contact precautions.[44,45] Patients may experience increased anxiety and depression and decreased levels of satisfaction under isolation precautions.[27,46]

A systematic review of 15 studies from 1989 to 2008[46] indicated four adverse outcomes related to contact precautions:
- less patient-to-health care provider contact,
- changes to systems of care that produce delays and more noninfectious adverse events,
- increased symptoms of depression and anxiety, and
- decreased satisfaction with care.

Although the majority of patients believe that contact precautions protect them and others, it is important to carefully consider whether contact precautions are necessary and to communicate the primary function of using contact precautions to the patient.[47]

By educating a patient who requires contact precautions and his or her family members, the perioperative nurse may be able to minimize feelings of isolation, depression, and anxiety. Nurses are in a position to evaluate patients for negative feelings, improve social contact, and provide education and frequent communication to the patient.

Recommendation III

Droplet precautions should be used throughout the perioperative environment (ie, preoperative, intraoperative, postoperative) when providing care to patients who are known or suspected to be infected with microorganisms that can be transmitted by large droplets.[1] *Amb*

Droplet precautions in addition to standard precautions reduce the risk of pathogens that spread through close respiratory or mucous membrane contact (eg, adenovirus, group A streptococcus, influenza, *Neisseria meningitides*, pertussis, rhinovirus).[1] Droplet precautions include donning PPE, considering patient placement to minimize contact with other patients, consulting with an infection preventionist, and placing a mask on the patient during transport.

Droplets in exhaled breath (ie, mouth or nose breathing, coughing, talking) may carry microorganisms that can be transmitted over short and long distances,[48] and infected droplets may originate during certain procedures (eg, suctioning, endotracheal induction, CPR).[1,5] During the 2003 SARS outbreak in Toronto, Canada, 26 health care providers contracted the virus from seven patients. Researchers concluded that close contact with the ill patients' airways (eg, during intubation, transportation) and failure to prevent exposure to respiratory secretions through infection control practices were associated with transmission.[49]

III.a. When a patient believed to have mumps, rubella, or pertussis enters the health care facility, droplet precautions should be implemented and followed, and only health care providers with presumptive immunity should be exposed to the patient.[50] *[1: Strong Evidence]*

III.b. Personal protective equipment should be worn in the perioperative setting as part of droplet precautions. *[1: Strong Evidence/Regulatory Requirement]*
The use of PPE protects the health care provider's mucous membranes, airway, skin, and clothing from coming into contact with blood, body fluids, and other potentially infectious materials.[1,4] (See Recommendation VI.)

III.b.1. Perioperative personnel should don surgical masks when in close contact with a patient who requires droplet precautions.[1]
Surgical masks prevent the transmission of large droplets (ie, greater than 5 microns) and, worn correctly, protect health care providers who are within close proximity of a patient who requires droplet precautions.[1] Masks serve as protection from infectious microorganisms from patients (eg, respiratory secretions, blood spatters, body fluid).

III.b.2. Health care providers should change PPE and clothing when they are exposed to patient secretions or droplets.
Changing PPE can help prevent cross-contamination of influenza viruses.[51]

III.c. Patients who require droplet precautions should be placed in a single-patient room before and after surgery. *[1: Strong Evidence]*
Single-patient placement in an isolation room helps prevent the spread of infection from patient to patient.[1,27,52] Special air handling and ventilation are not required as a part of droplet precautions.[1]

III.c.1. If single patient placement is not possible, the perioperative nurse should collaborate with the facility infection preventionist to establish optimal preoperative and postoperative placement for a patient who requires droplet precautions.[1]
The infection preventionist can help assess and mitigate the risks associated with non-isolation placement options (eg, cohorting, keeping the patient with an existing roommate) to minimize the potential for cross-contamination.

III.c.2. Patients who require droplet precautions should be placed at least 3 feet away from other patients.[1]
The defined risk area (ie, > 3 feet) around the patient is based on epidemiologic and simulated infection studies.[1]

III.c.3. If possible, draw curtains or close doors.
Curtains and doors help to separate the patients and reduce transmission of infectious organisms.

III.d. When transporting the patient from one area to another, the patient should wear a mask.[1] *[1: Strong Evidence]*
Masks prevent possible spread of infectious respiratory secretions from the patient to other individuals.

Recommendation IV

Airborne precautions should be used when providing care to patients who are known or suspected to be infected with microorganisms that can be transmitted by the airborne route.

Some procedures performed in the perioperative setting require access to the airway; therefore, special infection-control considerations for preventing transmission of airborne disease are necessary.[53] Airborne precautions in addition to standard precautions for the OR include consultation with an infection preventionist, respiratory protection, PPE, patient placement and transport precautions, administrative controls, and environmental controls.[9,53]

Airborne transmission can occur when small particles that contain infectious agents that remain infective over time and distance are inhaled.[1] This is specific to particles that are approximately 1 μm to 5 μm and that remain airborne for prolonged periods by normal air currents, which allow them to spread throughout a room or building.[53] The use of airborne precautions can help minimize transfer of diseases that are spread by the airborne route[54] (eg, *Mycobacterium tuberculosis* [TB], rubeola, Varicella zoster[1]).

IV.a. An infection preventionist should be consulted to determine necessary supplemental controls for patients requiring airborne isolation.[53] *[1: Strong Evidence]*

IV.b. When a patient suspected of measles infection enters the health care facility, all health care personnel should use respiratory protection, regardless of presumptive immunity, when providing care to the patient. *[1: Strong Evidence]*
Measles vaccination can fail and is ineffective for preventing measles about 1% of the time. Measles is highly contagious and transmission can occur anywhere from four days before presentation of a rash to four days after the rash resolves.[50]

IV.c. When a patient with confirmed or suspected varicella infection enters the health care facility, airborne and contact precautions should be implemented and followed, and only health care providers with evidence of immunity should provide care to the patient.[50] *[1: Strong Evidence]*

IV.d. Personal protective equipment should be worn in the perioperative setting as part of airborne precautions. *[1: Strong Evidence/Regulatory Requirement]*

The use of PPE protects the health care provider's mucous membranes, airway, skin, and clothing from coming into contact with blood, body fluids, and other potentially infectious materials.[1,4] (See Recommendation VI.)

IV.d.1. Perioperative personnel should don a surgical mask or N95 or higher level respirator, depending on disease-specific recommendations, before entering the room of a patient who requires airborne precautions.[1]

Wearing an N95 or higher level respirator, or a mask if a respirator is not available, reduces the risk of airborne transmission.[1]

IV.d.2. Respiratory protective devices worn during care of a patient with TB should be
- certified by the CDC/US National Institute for Occupational Safety and Health (NIOSH) as a nonpowered particulate filter respirator (N-, R-, or P-95, 99, or 100), including a disposable respirator or powered air-purifying respirator with high efficiency filters,[55] and
- available in different sizes and models to accommodate the different facial sizes and characteristics of health care providers.[53]

IV.e. An airborne infection isolation room should be used if available for patients who require airborne precautions, including during surgery and postoperative recovery.[1,53] *[1: Strong Evidence]*

Use of special air handling and ventilation systems such as an airborne infection isolation room helps prevent the spread of airborne pathogens, particularly TB, rubeola, and varicella zoster, and is recommended during procedures that can generate infectious aerosols (eg, endotracheal intubation, bronchoscopy, suctioning, autopsy procedures involving oscillating saws).[1(p31)]

IV.e.1. If no airborne infection isolation room is available, a portable anteroom system (PAS)-high-efficiency particulate air (HEPA) combination unit may be used.

A pilot study comparing freestanding HEPA filter units placed inside the OR with a novel PAS-HEPA combination unit that was placed outside the OR showed that the PAS-HEPA unit was more effective.[56] The PAS-HEPA unit achieved a downward evacuation of plume, away and toward the main entry door from the sterile field. Comparatively, the portable freestanding HEPA unit inside the OR moved the plume vertically upward and directly into the breathing zone where the surgical team would be during a procedure. Results indicated that the PAS-HEPA system effectively removed more than 94% of an initial release of at least 500,000 submicron particles per cubic foot within 20 minutes after release.

IV.f. When transporting the patient from an airborne infection isolation room to the OR, the patient should wear a mask if clinically appropriate.[1] Patients should be transported directly to the OR, bypassing the preoperative area, and transferred directly to an airborne infection isolation room in the postanesthesia care unit or other part of the hospital at the end of the procedure. *[1: Strong Evidence]*

IV.g. After cough-inducing procedures are performed in the OR, sufficient time should be allowed for 99% or more of airborne particles to be removed before sterile supplies are opened for subsequent patients. *[1: Strong Evidence]*

Performing cough-inducing procedures such as intubation, extubation, and bronchoscopy increases the likelihood that droplet nuclei will be expelled into the air.[53] For example, by waiting to place another patient in the room, the risk of airborne transmission of TB is reduced. The length of time required to expel more than 99% of airborne contaminants varies by the efficiency of the ventilation or filtration system.

IV.h. Elective surgery should be postponed for patients who have suspected or confirmed TB until the patient is determined to be noninfectious. If surgery cannot be postponed, perioperative personnel should follow airborne precautions and consult with an infection preventionist.[9,53] *[1: Strong Evidence]* Amb

Postponing elective surgery may prevent transmission of TB.

IV.h.1. A single-use, disposable bacterial filter should be placed between the anesthesia circuit and the patient's airway.

Placing a bacterial filter between the anesthesia circuit and the patient's airway prevents contamination of the anesthesia equipment and release of tubercle bacilli into the room.[9,53] The preferred filter will filter particles 0.3 μm or larger in size in both loaded and unloaded states and will have a filter efficiency of 95% (ie, filter penetration of < 5%) at the maximum design flow rates of the ventilator for the service life of the filter.[53]

IV.h.2. The patient should be intubated and extubated and placed for recovery in an airborne infection isolation room. If intubation or extubation must be performed in the OR, a

portable, industrial-grade HEPA filter should be used to supplement air cleaning in the following manner:
- position the unit near the patient's breathing zone,
- obtain engineering consultation to determine the appropriate placement,
- switch the portable unit off during the surgical procedure, and
- provide fresh air according to ventilation standards for the OR.[9]

Switching the unit off during the procedure is recommended because after the patient is intubated, the airway is circulating in a closed system; therefore, the portable units do not serve any purpose while the patient is intubated. Fresh air must be provided because portable units do not meet the requirements for the number of fresh air changes per hour.[9]

IV.h.3. If the patient is intubated or extubated in the OR, the OR doors should remain closed until adequate time has passed for air changes per hour to clean 99% of airborne particles from the air (eg, 15 air exchanges per hour for 28 minutes to remove 99.9% of airborne contaminants).[9]

IV.h.4. Standard cleaning and disinfection procedures should be followed after surgery on a patient who has TB, and should only be performed after the appropriate amount of time for air ventilation. Personal respiratory protective equipment is not necessary for cleaning an OR if the appropriate ventilation time is allowed. If room cleaning activities begin before the appropriate amount of time for air ventilation, cleaning personnel should wear N95 respirators or powered air-purifying respirators.[53]

IV.i. Administrative controls should be established to reduce the risk of TB exposure to patients and personnel. Administrative controls should include
- implementing work practices for managing patients with suspected or confirmed TB;
- ensuring potentially contaminated equipment (eg, endoscopes) is properly cleaned and sterilized or disinfected;
- training and educating health care providers about TB prevention, transmission, and symptoms;
- establishing a TB screening program to screen and evaluate health care providers who are at risk for TB or who might be exposed to *M tuberculosis*; and
- implementing a respiratory protection program for personnel requiring fit testing and certification to use an N95 respirator.[53]

[1: Strong Evidence]

IV.j. Environmental controls should be established to prevent the spread of airborne diseases. Environmental controls should include
- controlling the source of infection by using local exhaust ventilation (eg, hoods, tents, booths),[53]
- diluting and removing contaminated air with general ventilation,[53]
- controlling airflow to prevent contamination of air in areas adjacent to the source,[53]
- cleaning the air using HEPA filtration or ultraviolet germicidal irradiation,[53]
- using central wall suction units with inline filters to evacuate minimal surgical smoke,[9,57] and
- using a mechanical smoke evacuation system with HEPA filtration to manage large amounts of surgical smoke.[9]

[1: Strong Evidence]

The CDC recommends environmental controls to prevent the spread of airborne infections (eg, TB)[53] and to minimize exposure to laser plume that may contain infectious material (eg, human papilloma virus).[9]

Recommendation V

Health care personnel must follow the OSHA bloodborne pathogens standard when there is a risk of exposure to blood or other potentially infectious materials.[4]

Bloodborne pathogens are pathogenic microorganisms that are present in human blood and can cause disease (eg, hepatitis B, HIV).[4] Federal and state regulations and organizational standards[58,59] mandating bloodborne pathogen guidelines are intended to reduce health care provider exposure to bloodborne pathogens and to minimize the risk of infection.

There has been a focus on preventing bloodborne transmission of hepatitis B, hepatitis C, and HIV in particular.[1,19,60-62] These viruses are more easily transmitted parenterally or across mucous membranes.[20]

Methods for preventing bloodborne pathogen exposure include using PPE, implementing engineering and work practice controls, following infection prevention precautions, and establishing and following an infection control plan.

V.a. Health care personnel must wear PPE in the perioperative setting as part of the bloodborne pathogens standard.[4] [1: Strong Evidence]

The use of PPE protects the health care provider's mucous membranes, airway, skin, and clothing from coming into contact with blood, body fluids, and other potentially infectious materials.[1,4] Appropriate PPE does not permit blood or other potentially infectious materials to pass through to or reach the employee's work clothes, street clothes, undergarments, skin, eyes, mouth, or other mucous membranes under normal conditions of use and for the duration that the PPE is used.[4] (See Recommendation VI.)

TRANSMISSIBLE INFECTIONS

V.a.1. If a garment is penetrated by blood or other potentially infectious materials, the health care provider must remove the garment immediately or as soon as possible.[4]

V.a.2. Health care personnel must wear gloves when hand contact with blood, other potentially infectious materials, mucous membranes, or non-intact skin can be reasonably anticipated; when performing vascular access procedures; and when handling or touching contaminated items or surfaces.[4]

V.a.3. Health care personnel must wear masks in combination with eye protection devices whenever splashes, spray, spatter, or droplets of blood or other potentially infectious materials may be generated and eye, nose, or mouth contamination can be reasonably anticipated.[4]

Eye protection devices include goggles, glasses with solid side shields, and chin-length face shields.

V.a.4. Health care personnel must wear gowns, aprons, and other protective body clothing when exposure to blood or other potentially infectious materials is anticipated.[4]

V.a.5. Health care personnel must wear surgical caps or hoods and shoe covers or boots when gross contamination can be reasonably anticipated (eg, orthopedic surgery).[4]

V.b. Food and drink must not be taken into the semi-restricted or restricted areas of the perioperative suite. Food and drink must not be kept in refrigerators, freezers, shelves, or cabinets or on counter tops or work spaces where blood or other potentially infectious materials are present.[4] *[1: Regulatory Requirement]*

V.c. Perioperative personnel must use engineering and work practice controls.[4] *[1: Strong Evidence/Regulatory Requirement]*

Engineering controls isolate or remove the risk of exposure, and work practice controls reduce the likelihood of exposure by changing the method of performing a task.[4]

Engineering controls include
- needleless systems,[4,63,64]
- self-sheathing needles,[4] and
- sharps storage and disposal containers.[4]

Work practice controls include
- prohibiting risky handling of needles and sharps,
- prohibiting recapping of needles by a two-handed technique,[4]
- using a neutral zone or hands-free technique for passing sharps,[4,65] and
- double gloving during all surgical procedures (See Recommendation VI.b.).

V.d. Health care organizations must establish a written exposure control plan, make it accessible to employees, and review and update it at least annually.[4] *[1: Regulatory Requirement]*

Recommendation VI

Perioperative personnel must wear PPE when exposure to blood or other potentially infectious materials is anticipated.[4]

The OSHA standard requires employers to provide appropriate PPE to health care providers at no cost to reduce the risk of skin and mucous membrane exposure to blood, body fluids, and other potentially infectious materials.[4]

All health care providers are responsible for ensuring the safety of patients, other health care providers, their own family members, and the community.[66] According to the Workers' Family Protection Task Force, there are limited data to quantify household exposures to potentially infectious organisms; however, workers who may not exhibit negative effects from workplace exposure still may expose their family members by taking infectious pathogens home (eg, occupationally acquired hepatitis C or HIV). Existing standards that require employers and employees to reduce occupational risks (eg, using PPE, engineering controls) protect the workers' families as well.

It is the employer's responsibility to ensure that PPE is available and readily accessible, alternatives are available for employees with allergies, and that personnel use the appropriate PPE. Personal protective equipment includes gloves, gowns, eye protection, masks, and respirators.

VI.a. Gloves must be worn when hand contact with blood or other potentially infectious materials, mucous membranes, or non-intact skin can be reasonably anticipated,[4] including when
- performing vascular access procedures[3,4];
- coming into direct contact with patients who are colonized or infected with pathogens (eg, VRE, MRSA, respiratory syncytial virus)[27]; and
- handling or touching contaminated patient care items or environmental surfaces.[4]

[1: Strong Evidence/Regulatory Requirement]

Gloves help prevent health care providers' hands from becoming contaminated by patient blood, body fluids, and other potentially infectious materials.[3,4,26,32,67,68] Gloves have been found to protect health care providers' hands from VRE contamination[69] and to reduce the risks of sharps injuries.[70]

VI.a.1. Unsterile gloves should be visually inspected upon donning, before contact with potentially contaminated surfaces, and periodically throughout use.[71] After use, perioperative personnel should remove gloves, discard them, and perform hand hygiene.

VI.a.2. Sterile gloves should be visually inspected immediately upon donning and before contact with sterile supplies or the sterile field.

TRANSMISSIBLE INFECTIONS

Gloves may have perforations or tears that occur in the manufacturing process or as gloves are donned.

VI.a.3. Sterile gloves should be changed
- after each patient contact;
- when a visible defect is noted;
- when suspected or actual contamination occurs; and
- when a suspected or actual perforation occurs.[4,72,73]

Breaches in the glove barrier pose a risk for transmission of bloodborne pathogens during surgical procedures. Glove perforation also increases the risk of surgical site infection (SSI).[74]

Depending on the duration of wear, surgical gloves can develop microperforations that are not immediately recognizable to the wearer.[75-77] These perforations allow bacteria from the surgical site to pass through to the wearer's hands. One method for preventing this is to mandate regular glove changes in organizational policy. Changing gloves at regular intervals may decrease the incidence of glove perforation and bacterial contamination during surgical procedures.[73,77,78]

VI.a.4. Use of polyvinyl chloride or vinyl gloves should be limited to brief, low-risk exposures.

Research has shown that vinyl and polyvinyl gloves have a higher failure rate in use than nitrile or latex gloves.[71,79-81] In a study of 137 procedures, researchers noted higher microbial contamination of the health care providers' hands and a higher frequency of leaks with vinyl gloves compared to latex.[71] Similarly, a study of 886 examination gloves showed vinyl gloves were much more likely to leak than latex (51.3% vs 19.7%) as demonstrated by a standardized clinical protocol designed to mimic patient care activities.[79] Research also has indicated polyvinyl chloride gloves fail to protect against virus exposure 22% of the time.[82]

Comparisons of different glove types have supported the decreased durability of vinyl and polyvinyl chloride gloves. Researchers evaluated 2,000 gloves (ie, 800 latex, 800 vinyl, 400 nitrile) and tested them immediately out of the box and after manipulations designed to simulate in-use conditions.[81] Vinyl gloves failed 12% to 61% of the time, whereas latex and nitrile had failure rates of 0% to 4% and 1% to 3%, respectively.

Another comparison involving 5,510 medical examination gloves (1,464 nitrile, 1,052 latex, 1,006 copolymer, 1,988 vinyl) showed that vinyl and copolymer (ie, polyvinyl chloride) gloves were less effective barriers than latex and nitrile.[80] Results showed 8.2% failure rates for the vinyl and copolymer gloves compared to 1.3% for nitrile and 2.2% for latex.

VI.b. Perioperative team members should wear two pairs of surgical gloves, one over the other, during surgical and other invasive procedures with the potential for exposure to blood, body fluids, or other potentially infectious materials. When double gloves are worn, perforation indicator systems should be used. *[1: Strong Evidence]*

Glove barrier failure is a common occurrence in the perioperative setting. Glove failures can be caused by punctures, tears by sharp devices, or spontaneous failures. Breaches in the glove barrier pose a risk of transmission of bloodborne pathogens during surgery. Wearing double gloves helps prevent SSI and protect health care providers' hands.[83-89]

According to a study of 155 surgeons and residents in Canada, double gloving is an effective means to reduce the risk of percutaneous injury.[90] Double gloving also minimizes the amount of blood that is transferred to the health care provider's hands during a needlestick injury,[91] reduces the risk of glove perforation associated with lengthy surgical procedures,[92] and reduces the risk of perforation of the innermost glove.[85]

Double gloving or double gloving with an indicator glove system may increase the wearer's awareness of a perforation and thereby protect against exposure to bloodborne pathogens during surgery.[86,89,93,94] In one 24-month study,[86] researchers investigated the effects of double gloving with inner indicator gloves and found that the frequency of seeing blood on the hand after surgery was higher with single gloving than double gloving. They also noted that surgical team members were more likely to change their gloves during surgery when they double gloved with an indicator system compared with double gloving alone.

VI.b.1. When the invasive procedure is completed, perioperative personnel should remove both pairs of gloves, discard them, and perform hand hygiene.[2]

VI.c. Perioperative personnel must wear fluid-resistant attire during activities that generate splashes, spatter, sprays, or aerosols of blood or other potentially infectious materials.[4] *[1: Regulatory Requirement]*

The CDC recommends wearing fluid-resistant gowns for all patient contact.[1] Fluid-resistant attire protects health care providers' skin from being exposed to blood, body fluids, and other potentially infectious materials. Surgical scrub attire, laboratory coats, or jackets worn over personal clothing are not considered PPE.[1]

VI.d. Health care personnel must wear eye protection when splashes, spray, spatter, or droplets of blood or other potentially infectious materials can be reasonably anticipated.[4] *[1: Regulatory Requirement]*

The CDC recommends eye protection as part of standard precautions[1] and when there is a risk of infectious materials entering the eye.[95] Using eye protection helps prevent exposure to bloodborne pathogens and other diseases (eg, SARS, TB, *Neisseria meningitidis*) during aerosol-generating procedures, including bronchoscopy, endotracheal intubation, and open suctioning of the respiratory tract.[1]

Infectious diseases, including adenovirus, herpes simplex, *S aureus*, hepatitis B, hepatitis C, and HIV, can be transmitted through the mucous membranes of the eye (ie, conjunctiva).[95] These infectious agents can be introduced directly to the eye by blood splashes or respiratory droplets that are generated during coughing or suctioning or from touching the eyes with contaminated fingers or other objects.[95]

The type of eye protection that is necessary depends on the circumstances of exposure, other PPE that is being used, and personal vision needs; however, regular prescription eyeglasses and contact lenses are not considered eye protection.[95] Appropriate eye protection includes goggles, face shields, and full-face respirators. The CDC recommends selecting eye protection based on other PPE requirements to ensure proper fit and optimal protection.[95]

VI.d.1. Goggles should fit snugly, especially at the corners of the eye and across the brow, be indirectly vented, and have anti-fog properties.

Fitted, indirectly vented goggles with a manufacturer's anti-fog coating are the most reliable and practical means of protecting health care providers' eyes from splashes, sprays, and respiratory droplets. They can be fit over prescription glasses. Safety glasses do not provide splash or droplet protection and are not recommended for infection control purposes.[95]

VI.d.2. Face shields should be selected for circumstances where eye protection alone is not sufficient.

Face shields provide protection to the eyes and other areas of the face. Face shields that have crown and chin protection and wrap around the face to the point of the ear allow for the best face and eye protection from splashes and sprays. Although disposable face shields that fit loosely and are made of light-weight films with attached surgical masks are available, these may not provide complete protection.[95]

VI.d.3. Full facepiece elastomeric respirators and powered air-purifying respirators should be selected based on the respiratory hazard in an infection control situation.[95]

Full facepiece elastomeric respirators and powered air-purifying respirators provide highly effective eye protection in addition to respiratory protection.[95] These devices require prescription inserts for health care providers who wear glasses to avoid compromising the seal around the face. Another option for health care providers who wear prescription glasses is a powered air-purifying respirator that is designed with a loose-fitting face piece or with a hood that completely covers the head and neck.

VI.d.4. Eye protection should be removed by handling only the portion of the equipment that secures the device to the head.

By removing eye protection by the plastic temples, elasticized band, or ties rather than handling the front or sides, health care providers can minimize the risk of contamination of their hands.[95]

VI.d.5. Non-disposable eye protection should be placed in a designated receptacle for subsequent cleaning and disinfection, and health care providers should each be given their own eye protection when possible.[95]

VI.e. Perioperative personnel must wear surgical masks when splashes, spray, spatter, or droplets of blood or other potentially infectious materials may be generated and nose or mouth contamination can be reasonably anticipated.[4] *[1: Regulatory Requirement]*

Masks protect the mucous membranes of the nose and mouth, which are susceptible to infectious agents.[1,4] Masks are used to prevent contact with respiratory secretions or sprays of blood and body fluid as part of standard and droplet precautions.[1]

Splash injuries are common during endoscopic and laparoscopic urologic procedures, a fact that has implications for all minimally invasive procedures, according to a four-month study of 118 endoscopy procedures.[37] The investigators collected 236 masks from surgeons, surgical assistants, and perioperative nurses and analyzed them for blood macroscopically and using forensic techniques. Results indicated 48.5% of the surgeons' masks, 29.5% of the assistants' masks, and 31.8% of the nurses' masks were splashed with blood.

Masks also are used as part of sterile technique to protect patients from exposure to infectious agents that may be carried in the health care provider's mouth or nose.[1] Surgical masks have been shown to reduce bacterial contamination produced by dispersal of organisms from the wearer's upper airway[96] and are believed to protect the surgical site from becoming contaminated.[97] During cataract surgery, for example, there is significantly less bacterial contamination of the surgical site when the surgeon wears a face mask.[98] Visor masks are recommended as a standard practice during oral surgery when high-speed rotary instruments are used because these procedures result in splashing nearly 90% of the time.[38]

The Society for Cardiovascular Angiography and Interventions recommends wearing a mask to protect patients during cardiac catheterization procedures.[99] The Society noted that mask use has become more important with increased use of the catheterization laboratory as an interventional suite for device implantation. Significantly less bacterial contamination of the operative field during cardiac catheterization occurs when health care providers wear full masks compared to no masks, and there is a nonsignificant trend of increased bacterial colony counts when masks are worn below the nose as opposed to above the nose.[100]

The two types of masks available in health care settings are surgical masks and procedure masks. Surgical masks, which are evaluated by the US Food and Drug Administration for fluid resistance, bacterial filtration efficacy, differential pressure, and flammability, are appropriate for use as PPE in the perioperative setting.[1]

Whether to wear a mask or respirator depends on disease-specific recommendations,[101] but the CDC notes that it is good practice to don a mask within 6 to 10 feet of a patient or on entry to the patient's room when exposure to an "emerging or highly virulent pathogen" is likely.[1]

VI.e.1. Employers should provide masks in a variety of shapes (eg, molded, non-molded), sizes, filtration efficiencies, and methods of attachment (eg, ties, elastic, ear loops).
Providing several varieties may be necessary to meet individual health care providers' needs.[1]

VI.f. Perioperative personnel should wear N95 or higher level respirators during aerosol-generating procedures involving patients who have TB, SARS, or avian or pandemic influenza viruses.[1] *[1: Strong Evidence]*
Wearing an N95 or higher level respirator when caring for a patient who requires airborne precautions reduces the likelihood of airborne infection transmission.[1]
One review of 21 studies indicated that N95 respirators are more protective against influenza and similarly sized particles than surgical masks.[102] However, the investigators noted that additional research is needed to support the World Health Organization guidelines for wearing surgical masks for all patient care and N95 respirators for aerosol-generating procedures. In another review of 45 articles, researchers were unable to determine which specific hygienic measures were most effective in reducing MRSA rates, but they noted that a combination of measures—masks, gloves, gowns, and hand hygiene—are effective together.[103]

VI.g. Perioperative personnel must replace PPE and clothing as soon as possible after exposure to blood or other potentially infectious materials.[4] *[1: Regulatory Requirement]*
Replacing PPE and clothing after exposure to secretions and droplets that contain viruses is effective for preventing cross-infection.[51]

VI.h. Perioperative personnel must remove all PPE before leaving the work area and must place used PPE in an appropriately designated area or container for storage, washing, decontamination, or disposal.[4] After removing PPE, hand hygiene should be performed.[2] *[1: Regulatory Requirement]*

VI.h.1. Perioperative personnel should stand 3 feet away from the disposal container when removing soiled gloves.
One study of glove removal procedures indicated that when personnel stood 3 feet away from the garbage bin as opposed to 2 feet, there was less contamination on the cover of the bin and the front of the removed gloves.[104] There was no significant difference in hand contamination levels based on distance to the disposal container.

Recommendation VII

Perioperative personnel should take action to prevent the transmission of health care-acquired infections.

Several types of infections may be acquired in the perioperative setting and are affected by perioperative care, including SSIs, MDROs, central line-associated blood stream infections, and catheter-associated urinary tract infections. The entire perioperative team is responsible for collaborating to prevent these types of infections.

VII.a. Perioperative team members should adopt a systematic approach for reducing the risk of surgical site infections.[97] *[1: Strong Evidence]*
Despite advances in infection control practices (eg, improved OR ventilation, sterilization methods, barriers, surgical technique, antimicrobial prophylaxis), SSIs remain a substantial cause of morbidity and mortality among hospitalized patients.[97] Surgical site infections occur in 2% to 5% of US patients who undergo surgery in inpatient facilities for a total of approximately 500,000 SSIs each year, at a cost of up to $10 billion annually.[105] Furthermore, these infections are associated with seven to 10 additional postoperative days per SSI and increase the risk of death by as much as 11 times.

According to the Hospital Infection Control Practices Advisory Committee Guideline, SSI is the third most frequently reported health care-associated infection and accounts for between 14% and 16% of all health care-associated infections in hospitalized patients.[97] Among surgical patients, SSIs account for 38% of health care-associated infections, and 77% of deaths in surgical patients who develop an SSI are related to the infection.[97,105]

The pathogens that contribute most frequently to SSI include *S aureus*, coagulase-negative staphylococci, *Enterococcus* spp, and *Escherichia coli*, and increasingly include *Candida albicans* and MRSA.[97] Most SSIs are caused by the patient's endogenous flora (eg, gram-positive cocci, anaerobic bacteria, gram-negative aerobes), but they also can be caused by exogenous sources of pathogens such as members of the surgical team; the OR environment and air; and all devices, instruments, and materials that are brought to the sterile field.[97]

Surgical site infection prevention measures (ie, an action or a set of actions taken to reduce the risk of SSI) focus on reducing opportunities for microbial contamination of the patient's tissues or sterile surgical instruments. Specific methods for preventing SSI include adhering to sterile technique, implementing environmental cleaning protocols, using appropriate barriers and surgical attire, performing proper skin antisepsis and hand hygiene, minimizing traffic in the OR during surgical procedures, using adequate sterilization methods, treating carriers of *S aureus* preoperatively, and using preoperative antimicrobial prophylaxis.[97]

VII.a.1. Perioperative personnel should implement sterile technique when preparing, performing, or assisting with invasive procedures.[11,73,106]

Sterile technique performed by all perioperative team members is the foundation of SSI prevention.[97] Failure to adhere to the principles of asepsis is independently related to the risk of SSI.[1,73,107]

VII.a.2. A clean environment should be maintained.[11,97]

VII.a.3. Perioperative personnel should wear clean surgical attire.[22]

Although few controlled trials have evaluated whether the use of surgical attire has an effect on reducing SSIs, the Hospital Infection Control Practices Advisory Committee recommends the use of barriers (eg, scrub suits, masks, surgical caps, hoods, shoe covers, sterile gloves, gowns, drapes) to minimize the patient's exposure to the skin, mucous membranes, and hair of surgical team members.[97]

Wound infections may result when pathogens that adhere to the hair or scalp (eg, *S aureus*, Group A streptococcus, *Staphylococcus epidermidis*) are released into the operative air and settle into the surgical incision.[108-110]

VII.a.4. Preoperative skin antisepsis of the surgical site should be performed.[111]

Antiseptic skin preparation of the surgical site is intended to reduce the risk of postoperative SSI by removing soil and transient microorganisms from the skin; reducing the resident microbial count to subpathogenic levels in a short period and with the least amount of tissue irritation; and inhibiting rapid, rebound growth of microorganisms.

VII.a.5. Perioperative personnel should follow proper hand hygiene practices.[2]

Hand hygiene helps reduce the bacterial colony count on perioperative team members' hands and is believed to reduce the risk of SSI.[97,112] In one study, the introduction of a hand sanitizer with 70% isopropyl alcohol and 0.5% chlorhexidine gluconate and training perioperative team members on its use reduced SSI overall and superficial SSI in particular among patients undergoing neurosurgery.[113]

VII.a.6. Traffic in and out of the OR should be minimized during surgical procedures.[114]

The air in the OR may contain microbe-laden dust, lint, skin squames, or respiratory droplets, and the microbial level in the air is directly related to the number of people who are moving around in the room.[97]

VII.a.7. Perioperative personnel should provide reusable surgical items that are free of contamination at the time of use. Reusable surgical items should be subjected to cleaning and decontamination, followed by a disinfection or sterilization process.[115]

Inadequate sterilization of surgical instruments can contribute to SSI outbreaks.[97]

VII.a.8. Perioperative nurses should collaborate with medical colleagues to evaluate testing or decolonizing patients preoperatively for carriage of *S aureus* and using preoperative prophylaxis on carriers.

S aureus is carried in the nasal nares of 20% to 30% of healthy individuals, and this carriage has been found to be "the most powerful independent risk factor for SSI" in patients undergoing cardiothoracic surgery.[97] Among 135 orthopedic surgeons at a teaching hospital, 1.5% tested positive for MRSA and 35.7% tested positive for methicillin-sensitive *S aureus*.[116]

Mupirocin ointment may be an effective topical therapy for removing *S aureus* from the nares of colonized patients and health care providers, and the ointment can lower the risk of SSI when it is used on patients

TRANSMISSIBLE INFECTIONS

regardless of carrier status.[97,117] The evidence is conflicting, however. Another study failed to demonstrate an overall reduction in SSI when intranasal mupirocin was administered to carriers of *S aureus* preoperatively, and the study only showed a trend for decreased health care-associated infections caused by *S aureus*.[118]

Researchers in the Netherlands found that decontaminating endogenous microorganisms in the nasopharynx and oropharynx with chlorhexidine gluconate preoperatively reduces health care-associated infection after cardiac surgery.[119]

VII.a.9. Perioperative nurses should verify that preoperative antimicrobial prophylaxis is administered according to health care organization policy.

Surgical antimicrobial prophylaxis is a critically timed adjunct therapy intended to reduce the microbial burden of surgical contamination to a level that cannot overwhelm the patient's defenses.[97] The surgeon decides which antimicrobial agent to use by anticipating the surgical wound class for a given procedure. Comparisons of various antibiotics for short-term treatment have been shown to be equally effective against SSI in patients undergoing elective implant surgery[120] and orthopedic surgery.[121] To maximize the benefits of antimicrobial prophylaxis, the Hospital Infection Control Practices Advisory Committee[97] recommends

- using an antimicrobial agent for all procedures or classes of procedures for which use has been shown to reduce SSI rates or for procedures from which incisional or organ/space SSI would be catastrophic;
- using a medication that is safe, inexpensive, and bactericidal with an in vitro spectrum that covers the most probable intraoperative contaminants for the surgery;
- timing the initial dose of the medication so that a bactericidal concentration is established in serum and tissues by the time of the incision; and
- maintaining therapeutic antimicrobial levels in both serum and tissues during the procedure and until a few hours after the incision is closed.

The Society for Healthcare Epidemiology of America/Infectious Diseases Society of America practice recommendations[105] include

- delivering IV prophylaxis within one hour before the incision is made, or two hours for vancomycin and fluoroquinolones;
- using an antimicrobial agent that is consistent with published guidelines; and
- discontinuing use of the antimicrobial agent within 24 hours after surgery, or 48 hours for cardiothoracic procedures in adult patients.

VII.b. To limit or slow the spread of MDROs, perioperative personnel should collaborate with an infection preventionist to determine the best and safest plan for surgical patients who are diagnosed with an MDRO. [1: Strong Evidence]

Methicillin-resistant *S aureus* and VRE are not the only MDROs that present an infection prevention challenge. Other MDROs continue to emerge as a public health concern. Carbapenem-resistant Enterobacteriaceae has become a serious threat to public health. These organisms have the potential to spread and are associated with high mortality rates, and they often carry genes that cause high levels of resistance to many antimicrobial agents, leaving extremely limited options for treatment.[122,123]

When MDROs are introduced into a health care setting, several factors determine the likelihood of transmission and persistence of the resistant strain:

- vulnerability of patients (ie, patients in the hospital are more likely to get an infection because their immunity is weakened from the disease state),
- numbers of colonized patients,
- increased antimicrobial use, and
- effect of and adherence to prevention efforts.[27]

Successful approaches to preventing and controlling MDROs are often a combination of strategies,[27,124] including

- garnering administrative support (eg, commitment of fiscal and staffing resources, implementation of system changes, expert consultation, laboratory support, adherence monitoring, data analysis)[27,125];
- following and improving hand hygiene practices[13,27,34,41,69,126-130];
- using contact precautions until patients are culture negative[27,34,41,127];
- performing enhanced environmental cleaning[13,27,32,41,127];
- managing vascular and urinary catheters[27];
- preventing lower respiratory tract infection in intubated patients[27];
- accurately diagnosing infectious etiologies[27];
- following the recommendations of the CDC Campaign to Prevent Antimicrobial Resistance[27,131];
- limiting and carefully selecting antimicrobial agents[27,121,132-136];
- conducting MDRO surveillance as part of an MDRO control program[27,41,127,137,138];
- using active surveillance cultures[27,34,126];

- educating staff members to encourage behavior change through better understanding of MDROs[27,41,139]; and
- improving communication about patients with MDROs within and between health care facilities.[27]

Several studies also promote cohorting patients,[140,141] using designated beds or units, universal screening,[142] and closing units when necessary to control transmission of MDROs.[27]

VII.c. Perioperative personnel should implement CDC guidelines to prevent central line infections, including using sterile technique and maximal sterile barrier precautions (ie, hair covering, mask, sterile gown, sterile gloves, a sterile full body drape) when inserting central catheters.[143] *[1: Strong Evidence]*

Central line infections cause significant problems for patients and health care facilities in terms of increased length of stay and increased cost. It is a national imperative to eliminate central line-associated blood stream infection among patients, and the CDC Healthcare Infection Control Practices Advisory Committee has specific recommendations for all health care providers who insert central catheters, which includes anesthesia professionals. It is the perioperative nurses' responsibility to make sure this evidence-based guideline is followed to promote safety in all perioperative patients.[143]

One study from the United Kingdom demonstrated that 39% of hospital-acquired MRSA bacteremia cases were caused by a central line. The researchers recommended a focus of infection prevention efforts should be on improving insertion and care of central lines.[144]

Intraoperative stopcock contamination increases the rate of patient mortality, and patient and provider reservoirs contribute to 30-day postoperative infections, according to a multicenter study.[145] Researchers observed stopcock transmission events in 274 ORs and collected reservoir bacterial cultures. They identified stopcock contamination in 23% of procedures and concluded that although patients, provider hands, and the environment may have contributed to the transmission events, the environment was the most likely source. The researchers recommended designing multimodal programs to target each reservoir in parallel and introducing a comprehensive approach to reducing intraoperative bacterial contamination.

VII.d. Perioperative nurses should follow the CDC guidelines for the prevention of catheter-associated urinary tract infections[146] and the health care organization's policies and procedures for urinary catheter insertion to prevent urinary tract infections.

Catheter-associated urinary tract infections are considered health care-associated infections. They are preventable by following evidence-based recommendations.[146]

One UK study showed that 51% of hospital-acquired MRSA bacteremia cases were caused by urinary catheters. The researchers recommended focusing infection prevention efforts on improving the insertion and care of urinary catheters.[144] *[1: Strong Evidence]*

VII.d.1. Perioperative personnel should
- insert catheters only for medically indicated conditions;
- use urinary catheters for surgical patients only as necessary as opposed to routinely;
- document the date and time of catheter insertion and remove the catheter as soon as possible postoperatively, preferably within 24 hours;
- strictly follow sterile technique when placing a urinary catheter; and
- allow only trained persons who are familiar with correct sterile technique and maintenance to insert urinary catheters.

Recommendation VIII

Health care personnel should be immunized against vaccine-preventable diseases.

The CDC Advisory Committee for Immunization Practices recommends that health care providers receive immunizations if they come into contact with patients or infectious material from patients that may put them at risk for exposure and possible transmission of vaccine-preventable disease.[50] Including vaccinations as part of an organizational infection control and prevention program reduces the risk of occupationally acquired infections and, therefore, harm to patients from vaccine-preventable diseases.[4,50]

The CDC recommends that health care providers receive vaccinations for diseases for which routine vaccination or documentation of immunity is recommended because of risks in the workplace (ie, hepatitis B, seasonal influenza, measles, mumps, rubella, pertussis, varicella).[50]

VIII.a. Employers must make the hepatitis B vaccination series available to all perioperative employees whose work involves a reasonable risk of exposure to blood or other potentially infectious materials and must provide post-exposure evaluation and follow-up to all employees who have an exposure incident.[4,50] *[1: Regulatory Requirement]*

Hepatitis B is highly contagious and is transmitted via percutaneous exposure (eg, needlestick injury) or mucosal exposure to infected blood or body fluids. The risk of acquiring hepatitis B infection from occupational exposure depends on the frequency of percutaneous and mucosal exposure to blood or body fluids that contain the virus.[50] Risks to health care providers from sharps injuries and blood and body fluid exposure has been reduced as a result of widespread hepatitis B vaccination.[17]

Although rare, health care personnel who have hepatitis B or hepatitis C can transmit them to patients.[147]

VIII.a.1. Serologic testing should be repeated after hepatitis B vaccination for health care personnel who are at "high risk" of occupational percutaneous or mucosal exposure to blood or body fluids. If antibody levels are too low (< 10 mIU/mL), the health care provider should be revaccinated and tested again after completing the series.[50]

Performing serologic testing one to two months after the last dose of the vaccine helps determine whether there is a need for revaccination and guides post-exposure prophylaxis in the event of an exposure incident.[50]

VIII.a.2. In the event of blood or body fluid exposure (ie, percutaneous, ocular, mucous membrane, nonintact skin), the need for post-exposure prophylaxis should be evaluated immediately based on the hepatitis B surface antigen status of the source and the health care provider's vaccination history and vaccine-response status.[50]

VIII.b. All health care personnel who have no contraindications should receive annual influenza vaccinations. *[1: Strong Evidence]*

Health care providers are exposed to patients who have influenza and are therefore at risk of occupationally acquired influenza and transmitting the disease to patients and other providers.[50]

VIII.b.1. Health care organizations should implement strategies to improve influenza vaccination rates among perioperative personnel.

Strategies that can improve vaccination rates include
- establishing evidence-based educational and promotional programs to communicate about the disease and the vaccine,[50,148,149]
- capitalizing on the belief in ethical responsibility and protecting patients,[150]
- running a campaign that emphasizes the benefits of vaccination for personnel and patients,[50,151]
- implementing a vaccine declination policy,[50]
- encouraging senior medical staff members or opinion leaders to get vaccinated,[50]
- removing administrative barriers (eg, costs),[50,151]
- providing incentives for getting vaccinated,[50,151]
- providing the vaccine in locations and at times that are easily accessible to health care providers,[50,151] and
- monitoring and reporting provider vaccination rates.[50]

In January 2007, the Joint Commission began requiring accredited facilities to provide staff members, including volunteers and licensed independent practitioners, with influenza vaccinations and to report coverage levels.[50] As of January 2013, the Centers for Medicare & Medicaid Services will require acute care hospitals to report vaccination rates among providers as part of its hospital inpatient quality reporting program.[50]

Despite the fact that annual vaccination has been recommended for health care providers and is a high priority for reducing morbidity associated with the virus in health care settings, vaccination rates among health care providers still need to improve.[50,148,152]

According to a survey of 304 health care personnel at a German tertiary care university hospital, concern about adverse effects was a primary reason to avoid vaccination.[148] Health care providers who are less likely to get vaccinated include
- women[152];
- nurses, technicians, and administrative workers[152]; and
- those who did not receive a vaccine the previous year.[152]

According to a survey conducted across eight university medical centers in the Netherlands,[153] health care providers are more likely to get an influenza vaccination if they
- are older than 40 years of age,
- have a chronic illness,
- are aware of personal risk or the risk of infecting patients,
- trust that the vaccine is effective for reducing the risk of infecting patients,
- believe in the health care provider's responsibility to "do no harm" and ensure continuity of care, and
- have convenient access to the vaccine.

Social pressure for vaccination also increased the likelihood of health care providers getting vaccinated.

Health care personnel are more likely to accept the influenza vaccine if they have a desire to protect themselves or patients or have a perception that the vaccine is effective.[50]

Establishing a mandatory vaccination program is feasible and leads to high vaccination rates, as demonstrated by a five-year study conducted at a tertiary care center in Seattle, Washington.[154] In the first year of the program, 4,588 of 4,703 health care providers (97.6%) were vaccinated, and rates stayed above 98% for the subsequent four years. Of those who declined vaccination, 0.7% did so for religious reasons and were required to wear a mask during influenza season, and less than 0.2% opted to leave the facility. Although 72% of survey respondents at another facility in which mandatory vaccination was implemented reported feeling that the policy was "coercive," more than 90% agreed that the policy was ethically responsible and important for protecting patients and staff members.[150]

VIII.c. Perioperative personnel should have presumptive evidence of immunity to measles, mumps, and rubella, and this information should be documented and readily available in the health care setting.[50] *[1: Strong Evidence]*

Presumptive evidence includes written documentation of vaccination with two doses of measles-mumps-rubella vaccine administered at least 28 days apart, laboratory evidence of immunity, laboratory confirmation of disease, or birth before 1957.

Measles and mumps are highly contagious and can have serious consequences. Rubella was declared eliminated from the United States in 2004, but there is a risk of resurgence from importation.[50]

Exposure to measles, mumps, or rubella in the health care setting can be expensive and disruptive because of containment measures, necessary personnel furloughs or reassignments, and potential closures.[50]

VIII.d. Health care personnel should receive a single dose of tetanus toxoid, reduced diphtheria toxoid, and acellular pertussis (Tdap) as soon as feasible upon hire if they have not been vaccinated previously.[50] *[1: Strong Evidence]*

Pertussis (ie, whooping cough) is a highly contagious bacterial infection and is transmitted via contact and droplet routes.[50] Pertussis outbreaks in health care facilities can be costly in terms of personnel, testing, treatment, and prophylaxis, but adult vaccination may reduce the disease burden.[155] The Tdap vaccine protects against pertussis and reduces the risk of transmission to patients, other health care providers, family members, and the community.[50]

In October 2010, the CDC Advisory Committee for Immunization Practices recommended expanding the use of the Tdap vaccine.[156] According to CDC, although there is a high rate of coverage for pertussis vaccination in children, the disease is "poorly controlled in the United States;" Tdap coverage is 56% among adolescents and less than 6% among adults.[156]

VIII.d.1. Health care organizations should establish programs to increase Tdap vaccination among personnel, including providing convenient access to the vaccination, giving the vaccination free of charge, and educating health care providers about the benefits of vaccination.[50]

VIII.e. Health care organizations should ensure that all health care personnel have evidence of immunity to varicella, and providers who have no evidence of immunity should receive the varicella vaccine. This information should be documented and readily available in the health care setting.[50] *[1: Strong Evidence]*

Varicella is highly infectious and is transmitted via contact, droplet, and airborne routes. Primary infection usually results in lifetime immunity, and the US vaccination program that began in 1995 has led to greater than 85% declines in varicella incidence, hospitalizations, and deaths.[50]

Despite the reduced incidence, health care-associated transmission is still a risk and the disease can be fatal. Varicella is more likely to spread in hospital settings and long-term care facilities.[50] Varicella exposure among patients and health care providers can disrupt patient care and cost the facility in terms of identifying susceptible patients and staff members, managing those who are exposed, and mandating furloughs for exposed staff members.

VIII.e.1. When a patient with confirmed or suspected varicella infection enters the health care facility, airborne and contact precautions should be implemented and followed, and only health care providers with evidence of immunity should provide care to the patient.[50]

VIII.f. Health care organizations should review health care provider vaccination and immunity status at the time of hire and at least annually thereafter. *[1: Strong Evidence]*

Regularly reviewing vaccination and immunity status helps ensure that health care providers are up to date with respect to the recommended vaccines.[50]

VIII.f.1. All health care personnel should receive baseline TB screening upon hire. Follow-up testing should be performed in the case of exposure to TB.[53]

Recommendation IX

Activities of health care personnel with infections, exudative lesions, and nonintact skin should be restricted when these activities pose a risk of transmission of infection to patients and other health care providers. State, federal, and professional guidelines and strategies should be followed to determine the need for work restrictions for health care personnel with blood-borne infections.[20,28]

Restricting activities of personnel who have transmissible infections reduces transmission between providers and patients depending on the mode of transmission

TRANSMISSIBLE INFECTIONS

and epidemiology of the disease.[28] Infections that may require restrictions from providing direct patient care, entering the patient's environment, or handling instruments or devices that may be used during a surgical or invasive procedure include

- viral respiratory infections (eg, influenza, respiratory syncytial virus),[28]
- keratoconjunctivitis or purulent conjunctivitis caused by other microorganisms,[28]
- acute gastrointestinal illnesses (ie, vomiting or diarrhea with or without nausea, fever, or abdominal pain),[28,157]
- diphtheria (ie, identification as an asymptomatic carrier),[28]
- exudative lesions that cannot be contained (eg, eczema, impetigo, smallpox),[28,29,31,109]
- herpes simplex infections of the fingers or hands (ie, herpetic whitlow),[28]
- pediculosis,[28]
- scabies,[28] and
- meningococcal infection (ie, until 24 hours after the start of effective therapy).[28]

Work restrictions for health care personnel with bloodborne infections who provide direct patient care depend on several factors, including circulating viral burden and category of clinical activities.[20]

IX.a. An employee health nurse, infection preventionist, or physician should assess any health care provider with an infection, exudative lesions, or nonintact skin before he or she is allowed to return to work providing direct patient care or handling medical devices that are used in surgical or other invasive procedures. *[1: Strong Evidence]*

Medical clearance is necessary before health care providers who have an infection, exudative lesions, or nonintact skin can return to work with patients or other health care providers.[28]

IX.b. Health care personnel should report exposures as soon as they occur and infections as soon as the disease process is noted. *[1: Strong Evidence]*

Early self-reporting of exposures and infections helps prevent transmission to patients and other health care providers. Health care providers can be encouraged to self-report exposures or infections when facility policies are designed to prevent judgement or penalty (eg, loss of wages, benefits, job status) for self-reporting.[28,97]

IX.c. The health care organization should have a written policy regarding health care personnel who have a potentially transmissible infection. The policy should establish responsibility for reporting the condition, work restrictions, and guidelines for clearing the employee for work after an illness that required a restriction.[28,97] *[1: Strong Evidence]*

Recommendation X

Perioperative personnel should receive initial and ongoing education and complete competency verification of their understanding of the principles of infection prevention and the performance of standard, contact, droplet, and airborne precautions for prevention of transmissible infections and MDROs. *Amb*

Education and competency verification are prerequisites for ensuring standard and transmission-based precautions are understood and followed.[158] Ongoing development of knowledge and skills and documentation of personnel participation is a regulatory and accreditation requirement for both hospitals and ambulatory settings.[159-162]

Initial and ongoing education on infection prevention practices facilitate the development of knowledge, skills, and attitudes that affect safe patient care. Periodic education programs provide the opportunity to reinforce the principles of infection prevention, the necessary precautions to take when providing care to a patient who has a transmissible infection (eg, standards, contact, droplet, airborne), and the actions to take when a health care provider has a transmissible infection.

Competency verification measures individual performance; provides a mechanism for documentation; and verifies that perioperative personnel have an understanding of infection prevention, MDROs, and facility policies. Every nurse is personally accountable for maintaining competency validation.[163]

There are no universally accepted or mandated ways to perform or verify competency, and strategies differ between states. Some states mandate specific topics that affect public health (eg, bioterrorism) or that are specific to certain areas of nursing. The goal of competency verification is to reassure the public that nurses have the knowledge, skills, and judgment to provide safe and effective care.[164]

X.a. Education, training, and competency verification should address
- standard precautions;
- contact precautions;
- airborne precautions;
- droplet precautions;
- MDROs;
- procedures for transporting patients who require infection precautions;
- use of N95 or powered air-purifying respirators;
- bloodborne pathogens;
- double gloving;
- sharps safety; and
- perioperative considerations to prevent central line-associated blood stream infections, catheter-associated urinary tract infections, SSIs, and carbapenem-resistant Enterobacteriaceae.

[2: Moderate Evidence]

TRANSMISSIBLE INFECTIONS

Standard precautions are used for all patients in the perioperative setting, and transmission-based precautions can be modified depending on local conditions and patient characteristics (Table 1). Including each topic in education and training helps ensure appropriate follow-through in the event of a suspected or identified case of infection. Understanding the scientific premise of these precautions allows health care providers to follow and modify the precautions safely based on identified changes, resources, and health care settings.

X.b. Health care personnel who are occupationally exposed to blood or other potentially infectious materials must receive training before assignment to tasks where occupational exposure may occur, at least annually thereafter, and when changes to procedures or tasks affect occupational exposure.[4] *[1: Regulatory Requirement]*

Employers are responsible for providing training on the bloodborne pathogens standard during working hours at no cost to the employee. Employers are also responsible for ensuring employees participate in the training program and for offering materials in appropriate languages and at appropriate literacy levels.[4]

Providing the basis for the prevention of bloodborne pathogen exposure may instill an understanding of the processes that need to be followed and thereby prevent disease transmission. Education and training efforts are equally important in promoting awareness of hazards and acceptance of safe work and material-handling procedures in the workplace.[66] Educating employees on safe work practices (eg, using PPE) can help protect personnel, their family members, and the community from take-home transmissions.

X.b.1. Employee education must include
- an explanation of the modes of transmission of bloodborne pathogens and an explanation of the employer's exposure control plan;
- an explanation of the use and limitations of methods for reducing exposure (eg, engineering controls, work practices, PPE); and
- information on the hepatitis B vaccine, its efficacy and safety, the method of administration, and the benefits of vaccination.[4]

X.c. Perioperative personnel should receive education and competency validation on preventing the spread of MDROs as part of the health care organization's infection prevention program. Education should include
  ○ mechanisms of infection transmission,
  ○ case-based scenarios for managing infected patients,
  ○ participatory decision-making exercises about the implementation of precautions in addition to standard precautions, and
  ○ practice in the use of PPE for patients who require additional precautions.
[2: Moderate Evidence]

Implementing a mandatory, organization-wide infection-control program can significantly improve the rate of health care-associated MRSA infections.[139]

X.d. Perioperative personnel should participate in programs to educate health care personnel about the importance of being immunized against epidemiologically important pathogens. *[2: Moderate Evidence]*

Programs that deliver educational and promotional messages about the benefits of vaccination can improve vaccination rates among health care personnel.[151]

X.e. Health care personnel should be educated on the benefits of reporting infections, exudative lesions, and nonintact skin in a timely manner and on related work restrictions. *[1: Strong Evidence]*

Institutional policies and procedures that guide work restrictions because of infections are designed to protect patients. Health care providers have an ethical responsibility to promote their own health and well being, and a responsibility to remove themselves from care situations if it is clear that there is a significant risk to patients despite appropriate preventive measures.[20]

X.f. Health care personnel should receive education and training on the facility emergency preparedness plan. *[1: Strong Evidence]*

It is important for health care personnel to be prepared to respond to threats of intentionally released pathogens and to treat patients who are exposed to biological agents.[165]

X.g. Perioperative personnel should participate in educational programs to improve infection control practices. *[2: Moderate Evidence]*

Surgical teams at a large UK teaching hospital implemented a "clean practice protocol" that increased adherence to overall infection control practices from 63% to 89% in three months, as demonstrated by undisclosed infection-control audits held before and after the education protocol.[166] The protocol combined the use of a reminder poster and auditing several surgical units for activities related to hand decontamination, correct use of gloves, instrument cleaning, garment contamination, and notes contamination. After the audits and education, hand decontamination and the correct use of gloves and aprons improved significantly.

437

TRANSMISSIBLE INFECTIONS

Table 1. Guide for Perioperative Personnel Caring for Patients with Transmissible Infections[1]

Type of precaution	Type of organism/disease	Transport	Protection for unscrubbed personnel*	Preoperative area	Environmental measures
Contact	Draining abscess, infectious wounds, *Clostridium difficile*, acute viral infection, methicillin-resistant *Staphylococcus aureus* (MRSA), vancomycin-resistant Enterococci (VRE), vancomycin-intermediate/resistant *S aureus* (VISA/VRSA), extended-spectrum beta-lactamase (ESBL), multidrug-resistant pneumonia	Cover or contain the infected or colonized areas of the patient's body. Remove and dispose of contaminated personal protective equipment (PPE) and perform hand hygiene before transporting the patient. Don clean PPE to handle the patient at the transport destination.	Standard precautions plus the following: Wear gloves whenever touching the patient's skin or items that are in close proximity to the patient. Wear a gown when it can be anticipated that clothing will come into contact with the patient or contaminated environmental surfaces. Don a gown upon entry into the room, remove and perform hand hygiene before exiting.	Hold the patient in a single patient room if possible; otherwise keep ≥ 3 ft separation between patients.	Clean the room (eg, OR, airborne infection isolation room [AIIR]) immediately after patient use. Focus on frequently touched surfaces.
Droplet	Diphtheria, haemophilus influenza type b, seasonal influenza, pandemic influenza, meningococcal disease, mumps, mycoplasma pneumonia, group A streptococcus, pertussis, adenovirus, rubella	Instruct the patient to wear a mask and follow respiratory hygiene and cough etiquette. The transporter is not required to wear a mask.	Standard precautions plus the following: Wear a mask upon entry into the room.	Hold the patient in a single patient room if possible; otherwise keep ≥ 3 ft separation between patients. Draw a privacy curtain between beds to minimize the opportunity for close contact.	Routine
Airborne	Tuberculosis, disseminated herpes zoster, rubeola, monkeypox, smallpox, varicella zoster, chicken pox	Instruct the patient to wear a mask and follow respiratory hygiene and cough etiquette. Cover and contain affected skin lesions. The transporter is not required to wear a mask.	Standard precautions plus the following: Wear a fit-tested N95 or higher level respirator that is approved by the National Institute for Occupational Safety and Health.	Place the patient in an AIIR, if possible. Provide at least six (existing facility) or 12 (new construction/renovation) air changes per hour.	Consult an infection preventionist before patient placement to determine the safety of an alternative room that does not meet AIIR requirements. If an AIIR is not available, the OR should remain vacant postoperatively for the appropriate time to allow for a full exchange of air, generally one hour.

* "Unscrubbed personnel" include anesthesia professionals, the circulating RN, and preoperative and postanesthesthia care personnel.

Infection control professionals should modify or adapt this table according to local conditions and special patient considerations.

Reference
1. Siegel JD, Rhinehart E, Jackson M, Chiarello L; the Healthcare Infection Control Practices Advisory Committee. 2007 Guideline for Isolation Precautions: Preventing Transmission of Infectious Agents in Health Care Settings. Am J Infect Control. 2007;35(10 Suppl 2):S65-S164.

Recommendation XI

Documentation should reflect activities related to infection prevention. *Amb*

Documentation is a professional medicolegal standard.[167] Documentation related to infection prevention is applicable at the systems level and the patient care level. At the systems level, documentation serves as a basis for monitoring compliance, measuring performance, maintaining employee records, and logging exposure incidents. At the patient care level, documentation facilitates continuity of patient care through clear communication and supports collaboration between health care team members.

XI.a. Employers must maintain training records related to bloodborne pathogens for three years.[4] The records must include
- training dates,
- content or a summary of the training,
- names and qualifications of trainer(s), and
- names and job titles of trainees.

[1: Regulatory Requirement]

XI.b. All incidents of occupational exposure to blood or other potentially infectious materials must be documented.[4] Documentation should include
- the route of exposure;
- the circumstances associated with the exposure;
- the source individual's serological status, if known;
- the employee's name and social security number;
- the employee's hepatitis B vaccination status and other relevant medical information for both individuals, including vaccination dates and any medical records related to the employee's ability to receive vaccinations;
- results of all related examinations, medical tests, and post-exposure evaluation and follow-up procedures;
- a licensed health care professional's written opinion; and
- a copy of the information provided to the employee.

[1: Regulatory Requirement]

Documenting each exposure incident provides a record of the incident, what follow-through was taken, and the current status of the incident.

XI.b.1. Employers must maintain a sharps injury log to document all percutaneous injuries from contaminated sharps and must maintain the log in such a way that an injured employee's identification remains confidential.[4] At a minimum, a sharps injury log must include
- the type and brand of device involved in the incident,
- the department or work area where the exposure incident occurred, and

TRANSMISSIBLE INFECTIONS

- an explanation of how the incident occurred.

Some health care employers may be exempt from maintaining a sharps injury log. The requirement to establish and maintain a sharps injury log applies to any employer who is required to maintain a log of occupational injuries and illnesses under 29 CFR §1904.[4]

XI.b.2. Documentation related to exposure incidents must be maintained for the employee's duration of employment plus 30 years.[4]

XI.c. Records and results of TB screening should be maintained for each employee in the employee's health record.[53] If an employee has symptoms of TB, the symptoms should be recorded in the employee health record or medical record.[53] *[1: Strong Evidence]*

XI.d. Vaccination records should be maintained for each employee. All employee vaccinations should be documented in each employee's health record. Records of any vaccinations administered during employment should include
- the type of vaccine given;
- the date on which the vaccine is given;
- the name of the vaccine manufacturer and the lot number;
- any documented episodes of adverse reactions to a vaccination;
- the name, address, and title of the person who administered the vaccination; and
- the edition and distribution date of the language-appropriate vaccine information statement provided to the employee at the time of vaccination.[50]

[1: Strong Evidence]

Accurate vaccination records make it possible to quickly identify health care personnel who are susceptible to infection during an outbreak and can reduce costs and disruptions to health care operations.[50]

XI.d.1. Each employee's immunity status for vaccine-preventable diseases, including documented disease, vaccination history, and serology results, should be recorded in the employee's record.[50]

XI.d.2. The health care organization should use a secure computerized system to manage vaccination records for health care personnel.[50]

Computerized systems allow records to be retrieved easily and as needed.[50]

XI.e. Wound class should be documented according to the CDC Surgical Wound Classification system at the conclusion of the procedure.[97] *[1: Strong Evidence]*

The surgical wound classification system has been shown to be a predictor of the relative probability that a wound infection will

TRANSMISSIBLE INFECTIONS

occur.[97,168] In addition, the classification allows for comparison of wound infection rates associated with different surgical techniques, surgeons, and facilities. The comparison may be useful for research and also may serve to alert infection prevention personnel to wounds at increased risk for infection, enabling health care providers to implement appropriate surveillance and preventative measures.[97,168]

The definitions of the four CDC wound classifications are

- Class 1—Clean wounds: These are uninfected operative wounds in which no inflammation is encountered, and the respiratory, alimentary, genital, or uninfected urinary tracts are not entered. In addition, clean wounds are primarily closed, and, if necessary, drained with closed drainage (eg, Jackson-Pratt). Operative incisional wounds that follow nonpenetrating (blunt) trauma should be included in this category if they meet the criteria.
- Class 2—Clean-contaminated wounds: These are operative wounds in which the respiratory, alimentary, genital, or urinary tract is entered under controlled conditions and without unusual contamination. Specifically, operations involving the biliary tract, appendix, vagina, and oropharynx are included in this category, provided no evidence of infection or major break in technique is encountered (eg, spillage from the gastrointestinal tract).
- Class 3—Contaminated wounds: These include open, fresh, accidental wounds; operations with major breaks in sterile technique (eg, a procedure performed with unsterile instruments) or gross spillage from the gastrointestinal tract; and incisions in which acute, nonpurulent inflammation is encountered.
- Class 4—Dirty or infected wounds: These include old traumatic wounds with retained devitalized tissue and those that involve existing clinical infection or perforated viscera. This definition suggests that the organisms causing postoperative infection were present in the operative field before the operation.

XI.e.1. Perioperative nurses should use educational tools to assist in accurately identifying surgical wounds.

The AORN Surgical Wound Classification Decision Tree can help perioperative nurses accurately identify surgical wounds (Figure 1).

XI.f. Breaks in sterile technique should be documented per organization policy in consultation with infection prevention personnel.[73] *[1: Strong Evidence]*

Thoughtful assessment, collaboration with the surgeon and surgical team members, and the application of informed clinical judgment is required when determining whether contamination resulting from a break in sterile technique is significant enough for an infection to occur and the wound classification to be changed.

XI.g. Results of documented surveillance should be shared with perioperative personnel. *[1: Strong Evidence]*

Sharing documented surveillance can help to reduce morbidity and mortality.[169] Monitoring performance helps in assessing the effectiveness of quality improvement interventions, and sharing surveillance strategies and results helps in identifying best practices for implementing evidence-based guidelines for preventing health care-associated infections.

Surveillance of both process measures and the infection rates to which they are linked are important for evaluating how effective infection prevention efforts are and identifying what needs to be changed. Surveillance is an ongoing, systematic collection, analysis, interpretation, and dissemination of data based on infections occurring in the health care facility.[1]

Recommendation XII

Policies and procedures for the prevention and control of transmissible infections and MDROs should be developed, reviewed periodically, revised as necessary, and readily available within the practice setting. *Amb*

Policies and procedures assist in the development of patient safety, quality assessment, and performance improvement activities. Policies and procedures establish authority, responsibility, and accountability within the facility. They also serve as operational guidelines that are used to minimize patient risk factors for complications, standardize practice, direct perioperative personnel, and establish continuous performance improvement programs.

XII.a. Policies and procedures should be developed to guide, support, and monitor adherence to standard and transmission-based precautions, including systems that should be used to collect, analyze, and communicate information related to transmissible infections.[1] *[1: Strong Evidence]*

Definitive policies and procedures as part of an overall administrative strategy can demonstrate a commitment to preventing transmissible infections by incorporating infection control into the organizational objectives for patient and occupational safety.[1] Policies and procedures that guide and support patient care, treatment, and services are a regulatory and accreditation requirement for both hospitals and ambulatory settings.[1,161,162,170-173]

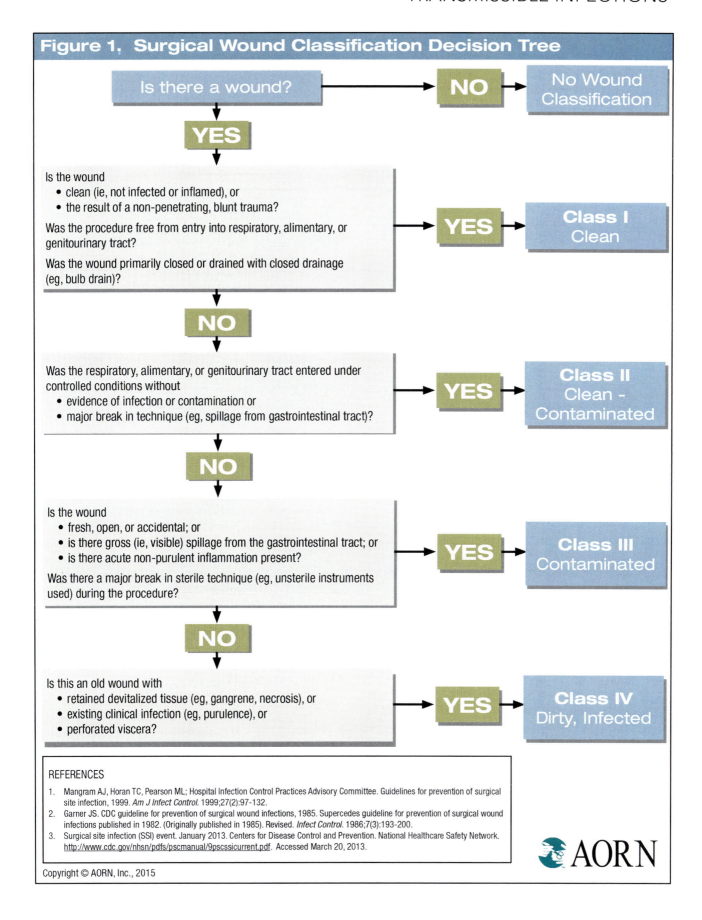

Figure 1. Surgical Wound Classification Decision Tree

TRANSMISSIBLE INFECTIONS

XII.a.1. Policies and procedures should be developed and implemented to address specific perioperative interventions to prevent SSIs, MDROs, central line-associated blood stream infections, and catheter-associated urinary tract infections.

XII.b. Policies and procedures designed to eliminate or minimize health care personnel exposure to blood and other potentially infectious materials must be developed and implemented.[4] *[1: Regulatory Requirement]*

A written exposure control plan that is consistent with federal, state, and local rules and regulations and that governs occupational exposure to bloodborne pathogens, is reviewed periodically, and is readily available in the practice setting promotes safety with medical devices and blood and body fluids.[4]

XII.c. Policies should be developed in accordance with federal and state guidelines and should be consistent with existing impaired-provider and disability guidelines to define work restrictions for health care providers who have infections, exudative lesions, and nonintact skin. The policies should include whether the employee
- has a viral burden above the recommended threshold for the relevant virus,
- has a medical condition or conditions that result in an inability to perform assigned tasks,
- has documented untoward events (eg, having transmitted hepatitis B, hepatitis C, or HIV),
- refuses or is unable to follow recommended guidelines to prevent transmission of infectious diseases, or
- is unable to perform regular duties, assuming that reasonable accommodation has been offered for the disability.[50]

[1: Strong Evidence]

XII.d. A comprehensive vaccination policy for all health care personnel should be developed and implemented.[50] The vaccination policy should include a method to ensure that
- all health care personnel are up to date with recommended vaccines,
- health care personnel vaccination and immunity status is reviewed at the time of hire and at least annually thereafter, and
- necessary vaccines are offered to employees in conjunction with routine annual disease-prevention measures (eg, influenza vaccination, TB testing).

[1: Strong Evidence]

XII.e. Policies and procedures should be developed based on federal and state guidelines to define emergency response to threats of intentionally released pathogens (eg, anthrax, botulism, plague, smallpox). *[1: Strong Evidence]*

Establishing policies and procedures for emergency preparedness guides health care providers in responding to intentionally released pathogens and treating patients who are exposed to biological agents.[165]

XII.f. Policies and procedures should include processes for initial education, training, ongoing competency verification, and annual review of issues dealing with infection transmission. *[5: No Evidence]*

Policies and procedures assist in the development of activities that support patient safety, quality assessment, and the establishment of guidelines for continuous performance improvement. Standardizing processes for performance expectations between perioperative settings facilitates continuity of care and reduces the risk of error when personnel rotate between areas.

Recommendation XIII

Perioperative team members should participate in a variety of quality assurance and performance improvement activities to monitor and improve the prevention of infections and MDROs. *Amb*

Quality assurance and performance improvement programs assist in evaluating the quality of patient care and the formulation of plans for corrective actions. These programs provide data that may be used to determine whether an individual organization is within benchmark goals and, if not, identify areas that may require corrective actions.

XIII.a. Process monitoring should be a part of every perioperative setting as part of an overall infection prevention program. Process monitoring should include[174]
- hand hygiene compliance,
- standard and transmissible infection precaution compliance,
- influenza vaccinations for personnel and patients,
- environmental cleaning practices, and
- central line and urinary catheter insertion practices.

[2: Moderate Evidence]

XIII.a.1. Perioperative nurses should assess and monitor cleaning and disinfection practices.

Monitoring cleaning and disinfection practices to ensure adherence can help control transmission of MDROs and other pathogens that may be residing in the environment.[11,175] The information obtained from assessments can be used to develop focused administrative and educational interventions that incorporate ongoing feedback to the environmental services personnel, to improve cleaning and disinfection practices in health care institutions.[10]

Compliance and adjunct monitoring after terminal cleaning can help prevent cross-contamination of areas that have or have had patients with MDROs.[27,175]

TRANSMISSIBLE INFECTIONS

XIII.a.2. Perioperative nurses should participate in quality improvement initiatives that promote understanding of and adherence to the principles of sterile technique.[73]

XIII.a.3. A quality improvement program for the use of indwelling urinary catheters and central lines should be developed and implemented.

Monitoring the use of indwelling catheters can reduce catheter-associated urinary tract infections.[146]

Quality improvement initiatives in which various strategies are "bundled" together may improve compliance with evidence-based recommended practices and reduce the incidence of central line-associated blood stream infections.[143]

XIII.a.4. A quality improvement program for the use of indwelling catheters should be developed and implemented.[143]

XIII.b. Quality indicators should be developed to measure improvement in the control and transmission of infectious diseases, including MDROs. Quality indicators for measuring the provision of safe patient care with regard to transmissible infections in the perioperative setting should include
- the rate of SSIs,
- the selection of antibiotics that are appropriate for surgery,
- the timing of antibiotic administration, and
- immunization rates of patients and personnel.

[1: Strong Evidence]

Quality indicators are measurable and demonstrate that facilities are using specific interventions to provide safe patient care.[176] According to the Agency for Healthcare Research and Quality, "An adequate quality indicator must have a sound clinical or empirical rationale for its use. It should measure an important aspect of quality that is subject to provider or health care system control."[176(p3)] Quality indicators are one response to the need for multidimensional, accessible quality measures that can be used to gauge performance in health care. The quality indicators are evidence-based and can be used to identify variations in the quality of care provided on both an inpatient and outpatient basis.

XIII.b.1. Perioperative personnel who contract an infection or have a communicable disease should report it to the designated responsible person.

Prompt reporting enables employers to provide timely and confidential evaluation, intervention, and testing, or appropriate prophylaxis.[1,28]

XIII.b.2. All exposure incidents (eg, needlesticks, blood exposures) must be reported according to health care organization policy and based on the OSHA bloodborne pathogens standard.[4]

Documenting all exposure incidents provides the employer with feedback regarding the circumstances of employee exposures. This information can be used to focus efforts on decreasing or eliminating specific circumstances or routes of exposures.[60]

XIII.b.3. Perioperative nurses should contribute to ongoing surveillance of proper use of PPE.

By monitoring the proper use of PPE, perioperative nurses can contribute to community safety by helping limit take-home transmissions of infectious and toxic agents.[66] To gather data on take-home transmissions, NIOSH has recommended expanding current surveillance programs, such as building on the existing NIOSH Sentinel Event Notification Surveillance for Occupational Risks programs for lead and pesticides, which would require prioritizing toxic agents and targeting surveillance in areas where workplace exposure is relatively common.

The NIOSH Task Force recommends, at a minimum,
- develop surveillance programs to document the effectiveness of control measures being used, including an assessment of the feasibility and effectiveness of alternative measures;
- assess the performance of existing protective clothing (eg, single-use disposable clothing, clothing that can be laundered) as barriers for chemical, biological, thermal, and physical hazards;
- assess the use and acceptance of PPE by workers;
- research and develop new types of materials for protective clothing and gloves, including evaluating performance and characteristics; and
- ensure that protective clothing is made available and designed to fit all workers.

XIII.c. Rates of transmissible infections and MDROs should be monitored, documented, and reported to the designated infection preventionist and quality assurance improvement manager and any other personnel deemed appropriate by the health care organization. Surveillance should include monitoring
- use of standard precautions, contact precautions, droplet precautions, and airborne precautions;
- outbreak-specific pathogens (eg, *N meningitides*);
- isolation precautions for MDROs, surveillance practices, and practitioner adherence[177];
- bloodborne pathogen exposures;
- use of PPE; and

TRANSMISSIBLE INFECTIONS

- health care personnel immunization rates. *[1: Strong Evidence]*

Surveillance is a critical component of any MDRO control program because it allows for the detection of newly emerging pathogens, helps identify epidemiologic trends (eg, single patient, clusters of patients), and measures the effectiveness of interventions.[27] Surveillance is important for follow-up with health care personnel who may have an infection or be colonized.[1]

XIII.d. Perioperative nurses should participate in surveillance programs for SSI. *[1: Strong Evidence]*

Routine review and interpretation of SSI rates may help detect significant increases or outbreaks and identify areas where additional resources might be needed to improve SSI rates.[105]

A successful surveillance program includes using epidemiologically sound infection definitions, surveillance methods, stratification of SSI rates according to risk factors associated with SSI development, and data feedback.[97] Using consistent definitions as part of an SSI surveillance program helps ensure accurate interpretation and reporting. The CDC's National Nosocomial Infections Surveillance system has developed standardized surveillance criteria for defining SSIs.[97]

Knowing what patient and surgery characteristics may influence the risk of SSI allows the surveillance team to stratify surgeries, makes surveillance data more comprehensible, and allows for targeted prevention measures.[97] According to the Hospital Infection Control Practices Advisory Committee, patient characteristics that may be associated with an increased risk of SSI include diabetes, cigarette smoking, systemic steroid use, obesity (ie, > 20% ideal body weight), extremes of age, poor nutritional status, and perioperative transfusion of certain blood products. Surgery characteristics that affect SSI incidence include preoperative antiseptic showering, preoperative hair removal, skin prep practices, preoperative hand and forearm antisepsis, management of infected or colonized perioperative team members, and antimicrobial prophylaxis.

XIII.d.1. Perioperative nurses should implement and record the measures related to Surgical Care Improvement Project (SCIP) initiatives according to health care organization policy.

As a national quality improvement initiative, SCIP is supported by more than 10 national organizations with the goal of improving surgical outcomes and significantly reducing surgical complications. Surgical Care Improvement Project measures are part of the Joint Commission's accountability measures.[178]

One study that involved Surgical Care Improvement Project initiatives showed the importance of following these standard guidelines to decrease the number of patients who experience an SSI.[179] Perioperative nurses can take an active role in implementing Surgical Care Improvement Project measures and reporting data to identify areas where improvements can be made.

XIII.d.2. The choice of which procedures to monitor should be made jointly by surgeons and infection prevention personnel. SSI surveillance should target high-risk procedures.[97]

XIII.d.3. When a cluster of SSIs involves an unusual organism, a formal epidemiologic investigation should be conducted.[97] *Amb*

Outbreaks and clusters of SSIs that involved unusual organisms (eg, *Clostridium perfringens*, *Legionella pneumophila*, *Legionelle dumoffii*, *Nocardia farcinica*, *Pseudomonas multivorans*, *Rhizopus oryzae*, *Rhodococcus bronchialis*) have been attributed to contaminated adhesive dressings, elastic bandages, colonized surgical personnel, tap water, and disinfectant solutions.[97]

XIII.e. Perioperative nurses should contribute to creating a culture of safety. *[1: Strong Evidence]*

A culture of safety is created through
- management initiatives that improve patient and health care personnel safety,
- health care personnel participation in safety planning,
- the availability of appropriate PPE for the identified tasks,
- the influence of group norms regarding appropriate safety practices, and
- the facility's socialization process for new hires.[1]

A culture of safety has a direct effect on preventing transmissible infections.[1]

Glossary

Airborne infection isolation: The isolation of patients infected with organisms spread via airborne droplet nuclei < 5 µm in diameter.

Airborne precautions: Precautions that reduce the risk of an airborne transmission of infectious airborne droplet nuclei (ie, small particle residue 5 microns or smaller). Airborne transmission refers to contact with infectious airborne droplet nuclei that can remain suspended in the air for extended periods of time or infectious dust particles that can be circulated by air currents.

Contact precautions: Precautions designed to reduce the risk of transmission of epidemiologically important microorganisms by direct or indirect contact.

Direct contact: Person-to-person contact resulting in physical transfer of infectious microorganisms between an infected or colonized person and a susceptible host.

Droplet precautions: Precautions that reduce the risk of large particle droplet (ie, 5 microns or larger) transmission of infectious agents.

Enhanced environmental cleaning: Environmental cleaning practices implemented to prevent the spread of infections or outbreaks, enhanced cleaning practices promote consistent and standardized cleaning procedures that extend beyond routine cleaning.

Exposure incident: A specific eye, mouth, other mucous membrane, non-intact skin, or parenteral contact with blood or other potentially infectious materials that results from the performance of an employee's duties.

Indirect contact: Contact of a susceptible host with a contaminated object (eg, instruments, hands).

Infection preventionist: A health care professional specializing in leading and directing infection prevention and control programs.

Isolation precautions: Special precautionary measures, practices, and procedures used in the care of patients with contagious or communicable diseases.

Personal protective equipment (PPE): Specialized equipment or clothing for eyes, face, head, body, and extremities; protective clothing; respiratory devices; and protective shields and barriers designed to protect the worker from injury or exposure to a patient's blood, tissue, or body fluids. Used by health care workers and others whenever necessary to protect themselves from the hazards of processes or environments, chemical hazards, or mechanical irritants encountered in a manner capable of causing injury or impairment in the function of any part of the body through absorption, inhalation, or physical contact.

Powered air-purifying respirator: A respirator that uses a battery-powered blower to move the air flow through the filters.

Procedure mask: A mask that covers the nose and mouth and is intended for use in general patient care situations. These masks generally attach to the face with ear loops rather than ties or elastic. Unlike surgical masks, procedure masks are not regulated by the US Food and Drug Administration.

Respirator: A personal protective device that is worn on the face, covers at least the nose and mouth, and is used to reduce the wearer's risk of inhaling hazardous airborne particles (including dust particles and infectious agents), gases, or vapors. Source: What is a respirator? NIOSH. http://www.cdc.gov/niosh/npptl/topics/respirators/disp_part/RespSource1.html. Accessed October 2, 2012.

Standard precautions: The primary strategy for successful infection control and reduction of worker exposure. Precautions used for care of all patients regardless of their diagnosis or presumed infectious status.

Surgical mask: A device worn over the mouth and nose by perioperative team members during surgical procedures to protect both the surgical patient and perioperative team members from transfer of microorganisms and body fluids. Surgical masks are also used to protect health care providers from contact with large infectious droplets (>5 mcm in size). According to draft guidance issued by the US Food and Drug Administration on May 15, 2003, surgical masks are evaluated using standardized testing procedures for fluid resistance, bacterial filtration efficiency, differential pressure (air exchange), and flammability to mitigate the risks to health associated with the use of surgical masks. These specifications apply to any masks that are labeled surgical, laser, isolation, or dental or medical procedure.

Transmission-based precautions: Precautions designed to be used with patients known or suspected to be infected or colonized with highly transmissible or epidemiologically important pathogens for which additional precautions are needed to prevent transmission in the practice setting.

References

1. Siegel JD, Rhinehart E, Jackson M, Chiarello L; Health Care Infection Control Practices Advisory Committee. 2007 Guideline for Isolation Precautions: Preventing Transmission of Infectious Agents in Health Care Settings. *Am J Infect Control.* 2007;35(10 Suppl 2): S65-S164. doi:10.1016/j.ajic.2007.10.007. [IVA]

2. Recommended practices for hand hygiene in the perioperative setting. In: *Perioperative Standards and Recommended Practices.* Denver, CO: AORN, Inc; 2012:73-86. [IVB]

3. World Health Organization. WHO Guidelines on Hand Hygiene in Health Care. Geneva, Switzerland: World Health Organization; 2009. [IVA]

4. Occupational Safety and Health Standards, Toxic and Hazardous Substances: Bloodborne Pathogens, 29 CFR §1910.1030 (2012). Occupational Safety and Health Administration. http://www.osha.gov/pls/oshaweb/owadisp.show_document?p_table=STANDARDS&p_id=10051. Accessed October 18, 2012.

5. Valenzuela TD, Hooton TM, Kaplan EL, Schlievert P. Transmission of "toxic strep" syndrome from an infected child to a firefighter during CPR. *Ann Emerg Med.* 1991;20(1):90-92. [VC]

6. Yu IT, Xie ZH, Tsoi KK, et al. Why did outbreaks of severe acute respiratory syndrome occur in some hospital wards but not in others? *Clin Infect Dis.* 2007;44(8):1017-1025. [IIB]

7. Stuart JM, Gilmore AB, Ross A, et al. Preventing secondary meningococcal disease in health care workers: recommendations of a working group of the PHLS meningococcus forum. *Commun Dis Public Health.* 2001;4(2):102-105. [IVA]

8. *Practice Guidance for Healthcare Environmental Cleaning.* Chicago, IL: American Society for Healthcare Environmental Services; 2008. [IVC]

9. Sehulster L, Chinn RY; CDC, HICPAC. Guidelines for environmental infection control in health-care facilities. Recommendations of CDC and the Healthcare Infection Control Practices Advisory Committee (HICPAC) [published correction appears in *MMWR Morb Mortal Wkly Rep.* 2003;52(42):1025-1026]. *MMWR Recomm Rep.* 2003;52(RR-10):1-42. [IVA]

10. Carling PC, Parry MF, Von Beheren SM; Healthcare Environmental Hygiene Study Group. Identifying opportunities to enhance environmental cleaning in 23 acute care hospitals. *Infect Control Hosp Epidemiol.* 2008;29(1):1-7. doi:10.1086/524329. [IIIB]

11. Recommended practices for environmental cleaning in the perioperative setting. In: *Perioperative Standards*

and *Recommended Practices*. Denver, CO: AORN, Inc; 2012:237-250. [IVB]

12. Mutters R, Nonnenmacher C, Susin C, Albrecht U, Kropatsch R, Schumacher S. Quantitative detection of *Clostridium difficile* in hospital environmental samples by real-time polymerase chain reaction. *J Hosp Infect*. 2009;71(1):43-48. doi:10.1016/j.jhin.2008.10.021. [IIIB]

13. Weber DJ, Rutala WA, Miller MB, Huslage K, Sickbert-Bennett E. Role of hospital surfaces in the transmission of emerging health care-associated pathogens: norovirus, *Clostridium difficile*, and Acinetobacter species. *Am J Infect Control*. 2010;38(5 Suppl 1):S25-S33. [VA]

14. Lessa FC, Gould PL, Pascoe N, et al. Health care transmission of a newly emergent adenovirus serotype in health care personnel at a military hospital in Texas, 2007. *J Infect Dis*. 2009;200(11):1759-1765. [IIIA]

15. Boyce JM, Pittet D; Healthcare Infection Control Practices Advisory Committee, HICPAC/SHEA/APIC/IDSA Hand Hygiene Task Force. Guideline for Hand Hygiene in Health-Care Settings. Recommendations of the Healthcare Infection Control Practices Advisory Committee and the HICPAC/SHEA/APIC/IDSA Hand Hygiene Task Force. Society for Healthcare Epidemiology of America/Association for Professionals in Infection Control/Infectious Diseases Society of America. *MMWR Recomm Rep*. 2002;51(RR-16):1-45. [IVA]

16. Guideline for medication safety. In: *Guidelines for Perioperative Practice*. Denver, CO: AORN, Inc; 2015:291-329. [IVB]

17. Perz JF, Thompson ND, Schaefer MK, Patel PR. US outbreak investigations highlight the need for safe injection practices and basic infection control. *Clin Liver Dis*. 2010;14(1):137-151. doi:10.1016/j.cld.2009.11.004. [VA]

18. Williams IT, Perz JF, Bell BP. Viral hepatitis transmission in ambulatory health care settings. *Clin Infect Dis*. 2004;38(11):1592-1598. doi:10.1086/420935. [VA]

19. Centers for Disease Control and Prevention (CDC). Transmission of hepatitis B and C viruses in outpatient settings—New York, Oklahoma, and Nebraska, 2000-2002. *MMWR Morb Mortal Wkly Rep*. 2003;52(38):901-906. [VA]

20. Henderson DK, Dembry L, Fishman NO, et al. SHEA guideline for management of healthcare workers who are infected with hepatitis B virus, hepatitis C virus, and/or human immunodeficiency virus. *Infect Control Hosp Epidemiol*. 2010;31(3):203-232. [IVA]

21. Young TN, Arens FJ, Kennedy GE, Laurie JW, Rutherford G. Antiretroviral post-exposure prophylaxis (PEP) for occupational HIV exposure. *Cochrane Database Syst Rev*. 2012;5. [IA]

22. Recommended practices for surgical attire. In: *Perioperative Standards and Recommended Practices*. Denver, CO: AORN, Inc; 2012:57-72. [IVB]

23. Neely AN, Maley MP. Survival of enterococci and staphylococci on hospital fabrics and plastic. *J Clin Microbiol*. 2000;38(2):724-726. [IIB]

24. Neely AN, Orloff MM. Survival of some medically important fungi on hospital fabrics and plastics. *J Clin Microbiol*. 2001;39(9):3360-3361. [IIIB]

25. Gastmeier P, Stamm-Balderjahn S, Hansen S, et al. How outbreaks can contribute to prevention of nosocomial infection: analysis of 1,022 outbreaks. *Infect Control Hosp Epidemiol*. 2005;26(4):357-361. doi:10.1086/502552. [VA]

26. Bhalla A, Pultz NJ, Gries DM, et al. Acquisition of nosocomial pathogens on hands after contact with environmental surfaces near hospitalized patients. *Infect Control Hosp Epidemiol*. 2004;25(2):164-167. doi:10.1086/502369. [IIB]

27. Siegel JD, Rhinehart E, Jackson M, Chiarello L; Healthcare Infection Control Practices Advisory Committee. *Management of Multidrug-Resistant Organisms in Healthcare Settings, 2006*. Atlanta, GA: Centers for Disease Control and Prevention; 2006. [IVA]

28. Bolyard EA, Tablan OC, Williams WW, Pearson ML, Shapiro CN, Deitchmann SD. Guideline for infection control in healthcare personnel, 1998. Hospital Infection Control Practices Advisory Committee. *Infect Control Hosp Epidemiol*. 1998;19(6):407-463. [IVA]

29. Wharton M, Strikas RA, Harpaz R, et al. Recommendations for using smallpox vaccine in a pre-event vaccination program. Supplemental recommendations of the Advisory Committee on Immunization Practices (ACIP) and the Healthcare Infection Control Practices Advisory Committee (HICPAC). *MMWR Recomm Rep*. 2003;52(RR-7):1-16. [IVA]

30. Sethi AK, Al-Nassir WN, Nerandzic MM, Bobulsky GS, Donskey CJ. Persistence of skin contamination and environmental shedding of *Clostridium difficile* during and after treatment of *C difficile* infection. *Infect Control Hosp Epidemiol*. 2010;31(1):21-27. [IIA]

31. Occelli P, Blanie M, Sanchez R, et al. Outbreak of staphylococcal bullous impetigo in a maternity ward linked to an asymptomatic healthcare worker. *J Hosp Infect*. 2007;67(3):264-270. [IIIB]

32. Duckro AN, Blom DW, Lyle EA, Weinstein RA, Hayden MK. Transfer of vancomycin-resistant enterococci via health care worker hands. *Arch Intern Med*. 2005;165(3):302-307. doi:10.1001/archinte.165.3.302. [IIIB]

33. Edgeworth JD. Has decolonization played a central role in the decline in UK methicillin-resistant *Staphylococcus aureus* transmission? A focus on evidence from intensive care. *J Antimicrob Chemother*. 2011;66(Suppl 2):ii41-ii47. [VA]

34. Boyce JM, Havill NL, Kohan C, Dumigan DG, Ligi CE. Do infection control measures work for methicillin-resistant *Staphylococcus aureus*? *Infect Control Hosp Epidemiol*. 2004;25(5):395-401. doi:10.1086/502412. [IIIB]

35. Mastoraki A, Douka E, Kriaras I, Stravopodis G, Saroglou G, Geroulanos S. Preventing strategy of multidrug-resistant *Acinetobacter baumanii* susceptible only to colistin in cardiac surgical intensive care units. *Eur J Cardiothorac Surg*. 2008;33(6):1086-1090. [IIIB]

36. Huskins WC, Huckabee CM, O'Grady NP, et al. Intervention to reduce transmission of resistant bacteria in intensive care. *N Engl J Med*. 2011;364(15):1407-1418. [IA]

37. Wines MP, Lamb A, Argyropoulos AN, Caviezel A, Gannicliffe C, Tolley D. Blood splash injury: an underestimated risk in endourology. *J Endourol*. 2008;22(6):1183-1187. [IIIB]

38. Ishihama K, Iida S, Koizumi H, et al. High incidence of blood exposure due to imperceptible contaminated splatters during oral surgery. *J Oral Maxillofac Surg*. 2008;66(4):704-710. [IIIB]

39. Vonberg RP, Kuijper EJ, Wilcox MH, et al. Infection control measures to limit the spread of *Clostridium difficile*. *Clin Microbiol Infect*. 2008;14(Suppl 5):2-20. doi:10.1111/j.1469-0691.2008.01992.x. [VA]

40. Datta R, Platt R, Yokoe DS, Huang SS. Environmental cleaning intervention and risk of acquiring multidrug-resistant organisms from prior room occupants. *Arch Intern Med*. 2011;171(6):491-494. doi:10.1001/archinternmed.2011.64. [IIB]

41. Rodríguez-Baño J, García L, Ramírez E, et al. Long-term control of hospital-wide, endemic multidrug-resistant *Acinetobacter baumannii* through a comprehensive

"bundle" approach. *Am J Infect Control*. 2009;37(9):715-722. [IIA]

42. Eckstein BC, Adams DA, Eckstein EC, et al. Reduction of *Clostridium difficile* and vancomycin-resistant Enterococcus contamination of environmental surfaces after an intervention to improve cleaning methods. *BMC Infect Dis*. 2007;7:61. [IIIA]

43. Jernigan JA, Siegman-Igra Y, Guerrant RC, Farr BM. A randomized crossover study of disposable thermometers for prevention of *Clostridium difficile* and other nosocomial infections. *Infect Control Hosp Epidemiol*. 1998;19(7):494-499. [IA]

44. Kirkland KB. Taking off the gloves: toward a less dogmatic approach to the use of contact isolation. *Clin Infect Dis*. 2009;48(6):766-771. doi:10.1086/597090. [VB]

45. Saint S, Higgins LA, Nallamothu BK, Chenoweth C. Do physicians examine patients in contact isolation less frequently? A brief report. *Am J Infect Control*. 2003;31(6):354-356. [IVA]

46. Morgan DJ, Diekema DJ, Sepkowitz K, Perencevich EN. Adverse outcomes associated with contact precautions: a review of the literature. *Am J Infect Control*. 2009;37(2):85-93. doi:10.1016/j.ajic.2008.04.257. [VA]

47. Zastrow RL. Emerging infections: the contact precautions controversy. *Am J Nurs*. 2011;111(3):47-53. [VB]

48. Papineni RS, Rosenthal FS. The size distribution of droplets in the exhaled breath of healthy human subjects. *J Aerosol Med*. 1997;10(2):105-116. [IIB]

49. Raboud J, Shigayeva A, McGeer A, et al. Risk factors for SARS transmission from patients requiring intubation: a multicentre investigation in Toronto, Canada. *PLoS ONE [Electronic Resource]*. 2010;5(5):e10717. [IIIA]

50. Advisory Committee on Immunization Practices; Centers for Disease Control and Prevention (CDC). Immunization of health-care personnel: recommendations of the Advisory Committee on Immunization Practices (ACIP). *MMWR Recomm Rep*. 2011;60(RR-7):1-45. [IVA]

51. Sakaguchi H, Wada K, Kajioka J, et al. Maintenance of influenza virus infectivity on the surfaces of personal protective equipment and clothing used in healthcare settings. *Environ Health Prev Med*. 2010;15(6):344-349. [IIIB]

52. Kilpatrick C, Prieto J, Wigglesworth N. Single room isolation to prevent the transmission of infection: Development of a patient journey tool to support safe practice. *Br J Infect Control*. 2008;9(6):19-25. [VB]

53. Centers for Disease Control and Prevention (CDC). Guidelines for preventing the transmission of *Mycobacterium tuberculosis* in health-care settings, 2005. *MMWR Morb Mortal Wkly Rep*. 2005;54(RR-17):1-140. [IVA]

54. Bassetti S, Bischoff WE, Walter M, et al. Dispersal of *Staphylococcus aureus* into the air associated with a rhinovirus infection. *Infect Control Hosp Epidemiol*. 2005;26(2):196-203. doi:10.1086/502526. [IIB]

55. Respirator trusted-source information. Centers for Disease Control and Prevention. http://www.cdc.gov/niosh/npptl/topics/respirators/disp_part/RespSource.html. Accessed October 26, 2012.

56. Olmsted RN. Pilot study of directional airflow and containment of airborne particles in the size of *Mycobacterium tuberculosis* in an operating room. *Am J Infect Control*. 2008;36(4):260-267. doi:10.1016/j.ajic.2007.10.028. [IIB]

57. Guideline for electrosurgery. In: *Guidelines for Perioperative Practice*. Denver, CO: AORN, Inc; 2015:121-138. [IVB]

58. Preventing the transmission of bloodborne pathogens information statement. American Academy of Orthopaedic Surgeons. http://www.aaos.org/about/papers/advistmt/1018.asp. Updated June 2008. Accessed October 26, 2012. [VA]

59. Association for Professionals in Infection Control and Epidemiology, Inc. APIC position paper: prevention of device-mediated bloodborne infections to health care workers. *Am J Infect Control*. 1998;26(6):578-580. [VA]

60. OSHA's bloodborne pathogens standard: analysis and recommendations. *Health Devices*. 1993;22(2):35-92.

61. Aarnio P, Laine T. Glove perforation rate in vascular surgery—a comparison between single and double gloving. *Vasa*. 2001;30(2):122-124. [IIIC]

62. Wilburn SQ. Needlestick and sharps injury prevention. *Online J Issues Nurs*. 2004;9(3):5. [VA]

63. Jagger J, Perry J, Gomaa A, Phillips EK. The impact of U.S. policies to protect healthcare workers from bloodborne pathogens: the critical role of safety-engineered devices. *J Infect Public Health*. 2008;1(2):62-71. doi:10.1016/j.jiph.2008.10.002. [VA]

64. Tuma S, Sepkowitz KA. Efficacy of safety-engineered device implementation in the prevention of percutaneous injuries: a review of published studies. *Clin Infect Dis*. 2006;42(8):1159-1170. doi:10.1086/501456. [IVA]

65. Vose JG, McAdara-Berkowitz J. Reducing scalpel injuries in the operating room. *AORN J*. 2009;90(6):867-872. doi:10.1016/j.aorn.2009.07.025. [VB]

66. Protecting workers' families: a research agenda report of the Workers' Family Protection Task Force [DHHS (NIOSH) publication number 2002-113]. http://www.cdc.gov/niosh/docs/2002-113. Accessed October 26, 2012. [VA]

67. Tenorio AR, Badri SM, Sahgal NB, et al. Effectiveness of gloves in the prevention of hand carriage of vancomycin-resistant enterococcus species by health care workers after patient care. *Clin Infect Dis*. 2001;32(5):826-829. doi:10.1086/319214. [IIB]

68. Daeschlein G, Kramer A, Arnold A, Ladwig A, Seabrook GR, Edmiston CE Jr. Evaluation of an innovative antimicrobial surgical glove technology to reduce the risk of microbial passage following intraoperative perforation. *Am J Infect Control*. 2011;39(2):98-103. doi:10.1016/j.ajic.2010.05.026. [IIB]

69. Hayden MK, Blom DW, Lyle EA, Moore CG, Weinstein RA. Risk of hand or glove contamination after contact with patients colonized with vancomycin-resistant enterococcus or the colonized patients' environment. *Infect Control Hosp Epidemiol*. 2008;29(2):149-154. [IIIA]

70. Kinlin LM, Mittleman MA, Harris AD, Rubin MA, Fisman DN. Use of gloves and reduction of risk of injury caused by needles or sharp medical devices in healthcare workers: results from a case-crossover study. *Infect Control Hosp Epidemiol*. 2010;31(9):908-917. doi:10.1086/655839. [IIIB]

71. Olsen RJ, Lynch P, Coyle MB, Cummings J, Bokete T, Stamm WE. Examination gloves as barriers to hand contamination in clinical practice. *JAMA*. 1993;270(3):350-353. [IIB]

72. Eklund AM, Ojajarvi J, Laitinen K, Valtonen M, Werkkala KA. Glove punctures and postoperative skin flora of hands in cardiac surgery. *Ann Thorac Surg*. 2002;74(1):149-153. [IIB]

73. Guideline for sterile technique. In: *Guidelines for Perioperative Practice*. Denver, CO: AORN, Inc; 2015:67-96. [IVA]

74. Misteli H, Weber WP, Reck S, et al. Surgical glove perforation and the risk of surgical site infection. *Arch Surg*. 2009;144(6):553-558. doi:10.1001/archsurg.2009.60. [IIIA]

75. Harnoss JC, Partecke LI, Heidecke CD, Hubner NO, Kramer A, Assadian O. Concentration of bacteria passing

through puncture holes in surgical gloves. *Am J Infect Control.* 2010;38(2):154-158. [IIA]

76. Hubner NO, Goerdt AM, Stanislawski N, et al. Bacterial migration through punctured surgical gloves under real surgical conditions. *BMC Infect Dis.* 2010;10:192. [IIC]

77. Partecke LI, Goerdt AM, Langner I, et al. Incidence of microperforation for surgical gloves depends on duration of wear. *Infect Control Hosp Epidemiol.* 2009;30(5):409-414. [IIIA]

78. Al-Maiyah M, Bajwa A, Mackenney P, et al. Glove perforation and contamination in primary total hip arthroplasty. *J Bone Joint Surg Br.* 2005;87(4):556-559. [IA]

79. Korniewicz DM, Kirwin M, Cresci K, et al. Barrier protection with examination gloves: double versus single. *Am J Infect Control.* 1994;22(1):12-15. [IIB]

80. Korniewicz DM, El-Masri M, Broyles JM, Martin CD, O'connell KP. Performance of latex and nonlatex medical examination gloves during simulated use. *Am J Infect Control.* 2002;30(2):133-138. [IIB]

81. Rego A, Roley L. In-use barrier integrity of gloves: latex and nitrile superior to vinyl. *Am J Infect Control.* 1999;27(5):405-410. [IIB]

82. Klein RC, Party E, Gershey EL. Virus penetration of examination gloves. *Biotechniques.* 1990;9(2):196-199. [IIB]

83. Tulipan N, Cleves MA. Effect of an intraoperative double-gloving strategy on the incidence of cerebrospinal fluid shunt infection. *J Neurosurg.* 2006;104(1 Suppl):5-8. doi:10.3171/ped.2006.104.1.5. [IIA]

84. Tanner J, Parkinson H. Surgical glove practice: the evidence. *J Perioper Pract.* 2007;17(5):216-218, 220-222, 224-225. [IA]

85. Tanner J, Parkinson H. Double gloving to reduce surgical cross-infection. *Cochrane Database Syst Rev.* 2009;1. [IA]

86. Korniewicz D, El-Masri M. Exploring the benefits of double gloving during surgery. *AORN J.* 2012;95(3):328-336. doi:10.1016/j.aorn.2011.04.027. [IIIB]

87. Berguer R, Heller PJ. Preventing sharps injuries in the operating room. *J Am Coll Surg.* 2004;199(3):462-467. doi:10.1016/j.jamcollsurg.2004.04.018. [VA]

88. Lancaster C, Duff P. Single versus double-gloving for obstetric and gynecologic procedures. *Am J Obstet Gynecol.* 2007;196(5):e36-e37. doi:10.1016/j.ajog.2006.08.045. [VA]

89. Laine T, Kaipia A, Santavirta J, Aarnio P. Glove perforations in open and laparoscopic abdominal surgery: the feasibility of double gloving. *Scand J Surg.* 2004;93(1):73-76. [IA]

90. Haines T, Stringer B, Herring J, Thoma A, Harris KA. Surgeons' and residents' double-gloving practices at 2 teaching hospitals in Ontario. *Can J Surg.* 2011;54(2):95-100. [IIIB]

91. Wittmann A, Kralj N, Kover J, Gasthaus K, Hofmann F. Study of blood contact in simulated surgical needlestick injuries with single or double latex gloving. *Infect Control Hosp Epidemiol.* 2009;30(1):53-56. doi:10.1086/593124. [IIA]

92. Myers DJ, Epling C, Dement J, Hunt D. Risk of sharp device-related blood and body fluid exposure in operating rooms. *Infect Control Hosp Epidemiol.* 2008;29(12):1139-1148. doi:10.1086/592091. [VA]

93. Florman S, Burgdorf M, Finigan K, Slakey D, Hewitt R, Nichols RL. Efficacy of double gloving with an intrinsic indicator system. *Surg Infect (Larchmt).* 2005;6(4):385-395. [IIB]

94. Duron JJ, Keilani K, Elian NG. Efficacy of double gloving with a coloured inner pair for immediate detection of operative glove perforations. *Eur J Surg.* 1996;162(12):941-944. [VB]

95. Eye safety: eye protection for infection control. NIOSH workplace safety and health topic. Centers for Disease Control and Prevention. http://www.cdc.gov/niosh/topics/eye/eye-infectious.html. Accessed October 26, 2012. [IVB]

96. Philips BJ, Fergusson S, Armstrong P, Anderson FM, Wildsmith JA. Surgical face masks are effective in reducing bacterial contamination caused by dispersal from the upper airway. *Br J Anaesth.* 1992;69(4):407-408. [IIC]

97. Mangram AJ, Horan TC, Pearson ML, Silver LC, Jarvis WR; Hospital Infection Control Practices Advisory Committee. Guideline for prevention of surgical site infection, 1999. *Infect Control Hosp Epidemiol.* 1999;20(4):250-278. doi:10.1086/501620. [IVA]

98. Alwitry A, Jackson E, Chen H, Holden R. The use of surgical facemasks during cataract surgery: is it necessary? *Br J Ophthalmol.* 2002;86(9):975-977. [IB]

99. Chambers CE, Eisenhauer MD, McNicol LB, et al. Infection control guidelines for the cardiac catheterization laboratory: society guidelines revisited. *Catheter Cardiovasc Interv.* 2006;67(1):78-86. doi:10.1002/ccd.20589. [IVA]

100. Berger SA, Kramer M, Nagar H, Finkelstein A, Frimmerman A, Miller HI. Effect of surgical mask position on bacterial contamination of the operative field. *J Hosp Infect.* 1993;23(1):51-54. [IIB]

101. Lipp A. The effectiveness of surgical face masks: what the literature shows. *Nurs Times.* 2003;99(39):22-24. [VB]

102. Gralton J, McLaws ML. Protecting healthcare workers from pandemic influenza: N95 or surgical masks? *Crit Care Med.* 2010;38(2):657-667. [VA]

103. Korczak D, Schöffmann C. Medical and health economic evaluation of prevention- and control measures related to MRSA infections or -colonisations at hospitals. *GMS Health Technol Assess.* 2010;6:Doc04. [IIIB]

104. Lai JY, Guo YP, Or PP, Li Y. Comparison of hand contamination rates and environmental contamination levels between two different glove removal methods and distances. *Am J Infect Control.* 2011;39(2):104-111. doi:10.1016/j.ajic.2010.06.007. [IIB]

105. Anderson DJ, Kaye KS, Classen D, et al. Strategies to prevent surgical site infections in acute care hospitals. *Infect Control Hosp Epidemiol.* 2008;29(Suppl 1):S51-S61. doi:10.1086/591064. [IVA]

106. Recommended practices for cleaning and care of surgical instruments and powered equipment. In: *Perioperative Standards and Recommended Practices.* Denver, CO: AORN, Inc; 2012:513-536. [IVB]

107. Beldi G, Bisch-Knaden S, Banz V, Muhlemann K, Candinas D. Impact of intraoperative behavior on surgical site infections. *Am J Surg.* 2009;198(2):157-162. [IA]

108. Dineen P, Drusin L. Epidemics of postoperative wound infections associated with hair carriers. *Lancet.* 1973;2(7839):1157-1159. [VA]

109. Mastro TD, Farley TA, Elliott JA, et al. An outbreak of surgical-wound infections due to group A streptococcus carried on the scalp. *N Engl J Med.* 1990;323(14):968-972. [IIIB]

110. Mase K, Hasegawa T, Horii T, et al. Firm adherence of *Staphylococcus aureus* and *Staphylococcus epidermidis* to human hair and effect of detergent treatment. *Microbiol Immunol.* 2000;44(8):653-656. [IIB]

111. Recommended practices for preoperative patient skin antisepsis. In: *Perioperative Standards and Recommended Practices.* Denver, CO: AORN, Inc; 2012:445-464. [IVB]

112. Carro C, Camilleri L, Traore O, et al. An in-use microbiological comparison of two surgical hand disinfection techniques in cardiothoracic surgery: hand rubbing versus hand scrubbing. *J Hosp Infect*. 2007;67(1):62-66. [IIIA]

113. Le TA, Dibley MJ, Vo VN, Archibald L, Jarvis WR, Sohn AH. Reduction in surgical site infections in neurosurgical patients associated with a bedside hand hygiene program in Vietnam. *Infect Control Hosp Epidemiol*. 2007;28(5):583-588. doi:10.1086/516661. [IIA]

114. Recommended practices for traffic patterns in the perioperative practice setting. In: *Perioperative Standards and Recommended Practices*. Denver, CO: AORN, Inc; 2012:95-98. [IVB]

115. Guideline for sterilization. In: *Guidelines for Perioperative Practice*. Denver, CO: AORN, Inc; 2015:665-692. [IVB]

116. Schwarzkopf R, Takemoto RC, Immerman I, Slover JD, Bosco JA. Prevalence of *Staphylococcus aureus* colonization in orthopaedic surgeons and their patients: a prospective cohort controlled study. *J Bone Joint Surg Am*. 2010;92(9):1815-1819. doi:10.2106/JBJS.I.00991. [IIA]

117. Ammerlaan HS, Kluytmans JA, Wertheim HF, Nouwen JL, Bonten MJ. Eradication of methicillin-resistant *Staphylococcus aureus* carriage: a systematic review. *Clin Infect Dis*. 2009;48(7):922-930. doi:10.1086/597291. [IA]

118. Konvalinka A, Errett L, Fong IW. Impact of treating *Staphylococcus aureus* nasal carriers on wound infections in cardiac surgery. *J Hosp Infect*. 2006;64(2):162-168. [IA]

119. Segers P, Speekenbrink RG, Ubbink DT, van Ogtrop ML, de Mol BA. Prevention of nosocomial infection in cardiac surgery by decontamination of the nasopharynx and oropharynx with chlorhexidine gluconate: a randomized controlled trial. *JAMA*. 2006;296(20):2460-2466. [IA]

120. Yinusa W, Onche II, Thanni LO. Short-term antibiotic prophylaxis in implant surgery: a comparison of three antibiotics. *Niger Postgrad Med J*. 2007;14(2):90-93. [IB]

121. Kato D, Maezawa K, Yonezawa I, et al. Randomized prospective study on prophylactic antibiotics in clean orthopedic surgery in one ward for 1 year. *J Orthop Sci*. 2006;11(1):20-27. doi:10.1007/s00776-005-0970-0. [IIB]

122. Centers for Disease Control and Prevention (CDC). Carbapenem-resistant Enterobacteriaceae containing New Delhi metallo-beta-lactamase in two patients – Rhode Island, March 2012. *MMWR Morb Mortal Wkly Rep*. 2012;61:446-448. [VA]

123. Healthcare-associated infections (HAIs). 2012 CRE toolkit – Guidance for control of carbapenem-resistant Enterobacteriaceae (CRE). Part 2: Regional CRE prevention. Centers for Disease Control and Prevention. http://www.cdc.gov/hai/organisms/cre/cre-toolkit/rCRE prevention-AppendixC.html. Accessed October 26, 2012. [IVA]

124. Fairclough SJ. Why tackling MRSA needs a comprehensive approach. *Br J Nurs*. 2006;15(2):72-75. [VA]

125. Larson EL, Quiros D, Giblin T, Lin S. Relationship of antimicrobial control policies and hospital and infection control characteristics to antimicrobial resistance rates. *Am J Crit Care*. 2007;16(2):110-120. [IIIA]

126. Ellingson K, Muder RR, Jain R, et al. Sustained reduction in the clinical incidence of methicillin-resistant *Staphylococcus aureus* colonization or infection associated with a multifaceted infection control intervention. *Infect Control Hosp Epidemiol*. 2011;32(1):1-8. [IIB]

127. Griffin FA. 5 Million Lives Campaign. Reducing methicillin-resistant *Staphylococcus aureus* (MRSA) infections. *Jt Comm J Qual Patient Saf*. 2007;33(12):726-731. [IVA]

128. Sroka S, Gastmeier P, Meyer E. Impact of alcohol hand-rub use on methicillin-resistant *Staphylococcus aureus*: an analysis of the literature. *J Hosp Infect*. 2010;74(3):204-211. doi:10.1016/j.jhin.2009.08.023. [VC]

129. Miyachi H, Furuya H, Umezawa K, et al. Controlling methicillin-resistant *Staphylococcus aureus* by stepwise implementation of preventive strategies in a university hospital: impact of a link-nurse system on the basis of multidisciplinary approaches. *Am J Infect Control*. 2007;35(2):115-121. [IIIB]

130. Hsu J, Abad C, Dinh M, Safdar N. Prevention of endemic healthcare-associated Clostridium difficile infection: reviewing the evidence. *Am J Gastroenterol*. 2010;105(11):2327-2339. doi:10.1038/ajg.2010.254. [IVA]

131. Salgado CD, O'Grady N, Farr BM. Prevention and control of antimicrobial-resistant infections in intensive care patients. *Crit Care Med*. 2005;33(10):2373-2382. [VA]

132. Tyllianakis ME, Karageorgos ACh, Marangos MN, Saridis AG, Lambiris EE. Antibiotic prophylaxis in primary hip and knee arthroplasty: comparison between cefuroxime and two specific antistaphylococcal agents. *J Arthroplasty*. 2010;25(7):1078-1082. doi:10.1016/j.arth.2010.01.105. [IB]

133. Zilberberg MD, Chen J, Mody SH, Ramsey AM, Shorr AF. Imipenem resistance of Pseudomonas in pneumonia: a systematic literature review. *BMC Pulm Med*. 2010;10:45. doi:10.1186/1471-2466-10-45. [VA]

134. Tacconelli E. Antimicrobial use: risk driver of multidrug resistant microorganisms in healthcare settings. *Curr Opin Infect Dis*. 2009;22(4):352-358. doi:10.1097/QCO.0b013e32832d52e0. [VA]

135. Tacconelli E, De Angelis G, Cataldo MA, Pozzi E, Cauda R. Does antibiotic exposure increase the risk of methicillin-resistant *Staphylococcus aureus* (MRSA) isolation? A systematic review and meta-analysis. *J Antimicrob Chemother*. 2008;61(1):26-38. [VB]

136. Davey P, Brown E, Fenelon L, et al. Interventions to improve antibiotic prescribing practices for hospital inpatients. *Cochrane Database Syst Rev*. 2009;1. [IA]

137. Rodríguez-Baño J, García L, Ramírez E, et al. Long-term control of endemic hospital-wide methicillin-resistant *Staphylococcus aureus* (MRSA): the impact of targeted active surveillance for MRSA in patients and healthcare workers. *Infect Control Hosp Epidemiol*. 2010;31(8):786-795. [IIA]

138. Warren DK, Guth RM, Coopersmith CM, Merz LR, Zack JE, Fraser VJ. Impact of a methicillin-resistant *Staphylococcus aureus* active surveillance program on contact precaution utilization in a surgical intensive care unit. *Crit Care Med*. 2007;35(2):430-434. [IIA]

139. Lee TC, Moore C, Raboud JM, et al. Impact of a mandatory infection control education program on nosocomial acquisition of methicillin-resistant *Staphylococcus aureus*. *Infect Control Hosp Epidemiol*. 2009;30(3):249-256. [IIA]

140. Rosenberger LH, Hranjec T, Politano AD, et al. Effective cohorting and "superisolation" in a single intensive care unit in response to an outbreak of diverse multi-drug-resistant organisms. *Surg Infect (Larchmt)*. 2011;12(5):345-350. doi:10.1089/sur.2010.076. [IIIB]

141. Curran ET, Hamilton K, Monaghan A, McGinlay M, Thakker B. Use of a temporary cohort ward as part of an intervention to reduce the incidence of methicillin-resistant *Staphylococcus aureus* in a vascular surgery ward. *J Hosp Infect*. 2006;63(4):374-379. doi:10.1016/j.jhin.2006.02.017. [IIIA]

142. Murthy A, De Angelis G, Pittet D, Schrenzel J, Uckay I, Harbarth S. Cost-effectiveness of universal MRSA

screening on admission to surgery. *Clin Microbiol Infect.* 2010;16(12):1747-1753. [IIIB]

143. O'Grady NP, Alexander M, Burns LA, et al. Guidelines for the prevention of intravascular catheter-related infections. *Am J Infect Control.* 2011;39(4 Suppl 1):S1-S34. doi:10.1016/j.ajic.2011.01.003. [IVA]

144. Carnicer-Pont D, Bailey KA, Mason BW, Walker AM, Evans MR, Salmon RL. Risk factors for hospital-acquired methicillin-resistant *Staphylococcus aureus* bacteraemia: a case-control study. *Epidemiol Infect.* 2006;134(6):1167-1173. [IIB]

145. Loftus RW, Brown JR, Koff MD, et al. Multiple reservoirs contribute to intraoperative bacterial transmission. *Anesth Analg.* 2012;114(6):1236-1248. doi:10.1213/ANE.0b013e31824970a2. [IIA]

146. Gould CV, Umscheid CA, Agarwal RK, Kuntz G, Pegues DA; Healthcare Infection Control Practices Advisory Committee. Guideline for prevention of catheter-associated urinary tract infections 2009. *Infect Control Hosp Epidemiol.* 2010;31(4):319-326. doi:10.1086/651091. [VA]

147. Carlson AL, Perl TM. Health care workers as source of hepatitis B and C virus transmission. *Clin Liver Dis.* 2010;14(1):153-168. [VA]

148. Ehrenstein BP, Hanses F, Blaas S, Mandraka F, Audebert F, Salzberger B. Perceived risks of adverse effects and influenza vaccination: A survey of hospital employees. *Eur J Public Health.* 2010;20(5):495-499. [IIIB]

149. Pearson ML, Bridges CB, Harper SA; Healthcare Infection Control Practices Advisory Committee (HICPAC), Advisory Committee on Immunization Practices (ACIP). Influenza vaccination of health-care personnel: recommendations of the Healthcare Infection Control Practices Advisory Committee (HICPAC) and the Advisory Committee on Immunization Practices (ACIP) [published correction appears in *MMWR Recomm Rep.* 2006;10;55(9):252]. *MMWR Recomm Rep.* 2006;55(RR-2):1-16. [IVA]

150. Feemster KA, Prasad P, Smith MJ, et al. Employee designation and health care worker support of an influenza vaccine mandate at a large pediatric tertiary care hospital. *Vaccine.* 2011;29(9):1762-1769. [IIIB]

151. Llupia A, Garcia-Basteiro AL, Olive V, et al. New interventions to increase influenza vaccination rates in health care workers. *Am J Infect Control.* 2010;38(6):476-481. [IIB]

152. Amodio E, Anastasi G, Marsala MGL, Torregrossa MV, Romano N, Firenze A. Vaccination against the 2009 pandemic influenza A (H1N1) among healthcare workers in the major teaching hospital of Sicily (Italy). *Vaccine.* 2011;29(7):1408-1412. [IIIB]

153. Hopman CE, Riphagen-Dalhuisen J, Looijmans-van den Akker I, et al. Determination of factors required to increase uptake of influenza vaccination among hospital-based healthcare workers. *J Hosp Infect.* 2011;77(4):327-331. [IIIB]

154. Rakita RM, Hagar BA, Crome P, Lammert JK. Mandatory influenza vaccination of healthcare workers: a 5-year study. *Infect Control Hosp Epidemiol.* 2010;31(9):881-888. [IIIB]

155. Leekha S, Thompson RL, Sampathkumar P. Epidemiology and control of pertussis outbreaks in a tertiary care center and the resource consumption associated with these outbreaks. *Infect Control Hosp Epidemiol.* 2009;30(5):467-473. [IIIB]

156. Centers for Disease Control and Prevention (CDC). Updated recommendations for use of tetanus toxoid, reduced diphtheria toxoid and acellular pertussis (Tdap) vaccine from the Advisory Committee on Immunization Practices, 2010. *MMWR Morb Mortal Wkly Rep.* 2011;60(1):13-15. [IVA]

157. Johnston CP, Qiu H, Ticehurst JR, et al. Outbreak management and implications of a nosocomial norovirus outbreak. *Clin Infect Dis.* 2007;45(5):534-540. [IIIB]

158. Kak N, Burkhalter B, Cooper M-A. Measuring the competence of healthcare providers [Issue paper]. Bethesda, MD: US Agency for International Development; 2001. http://www.hciproject.org/sites/default/files/Measuring%20the%20Competence%20of%20HC%20Providers_QAP_2001.pdf. Accessed October 26, 2012. [VA]

159. HR.01.05.03: Staff participate in ongoing education and training. In: *Comprehensive Accreditation Manual: CAMH for Hospitals.* Oakbrook Terrace, IL: The Joint Commission; 2012.

160. HR.01.05.03: Staff participate in ongoing education and training. In: *Comprehensive Accreditation Manual for Ambulatory Care.* Oakbrook Terrace, IL: Joint Commission; 2012.

161. Centers for Medicare & Medicaid Services. *State Operations Manual Appendix A—Survey Protocol, Regulations and Interpretive Guidelines for Hospitals.* Rev. 78; 2011.

162. Centers for Medicare & Medicaid Services. *State Operations Manual Appendix L: Guidance for Surveyors: Ambulatory Surgical Centers.* Rev. 76; 2011.

163. Sportsman S. Competency education and validation in the United States: what should nurses know? *Nurs Forum.* 2010;45(3):140-149. doi:10.1111/j.1744-6198.2010.00183.x. [VA]

164. Jordan C, Thomas MB, Evans ML, Green A. Public policy on competency: how will nursing address this complex issue? *J Contin Educ Nurs.* 2008;39(2):86-91. [VA]

165. Bioterrorism agents/diseases: emergency preparedness and response. Centers for Disease Control and Prevention. http://www.bt.cdc.gov/agent/agentlist.asp. Accessed October 26, 2012. [IVA]

166. Howard DP, Williams C, Sen S, et al. A simple effective clean practice protocol significantly improves hand decontamination and infection control measures in the acute surgical setting. *Infection.* 2009;37(1):34-38. [IIB]

167. Guideline for perioperative health care information management. In: *Guidelines for Perioperative Practice.* Denver, CO: AORN, Inc; 2015:491-512. [IVB]

168. Simmons BP. Guideline for prevention of surgical wound infections. *Am J Infect Control.* 1983;11(4):133-143. [IVB]

169. Yokoe DS, Classen D. Improving patient safety through infection control: a new healthcare imperative. *Infect Control Hosp Epidemiol.* 2008;29(Suppl 1):S3-S11. doi:10.1086/591063. [IVA]

170. Governance. In: *2012 Accreditation Handbook for Ambulatory Health Care.* Skokie, IL: Accreditation Association for Ambulatory Health Care; 2012:20-27.

171. Personnel: personnel records. In: *Procedural Standards and Checklist for Accreditation Ambulatory Facilities.* Version 1. Gurnee, IL: American Association for Accreditation of Ambulatory Facilities; 2008:51-52.

172. LD.04.01.07: The hospital has policies and procedures that guide and support patient care, treatment, and services. In: *Hospital Accreditation Standards 2012.* Oakbrook Terrace, IL: Joint Commission on Resources; 2012.

173. LD.04.01.07: The organization has policies and procedures that guide and support patient care, treatment, or services. In: *Standards for Ambulatory Care 2012: Standards, Elements of Performance Scoring Accreditation*

Polices. Oakbrook Terrace, IL: The Joint Commission; 2012.

174. National action plan to prevent healthcare-associated infections: roadmap to elimination. US Department of Health & Human Services. http://www.hhs.gov/ash/initiatives/hai/actionplan/. Accessed October 26, 2012. [VA]

175. Carling PC, Bartley JM. Evaluating hygienic cleaning in health care settings: what you do not know can harm your patients. *Am J Infect Control*. 2010;38(5 Suppl 1):S41-S50. doi:10.1016/j.ajic.2010.03.004. [IIB]

176. Farquhar M. AHRQ quality indicators. In: Hughes RG, ed. *Patient Safety and Quality: An Evidence-Based Handbook for Nurses*. Rockville MD: Agency for Healthcare Research and Quality; 2008:41-67. http://purl.access.gpo.gov/GPO/LPS93676. Accessed October 26, 2012. [IA]

177. Larson EL, Cohen B, Ross B, Behta M. Isolation precautions for methicillin-resistant *Staphylococcus aureus*: electronic surveillance to monitor adherence. *Am J Crit Care*. 2010;19(1):16-26. doi:10.4037/ajcc2009467. [IVA]

178. Accountability measures. Joint Commission. http://www.jointcommission.org/accountability_measures.aspx. Accessed October 26, 2012.

179. Rosenberger LH, Politano AD, Sawyer RG. The surgical care improvement project and prevention of post-operative infection, including surgical site infection. *Surg Infect (Larchmt)*. 2011;12(3):163-168. doi:10.1089/sur.2010.083. [VA]

Acknowledgments

Lead Author
Lisa Spruce, DNP, RN, ACNS, ACNP, ANP, CNOR
Director of Evidence-based Perioperative Practice
AORN Nursing Department
Denver, Colorado

Contributing Authors
Ramona Conner, MSN, RN, CNOR
Manager, Standards and Guidelines
AORN Nursing Department
Denver, Colorado

Kimberly J. Retzlaff
Managing Editor
AORN Publications Department
Denver, Colorado

The authors and AORN thank George Allen, PhD, MS, RN, CNOR, CIC, Director Infection Control, Downstate Medical Center and Clinical Assistant Professor, SUNY College of Health Related Professions, Brooklyn, New York; Hudson Garret, Jr., PhD, MSN, MPH, FNP-BC, Senior Director, Clinical Affairs, PDI Healthcare, Atlanta, Georgia; Marcia R. Patrick, MSN, RN, CIC, Association for Professionals in Infection Control and Epidemiology liaison to the AORN Recommended Practices Advisory Board and Independent Consultant, Tacoma, Washington; and Rebecca Saxton, PhD, RN, CNOR, CNE, Associate Professor, Research College of Nursing, Director, Center for Nursing Research and Innovation, Kansas City, Missouri, for their assistance in developing this guideline.

Publication History

Originally published February 1993, *AORN Journal*, as "Recommended practices for universal precautions in the perioperative practice setting."

Revised November 1998 as "Recommended practices for standard and transmission-based precautions in the perioperative practice setting"; published February 1999, *AORN Journal*. Reformatted July 2000.

Approved June 2006, AORN Board of Directors, as "Recommended practices for prevention of transmissible infections in perioperative practice settings." Published in *Standards, Recommended Practices, and Guidelines*, 2007 edition.

Revised and reformatted December 2012 for online publication in *Perioperative Standards and Recommended Practices*.

Evidence ratings revised 2013 to conform to the AORN Evidence Rating Model.

Minor editing revisions made in November 2014 for publication in *Guidelines for Perioperative Practice*, 2015 edition.

AMBULATORY SUPPLEMENT: TRANSMISSIBLE INFECTIONS

Recommendation III

Droplet precautions should be used throughout the perioperative environment (ie, preoperative, intraoperative, postoperative) when providing care to patients who are known or suspected to be infected with microorganisms that can be transmitted by large droplets.[A1]

Amb The facility should screen individuals for infectious agents (eg, influenza, pertussis) transmitted by droplets.[A1] Identification of infected individuals before their admission to the ambulatory surgery center (ASC) may prevent infection transmission.[A1]

Recommendation IV

Airborne precautions should be used when providing care to patients who are known or suspected to be infected with microorganisms that can be transmitted by the airborne route.

IV.h. Elective surgery should be postponed for patients who have suspected or confirmed [tuberculosis] TB until the patient is determined to be noninfectious. If surgery cannot be postponed, perioperative personnel should follow airborne precautions and consult with an infection preventionist.

Amb Personnel in an ASC that provides care to patients with confirmed or suspected TB should follow recommendation IV.

Amb Unless the facility has the capability of establishing a negative pressure room, patients with suspected or confirmed cases of TB should be transferred to or re-scheduled at a facility with a negative pressure room. A negative pressure airborne infection isolation room and a respiratory protection program are needed for airborne infection isolation. Airborne infection isolation is needed for any patient with suspected or confirmed active pulmonary TB.[A1-A3]

Recommendation X

Perioperative personnel should receive initial and ongoing education and competency validation of their understanding of the principles of infection prevention and the performance of standard, contact, droplet, and airborne precautions for prevention of transmissible infections and [multidrug-resistant organisms] MDROs.

Amb An ASC that is certified by the Centers for Medicare & Medicaid Services (CMS) must designate a staff member trained in infection prevention to lead the facility's infection prevention program.[A4]

> **Interpretive Guidelines: §416.51(b)(1)**
>
> *The ASC must designate in writing, a qualified licensed health care professional who will lead the facility's infection control program. The ASC must determine that the individual has had training in the principles and methods of infection control.*
>
> Interpretative Guidelines: §416.51(b)(1). In: Centers for Medicare & Medicaid Services. *State Operations Manual Appendix A—Survey Protocol, Regulations and Interpretive Guidelines for Hospitals.* Rev. 89; 2013.

Amb Ambulatory surgery center personnel, including
- medical personnel,
- nursing personnel,
- personnel responsible for on-site sterilization/high-level disinfection processes, and
- environmental services personnel

should receive infection prevention education.[A5]

Amb Infection prevention education should be conducted
- upon hire,
- annually, and
- periodically as needed.[A5]

Recommendation XI

Documentation should reflect activities related to infection prevention.

Amb A CMS-certified facility's infection prevention program must document the process of consideration, selection, and implementation of a nationally recognized infection control guideline,[A4] such as the AORN *Perioperative Standards and Recommended Practices.*[A6]

Amb Supporting documentation for the surgical site infection tracking and surveillance program should be maintained.[A5]

Amb Infection prevention education records should be maintained for all personnel.[A7]

Recommendation XII

Policies and procedures for the prevention and control of transmissible infections and MDROs should be developed, reviewed periodically, revised as necessary, and readily available within the practice setting.

AMBULATORY SUPPLEMENT: TRANSMISSIBLE INFECTIONS

Amb The infection prevention policy and procedure must comply with the state's reporting requirements for notifiable diseases.[A5,A8]

Recommendation XIII

Perioperative team members should participate in a variety of quality assurance and performance improvement activities to monitor and improve the prevention of infections and MDROs.

Amb A risk assessment should be conducted as part of the infection prevention plan. There are diverse floor plans and environmental controls in ASCs that may present challenges to supporting current infection prevention practices.

Amb The patient population and community served should be part of the risk assessment.

Amb The ASC must have a program to control and investigate infectious and communicable diseases.[A8]

Amb The infection prevention program should include surgical site infection (SSI) surveillance.[A8]

Amb A CMS-certified facility is required to have a process to follow up on each patient after discharge to identify and track infections associated with the patient's stay in the ASC.[A9]

The information should include
- a report of any SSI,
- identification details (eg, culture),
- symptoms,
- treatment, and
- prescribed antibiotics.[A5]

XIII.d.3. When a cluster of SSIs involves an unusual organism, a formal epidemiologic investigation should be conducted.[A10]

Amb An outbreak investigation should be conducted if there is an unexpected increase in infections.[A11]

Amb A multidisciplinary team should be assembled to conduct the investigation.

Amb Resources for conducting an investigation may include
- an infectious disease physician,
- the state department of health, and
- the Centers for Disease Control and Prevention.

Amb A facility participating in the CMS Ambulatory Surgical Quality Reporting Program must report influenza vaccination data for health care personnel (eg, employees, licensed independent practitioners, students, volunteers).[A12]

Glossary

Surveillance: The ongoing collection of data that pertains to occurrence of a specific disease or health care concern of interest (eg, surgical site infection, hand hygiene compliance) and the analysis, interpretation, and then dissemination of this data analysis to those who are responsible for implementing measures to control the disease or health problem.

References

A1. Siegel JD, Rhinehart E, Jackson M, Chiarello L; Health Care Infection Control Practices Advisory Committee. 2007 Guideline for Isolation Precautions: Preventing Transmission of Infectious Agents in Health Care Settings. *Am J Infect Control.* 2007;35(10 Suppl 2): S65-S164. doi:10.1016/j.ajic.2007.10.007. [IVA]

A2. Bennett G, Kassai M. Isolation precautions: special applications in ambulatory surgery settings. In: *Infection Prevention Manual for Ambulatory Surgery Centers.* Rome, GA: ICP Associates, Inc; 2011:Section 4:15.

A3. Jensen PA, Lambert LA, Iademarco MF, Ridzon R; CDC. Guidelines for preventing the transmission of *Mycobacterium tuberculosis* in health-care settings, 2005. *MMWR Recomm Rep.* 2005;54(RR17):1-141. http://www.cdc.gov/mmwr/preview/mmwrhtml/rr5417a1.htm?s_cid=rr5417a1_e. Accessed October 24, 2013.

A4. §416.51(b) Standard: Infection control program. In: Centers for Medicare & Medicaid Services. *State Operations Manual Appendix L—Guidance for Surveyors: Ambulatory Surgical Centers.* Rev. 89; 2013. http://www.cms.gov/Regulations-and-Guidance/Guidance/Manuals/downloads/som107ap_l_ambulatory.pdf. Accessed October 18, 2013.

A5. Exhibit 351: ASC Infection Control Surveryor Worksheet (Rev. 84, Issued: 06-07-13, Effective: 06-07-13, Implementation: 06-07-13). Centers for Medicare & Medicaid Services. http://www.cms.gov/Regulations-and-Guidance/Guidance/Manuals/downloads/som107_exhibit_351.pdf. Accessed October 18, 2013.

A6. *Perioperative Standards and Recommended Practices.* Denver, CO: AORN, Inc; 2013.

A7. Occupational Safety and Health Standards, Toxic and Hazardous Substances: Bloodborne Pathogens, 29 CFR §1910.1030. Occupational Safety and Health Administration. https://www.osha.gov/pls/oshaweb/owadisp.show_document?p_table=standards&p_id=10051. Accessed October 18, 2013.

A8. Interpretative Guidelines: §416.51(b)(3). In: Centers for Medicare & Medicaid Services. *State Operations Manual Appendix L—Guidance for Surveyors: Ambulatory Surgical Centers.* Rev. 89; 2013. http://www.cms.gov/Regulations-and-Guidance/Guidance/Manuals/downloads/som107ap_l_ambulatory.pdf. Accessed October 18, 2013.

A9. Survey Procedures: §416.51(b)(3). In: Centers for Medicare & Medicaid Services. *State Operations Manual Appendix L—Guidance for Surveyors: Ambulatory Surgical Centers.* Rev. 89; 2013. http://www.cms.gov/Regulations-and-Guidance/Guidance/Manuals/downloads/som107ap_l_ambulatory.pdf. Accessed October 18, 2013.

A10. Mangram AJ, Horan TC, Pearson ML, Silver LC, Jarvis WR; Hospital Infection Control Practices Advisory Committee. Guideline for prevention of surgical site infection, 1999. Infect Control Hosp Epidemiol. 1999;20(4):250-278. doi:10.1086/501620. [IVA]

A11. *APIC Text of Infection Control & Epidemiology.* 3rd ed. Vol 1. Essential Elements. Washington, DC: Association for Professionals in Infection Control & Epidemiology, Inc; 2009.

A12. Centers for Medicare & Medicaid Services. *Ambulatory Surgical Center Quality Reporting Program Quality Measures Specifications Manual.* Version 3. July 2013. QualityNet. http://qualitynet.org/dcs/ContentServer?c=

AMBULATORY SUPPLEMENT: TRANSMISSIBLE INFECTIONS

Page&pagename=QnetPublic%2FPage%2FQnetTier2&cid=1228772475754. Accessed October 18, 2013.

Resources

Outbreak Database. http://www.outbreak-database.com. Accessed October 18, 2013.

Steps of an outbreak investigation. Centers for Disease Control and Prevention. http://www.cdc.gov/excite/classroom/outbreak/steps.htm. Accessed October 18, 2013.

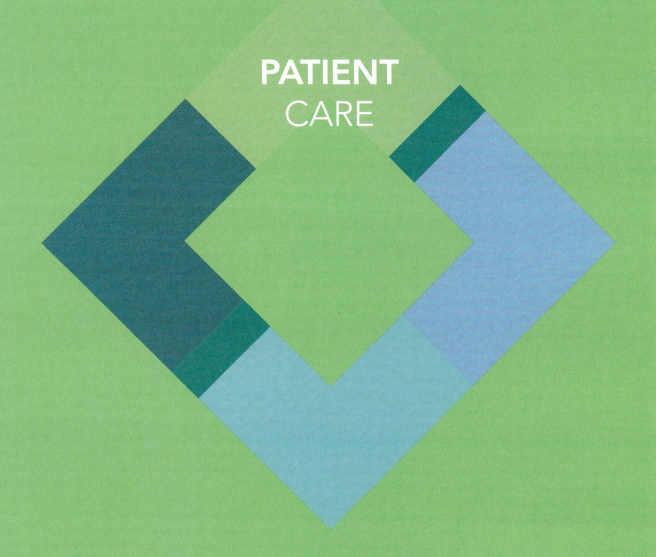

GUIDELINE FOR COMPLEMENTARY CARE INTERVENTIONS

The Guideline for Complementary Care Interventions has been approved by the AORN Guidelines Advisory Board. It was presented as a proposed guideline for comments by members and others. The guideline is effective January 15, 2015. The recommendations in this guideline are intended to be achievable and represent what is believed to be an optimal level of practice. Policies and procedures will reflect variations in practice settings and/or clinical situations that determine the degree to which the guideline can be implemented. AORN recognizes the many diverse settings in which perioperative nurses practice; therefore, this guideline is adaptable to all areas where operative and other invasive procedures may be performed.

Purpose

This document provides guidance for perioperative registered nurses (RNs) when complementary care interventions are implemented in the perioperative setting. This document includes guidance for music therapy, hypnosis, massage, acupuncture and acupressure, aromatherapy, Reiki, and guided imagery for patients before, during, or after surgery. The goal of complementary care interventions is to minimize the anxiety and pain of the perioperative patient.

Surgical patients experience high levels of anxiety.[1] Reasons for this anxiety include fear of surgery, anesthesia, loss of control, and disease.[2] The percentage of adult surgical patients who experience anxiety ranges from 11% to as high as 80%.[2] Anxiety can have negative effects on pain management.[3-5] An anxious patient may require more anesthetics and more opioids to relieve pain.[2]

Mitchell[6,7] surveyed 214 surgical outpatients to evaluate the effect of the clinical environment on the anxiety of patients who are scheduled to receive local or regional anesthesia. Seventy-seven percent of the patients surveyed reported that they experienced some degree of anxiety, as rated on a 5-point Likert-type scale that ranged from "feeling a little anxious" to "extremely anxious," on the day of their procedure. The highest percentage of patients (47%) reported feeling a little anxious.

The ability to provide complementary care interventions depends on several factors, including the patient's acceptance and engagement; the clinical experience, education, and competency of the perioperative team to provide complementary care interventions; and procedural and facility constraints. Complementary care may not be feasible or appropriate for every patient.

The topics of animal therapy, natural hormones, and dietary supplements as complementary care interventions are outside the scope of this document.

Evidence Review

On April 15, 2013, a medical librarian conducted a systematic search of the databases MEDLINE®, CINAHL®, and the Cochrane Database of Systematic Reviews for meta-analyses, systematic reviews, randomized controlled and non-randomized trials and studies, case reports, reviews, and guidelines from government agencies and standards-setting bodies. The librarian also searched the Scopus® database, although not systematically. Searches were limited to literature published in English since January 2006. At the time of the initial searches, the librarian established weekly alerts on the search topics and until July 2014, presented relevant results to the lead author. During the development of this guideline, the author requested supplementary literature searches and additional literature that either did not fit the original search criteria or was discovered during the evidence-appraisal process.

The lead author's original search request for literature related to moderate sedation and local anesthesia yielded 862 sources deemed appropriate for consideration in guidelines on those topics. Of these, 59 were identified as relevant to complementary care interventions (Figure 1). Search terms that yielded these results included *sedation, conscious sedation, moderation sedation, topical anesthesia, local anesthesia, local infiltration, anxiety, anti-anxiety agents, analgesia, surgical procedures, perioperative nursing,* and *nurse's role*. The literature scope was not expanded to the terms *complementary care, integrative medicine, complementary alternative medicine, healing touch, therapeutic touch, reflexology, herbal medicine, nausea,* or *vomiting*. Future review and update of this document will include a literature search that includes these terms.

Excluded were non-peer-reviewed publications and studies on the topics of pet therapy, natural hormones, and dietary supplements. Low-quality evidence was excluded when higher-quality evidence was available.

Included articles were independently evaluated and critically appraised according to the strength and quality of the evidence. Articles identified by the search were provided to the project team for evaluation. The team consisted of the lead author and four evidence appraisers. The lead author divided the search results and assigned members of the team to review and critically appraise each article using the AORN Research or Non-Research Evidence Appraisal Tools as appropriate. The literature was independently evaluated and appraised according to the strength and quality of the evidence. Each article was

COMPLEMENTARY CARE INTERVENTIONS

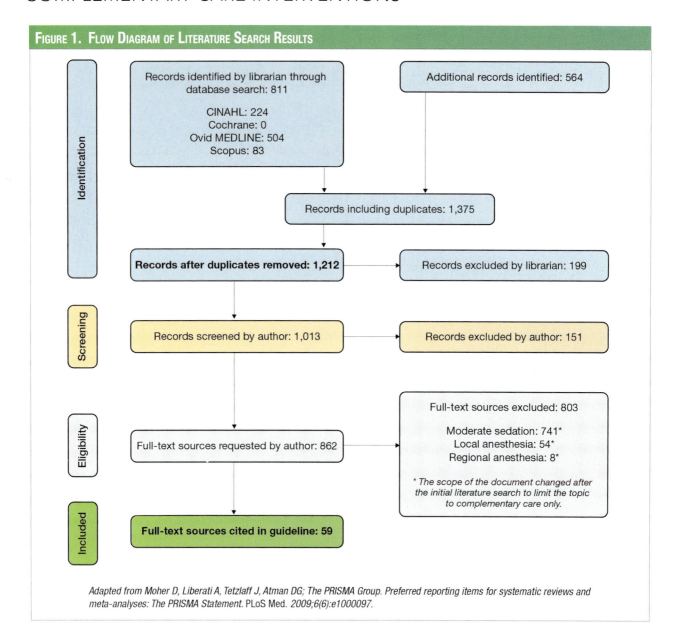

Figure 1. Flow Diagram of Literature Search Results

Adapted from Moher D, Liberati A, Tetzlaff J, Atman DG; The PRISMA Group. Preferred reporting items for systematic reviews and meta-analyses: The PRISMA Statement. PLoS Med. 2009;6(6):e1000097.

then assigned an appraisal score. The appraisal score is noted in brackets after each reference, as applicable.

The collective evidence supporting each intervention within a specific recommendation was summarized, and the AORN Evidence-Rating Model was used to rate the strength of the evidence. Factors considered in review of the collective evidence were the quality of the evidence, the quantity of similar evidence on a given topic, and the consistency of evidence supporting a recommendation. The evidence rating is noted in brackets after each intervention.

Note: The evidence summary table is available at http://www.aorn.org/evidencetables/.

Editor's note: MEDLINE is a registered trademark of the US National Library of Medicine's Medical Literature Analysis and Retrieval System, Bethesda, MD. CINAHL, Cumulative Index to Nursing and Allied Health Literature, is a registered trademark of EBSCO Industries, Birmingham, AL. Scopus is a registered trademark of Elsevier B.V., Amsterdam, The Netherlands.

Recommendation I

The perioperative team can implement music interventions.

The collective body of evidence strongly supports the use of music to relieve anxiety during surgical and other invasive procedures.[1,3,8-34]

Sixteen studies,[3,10-16,18,19,21,24-26,34,35] three systematic reviews,[8,23,36] an integrative review,[1] and five literature reviews[27-29,31,33] evaluated the ability of music interventions to reduce patient anxiety, pain, and stress before, during, and after operative and other invasive procedures. Thirteen studies found that music was an effective intervention to reduce anxiety levels in the surgical and invasive procedure areas. Three studies found that a music intervention did not have a significant

COMPLEMENTARY CARE INTERVENTIONS

effect on anxiety levels but that music contributed to an overall favorable patient experience.[15,19,25]

The limitations of the evidence are that few studies have explored the feasibility of incorporating music into everyday practice. Further research is needed to define feasibility of using music therapy in the perioperative area.

The benefits of using music therapy outweigh the harms. The benefits include a possible reduction in the patient's anxiety.

I.a. The perioperative team can implement music interventions across the perioperative continuum of care. *[1: Strong Evidence]*

The collective evidence indicates that music is effective in decreasing patient anxiety and pain in all phases of perioperative care.

Nilsson[8] conducted a systematic review of the anxiety- and pain-reducing effects of music interventions. In the 42 randomized controlled trials (RCTs) reviewed, 3,936 patients had elective surgeries of various types (eg, gynecological, orthopedic, general, cardiac, urologic). The timing of the music intervention was preoperative, intraoperative, postoperative, a combination of two of these periods, or a combination of all three periods. The author concluded that music interventions could reduce anxiety, pain, the use of sedatives and analgesics, heart rate, blood pressure, respiratory rate, and blood cortisol levels.

Johnson et al[16] evaluated the anxiety levels of 119 female patients undergoing outpatient gynecological surgery in an experimental three-group design of music with headphones, headphones only, and usual care. The researchers measured preoperative and postoperative anxiety levels using the Rapid Assessment Anxiety tool. The music-with-headphones and headphones-only interventions continued from the preoperative area, through surgery, and into the postanesthesia care unit until the patient's Aldrete level of consciousness equaled 2. After surgery, the music group experienced the lowest anxiety scores among the patients who had reported moderate to high anxiety levels before surgery. The researchers concluded that music is an easy and inexpensive intervention to reduce anxiety.

In an RCT, Hook et al[18] examined the effect of music on reducing preoperative and postoperative anxiety and postoperative pain and distress in 102 female surgical patients. The researchers used a pretest-posttest design to measure anxiety with the State-Trait Anxiety Inventory (STAI) and a visual analog scale (VAS). The researchers also used the VAS to measure postoperative pain sensation and pain distress.

The control and experimental groups received standard preoperative and postoperative nursing and medical care. The experimental group listened to 30 minutes of music twice before and six times after surgery at defined intervals. The experimental music group had a significant change in postoperative anxiety and postoperative pain. The findings suggested that music is a nonpharmacological, complementary, noninvasive intervention to reduce anxiety and postoperative pain.[18]

Binns-Turner et al[3] evaluated the effect of music provided throughout the preoperative, intraoperative, and postoperative periods on anxiety, pain, heart rate, and mean arterial pressure (MAP). A convenience sample of 30 women

Pain and Anxiety Measurement Instruments

The State-Trait Anxiety Inventory (STAI)
- Psychological inventory that measures two types of anxiety:
  - state measures anxiety about an event
  - trait measures anxiety as a characteristic
- Based on a 4-point Likert scale
- Consists of 40 items on a self-report basis
- Total scores range from 20 to 80
  - High anxiety: 60-80
  - Moderate anxiety: 40-59
  - Mild anxiety: 20-39

Visual Analog Score (VAS)
- A measurement instrument that assesses a characteristic that cannot be directly measured and that ranges across a continuum.
- An example is the amount of pain a patient experiences—it can range from no pain to extreme pain.
- The VAS is a horizontal line 100 mm in length with "no pain" at one end and "extreme pain" at the other end.

Examples of a VAS

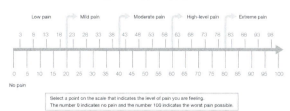

A variation is the use of faces to gauge the level of pain.

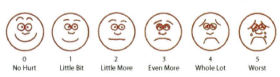

Wong-Baker FACES Pain Rating Scale. In: Hockenberry MJ, Wilson D. *Wong's Essentials of Pediatric Nursing.* 8th ed. St Louis, MO: Mosby; 2009. Used with permission. Copyright Mosby.

undergoing a mastectomy for a breast malignancy were randomly assigned to either a control group or a music therapy group. The control group received standard care and the intervention group listened to music with earphones throughout the perioperative period. The researchers measured anxiety, pain, heart rate, and MAP before and after surgery. Anxiety was measured using the Spielberger State Anxiety Scale, and pain was measured with a VAS. The findings included a statistically significant difference in MAP, anxiety scores, and pain scores between the control group and the music intervention groups. The intervention group's anxiety, pain, and MAP were significantly lower or improved after surgery. Limitations of the study included that the sample was a small, convenience sample.

A systematic Cochrane review,[23] six RCTs,[10-12,14,26,35] and an integrative review[1] evaluated the effect of music in reducing anxiety levels in the preoperative area.

In an RCT, Bringman et al[14] studied the preoperative anxiety levels of 327 patients undergoing elective surgery. In the preoperative area, a music therapist randomly assigned patients to either listen to relaxing music with earphones or receive an oral dose of midazolam 0.05 mg/kg to 0.1 mg/kg. Patients completed the STAI before and after the interventions. The STAI scale ranges from 20 to 80. The mean STAI anxiety score of the control group ranged from 37.63 to 44.43. The anxiety scores of the music intervention group decreased by 5.72 units on the STAI compared with the scores of the standard care control group. The researchers concluded that relaxing music decreased preoperative anxiety to a greater extent than oral midazolam and that listening to music has no adverse effects. The authors concluded that the use of preoperative, relaxing music should be supported to reduce preoperative anxiety.

Lee et al[11] conducted an RCT that compared the effectiveness of music played via headphones, music broadcast via room speakers, or no music to reduce preoperative patients' anxiety while they waited for surgery. The sample size was 167 patients. The researchers used the VAS to measure anxiety subjectively on a scale of "not anxious" to "extremely anxious." The heart rate variability (HRV) tool was used to measure anxiety objectively by identifying the effect of mental stress on the autonomic control of the heart rate. There was not a significant difference in the HRV in the three groups. The VAS levels for the two music groups were reduced after the music interventions. The researchers concluded that music via either headphones or speakers was effective in reducing preoperative anxiety.

Lee et al[26] conducted another RCT of 140 patients that compared listening to relaxing music via headphones for 10 minutes with listening to no music in the preoperative area. Anxiety levels were measured with VAS scores and HRV monitoring. The experimental group's VAS scores were significantly decreased after they listened to the music. The control group's VAS scores increased after 10 minutes of rest. The heart rate decrease in the experimental group was significantly greater than that in the control group. The researchers concluded that listening to music was an effective way to decrease the anxiety of preoperative patients. In addition, the researchers concluded the HRV assessment is an objective way for nurses to measure patient's preoperative anxiety when a patient cannot express subjective feelings.

El-Hassan et al[12] conducted a prospective RCT of 180 endoscopy patients to determine whether music reduced their preoperative anxiety. The anxiety levels of the music intervention group were measured with the STAI before and after the intervention (ie, listening to music for 15 minutes). The anxiety levels of the control group receiving standard care with no music were measured with the STAI after admission to the pre-endoscopy area and 15 minutes later. The intervention group listened to self-selected music for 15 minutes with headphones before the endoscopy procedure. The control group received the same care as the intervention group with the exception of listening to music. The researchers found a significant reduction in the postintervention anxiety scores of the group that listened to self-selected music. The researchers concluded that music is a simple way to improve well-being in preprocedure patients.

Ni et al[35] randomly assigned 172 adult surgical outpatients into one of two groups to evaluate the effect of music on preoperative anxiety and vital signs. The experimental group listened to music through headphones for 20 minutes before surgery and the control group received routine nursing care. Vital signs (ie, blood pressure, heart rate) and STAI anxiety levels were measured before and after the interventions. The STAI score of the music group decreased by 5.83 units. The STAI score of the control group decreased by 1.72 units. The difference between the music group's postintervention STAI scores for anxiety and the control's group's scores was statistically significant. Blood pressure and heart rate decreased in both groups. The researchers concluded that a music intervention might lower preoperative anxiety levels, blood pressure, and heart rate.

A Cochrane systematic review by Bradt et al[23] evaluated the effects of music interventions on preoperative patient anxiety. The review included 26 randomized and quasi-randomized trials with 2,051 participants and compared music interventions with standard preoperative care to standard care alone. The anxiety scores of the music intervention group decreased by 5.72 units on the STAI compared with the scores of the standard care group. The researchers concluded that listening to music might decrease preoperative patient anxiety. These findings are consistent with three other Cochrane reviews[37-39] that evaluated the use of music to reduce medical patients' anxiety.

Using an RCT design, Arslan et al[10] studied preoperative anxiety levels in men undergoing urogenital surgery. The experimental group participants listened to their choice of music through earphones for 30 minutes before surgery. The control group received routine preoperative care and 30 minutes of rest. Anxiety levels were measured with the STAI preintervention and postintervention. The experimental group had significantly lower postintervention anxiety scores and the control group had significantly increased postintervention anxiety scores. The researchers concluded that offering music to preoperative patients is an independent nursing intervention that may reduce anxiety levels.

An integrative review by Pittman and Kridli[1] analyzed 11 experimental and nonexperimental research studies that compared listening to music to no music and used the STAI preintervention and postintervention to measure anxiety levels. After a review of the 11 studies, the authors found that in three studies listening to music lowered blood pressure; three studies demonstrated a relationship between listening to music and decreased heart rates; and two studies provided evidence of a decreased respiratory rate after participants listened to music. The reviewers concluded that nurses can use music interventions to establish a calm, relaxing preoperative environment that supports reducing anxiety.

Seven RCTs,[13,15,17,19,21,34,40] a systematic review with meta-analysis,[9] and one quasi-experimental study[24] examined the effect of music on anxiety levels during surgery (ie, peripheral vascular, gynecological, urological, plastic, gastroenterological) and invasive procedures (ie, interventional radiology, angiography).

In a prospective RCT of 40 patients, Jiménez-Jiménez et al[17] compared patients undergoing peripheral vascular surgery who received routine intraoperative care with patients who listened to music through headphones during the procedure. The researchers used the STAI to measure anxiety before and after surgery. The anxiety and stress feelings scores were significantly lower in the music therapy group after surgery.

In a systematic review with meta-analysis of eight studies with 722 patients who underwent colonoscopy, Tam et al[9] examined the effect of listening to music during surgery. They concluded that listening to music reduced anxiety, procedure time, and the amount of sedation used.

Zhang et al[40] assessed male patient anxiety and pain during flexible cystoscopy procedures. The patients were randomly assigned to either the experimental group that listened to music of their choice or the control group that did not listen to music. The researchers measured anxiety levels with the STAI-state (STAI-s) before and after the procedure. Pain levels were assessed postoperatively using the VAS. The difference in the mean pain and postprocedure anxiety levels were statistically significant in the experimental group. The researchers concluded that patients listening to music experienced less discomfort and anxiety and that music was a simple, nonpharmocological intervention to increase patient satisfaction.

Yeo et al[21] randomly assigned 70 male patients undergoing rigid cystoscopy into one of two groups. The experimental group listened to classical music during the procedure and the control group did not listen to music. Before and after surgery, anxiety levels were measured with the STAI, and pain and satisfaction were measured with a VAS. The music group had significantly less anxiety and pain, higher satisfaction scores, and lower postprocedure pulse rates and systolic blood pressures. Limitations of the study were a small sample size and that the study was not blinded to the patient or the surgeon.

Sadideen et al[24] studied anxiety and satisfaction levels in patients undergoing plastic surgery under local anesthesia. The intervention group listened to music via speakers in the OR. The control group did not have music played in the OR. Objective measures of anxiety were VAS scores and respiratory rate. The researchers quantified patients' satisfaction using a 5-point Likert scale. Measurements were taken before the procedure started and on completion. After surgery, the music group had lower VAS scores and respiratory rates. The difference in the satisfaction scores between the two groups was not statistically significant.

Two RCTs studied the effect of music on anxiety levels of patients undergoing coronary angiography procedures.[13,34] Weeks and Nilsson[34] randomly assigned 98 patients to one of three groups. Patients listened to music through an audio pillow, music through the loud speaker, or no music. Patients in the two music groups had a significant reduction in anxiety levels compared with the control group.

Doğan and Senturan[13] randomly assigned 100 patients to an experimental group that listened to music during the procedure and 100 patients to a control group that received standard care. The anxiety levels of the experimental group decreased more significantly than those of the control group.

McLeod[25] studied the effectiveness of music on patient anxiety levels during minor plastic surgery procedures. The Speilberger STAI questionnaire was used to assess the anxiety of 80 patients before and after surgery. Forty patients in the experimental group listened to self-selected music during surgery, and the 40 patients in the control group received standard care with no music. Statistical analysis of the STAI scores demonstrated that there was not a significant difference in the anxiety scores between the experimental group that listened to music and the control group. The researchers reported that the patients seemed to enjoy the music.

Nilsson et al[19] and Kulkarni et al[15] evaluated the effect of music on patient anxiety during interventional radiology procedures. Both studies found that there was not a significant difference in the anxiety levels between the music intervention groups or the control groups.

I.a.1. The perioperative RN should assess the patient's acceptance of and willingness to use music as a complementary intervention and should obtain consent. *[4: Benefits Balanced with Harms]*

I.a.2. The perioperative RN should solicit the patient's music preference (eg classical, easy listening). *[4: Benefits Balanced with Harms]*

I.a.3. When music therapy is used, the patient should use personal listening devices (eg, head phones, ear buds) when feasible. *[4: Benefits Balanced with Harms]*

The use of personal listening devices limits noise and distraction in the perioperative setting.

Recommendation II

The perioperative team can implement preoperative or postoperative massage therapy.

The collective body of evidence supports the use of massage to relieve anxiety during surgical and other invasive procedures.[41-43] Two RCTs and one quasi-experimental study investigated massage as an intervention to reduce patient anxiety.[41-43]

The limitations of the evidence are that few studies have explored the feasibility of incorporating massage into everyday practice and the competency of perioperative nurses to implement massage techniques. Further research is needed.

The benefits of using massage outweighs the harms. The benefits include a potential reduction in the patient's anxiety.

II.a. Massage therapy techniques can be used. *[2: Moderate Evidence]*

Wentworth et al[41] assessed the effect of a 20-minute massage session on patients' pain, anxiety, and tension before an invasive cardiovascular procedure. The study method was an experimental pretest-posttest design with random assignment of 130 patients. The control group received standard care with relaxation time and the intervention group received hands-on massage 30 minutes before the procedure. The researchers measured pain, anxiety, and tension levels with a VAS before the intervention and after the procedure. Mean results for patients in the massage intervention group indicated a significant decrease in pain, muscle tension, and anxiety from before the massage therapy to after the massage therapy. The mean results for patients in the standard care group indicated an insignificant change in pain, muscle tension, and anxiety before and after standard care. The researchers' findings suggest that massage therapy can be delivered to patients before an invasive procedure and that massage is an effective technique for reducing pain, tension, and anxiety.

In an RCT, Rosen et al[43] studied the effectiveness of massage therapy to reduce pain and anxiety in patients with cancer undergoing surgical placement of a vascular access device. The intervention group received massage therapy for two 20-minute sessions, one before and one after surgery. The control group received structured attention. Anxiety and pain were measured with the STAI before surgery and after each intervention. The massage group had a statistically significant decrease in anxiety after the first massage compared with the control group.

Using a quasi-experimental design with pretest and posttest evaluations and non-random assignment, Brand et al[42] studied the effect of hand massage in reducing preoperative patient anxiety in an ambulatory surgery center. Anxiety levels were measured using a VAS. A certified massage therapist trained three nurses to perform the hand massage procedure. The intervention group received a five-minute massage on each hand, and the control group received standard care. The intervention group had a significant decrease in postintervention anxiety scores. The control group's anxiety scores decreased, but the decrease was not statistically significant. An unexpected finding of this study was that the hand massage facilitated the IV start.

II.a.1. The perioperative RN should assess the patient's acceptance of and willingness to use massage as a complementary intervention and should obtain consent. *[4: Benefits Balanced with Harms]*

II.a.2. Perioperative RNs who provide massage interventions (eg, hand rubs) should receive education and complete competency verification activities on the principles and techniques of massage therapy that are in compliance with state regulation.

COMPLEMENTARY CARE INTERVENTIONS

Licensure may be required by the state for providers of some massage therapies. *[4: Benefits Balanced with Harms]*

Recommendation III

The perioperative team can implement preoperative acupuncture and acupressure.

The collective body of evidence supports the use of acupuncture and acupressure to relieve anxiety during surgical and other invasive procedures.[44-47]

The limitations of the evidence are that few studies have explored the feasibility of incorporating acupuncture and acupressure into everyday practice and the competency of perioperative nurses to implement these holistic measures. Further research is needed.

The benefits of using acupressure and acupuncture outweigh the harms. The benefits include a potential reduction in the patient's anxiety.

III.a. Acupuncture can be implemented before surgery. *[2: Moderate Evidence]*

Two RCTs investigated the effect of acupuncture on preoperative patient anxiety levels.[44,46] Acar et al[44] investigated the effect of ear-press needle acupuncture on the Yintang point to decrease preoperative anxiety in a prospective randomized single-blind controlled study. Patient anxiety was measured before and after the interventions with the STAI and the bispectral index (BIS). The BIS uses electroencephalogram-derived data intraoperatively to monitor the depth of anesthesia. The BIS is also used to monitor sedation in the intensive care unit and during monitored anesthesia care and has been used preoperatively to assess anxiety.

The experimental group received acupuncture at the Yintang point, which is at the root of the nose and between the eyebrows. The control group received sham acupuncture at a nonacupoint 2 cm lateral to the distal end of the right eyebrow. The BIS values were significantly lower in the acupuncture group at two minutes to 20 minutes compared with the sham site group. The mean STAI-s scores decreased in the acupuncture group. The researchers concluded that the lower BIS and STAI scores indicated the patients were calmer and more relaxed and that acupuncture at the Yintang point significantly decreased preoperative patient anxiety.[44]

Wu et al[46] compared the effectiveness of body acupuncture to auricular acupuncture on preoperative patient anxiety in a blinded RCT. Ambulatory surgery patients were randomly assigned to either the body acupuncture intervention or the ear acupuncture intervention. The researchers measured anxiety levels using the ZUNG Self-Rating Anxiety Scale before and after the interventions. Both acupuncture methods decreased the anxiety of the preoperative patients, but the reductions did not reach statistical significance.

III.a.1. The perioperative RN should assess the patient's acceptance of and willingness to use acupuncture as a complementary intervention and should obtain consent. *[4: Benefits Balanced with Harms]*

III.a.2. Acupuncture should be performed by licensed acupuncturist as required by state regulation. *[4: Benefits Balanced with Harms]*

III.b. Acupressure can be implemented before surgery. *[2: Moderate Evidence]*

Use of acupressure before surgery is supported by one RCT.[45] Valiee et al[45] investigated the effect of acupressure on preoperative patient anxiety levels. Anxiety levels were measured using a standard VAS and vital signs (ie, blood pressure, heart rate, respiratory rate). The experimental group received acupressure on the correct acupoints, and the control group received acupressure on sham points. The postintervention anxiety levels decreased 21% for the acupressure group and 6.1% for the placebo group. The researchers concluded that results of the study support the use of acupressure to reduce preoperative anxiety. The acupressure intervention on the third eye and Shen Men points can be performed by a trained patient or a health care professional.

III.b.1. The perioperative RN should assess the patient's acceptance of and willingness to use acupressure as a complementary intervention and should obtain consent. *[4: Benefits Balanced with Harms]*

III.b.2. Acupressure practitioners should receive education and complete competency verification activities on the principles and techniques of acupressure. *[4: Benefits Balanced with Harms]*

Recommendation IV

The perioperative team can implement preoperative aromatherapy.

Aromatherapy is based on the use of oils extracted from aromatic plants with medicinal qualities.[2] The collective body of evidence supports the use of aromatherapy to relieve anxiety during surgical and other invasive procedures.[2,36,48,49]

Four RCTs studied aromatic agents (ie, essential oil of lavandin, lavandula, essential oil of lavender, neroli oil) to reduce preoperative anxiety levels.[2,36,48,49]

The limitations of the evidence are that few studies have explored the feasibility of incorporating aromatherapy into everyday practice and the competency of perioperative nurses to use aromatherapy. Further research is needed.

The benefits of using aromatherapy outweigh the harms. The benefits include a potential reduction in the patient's anxiety.

COMPLEMENTARY CARE INTERVENTIONS

IV.a. Aromatic essential oils can be used. *[2: Moderate Evidence]*

Braden et al[48] evaluated the ability of the essential oil lavandin to reduce preoperative anxiety. Anxiety levels were measured with the VAS on admission and before the patient was taken to the operating room (OR). A total of 150 patients were randomly assigned to one of three groups. The control group received standard care. The jojoba oil group received the oil on a cotton ball for olfactory application; the oil was applied to the pedal pulse point and covered with a bandage for absorption. The undiluted lavandin group received the oil on a cotton ball for olfactory application; the oil was applied to the pedal pulse point and covered with a bandage for absorption. The anxiety scores of the lavandin oil group were lower at the time of transfer to the OR but the difference was not statistically significant.

Fayazi et al[2] investigated the effect of inhalation aromatherapy to reduce patients' preoperative anxiety. The aromatherapy intervention was two drops of lavandula oil on a handkerchief that was inhaled for 20 minutes. The placebo group inhaled two drops of water on the handkerchief for 20 minutes. Anxiety levels were measured with the STAI before and after the interventions. The mean level of anxiety in the experimental group was 51 before the intervention of inhaling the lavandula oil and 38.61 after the intervention. The mean level of anxiety in the control group was 50.67 before the placebo intervention and 49.53 after the intervention. The mean difference in the STAI scores before and after the interventions was 12.34 for the lavandula group and 2.42 for the control group. The lavandula group's anxiety decreased from moderate to mild anxiety. The placebo group's anxiety level remained at a moderate level. The difference between the two groups was statistically significant. The researchers concluded that nurses could use aromatherapy as an intervention to reduce patients' preoperative anxiety.

Two RCTs studied aromatherapy to reduce patient anxiety levels in gastroenterology procedures.[36,49] Hoya et al[36] studied the optimal soothing environment (OSE) as a nonpharmacological intervention to reduce anxiety before gastroscopy procedures. The OSE intervention included an essential oil burner with lavender essential oil and a DVD with soothing natural environmental images and sounds. The control group received standard care. Anxiety levels of both groups were measured on arrival, before the procedure, and after the procedure with the FACES Scale, a type of VAS. The anxiety level of the control group increased before the gastroscopy procedure. The anxiety level of the OSE group did not increase before the gastroscopy. The researchers concluded that the OSE intervention was effective for reducing anxiety and that nurses could use this therapy to promote health and wellness.

Hu et al[49] investigated the effect of aromatherapy on anxiety, stress, and physiological parameters of patients undergoing colonoscopy. Anxiety levels were measured with the STAI-s before aromatherapy and after the colonoscopy. Pain levels were measured with a VAS. Heart rate, respiratory rate, and blood pressure were measured before aromatherapy and after the colonoscopy. The experimental group inhaled 50 mL of neroli oil on a piece of gauze in a hand-held nebulizer. The control group inhaled 50 mL of sunflower oil on a piece of gauze in a hand-held nebulizer. The STAI scores of the aromatherapy group decreased 11 points which was statistically significant. The STAI scores of the control group decreased 7 points which was not statistically significant. The difference between the anxiety scores of the two groups was not a significant. The researchers concluded that aromatherapy before colonoscopy procedures can have an effect on anxiety and physiological parameters (eg, blood pressure), and aromatherapy is a safe and inexpensive preprocedure technique.

IV.a.1. Aromatherapy should be provided in a manner that will limit exposure of the aromatic essential oils to the intended patient. *[4: Benefits Balanced with Harms]*

Other occupants (eg, patients, visitors, personnel) of the area may be sensitive to the aromatic essential oils.

IV.a.2. The perioperative RN should assess the patient's acceptance of and willingness to use aromatherapy as a complementary intervention and should obtain consent. *[4: Benefits Balanced with Harms]*

IV.a.3. Perioperative RNs who implement aromatherapy should receive education and complete competency verification activities on the principles and techniques of aromatherapy. *[4: Benefits Balanced with Harms]*

Recommendation V

The perioperative team can implement patient hypnosis before, during, and after the surgical procedure.

The collective body of evidence supports the use of hypnosis to relieve anxiety and pain during surgical and other invasive procedures.[50-54] Three RCTs[50,51,54] and a case-controlled study[52] evaluated the use of hypnosis to reduce anxiety and pain.

The limitations of the evidence are that few studies have explored the feasibility of incorporating hypnosis into everyday practice and the competency of perioperative nurses to implement hypnosis. Further research is needed.

COMPLEMENTARY CARE INTERVENTIONS

The benefits of using hypnosis outweigh the harms. Benefits include a potential reduction in the patient's anxiety and pain.

V.a. Patient hypnosis therapy can be used. *[2: Moderate Evidence]*

In an RCT, Lang et al[51] studied the use of self-hypnotic relaxation to reduce anxiety and pain during percutaneous tumor treatment by transcatheter embolization or radio-frequency ablation in 201 patients. The self-hypnotic relaxation treatment was compared to standard care, and empathetic attention. The standard care group consisted of 70 patients, the empathy group consisted of 65 patients, and the hypnosis group consisted of 66 patients. The hypnosis group had less pain and anxiety and used less medication than the standard care and empathy groups. The researchers concluded that procedural hypnosis that included empathetic attention reduced pain, anxiety, and medication use. Empathetic attention without hypnosis did not help the patients with self-coping strategies and could result in more adverse events.

Schnur et al[54] used an RCT design to study 90 patients undergoing excisional breast biopsy. Patients received either a 15-minute hypnosis session before surgery or a 15-minute attention control session before surgery. The VAS and the short version of the Profile of Mood States (SV-POMS) were used to measure patients' distress before and after surgery. The hypnosis intervention group experienced significantly lower mean values of emotional upset measured by the VAS before surgery. After hypnosis, compared with the control group, the patients in the hypnosis group had significantly lower mean levels of emotional upset and depressed mood as measured by the VAS, significantly lower levels of anxiety as measured by the SV-POMS, and significantly higher levels of relaxation as measured by the VAS. The researchers concluded that a brief hypnosis session before surgery is an effective technique to decrease patient distress before an excisional breast biopsy when many patients have a high level of anxiety.

In an RCT, Marc et al[50] studied women's satisfaction with using a hypnotic intervention to reduce anxiety and pain during an outpatient gynecology procedure. A total of 350 patients were randomly assigned to either a short, standardized hypno-analgesia intervention or standard care. Ninety-seven percent of the hypnosis group reported that they would recommend the technique to a friend having a similar procedure. All but one patient in the 172-patient intervention group appreciated the hypnosis experience. The hypnosis group required less pain medication than the control group. The researchers did not comment on postprocedure anxiety levels.

Abdeshahi et al[52] conducted a case-controlled study to evaluate the effect of hypnosis on pain, anxiety, and hemorrhage during the extraction of third molars. The patients served as their own control group by undergoing extraction of the molars on one side under hypnosis and the opposite side under local anesthesia. There was a significant difference in pain scores at five and 12 hours after surgery, with the hypnosis group taking less analgesic medications. There was significantly greater hemorrhage in the local anesthetic group (41.7%) compared with the hypnosis group (20.8%) at five hours after surgery. Anxiety scores were not reported. The researchers concluded that hypnosis is an adjunct technique to treat anxious patients when conventional methods cannot be used and the practitioner is experienced in the technique.

V.a.1. The perioperative RN should assess the patient's acceptance of and willingness to use hypnosis as a complementary intervention and should obtain consent. *[4: Benefits Balanced with Harms]*

V.a.2. Perioperative RNs who implement hypnosis therapy should receive education and complete competency verification activities on the principles and techniques of hypnosis. *[4: Benefits Balanced with Harms]*

Recommendation VI

The perioperative team can implement preoperative Reiki therapy.

Reiki is an ancient Tibetan technique and healing practice.[55] The Reiki practitioner gently lays his or her hands on or above 12 strategic areas on the patient's body.[55] The Reiki practitioner's energy is thought to promote healing and bring harmony to the patient's energy field.[56]

The collective body of evidence supports that Reiki has a minimal effect in relieving anxiety.[55,56] Two studies investigated the use of Reiki in the gastroenterology procedure area.[55,56]

The limitations of the evidence are that few studies have explored the feasibility of incorporating Reiki by competent practitioners into everyday practice. Further research is needed.

The benefits of using Reiki outweigh the harms. Benefits include a potential reduction in the patient's anxiety and pain.

VI.a. Reiki therapy performed by a Reiki practitioner can be used. *[3: Limited Evidence]*

Bourque et al[56] conducted a pilot study to determine whether the use of Reiki before a surgical procedure would decrease the amount of meperidine required during the procedure. To determine the average dose of meperidine used during the procedure, the investigators conducted a chart review of 30 patients undergoing screening colonoscopy. The average dose of meperidine was 50 mg. The control group were patients in the chart review. The experimental group of 25 patients received Reiki 10 minutes before the start of the colonoscopy. Five patients were randomly chosen to receive placebo Reiki which did not involve the proper hand positions, symbols, or energy transfers.

There was not a significant difference in the amount of meperidine used by the Reiki group, the placebo Reiki group, or the chart review group. Four patients in the Reiki group received less than the average 50 mg dose. No patients in the chart review group or the placebo Reiki group received less than 50 mg of meperidine. The researchers concluded that Reiki could potentially reduce the amount of medication needed during screening colonoscopy.[56]

Hulse et al[55] conducted a pilot study to investigate the use of Reiki before colonoscopy to reduce anxiety and medication use during the procedure. A prospective nonblinded partially randomized patient preference design was used in the study. The study was partially randomized because patients assigned to the control group asked to be part of the Reiki group.

The experimental group received 15 minutes of a modified Reiki intervention by a Reiki-trained nurse. The control group received standard care. Baseline, postintervention, and postcolonoscopy measures of pain and anxiety were collected with a self-report instrument developed by the nurse principal investigator. The Reiki group did not have statistically significant reductions in pain and blood pressure. The Reiki group did have statistically significant reductions in heart rate, respirations, and self-reported anxiety after the intervention compared with baseline values. The researchers concluded that anxious people are more likely to participate in adjunctive therapies. Limitations of this pilot study were that the principal investigator was not blinded to the group assignments; the sample size was small; and a non-validated pain and anxiety instrument was used.

VI.a.1. The perioperative RN should assess the patient's acceptance of and willingness to use Reiki as a complementary intervention and should obtain consent. *[4: Benefits Balanced with Harms]*

VI.a.2. Reiki practitioners should receive education and complete competency verification activities on the principles and techniques of Reiki therapy. *[4: Benefits Balanced with Harms]*

Recommendation VII

Additional complementary care interventions can be used.

Three studies of other holistic interventions (eg, guided imagery,[57] relaxation tapes,[58] essential oils[59]) evaluated measures to reduce surgical patients' anxiety and pain. The collective body of evidence supports the use of these holistic care interventions to relieve anxiety during surgical and other invasive procedures.[57-59]

The limitations of the evidence are that few studies have explored the feasibility of incorporating holistic measures into everyday practice and the competency of perioperative nurses to implement holistic measures. Further research is needed.

The benefits of using holistic interventions outweigh the harms. Benefits include a potential reduction in the patient's anxiety and pain.

VII.a. Guided imagery can be used. *[2: Moderate Evidence]*

In a randomized single-blinded study, Gonzales et al[57] evaluated the effect of guided imagery on the anxiety and pain of adult patients undergoing same-day surgery. Patients were randomly assigned to one of two groups. Patients in the experimental group listened to a guided imagery compact disc with headphones for 28 minutes before surgery and throughout induction. Patients in the control group had 28 minutes of quiet before surgery and no intervention.

Baseline anxiety was measured using the Amsterdam Preoperative Anxiety and Information Scale (APAIS) and the vertical VAS (vVAS). The APAIS and vVAS data collection continued after surgery with measurements at one and two hours after surgery in the postanesthesia care unit and the ambulatory procedure unit until discharge. There was a significant decrease in the postoperative anxiety levels of the experimental group. The reduction in the pain levels of the experimental group approached statistical significance. The researchers concluded that guided imagery could be useful in the ambulatory surgery area to reduce preoperative anxiety and postoperative pain but that further research is needed.[57]

VII.a.1. The perioperative RN should assess the patient's acceptance of and willingness to use guided imagery as a complementary intervention and should obtain consent. *[4: Benefits Balanced with Harms]*

VII.a.2. Perioperative RNs who implement guided imagery should receive education and complete competency verification activities on the principles and techniques of guided imagery. *[4: Benefits Balanced with Harms]*

VII.b. Relaxation tapes can be used. *[2: Moderate Evidence]*

Ko and Lin[58] used a pretest-posttest design to evaluate the effects of a relaxation tape on the anxiety levels of 80 surgical patients. Before surgery, the patients listened to a 10-minute tape that included a five-minute preparation period of deep breathing followed by a five-minute period of guided imagery, meditation, and recovery. The researchers used the STAI to measure anxiety before and after the patients listened to the tape. The pretest-posttest STAI scores changed significantly, with female patients having a greater reduction in anxiety than the male patients. The results indicated that relaxation tapes could reduce the anxiety levels of surgical patients. A limitation of the study was the use of a convenience sample with no matched control group.

VII.b.1. The perioperative RN should assess the patient's acceptance of and willingness to use relaxation tapes as a complementary intervention and should obtain consent. *[4: Benefits Balanced with Harms]*

VII.c. Oral essential oils can be used. *[1: Strong Evidence]*

Akhlaghi et al[59] studied 60 minor surgery patients using a double-blind design. A psychologist measured the baseline anxiety using the STAI and the APAIS. The patients received an oral premedication two hours before surgery. The experimental group received Citrus aurantium blossom distillate 1 mL/kg. The control group received a placebo of saline solution 1 mL/kg. A psychologist measured anxiety levels two hours after administration of the premedication and before induction of anesthesia. The researchers analyzed both the STAI-s and APAIS scores and concluded that the experimental group had significantly less anxiety than the control group. The researchers concluded Citrus aurantium blossom distillate may reduce outpatient preoperative anxiety and that there may be a role for herbal medicine as a premedication.

VII.c.1. The perioperative RN should assess the patient's acceptance of and willingness to use oral essential oils as a complementary intervention and should obtain consent. *[4: Benefits Balanced with Harms]*

VII.c.2. Perioperative RNs who provide oral essential oils should receive education and complete competency verification activities on the principles and techniques of essential oils. *[4: Benefits Balanced with Harms]*

Glossary

State-Trait Anxiety Inventory (STAI): A tool used to measure anxiety. The state score measures how a person feels at a specific moment in time. The trait score measures how a person feels generally.

Visual analog scale (VAS): A measure of pain intensity that consists of a line 100 mm long, with two descriptors representing extremes of pain intensity from no pain to extreme pain at each end of the scale. Patients rate their pain intensity by making a mark somewhere on the line that represents their pain intensity, and the VAS is scored by measuring the distance from the "no pain" end of the line. A variaton is the use of 6 different faces that represent a pain level from zero to 10.

References

1. Pittman S, Kridli S. Music intervention and preoperative anxiety: an integrative review. *Int Nurs Rev.* 2011;58(2):157-163. [IIB]
2. Fayazi S, Babashahi M, Rezaei M. The effect of inhalation aromatherapy on anxiety level of the patients in preoperative period. *Iran J Nurs Midwifery Res.* 2011;16(4):278-283. [IB]
3. Binns-Turner PG, Wilson LL, Pryor ER, Boyd GL, Prickett CA. Perioperative music and its effects on anxiety, hemodynamics, and pain in women undergoing mastectomy. *AANA J.* 2011;79(4 Suppl):S21-S27. [IIB]
4. Sadati L, Pazouki A, Mehdizadeh A, Shoar S, Tamannaie Z, Chaichian S. Effect of preoperative nursing visit on preoperative anxiety and postoperative complications in candidates for laparoscopic cholecystectomy: a randomized clinical trial. *Scand J Caring Sci.* 2013;27(4):994-998. [IB]
5. Pinto PR, McIntyre T, Nogueira-Silva C, Almeida A, Araujo-Soares V. Risk factors for persistent postsurgical pain in women undergoing hysterectomy due to benign causes: a prospective predictive study. *J Pain.* 2012;13(11):1045-1057. [IIIA]
6. Mitchell M. Patient anxiety and conscious surgery. *J Perioper Pract.* 2009;19(6):168-173. [IIIB]
7. Mitchell M. Conscious surgery: influence of the environment on patient anxiety. *J Adv Nurs.* 2008;64(3):261-271. [IIIB]
8. Nilsson U. The anxiety- and pain-reducing effects of music interventions: a systematic review. *AORN J.* 2008;87(4):780-807. [IA]
9. Tam WW, Wong EL, Twinn SF. Effect of music on procedure time and sedation during colonoscopy: a meta-analysis. *World J Gastroenterol.* 2008;14(34):5336-5343. [IA]
10. Arslan S, Özer N, Özyurt F. Effect of music on preoperative anxiety in men undergoing urogenital surgery. *Aust J Adv Nurs.* 2008;26(2):46-54. [IA]
11. Lee KC, Chao YH, Yiin JJ, Chiang PY, Chao YF. Effectiveness of different music-playing devices for reducing preoperative anxiety: a clinical control study. *Int J Nurs Stud.* 2011;48(10):1180-1187. [IB]
12. El-Hassan H, McKeown K, Muller AF. Clinical trial: music reduces anxiety levels in patients attending for endoscopy. *Aliment Pharmacol Ther.* 2009;30(7):718-724. [IA]
13. Dogan MV, Leman S. The effect of music therapy on the level of anxiety in the patients undergoing coronary angiography. *Open J Nurs.* 2012;2(3):165-169. [IB]
14. Bringman H, Giesecke K, Thorne A, Bringman S. Relaxing music as pre-medication before surgery: a randomised controlled trial. *Acta Anaesthesiol Scand.* 2009;53(6):759-764. [IA]
15. Kulkarni S, Johnson PC, Kettles S, Kasthuri RS. Music during interventional radiological procedures, effect on sedation, pain and anxiety: a randomised controlled trial. *Br J Radiol.* 2012;85(1016):1059-1063. [IB]
16. Johnson B, Raymond S, Goss J. Perioperative music or headsets to decrease anxiety. *J PeriAnesth Nurs.* 2012;27(3):146-154. [IA]
17. Jiménez-Jiménez M, Garcia-Escalona A, Martin-Lopez A, De Vera-Vera R, De Haro J. Intraoperative stress and anxiety reduction with music therapy: a controlled randomized clinical trial of efficacy and safety. *J Vasc Nurs.* 2013;31(3):101-106. [IA]
18. Hook L, Sonwathana P, Petpichetchian W. Music therapy with female surgical patients: effect on anxiety and pain. *Thai J Nurs Res.* 2008;12(4):259-271. [IA]

19. Nilsson U, Lindell L, Eriksson A, Kellerth T. The effect of music intervention in relation to gender during coronary angiographic procedures: a randomized clinical trial. *Eur J Cardiovasc Nurs*. 2009;8(3):200-206. [IB]

20. Ottaviani S, Bernard JL, Bardin T, Richette P. Effect of music on anxiety and pain during joint lavage for knee osteoarthritis. *Clin Rheumatol*. 2012;31(3):531-534. [IB]

21. Yeo JK, Cho DY, Oh MM, Park SS, Park MG. Listening to music during cystoscopy decreases anxiety, pain, and dissatisfaction in patients: a pilot randomized controlled trial. *J Endourol*. 2013;27(4):459-462. [IC]

22. Wu J, Chaplin W, Amico J, et al. Music for surgical abortion care study: a randomized controlled pilot study. *Contraception*. 2012;85(5):496-502. [IC]

23. Bradt J, Dileo C, Shim M. Music interventions for preoperative anxiety. *Cochrane Database Syst Rev*. 2013;6:006908. [IIA]

24. Sadideen H, Parikh A, Dobbs T, Pay A, Critchley PS. Is there a role for music in reducing anxiety in plastic surgery minor operations? *Ann R Coll Surg Engl*. 2012;94(3):152-154. [IIB]

25. Mcleod Roddy. Evaluating the effect of music on patient anxiety during minor plastic surgery. *J Perioper Pract*. 2012;22(1):14-18. [IIC]

26. Lee KC, Chao YH, Yiin JJ, Hsieh HY, Dai WJ, Chao YF. Evidence that music listening reduces preoperative patients' anxiety. *Biol Res Nurs*. 2012;14(1):78-84. [IB]

27. Moris DN, Linos D. Music meets surgery: two sides to the art of "healing." *Surg Endosc*. 2013;27(3):719-723. [VA]

28. Beccaloni AM. The medicine of music: a systematic approach for adoption into perianesthesia practice. *J PeriAnesth Nurs*. 2011;26(5):323-330. [VB]

29. Wakim JH, Smith S, Guinn C. The efficacy of music therapy. *J PeriAnesth Nurs*. 2010;25(4):226-232. [VC]

30. Selimen D, Andsoy II. The importance of a holistic approach during the perioperative period. *AORN J*. 2011;93(4):482-490. [VB]

31. Gooding L, Swezey S, Zwischenberger JB. Using music interventions in perioperative care. *South Med J*. 2012;105(9):486-490. [VB]

32. Kim YK, Kim SM, Myoung H. Musical intervention reduces patients' anxiety in surgical extraction of an impacted mandibular third molar. *J Oral Maxillofac Surg*. 2011;69(4):1036-1045. [IB]

33. Matsota P, Christodoulopoulou T, Smyrnioti ME, et al. Music's use for anesthesia and analgesia. *J Altern Complement Med*. 2013;19(4):298-307. [VA]

34. Weeks BP, Nilsson U. Music interventions in patients during coronary angiographic procedures: a randomized controlled study of the effect on patients' anxiety and well-being. *Eur J Cardiovasc Nurs*. 2011;10(2):88-93. [IC]

35. Ni CH, Tsai WH, Lee LM, Kao CC, Chen YC. Minimising preoperative anxiety with music for day surgery patients—a randomised clinical trial. *J Clin Nurs*. 2012;21(5):620-625. [IA]

36. Hoya Y, Matsumura I, Fujita T, Yanaga K. The use of nonpharmacological interventions to reduce anxiety in patients undergoing gastroscopy in a setting with an optimal soothing environment. *Gastroenterol Nurs*. 2008;31(6):395-399. [IC]

37. Bradt J, Dileo C, Grocke D. Music interventions for mechanically ventilated patients. *Cochrane Database Syst Rev*. 2010;(12):CD006902. [IIA]

38. Bradt J, Dileo C, Grocke D, Magill L. Music interventions for improving psychological and physical outcomes in cancer patients. *Cochrane Database Syst Rev*. 2011;(8):CD006911. [IIA]

39. Bradt J, Dileo C, Potvin N. Music for stress and anxiety reduction in coronary heart disease patients. *Cochrane Database Syst Rev*. 2013;12:CD006577. [IIA]

40. Zhang ZS, Wang XL, Xu CL, et al. Music reduces panic: an initial study of listening to preferred music improves male patient discomfort and anxiety during flexible cystoscopy. *J Endourol*. 2014;28(6):739-744. [IA]

41. Wentworth LJ, Briese LJ, Timimi FK, et al. Massage therapy reduces tension, anxiety, and pain in patients awaiting invasive cardiovascular procedures. *Prog Cardiovasc Nurs*. 2009;24(4):155-161. [IB]

42. Brand LR, Munroe DJ, Gavin J. The effect of hand massage on preoperative anxiety in ambulatory surgery patients. *AORN J*. 2013;97(6):708-717. [IIB]

43. Rosen J, Lawrence R, Bouchard M, Doros G, Gardiner P, Saper R. Massage for perioperative pain and anxiety in placement of vascular access devices. *Adv Mind Body*. 2013;27(1):12-23. [IB]

44. Acar HV, Cuvas O, Ceyhan A, Dikmen B. Acupuncture on Yintang point decreases preoperative anxiety. *J Altern Complement Med*. 2013;19(5):420-424. [IA]

45. Valiee S, Bassampour SS, Nasrabadi AN, Pouresmaeil Z, Mehran A. Effect of acupressure on preoperative anxiety: a clinical trial. *J PeriAnesth Nurs*. 2012;27(4):259-266. [IB]

46. Wu S, Liang J, Zhu X, Liu X, Miao D. Comparing the treatment effectiveness of body acupuncture and auricular acupuncture in preoperative anxiety treatment. *J Res Med Sci*. 2011;16(1):39-42. [IC]

47. Liodden I, Norheim AJ. Acupuncture and related techniques in ambulatory anesthesia. *Curr Opin Anaesthesiol*. 2013;26(6):661-668. [VB]

48. Braden R, Reichow S, Halm MA. The use of the essential oil lavandin to reduce preoperative anxiety in surgical patients. *J PeriAnesth Nurs*. 2009;24(6):348-355. [IA]

49. Hu PH, Peng YC, Lin YT, Chang CS, Ou MC. Aromatherapy for reducing colonoscopy related procedural anxiety and physiological parameters: a randomized controlled study. *Hepatogastroenterology*. 2010;57(102-103):1082-1086. [IC]

50. Marc I, Rainville P, Masse B, et al. Women's views regarding hypnosis for the control of surgical pain in the context of a randomized clinical trial. *J Womens Health*. 2009;18(9):1441-1447. [IB]

51. Lang EV, Berbaum KS, Pauker SG, et al. Beneficial effects of hypnosis and adverse effects of empathic attention during percutaneous tumor treatment: when being nice does not suffice. *J Vasc Interv Radiol*. 2008;19(6):897-905. [IA]

52. Abdeshahi SK, Hashemipour MA, Mesgarzadeh V, Shahidi Payam A, Halaj Monfared A. Effect of hypnosis on induction of local anaesthesia, pain perception, control of haemorrhage and anxiety during extraction of third molars: a case-control study. *J Craniomaxillofac Surg*. 2013;41(4):310-315. [IIB]

53. Flory N, Martinez Salazar GM, Lang EV. Hypnosis for acute distress management during medical procedures. *Int J Clin Exp Hypn*. 2007;55(3):303-317. [VB]

54. Schnur JB, Bovbjerg DH, David D, et al. Hypnosis decreases presurgical distress in excisional breast biopsy patients. *Anesth Analg*. 2008;106(2):440-444. [IB]

55. Hulse RS, Stuart-Shor EM, Russo J. Endoscopic procedure with a modified Reiki intervention: a pilot study. *Gastroenterol Nurs*. 2010;33(1):20-26. [IC]

56. Bourque AL, Sullivan ME, Winter MR. Reiki as a pain management adjunct in screening colonoscopy. *Gastroenterol Nurs*. 2012;35(5):308-312. [IIC]

57. Gonzales EA, Ledesma RJ, McAllister DJ, Perry SM, Dyer CA, Maye JP. Effects of guided imagery on postoperative outcomes in patients undergoing same-day surgical procedures: a randomized, single-blind study. *AANA J.* 2010;78(3):181-188. [IB]

58. Ko YL, Lin PC. The effect of using a relaxation tape on pulse, respiration, blood pressure and anxiety levels of surgical patients. *J Clin Nurs.* 2012;21(5-6):689-697. [IIIB]

59. Akhlaghi M, Shabanian G, Rafieian-Kopaei M, Parvin N, Saadat M, Akhlaghi M. Citrus aurantium blossom and preoperative anxiety. *Rev Bras Anestesiol.* 2011;61(6):702-712. [IA]

Acknowledgements

LEAD AUTHOR
Mary J. Ogg, MSN, RN, CNOR
Perioperative Nursing Specialist
AORN Nursing Department
Denver, Colorado

CONTRIBUTING AUTHOR
Ramona L. Conner, MSN, RN, CNOR
Manager, Standards and Guidelines
AORN Nursing Department
Denver, Colorado

The authors and AORN thank Lisa Spruce, DNP, RN, ACNS, ACNP, ANP, CNOR, Director of Evidence-based Perioperative Practice, AORN, Inc, Denver, Colorado; Elayne Kornblatt Phillips, PhD-BSN, MPH, RN, Clinical Associate Professor, University of Virginia, Charlottesville; Melanie F. Sandoval, PhD, RN, Research Nurse Scientist, Perioperative Services, University of Colorado, Aurora; and Deborah S. Hickman, MS, RN, CNOR, CRNFA, Director, Renue Plastic Surgery, Brunswick, Georgia, for their assistance in developing this guideline.

PUBLICATION HISTORY
Originally published in *Guidelines for Perioperative Practice*, 2015 edition.

COMPLEMENTARY CARE INTERVENTIONS

GUIDELINE FOR PREVENTION OF DEEP VEIN THROMBOSIS

The Guideline for Prevention of Deep Vein Thrombosis was developed by the AORN Recommended Practices Committee and was approved by the AORN Board of Directors. It was presented as proposed recommendations for comments by members and others. The guideline is effective March 1, 2011. The recommendations in the guideline are intended to be achievable and represent what is believed to be an optimal level of practice. Policies and procedures will reflect variations in practice settings and/or clinical situations that determine the degree to which the guideline can be implemented. AORN recognizes the various settings in which perioperative nurses practice; therefore, this guideline is adaptable to various practice settings. These practice settings include traditional operating rooms (ORs), ambulatory surgery centers, physicians' offices, cardiac catheterization laboratories, endoscopy suites, radiology departments, and all other areas where operative and other invasive procedures may be performed.

Purpose

This guideline provides a framework for developing a protocol for deep vein thrombosis (DVT) prevention. The document provide guidance for administering pharmacologic and/or mechanical DVT prophylaxis and for patient and health care personnel education. Although the prevention of DVT and pulmonary embolism (PE) should be a priority of the entire health care organization, the particular risks facing perioperative patients makes it imperative that perioperative RNs take an active role in DVT prevention. The patient in the perioperative environment may present with or encounter one or more of the three primary causative factors of DVT formation (ie, venous stasis, vessel wall injury, hypercoagulability).[1] The risk for DVT may be elevated for all perioperative patients, including children, because of immobility, tissue trauma, and surgical positioning requirements.[1-8] Deep vein thrombosis usually occurs in the lower extremities but also may occur in the upper extremities.[9] Prevention of DVT reduces the potential for associated complications such as post-thrombotic syndrome and PE.[10,11]

The perioperative nursing care interventions related to the treatment of complications of DVT (eg, venous stasis ulcers or their postoperative treatment, post-thrombotic syndrome, PE) are beyond the scope of this document. The choice of DVT prophylaxis is a medical decision and is beyond the scope of this document.

Recommendation I

A health care organization-wide protocol for the prevention of DVT that includes care of the perioperative patient should be developed and implemented.[12,13]

Using an organization-wide protocol developed from evidence-based, professional guidelines and providing alternative treatment considerations prompts health care providers to give consistent and appropriate DVT prophylactic care.[13] In a study of 150 hospitals, Maynard concluded that a protocol including a risk assessment and physician orders for venous thromboembolism (VTE) prevention accelerated improvements in VTE prophylaxis efforts.[14] Integration of the health care organization's protocol into all physician orders provides consistency between all care providers and increases use of the protocol.[12,13,15]

I.a. The health care organization-wide DVT protocol should be developed by a multidisciplinary team that includes key stakeholders including, but not limited to,
- RNs;
- physicians;
- anesthesia professionals;
- pharmacists; and
- personnel from
  - quality/risk management,
  - information technology (IT), and
  - administration.[13]

Key stakeholders' acceptance of the protocol is improved if they are involved in the decision-making process.[13] Each key stakeholder provides knowledge and expertise according to his or her area of practice and responsibility. The perioperative RN is a key stakeholder as a primary professional involved in implementing the protocol in the perioperative area and provides evidence-based references related to the safety, effectiveness, efficiency, and financial considerations of DVT prophylactic measures.[16,17] Physicians representing each medical specialty can be resources for the evidence-based DVT prevention protocols developed by their medical specialty organizations.[8,14,18-20] Representatives from IT provide expertise in using technology to gather necessary data for use in the quality improvement program and by creating electronic programs that support protocol implementation. Administrative representatives approve the financial resources necessary to support the measures used in the protocol.

DEEP VEIN THROMBOSIS

I.b. The DVT protocol should
- be supported by an evidence-based model (eg, risk-based, group-specific);
- be accessible to all health care providers;
- contain links to evidence-based treatment options;
- provide alternatives to suggested treatment;
- list contraindications;
- be simple to apply; and
- apply to all patients within the health care organization's scope of service. [12-14,17]

A standardized protocol can be easier to approve, put into action, and modify as necessary.[13] Use of an evidence-based model (eg, risk-based, group-specific) facilitates consistency in treatment and promotes adherence to the protocol.[12] An evidence-based model is based on validated research studies and links patient-related criteria (eg, patient-specific risk factors, the reason for admission) to the preferred prophylactic method.[13,14,17] One example of a risk-based protocol defines a value for each prophylactic measure and a value for each patient-specific risk factor. The appropriate prophylactic measure is determined by summing the patient-specific risk factors values and connecting that number to the value assigned to the prophylactic measure.[21] Another risk-based protocol groups predetermined risk factors into categories such as a level one, two, or three. The appropriate prophylactic measure is determined by placing the patient into the appropriate group based on the patient's risk factors.[22] A group-specific protocol initially determines the type of prophylaxis based on the reason for hospitalization. This initial determination may be changed when other risk factors identified during the assessment are included.[12]

I.b.1. The DVT protocol should include the use of a computer-generated alert identifying the patient at risk for developing a DVT. The alert is created by compiling the information from the patient assessment to produce a clinical decision support tool. When computerized documentation is not available, the patient assessment form should highlight those items, or groups of items, that indicate risk for developing a DVT and a consistent order set should be used.

The computer-generated alert was shown in one study to improve the rate of prophylaxis from 1.5% to 10% for mechanical and from 13% to 23.6% for pharmacological prophylaxis. The population in this study consisted of 1,255 patients in the intervention group and 1,251 patients in the control group.[15]

O'Connor et al[23] compared the number of patients receiving DVT prophylaxis when handwritten orders were used compared to when order sets were used. A random review of charts during an eight-month period (N = 291) showed that DVT prophylaxis was ordered for 35.6% of patients when order sets were used compared to 10% of patients when handwritten orders were used.[23]

Maynard et al demonstrated in a sample of 30,850 admissions that adequate prophylaxis improved from 58% in 2005 to 93% in 2007 with the use of a standardized prevention protocol and order set.[22] A review of the literature by Maynard et al also supported the effectiveness of a computer-generated alert and a consistent order set.[14]

The American College of Chest Physicians' evidence-based recommendations include the use of a computer decision support system.[12]

I.b.2. The DVT protocol should include a start time (eg, upon admission, preoperatively, postoperatively) for all types of prophylaxis based on the clinical condition of the patient.

Preoperative initiation of DVT prophylaxis is listed as criteria in clinical trials and listed as a requirement in evidence-based guidance statements.[12,24-27] The risk of DVT formation begins with preoperative immobility and continues throughout the intraoperative phase of care and is decreased by preoperative initiation of DVT prophylaxis. Some prophylactic measures, such as pharmacological methods, may be contraindicated because of the increased risk of bleeding and may need to be started postoperatively.[12]

I.c. The organization-wide protocol should include specific DVT prevention measures that address perioperative-associated DVT risk factors including, but not limited to,
- positioning;
- compression of tissue caused by retraction; and
- use of a pneumatic tourniquet, especially during prolonged periods of inflation.

Specific DVT prevention measures are needed during the perioperative patient care period, which may not be applicable to other areas of the organization. Patient positioning for the surgical procedure, such as the reverse Trendelenburg position (ie, the patient's head is positioned above heart level) and other positions that cause flexion and internal rotation of the hip and knee, can cause venous stasis. Venous stasis also can be caused by tissue compression resulting from retraction.[2,12,28] Tourniquet pressure can cause venous stasis or congestion by prohibiting venous return.[29]

Recommendation II

The perioperative RN should complete a preoperative patient assessment to determine DVT risk factors.

The preoperative nursing assessment provides information necessary to determine the individual patient risk factors for DVT and identify the appropriate DVT prophylaxis measures.

II.a. The preoperative patient DVT risk factor assessment should include, but not be limited to, the following[12,17,30]:
- Venous stasis:
  - age greater than 40 years;
  - cancer (eg, active or occult) and associated therapy;
  - history of cardiac disease;
  - obesity;
  - pregnancy and the postpartum period;
  - prolonged bed rest or immobilization;
  - prolonged travel (ie, between four to 10 hours within the previous eight weeks);
  - surgery lasting longer than 30 minutes; and
  - varicose veins.
- Vessel wall injury:
  - cancer (eg, active or occult) and associated therapy;
  - central venous catheters;
  - extensive burns;
  - previous history of DVT or stroke;
  - surgery; and
  - trauma (eg, major trauma, lower-extremity injury).
- Hypercoagulability:
  - cancer (eg, active or occult) and associated therapy;
  - inherited or acquired thrombophilia (ie, conditions in which the blood coagulates faster than normal);
  - oral contraceptive use or hormone replacement therapy;
  - pregnancy and the postpartum period; and
  - trauma (eg, major trauma, lower-extremity injury).
- Other:
  - acute medical illness,
  - acute infectious processes,
  - inflammatory conditions, and
  - smoking.

The risk factor grouping of venous stasis, vessel wall injury, and hypercoagulability is frequently referred to in the literature as Virchow's Triad. Published reviews of the literature have indicated that patients with these risk factors exhibit a greater potential for DVT formation.[1,12,17,30,31]

II.b. The perioperative RN should consult and collaborate with surgical team members and members of other disciplines as appropriate regarding the need for and selection of prophylaxis based on the organizational protocol and the individual patient's DVT risk factor assessment.

The perioperative RN has a professional responsibility to advocate for the patient during the entire perioperative period by consulting and collaborating with other professional colleagues regarding patient care.[16,17]

Recommendation III

The perioperative RN should implement specific interventions when the patient is receiving mechanical DVT prophylaxis.

Mechanical prophylaxis may be used throughout the perioperative period for various procedures, and specific interventions are necessary to decrease potential complications. Mechanical prophylaxis includes early ambulation, active and passive foot and ankle exercises, and the use of graduated compression stockings and intermittent pneumatic compression devices.[17] *The American College of Chest Physicians Evidence-Based Clinical Based Guidelines,* 8th edition, states that mechanical prophylaxis has been shown to reduce the risk of DVT, may improve the effectiveness of pharmacological prophylaxis, may be used in patients with a high risk of bleeding, and may reduce leg swelling.[12]

III.a. The perioperative RN should instruct the patient to perform foot and ankle exercises preoperatively.

Foot and ankle exercises create natural muscle compression of the venous system of the legs, decreasing venous stasis.

III.b. The perioperative RN should implement specific activities when the patient is receiving mechanical DVT prophylaxis using intermittent pneumatic compression devices.

Researchers suggest that intermittent pneumatic compression devices reduce venous stasis by improving venous return from the lower extremities.[24] Several intermittent pneumatic compression devices, with a wide variety of design features providing inflation on the foot, calf, or entire leg have been cleared by the US Food and Drug Administration. The devices generally consist of wraps (eg, thigh- or knee-length, foot sleeves) that are placed on the legs or feet; tubing that connects the wrap to the pump; and a pump. The wrap may consist of single or multiple chambers. The chambers may be inflated as a single unit or sequentially and may be cycled using a preset timing device or manual timing device. The compression system also may feature technology allowing the inflation to be synchronized to the patient's respiration-related venous phasic flow, or customized inflation based on the patient's individual venous refill time.[32] The pump may be mobile or stationary.[24]

Foot inflation devices simulate natural walking by providing compression to the plantar venous plexus. Calf and thigh devices work via a milking action that increases the velocity of venous return, enhances fibrinolysis, and increases the release of endothelial-derived relaxing factors and urokinase.[7,12,24] These relaxing factors and urokinase assist in preventing or inhibiting thrombosis development and enhance thrombolysis (ie, clot destruction) during thrombosis formation.[24]

In a study of 502 total hip arthroplasties, Hooker et al concluded that intraoperative and postoperative thigh-high intermittent pneumatic compression is an effective prophylactic measure.[33] Woolson studied 322 patients and came to a similar conclusion.[34] In another study (N = 3,016), Sugano et al concluded that mechanical DVT prophylaxis is safe and effective for elective hip surgeries.[35]

III.b.1. The perioperative RN should assess the patient for and report to the physician any contraindications or possible complications related to use of the intermittent pneumatic compression device.

Contraindications include, but are not limited to,
- conditions affecting the lower extremity (eg, dermatitis, gangrene, extreme leg deformity, untreated infected wounds, injuries, or surgical sites);
- conditions compromising lower extremity venous flow (eg, severe arteriosclerosis, other ischemic vascular disease, massive leg edema);
- sensitivity to latex, unless wraps and tubing are latex free; and
- severe congestive heart failure.[36]

Complications include, but are not limited to,
- compartment syndrome;
- latex sensitivity or allergy, unless the wraps and tubing are latex-free;
- peroneal nerve palsy; and
- skin injury.[24]

III.b.2. Intermittent pneumatic compression wraps should be applied according to the manufacturer's written instructions.

III.b.3. When the manufacturer's written instructions for use require the use of stockinet, elastic hose, or other material under the device wraps, the material should be wrinkle-free when applied to the skin.

Stockinet, elastic hose, or other materials may be recommended by some manufacturers for skin protection under the device wraps. Smooth, wrinkle-free under-wrap material may reduce the risk of skin injury.

III.b.4. During application, the device or wrap tubing should be placed external to the wrap and away from locations that may create a pressure injury.

Placement of the device or wrap tubing between the patient's skin and the device wrap may lead to a pressure injury.

III.b.5. The perioperative RN should reassess and verify that the intermittent pneumatic compression device and wraps are operating and are positioned properly after the patient is transferred to the OR bed.

III.b.6. The perioperative RN should reassess the wraps for proper placement if the patient's position is changed during the surgical procedure.

Reassessment of proper placement of wraps after the patient's position is changed is needed to verify proper device placement and correct function.

III.b.7. The intermittent pneumatic compression device should remain on during the intraoperative and immediate postoperative period except for very brief periods of time, when removal is necessitated by patient care needs.[12]

III.b.8. The DVT protocol should specify when the wraps should be disconnected from the pump and when a patient skin assessment should be performed (eg, ambulation, before discharge, transfer of care). If evidence of complications is present, the perioperative RN should document the information and report it to the physician.

III.c. The perioperative RN should implement specific activities when the patient is receiving mechanical DVT prophylaxis using graduated compression stockings.

Graduated compression stockings, either thigh-high or knee-high in length, are frequently used intraoperatively and postoperatively. The stockings are thought to work by applying a constant graduated pressure to the leg, thereby reducing the venous diameter and venous stasis.[37,38] Conflicting evidence exists regarding which length of stocking, thigh- or knee-length, provides the greatest efficacy.[26,38-42]

III.c.1. The perioperative RN should assess the patient for contraindications or possible complications related to the use of graduated compression stockings.

Contraindications include, but are not limited to,
- ankle-brachial pressure index < 0.8 mm Hg;
- arteriosclerosis;
- cellulitis in lower extremities;
- dermatitis in lower extremities;
- latex allergy or sensitivity, unless stockings are latex-free;
- leg edema;
- leg ulcers;
- peripheral vascular disease;
- presence of infectious processes;
- recent surgical graft;
- severe peripheral neuropathy; and

DEEP VEIN THROMBOSIS

- thigh circumference exceeds the limit defined by the stocking manufacturer directions for use.[38,42,43]

Complications include, but are not limited to,
- ischemia;
- latex allergy or sensitivity, unless stockings are latex-free;
- numbness and tingling; and
- skin injury.[42,43]

III.c.2. Graduated compression stockings should be properly fitted to the individual patient. The patient's legs should be measured separately and according to the manufacturer's instructions.[42,44]

When stockings are too tight, venous return may be decreased and lead to venous pooling and clot formation. In addition, stockings that are too tight may cause the development of peroneal nerve palsy associated with increased direct pressure on the peroneal nerve.[45] When stockings are too loose, they may not provide the effective gradient compression required for DVT prevention. Measuring each of the patient's legs is necessary because there may be enough variability in circumference to require a different stocking size for each leg.[44]

III.c.3. Graduated compression stockings should be applied according to the manufacturer's written instructions, which may include verifying that the
- stockings are not rolled up or down;
- stockings are smooth when fitted;
- toe holes lie underneath the toes;
- heel patches are in the correct position; and
- thigh gussets are positioned on the patient's inner thighs.[42,43,45]

Skin breakdown or a tourniquet effect can be created by graduated compression stockings, if not applied correctly.[42-45]

III.c.4. The perioperative RN should verify that the graduated compression stockings have not rolled up the foot or down the leg during transfer to and from the OR bed or during procedural positioning.

When the graduated compression stockings are allowed to roll up the foot or down the patient's leg, a tourniquet effect can be created and may lead to the formation of a DVT, arterial ischemia, gangrene, and necrosis by constricting blood flow.[42,45]

III.d. As soon as possible postoperatively, the perioperative RN should assist the patient with ambulation if appropriate and should assist with foot and ankle exercises for the patient who is unable to ambulate.

Early ambulation and foot and ankle exercises create natural compression of the venous system and decrease venous stasis. These exercises alone are not adequate to prevent venous stasis in most hospitalized patients; therefore, supplemental mechanical or pharmacological prophylaxis may be required.[12]

Recommendation IV

The perioperative RN should implement specific interventions when the patient is receiving pharmacologic DVT prophylaxis.

Specific interventions are necessary to decrease the risk of potential complications from pharmacologic prophylaxis that may be used throughout the perioperative period. Pharmacologic prophylaxis consists of anticoagulant medications that inhibit blood clotting. The pharmacologic regimen may consist of medications such as warfarin; synthetic pentasacchride (ie, foundaparinux); low molecular weight heparin; and low-dose heparin.

IV.a. The perioperative RN should assess the patient for contraindications or the risk of possible complications related to pharmacologic DVT prophylaxis.

Contraindications include, but are not limited to,
- complex trauma injuries;
- hemorrhage;
- infective endocarditis;
- neurosurgery;
- ocular surgery;
- pregnancy;
- recent intracranial, gastric, or genitourinary bleeding;
- recent surgery (ie, within two days); and
- recent lumbar puncture or neuraxial (ie, spinal, epidural) anesthesia or analgesia (ie, within 24 hours).[12,46-48]

Complications include, but are not limited to,
- bleeding,
- compartment syndrome,
- hematoma formation,
- heparin-induced thrombocytopenia,
- osteoporosis and osteopenia,
- skin necrosis,
- thrombocytopenia, and
- urticaria at injection sites.[4,12]

IV.b. Pharmacologic DVT prophylaxis should be administered in accordance with the "AORN guidance statement: Safe medication practices in perioperative settings across the life span."[49]

Recommendation V

The perioperative RN should provide the patient and his or her designated caregiver(s) instructions regarding prevention of DVT and the prescribed prophylactic measures.

473

DEEP VEIN THROMBOSIS

Education related to DVT prevention and the prescribed prophylactic measures may improve patient compliance and acceptance.[17,30,42,50]

V.a. The patient receiving mechanical prophylaxis and his or her designated caregiver(s) should receive preoperative and postoperative instructions including, but not limited to, the following topics
- the mechanism of mechanical prophylaxis;
- the importance of compliance;
- the importance of wearing properly sized, graduated compression stockings;
- removal and proper reapplication of the intermittent compression device immediately after ambulation; and
- proper application, removal, and reapplication of graduated compression stockings.[17,42-44]

Education assists the patient in understanding the potential complications of mechanical prophylaxis, as well as the importance of compliance with its correct use.[42,45,50]

V.b. The patient receiving pharmacologic prophylaxis and his or her designated caregiver(s) should receive preoperative and postoperative instructions including, but not limited to, the importance of
- follow-up appointments, including where and when they should occur;
- continuing medication post-discharge for the duration prescribed;
- following through with laboratory work at periodic intervals;
- avoiding certain activities (eg, contact sports);
- not using over-the-counter medications (eg, aspirin, ibuprofen);
- using a soft toothbrush;
- using an electric razor;
- reporting any unusual bruising;
- obtaining a medical alert bracelet;
- being aware of medication and food interactions, including herbal and other over-the-counter preparations (eg, ginger, ginkgo biloba, ginseng, feverfew, St John's wort, green tea); and
- informing health care workers about pharmacologic prophylaxis before undergoing any procedures (eg, dental work, laboratory tests).[17,51]

V.c. Before a patient is discharged, the perioperative RN should provide the patient and his or her designated caregiver(s) with instructions on the prevention of DVT including, but not limited to,
- current and future risk factors;
- maintaining adequate hydration;
- common signs and symptoms of DVT or PE (eg, leg pain, swelling, unexplained shortness of breath, wheezing, chest pain, palpitations, anxiety, sweating, coughing up blood);
- avoiding clothing that constricts the lower extremities;
- participating in physical exercise as indicated;
- performing active and passive range of motion, especially of the lower extremities, as indicated;
- avoiding sitting with knees bent or legs crossed for long periods of time;
- elevating legs when sitting;
- avoiding sitting or standing for long periods of time;
- complying with all forms of DVT prophylaxis;
- performing frequent coughing and deep breathing exercises and changing position when in bed;
- avoiding raising the knee gatch of the bed during inpatient care;
- alerting other patient care providers to the patient's history of DVT and current prophylactic measures; and
- the physiology of blood flow and clot formation.[17,52]

Education provides the patient with an awareness of DVT prevention measures and the signs and symptoms of DVT that should be reported to the physician.[17,53] Deep vein thrombosis frequently develops or becomes evident after the patient is discharged. This is supported by a study of 5,451 patients with DVT, nearly half of whom were diagnosed as outpatients, which indicates that more than half of those patients waited three or more days after the onset of symptoms to seek treatment.[52]

Recommendation VI

Personnel should receive initial education and competency validation, as applicable to their roles, on patient care measures to prevent DVT.

Initial and ongoing education of perioperative personnel on the prevention of DVT, the risk to the patient, and appropriate methods of prophylaxis facilitates the development of knowledge, skills, and attitudes that affect safe patient care.

VI.a. Perioperative RNs and all patient care personnel should receive initial education, competency validation, and current information on
- DVT prevention protocols and updates;
- DVT prevention policies and procedures and updates;
- DVT risk factors;
- perioperative-specific preventive measures; and
- the correct application and use of mechanical prophylactic measures (eg, contraindications, signs and symptoms of complications).

VI.b. Perioperative RNs should receive initial education and competency validation, as well as seek evidence-based knowledge, on
- the pathophysiology of DVT and PE;

- contraindications and complications for each category of prophylaxis;
- the selection of prophylactic measures; and
- the administration of pharmacologic prophylaxis.

Perioperative RNs have a professional responsibility to incorporate research findings into practice.[16] Methods of DVT prophylaxis are evolving and new information is being published periodically.

Recommendation VII

Documentation should include a patient assessment, plan of care, nursing diagnoses, and identification of desired outcomes and interventions, as well as an evaluation of the patient's response to the care provided.

Documentation serves as a method of communication among all care providers involved in planning, implementing, and evaluating patient care. Documenting nursing activities provides a description of the perioperative nursing care administered and the status of patient outcomes on transfer of care.

VII.a. Documentation should be recorded in a manner consistent with the health care organization's policies and procedures and should include, but not be limited to,
- results of the nursing assessment including risk factors and complications, if present;
- application and removal times for all mechanical prophylactic measures;
- the type and size of wrap or graduated compression stockings applied;
- the identifier and settings of the mechanical unit, if applicable;
- the time, route, and dosage of all pharmacologic prophylaxis;
- the reason for any variance from the protocol; and
- responses to complications, if present.

Recommendation VIII

Policies and procedures for DVT prophylaxis should be developed, reviewed periodically, revised as necessary, and readily available in the practice setting.

Policies and procedures assist in the development of patient safety, quality assessment, and improvement activities. Policies and procedures establish authority, responsibility, and accountability within the facility. They also serve as operational guidelines that are used to minimize patient risk factors for complications, standardize practice, direct staff members, and establish continuous performance improvement programs.

VIII.a. The health care organization's policies and procedures regarding use of mechanical prophylaxis units must be in compliance with the Safe Medical Devices Act of 1990, as amended in March 2000.[54]

VIII.a.1. When patient or personnel injuries or equipment failures occur, the mechanical prophylaxis unit and its components should be removed from service and all components retained, if possible.

Retaining the unit and its components allows for a complete systems check to determine possible reasons for the failure.

VIII.b. Policies and procedures for preventing DVT should include the steps required for initiating and implementing the DVT protocol and reporting and responding to adverse events.[49]

Recommendation IX

A quality improvement program should be in place to evaluate the outcomes of DVT prophylaxis (eg, DVT rate) and protocol compliance.

The Agency for Healthcare Research and Quality states that quality and performance improvement programs assist in evaluating the quality of patient care and the formulation of plans for corrective actions. These programs provide data that may be used to determine whether an individual organization is within benchmark goals and, if not, identify areas that may require corrective actions.[13]

IX.a. The quality improvement program should include a study time frame (eg, six months before and six months after a change has been instituted) and should
- compare the health care organization's DVT prevention protocol to current research and established, research-based guidelines;
- determine the health care organization's DVT prevention protocol rate of use;
- determine and explore barriers to the use of the protocol; and
- determine the rate of readmissions for DVT or complications related to DVT.[13,14]

Establishing a time frame assists in determining a baseline for comparison. Measuring the rate of readmissions helps to determine the effectiveness of the DVT prevention protocol. Determining the rate of use and the barriers to use assists with refinement of the protocol and ideally leads to an increase in protocol compliance and an improvement in patient outcomes.[13,14]

References

1. Ahonen J. Day surgery and thromboembolic complications: time for structured assessment and prophylaxis. *Curr Opin Anaesthesiol.* 2007;20(6):535-539.

2. Heck CA, Brown CR, Richardson WJ. Venous thromboembolism in spine surgery. *J Am Acad Orthop Surg.* 2008;16(11):656-664.

3. Osborne NH, Wakefield TW, Henke PK. Venous thromboembolism in cancer patients undergoing major surgery. *Ann Surg Oncol.* 2008;15(12):3567-3578.

4. Rawat A, Huynh TT, Peden EK, Kougias P, Lin PH. Primary prophylaxis of venous thromboembolism in surgical patients. *Vasc Endovascular Surg.* 2008;42(3):205-216.

5. Jackson PC, Morgan JM. Perioperative thromboprophylaxis in children: development of a guideline for management. *Paediatr Anaesth.* 2008;18(6):478-487.

6. Squizzato A, Venco A. Thromboprophylaxis in day surgery. *Int J Surg.* 2008;6 Suppl 1:S29-30.

7. Mayle RE Jr, DiGiovanni CW, Lin SS, Tabrizi P, Chou LB. Current concepts review: venous thromboembolic disease in foot and ankle surgery. *Foot Ankle Int.* 2007;28(11):1207-1216.

8. Forrest JB, Clemens JQ, Finamore P, et al. AUA Best Practice Statement for the prevention of deep vein thrombosis in patients undergoing urologic surgery. *J Urol.* 2009;181(3):1170-1177.

9. Arnhjort T, Persson LM, Rosfors S, Ludwigs U, Larfars G. Primary deep vein thrombosis in the upper limb: A retrospective study with emphasis on pathogenesis and late sequelae. *Eur J Intern Med.* 2007;18(4):304-308.

10. Prandoni P, Kahn SR. Post-thrombotic syndrome: prevalence, prognostication and need for progress. *Br J Haematol.* 2009;145(3):286-295.

11. Wille-Jorgensen P, Jorgensen LN, Crawford M. Asymptomatic postoperative deep vein thrombosis and the development of postthrombotic syndrome. A systematic review and meta-analysis. *Thromb Haemost.* 2005;93(2):236-241.

12. Geerts WH, Bergqvist D, Pineo G F, et al. Prevention of venous thromboembolism: American College of Chest Physicians Evidence-Based Clinical Practice Guidelines (8th Edition). *Chest.* 2008;133(6 Suppl):381S-453S.

13. Preventing hospital-acquired venous thromboembolism: a guide for effective quality improvement. Agency for Healthcare Research and Quality. http://www.ahrq.gov/QUAL/vtguide/. Accessed February 14, 2011.

14. Maynard G, Stein J. Designing and implementing effective venous thromboembolism prevention protocols: lessons from collaborative efforts. *J Thromb Thrombolysis.* 2010;29(2):159-166.

15. Kucher N, Koo S, Quiroz R, et al. Electronic alerts to prevent venous thromboembolism among hospitalized patients. *N Engl J Med.* 2005;352(10):969-977.

16. Standards of perioperative nursing. In: *Perioperative Standards and Recommended Practices.* Denver, CO: AORN, Inc; 2010: 9-27.

17. Barnett JS, DeCarlo LJ. Incidence of deep venous thrombosis in the surgical patient population and prophylactic measures to reduce occurrence. *Perioper Nurs Clin.* 2008;3(4):367-382.

18. Committee on Practice Bulletins—Gynecology American College of Obstetricians and Gynecologists. ACOG practice bulletin No. 84: prevention of deep vein thrombosis and pulmonary embolism. *Obstet Gynecol.* 2007;110(2 Pt 1):429-440.

19. Richardson W, Apelgren K, Earle D, Fanelli R. Guidelines for deep venous thrombosis prophylaxis during laparoscopic surgery. *Surg Endosc.* 2007;21(12):2331-2334.

20. Parvizi J, Azzam K, Rothman RH. Deep venous thrombosis prophylaxis for total joint arthroplasty: American Academy of Orthopaedic Surgeons guidelines. *J Arthroplasty.* 2008;23(7 Suppl):2-5.

21. Caprini JA. Risk assessment as a guide to thrombosis prophylaxis. *Curr Opin Pulm Med.* 2010;16(5):448-452.

22. Maynard GA, Morris TA, Jenkins IH, et al. Optimizing prevention of hospital-acquired venous thromboembolism (VTE): prospective validation of a VTE risk assessment model. *J Hosp Med.* 2010;5(1):10-18.

23. O'Connor C, Adhikari NK, DeCaire K, Friedrich JO. Medical admission order sets to improve deep vein thrombosis prophylaxis rates and other outcomes. *J Hosp Med.* 2009;41(2):81-89.

24. Colwell CW Jr, Froimson MI, Mont MA, et al. Thrombosis prevention after total hip arthroplasty: a prospective, randomized trial comparing a mobile compression device with low-molecular-weight heparin. *J Bone Joint Surg Am.* 2010;92(3):527-535.

25. Johanson NA, Lachiewicz PF, Lieberman J R, et al. Prevention of symptomatic pulmonary embolism in patients undergoing total hip or knee arthroplasty. *J Am Acad Orthop Surg.* 2009;17(3):183-196.

26. Venous thromboembolism: reducing the risk of venous thromboembolism (deep vein thrombosis and pulmonary embolism) in inpatients undergoing surgery. National Institute for Helth and Clinical Excellence. http://guidance.nice.org.uk/CG46. Accessed February 14, 2011.

27. National Quality Forum. National Voluntary Consensus Standards for Prevention and Care of Venous Thromboembolism: Additional Performance Measures. 2008.

28. Recommended practices for positioning the patient in the perioperative practice setting. In: *Perioperative Standards and Recommended Practices.* Denver, CO: AORN, Inc; 2010: 327-350.

29. Recommended practices for the use of the pneumatic tourniquet in the perioperative practice setting. In: *Perioperative Standards and Recommended Practices.* Denver, CO: AORN, Inc; 2010: 175-188.

30. Kehl-Pruett W. Deep vein thrombosis in hospitalized patients: a review of evidence-based guidelines for prevention. *Dimens Crit Care Nurs.* 2006;25(2):53-59.

31. Acute Pulmonary Embolism (Helical CT): eMedicine. http://emedicine.medscape.com/article/361131-overview. Accessed February 14, 2011.

32. Intermittent pneumatic compression devices. *Health Devices.* 2007;36(6):177-204.

33. Hooker JA, Lachiewicz PF, Kelley SS. Efficacy of prophylaxis against thromboembolism with intermittent pneumatic compression after primary and revision total hip arthroplasty. *J Bone Joint Surg Am.* 1999;81(5):690-696.

34. Woolson ST. Intermittent pneumatic compression prophylaxis for proximal deep venous thrombosis after total hip replacement. *J Bone Joint Surg Am.* 1996;78(11):1735-1740.

35. Sugano N, Miki H, Nakamura N, Aihara M, Yamamoto K, Ohzono K. Clinical efficacy of mechanical thromboprophylaxis without anticoagulant drugs for elective hip surgery in an Asian population. *J Arthroplasty.* 2009;24(8):1254-1257.

36. Bonner L, Coker E, Wood L. Preventing venous thromboembolism through risk assessment approaches. *Br J Nurs.* 2008;17(12):778-782.

37. Morris RJ, Woodcock JP. Intermittent pneumatic compression or graduated compression stockings for deep vein thrombosis prophylaxis? A systematic review of direct clinical comparisons. *Ann Surg.* 2010;251(3):393-396.

38. Autar R. A review of the evidence for the efficacy of anti-embolism stockings (AES) in venous thromboembolism (VTE) prevention. *J Orthop Nurs.* 2009;13(1):41-49.

39. The CLOTS (Clots in Legs Or sTockings after Stroke) trial collaboration. Thigh-length versus below-knee stockings for deep venous thrombosis prophylaxis

after stroke: a randomized trial. *Ann Intern Med.* 2010;153(9):553-562.

40. Morris RJ, Woodcock JP. Evidence-based compression: prevention of stasis and deep vein thrombosis. *Ann Surg.* 2004;239(2):162-171.

41. Sajid MS, Tai NR, Goli G, Morris RW, Baker DM, Hamilton G. Knee versus thigh length graduated compression stockings for prevention of deep venous thrombosis: a systematic review. *Eur J Vasc Endovasc Surg.* 2006;32(6):730-736.

42. Winslow EH, Brosz DL. Graduated compression stockings in hospitalized postoperative patients: correctness of usage and size. *Am J Nurs.* 2008;108(9):40-51.

43. Welch E. The assessment and management of venous thromboembolism. *Nurs Stand.* 2006;20(28):58-66.

44. Walker L, Lamont S. Graduated compression stockings to prevent deep vein thrombosis. *Nurs Stand.* 2008;22(40):35-38.

45. Van Wicklin SA, Ward KS, Cantrell SW. Implementing a research utilization plan for prevention of deep vein thrombosis. *AORN J.* 2006;83(6):1353-1368.

46. Horlocker TT, Wedel DJ, Rowlingson JC, et al. Regional anesthesia in the patient receiving antithrombotic or thrombolytic therapy: American Society of Regional Anesthesia and Pain Medicine Evidence-Based Guidelines (Third Edition). *Reg Anesth Pain Med.* 2010;35(1):64-101.

47. Mood GR, Tang WHW, Perioperative DVT Prophylaxis: eMedicine. http://emedicine.medscape.com/article/284371-overview. Accessed February 14, 2011.

48. Huntington S, Acomb C. Reducing the risk of thromboembolic events with warfarin. *Br J Card Nurs.* 2008;3(6):248-263.

49. AORN guidance statement: safe medication practices in perioperative settings across the life span. in: *Perioperative Standards and Recommended Practices.* Denver, CO: AORN, Inc; 2010: 665-672.

50. Stewart D, Zalamea N, Waxman K, Schuster R, Bozuk M. A prospective study of nurse and patient education on compliance with sequential compression devices. *Am Surg.* 2006;72(10):921-923.

51. Pruitt B, Lawson R. What you need to know about venous thromboembolism. *Nurs.* 2009;39(4):22- 28.

52. Goldhaber SZ, Tapson VF, DVT FREE Steering Committee. A prospective registry of 5,451 patients with ultrasound-confirmed deep vein thrombosis. *Am J Cardiol.* 2004;93(2):259-262.

53. Arcelus JI, Kudrna JC, Caprini JA. Venous thromboembolism following major orthopedic surgery: what is the risk after discharge? *Orthop.* 2006;29(6):506-516.

54. Medical device reporting: manufacturer reporting, importer reporting, user facility reporting, distributor reporting. Food and Drug Administration, HHS. Final rule. *Fed Regist.* 2000;65(17):4112-4121.

Acknowledgments

LEAD AUTHOR
Byron Burlingame, MS, RN, CNOR
Perioperative Nursing Specialist
AORN Center for Nursing Practice
Denver, CO

CONTRIBUTING AUTHORS
Sharon Van Wicklin, MSN, RN, CNOR, CRNFA, CPSN, PLNC
Perioperative Nursing Specialist
AORN Center for Nursing Practice
Denver, CO

David L. Feldman, MD, MBA, CPE, FACS
American College of Surgeons

Patricia Graybill-D'Ercole, MSN, RN, CNOR, CRCST
Nurse Manager
Wellspan Health/York Hospital
York, Pennsylvania

PUBLICATION HISTORY
Originally published March 2011 online in *Perioperative Standards and Recommended Practices.*

Reformatted September 2012 for publication in *Perioperative Standards and Recommended Practices,* 2013 edition.

Minor editing revisions made in November 2014 for publication in *Guidelines for Perioperative Practice,* 2015 edition.

DEEP VEIN THROMBOSIS

PATIENT CARE

GUIDELINE FOR PREVENTION OF UNPLANNED PERIOPERATIVE HYPOTHERMIA

The Guideline for Prevention of Unplanned Perioperative Hypothermia was developed by the AORN Recommended Practices Committee and was approved by the AORN Board of Directors. It was presented as proposed recommendations for comments by members and others. The guideline is effective January 1, 2008. The recommendations in the guideline are intended to be achievable and represent what is believed to be an optimal level of practice. Policies and procedures will reflect variations in practice settings and/or clinical situations that determine the degree to which the guideline can be implemented. AORN recognizes the various settings in which perioperative registered nurses practice; therefore, this guideline is adaptable to various practice settings. Practice settings include traditional operating rooms, ambulatory surgery centers, physicians' offices, cardiac catheterization suites, endoscopy suites, radiology departments, and all other areas where operative and other invasive procedures may be performed.

Purpose

This document provides guidance to perioperative registered nurses in optimizing patient care practices to maintain normothermia and prevent unplanned hypothermia. Hypothermia, defined as a core body temperature less than 36° C (96.8° F), presents a constant challenge for perioperative registered nurses because many surgical patients are at risk for unplanned hypothermia during surgery. There are three phases of unplanned hypothermia: the redistribution phase, the linear decrease phase, and the thermal plateau phase. This guideline focuses on the prevention of the redistribution phase of unplanned hypothermia. Planned or therapeutic hypothermia is outside the scope of this document.

In the redistribution phase of unplanned hypothermia, a rapid shift of body heat from the body's core to its periphery occurs, resulting in a core temperature drop of approximately 1.6° C (2.7° F) during the first hour after induction of anesthesia.[1,2] The initial temperature drop of the redistribution phase is followed by a slow linear decrease phase during the second and subsequent hours of anesthesia, in which heat loss exceeds the body's ability to metabolically produce heat. In this second phase, warming the patient can effectively limit further heat loss. After approximately three to five hours of anesthesia, the patient's core temperature often plateaus and is characterized by a core body temperature that remains constant, even during prolonged surgery.[3,4]

Unplanned hypothermia is among the most common complications of surgery. It results from anesthesia-induced thermoregulation impairment and the heat loss inherent to surgery and the surgical environment.[5] The risk of hypothermia is greater in some patients (eg, neonates,[6,7] trauma patients,[8] patients with extensive burns[9]). All patients, however, are at risk of hypothermia as the duration of anesthesia time increases.[1,2,10,11]

Randomized clinical trials have demonstrated that mild hypothermia increases the incidence of serious adverse consequences including surgical site infections[12] and adverse cardiac events including ventricular tachycardia.[13,14] In trauma patients, hypothermia is associated with increased mortality.[15] Mild hypothermia inhibits platelet activation, resulting in increased blood loss.[16,17] A 2° C (3.6° F) drop in temperature increases blood loss by approximately 500 mL.[18] Mild hypothermia also alters medication metabolism and increases the duration of muscle relaxant action.[19,20] Hypothermia extends postanesthesia recovery time[21,22] and prolongs hospitalization.[12,23] The risk of these complications is considered greater for frail, elderly patients undergoing extensive surgery than it is for young, generally healthy patients undergoing comparatively minor procedures.[24]

Recommendation I

The perioperative registered nurse should assess the patient for risk of unplanned perioperative hypothermia.

I.a. Perioperative registered nurses should evaluate the patient's risk for unplanned hypothermia. Sources of data include chart review, physical assessment and patient interview, and review of the anesthesia planned and proposed surgical procedure.

I.b. Infancy or neonatal status should be considered. Neonates and infants are more susceptible to hypothermia than adults because they have a high ratio of body surface area to weight, which leads to more heat loss through their skin.[6,7] Studies show that greater temperature decreases occurred in infants and neonates when undergoing major surgery involving an open procedure.[7]

I.c. The extent and severity of a patient's traumatic injuries should be considered.

HYPOTHERMIA

Patients with severe traumatic injuries are more likely to be hypothermic upon hospital admission and are at high risk of development of unplanned perioperative hypothermia. Between 21% and 50% of severely injured trauma patients become hypothermic.[8] Predisposing factors include exposure in the field, blood loss and shock, rapid infusions of cool fluids, removal of clothing, and impaired heat production. Hypothermia triggers a cascade of coagulopathy and acidosis. Studies have consistently found that hypothermia increases the risk of death in trauma patients.[15,25,26] In one large study more than half of the hypothermic trauma patients died.[27]

I.d. The extent and severity of any patient burns should be considered.

Patients with extensive burns lose body heat readily by radiation from burned tissue and convection when tissue is exposed to air currents. Burned patients are at high risk for unplanned hypothermia. The threshold for physiologic response to external temperature is set higher in these patients, triggering a metabolic response to cold at higher ambient temperatures than in unburned patients. The set point is estimated to be 0.03° C higher for each percent of total body surface area burned (eg, 50% burn = 1.5° C higher set point).[9] The natural insulating effect of skin is also impaired. The higher set point, combined with the lack of insulation, places patients with severe burns at high risk for hypothermia.

I.e. The type and duration of planned anesthesia should be reviewed.

Hypothermia in the operating room results from impaired thermoregulation induced by anesthetic agents and exposure to the relatively cool environment. General or major regional anesthesia (eg, epidural, spinal) for periods longer than one hour induces hypothermia. General anesthetics inhibit tonic vasoconstriction and cause vasodilatation. This results in a shift of heat from the body's core to its periphery and a drop in core temperature of approximately 1.6° C over the first hour after induction. During the subsequent two hours of anesthesia time, core temperature continues to decrease an additional 1.1° C.[1] Epidural and spinal anesthesia decrease the vasoconstriction and shivering to a slightly lesser degree, depending on the level of the block.[28,29]

I.f. Perioperative registered nurses should be aware of factors influencing the severity of potential hypothermia in patients under general or major regional anesthesia. These factors include, but are not limited to, the following:

I.f.1. **Older adults.** In a case control study of adult general surgery patients, increased age was found to be a predictive risk factor for perioperative hypothermia.[30] This has been found in patients receiving either general or epidural anesthesia,[31] or spinal anesthesia.[32] Older patients lose heat more rapidly than younger adults due to decreased fat or muscle mass and changes in vascular tone that inhibit vasoconstriction and decrease heat production.[32] Older patients' thermoregulatory defenses are also impaired more than younger patients by general[11] and neuraxial[33] anesthesia.

I.f.2. **Body weight.** Low body weight has been identified as a risk factor for perioperative hypothermia in general surgery patients.[30] Thin patients have a large body-surface-area-to-weight ratio and limited insulation to prevent heat loss. Obese patients have a high weight-to-body-surface ratio and maintain peripheral tissues at high temperatures due to high body fat and a consistent vasodilated state in the time before induction of anesthesia. These patients generally have low core-to-peripheral temperature gradients and little redistribution hypothermia.[34]

I.f.3. **Metabolic disorders.** Some metabolic disorders inhibit thermoregulation by impeding heat production or physiologic responses to changes in external temperatures. Central nervous system dysfunctions may cause insufficient thermoregulation. Cardiovascular diseases may cause peripheral vasoconstriction. Hypothyroidism and hypopituitarism may inhibit heat production. Patients with diabetic neuropathies have been found to have lower core body temperature after two hours of anesthesia than generally healthy adults undergoing similar surgery.[35]

I.f.4. **Chronic treatment with antipsychotics or antidepressants.** Antipsychotics impair the central thermoregulatory effect of the hypothalamus, resulting in decreased heat production and increased heat loss.[36] The cause of thermoregulation impairment during anesthesia in chronically depressed patients remains unclear.[37]

I.f.5. **Use of a pneumatic tourniquet.** Pneumatic tourniquets help prevent hypothermia while inflated; however, they cause abrupt hypothermia when released. Pneumatic tourniquets reduce hypothermia by preventing blood and heat exchange between the isolated extremity and the remainder of the body. More metabolic heat is thus conserved in the core thermal compartment. Upon release of the tourniquet, a redistribution of heat from the core to the extremity results in a rapid decrease in core temperature.[38-41]

I.f.6. **Cold surgical environment.** Environmental temperature determines the rate at which metabolic heat is lost through radiation and convection from the skin, and by evaporation of skin-preparation solutions.[4,42]

I.f.7. **Open-cavity surgery.** There is substantial heat loss into the relatively cool environment of the operating room from surgical incisions. This decrease in core temperature is more pronounced during large open-cavity procedures than small-cavity procedures.[4,43]

I.f.8. **Infusions of cool fluids, blood, and blood products.** A unit of refrigerated blood or one liter of crystalloid solution administered at ambient temperature decreases mean body temperature approximately 0.25° C in a 70-kg patient.[44]

I.f.9. **Cool irrigation solutions in body cavities.** Irrigation solutions placed into the abdomen, pelvis, or thorax enhance heat transfer from the body core to the solution and increase heat loss.

I.g. Patients' preoperative baseline temperature should be assessed. When preoperative hypothermia is identified, interventions should be undertaken to normalize patients' core temperature before surgery when possible. Preexisting hypothermia is considered one of the most significant contributing factors to intraoperative hypothermia.[6]

Recommendation II

The perioperative registered nurse should develop a plan of care to minimize the risk of unplanned perioperative hypothermia in patients identified at risk.

II.a. The perioperative registered nurse should establish expected outcomes and collaborate with anesthesia care providers in the selection of appropriate temperature monitoring technology and interventions to reduce the risk of unplanned hypothermia.

II.b. The perioperative registered nurse should identify and assure the availability of temperature monitoring technology and patient warming equipment and supplies, as needed, and adjust environmental conditions according to individualized patient needs.[45]

Recommendation III

Equipment to monitor core temperature should be selected based upon reliability and access to the route.

III.a. The perioperative registered nurse should ensure that equipment to monitor the patient's temperature is readily available. Temperature monitoring devices that provide the most accurate and consistent readings during each phase of perioperative care should be selected. The selection of the best monitoring device should depend upon the accuracy of measuring core body temperature, reliability of the device, accessibility of the monitoring site, patient safety, and ease of use. The ideal thermometer should be accurate within +/− 0.1° C and not sensitive to outside temperature influences.[46] The device should accurately identify temperatures that are above and below normal.

III.a.1. There are four reliable sites for measurement of core temperature:
- **Tympanic membrane.** The tympanic membrane temperature, measured by a thermocouple, is the preferred method in many preoperative and postoperative areas.[47,48] This method is noninvasive, and the monitoring site receives blood supply from the carotid artery, which supplies the thermoregulatory center of the hypothalamus.
- **Distal esophagus.** The distal esophagus is considered a desirable site to measure temperature, particularly in the operating room, and is less prone to artifact than most others. It is an alternative to the pulmonary artery and is widely used intraoperatively. Placement of the probe in the lower fourth of the esophagus prevents artifactual cooling of the probe by respiratory gases.[48]
- **Nasopharynx.** The nasopharynx is another reliable monitoring site for intraoperative measurement because it approximates core temperature.[48] A thermistor probe is inserted through the nares to the nasopharynx. Measurements may be influenced by the temperature of inspired gases and often are 0.5° C lower than pulmonary artery temperatures.[49,50]
- **Pulmonary artery.** The most accurate measurement of core body temperature is through the pulmonary artery, which is bathed in blood from the core.[48] This invasive form of monitoring, however, is not justified solely for temperature assessment.

III.a.2. Less reliable sites for estimating core temperature include the following:
- **Axillary.** Temperatures can be measured through a thermocouple or an infrared axillary reading. Axillary temperatures are not accurate.[51-58] Readings have been found to be significantly lower than pulmonary artery measurements.[52] Accuracy of readings in pediatric patients has been shown to decrease as temperature increases.[55]
- **Bladder.** Temperatures can be measured using urinary catheters containing temperature transducers. Bladder temperatures are close to core temperature, but

HYPOTHERMIA

the accuracy of the measurement decreases during cardiopulmonary bypass,[59] when the patient is hypothermic and urinary output is lower,[50] and during lower abdominal surgery. This method is a better approximation of core temperature than rectal or axillary methods.[59]

- **Oral.** A systematic review of research studies comparing oral temperatures taken at the posterior sublingual site found that in the absence of a pulmonary catheter, this method provides a reliable estimate of core temperature, even in intubated patients.[48] This method does not detect malignant hyperthermia, however, and is not recommended for intraoperative use.
- **Rectal.** Temperatures taken by the rectal route are directly related to the area's blood flow, and measurements seriously lag behind core temperatures.[50,60] This method of measurement does not appropriately detect malignant hyperthermia and is not a good alternative for general use.[61,62]
- **Skin.** Skin temperature may be measured using a crystal skin-surface thermometer. Studies have demonstrated that peripheral skin temperature correlates poorly with core temperature.[58,63] A recent study found that redistribution of body heat has little effect on the core-to-forehead temperature difference.[64]
- **Temporal artery.** Temporal artery temperature may be measured noninvasively with a scanner probe attached to the forehead. The temporal artery is a branch of the carotid artery and provides a measurement of core temperature; however, this method has been found to be unreliable.[65-67]

III.b. Equipment selected for measuring temperature should be free of mercury. Mercury is a heavy metal that can cause serious adverse health consequences, including chromosomal abnormalities. Environmental contamination can cause harmful effects on wildlife. Mercury thermometers are identifiable by the liquid mercury bubble used for reading the thermometer. Disposal of mercury is regulated by the Resource Conservation and Recovery Act.[68,69]

III.c. Temperature monitoring devices should be used according to the manufacturers' written instructions. Manufacturers' instructions provide details that may enhance the reliability of measurements.

Recommendation IV

The core temperature of patients at risk for unplanned hypothermia should be monitored preoperatively, intraoperatively, and postoperatively.

Monitoring patient temperature alerts the provider to the need for preventive or corrective action. Changes can be a decrease in core temperature or an increase in temperature associated with application of a heating device or inflation of a pneumatic tourniquet. It is important to measure core temperature because peripheral temperature is often significantly different from core temperature. The perception of cold is an inadequate measure. For example, hypothermia during regional anesthesia may not trigger a perception of cold by the patient.[62]

IV.a. The patient's temperature should be assessed preoperatively. Assessment of the patient's temperature preoperatively provides a baseline for planning patient care. This assessment alerts care providers of the need to treat preexisting hypothermia or to avoid overheating the patient with an elevated temperature.

IV.b. The patient's core body temperature should be monitored intraoperatively. Intraoperative temperature monitoring is used to provide information to prevent or mitigate hypothermia and to avoid overheating.

IV.c. The temperature of patients should be monitored when undergoing general anesthesia that exceeds 30 minutes and during regional anesthesia when changes are anticipated or suspected.[62]

IV.c.1. The American Society of Anesthesiologists (ASA) recommends that temperature be continually evaluated and monitored "when clinically significant changes in body temperature are intended, anticipated, or suspected."[70]

IV.c.2. The American Association of Nurse Anesthetists recommends monitoring body temperature continuously in pediatric patients receiving general anesthesia and, when indicated, on all patients.[71]

IV.d. The patient's core body temperature should be evaluated postoperatively. The patient's postoperative core temperature provides a basis for evaluation of the effectiveness of intraoperative measures to prevent unplanned hypothermia and provides data to guide the postoperative plan of care.

IV.e. Abnormal patient temperatures should be communicated to the appropriate patient care providers. Managing the patient's temperature requires a coordinated effort among members of the entire perioperative team.

Recommendation V

Interventions should be implemented to prevent unplanned hypothermia.

V.a. Prewarming the patient for a minimum of 15 minutes immediately prior to induction of anesthesia should be considered for patients at risk of unplanned hypothermia. Warming the patient's skin and peripheral tissues before induction of general or major regional anesthesia prevents redistribution hypothermia. The temperature of the peripheral tissues is increased and vasodilatation triggered. This results in a smaller core to periphery temperature gradient and minimizes the effect of anesthesia-induced vasodilatation.

In a randomized clinical trial of patients undergoing cesarean section, 15 minutes of prewarming and intraoperative forced-air warming resulted in a higher core body temperature in both patients and their infants.[72] In outpatients, 15 minutes of forced-air prewarming resulted in higher core body temperatures upon arrival in the postanesthesia care unit, when compared to prewarming with warm cotton blankets.[73] In a study of volunteers, 30 minutes of forced-air warming resulted in an increase in peripheral temperature determined to be more than the amount typically redistributed from core to periphery under anesthesia.[74]

V.b. Patients should be kept normothermic intraoperatively. Patients who remain normothermic intraoperatively experience fewer adverse outcomes. Insulating blankets (eg, cotton, reflective) reduce heat loss by 30%,[75,76] but this is usually insufficient to prevent hypothermia in anesthetized patients.[77] Circulating fluid mattresses under the patient are nearly ineffective at minimizing the risk of hypothermia.[62,78-81] The patient's body weight, in combination with the heat of the fluid mattress, increases the risk of pressure ulcer or necrosis.[62]

V.c. Effective methods of preventing unplanned hypothermia should be used. These methods involve skin surface warming including, but not limited to, the following:

- **Forced-air warming** is safe and the most widely used skin surface warming method. The efficacy of forced-air warming in preventing unplanned hypothermia has been proven in many clinical trials.[11,81-86] The method is effective in neonates,[87] pediatric patients,[85] and morbidly obese patients.[88] Forced-air warming has also been found to be effective in rewarming patients after cardiopulmonary bypass.[89-91] Forced-air warming does not increase the risk of wound contamination.[83,92]
- **Circulating-water garments** circulate warm water through a special, segmented, conductive-heating garment wrapped around the patient. This method has been found to effectively transfer heat to the patient and maintains normothermia in adult[93-97] and pediatric patients.[98] Circulating-water garments maintained normothermia better than a combination of water blanket and fluid warmer in patients undergoing on-pump[96] or off-pump[94,95] cardiopulmonary bypass. Studies have shown that more heat is transferred to the patient by a circulating water garment than forced-air warming.[97] Compared to an upper body forced-air blanket, normothermia was maintained better using the circulating-water garments in patients undergoing abdominal surgery.[99] Circulating-water garments have also been found to effectively rewarm patients after cardiopulmonary bypass[94,100,101] and to rewarm hypothermic patients better than a full-body forced-air blanket.[97]
- **Energy transfer pads** circulate water through a set of heat-exchange pads that adhere to the patient's skin. Energy transfer pads have been found to be an effective tool to reduce intraoperative hypothermia during off-pump cardiac surgery.[102]

V.d. Warming intravenous (IV) fluids should be considered only if large volumes (ie, more than 2 liters/hour for adults) are being administered. Warming IV fluids to near 37° C (98.6° F) prevents heat loss from the administration of cold IV fluids and should be considered as an adjunct to skin surface warming. When less than 2 liters of volume is given, fluid warming is of limited value because fluid-induced cooling is minimal. In studies of patients undergoing major surgery, the combination of forced-air warming and fluid warming decreased the risk of hypothermia more than forced-air warming alone.[103,104] In one study, however, the average temperature in patients in both groups was normothermic.[104] Fluid warming is not a substitute for forced-air warming, which usually transfers far more heat, and warmed fluids alone will not usually keep patients normothermic.[60,104,105] When fluids are being warmed, technology designed for this purpose should be used according to the manufacturers' written instructions.

V.e. Warming irrigation solutions to be used inside the abdomen, pelvis, or thorax should be considered. Warmed irrigation fluid [near 37° C (98.6° F)] should be used as an adjunct therapy to decrease heat loss, but it is insufficient alone to prevent hypothermia. In a study of patients undergoing laparoscopy without forced-air warming, patients receiving warmed irrigation solutions maintained higher core body temperatures than those receiving room temperature solutions;[24,106] however, warmed irrigation fluids alone did

HYPOTHERMIA

not prevent hypothermia.[106] No improvement in body temperature was found when using warmed irrigation during arthroscopic surgery.[107] When using warmed irrigation solutions, the temperature of the solution should be measured with a thermometer at the point of use and verified before instillation. Irrigating with hot solutions has resulted in patient injuries.

V.f. Increasing the room temperature should be considered when active skin warming is not feasible, or in addition to active skin warming in cases where active skin warming alone is insufficient. When a large surface area must be exposed for the surgical procedure, forced-air warming may not be sufficient. For these patients, the severity of hypothermia may be reduced by raising the room temperature to more than 23° C (73.4° F).[62,108] In orthopedic procedures, normothermia was successfully maintained without forced-air warming when the room temperature remained above 26° C (78.8° F).[109]

V.g. Equipment to humidify warm anesthetic gases should be available for pediatric patients. Less than 10% of metabolic heat is lost through the respiratory tract, and heating and humidification of the airway have little effect on core temperature.[62] This intervention is more effective in infants and children.[110] This method transfers much less heat than forced air and should not be used in lieu of forced-air warming.

V.h. Skin preparation solutions should be used at a temperature recommended by the solution manufacturer. Heating some skin preparation agents may increase the risk of a chemical or thermal burn. Heating flammable antimicrobial skin preparation agents creates a fire hazard. Manufacturers' written instructions provide guidance for the appropriate storage temperature.

V.i. Additional precautions should be taken to prevent unplanned hypothermia in infants and neonates.

V.i.1. The room should be prewarmed and maintained higher than 26° C (78.8° F).[62] In a study of anesthetized neonates and infants, operating room temperatures less than 23° C (73.4° F) increased the risk of hypothermia by 1.96 times.[7]

V.i.2. Skin exposure should be minimized and limited in time as much as possible.

V.i.3. Equipment should be available to humidify and warm the airway. Active humidification and heating of inspired gases has been found to result in a 0.25° to 0.5° C higher core temperature in infants.[110,111]

V.i.4. Equipment should be available to warm IV fluids.[112]

V.i.5. Irrigation fluids should be warmed to normal body temperature (37° C [98.6° F]) and the fluid temperature verified before use. Instillation of warmed irrigation fluids minimizes heat lost through radiation.

V.i.6. Patient temperature should be monitored continuously intraoperatively. An infant's temperature decreases within 10 minutes after induction of anesthesia.[7] Vigorous warming may cause hyperthermia. Continuous monitoring provides early identification of temperature changes, including hyperthermia caused by overheating.

V.j. Additional precautions should be taken to prevent unplanned hypothermia in patients with severe trauma.

V.j.1. Patients with severe trauma are at risk of hypothermia. In this patient population, hypothermia is associated with increased risk of death.[113] The patient may be hypothermic upon arrival in the perioperative area. Forced-air warming may not be appropriate because of the amount of tissue exposed for the surgical procedure. Extra measures are required to minimize heat loss if forced-air warming is contraindicated and may be necessary in addition to forced-air warming.

V.j.2. The room temperature should be prewarmed higher than 29.4° C (85° F).[45,114]

V.j.3. The room temperature should be maintained higher than 29.4° C (85° F) until active warming devices achieve normothermia.[45,114]

V.j.4. Equipment should be available to warm IV fluids. Large volumes of fluids may be given rapidly to stabilize the patient. Warming these fluids minimizes heat lost through radiation.

V.j.5. Irrigation fluids should be warmed to normal body temperature (ie, 37° C [98.6° F]).

V.j.6. Equipment should be available to humidify and warm the airway.

V.j.7. Patient temperature should be monitored continuously intraoperatively.

V.k. Additional precautions should be taken to prevent unplanned hypothermia in patients with extensive burns.

V.k.1. Forced-air warming should be used when feasible. It may not be feasible for patients with extensive burns, however, when a large amount of tissue must be exposed for the surgical procedure. Extra measures are required for extensive burns to minimize heat loss.

V.k.2. The room temperature should be prewarmed and maintained higher than 29.4° C (85° F). High ambient temperatures minimize heat loss through radiation and convection.

HYPOTHERMIA

V.k.3. Body surfaces not involved in the surgical procedure should be covered. Covering these surfaces minimizes heat lost through convection.

V.k.4. Equipment should be available to warm IV fluids.

V.k.5. Irrigation fluids should be warmed to near 37° C (98.6° F).

V.k.6. Equipment should be available to warm and humidify anesthetic gases.

V.k.7. Intraoperative patient temperature should be monitored continuously.

Recommendation VI

Warming devices should be used in a manner that minimizes the potential for patient injuries.

VI.a. Prewarming and continued normothermia management must be provided using only US Food and Drug Administration (FDA)-cleared devices.

VI.b. Intravenous fluid bags or irrigation bottles of heated fluid should not be used to warm patients' skin. In 1994, the ASA Closed Claims Project reported that 52% of burn injuries in the operating room were associated with the use of unapproved devices. Sixty-four percent of these injuries resulted from using heated IV fluid bags to warm patients' skin.[115]

VI.c. Warming devices should be used in accordance with manufacturers' written instructions and in a manner that minimizes the potential for injury. Forced-air warming technology should be used only with the appropriate blanket attached to the hose. The hose end has a dangerously high air temperature, and the blanket serves to disperse this heat. Using the air unit without a blanket has resulted in serious burns.[116,117] Intravenous fluid should be warmed only by technology designed for this purpose, at temperatures recommended by the fluid manufacturer.

VI.d. Ischemic tissue should never be heated. Heat is inadequately distributed in ischemic tissue, and application of heat increases the risk of thermal injury.

Recommendation VII

Competency

Personnel should receive initial education and competency validation and updates on the prevention of unplanned hypothermia and the use of warming equipment.

VII.a. Personnel providing perioperative patient care should be knowledgeable about principles of thermoregulation, risks and consequences of hypothermia, correct use of temperature measurement technology, and measures to minimize the risk of unplanned hypothermia. Personnel should be instructed in the proper operation, care, and handling of warming devices and accessories before use. Initial education of the underlying principles of unplanned hypothermia provides direction for personnel in providing safe care. Additional, periodic educational programs provide reinforcement of these principles and new information on changes in technology, its application, compatibility of equipment and accessories, and potential hazards.

VII.b. Administrative personnel should assess and document annual competency of personnel in prevention of unplanned hypothermia and safe use of warming devices and accessories according to hospital and department policy. Incorrect use of warming devices can result in serious injury to patients. Competency assurance verifies that personnel have a basic understanding of thermoregulation, risks of unplanned hypothermia, and safe use of warming equipment. This knowledge is essential to minimizing the risks of misuse of the equipment and to providing safe care.

Recommendation VIII

Documentation

Patient assessments, the plan of care, interventions implemented, and evaluation of care to prevent unplanned perioperative hypothermia should be documented.

VIII.a. Documentation should include a patient assessment, a plan of care, nursing diagnoses, identification of desired outcomes, interventions, and an evaluation of the patient's response to care provided. The Perioperative Nursing Data Set (PNDS), the uniform perioperative nursing vocabulary, should be used to document patient care and to develop policies and procedures related to prevention of unplanned perioperative hypothermia.

VIII.a.1. Potential diagnoses include
- risk for imbalanced body temperature,
- ineffective thermoregulation, and
- hypothermia.[45]

VIII.a.2. An expected outcome of primary importance to these recommended practices is "The patient is at or returning to normothermia at the conclusion of the immediate postoperative period." This outcome falls within the physiologic domain.[45]

VIII.a.3. Interventions that may lead to the desired outcome include the following: assesses risks for unplanned hypothermia; implements thermoregulation measures; monitors body temperature; and evaluates response to thermoregulation measures.[45]

VIII.b. The patient's temperature and the interventions taken to protect him or her from unplanned hypothermia should be documented in the

HYPOTHERMIA

perioperative record. Documentation should include, but not be limited to,
- preoperative assessment with baseline temperature measure;
- plan of care for prevention of hypothermia;
- patient temperature measurements taken throughout perioperative care;
- use of temperature-regulating devices, including identification of the unit and temperature settings used;
- other thermoregulation interventions; and
- postoperative outcome evaluation.

Recommendation IX

Policies and Procedures
Policies and procedures for prevention of unplanned hypothermia should be developed in collaboration with anesthesia care providers, reviewed periodically, revised as necessary, and readily available in the practice setting.

IX.a. This guideline should be used for the development of policies and procedures in the perioperative practice setting. Policies and procedures establish authority, responsibility, and accountability within the facility. They also serve as operational guidelines.

IX.b. Policies and procedures for prevention of unplanned hypothermia should be developed and include, but not be limited to,
- preoperative, intraoperative, and postoperative patient assessments;
- interventions to be employed;
- documentation of care provided;
- use, care, and cleaning of equipment;
- maintenance of equipment;
- reporting and removal from service of malfunctioning equipment;
- reporting of incidence of hypothermia or injuries; and
- competency verification.

IX.c. Policies and procedures should be reviewed and revised at regularly scheduled intervals and be readily available in the practice setting.

Recommendation X

Quality
A quality improvement/management program should be in place to evaluate the structure, process, and outcomes of interventions used to protect patients from unplanned perioperative hypothermia.

X.a. Unplanned hypothermia should be evaluated as part of the perioperative quality management program. The patient outcomes of preventive measures should be evaluated. Outcomes in high-risk populations should be included (eg, neonates, infants, severe trauma, burn patients). The Surgical Care Improvement Project includes "colorectal surgery patients with immediate postoperative normothermia" as an evidence-based indicator of quality.[118]

X.b. Measures should be implemented as necessary to minimize the incidence of unplanned hypothermia. Corrective measures may include increasing the availability of warming equipment and educational programs, and providing clinicians with feedback about outcomes.

X.c. Adverse events related to warming devices should be reported through the facility's incident reporting system and investigated in compliance with the Safe Medical Devices Act of 1990, amended in March 2000.[119]

X.d. Adverse events should be investigated and analyzed to minimize the risk of recurrence. An injury related to the use of a warming device must be reported to the FDA. Serious injuries and deaths must be reported to the FDA and manufacturer within 10 days. Device identification, maintenance and service information, and adverse event information should be included in the report from the practice setting. Retaining the equipment and accessories allows for a complete evaluation and facilitates determination of the cause of the injury. Semiannual reports must be submitted to the FDA as follow-up to any adverse event report submitted during the previous six-month period.

Glossary

Active skin warming: The application of conductive, convective, or radiative warming to the skin.

Ambient temperature: The temperature of the immediate environment, usually ranging from 20° C to 25° C (68° F to 77° F).

Circulating-fluid garment: A microprocessor-controlled heating and cooling device with temperature sensors; skin thermistor; and a specially designed, segmented garment that wraps around the patient.

Core temperature: The temperature of the thermal compartment of the body containing highly perfused tissues and major organs.

Energy transfer pads: A servo-regulated system circulating temperature-controlled water through energy transfer pads adhered to the patient's skin and used to cool or warm the patient.

Forced-air warming: Convection warming technology dispersing a blanket of warm air over the patient's skin in a controlled manner.

Infant: A child one month after birth to approximately 12 months of age.

Mild hypothermia: A core temperature between 34° C to 36° C (93.2° F to 96.8° F).[24]

Neonate: An infant from birth to 28 days of age.

Neuraxial anesthesia: Spinal or epidural regional nerve blocks.

Normothermia: A core temperature between 36° C to 38° C (96.8° F to 100.4° F).

Passive insulation: Method of containing body heat and insulate the body from heat loss through radiation (eg, blankets, clothing).

Redistribution hypothermia: A decrease in body temperature occurring as heat is exchanged from the body's core compartment to the peripheral tissues.

Thermistor: An electrical resistor using a semiconductor whose resistance varies sharply in a known manner with the temperature.

Thermocouple: A device for measuring temperature in which a pair of wires of dissimilar metals is joined and the free ends connected to an instrument that measures the difference in potential created at the junction of the two metals.

Thermometer: An instrument for measuring temperature.

Thermostat: A device that automatically establishes and maintains a desired temperature.

References

1. Matsukawa T, Sessler DI, Christensen R, Ozaki M, Schroeder M. Heat flow and distribution during epidural anesthesia. *Anesthesiology.* 1995;83:961-967.
2. Matsukawa T, Sessler DI, Sessler AM, Schroeder M, Ozaki M, Kurz A, Cheng C. Heat flow and distribution during induction of general anesthesia. *Anesthesiology.* 1995;82:662-673.
3. Buggy DJ, Crossley AW. Thermoregulation, mild perioperative hypothermia and postanaesthetic shivering. *Br J Anaesth.* 2000;84:615-628.
4. Sessler DI. Perioperative heat balance. *Anesthesiology.* 2000;92:578-596.
5. Sessler DI. Perioperative thermoregulation and heat balance. *Ann N Y Acad Sci.* 1997;813:757-777.
6. Macario A, Dexter F. What are the most important risk factors for a patient's developing intraoperative hypothermia? *Anesth Analg.* 2002;94:215-220.
7. Tander B, Baris S, Karakaya D, Ariturk E, Rizalar R, Bernay F. Risk factors influencing inadvertent hypothermia in infants and neonates during anesthesia. *Paediatr Anaesth.* 2005;15:574-579.
8. Tisherman S. Hypothermia, cold injury, and drowning. In: Peitzman A, Rhodes M, Schwab C, Yealy D, Fabian T, eds. *The Trauma Manual,* 2nd ed. Philadelphia: Lippincott, Williams, & Wilkins; 2002:404-410.
9. Caldwell FT, Jr., Wallace BH, Cone JB. The effect of wound management on the interaction of burn size, heat production, and rectal temperature. *J Burn Care Rehabil.* 1994;15:121-129.
10. Sessler DI, Moayeri A, Stoen R, Glosten B, Hynson J, McGuire J. Thermoregulatory vasoconstriction decreases cutaneous heat loss. *Anesthesiology.* 1990;73:656-660.
11. Kurz A, Plattner O, Sessler DI, Huemer G, Redl G, Lackner F. The threshold for thermoregulatory vasoconstriction during nitrous oxide/isoflurane anesthesia is lower in elderly than in young patients. *Anesthesiology.* 1993;79:465-469.
12. Kurz A, Sessler DI, Lenhardt R. Perioperative normothermia to reduce the incidence of surgical-wound infection and shorten hospitalization. Study of Wound Infection and Temperature Group. *N Engl J Med.* 1996;334:1209-1215.
13. Flores-Maldonado A, Guzman-Llanez Y, Castaneda-Zarate S, Pech-Colli J, Alvarez-Nemegyei J, Cervera-Saenz M, Canto-Rubio A, Terrazas-Olguin MA. Risk factors for mild intraoperative hypothermia. *Arch Med Res.* 1997;28:587-590.
14. Frank SM, Beattie C, Christopherson R, Norris EJ, Perler BA, Williams GM, Gottlieb SO. Unintentional hypothermia is associated with postoperative myocardial ischemia. The Perioperative Ischemia Randomized Anesthesia Trial Study Group. *Anesthesiology.* 1993;78:468-476.
15. Gentilello LM, Jurkovich GJ, Stark MS, Hassantash SA, O'Keefe GE. Is hypothermia in the victim of major trauma protective or harmful? A randomized, prospective study. *Ann Surg.* 1997;226:439-447; discussion 447-439.
16. Michelson AD, MacGregor H, Barnard MR, Kestin AS, Rohrer MJ, Valeri CR. Reversible inhibition of human platelet activation by hypothermia in vivo and in vitro. *Thromb Haemost.* 1994;71:633-640.
17. Reed RL, 2nd, Johnson TD, Hudson JD, Fischer RP. The disparity between hypothermic coagulopathy and clotting studies. *J Trauma.* 1992;33:465-470.
18. Schmied H, Kurz A, Sessler DI, Kozek S, Reiter A. Mild hypothermia increases blood loss and transfusion requirements during total hip arthroplasty. *Lancet.* 1996;347:289-292.
19. Heier T, Caldwell JE. Impact of hypothermia on the response to neuromuscular blocking drugs. *Anesthesiology.* 2006;104:1070-1080.
20. Leslie K, Sessler DI, Bjorksten AR, Moayeri A. Mild hypothermia alters propofol pharmacokinetics and increases the duration of action of atracurium. *Anesth Analg.* 1995;80:1007-1014.
21. Kurz A, Sessler DI, Narzt E, Bekar A, Lenhardt R, Huemer G, Lackner F. Postoperative hemodynamic and thermoregulatory consequences of intraoperative core hypothermia. *J Clin Anesth.* 1995;7:359-366.
22. Lenhardt R, Marker E, Goll V, Tschernich H, Kurz A, Sessler DI, Narzt E, Lackner F. Mild intraoperative hypothermia prolongs postanesthetic recovery. *Anesthesiology.* 1997;87:1318-1323.
23. Frank SM, Fleisher LA, Breslow MJ, Higgins MS, Olson KF, Kelly S, Beattie C. Perioperative maintenance of normothermia reduces the incidence of morbid cardiac events. A randomized clinical trial. *JAMA.* 1997;277:1127-1134.
24. Sessler DI. Complications and treatment of mild hypothermia. *Anesthesiology.* 2001;95:531-543.
25. Jurkovich GJ, Greiser WB, Luterman A, Curreri PW. Hypothermia in trauma victims: an ominous predictor of survival. *J Trauma.* 1987;27:1019-1024.
26. Luna GK, Maier RV, Pavlin EG, Anardi D, Copass MK, Oreskovich MR. Incidence and effect of hypothermia in seriously injured patients. *J Trauma.* 1987;27:1014-1018.
27. Rutherford EJ, Fusco MA, Nunn CR, Bass JG, Eddy VA, Morris JA, Jr. Hypothermia in critically ill trauma patients. *Injury.* 1998;29:605-608.
28. Sessler DI, Moayeri A. Skin-surface warming: heat flux and central temperature. *Anesthesiology.* 1990;73:218-224.
29. Kurz A, Sessler DI, Schroeder M, Kurz M. Thermoregulatory response thresholds during spinal anesthesia. *Anesth Analg.* 1993;77:721-726.
30. Kasai T, Hirose M, Yaegashi K, Matsukawa T, Takamata A, Tanaka Y. Preoperative risk factors of intraoperative hypothermia in major surgery under general anesthesia. *Anesth Analg.* 2002;95:1381-1383.
31. Frank SM, Shir Y, Raja SN, Fleisher LA, Beattie C. Core hypothermia and skin-surface temperature gradients. Epidural versus general anesthesia and the effects of age. *Anesthesiology.* 1994;80:502-508.
32. Frank SM, Raja SN, Bulcao C, Goldstein DS. Age-related thermoregulatory differences during core cooling in humans. *Am J Physiol Regul Integr Comp Physiol.* 2000; 279:R349-354.

33. Vassilieff N, Rosencher N, Sessler DI, Conseiller C. Shivering threshold during spinal anesthesia is reduced in elderly patients. *Anesthesiology.* 1995;83:1162-1166.

34. Kurz A, Sessler DI, Narzt E, Lenhardt R, Lackner F. Morphometric influences on intraoperative core temperature changes. *Anesth Analg.* 1995;80:562-567.

35. Kitamura A, Hoshino T, Kon T, Ogawa R. Patients with diabetic neuropathy are at risk of a greater intraoperative reduction in core temperature. *Anesthesiology.* 2000;92:1311-1318.

36. Kudoh A, Takase H, Takazawa T. Chronic treatment with antipsychotics enhances intraoperative core hypothermia. *Anesth Analg.* 2004;98:111-115.

37. Kudoh A, Takase H, Takazawa T. Chronic treatment with antidepressants decreases intraoperative core hypothermia. *Anesth Analg.* 2003;97:275-279.

38. Estebe JP, Le Naoures A, Malledant Y, Ecoffey C. Use of a pneumatic tourniquet induces changes in central temperature. *Br J Anaesth.* 1996;77:786-788.

39. Sanders BJ, D'Alessio JG, Jernigan JR. Intraoperative hypothermia associated with lower extremity tourniquet deflation. *J Clin Anesth.* 1996;8:504-507.

40. Akata T, Kanna T, Izumi K, Kodama K, Takahashi S. Changes in body temperature following deflation of limb pneumatic tourniquet. *J Clin Anesth.* 1998;10:17-22.

41. Bloch EC, Ginsberg B, Binner RA, Jr., Sessler DI. Limb tourniquets and central temperature in anesthetized children. *Anesth Analg.* 1992;74:486-489.

42. Sessler DI, Sessler AM, Hudson S, Moayeri A. Heat loss during surgical skin preparation. *Anesthesiology.* 1993;78:1055-1064.

43. Roe CF. Effect of bowel exposure on body temperature during surgical operations. *Am J Surg.* 1971; 122:13-15.

44. Sessler DI. Consequences and treatment of perioperative hypothermia. *Anesthesiology Clinics of North America.* 1994;23:425-456.

45. Felciano D. Abdominal vascular injury. In: Moore E, Feliciano D, Mattox K, eds. *Trauma.* 5th ed. New York, NY: McGraw-Hill; 2002:755-880.

46. Moran DS, Mendal L. Core temperature measurement: methods and current insights. *Sports Med.* 2002; 32:879-885.

47. American Society of PeriAnesthesia Nurses. Clinical guideline for the prevention of unplanned perioperative hypothermia. *J Perianesth Nurs.* 2001;16:305-314.

48. Hooper VD, Andrews JO. Accuracy of noninvasive core temperature measurement in acutely ill adults: the state of the science. *Biol Res Nurs.* 2006;8:24-34.

49. Ilsley AH, Rutten AJ, Runciman WB. An evaluation of body temperature measurement. *Anaesth Intensive Care.* 1983;11:31-39.

50. Holtzclaw BJ. Monitoring body temperature. *AACN Clin Issues Crit Care Nurs.* 1993;4:44-55.

51. Bailey J, Rose P. Axillary and tympanic membrane temperature recording in the preterm neonate: a comparative study. *J Adv Nurs.* 2001;34:465-474.

52. Erickson RS, Kirklin SK. Comparison of ear-based, bladder, oral, and axillary methods for core temperature measurement. *Crit Care Med.* 1993;21:1528-1534.

53. Giuffre M, Heidenreich T, Carney-Gersten P, Dorsch JA, Heidenreich E. The relationship between axillary and core body temperature measurements. *Appl Nurs Res.* 1990;3:52-55.

54. Hicks MA. A comparison of the tympanic and axillary temperatures of the preterm and term infant. *J Perinatol.* 1996;16:261-267.

55. Jean-Mary MB, Dicanzio J, Shaw J, Bernstein HH. Limited accuracy and reliability of infrared axillary and aural thermometers in a pediatric outpatient population. *J Pediatr.* 2002;141:671-676.

56. Jensen BN, Jensen FS, Madsen SN, Lossl K. Accuracy of digital tympanic, oral, axillary, and rectal thermometers compared with standard rectal mercury thermometers. *Eur J Surg.* 2000;166:848-851.

57. Weiss ME, Richards MT. Accuracy of electronic axillary temperature measurement in term and preterm neonates. *Neonatal Netw.* 1994;13:35-40.

58. Cork RC, Vaughan RW, Humphrey LS. Precision and accuracy of intraoperative temperature monitoring. *Anesth Analg.* 1983;62:211-214.

59. Lefrant JY, Muller L, de La Coussaye JE, Benbabaali M, Lebris C, Zeitoun N, Mari C, Saissi G, Ripart J, Eledjam JJ. Temperature measurement in intensive care patients: comparison of urinary bladder, oesophageal, rectal, axillary, and inguinal methods versus pulmonary artery core method. *Intensive Care Med.* 2003;29:414-418.

60. Lenhardt R. Monitoring and thermal management. *Best Pract Res Clin Anaesthesiol.* 2003;17:569-581.

61. Iaizzo PA, Kehler CH, Zink RS, Belani KG, Sessler DI. Thermal response in acute porcine malignant hyperthermia. *Anesth Analg.* 1996;82:782-789.

62. Sessler DI. Temperature Monitoring. In: Miller RD, ed. *Miller's Anesthesia.* 6th ed. Philadelphia, PA: Elsevier; 2005:1571-1597.

63. Bissonnette B, Sessler DI, LaFlamme P. Intraoperative temperature monitoring sites in infants and children and the effect of inspired gas warming on esophageal temperature. *Anesth Analg.* 1989;69:192-196.

64. Ikeda T, Sessler DI, Marder D, Xiong J. Influence of thermoregulatory vasomotion and ambient temperature variation on the accuracy of core-temperature estimates by cutaneous liquid-crystal thermometers. *Anesthesiology.* 1997;86:603-612.

65. Hebbar K, Fortenberry JD, Rogers K, Merritt R, Easley K. Comparison of temporal artery thermometer to standard temperature measurements in pediatric intensive care unit patients. *Pediatr Crit Care Med.* 2005;6:557-561.

66. Suleman MI, Doufas AG, Akca O, Ducharme M, Sessler DI. Insufficiency in a new temporal-artery thermometer for adult and pediatric patients. *Anesth Analg.* 2002;95:67-71.

67. Greenes DS, Fleisher GR. Accuracy of a noninvasive temporal artery thermometer for use in infants. *Arch Pediatr Adolesc Med.* 2001;155:376-381.

68. AORN guidance statement: environmental responsibility. In: *Standards, Recommended Practices, and Guidelines.* 2006 ed. Denver: AORN, Inc; 2006:243-250.

69. U.S. Environmental Protection Agency. Mercury. Available at: http://www.epa.gov/mercury/index.htm. Accessed August 26, 2006.

70. American Society of Anesthesiologists. Standards for basic anesthetic monitoring. Available at: http://www.asahq.org/publicationsAndServices/standards/02.pdf. Accessed August 26, 2006.

71. Scope and standards for nurse anesthesia practice. *Professional Practice Manual for the Certified Registered Nurse Anesthetist.* Park Ridge, IL: American Association of Nurse Anesthetists; 1996:1-4.

72. Horn EP, Schroeder F, Gottschalk A, Sessler DI, Hiltmeyer N, Standl T, Schulte am Esch J. Active warming during cesarean delivery. *Anesth Analg.* 2002;94:409-414.

73. Fossum S, Hays J, Henson MM. A comparison study on the effects of prewarming patients in the outpatient surgery setting. *J Perianesth Nurs.* 2001;16:187-194.

74. Sessler DI, Schroeder M, Merrifield B, Matsukawa T, Cheng C. Optimal duration and temperature of prewarming. *Anesthesiology.* 1995;82:674-681.

75. Sessler DI, Schroeder M. Heat loss in humans covered with cotton hospital blankets. *Anesth Analg.* 1993;77:73-77.

76. Sessler DI, McGuire J, Sessler AM. Perioperative thermal insulation. *Anesthesiology.* 1991;74:875-879.

77. Ng SF, Oo CS, Loh KH, Lim PY, Chan YH, Ong BC. A comparative study of three warming interventions to determine the most effective in maintaining perioperative normothermia. *Anesth Analg.* 2003;96:171-176.

78. Matsuzaki Y, Matsukawa T, Ohki K, Yamamoto Y, Nakamura M, Oshibuchi T. Warming by resistive heating maintains perioperative normothermia as well as forced air heating. *Br J Anaesth.* 2003;90:689-691.

79. Morris RH, Kumar A. The effect of warming blankets on maintenance of body temperature of the anesthetized, paralyzed adult patient. *Anesthesiology.* 1972;36:408-411.

80. Negishi C, Hasegawa K, Mukai S, Nakagawa F, Ozaki M, Sessler DI. Resistive-heating and forced-air warming are comparably effective. *Anesth Analg.* 2003;96:1683-1687.

81. Hynson JM, Sessler DI. Intraoperative warming therapies: a comparison of three devices. *J Clin Anesth.* 1992;4:194-199.

82. Borms SF, Engelen SL, Himpe DG, Suy MR, Theunissen WJ. Bair hugger forced-air warming maintains normothermia more effectively than thermo-lite insulation. *J Clin Anesth.* 1994;6:303-307.

83. Huang JK, Shah EF, Vinodkumar N, Hegarty MA, Greatorex RA. The Bair Hugger patient warming system in prolonged vascular surgery: an infection risk? *Crit Care.* 2003;7:R13-16.

84. Lamb FJ, Rogers R. Forced-air warming maintains normothermia during orthotopic liver transplantation. *Anaesthesia.* 1995;50:745.

85. Murat I, Berniere J, Constant I. Evaluation of the efficacy of a forced-air warmer (Bair Hugger) during spinal surgery in children. *J Clin Anesth.* 1994;6:425-429.

86. Russell SH, Freeman JW. Prevention of hypothermia during orthotopic liver transplantation: comparison of three different intraoperative warming methods. *Br J Anaesth.* 1995;74:415-418.

87. Komatsu H, Chujo K, Ogli K. Forced-air warming system for perioperative use in neonates. *Paediatr Anaesth.* 1996;6:427-428.

88. Mason DS, Sapala JA, Wood MH, Sapala MA. Influence of a forced air warming system on morbidly obese patients undergoing Roux-en-Y gastric bypass. *Obes Surg.* 1998;8:453-460.

89. Janke EL, Pilkington SN, Smith DC. Evaluation of two warming systems after cardiopulmonary bypass. *Br J Anaesth.* 1996;77:268-270.

90. Rajek A, Lenhardt R, Sessler DI, Brunner G, Haisjackl M, Kastner J, Laufer G. Efficacy of two methods for reducing postbypass afterdrop. *Anesthesiology.* 2000;92:447-456.

91. Mort TC, Rintel TD, Altman F. The effects of forced-air warming on postbypass central and skin temperatures and shivering activity. *J Clin Anesth.* 1996;8:361-370.

92. Zink RS, Iaizzo PA. Convective warming therapy does not increase the risk of wound contamination in the operating room. *Anesth Analg.* 1993;76:50-53.

93. Hofer CK, Worn M, Tavakoli R, Sander L, Maloigne M, Klaghofer R, Zollinger A. Influence of body core temperature on blood loss and transfusion requirements during off-pump coronary artery bypass grafting: a comparison of 3 warming systems. *J Thorac Cardiovasc Surg.* 2005;129:838-843.

94. Nesher N, Insler SR, Sheinberg N, Bolotin G, Kramer A, Sharony R, Paz Y, Pevni D, Loberman D, Uretzky G. A new thermoregulation system for maintaining perioperative normothermia and attenuating myocardial injury in off-pump coronary artery bypass surgery. *Heart Surg Forum.* 2002;5:373-380.

95. Nesher N, Uretzky G, Insler S, Nataf P, Frolkis I, Pineau E, Cantoni E, Bolotin G, Vardi M, Pevni D, Lev-Ran O, Sharony R, Weinbroum AA. Thermo-wrap technology preserves normothermia better than routine thermal care in patients undergoing off-pump coronary artery bypass and is associated with lower immune response and lesser myocardial damage. *J Thorac Cardiovasc Surg.* 2005;129:1371-1378.

96. Nesher N, Wolf T, Kushnir I, David M, Bolotin G, Sharony R, Pizov R, Uretzky G. Novel thermoregulation system for enhancing cardiac function and hemodynamics during coronary artery bypass graft surgery. *Ann Thorac Surg.* 2001;72:S1069-1076.

97. Taguchi A, Ratnaraj J, Kabon B, Sharma N, Lenhardt R, Sessler DI, Kurz A. Effects of a circulating-water garment and forced-air warming on body heat content and core temperature. *Anesthesiology.* 2004;100:1058-1064.

98. Nesher N, Wolf T, Uretzky G, Oppenheim-Eden A, Yussim E, Kushnir I, Shoshany G, Rosenberg B, Berant M. A novel thermoregulatory system maintains perioperative normothermia in children undergoing elective surgery. *Paediatr Anaesth.* 2001;11:555-560.

99. Janicki PK, Higgins MS, Janssen J, Johnson RF, Beattie C. Comparison of two different temperature maintenance strategies during open abdominal surgery: upper body forced-air warming versus whole body water garment. *Anesthesiology.* 2001;95:868-874.

100. Motta P, Mossad E, Toscana D, Lozano S, Insler S. Effectiveness of a circulating-water warming garment in rewarming after pediatric cardiac surgery using hypothermic cardiopulmonary bypass. *J Cardiothorac Vasc Anesth.* 2004;18:148-151.

101. Nesher N, Zisman E, Wolf T, Sharony R, Bolotin G, David M, Uretzky G, Pizov R. Strict thermoregulation attenuates myocardial injury during coronary artery bypass graft surgery as reflected by reduced levels of cardiac-specific troponin I. *Anesth Analg.* 2003;96:328-335.

102. Grocott HP, Mathew JP, Carver EH, Phillips-Bute B, Landolfo KP, Newman MF. A randomized controlled trial of the Arctic Sun Temperature Management System versus conventional methods for preventing hypothermia during off-pump cardiac surgery. *Anesth Analg.* 2004;98:298-302.

103. Camus Y, Delva E, Cohen S, Lienhart A. The effects of warming intravenous fluids on intraoperative hypothermia and postoperative shivering during prolonged abdominal surgery. *Acta Anaesthesiol Scand.* 1996;40:779-782.

104. Smith CE, Desai R, Glorioso V, Cooper A, Pinchak AC, Hagen KF. Preventing hypothermia: convective and intravenous fluid warming versus convective warming alone. *J Clin Anesth.* 1998;10:380-385.

105. Sessler DI. Mild perioperative hypothermia. *N Engl J Med.* 12 1997;336:1730-1737.

106. Moore SS, Green CR, Wang FL, Pandit SK, Hurd WW. The role of irrigation in the development of hypothermia during laparoscopic surgery. *Am J Obstet Gynecol.* 1997;176:598-602.

107. Kelly JA, Doughty JK, Hasselbeck AN, Vacchiano CA. The effect of arthroscopic irrigation fluid warming on body temperature. *J Perianesth Nurs.* 2000;15:245-252.

108. Morris RH. Influence of ambient temperature on patient temperature during intraabdominal surgery. *Ann Surg.* 1971;173:230-233.

109. El-Gamal N, El-Kassabany N, Frank SM, Amar R, Khabar HA, El-Rahmany HK, Okasha AS. Age-related thermoregulatory differences in a warm operating room

110. Bissonnette B, Sessler DI. Passive or active inspired gas humidification increases thermal steady-state temperatures in anesthetized infants. *Anesth Analg.* 1989;69:783-787.

111. Bissonnette B, Sessler DI, LaFlamme P. Passive and active inspired gas humidification in infants and children. *Anesthesiology.* 1989;71:350-354.

112. Bissonnette B. Temperature monitoring in pediatric anesthesia. *Int Anesthesiol Clin.* Summer 1992;30:63-76.

113. Hildebrand F, Giannoudis PV, van Griensven M, Chawda M, Pape HC. Pathophysiologic changes and effects of hypothermia on outcome in elective surgery and trauma patients. *Am J Surg.* 2004;187:363-371.

114. Rodrick M, Krugh J, Hanson W. Anesthesia for the trauma patient. In: Peitzman A, Rhodes M, Schwab C, Yealy D, Fabian T, eds. *The Trauma Manual.* 2nd ed. Philadelphia, PA: Lippincott, Williams & Wilkins; 2002: 386-395.

115. Cheney FW, Posner KL, Caplan RA, Gild WM. Burns from warming devices in anesthesia. A closed claims analysis. *Anesthesiology.* 1994;80:806-810.

116. Misusing forced-air hyperthermia units can burn patients. *Health Devices.* (17-950).

117. U.S. Food and Drug Administration. Burns from misuse of forced-air warming devices. Available at: http://www.fda.gov/cdrh/psn/show9.html. Accessed August 26, 2006.

118. Surgical Care Improvement Project. Available at: http://www.medqic.org/dcs/ContentServer?cid=1122904 930422&pagename=Medqic%2FContent%2FParent Shel lTemplate&parentName=Topic&c=MQParents. Accessed August 27, 2006.

119. Medical device reporting: Manufacturer reporting, importer reporting, user facility reporting, distributor reporting. *Federal Register.* Jan 26, 2000;65:4112-4121.

Publication History

Originally published in *Perioperative Standards and Recommended Practices,* 2008 edition.

Minor editing revisions made to omit PNDS codes; reformatted September 2012 for publication in *Perioperative Standards and Recommended Practices,* 2013 edition.

Minor editing revisions made in November 2014 for publication in *Guidelines for Perioperative Practice,* 2015 edition.

GUIDELINE FOR HEALTH CARE INFORMATION MANAGEMENT

The Guideline for Health Care Information Management has been approved by the AORN Recommended Practices Advisory Board. It was presented as proposed recommendations for comments by members and others. The guideline is effective December 1, 2011. The recommendations in the guideline are intended to be achievable and represent what is believed to be an optimal level of practice. Policies and procedures will reflect variations in practice settings and/or clinical situations that determine the degree to which the guideline can be implemented. AORN recognizes the various settings in which perioperative nurses practice; therefore, this guideline is adaptable to various practice settings. These practice settings include traditional operating rooms (ORs), ambulatory surgery centers, physicians' offices, cardiac catheterization laboratories, endoscopy suites, radiology departments, and all other areas where operative and other invasive procedures may be performed.

Purpose

This document provides guidance to assist perioperative nurses in documenting and managing patient care information within the perioperative practice setting. Highly reliable data collection is not only necessary to chronicle the patient response to nursing interventions, but also to demonstrate the health care organization's progress toward quality care outcomes. Health care data collection and retention is rapidly transitioning from traditional paper formats to standardized electronic applications that incorporate criteria from statutes and regulations, accreditation requirements, and standards setting bodies. Whether patient data are captured using paper or electronic formats, the nursing process should be completed for each surgical or procedural intervention performed.[1,2] The nursing process is a formalized systematic approach to providing and documenting patient care and is embedded within perioperative patient care workflow (ie, clinical workflow). Comprehensive perioperative documentation accurately reflects the patient experience and is essential for the continuity of goal-directed nursing care and for effective comparison of realized versus anticipated patient outcomes.[3,4]

This document should be viewed as a conceptual outline that can be used to create a comprehensive documentation platform. It is not inclusive of all documentation elements, nor should it be seen as the only guideline that may be used when developing or revising a clinical documentation system.

Recommendation I

The patient's health care record should reflect the perioperative patient's plan of care, including assessment, nursing diagnosis, outcome identification, planning, implementation, and evaluation of progress toward the outcome.[1,3-5]

The nursing process provides the guiding framework for documenting perioperative nursing care. When the nursing process is used in perioperative practice settings, it demonstrates the critical-thinking skills practiced by the registered nurse (RN) in caring for the patient undergoing surgical and other procedural interventions.[1,3,6-8] Documentation includes related information about the patient's current and past health status, nursing diagnoses and interventions, expected patient outcomes, and evaluation of the patient's response to perioperative nursing care.[5,9,10]

I.a. The perioperative RN conducts a patient assessment (eg, physical, psychosocial, cultural, spiritual) and should record the findings in the patient health care record before the surgical or other invasive procedure.[1,4]

The patient assessment forms a baseline for identifying the patient's health status, developing nursing diagnoses, and establishing an individualized plan of care. Concurrent reassessment throughout the patient's perioperative experience contributes to continuity in the delivery of care.[1,3,5,10]

Intraoperative nursing interventions for inpatient and ambulatory settings are embedded within the delivery of care but are not consistently reflected in clinical documentation.[7] In a systematic review of nursing documentation literature, inadequacies in the use of nursing process structure within clinical documentation resulted in one or more deficiencies in the application of the assessment process.[11] Using the structured data elements (eg, Perioperative Nursing Data Set [PNDS]) that include nursing diagnoses, interventions, and outcomes in clinical documentation demonstrates nursing contributions to patient outcomes and represents professional nursing practice.[7,8]

I.b. The health care record should include the nursing interventions performed and the time performed, the location of care, and the person performing the care.[4,5,12,13]

Clinical judgments are based on actual or potential patient problems (eg, nursing diagnoses), which determine the nursing interventions to be implemented to achieve expected

INFORMATION MANAGEMENT

perioperative patient outcomes.[1,10,14] Documenting nursing interventions promotes continuity of patient care and improves the exchange of patient care information between health care team members.[4,5]

I.c. Expected and interim patient outcomes that are identified by the perioperative RN should be recorded in the patient health care record.[10]

The goals for nursing interventions are to prevent potential patient injury or complications and treat actual patient problems (eg, nursing diagnoses). Identified nursing diagnoses contribute to interim and expected patient outcomes for the planned operative or procedural intervention. Research also indicates that nurses who associate the patient diagnoses with planned interventions are more outcome focused than task oriented.[15]

I.d. The patient health care record should reflect continuous reassessment and evaluation of perioperative nursing care and the response to implemented nursing interventions.[1,3,5,16]

The nursing process directs perioperative nurses to evaluate the effectiveness of nursing interventions toward attaining desired patient outcomes. The evaluation process provides information for continuity of care, performance improvement activities, perioperative nursing research, and management of risk. Documentation provides a mechanism for comparing actual versus expected outcomes.[1,3,5]

I.d.1. Patient data must be collected concurrently with each assessment, reassessment, or evaluation and recorded in the patient health care record.[17,18]

Continuous evaluation of the patient's condition establishes a baseline to determine fluctuations in the patient's status.[1,3,12,13,19] Appropriately captured patient data contribute to a centralized repository that members of the health care team can use to monitor the patient's status, coordinate prescribed treatments, and evaluate the effectiveness of care rendered.[4,16,20]

Recommendation II

Perioperative nursing documentation should be synchronized with the nursing work flow.[21-23]

Nursing work flow represents the cognitive process of nursing care activities and establishes the process for patient care data collection. Documentation of nursing activities is dictated by health care organization policy and regulatory and accrediting agency requirements and is necessary to inform other health care professionals involved in the patient's care. To accurately represent the patient experience and promote quality delivery of care, data aggregation should be coordinated with clinical work flow.[8,21-25] Incorporating nursing process work flow into the framework of clinical documentation platforms has been shown to improve documentation completeness and compliance with regulatory requirements.[26]

II.a. Clinical documentation should facilitate data capture using a format designed to support clinical work flow activities while eliminating redundancy in data entry.[2,22,25,27]

The burden of clinical documentation has been associated with decreased nursing attention to patient care activities and has been shown to affect patient safety.[28] Work inefficiencies, such as how or where clinical data are captured within perioperative documentation systems, have a negative correlation on clinical reasoning and decision making.[14,23,24,29,30] Interruption of established clinical processes competes for cognitive resources and may contribute to an adverse event or patient harm by reducing situational awareness.[31-34] Redundancy in the design of documentation activities further reduces the nurse's ability to focus on the clinical environment and may pose a risk for error.[27] When processes are simplified and data capture is standardized and organized, there is a reduction in the reliance on memory to complete tasks, thereby eliminating potential harmful events.[23,25,29]

An observational study on nursing work flow examined the percentage of time nurses dedicated to patient care and documentation activities.[35] The study identified that nursing time is focused primarily on patient care (eg, assessment, interventions) with documentation being completed in intervals and not concurrently with patient care. This, with the frequency of switching between nursing activities (ie, patient care, documentation), was correlated with nursing cognitive disruption, which resulted in slower performance and raised the potential for error.

A follow-up observational and randomized investigation examined the effect of new electronic documentation implementation on nursing activities and work flow. Findings indicated that the repeated clustering of patient care and documentation activities, though evenly distributed, affected nursing work flow by increasing the amount of time dedicated to electronic documentation without negatively affecting direct patient care time.[36]

II.a.1. Clinical documentation should reflect patient-focused care.[37-40]

Perioperative RNs provide patient-focused interventions that should be incorporated into the patient health care record.[41] Clinical (eg, nursing) documentation systems often do not support health care personnel in accommodating the specific needs of the individual (eg, teaching needs, age-specific criteria, self-care requirements).[37,42,43] Two research studies highlight the discrepancy

INFORMATION MANAGEMENT

between quality of care delivered and what is captured in documentation.[44,45] Health care currently relies on the technology-centered medical model of care, which often does not replicate patient-centric, evidence-based care within documentation platforms.

II.a.2. Perioperative RNs should evaluate perioperative electronic documentation systems for their effect on clinical work flow and patient safety, and their ability to accommodate the objectives of the implementation site.[11,21,22,30,46] Clinical information systems should address
- clinical work flow,[21,22,24-26,47-49]
- information needs of the patient care environment,[38]
- patient population characteristics,[37,39,42] and
- clinician and provider usability requirements.[26,34,48,50]

Effective information systems collect, store, and organize patient information to allow real-time updates, support clinical decision making, and be accessible to health care professionals when needed.[51-55] Research on the effect of health information technology implementation has shown that changes in contextual clinical work processes made to accommodate clinical information systems have both positive and negative influence on clinical work flow and patient safety.[23,34,35,43,50] Technology implementation with the most positive effects on clinical work flow, data availability, patient outcomes, and health care provider satisfaction occurs when clinicians are involved in the selection and implementation of the information system.[44,46,56]

Recommendation III

Electronic perioperative nursing documentation should use structured vocabulary (eg, PNDS) inclusive of the nursing process work flow with discrete representation of each phase of the perioperative patient care continuum (ie, preadmission, preoperative, intraoperative, postoperative).[26,57]

The use of structured vocabulary facilitates the capture of expressed observations, treatments, and patient responses within the clinical domain of care. Structured vocabulary describes patient care using controlled (ie, standardized) and unambiguous terms that are interpreted with consistent meaning between health care clinicians.[26,58] Patient information gathered from the collection of standardized data creates the knowledge perioperative RNs use to provide individualized patient care. The synthesis of knowledge for patient care interventions is in turn documented, resulting in the wisdom of perioperative nursing practice.[59,60]

III.a. The PNDS should be incorporated into the documentation platform.[7,61,62]

The PNDS is a controlled, structured, and coded nursing language that describes perioperative nursing influence on the effectiveness and safety of patient care delivery, and the contributions of perioperative nursing toward patient outcomes. Clinical documentation systems incorporating standardized language provide patient care data that can be aggregated and analyzed to determine clinical efficiencies, examine operational metrics, and facilitate new evidence for sustainable improvements in health care quality.[21,61,63]

III.a.1. Each phase of perioperative nursing documentation should incorporate nursing process work flow and require unambiguous representation of the patient experience.[64-68]

The phases of perioperative patient care collectively represent the unique domain of perioperative nursing. Standardization of patient care information improves the quality of the data[69] and can be used to support the extraction and interpretation of data for
- clinical decision support,[70,71]
- improved quality metrics,[26,71,72]
- information exchange,[71,72]
- research,[72,73]
- policy making,[26,72] and
- nursing visibility.[7,8,26,57,58,61,64,74-76]

III.b. The health care organization should implement a documentation system that includes a standardized perioperative electronic framework.

Standardization in documentation platforms promotes uniformity in comprehensive patient care data capture between health care organizations and creates a foundation for sharing health care data. The burgeoning cost of health care and the drive for improved quality have created urgency for implementation of electronic medical records (EMRs) and interoperable electronic health record (EHR) systems.[77-79] Adoption of EHR systems is a component of the American Recovery and Reinvestment Act (ARRA) of 2009 to facilitate access to quality care and improved patient safety[80] through high-reliability processes using data analysis to evaluate performance and outcomes.[81] Data quality facilitated by the adoption of an EHR and established by compliance with laws, clinical practice standards, and national quality measures adds to the relevance in efficiency benchmarks. The adoption of EHR technology also will lead to quantifiable improvements in reducing the time required for patient care data capture by nurses.[47,72,78,82]

Inpatient and ambulatory EHR implementation has been stimulated by the ARRA incentives for EHR adoption and subsequent analysis and dissemination of performance metrics.[71] Achieving success with the national Health

INFORMATION MANAGEMENT

Information Technology for Economic and Clinical Health (HITECH) agenda for comparative analysis between health care organizations may be accomplished by implementing an electronic documentation framework embedded with standardized sets of documentation values that are applicable across multiple perioperative settings to increase the confidence in data quality and research validity.[69,72,83]

Recommendation IV

Perioperative nursing documentation should be structured to meet professional and regulatory compliance requirements for a comprehensive representation of patient care.[66,84-87]

Patient care information collected and entered into the health care record is a tool for monitoring and evaluating the patient's health status and response to care, a resource to evaluate compliance with regulatory requirements, and a method to equate provision of services for reimbursement.[4,5,8]

IV.a. Perioperative nursing documentation should correspond to the elements of regulatory statutes, health care accreditation measures, national practice standards, and mandatory quality and reimbursement for quality performance criteria.

Clinical documentation serves as the legal record of care delivery and assists with cross-disciplinary patient care coordination.[5,84,88]

IV.a.1. The components for clinical documentation should include the following:
- "assessments;
- clinical problems;
- communications with other health care professionals regarding the patient;
- communication with and education of the patient, the patient's family members, the patient's designated support person, and other third parties;
- medication records (MAR);
- order acknowledgement, implementation, and management;
- [patient care interventions];
- patient clinical parameters;
- patient responses and outcomes, including changes in the patient's status; and
- plans of care that reflect the social and cultural framework of the patient."[8]

IV.a.2. Perioperative nursing documentation should correspond to professional guidelines and standards. The following organizations' guidelines and standards should be incorporated into the clinical documentation platform:
- AORN,
- American Association of Blood Banks (AABB),
- Agency for Healthcare Research and Quality (AHRQ),
- American National Standards Institute (ANSI),
- American Society of Anesthesiologists (ASA),
- Association for the Advancement of Medical Instrumentation (AAMI),
- American Association of Anesthesia Clinical Directors (AACD),
- Association of PeriAnesthesia Nurses (ASPAN),
- Institute for Safe Medication Practices (ISMP),
- Malignant Hyperthermia Association of the United States (MHAUS),
- National Fire Protection Agency (NFPA),
- National Institute for Occupational Safety and Health (NIOSH),
- National Quality Forum (NQF),
- US Pharmacopeia (USP), and
- United Network for Organ Sharing (UNOS).

Examples of guidance from professional standards setting agencies that may be considered for incorporation into perioperative documentation include
- the AACD Glossary of Times,
- national patient safety guidelines,
- organ and tissues tracking guidelines,
- perioperative recommendations for safe patient care, and
- safe medication administration guidelines.

As licensed health care professionals, perioperative RNs have a responsibility to maintain the established standards of perioperative nursing care. The standards of nursing practice require documentation to be based on the patient's condition or needs and the relationship to the proposed intervention, and have relevance to the period of patient care (eg, preadmission testing, preoperative, intraoperative, and postoperative care).[1,3,5,8] National practice standards cross all disciplines of nursing care and are applicable to perioperative nursing.

IV.a.3. Perioperative nursing documentation should correspond to established guidelines for perioperative nursing care.[89] Elements of perioperative guidelines that should be incorporated into clinical documentation include
- aseptic technique maintenance[65,90-93];
- local anesthesia administration[85,94-104];
- medication administration practices (eg, use of abbreviations)[20,94-96,101,105-111];
- moderate sedation/analgesia administration[85,95-104,112,113];
- patient care considerations (eg, latex allergy, implanted electronic device, dentures)[19,65,66,87,95,101,114-119];
- patient positioning[65,85,97,101,116,120,121];

INFORMATION MANAGEMENT

- patient information exchange[19,66,85,86,97,101,103,104,119,122-128];
- safety precautions including
  - electrical,[101,119,129-133]
  - environment of care preparation (eg, device alarms, blanket warmer temperatures),[65,98,131,134-137]
  - equipment use (eg, laser, MRI),[41,120,138,139]
  - fire prevention,[65,101,108,124,129,134,139-142]
  - human tissue procurement, processing, and preservation,[65,101,103,104,124,143-148]
  - infection prevention,[65,97,101,108,109,111,112,137,149-155]
  - tissue protection,[97,101,108,124,139,141,156-158]
  - radiation exposure prevention,[156]
  - retained surgical items prevention,[101,159,160]
  - correct site, side, person surgery processes,[19,65,66,78,87,99,103,104,108,118,119,121,124,161-167] and
  - skin preparation and antisepsis[65,85,95,97,98,100-102,108,110,113,140,150,154,168-171];
- specimens and tissues[65,87,97,101-103,124,144-147,160,166];
- sterilization/disinfection practices[65,97,101,102,113,114,126,129,131,134,140,142,152,166,172-178]; and
- traffic control measures.[65,102,134,140,149,152,176]

The AORN guidelines for perioperative practice are nationally recognized as the standard of care for all operative or invasive procedure patient care settings. Perioperative guidelines are not mandatory nursing care criteria but have been incorporated into regulatory and other standards setting agencies' guidelines and have been used to support judicial decisions.[179-185]

IV.a.4. Perioperative nursing documentation should correspond to local, state, and national regulatory requirements.

State and federal regulations are a collection of general and permanent rules (ie, laws) established to protect the welfare of the public and fortify the guiding principles of the nation. Many statutes or laws are established at the national level and may be amplified at the state level. The amplified statute would become the mandatory authority for the state. An example of this would be document retention requirements that vary between states. Failure to comply with the final law-making authority could result in monetary penalties or incarceration of the offending body. Agencies with regulatory authority include

- Centers for Medicare & Medicaid Services (CMS),
- Department of Health and Human Services (HHS),
- Occupational Safety and Health Administration (OSHA), and
- US Food and Drug Administration (FDA).

Criteria identified by national regulatory agencies for patient care documentation include

- allergies,[65,66,84,87,88,168,186]
- cultural variables,[66,84,88,99,118,187]
- equipment used for patient care (eg, type, model number),[65,66,85,86,98,117,118,129,130,160,168,186,188]
- names of legal guardian(s) and patient support person(s),[65,86,99,118,186]
- nutritional considerations,[66,86,87,186]
- ordered tests and services provided,[65,66,117,189]
- patient and family education,[66,84,88,118,151,186]
- patient identifiers and demographics,[65,66,87,117,160,163]
- patient attributes and status,[65,66,84,85,87,90,118,162,163,186,190]
- safety precautions,[65,84,88,129,155,189]
- surgical consent(s),[65,66,118,163] and
- surgical implants and explants.[65,66,84,88,117,146,188,191,192]

IV.a.5. Perioperative nursing documentation should correspond to health care accreditation organization requirements.

Compliance with state or national health care accreditation agency criteria is mandatory for organizations seeking CMS reimbursement or striving to meet established patient safety goals. Accrediting bodies review documentation for compliance to the minimum standards on an element of performance. The following accreditation agencies have deemed status:

- American Association for Accreditation of Ambulatory Surgery Facilities, Inc (AAAASF),[132]
- Accreditation Association for Ambulatory Health Care, Inc (AAAHC),[111]
- State CMS,[193]
- DNV Healthcare, Inc (DNV),[194]
- Healthcare Facilities Accreditation Program (HFAP),[195] and
- The Joint Commission.[196,197]

Elements of performance identified by accreditation agencies may include evidence of

- blood and tissue tracking;
- compliance with The Joint Commission's National Patient Safety Goals;
- elimination of nationally identified unacceptable abbreviations, acronyms, and symbols;
- hand off communications;
- identification of implantable objects;
- identification of designated support person(s);
- infection control practices;
- medication reconciliation;
- patient care elements (eg, care plans, tests, services provided);

495

INFORMATION MANAGEMENT

- pain management interventions;
- patient and family member education;
- patient demographics; and
- presence of current history and physical.

IV.a.6. Perioperative nursing documentation should incorporate mandatory reporting and reimbursement for quality performance criteria.

To improve population health, the US government is coordinating evidence-based standards development to be incorporated into the national agenda on health care reform. These efforts are incentivized through inclusion within CMS reimbursement programs and made public through national reporting forums (eg, Hospital Compare[198]). Agencies responsible for national standards development or reimbursement for quality performance criteria include, but are not limited to, the following:
- Centers for Disease Control (CDC),
- NQF, and
- AHRQ.

Measurement criteria for quality performance reimbursement are included in the following regulations and criteria:
- Ambulatory Surgical Center Payment System (ASCPS),[199]
- Deficit Reduction Act of 2005,[160]
- Hospital Inpatient Prospective Payment System (IPPS),[199]
- Hospital Outpatient Prospective Payment System (OPPS),[199]
- Surgical Care Improvement Project (SCIP),[200] and
- Value-based Purchasing (VBP).[201,202]

IV.a.7. Perioperative documentation should include all patient care orders occurring in the perioperative patient care setting.[66] Patient care orders are to be entered into the clinical documentation system as close to the time when the order is communicated or intervention is initiated. All orders, including verbal orders, standing orders, orders included on surgeon preference cards, and order sets must be dated, timed, and authenticated by the ordering health care practitioner with prescriptive authority.[66,196,203-205] Verbal orders must be documented when they are communicated and verified using a read-back process that involves the ordering health care practitioner.[206-209]

Using standing orders and preprinted order sets has been shown to reduce medication errors and improve documentation compliance.[210] To prevent patient harm from outdated, incomplete, or erroneous entries, well-constructed standing orders and preprinted order sets should

- avoid the use of unacceptable abbreviations,
- eliminate trailing zeros in medication dosages,
- use standardized names and terms to describe treatments and interventions (eg, brand vs generic medications, device instructions), and
- be reviewed frequently by the attending surgeon for accuracy of information for the intended procedure.[206-208,211]

IV.a.8. The patient care record must include a complete and accurate informed patient consent for each surgical or invasive procedure to be performed.[66,99,163] The informed consent process must be documented for procedures and treatments that are identified in the health care facility's medical staff policies as requiring informed consent.[66,84,163] Unless designated as an emergency situation in the health care facility's informed consent policy, a "properly executed informed consent"[99] must include
- the name of the health care facility providing the surgery or invasive procedure;
- the specific name of the intervention to be performed;
- indications for the proposed intervention;
- the name of the responsible health care provider performing the intervention;
- a statement identifying the risks and benefits associated with the proposed intervention and indication of discussion with the patient or patient's legal representative;
- the signature of the patient or the patient's legal representative;
- the date and time the patient or the patient's legal representative signed the informed consent document;
- the date and time, and signature of the person who witnessed the patient or the patient's legal representative signing the informed consent document; and
- the signature of the responsible health care provider who executed the informed consent discussion with the patient or the patient's legal representative.[84,87,88]

Additional content that may be identified on the informed consent document and may be regulated by state statutes and administrative rules includes
- identification of assisting physicians including, but not limited to, medical residents who will be contributing significantly to the proposed intervention and
- identification of assisting health care personnel who are not physicians but who are performing within their scope of practice (eg, registered nurse first assistant [RNFA], nurse practitioner) and who

INFORMATION MANAGEMENT

will be contributing significantly to the proposed intervention.[84,87,88]

The patient or the patient's legal representative is entitled to participate in the informed decision-making process for planning care and treatment, including the right to request or refuse treatment.[99,204]

IV.a.9. Individuals participating in the patient's perioperative care, as well as those not directly involved in the scheduled surgical or procedural intervention (eg, x-ray technicians, industry representatives, approved observers), must be recorded in the patient health care record.[66,99,204] Documentation must include the names, roles, and credentials of individuals participating in the patient's perioperative care experience and may include[84,88]
- surgical or procedural patient care team members,
- identified legal representatives,
- identified patient support person(s),
- recipients of patient care information on behalf of the patient,
- health care professionals contributing to the patient's care (eg, pathologist, approved health care student), and
- law enforcement officers (eg, prison guards).

A comprehensive patient-centric record of care reflects interactions between the patient's health care team and those individuals legally representing or providing physical, spiritual, or other support services to the patient.[84,88] Documentation of interactions provides the groundwork for transparency in care planning through effective representation of the patient's involvement in the plan of care and contributions made toward the treatment plan.

IV.b. Clinical documentation platforms (ie, paper, electronic) should support the collection of tailored health care information using a format that accommodates and is customized to the clinical environment.[42,43] Formats selected for the collection of tailored patient care information should be established based on nationally recognized standards of practice that outline the nurse's responsibilities to the patient.[12]

Tailoring patient health information allows the collection of unique patient care data (eg, communicable diseases, responses to medications, psychosocial considerations) that may affect the planned operative or other invasive procedure. The collection of tailored health care information is standardized to the clinical setting (eg, surgical versus interventional radiology) but may vary by the requirements of the environment where perioperative care is delivered (eg, pediatric hospital, cancer treatment center, ambulatory surgery center).[42,43]

IV.b.1. Charting by exception processes should be well constructed and reviewed by the health care organization's risk management and legal representatives.[80]

Charting by exception, also known as variance charting,[212] has been successfully implemented using a well-researched and -designed documentation system.[213] A well-designed documentation system corresponds to the health care organization's policy for charting by exception and allows for an undisputable description of the patient condition. Charting by exception may lead to litigious situations when organizational policy has not been well formulated or updated for changes in statutory requirements or when the nurse has not followed the established guidance for charting by exception.[12,16,184,214]

The minimum criteria for charting by exception include[12,212,214-217]
- identifying objective physical assessment criteria for the patient population being served (eg, endoscopy population, orthopedic population);
- identifying and defining what constitutes normal findings;
- describing the process for documenting normal findings (eg, "within normal limits");
- describing the process for identifying, describing, and documenting objective abnormal or key findings;
- listing the practice standards, care guidelines, and clinical pathways used to guide patient care;
- listing a rationale, including decisions and interventions, for deviations from established guidance for patient care;
- setting the frequency of documentation entries; and
- adhering to state or national statutory requirements (eg, record authentication).

IV.c. Cognitive processes used in patient care should be supported by clinical support technologies that are embedded within electronic clinical documentation systems.[23,218,219]

The processes within perioperative patient care are classified as cognitive performance or the intellectual processing of information to complete a finite task.[218] Multitasking, environmental stimulation, and availability of information contribute to the nurse's ability, or inability, to accommodate needed adjustments in patient care activities. Poorly designed clinical information systems, those not conforming to national data standards, and those without consideration of clinical work flow and work process requirements may contribute to patient harm.[23,24,30,218-220]

Conversely, clinical information systems that incorporate technology innovations (eg, order entry, decision support, clinical alerts)

INFORMATION MANAGEMENT

and support the cognitive processes of patient care are believed to enhance health care worker performance and result in improved patient safety and quality patient outcomes.[23,24,52,218-220]

Recommendation V

Patient care information must be secure, held confidential, and protected from unauthorized disclosure.[221]

The Health Insurance Portability and Accountability Act (HIPAA) of 1996 guarantees the privacy of individuals receiving health services and the confidentiality of "individually identifiable health information."[222] Updated to correspond with the HITECH Act, HIPAA now includes security standards for protecting electronic health information (ie, Security Rule) and regulations that specify compliance, investigation, payments, and penalties (ie, Enforcement Rule) that were established in 1996.[221]

V.a. Access to patient health information should be limited to authorized individuals based on the health care role (eg, surgeon, RN, perfusionist), responsibility, and function (eg, postanesthesia care unit RN assisting in the endoscopy unit).[223-225] Risk-reduction strategies to proactively mitigate potential access violations should include[225-228]
- establishing perioperative information management policies that include remote access protocols, on/off site information storage practices, and employee exit strategies that are reviewed frequently and updated as the environment changes (eg, new regulations, transitions from paper to electronic documentation platforms);
- identifying procedures for the use of mobile devices (eg, cell phone, tablet technologies, video imaging) within the perioperative care environment;
- establishing awareness and sensitivity to data security and privacy by reinforcing the existing health care organization's information security policy for monitoring and auditing access to patient health information;
- restricting access to electronic health information to users with individualized, unique authorization credentials that are associated with time-sensitive passwords using alphanumeric-symbol combinations; and
- holding annual, competency-based education programs on information access and sharing for all employees within the perioperative care environment.

Controlling access to the patient's health information prevents privacy and security breaches for HIPAA covered entities.[221,223,224] The health care organization has a legal responsibility to create procedures to circumvent unauthorized access to sensitive patient health information and to execute a plan for data breach notification practices should a breach occur.[221,222,229,230]

V.b. Perioperative health care workers should be familiar with the health care organization's information policies before sharing electronic patient information. Considerations for recipients of electronic health information that should be incorporated into the organization's information policies include[228,229,231] ensuring that
- electronic patient health information, either to or from outside organizations or with the patient, meets current requirements for information exchange and security (eg, malware protection),
- validation occurs for original source authenticity and the accuracy of transmitted information, and
- electronically transmitted content is evaluated for potential corruption.

Electronic transmissions of patient health information is held to the same privacy and security criteria as facility-based EHRs. Sensitive patient information in paper, electronic text, or image formatting can be exposed to unintended or unauthorized disclosure without proper sharing safeguards in place.[80,221,222,224,231] Electronic transmission of patient health information by fax, e-mail, mobile storage media, or other formats may introduce malicious software into the health care information system.

V.b.1. Recipients of electronic patient health information should validate original source authenticity and accuracy of information and evaluate content for potential corruption.[228,229,231]

V.b.2. The patient must have a signed consent for release of information in the health care record before graphic imaging takes place and before the release of patient specific information, including remote access to and relocation of health information from the treating organization.[163,221,222,228,232-237] Non-consented disclosure of sensitive patient health information requires execution of the data breach notification process by the health care organization.[221,222,230,238] To complete full disclosure and reporting, the organization's information technology and risk management personnel should collaborate to discover all patient care records that were involved in the non-consented disclosure.[238]

V.c. Documentation entries made into the patient health care record must include an authentication process at the completion of the documentation process or according to the organization's established policies.[66,85,227,239,240,241] Health care records must accurately reflect the patient care experience, be promptly completed, and be associated with an author identification procedure to ensure the integrity of the content.[66,87,242] The authentication process may include, but is not limited to, the following[227,243,244]:

INFORMATION MANAGEMENT

- using an electronic or digital signature or a code key in the format designated by the health care organization as the legal representation of an individual's written signature for the EHR.
- completing a pen-to-paper signature, using initials with a signature legend on the same document, or a rubber signature stamp for paper-based documentation platforms (eg, faxed, scanned documents) and as permitted by the health care organization's policy.
  - Initials with a signature legend should be avoided on narrative documentation (eg, comments, patient quotes, consultation), assessment data collection, or when a signature is required by law (eg, patient informed consent).
  - Digitized inked signatures (ie, signature image) should only be used when deemed acceptable by the health care organization and allowed by state or federal reimbursement regulations.
- using a countersignature demonstrating accuracy of content entered into a patient health care record; once countersigned, the content is legally considered the cosigner's entry (eg, nursing student entry).

Authentication identifies the author of the documentation entry and indicates responsibility for the interventions performed and patient information collected. Authentication legally binds the owner of the signature with the responsibility for accuracy of the content within the document.[227]

V.c.1. Authentication of verbal orders must occur within the time frame specified by state statutory guidelines. If state law does not specify a time frame, the federal mandate applies for verbal orders to be authenticated by the responsible physician within 48 hours of entering the order.[66]

V.d. The patient care record must be retained in the original or a legally reproducible format for the minimum allocation of time dictated by federal regulations and state statutes of limitations. Organizational policies may address other time frames for record retention based on the patient population served (eg, pediatrics, cancer treatment), facility demographics (eg, research, trauma, academic), media used to store patient data (eg, paper, microfilm, optical disc), or operational requirements (eg, regulatory compliance).[66,87,227,242,245-247]

The American Health Information Management Association (AHIMA) recommends retaining operative indexes for a minimum of 10 years and the register of surgical procedures permanently.[245] The minimum retention guidelines for perioperative information according to US Federal regulations are detailed in Table 1.

V.e. Electronic documentation platforms should have an alternate data entry and backup process.[248] Perioperative services should formalize a thorough downtime process addressing hardware, operating system, and network disruptions to preserve data accuracy and uninterrupted health care processes. Downtime planning should incorporate strategies to
  - facilitate an uninterrupted patient care schedule (eg, paper forms, documentation backup media),
  - identify changes to existing work flows (eg, how new orders are communicated, clinical resources),
  - recover potential loss of patient care data, and
  - incorporate patient care data that are captured using alternate documentation platforms (eg, paper forms) into the electronic information system.[31,248,249]

Perioperative personnel with system access responsibilities should receive ongoing education on the policies, procedures, and alternate work flows associated with the downtime or technology performance issues.[31,248,249]

Backup processes will mitigate interruptions in patient care caused by technology failures. Dependance on technology can significantly influence the effectiveness and efficiency of patient care delivery.

Recommendation VI

Modifications to existing content in the patient health care record must comply with relevant federal and state regulations, health care accreditation requirements, and national practice guidelines.[8,227] Amendments, corrections, or addendums to the patient care record should only occur to present an accurate description of the care provided or to protect the patient's interest.[4,250]

The patient care record is a legal representation of services provided by the health care organization. Perioperative nurses are obligated to accurately represent the patient's care within the health care record.[66,87,242] Using inappropriate methods to correct, clarify, or change existing entries in the patient health care record may expose the health care organization or clinicians to liability for falsification of patient care information.[8,12,16]

VI.a. The health care organization's information management policy should outline the processes to make legally acceptable modifications to the patient care record.

Corrections, amendments, and addendums that are completed are limited by the functionality of the documentation platform used.[227,250]

VI.a.1. Amendments or addendums to the patient care record should follow established organizational policies and procedures. Corrections, amendments, and addendums in paper records should be performed by[4,227]

INFORMATION MANAGEMENT

TABLE 1. US Federal Minimum Retention Guidelines

Documentation type	Retention period	Source
Ambulatory surgical services	Not specified	42 CFR §416.47 Condition of participation: Medical records[1]
Hospitals	5 years from the date of discharge	42 CFR §482.24(b)(1) Condition of participation: Medical record services[2]
Hospitals, critical access	6 years from date of last entry or longer as mandated by state statutory guidelines or as necessary for legal proceedings	42 CFR §485.638 Condition of participation: Clinical records[3]
Department of Veterans Affairs operation log file (including type of operation, date, patient's name, surgeon, assistant scrub nurse [scrub person], sponge count, anesthetist, agent, method, preoperative and postoperative diagnoses, complications, and other information)	Destroy after 20 years	National Archives Job No. N1-015-94-2, Item 1[4]
Department of Veterans Affairs (date the surgery was performed, members of the surgical and nursing teams, and other information pertaining to the surgery of a patient)	Destroy after 3 years	National Archives Job No. N1-015-94-2, Item 2[5]

References
1. Centers for Medicare & Medicaid Services. 42 CFR §416.47: Condition of participation: Medical records. 2010.
2. Centers for Medicare & Medicaid Services. 42 CFR §482.24: Condition of participation: Medical record services. 2010.
3. Centers for Medicare & Medicaid Services. 42 CFR §485.638: Conditions of participation: Clinical records. 2010.
4. Veterans Health Administration Records Control Schedule 10-1. Washington, DC. Veterans Health Administration; 2011. http://www1.va.gov/vhapublications/RCS10/rcs10-1.pdf. Accessed October 20, 2011.
5. Veterans Health Administration Records Control Schedule 10-1. Washington, DC. Veterans Health Administration; 2011. http://www1.va.gov/vhapublications/RCS10/rcs10-1.pdf. Accessed October 20, 2011.

- placing a single line through the incorrect entry, being careful not to obliterate the inaccurate information;
- writing "error," "mistaken entry," or "omit" next to the incorrect text as determined by organizational policy;
- providing the rationale for the correction above the inaccurate entry if room is available or adding it to the margin of the document;
- signing and dating the entry; and
- entering the correct information in the next available space or adjacent to the acknowledged inaccurate information.

VI.a.2. Corrections, amendments, and addendums in EHRs should[80,227,250]
- have versioning or "track corrections" function (eg, electronic strike-through with time stamp) to identify the alterations made to an entry that has been authenticated;
- automatically date-, time-, and author-stamp each entry;
- generate a symbol or other notation to identify when an alteration has been made to existing content by creating a new version of the document;
- retain and link the original document version to the newly created version; and
- reflect corrections made to the EHR on the paper copy.

Additionally,
- corrections completed after a final signature or authentication process has occurred will comply with the functionality of the information system and established organizational policies and procedures,
- corrections completed before the final signature or authentication process may not be classified as a "correction" according to organizational policy and the information system that is in place,
- addendums should be completed where the original document was created using the source information system when available and should be reflected in the permanent patient care record or data repository system, and
- deletions and retractions of content from a closed EHR system should be made according to organizational policies and procedures and the functionality of the information system that is in place.

Recommendation VII

Perioperative personnel should receive initial and ongoing education related to accurately documenting patient care and should demonstrate competency in documentation processes and best practices to maintain security and privacy of patient care information.[8,80,251,252]

Initial and periodic competency-based education programs made available to maintain proficiency in the application of knowledge and use of the documentation platform improve the effectiveness of documentation practices and reinforce strategies to avert unintentional disclosure of patient care information.

VII.a. A review of the health care organization's policies for information management and the procedures for documentation processes and activities should be incorporated into orientation and ongoing education for personnel within the perioperative care environment.

Perioperative personnel receiving ongoing education and periodic review of policies and procedures develop the knowledge, skills, and attitudes that affect patient outcomes.

VII.a.1. Perioperative nurses should have knowledge of the significance and use of structured vocabularies for clinical documentation. Minimum education criteria on structured terminologies include
- the value structured terminology brings to clinical documentation;
- an overview of the PNDS;
- the contributions of the PNDS to perioperative nursing practice and patient outcomes; and
- how standardized documentation facilitates benchmarks, comparative analysis, and efficiency reporting.

VII.a.2. Minimum education and competency activities for perioperative RNs should include reviewing
- national and organizational documentation standards, guidelines, and requirements;
- procedures for completing amendments, addendums, and corrections;
- procedures for sharing patient information securely while maintaining patient privacy;
- procedures for initiating breach notification;
- compliance requirements for health care data capture; and
- legal implications for failure to comply with documentation standards.

Additional education and competency considerations for users of perioperative information systems, a component of the EHR, should also incorporate the following minimum skills by demonstrating
- accessing and closing the patient care record;

INFORMATION MANAGEMENT

- information system's functionality (eg, data entry, order acknowledgment);
- authentication processes;
- downtime procedures including alternate work flows to accommodate patient care; and
- compliance requirements for health care data capture.

Recommendation VIII

Policies and procedures related to perioperative information management should be developed, reviewed annually, revised as needed to accommodate changes in practice and documentation standards, and be readily available in the practice setting.

Policies and procedures establish authority, responsibility, and accountability and serve as operational guidelines that are used to minimize patient risk factors, standardize practice, direct health care personnel, and establish guidelines for continuous performance improvement activities. As new evidence emerges, policies and procedures will evolve to accommodate best practices and technology developments.

VIII.a. The perioperative services information management policy should complement and reinforce existing organization-wide policies (ie, risk management, quality improvement, health information privacy and security) and include the unique considerations of the perioperative care environment.

A collaborative approach to policy development and the provision of access to policies for all health care personnel will result in improved communications and compliance to established practices within the health care organization.

VIII.a.1. Information management policies and documentation procedures for EHR systems should include guidance on[250]
- forwarding addendums to each destination where patient information is retained,
- editing content before a final signature or authentication process occurs,
- using cut-copy-paste and "carry forward" functionality to populate the patient care record,
- completing corrections in an active or locked patient care record,
- rectifying a misidentification of patient health information (ie, wrong name association),
- amending clinical content in an active or locked patient care record,
- completing a delayed entry and updating the long-term record or data repository,
- deleting or retracting information from a locked patient care record while maintaining the integrity of the record, and

INFORMATION MANAGEMENT

- defining components that are required for record completion.

VIII.a.2. Policies and procedures must include information on data privacy and security and identify risk-reduction strategies to proactively mitigate potential violations of patient health information access.[221] Risk-reduction strategies should include[225-228]
- establishing remote access protocols, on/off site information storage practices, and employee exit strategies to protect patient health information;
- frequently reviewing and updating policies as the health care information environment changes (eg, new regulations, transitions from paper to electronic documentation platforms);
- identifying procedures for using mobile devices (eg, cell phone, tablet technologies, video imaging) within the perioperative care environment;
- reinforcing the existing health care organization's information security policy for monitoring and auditing access to patient health information within the perioperative care environment;
- restricting access to electronic health information by user type with individualized unique authorization credentials associated with time-sensitive passwords using alpha-numeric-symbol combinations; and
- holding annual competency-based education programs on information access and sharing for all employees within the perioperative care environment.

Recommendation IX

A quality management program should be established to ensure the integrity of the data within the patient health care record.

A fundamental precept for the professional perioperative nurse is the responsibility to provide safe, high-quality nursing care to patients undergoing operative and other invasive procedures.[3] Regularly monitoring and validating documentation processes is necessary for variance reporting, which supports process and performance measurement to quantify organizational effectiveness and nursing influence on patient outcomes.[8]

IX.a. Perioperative personnel should participate in the organization-wide clinical documentation improvement (CDI) program.

Participation in a CDI program facilitates data and documentation analysis while providing a structured framework to achieve consistency in quality processes that affect patient satisfaction, accreditation standing, and reimbursement status.[253] Representation in the CDI program ensures concerns specific to perioperative practice parameters are addressed and that areas for improvement are identified.

IX.a.1. Minimum criteria that should be reviewed for a perioperative CDI program should include[227,252]
- use of unacceptable abbreviations,
- timeliness and chronology of patient information,
- legibility,
- use of vague or generalized language,
- blank spaces or data fields,
- content omissions (eg, missing informed consent),
- delayed entries (eg, next day entry),
- inconsistencies (eg, conflicting assessment findings, procedure start times),
- inappropriate information (eg, communications with attorneys),
- authentication of verbal orders,
- absence of signatures or countersignature,
- appropriate documentation practices (eg, charting by exception/variance charting), and
- alterations to clinical content.

IX.b. Validation procedures for the perioperative information system should be incorporated into the quality management program. Data quality may be ensured by periodically evaluating the information system for the integrity of
- collected patient care information,
- report generation,
- file storage and retrieval,
- data security, and
- control for document versioning.[227,250,251]

Validation procedures for the perioperative information system should be incorporated into the health care organization's comprehensive strategies for EHR system security and maintenance.

Perioperative information systems are complex systems that contribute to improved care or may add to error-prone documentation processes.[32,251,254] Validation procedures help to maintain the integrity of patient health information.

IX.b.1. Routine audits should be performed as a part of a quality-driven information management program. Audit trails should be retained and placed on a retention schedule following the state statute of limitations and needs of the health care organization.[227,255] Audit trails may include[227,255]
- paper-based sign-out processes,
- logbook activities,
- EHR access and operations performed,
- electronic tracking system, and
- data mining activities.

Auditing procedures help to establish user and organizational accountability for

INFORMATION MANAGEMENT

IX.b.2. Perioperative information systems should be included in the organizational information technology risk mitigation plan.[251] Collaborating with the organization's risk manger, information services department, and engineering department, perioperative nursing leaders should coordinate efforts to plan for
- perioperative information system upgrades and maintenance;
- system redundancies (eg, remote patient care record access, backup generators);
- unanticipated access to and theft of patient health care information; and
- organizational information technology network infrastructure maintenance, upgrades, and conversions on the perioperative information system.[251]

Proactive contingency planning for information system failures and disaster response procedures will help maintain continuity in patient care activities.

Glossary

Addendum: New documentation used to add information to an original documentation entry of patient health information.

American Recovery and Reinvestment Act (ARRA): An economic stimulus package enacted by the US Congress in 2009 with a defined purpose to stimulate jobs, investments, and consumer spending. ARRA contains provisions for improved health care quality through the use of health information technology. (Source: American Recovery and Reinvestment Act – H.R.1. http://frwebgate.access.gpo.gov/cgi-bin/getdoc.cgi?dbname=111_cong_bills&docid=f:h1enr.pdf. Accessed October 20, 2011.)

Amendments: Additional documentation completed to clarify a preexisting entry of patient health information.

Authentication: A security measure to establish the validity of an electronic transmission, message, or original source (eg, author) or to verify the authorization of an individual to receive specific information. Authentication is used to confirm that an individual or system is who or what it claims to be.

Clinical information systems: Computer technology used in the patient care environment for collecting patient health care information.

Clinical support technologies: Assorted technologies used in the patient care environment to facilitate the clinician's ability to provide safe, comprehensive interventions for delivery of quality health care.

Code key: A computer code used to authenticate entries in an electronic health record as permitted by state, federal, and reimbursement regulations.

Controlled terminology: Terminology developed according to specific characteristics so that each data element is expressed as a single, clear, and unambiguous concept. Controlled terminology concepts maintain their meaning permanently.

Corrections: A change made to the documented patient health information meant to clarify the entry after the document has been authenticated.

Customize: To specifically select or set preferences or options for health care information.

Data mining: The process of extracting and analyzing data for usable information from relationships, patterns, information clusters, and data trends. The new information may be used for predictive modeling in decision support processes for clinical, operational, and research utilization.

Data quality: Data remaining unchanged from its original meaning; it is complete, correct, comprehensive, and consistent for the intended use.

Data repository: A central location where health care data (eg, clinical, financial, operational) and files are stored and maintained for later retrieval and use.

Deemed status: The "deeming" authority granted to national accreditation organizations (eg, The Joint Commission, DNV-Hospital Accreditation) by the Centers for Medicare & Medicaid Services (CMS) to determine, on CMS's behalf, whether a health care provider organization is in compliance with the regulations to provide and receive payment for Medicare services. Six areas are deemable: quality assurance, antidiscrimination, access to services, confidentiality and accuracy of enrollee records, information on advance directives, and provider participation rules.

Digital signature: A cryptographic signature (ie, digital key) used to authenticate the user, provide legal ownership, and ensure integrity of the unit of information.

Digitized inked signatures: A handwritten signature using a pen pad to create an electronic representation of the actual signature.

Downtime: Periods of time when the clinical information system (ie, electronic health record) is unavailable because of scheduled maintenance or upgrade, technology failure, power outage, or other unscheduled event.

Electronic health record: An electronic record of health-related information for an individual that conforms to nationally recognized interoperability standards and that can be created, managed, and consulted by authorized clinicians and staff members across more than one health care organization.

Electronic medical records: Electronic records of health-related information for individuals that can be created, gathered, managed, and consulted by authorized clinicians and staff members within one health care organization.

Electronic signature: The technology-neutral electronic process used to sign (ie, attest) content for authorship and legal responsibility for a section of information. The electronic signature format is determined by the technology used to collect or create the signature.

Health Information Technology for Economic and Clinical Health (HITECH): A component of the American Recovery and Reinvestment Act of 2009 addressing

INFORMATION MANAGEMENT

the use of electronic health information technology to improve health care quality, coordination of care, and health information privacy and security.

Integrity: The accuracy, consistency, and reliability of information content, processes, and systems.

Interoperable: The ability for health information systems to exchange or share health information within and across organizational boundaries.

Malware: Software considered harmful to a computer system including, but not limited to, the following: viruses, worms, trojan horses, spyware, and unauthorized adware.

Signature legend: A document that identifies an author's full signature and title when initials are used to authenticate entries in the health care record.

Tailored health care information: The unique patient characteristics based on multiple factors influencing health status and health behaviors and collected to inform individualized nursing interventions.

Versioning: The process of assigning a unique version name or number to an electronic heath record and used to identify revisions occurring to previously documented content.

References

1. *Nursing: Scope and Standards of Practice.* Silver Spring, MD: American Nurses Association; 2010.
2. Gugerty B, Maranda MJ, Beachley M, et al. *Challenges and Opportunities in Documentation of the Nursing Care of Patients.* Baltimore, MD: Maryland Nursing Workforce Commission, Documentation Work Group; 2007.
3. Standards of perioperative nursing. In: *Perioperative Standards and Recommended Practices.* Denver, CO: AORN, Inc; 2010: 9-27.
4. Iyer PW, Koob SL. Nursing documentation. In: Iyer PW, Levin BB, Agosto M, eds. *Nursing Malpractice.* Tucson, AZ: Lawyers and Judges Pub Co; 2007: 181-227.
5. *Complete Guide to Documentation.* Philadelphia, PA: Wolters Kluwer Health/Lippincott Williams & Wilkins; 2008.
6. *Nursing's Social Policy Statement: The Essence of the Profession.* Silver Spring, MD: American Nurses Association; 2010.
7. Beyea SC. Describing professional nursing through a universal record in perioperative settings. *Int J Nurs Terminol Classif.* 2003;14(4):23.
8. *ANA Principles for Documentation.* Silver Spring, MD: American Nurses Association; 2010.
9. Kuc JA. Perioperative records. In: Iyer PW, Levin BL, Shea MA, eds. *Medical Legal Aspects of Medical Records.* Tucson, AZ: Lawyers & Judges Publishing Company; 2006: 657-677.
10. Junttila K, Hupli M, Salanterä S. The use of nursing diagnoses in perioperative documentation. *Int J Nurs Terminol Classif.* 2010;21(2):57-68.
11. Wang N, Hailey D, Yu P. Quality of nursing documentation and approaches to its evaluation: a mixed-method systematic review. *J Adv Nurs.* 2011;67(9):1858-1875. doi:10.1111/j.1365-2648.2011.05634.x; 10.1111/j.1365-2648.2011.05634.x.
12. Ferrell KG. Documentation, part 2: the best evidence of care. Complete and accurate charting can be crucial to exonerating nurses in civil lawsuits. *Am J Nurs.* 2007;107(7):61-64. doi:10.1097/01.NAJ.0000279271.41357.fa.
13. McGeehan R. Best practice in record-keeping. *Nurs Stand.* 2007;21(17):51.
14. Potter P, Wolf L, Boxerman S, et al. Understanding the cognitive work of nursing in the acute care environment. *J Nurs Adm.* 2005;35(7-8):327-335.
15. Micek WT, Berry L, Gilski D, Kallenbach A, Link D, Scharer K. Patient outcomes: the link between nursing diagnoses and interventions. *J Nurs Adm.* 1996;26(11):29-35.
16. Monarch K. Documentation, part 1: principles for self-protection. Preserve the medical record—and defend yourself. *Am J Nurs.* 2007;107(7):58-60. doi:10.1097/01.NAJ.0000279270.41357.b3.
17. Provision of care, treatment, and services. PC.02.02.01. In: *2011 Comprehensive Accreditation Manual for Hospitals.* Oakbrook Terrace, IL: Joint Commission Resources; 2011.
18. Provision of care, treatment, and services. PC.02.02.01. In: *2011 Comprehensive Accreditation Manual for Ambulatory Care.* Oakbrook Terrace, IL: Joint Commission Resources; 2011.
19. AORN guidance statement: Preoperative patient care in the ambulatory surgery setting. In: *Perioperative Standards and Recommended Practices.* Denver, CO: AORN, Inc; 2011: 227-232.
20. AORN guidance statement: Postoperative patient care in the ambulatory surgery setting. In: *Perioperative Standards and Recommended Practices.* Denver, CO: AORN, Inc; 2011: 219-226.
21. Whittenburg L. Workflow viewpoints: analysis of nursing workflow documentation in the electronic health record. *J Healthc Inf Manag.* 2010;24(3):71-75.
22. Lee S, McElmurry B. Capturing nursing care workflow disruptions: comparison between nursing and physician workflows. *Comput Inform Nurs.* 2010;28(3):151-159. doi:10.1097/NCN.0b013e3181d77d3e.
23. Karsh BT, Holden RJ, Alper SJ, Or CK. A human factors engineering paradigm for patient safety: designing to support the performance of the healthcare professional. *Qual Saf Health Care.* 2006;15 (Suppl 1):i59-65. doi:10.1136/qshc.2005.015974.
24. Institute of Medicine; Page A, eds. *Keeping Patients Safe: Transforming the Work Environment of Nurses.* Washington, DC: National Academies Press; 2004.
25. Keohane CA, Bane AD, Featherstone E, et al. Quantifying nursing workflow in medication administration. *J Nurs Adm.* 2008;38(1):19-26.
26. Häyrinen K, Lammintakanen J, Saranto K. Evaluation of electronic nursing documentation—nursing process model and standardized terminologies as keys to visible and transparent nursing. *Int J Med Inform.* 2010;79(8):554-564.
27. Capuano T, Bokovoy J, Halkins D, Hitchings K. Work flow analysis: eliminating non-value-added work. *J Nurs Adm.* 2004;34(5):246-256.
28. Hendrich A, Chow M, Skierczynski B, Lu Z. A 36-hospital time and motion study: how do medical-surgical nurses spend their time? *Permanente J.* 2008;12(3):25-34.
29. Benner P, Sheets V, Uris P, Malloch K, Schwed K, Jamison D. Individual, practice, and system causes of errors in nursing: a taxonomy. *J Nurs Adm.* 2002;32(10):509-523.
30. Ammenwerth E, Eichstadter R, Haux R, Pohl U, Rebel S, Ziegler S. A randomized evaluation of a computer-based nursing documentation system. *Methods Inf Med.* 2001;40(2):61-68.
31. Bloomrosen M, Starren J, Lorenzi NM, Ash JS, Patel VL, Shortliffe EH. Anticipating and addressing

the unintended consequences of health IT and policy: a report from the AMIA 2009 Health Policy Meeting. *J Am Med Inform Assoc.* 2011;18(1):82-90. doi:10.1136/jamia.2010.007567.

32. Clancy CM. Nursing, system design, and health care quality. *AORN J.* 2009;90(4):581-583. doi:10.1016/j.aorn.2009.09.008.

33. Ash JS, Berg M, Coiera E. Some unintended consequences of information technology in health care: the nature of patient care information system-related errors. *J Am Med Inform Assoc.* 2004;11(2):104-112. doi:10.1197/jamia.M1471.

34. Harrison MI, Koppel R, Bar-Lev S. Unintended consequences of information technologies in health care—an interactive sociotechnical analysis. *J Am Med Inform Assoc.* 2007;14(5):542-549. doi:10.1197/jamia.M2384.

35. Cornell P, Herrin-Griffith D, Keim C, et al. Transforming nursing workflow, part 1: the chaotic nature of nurse activities. *J Nurs Adm.* 2010;40(9):366-373. doi:10.1097/NNA.0b013e3181ee4261.

36. Cornell P, Riordan M, Herrin-Griffith D. Transforming nursing workflow, part 2: the impact of technology on nurse activities. *J Nurs Adm.* 2010;40(10):432-439. doi:10.1097/NNA.0b013e3181f2eb3f.

37. Irwin RS, Richardson ND. Patient-focused care: using the right tools. *Chest.* 2006;130(1 Suppl):73S-82S. doi:10.1378/chest.130.1_suppl.73S.

38. Allan J, Englebright J. Patient-centered documentation: an effective and efficient use of clinical information systems. *J Nurs Adm.* 2000;30(2):90-95.

39. Nailon RE. The assessment and documentation of language and communication needs in healthcare systems: current practices and future directions for coordinating safe, patient-centered care. *Nurs Outlook.* 2007;55(6):311-317. doi:10.1016/j.outlook.2007.04.005.

40. Institute of Medicine. *Crossing the Quality Chasm: A New Health System for the 21st Century.* Washington, DC: National Academies Press; 2001. http://www.nap.edu/openbook.php?record_id=10027. Accessed October 6, 2011.

41. Recommended practices for the use of the pneumatic tourniquet in the perioperative practice setting. In: *Perioperative Standards and Recommended Practices.* Denver, CO: AORN, Inc; 2011: 177-190.

42. Spooner SA; Council on Clinical Information Technology. Special requirements of electronic health record systems in pediatrics. *Pediatrics.* 2007;119(3):631-637. doi:10.1542/peds.2006-3527.

43. Park EJ, McDaniel A, Jung MS. Computerized tailoring of health information. *Comput Inform Nurs.* 2009;27(1):34-43. doi:10.1097/NCN.0b013e31818dd396.

44. Payne TH, tenBroek AE, Fletcher GS, Labuguen MC. Transition from paper to electronic inpatient physician notes. *J Am Med Inform Assoc.* 2010;17(1):108-111. doi:10.1197/jamia.M3173.

45. Korst LM, Eusebio-Angeja AC, Chamorro T, Aydin CE, Gregory KD. Nursing documentation time during implementation of an electronic medical record. *J Nurs Adm.* 2003;33(1):24-30.

46. Urquhart C, Currell R, Grant MJ, Hardiker NR. Nursing record systems: effects on nursing practice and healthcare outcomes. *Cochrane Database Syst Rev.* 2009;(1). doi:10.1002/14651858.CD002099.pub2.

47. Mahler C, Ammenwerth E, Wagner A, et al. Effects of a computer-based nursing documentation system on the quality of nursing documentation. *J Med Syst.* 2007;31(4):274-282.

48. Poissant L, Pereira J, Tamblyn R, Kawasumi Y. The impact of electronic health records on time efficiency of physicians and nurses: a systematic review. *J Am Med Inform Assoc.* 2005;12(5):505-516. doi:10.1197/jamia.M1700.

49. Stead WW, Lin HS, eds. *Computational Technology for Effective Health Care: Immediate Steps and Strategic Directions.* Washington, DC: National Academies Press; 2009. http://www.nap.edu/openbook.php?record_id=12572&page=R1. Accessed October 6. 2011.

50. Asaro PV, Boxerman SB. Effects of computerized provider order entry and nursing documentation on workflow. *Acad Emerg Med.* 2008;15(10):908-915. doi:10.1111/j.1553-2712.2008.00235.x.

51. Manasse HR Jr. Not too perfect: hard lessons and small victories in patient safety. *Am J Health Syst Pharm.* 2003;60(8):780-787.

52. Amarasingham R, Plantinga L, Diener-West M, Gaskin DJ, Powe NR. Clinical information technologies and inpatient outcomes: a multiple hospital study. *Arch Intern Med.* 2009;169(2):108-114. doi:10.1001/archinternmed.2008.520.

53. Shojania KG, Jennings A, Mayhew A, Ramsay CR, Eccles MP, Grimshaw J. The effects of on-screen, point of care computer reminders on processes and outcomes of care. *Cochrane Database Syst Rev.* 2009;3(3):CD001096. doi:10.1002/14651858.CD001096.pub2.

54. Institute of Medicine. *The Future of Nursing: Leading Change, Advancing Health.* Washington, DC: National Academies Press; 2011. http://books.nap.edu/openbook.php?record_id=12956. Accessed October 6, 2011.

55. Previte JP. Information and communication system implementation in anesthesia. *Int Anesthesiol Clin.* 2006;44(1):179-197.

56. American Academy of Nursing. Position statement: use of electronic information for health and health care. 2008. http://www.aannet.org/files/public/EMR%20Position%20Statement%20Recommendation%20Post%20NIEP.doc. Accessed October 10, 2011.

57. Kim H, Dykes P, Mar P, Goldsmith D, Choi J, Goldberg H. Towards a standardized representation to support data reuse: representing the ICNP semantics using the HL7 RIM. *Stud Health Technol Inform.* 2009;146:308-313.

58. Zielstorff RD. Characteristics of a good nursing nomenclature from an informatics perspective. *Online J Issues Nurs.*1998;3(2).

59. *Nursing Informatics: Scope and Standards of Practice.* Silver Spring, MD: American Nurses Association; 2008.

60. Graves JR, Corcoran S. The study of nursing informatics. *Image J Nurs Sch.* 1989;21(4):227-231.

61. Petersen C, ed. *Perioperative Nursing Data Set.* 3rd ed. Denver, CO: AORN, Inc; 2011.

62. Beyea SC. Standardized language — making nursing practice count. *AORN J.* 1999;70(5):831-838.

63. Lundberg C, Warren J, Brokel J, et al. Selecting a standardized terminology for the electronic health record that reveals the impact of nursing on patient care. *Online J Nurs Inform.* 2008;12(2). http://www.ojni.org/12_2/lundberg.pdf. Accessed October 6, 2011.

64. Saba VK, Taylor SL. Moving past theory: use of a standardized, coded nursing terminology to enhance nursing visibility. *Comput Inform Nurs.* 2007;25(6):324-333. doi:10.1097/01.NCN.0000299654.13777.9f.

65. Centers for Medicare & Medicaid Services. Department of Health and Human Services. Condition of participation: Surgical services. 42 CFR §482.51. http://edocket.access.gpo.gov/cfr_2004/octqtr/pdf/42cfr482.51.pdf. Revised November 27, 2007. Accessed October 6, 2011.

INFORMATION MANAGEMENT

66. Centers for Medicare & Medicaid Services. Department of Health and Human Services. Condition of participation: Medical record services. 42 CFR §482.24. http://edocket.access.gpo.gov/cfr_2004/octqtr/pdf/42cfr482.24.pdf. Revised November 27, 2007. Accessed October 6, 2011.

67. Record of care, treatment, and services. RC.01.01.01. The hospital maintains complete and accurate medical records for each individual patient. In: *Comprehensive Accreditation Manual for Hospitals.* Oakbrook Terrace, IL: Joint Commission Resources; 2011.

68. Record of care, treatment, and services. RC.02.01.01. The medical record contains information that reflects the patient's care, treatment, and services. In: *Comprehensive Accreditation Manual for Hospitals.* 2011 ed. Oakbrook Terrace, IL: Joint Commission Resources; 2011.

69. Westra BL, Subramanian A, Hart CM, et al. Achieving "meaningful use" of electronic health records through the integration of the Nursing Management Minimum Data Set. *J Nurs Adm.* 2010;40(7-8):336-343. doi:10.1097/NNA.0b013e3181e93994.

70. Mangalmurti SS, Murtagh L, Mello MM. Medical malpractice liability in the age of electronic health records. *N Engl J Med.* 2010;363(21):2060-2067. doi:10.1056/NEJMhle1005210.

71. Electronic health record incentive program. Final rule. *Fed Regist.* 2010;75(144):44314-44588. 42 CFR §412, 413, 422, et al. http://edocket.access.gpo.gov/2010/pdf/2010-17207.pdf. Accessed October 18, 2011.

72. Häyrinen K, Saranto K, Nykanen P. Definition, structure, content, use and impacts of electronic health records: a review of the research literature. *Int J Med Inform.* 2008;77(5):291-304. doi:10.1016/j.ijmedinf.2007.09.001.

73. Hyun S, Bakken S. Toward the creation of an ontology for nursing document sections: mapping section names to the LOINC semantic model. *AMIA Annu Symp Proc.* 2006:364-368.

74. Executive summary. In: *Health Information Technology Automation of Quality Measure: Quality Data Set and Data Flow.* Washington, DC: National Quality Forum; 2009:iii-vi.

75. Kahn MG, Ranade D. The impact of electronic medical records data sources on an adverse drug event quality measure. *J Am Med Inform Assoc.* 2010;17(2):185-191. doi:10.1136/jamia.2009.002451.

76. Goossen WT, Ozbolt JG, Coenen A, et al. Development of a provisional domain model for the nursing process for use within the Health Level 7 reference information model. *J Am Med Inform Assoc.* 2004;11(3):186-194. doi:10.1197/jamia.M1085.

77. Jha AK, DesRoches CM, Campbell EG, et al. Use of electronic health records in U.S. hospitals. *N Engl J Med.* 2009;360(16):1628-1638. doi:10.1056/NEJMsa0900592.

78. Brown DS, Donaldson N, Burnes Bolton L, Aydin CE. Nursing-sensitive benchmarks for hospitals to gauge high-reliability performance. *J Healthc Qual.* 2010;32(6):9-17. doi:10.1111/j.1945-1474.2010.00083.x.

79. US Department of Health and Human Services. *Report to Congress: Medicare Ambulatory Surgical Center Value-Based Purchasing Implementation Plan.* Washington, DC: Centers for Medicare & Medicaid Services; 2011. http://www.cms.gov/ASCPayment/downloads/C_ASC_RTC%202011.pdf. Accessed October 7, 2011.

80. ECRI. Electronic health records. *Healthcare Risk Control.* 2011;2(Medical Records 1.1).

81. Hines S, Luna K, Lofthus J, et al. *Becoming a High Reliability Organization: Operational Advice for Hospital Leaders.* Rockville, MD: Agency for Healthcare Research and Quality; 2008.

82. Thompson D, Johnston P, Spurr C. The impact of electronic medical records on nursing efficiency. *J Nurs Adm.* 2009;39(10):444-451. doi:10.1097/NNA.0b013e3181b9209c.

83. Shekelle PG, Morton SC, Keeler EB, et al. *Costs and Benefits of Health Information Technology.* Rockville, MD: Agency for Healthcare Research and Quality; April 2006.

84. Centers for Medicare & Medicaid Services. Department of Health and Human Services. Conditions for participation for hospitals. 42 CFR §482. http://www.access.gpo.gov/nara/cfr/waisidx_10/42cfr482_10.html. Accessed October 7, 2011.

85. Centers for Medicare & Medicaid Services. Department of Health and Human Services. Condition of participation: nursing services. 42 CFR §482.23. Revised November 27, 2007. http://edocket.access.gpo.gov/cfr_2010/octqtr/pdf/42cfr482.23.pdf. Accessed October 7, 2011.

86. Centers for Medicare & Medicaid Services. Department of Health and Human Services. Condition for coverage — nursing services. 42 CFR §416.46. http://edocket.access.gpo.gov/cfr_2010/octqtr/pdf/42cfr416.46.pdf. Accessed October 7, 2011.

87. Centers for Medicare & Medicaid Services. Department of Health and Human Services. Condition of participation: medical records. 42 CFR §416.47. http://edocket.access.gpo.gov/cfr_2010/octqtr/pdf/42cfr416.47.pdf. Accessed October 7, 2011.

88. Centers for Medicare & Medicaid Services. Department of Health and Human Services. Ambulatory surgical services. 42 CFR §416. http://www.access.gpo.gov/nara/cfr/waisidx_10/42cfr416_10.html. Accessed October 7, 2011.

89. *Perioperative Standards and Recommended Practices.* Denver, CO: AORN, Inc; 2011.

90. Centers for Medicare & Medicaid Services. Department of Health and Human Services. Conditions for coverage—infection control. 42 CFR §416.51. http://edocket.access.gpo.gov/cfr_2010/octqtr/pdf/42cfr416.51.pdf. Accessed October 7, 2011.

91. National Patient Safety Goal. NPSG.07.05.01. Implement evidence-based practices for preventing surgical site infections. In: *Comprehensive Accreditation Manual for Hospitals.* Oakbrook Terrace, IL: Joint Commission Resources; 2011.

92. Infection prevention and control. Standard IC.01.05.01. The hospital has an infection prevention and control plan. In: *Comprehensive Accreditation Manual for Hospitals.* Oakbrook Terrace, IL: Joint Commission Resources; 2011.

93. Infection prevention and control. Standard IC.02.01.01. Hospital leaders allocate needed resources for the infection prevention and control program. In: *Comprehensive Accreditation Manual for Hospitals.* Oakbrook Terrace, IL: Joint Commission Resources; 2011.

94. Recommended practices for managing the patient receiving local anesthesia. In: *Perioperative Standards and Recommended Practices.* Denver, CO: AORN, Inc; 2011: 321-326.

95. Recommended practices for medication safety. In: *Perioperative Standards and Recommended Practices.* Denver, CO: AORN, Inc. In press.

96. Krenzischek DA, Wilson L; ASPAN. ASPAN pain and comfort clinical guideline. *J Perianesth Nurs.* 2003;18(4):232-236.

97. Practice recommendation 2: components of initial, ongoing, and discharge assessment and management. In: *Perianesthesia Nursing Standards and Practice*

Recommendations 2010-2012. Cherry Hill, NJ: American Society of PeriAnesthesia Nurses; 2010: 73-78.

98. Centers for Medicare & Medicaid Services. Department of Health and Human Services. Condition for coverage—pharmaceutical services. 42 CFR §416.48. http://edocket.access.gpo.gov/cfr_2010/octqtr/pdf/42cfr416.48.pdf. Accessed October 7, 2011.

99. Centers for Medicare & Medicaid Services. Department of Health and Human Services. Condition of participation: patient's rights. 42 CFR §482.13. http://edocket.access.gpo.gov/cfr_2010/octqtr/pdf/42cfr482.13.pdf. Accessed October 7, 2011.

100. Medication management. In: *Comprehensive Accreditation Manual for Hospitals.* Oakbrook Terrace, IL: Joint Commission Resources; 2011: MM-1–MM-23.

101. Provision of care, treatment, and services. In: *Comprehensive Accreditation Manual for Hospitals.* Oakbrook Terrace, IL: Joint Commission Resources; 2011: PC-1–PC-66.

102. Standard 5.001: Facility safety manual. In: *Medicare Standards and Checklist for Accreditation of Ambulatory Surgery Facilities.* Gurnee, IL: American Association for Accreditation of Ambulatory Surgery Facilities; 2005: 24-29.

103. Standard 04: Quality of care provided. In: *Accreditation Handbook for Ambulatory Health Care.* Skokie, IL: Accreditation Association for Ambulatory Health Care; 2009: 32-33.

104. Standard 06: Clinical records and health information. In: *Accreditation Handbook for Ambulatory Health Care.* Skokie, IL: Accreditation Association for Ambulatory Health Care; 2009:38-39.

105. AORN guidance statement: "do-not-use" abbreviations, acronyms, dosage designations, and symbols. In: *Perioperative Standards and Recommended Practices.* Denver, CO: AORN, Inc; 2011: 487-490.

106. AORN position statement on preventing wrong-patient, wrong-site, wrong-procedure events. AORN. http://www.aorn.org/PracticeResources/AORNPositionStatements/PositionCorrectSiteSurgery. Accessed October 7, 2011.

107. AORN position statement on pediatric medication safety. In: *Perioperative Standards and Recommended Practices.* Denver, CO: AORN, Inc; 2010: 737-738.

108. Recommended practices for preoperative patient skin antisepsis. In: *Perioperative Standards and Recommended Practices.* Denver, CO: AORN, Inc; 2011: 361-380.

109. Rights and responsibilities of the individual. In: *Comprehensive Accreditation Manual for Hospitals.* Oakbrook Terrace, IL: Joint Commission Resources; 2011:RI-1–RI-18.

110. National Patient Safety Goal. NPSG Goal 8: accurately and completely reconcile medications across the continuum of care. In: *Comprehensive Accreditation Manual for Hospitals.* Oakbrook Terrace, IL: Joint Commission Resources; 2011.

111. Accreditation Association for Ambulatory Health Care. http://www.aaahc.org/eweb/StartPage.aspx. Accessed October 11, 2011.

112. Recommended practices for prevention of transmissible infections in the perioperative practice settings. In: *Perioperative Standards and Recommended Practices.* Denver, CO: AORN, Inc; 2011: 291-302.

113. Standard 310: PACU rooms. In: *Regular Standards and Checklist for Accreditation of Ambulatory Surgery Facilities.* Gurnee, IL: American Association for Accreditation of Ambulatory Surgery Facilities; 2007: 22-23.

114. AORN malignant hyperthermia guideline. In: *Perioperative Standards and Recommended Practices.* Denver, CO: AORN, Inc; 2011: 541-576.

115. AORN guidance statement: Care of the perioperative patient with an implanted electronic device. In: *Perioperative Standards and Recommended Practices.* Denver, CO: AORN, Inc; 2011: 503-524.

116. Recommended practices for prevention of deep vein thrombosis. In: *Perioperative Standards and Recommended Practices.* Denver, CO: AORN, Inc; 2011: e1-e11.

117. Centers for Medicare & Medicaid Services. Department of Health and Human Services. Condition of participation: laboratory services. 42 CFR §482.27. http://edocket.access.gpo.gov/cfr_2010/octqtr/pdf/42cfr482.27.pdf. Accessed October 7, 2011.

118. Centers for Medicare & Medicaid Services. Department of Health and Human Services. Condition of participation: patient admission, assessment and discharge. 42 CFR §416.52. http://edocket.access.gpo.gov/cfr_2010/octqtr/pdf/42cfr416.52.pdf. Accessed October 7, 2011.

119. Record of care, treatment, and services. In: *Comprehensive Accreditation Manual for Hospitals.* Oakbrook Terrace, IL: Joint Commission Resources; 2011:RC-1–RC-14.

120. Recommended practices for positioning the patient in the perioperative practice setting. In: *Perioperative Standards and Recommended Practices.* Denver, CO: AORN, Inc; 2011: 337-360.

121. Universal Protocol for Preventing Wrong Site, Wrong Procedure, and Wrong Person Surgery. In: *Comprehensive Accreditation Manual for Hospitals.* Oakbrook Terrace, IL: Joint Commission Resources; 2011:NPSG-12–NPSG-24.

122. Recommended practices for transfer of patient care information. In: *Perioperative Standards and Recommended Practices.* Denver, CO: AORN, Inc; 2011: 381-388.

123. Standards of perioperative nursing. In: *Perioperative Standards and Recommended Practices.* Denver, CO: AORN, Inc; 2011: 3-52.

124. Standard 10: Surgical and related services. In: *Accreditation Handbook for Ambulatory Health Care.* Skokie, IL: Accreditation Association for Ambulatory Health Care; 2009: 50-54.

125. Standard 17: Behavioral health services. In: *Accreditation Handbook for Ambulatory Health Care.* Skokie, IL: Accreditation Association for Ambulatory Health Care; 2009: 64.

126. Standard 8.000: Operating room suite operations & management. In: *Medicare Standards and Checklist for Accreditation of Ambulatory Surgery Facilities.* Gurnee, IL: American Association for Accreditation of Ambulatory Surgery Facilities; 2005: 35-41.

127. Standard 630: Laboratory, pathology, x-ray, consultation and treating physician reports. In: *Regular Standards and Checklist for Accreditation of Ambulatory Surgery Facilities.* Gurnee, IL: American Association for Accreditation of Ambulatory Surgery Facilities; 2007: 33-34.

128. Standard 4.007: X-ray reports. In: *Medicare Standards and Checklist for Accreditation of Ambulatory Surgery Facilities.* Gurnee, IL: American Association for Accreditation of Ambulatory Surgery Facilities; 2005:20.

129. Centers for Medicare & Medicaid Services. Department of Health and Human Services. Condition of participation: Physical environment. 42 CFR §482.41. http://edocket.access.gpo.gov/cfr_2010/octqtr/pdf/42cfr482.41.pdf. Accessed October 7, 2011.

130. Centers for Medicare & Medicaid Services. Department of Health and Human Services. Condition for coverage—Environment. 42 CFR §416.44. http://edocket.access.gpo.gov/cfr_2010/octqtr/pdf/42cfr416.44.pdf. Accessed October 6, 2011.

131. Environment of care. In: 2011 *Comprehensive Accreditation Manual for Hospitals.* Oakbrook Terrace, IL: Joint Commission Resources; 2011.

132. American Association for Accreditation of Ambulatory Surgery Facilities. http://www.aaaasf.org/. Accessed October 6, 2011.

133. Standard 10.Q: Surgical and related services. In: *Accreditation Handbook for Ambulatory Health Care.* Skokie, IL: Accreditation Association for Ambulatory Health Care, Inc; 2009: 51.

134. Recommended practices for a safe environment of care. In: *Perioperative Standards and Recommended Practices.* Denver, CO: AORN, Inc; 2011: 215-236.

135. Recommended practices for electrosurgery. In: *Perioperative Standards and Recommended Practices.* Denver, CO: AORN, Inc; 2011: 99-118.

136. AORN latex guideline. In: *Perioperative Standards and Recommended Practices.* Denver, CO: AORN, Inc; 2011: 525-540.

137. Quality Indicators. Agency for Healthcare Research and Quality. http://www.qualityindicators.ahrq.gov/. Published November 2000. Updated August 2011. Accessed October 6, 2011.

138. Recommended practices for minimally invasive surgery. In: *Perioperative Standards and Recommended Practices.* Denver, CO: AORN, Inc; 2011: 143-176.

139. Recommended practices for laser safety in perioperative practice settings. In: *Perioperative Standards and Recommended Practices.* Denver, CO: AORN, Inc; 2011: 125-142.

140. Infection prevention and control. In: 2011 *Comprehensive Accreditation Manual for Hospitals.* Oakbrook Terrace, IL: Joint Commission Resources; 2011.

141. Standard 410: General Safety in the Facility. General. In: *Regular Standards and Checklist for Accreditation of Ambulatory Surgery Facilities.* Gurnee, IL: American Association for Accreditation of Ambulatory Surgery Facilities; 2007:25.

142. *ANSI/AAMI ST79:2006 and A1:2008, A2:2009: Comprehensive Guide to Steam Sterilization and Sterility Assurance in Health Care Facilities.* Arlington, VA: Association for the Advancement of Medical Instrumentation; 2009.

143. Recommended practices for surgical tissue banking. In: *Perioperative Standards and Recommended Practices.* Denver, CO: AORN, Inc; 2011: 201-214.

144. Recommended practices for the care and handling of specimens in the perioperative environment. In: *Perioperative Standards and Recommended Practices.* Denver, CO: AORN, Inc; 2011: 283-290.

145. Standardized packaging, labeling and transporting of organs, vessels, and tissue typing materials. Organ Procurement and Transplantation Network. http://optn.transplant.hrsa.gov/PoliciesandBylaws2/policies/pdfs/policy_17.pdf. Updated June 29, 2011. Accessed October 6, 2011.

146. Centers for Medicare & Medicaid Services. Department of Health and Human Services. Condition of participation: organ, tissue, and eye procurement. 24 CFR §482.45. http://ecfr.gpoaccess.gov/cgi/t/text/text-idx?c=ecfr&sid=161a6bff7c036b1836ab37d4d1604d53&rgn=div8&view=text&node=42:5.0.1.1.1.3.4.13&idno=42. Published June 22, 1998. Accessed October 6, 2011.

147. US Department of Labor, Occupational Safety and Health Standards. Bloodborne pathogens. 29 CFR §1910.1030. http://www.osha.gov/pls/oshaweb/owadisp.show_document?p_table=standards&p_id=10051. Accessed October 6, 2011.

148. Transplant safety. In: 2011 *Comprehensive Accreditation Manual for Hospitals.* Oakbrook Terrace, IL: Joint Commission Resources; 2011.

149. Recommended practices for traffic patterns in the perioperative practice setting. In: *Perioperative Standards and Recommended Practices.* Denver, CO: AORN, Inc; 2011: 95-98.

150. Mangram AJ, Horan TC, Pearson ML, Silver LC, Jarvis WR. Guideline for prevention of surgical site infection, 1999. *Infect Control Hosp Epidemiol.* 1999;20(4):247-278. doi:10.1086/501620.

151. Centers for Medicare & Medicaid Services. Department of Health and Human Services. Condition of participation: discharge planning. 42 CFR §482.43. http://edocket.access.gpo.gov/cfr_2010/octqtr/pdf/42cfr482.43.pdf. Accessed October 6, 2011.

152. National Patient Safety Goal 7: reduce the risk of health care–associated infections. In: *2011 Comprehensive Accreditation Manual for Hospitals.* Oakbrook Terrace, IL: Joint Commission Resources; 2011.

153. SCIP-Inf-4: Cardiac surgery patients with controlled 6 a.m. postoperative blood glucose. In: *The Specifications Manual for National Hospital Inpatient Quality Measures.* Version 3.3. Centers for Medicare & Medicaid Services and Joint Commission; 2011.

154. SCIP-Inf-6: Surgery patients with appropriate hair removal. In: *The Specifications Manual for National Hospital Inpatient Quality Measures.* Version 3.3. Centers for Medicare & Medicaid Services and Joint Commission; 2011.

155. *Guide to Patient Safety Indicators.* Version 3.1. Rockville, MD: Department of Health and Human Services Agency for Healthcare Research and Quality; 2007.

156. Recommended practices for reducing radiological exposure in the perioperative practice setting. In: *Perioperative Standards and Recommended Practices.* Denver, CO: AORN, Inc; 2011: 251-262.

157. ANSI Z136.4-2010: American National Standard Recommended Practice for Laser Safety Measurements for Hazard Evaluation. Orlando, FL: Laser Institute of America; 2010.

158. ANSI Z136.7-2008: American National Standard for Testing and Labeling of Laser Protective Equipment. Orlando, FL: Laser Institute of America; 2008.

159. Recommended practices for prevention of retained surgical items. In: *Perioperative Standards and Recommended Practices.* Denver, CO: AORN, Inc; 2011: 263-282.

160. 109th US Congress. Deficit Reduction Act of 2005. Pub L 109-171. February 8, 2006. http://frwebgate.access.gpo.gov/cgi-bin/getdoc.cgi?dbname=109_cong_public_laws&docid=f:publ171.109.pdf. Accessed October 6, 2011.

161. AORN guidance statement: creating a patient safety culture. In: *Perioperative Standards and Recommended Practices.* Denver, CO: AORN, Inc; 2011: 577-582.

162. Centers for Medicare & Medicaid Services. Department of Health and Human Services. Condition of participation: medical staff. 42 CFR §482.22. http://edocket.access.gpo.gov/cfr_2004/octqtr/pdf/42cfr482.23.pdf. Accessed October 6, 2011.

163. Centers for Medicare & Medicaid Services. Department of Health and Human Services. Condition for coverage—surgical services. 42 CFR §416.42. http://www.gpo.gov/fdsys/pkg/CFR-2010-title42-vol3/pdf/CFR-2010-title42-vol3-sec416-42.pdf. Published 2010. Accessed October 7, 2011.

INFORMATION MANAGEMENT

164. Centers for Medicare & Medicaid Services. Department of Health and Human Services. Condition for coverage—laboratory and radiologic services. 42 CFR §416.49. http://edocket.access.gpo.gov/cfr_2010/octqtr/pdf/42cfr416.49.pdf. Published 2010. Accessed October 7, 2011.

165. Standard 1010: Anesthesia. Pre-anesthesia care. In: *Regular Standards and Checklist for Accreditation of Ambulatory Surgery Facilities.* 11th ed. Gurnee, IL: American Association for Accreditation of Ambulatory Surgery Facilities; 2007: 50-51.

166. Standard 4.020: Additional Medicare standards. In: *Medicare Standards and Checklist for Accreditation of Ambulatory Surgery Facilities.* 3rd ed. Gurnee, IL: American Association for Accreditation of Ambulatory Surgery Facilities; 2005: 22-24.

167. Standard 4.003: Patient charts. Medical history. In: *Medicare Standards and Checklist for Accreditation of Ambulatory Surgery Facilities.* 3rd ed. Gurnee, IL: American Association for Accreditation of Ambulatory Surgery Facilities; 2005: 19.

168. Centers for Medicare & Medicaid Services. Department of Health and Human Services. Condition of participation: pharmaceutical services. 42 CFR §482.25. http://edocket.access.gpo.gov/cfr_2010/octqtr/pdf/42cfr482.25.pdf. Published 2010. Accessed October 7, 2011.

169. National Patient Safety Goal. NPSG 2: Improve the effectiveness of communication among caregivers. In: *2011 Comprehensive Accreditation Manual for Hospitals.* Oakbrook Terrace, IL: Joint Commission Resources; 2011.

170. Standard 04.E. Quality of care provided. In: *Accreditation Handbook for Ambulatory Health Care.* 2009 ed. Skokie, IL: Accreditation Association for Ambulatory Health Care, Inc; 2009: 32.

171. Standard 06K. Clinical records and health information. In: *Accreditation Handbook for Ambulatory Health Care.* Skokie, IL: Accreditation Association for Ambulatory Health Care, Inc; 2009:38-39.

172. Recommended practices for high-level disinfection. In: *Perioperative Standards and Recommended Practices.* Denver, CO: AORN, Inc; 2011: 399-414.

173. Recommended practices for sterilization in the perioperative practice setting. In: *Perioperative Standards and Recommended Practices.* Denver, CO: AORN, Inc; 2011: 463-486.

174. Standard 230. Operating room policy, environment and procedures. Procedures — sterilization. In: *Regular Standards and Checklist for Accreditation of Ambulatory Surgery Facilities.* 11th ed. Gurnee, IL: American Association for Accreditation of Ambulatory Surgery Facilities; 2007: 14.

175. Standard 9.001. Requirements for facility classification. In: *Medicare Standards and Checklist for Accreditation of Ambulatory Surgery Facilities.* 3rd ed. Gurnee, IL: American Association for Accreditation of Ambulatory Surgery Facilities; 2005: 42-45.

176. Standard 10M. In: *2009 Accreditation Handbook for Ambulatory Health Care.* Skokie, IL: Accreditation Association for Ambulatory Health Care, Inc; 2009: 51.

177. Recommended practices for the prevention of unplanned perioperative hypothermia. In: *Perioperative Standards and Recommended Practices.* Denver, CO: AORN, Inc; 2011: 307-320.

178. Clinical practice guideline 1: ASPAN's evidence-based clinical practice guideline for the promotion of perioperative normothermia. In: *Perianesthesia Nursing Standards and Practice Recommendations 2010-2012.* Cherry Hill, NJ: American Society of PeriAnesthesia Nurses; 2010: 24-45.

179. Preventing the retention of foreign objects during interventional radiology procedures. *Pa Patient Saf Advis.* 2008;5(1):24-27.

180. Sales representatives and other outsiders in the OR. *Oper Room Risk Manag.* 2007; 2(Quality Assurance/Risk Management 7):1-9.

181. Use of blunt-tip suture needles to decrease percutaneous injuries to surgical personnel: safety and health information bulletin. Atlanta, GA. National Institute for Occupational Safety and Health; 2007: http://www.cdc.gov/niosh/docs/2008-101/. Accessed October 20, 2011.

182. Rutala WA, Weber DJ; Healthcare Infection Control Practices Advisory Committee (HICPAC). *Guideline for Disinfection and Sterilization in Healthcare Facilities, 2008.* Atlanta, GA: Centers for Disease Control and Prevention; 2008.

183. *Pommier v ABC Insurance Company,* 715 So2d 1270, 1297-1342 (La.App.3dCir. 1998).

184. *Lama v Borras,* 1994 16 F3d 473 (United States Court of Appeals, First Circuit, February 25, 1994). http://law.justia.com/cases/federal/appellate-courts/F3/16/473/491880/. Accessed October 20, 2011.

185. *Ledesma v Shashoua,* 2007 WL 2214650 (Tex App, August 3, 2007). http://www.nalnc.org/lnc_court_cases/Ledesma%20v.%20Shashoua.htm. Accessed October 20, 2011.

186. Centers for Medicare & Medicaid Services. Department of Health and Human Services. Condition of participation: Anesthesia services. 42 CFR §482.52. Published 2009.

187. Centers for Medicare & Medicaid Services. Department of Health and Human Services. Condition of participation: food and dietetic services. 42 CFR §482.28.

188. US Food and Drug Administration. Department of Health and Human Services. Medical device tracking requirements. 21 CFR §821. Updated April 2010. Accessed May 20, 2010.

189. Centers for Medicare & Medicaid Services. Department of Health and Human Services. Condition of participation: radiologic services. 42 CFR §482.26. Published 2010.

190. Social Security Act, 42 USC 1396d §1905, Pub L No. 74-271.

191. Medical device tracking; guidance for industry and FDA staff. US Food and Drug Administration. 2010. http://www.fda.gov/MedicalDevices/DeviceRegulationandGuidance/GuidanceDocuments/ucm071756.htm. Accessed October 20, 2011.

192. Food and Drug Administration Modernization Act of 1997, S 830, 105th Cong, 1st Sess (1997), Pub L No 105-115.

193. Overview certification & compliance. Centers for Medicare & Medicaid Services. Updated December 14, 2005. http://www.cms.gov/certificationandcomplianc/01_overview.asp?. Accessed October 20, 2011.

194. About DNV accreditation. DNV. http://www.dnvaccreditation.com/pr/dnv/about.aspx. Accessed October 20, 2011.

195. Overview. Healthcare Facilities Accreditation Program. http://www.hfap.org/about/overview.aspx. Accessed October 20, 2011.

196. *2011 Comprehensive Accreditation Manual for Hospitals.* Oakbrook Terrace, IL: Joint Commission Resources; 2011.

197. *2011 Comprehensive Accreditation Manual for Ambulatory Care.* Oakbrook Terrace, IL: Joint Commission Resources; 2011.

198. Hospital compare. US Department of Health and Human Services. http://www.hospitalcompare.hhs.gov/. Accessed October 20, 2011.

INFORMATION MANAGEMENT

199. US Department of Health and Human Services. Ambulatory surgical center payment system and CY 2011 payment rates. *Fed Regist.* 2010;75(226):71799-72580. http://edocket.access.gpo.gov/2010/pdf/2010-27926.pdf. Accessed October 20, 2011.

200. Surgical Care Improvement Project. http://www.qualitynet.org/dcs/ContentServer?c=Page&pagename=QnetPublic%2FPage%2FQnetTier2&cid=1141662756099. Accessed October 20, 2011.

201. US Department of Health and Human Services. Medicare program: hospital inpatient value-based purchasing program. *Fed Regist.* 2011;76(9):2454-2491. http://www.gpo.gov/fdsys/pkg/FR-2011-01-13/pdf/2011-454.pdf. Accessed October 20, 2011.

202. 2010 ORYX Performance Measure Reporting Requirements for Hospitals and Guidelines for Measure Selections. 2010. http://www.jointcommission.org/assets/1/18/2010_ORYX_Performance_Measure_Reporting_Requirements.pdf. Accessed October 20, 2011.

203. Straube BM. Letter to David T. Tayloe Jr. [written communication]. Baltimore, MD: Department of Health & Human Services; 2010. http://practice.aap.org/public/Straube%20Letter%20to%20Tayloe.PDF. Accessed September 30, 2011.

204. Centers for Medicare & Medicaid Services. US Department of Health and Human Services. Condition for coverage—patient rights. 42 CFR §416.50. Published 2010.

205. Record of care, treatment, and services. RC.02.03.07. Qualified staff receive and record verbal orders. In: *2011 Comprehensive Accreditation Manual for Ambulatory Care.* Oakbrook Terrace, IL: Joint Commission Resources; 2011.

206. Dawson A, Orsini MJ, Cooper MR, Wollenburg K. Medication safety—reliability of preference cards. *AORN J.* 2005;82(3):399.

207. Cole LM. Med report. Documenting to reduce medication errors. *OR Nurse.* 2008;2(7):17-19.

208. Medication management. MM.04.01.0. Medication orders are clear and accuarate. In: *2011 Comprehensive Accreditation Manual for Hospitals.* Oakbrook Terrace, IL: Joint Commission Resources; 2011.

209. Medication management. MM.04.01.01. Medication orders are clear and accurate. In: *2011 Comprehensive Accreditation Manual for Ambulatory Care.* Oakbrook Terrace, IL: Joint Commission Resources; 2011.

210. Broussard M, Bass PF 3rd, Arnold CL, McLarty JW, Bocchini JA Jr. *J Pediatr.* 2009;154(6):865-868. doi:10.1016/j.jpeds.2008.12.022.

211. Stevenson JG, Brunetti L, Santell JP, Hicks RW. USP medication safety forum. The impact of abbreviations on patient safety. *Joint Comm J Qual Patient Saf.* 2007;33(9):576-583.

212. Smith L. How to chart by exception. *Nursing.* 2002;32(9):30.

213. Noone JM. How to chart by exception. *J Nurs Adm.* 2000;30(7-8):342-343.

214. Murphy EK. Charting by exception. *AORN J.* 2003;78(5):821-823.

215. Anderson LA, Schramm CA. Adapting charting by exception to the perianesthesia setting. *J Perianesth Nurs.* 1999;14(5):260-269.

216. Short MS. Charting by exception on a clinical pathway. *Nurs Manage.* 1997;28(8):45-46.

217. Samuels JG. Abstracting pain management documentation from the electronic medical record: comparison of three hospitals. *Appl Nurs Res.* In press. doi:10.1016/j.apnr.2010.05.001.

218. Holden RJ. Cognitive performance-altering effects of electronic medical records: an application of the human factors paradigm for patient safety. *Cogn Technol Work.* 2011;13(1):11-29.

219. *Driving Quality and Performance Measurement—A Foundation for Clinical Decision Support: A Consensus Report.* Washington, DC: National Quality Forum; 2010.

220. Committee on Data Standards for Patient Safety, Board on Health Care Services, Institute of Medicine of the National Academies. *Key Capabilities of an Electronic Health Record System: Letter Report.* Washington, DC: National Academies Press; 2003.

221. Modifications to the HIPAA Privacy, Security, and Enforcement Rules Under the Health Information Technology for Economic and Clinical Health Act: Proposed Rule. *Fed Regist.* 2010;75(134):40868-40924. Codified at 45 CFR §160 and §164. http://edocket.access.gpo.gov/2010/pdf/2010-16718.pdf. Accessed October 11, 2011.

222. Health Insurance Portability and Accountability Act of 1996, 42 USC §201 (1996), Pub L No. 104-191, 110 Stat 1936.

223. Nelson ML. HIE provider verification: the privacy and security elephant in the room. *JHIM.* 2011;25(1):44-47.

224. Walsh D, Passerini K, Varshney U, Fjermestad J. Safeguarding patient privacy in electronic healthcare in the USA: the legal view. *Int J Electron Healthc.* 2008;4(3-4):311-326.

225. Malin B, Airoldi E. Confidentiality preserving audits of electronic medical record access. *Stud Health Technol Inform.* 2007;129(Pt 1):320-324.

226. *2010 HIMSS Analytics Report: Security of Patient Data Commissioned by Kroll's Fraud Solutions.* Chicago, IL: HIMSS Analytics; 2010.

227. AHIMA e-HIM Work Group on Maintaining the Legal EHR. Maintaining a legally sound health record: paper and electronic. *J AHIMA.* 2005;76(10):64A-L.

228. Kane B, Sands DZ. Guidelines for the clinical use of electronic mail with patients. The AMIA Internet Working Group, Task Force on Guidelines for the Use of Clinic-Patient Electronic Mail. *J Am Med Inform Assoc.* 1998;5(1):104-111.

229. US Department of Health and Human Services. *Nationwide Privacy and Security Framework for Electronic Exchange of Individually Identifiable Health Information.* Washington, DC: Office of the National Coordinator for Health Information Technology; 2008. http://healthit.hhs.gov/portal/server.pt/gateway/PTARGS_0_10731_848088_0_0_18/NationwidePS_Framework-5.pdf. Accessed October 11, 2011.

230. US Federal Trade Commission. Health breach notification rule. 16 CFR §318 (2009). http://ecfr.gpoaccess.gov/cgi/t/text/text-idx?c=ecfr&tpl=/ecfrbrowse/Title16/16cfr318_main_02.tpl. Accessed October 11, 2011.

231. Connecting for Health Work Group on Consumer Access Policies for Networked Personal Health Information. *Security and Systems Requirements.* New York, NY: Markle Foundation; 2008.

232. Centers for Medicare & Medicaid Services. Department of Health and Human Services. Condition of participation: surgical services. Standard: delivery of service. 42 CFR §482.51(b) (2004). http://edocket.access.gpo.gov/cfr_2010/octqtr/pdf/42cfr482.51.pdf. Accessed October 11, 2011.

233. Condition for Coverage—Medical Records. Standard: Form and Content of Record. 42 CFR §416.47(b). In: *State Operations Manual Appendix L - Guidance for Surveyors: Ambulatory Surgical Centers.* Rev.56, issued December 30, 2009. Baltimore, MD: Centers for Medicare & Medicaid Services; 2009. http://cms.gov/manuals/Downloads/som107ap_l_ambulatory.pdf. Accessed October 11, 2011.

234. Rights and responsibilities of the individual. RI.01.03.01. The hospital honors the patient's right to give or withhold informed consent. In: *2011 Comprehensive Accreditation Manual for Ambulatory Care*. Oakbrook Terrace, IL: Joint Commission Resources; 2011.

235. Rights and responsibilities of the individual. RI.01.03.03. The hospital honors the patient's right to give or withhold informed consent to produce or use recordings, films, or other images of the patient for purposes other than his or her care. In: *2011 Comprehensive Accreditation Manual for Ambulatory Care*. Oakbrook Terrace, IL: Joint Commission Resources; 2011.

236. Rights and responsibilities of the individual. RI.01.03.01. The hospital honors the patient's right to give or withhold informed consent. In: *2011 Comprehensive Accreditation Manual for Hospitals*. Oakbrook Terrace, IL: Joint Commission Resources; 2011.

237. Rights and responsibilities of the individual. RI.01.03.03. The hospital honors the patient's right to give or withhold informed consent to produce or use recordings, films, or other images of the patient for purposes other than his or her care. In: *2011 Comprehensive Accreditation Manual for Hospitals*. Oakbrook Terrace, IL: Joint Commission Resources; 2011.

238. The AMA Code of Medical Ethics' opinion on computerized medical records. *AMA J Ethics*. 2011;13(3):161-162.

239. Record of care, treatment, and services. RC.01.02.01. Entries in the medical record are authenticated. In: *2011 Comprehensive Accreditation Manual for Ambulatory Care*. Oakbrook Terrace, IL: Joint Commission Resources; 2011.

240. Record of care, treatment, and services. RC.01.04.01. The hospital audits its medical records. In: 2011 Comprehensive Accreditation Manual for Hospitals. Oakbrook Terrace, IL: Joint Commission Resources; 2011.

241. Electronic health record incentive program: final rule. *Fed Regist*. 2010;75(144):44314-44588. Codified at 42 CFR §412, 413, 422, et al. http://edocket.access.gpo.gov/2010/pdf/2010-17207.pdf. Accessed October 21, 2011.

242. Centers for Medicare & Medicaid Services. Department of Health and Human Services. Conditions of participation: clinical records. 42 CFR §485.638. http://www.gpo.gov/fdsys/pkg/CFR-2010-title42-vol5/pdf/CFR-2010-title42-vol5-sec485-638.pdf. Accessed October 11, 2011.

243. Electronic Signatures in Global and National Commerce Act. Pub L No. 106-229, 114 Stat 464.

244. US Food and Drug Administration. Department of Health and Human Services. Electronic records; electronic signatures. 21 CFR §11. Revised 2010.

245. *Practice Brief: Retention of Health Information (Updated)*. Chicago, IL: American Health Information Management Association; 2002.

246. Record of care, treatment, and services. RC.01.05.01. The hospital retains its medical records. In: *2011 Comprehensive Accreditation Manual for Hospitals*. Oakbrook Terrace, IL: Joint Commission Resources; 2011.

247. Record of care, treatment, and services. RC.01.05.01. The hospital retains its medical records. In: *2011 Comprehensive Accreditation Manual for Ambulatory Care*. Oakbrook Terrace, IL: Joint Commission Resources; 2011.

248. Campbell EM, Sittig DF, Guappone KP, Dykstra RH, Ash JS. Overdependence on technology: an unintended adverse consequence of computerized provider order entry. *AMIA Annu Symp Proc*. 2007:94-98.

249. Agrawal A, Glasser AR. Barcode medication. Administration implementation in an acute care hospital and lessons learned. *J Healthc Inf Manag*. 2009;23(4):24-29.

250. *Amendments, Corrections, and Deletions in the Electronic Health Record Toolkit*. Chicago, IL: American Health Information Management Association; 2009.

251. ECRI. Electronic health records. *Oper Room Risk Manag*. 2007;1A(Medical Records 7):1-23.

252. ECRI. Medical records. *Oper Room Risk Manag*. 2008;1(Medical Records 3):1-16.

253. Russo R, American Health Information Management Association. *Clinical Documentation Improvement*. Chicago, IL: American Health Information Management Association; 2010.

254. Magrabi F, Ong M, Runciman W, Coiera E. An analysis of computer-related patient safety incidents to inform the development of a classification. *J Am Med Inform Assoc*. 2010;17(6):663-670. doi:10.1136/jamia.2009.002444.

255. Nunn S. Managing audit trails. *J AHIMA*. 2009;80(9):44-45.

Acknowledgments

Lead Author
Sharon Giarrizzo-Wilson, MS, RN-BC, CNOR
Informatics Nurse Specialist
AORN, Inc
Denver, Colorado

Contributing Authors
Christine A. Anderson, PhD, RN
Educator/Staff Development
University of Michigan School of Nursing
Ypsilanti, Michigan

Antonia B. Hughes, MA, BSN, RN, CNOR
Perioperative Education Specialist
Baltimore Washington Medical Center
Edgewater, Maryland

Cathy A. Klein, JD, MSN, MSEd, RN-C
Attorney and Counselor at Law
Greenwood Village, CO

Publication History
Originally published March 1982, *AORN Journal*, as "Recommended practices for documentation of perioperative nursing care."

Format revision July 1982.

Revised March 1987; revised September 1991; revised November 1995; published June 1996.

Revised; published January 2000, *AORN Journal*. Reformatted July 2000.

Revised November 2011; published online as "Recommended practices for perioperative health care information management" in *Perioperative Standards and Recommended Practices*.

Reformatted September 2012 for publication in *Perioperative Standards and Recommended Practices*, 2013 edition.

Minor editing revisions made in November 2014 for publication in *Guidelines for Perioperative Practice*, 2015 edition.

INFORMATION MANAGEMENT

GUIDELINE FOR CARE OF THE PATIENT RECEIVING LOCAL ANESTHESIA

The Guideline for Care of the Patient Receiving Local Anesthesia has been approved by the AORN Guidelines Advisory Board. It was presented as a proposed guideline for comments by members and others. The guideline is effective January 15, 2015. The recommendations in this guideline are intended to be achievable and represent what is believed to be an optimal level of practice. Policies and procedures will reflect variations in practice settings and/or clinical situations that determine the degree to which the guideline can be implemented. AORN recognizes the many diverse settings in which perioperative nurses practice; therefore, this guideline is adaptable to all areas where operative and other invasive procedures may be performed.

Purpose

This document provides guidance for the perioperative registered nurse (RN) caring for a patient who is receiving local anesthesia by injection, infiltration, or topical application. This document includes guidance for patient assessment, patient monitoring, recognition and treatment of local anesthetic systemic toxicity (LAST), assessment for local anesthetic allergies, and documentation of patient care. It is not the intent of this guideline to address situations that require the services of an anesthesia professional or to substitute the services of a perioperative RN in those situations that require the services of an anesthesia professional.

The goal of the perioperative team is to provide safe care without causing undue pain and anxiety to the patient receiving local anesthesia. Local anesthesia is safe and effective although, rarely, a patient may have a toxic systemic or allergic reaction to the local anesthetic. Local anesthetic systemic toxicity occurs as serum levels of the local anesthetic increase. The symptoms of LAST may present as central nervous system (CNS) or cardiovascular system (CVS) complications or both.[1-7] Although the incidence of LAST is rare,[8-11] the consequences may be severe, potentially resulting in death. Allergic reactions to local anesthetics are also rare, occurring in less than 1% of all patients who receive a local anesthetic.[12,13]

Moderate sedation analgesia and regional anesthesia are outside the scope of this document.

Evidence Review

On April 15, 2013, a medical librarian conducted a systematic search of the databases MEDLINE®, CINAHL®, and the Cochrane Database of Systematic Reviews for meta-analyses, systematic reviews, randomized controlled and non-randomized trials and studies, case reports, reviews, and guidelines from government agencies and standards-setting bodies. The librarian also searched the Scopus® database, although not systematically. The search was limited to literature published in English since January 2006. At the time of the initial search, the librarian established weekly alerts on the search topics and until July 2014, presented relevant results to the lead author. During the development of this guideline, the author requested supplementary literature searches and additional literature that either did not fit the original search criteria or was discovered during the evidence-appraisal process.

Although the lead author's original search request encompassed both moderate sedation and local anesthesia, only literature relevant to the care and management of patients receiving local anesthesia was considered for inclusion in this document. Of the 862 sources deemed appropriate for consideration in the areas of moderate sedation and local anesthesia, 63 were identified as relevant to local anesthesia (Figure 1). Germane search terms included *surgical procedures, analgesia, local anesthesia, topical anesthesia, local infiltration, lidocaine, bupivacaine, anxiety, anti-anxiety agents, drug hypersensitivity, allergy, anaphylaxis, risk assessment, physical examination, vital signs, blood pressure, blood pressure determination, pulse, physiologic monitoring, advanced cardiac life support, ACLS, nurse's role,* and *perioperative nursing*.

Excluded were non-peer-reviewed publications and studies that addressed moderate sedation, regional anesthesia, pediatric patients, or pregnant patients. Low-quality evidence was excluded when higher-quality evidence was available.

Articles identified in the search were provided to the lead author and divided and assigned to four evidence reviewers for review and critical appraisal using the AORN Research or Non-Research Evidence Appraisal Tools as appropriate. The lead author and the evidence reviewers independently evaluated and appraised the literature according to the strength and quality of the evidence. Each article was then assigned an appraisal score determined by consensus. The appraisal score is noted in brackets after each reference, as applicable.

The evidence supporting each intervention and activity statement within a specific recommendation was summarized, and the AORN Evidence-Rating Model was used to rate the strength of the collective evidence. Factors considered in review of the collective evidence were the quality of evidence, the quantity of similar evidence on a given topic, and the consistency of evidence supporting a recommendation. The evidence rating is noted in brackets after each intervention.

LOCAL ANESTHESIA

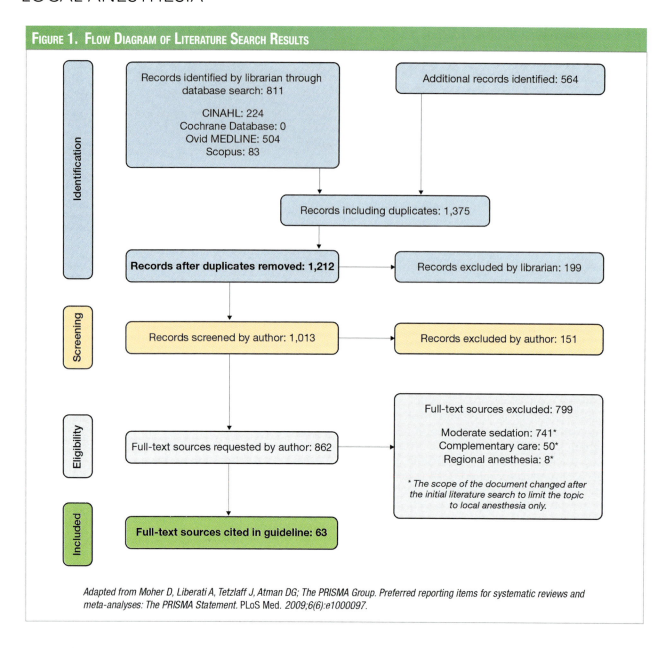

Figure 1. Flow Diagram of Literature Search Results

Adapted from Moher D, Liberati A, Tetzlaff J, Atman DG; The PRISMA Group. Preferred reporting items for systematic reviews and meta-analyses: The PRISMA Statement. PLoS Med. 2009;6(6):e1000097.

Note: The evidence summary table is available at http://www.aorn.org/evidencetables/.

Editor's note: MEDLINE is a registered trademark of the US National Library of Medicine's Medical Literature Analysis and Retrieval System, Bethesda, MD. CINAHL, Cumulative Index to Nursing and Allied Health Literature, is a registered trademark of EBSCO Industries, Birmingham, AL. Scopus is a registered trademark of Elsevier B.V., Amsterdam, The Netherlands.

Recommendation I

The perioperative RN should perform a preoperative nursing assessment for the patient who will receive local anesthesia.

Patient assessment before an intervention is a standard of perioperative nursing practice.[14] The American Nurses Association's *Nursing: Scope and Standards of Practice*[15] and the AORN "Standards of perioperative nursing"[14] direct the RN to collect patient health data that are relevant to the patient's care.

The collective evidence suggests that the preoperative patient assessment should include of a review of the patient's history that includes the cardiac, renal, and hepatic systems.[7,10,16] In addition to the total dose of the local anesthetic, cardiac, renal, or hepatic dysfunction are factors to consider when calculating local anesthetic plasma levels.[1,7,10,16]

The benefits of performing a nursing assessment outweigh the harms. Benefits include the ability to identify allergies and comorbid conditions that might affect the absorption of the local anesthetic; obtain baseline measures of vital signs, pain, and anxiety; and evaluate the patient's level of consciousness.

A limitation of the evidence is that no research studies were found that addressed preoperative nursing assessment of the patient receiving local anesthesia. Research is needed to define the exact elements that should be assessed before surgery.

I.a. The preoperative nursing assessment should include a review of the patient's
- allergies and sensitivities (eg, medications, tape, latex)[17];
- age;
- height, weight, and body mass index;
- current medications and use of alternative/complementary therapies[18];
- NPO status[19];
- medical history (eg, history and physical, progress note)[7,19];
- laboratory test results[17];
- diagnostic test results[17];
- baseline cardiac status (eg, heart rate, blood pressure)[6,17];
- baseline respiratory status (eg, rate, rhythm, blood oxygen level [SpO_2])[17];
- baseline skin condition for integrity (eg, rash, breaks, ecchymosis)[17];
- baseline neurological status[6,17];
- sensory impairments (eg, visual, auditory)[17];
- ability to tolerate the required operative position with draping for the duration of the procedure[17];
- level of anxiety[17];
- level of pain[17];
- perceptions of surgery[17]; and
- need for intravenous access.

[2: Moderate Evidence]

The collective evidence indicates that preoperative patient assessment provides important information regarding underlying conditions (eg, cardiac,[1,3,6,7,8,10,20,21] hepatic,[1,3,6,8,20] renal[3,20]) that may affect the patient's ability to metabolize the local anesthetic and place him or her at risk for developing LAST.[6] Preoperative vital signs provide a baseline reference for comparison if there is an adverse reaction to the local anesthetic. A systematic review[8] and seven literature reviews[1,3,6,7,10,20,21] describe underlying conditions that place a patient at increased risk for developing LAST.

I.b. The perioperative RN should use a physical acuity assessment tool (eg, the American Society of Anesthesiologists Physical Status Classification [Table 1][19,22] to determine patient acuity.
[2: Moderate Evidence]

Use of a physical assessment tool with inter-rater reliability provides an objective and consistent means for assessing the patient's acuity.

I.b.1. If the perioperative RN identifies a concern regarding the patient's acuity, the RN should consult with the physician to determine the plan of care. [4: Benefits Balanced with Harms]

I.c. Based on the patient assessment (ie, acuity, anxiety level), the type of procedure,[23,24] and the health care organization policy,[14] the perioperative RN should identify the personnel needed to implement the plan of care (eg, an additional RN to monitor). At a minimum, one perioperative RN circulator should be dedicated to each patient undergoing an operative or other invasive procedure and should be present during that patient's entire intraoperative experience.[25]
[2: Moderate Evidence]

AORN is committed to the provision of safe perioperative nursing care by ensuring that every patient undergoing an operative or other invasive procedure is cared for by minimum of one RN in the circulating role. The perioperative RN works collaboratively with other perioperative professionals (eg, surgeons, anesthesia professionals, surgical technologists) to meet patient needs, the perioperative RN is accountable for the patient's outcomes resulting from the nursing care provided during the operative or other invasive procedure. Using clinical knowledge, judgment, and clinical-reasoning skills based on scientific principles, the perioperative RN plans and implements nursing care to address the physical, psychological, and spiritual responses of the patient undergoing an operative or other invasive procedure.[25]

TABLE 1. Physical Status Classification

Status	Definition of patient status	Example
P1	A normal healthy patient	No physiologic, psychological, biochemical, or organic disturbance.
P2	A patient with mild systemic disease	Cardiovascular disease, asthma, chronic bronchitis, obesity, or diabetes mellitus.
P3	A patient with severe systemic disease	Cardiovascular or pulmonary disease that limits activity; severe diabetes with systemic complications; history of myocardial infarction, angina pectoris, or poorly controlled hypertension.
P4	A patient with severe systemic disease that is a constant threat to life	Severe cardiac, pulmonary, renal, hepatic, or endocrine dysfunction.
P5	A moribund patient who is not expected to survive without the operation	Surgery is done as a last recourse or resuscitative effort; major multi-system or cerebral trauma, ruptured aneurysm, or large pulmonary embolus.
P6	A declared brain-dead patient whose organs are being removed for donor purposes	

Reproduced with permission from the American Society of Anesthesiologists, Park Ridge, IL.

A practice guideline by the American Society of Anesthesiologists (ASA)[23] and one literature review[24] support the need for adequate staffing. The number and qualifications of nurses are not delineated in the literature for the care of the patient receiving a local anesthetic. This issue warrants further research. The ASA practice guideline states that there should be an adequate number of personnel (eg, licensed and qualified nurses) to meet the patient's needs for all procedures performed.[23] The literature review supports the practice guideline and recommends adequate staffing levels.[24]

Recommendation II

The perioperative RN should monitor and document the patient's physiological and psychological responses, identify nursing diagnoses based on assessment of the data, and implement the plan of care.

Patient assessment, diagnosis, and implementation are standards of perioperative nursing practice.[14] The American Nurses Association's *Nursing: Scope and Standards of Practice*[15] and the AORN "Standards of perioperative nursing"[14] direct the RN to collect patient health data that are relevant to the patient's situation (eg, surgical or invasive procedure), analyze the assessment data, and implement nursing interventions.

Monitoring of the patient's physiological and psychological status may lead to early detection of potential complications.[19] Changes in the patient's cardiac rhythm and rate, blood pressure, and mental status may be early manifestations of LAST.

Monitoring parameters and frequency are unresolved issues that warrant further research. Clark[6] advocated for monitoring vital signs before the procedure and then at five-minute intervals. Kosh et al[28] recommended taking the vital signs before patient discharge.

The collective evidence supports monitoring and interpreting the patient's physiological and psychological responses while he or she is receiving a local anesthetic during a procedure. One practice guideline[16] and nine literature reviews[1,4,5,7,11,20,26-28] describe the signs and symptoms of LAST.

The limitations of the evidence are that no studies were found that identify the parameters that should be monitored or the optimal frequency for monitoring. Further research is needed.

The benefits of patient monitoring outweigh the harms. Benefits include early detection of symptoms of LAST or allergic reaction, pain, and anxiety.

II.a. The perioperative RN should determine data collection priorities based on the patient's condition and needs and the procedure to be performed. Data collection should include the parameters to be monitored (eg, heart rate and rhythm, blood pressure, level of consciousness), the frequency (eg, baseline,[6] after local anesthetic administration, every five[6] to 15 minutes, postprocedure,[28] before discharge[29]), and documentation. *[2: Moderate Evidence]*

In the case of *Messer v Martin*, the court upheld the standard of care to monitor the patient's vital signs during and after a procedure performed with the patient under local anesthesia. In this case, a patient underwent a surgical procedure with local anesthesia and then fainted in the elevator after leaving the clinic. The patient filed suit against the physician, the clinic, and the professional liability carrier for neglecting to monitor the patient's postoperative vital signs and was granted summary judgment. An expert RN witness stated in a deposition that the standard of care was to monitor the patient's vital signs. The assigned nurse failed to monitor the vital signs during or after the procedure.[29]

II.a.1. Baseline patient monitoring[7] and documentation should include
- pulse,
- blood pressure,[6,28]
- respiratory rate,[19]
- SpO_2 by pulse oximetry,[6,19]
- pain level,
- anxiety level, and
- level of consciousness.[6,28]

[2: Moderate Evidence]

II.a.2. Intraoperative and postoperative patient monitoring[7] and documentation should include
- pain level,
- anxiety level, and
- level of consciousness.[6,28]

[2: Moderate Evidence]

II.a.3. Intraoperative and postoperative patient monitoring[7] and documentation may include
- pulse,
- blood pressure,[6,28]
- heart rhythm and rate,
- respiratory rate,[19] and
- SpO_2 by pulse oximetry.[6,19]

[2: Moderate Evidence]

Recommendation III

The perioperative RN should receive initial and ongoing education and competency verification on his or her understanding of local anesthesia pharmacology, calculation of total dose, contraindications, desired effects, adverse effects, and resuscitation.

The collective evidence supports that perioperative RNs should have knowledge of the local anesthetic medication's indications for use, contraindications, desired effects, and adverse effects. Local anesthetics produce the desired effect of pain relief by preventing the generation and conduction of nerve impulses by the peripheral nervous system and the CNS.[1,11,30] Although LAST and allergic reactions are rare events, early detection and treatment can lead to a better outcome for the patient. Early recognition of an adverse

Table 2. Local Anesthetic Classification, Onset, and Duration

Local Anesthetic	Classification	Onset	Duration
Bupivacaine[1]	Aminoamide	Slow	Long
Lidocaine[1]	Aminoamide	Fast	Medium
Mepivacaine[1]	Aminoamide	Fast	Medium
Prilocaine[2]	Aminoamide	Fast	Medium
Procaine[2]	Aminoester	Slow	Short
Ropivacaine[1]	Aminoamide	Slow	Long
Tetracaine[1]	Aminoester	Slow	Long

References
1. Culp Jr WC, Culp WC. Practical application of local anesthetics. *J Vasc Interv Radiol.* 2011;22(2):111-118.
2. Jackson T, McLure HA. Pharmacology of local anesthetics. *Ophthalmol Clin North Am.* 2006;19(2):155-161.

reaction that could lead to LAST,[16] cessation of the local anesthetic injection, and treatment may prevent symptom progression.[4,10]

The limitations of the evidence are that no studies were found that have investigated the perioperative RN's knowledge of local anesthetics as a risk factor for the patient's development of LAST or allergic reaction. Further research is needed to define the role of the perioperative RN in early detection of LAST and adverse medication reactions (eg, allergy).

The benefits of the perioperative RN knowing the local anesthetic medication's indications for use, contraindications, desired effects, and adverse effects outweigh the harms. Benefits include the potential for early detection and treatment of LAST and allergic reactions.

III.a. The perioperative RN should receive initial and ongoing education and competency verification on the local anesthetic recommended dose, onset, and duration of action.[18]

Four literature reviews[1,4,11,30] describe local anesthetic duration and onset. Local anesthetics have different durations of action depending on their affinity for protein and the length of time the local anesthetic is near the neural fibers.[1,30] Constriction of the blood vessels in the area delays absorption. Adding a vasopressor (eg, epinephrine) to the local anesthetic will delay absorption and prolong the effect.[4,30]

Local anesthetics can be classified into two groups: aminoamide and aminoester.[1,11] The local anesthetic's molecular structure determines its classification.[1,11] The aminoamide group includes lidocaine, bupivacaine, mepivacaine, and prilocaine.[11] The aminoester group includes tetracaine[1] and procaine.[11] Local anesthetics differ in the time to onset of action and duration (Table 2).[1,11]

III.a.1. Before administration of the local anesthetic, the perioperative RN should verify the correct dosing parameters and identify the patient-specific maximum dose by consulting either the health care organization's medication formulary, a pharmacist, a physician, or the product information sheet or other published reference material.[18] *[2: Moderate Evidence]*

Estimating the maximum dosage before administration of the local anesthetic,[7] using the smallest amount of local anesthetic to achieve the desired effect,[16] injecting the medication incrementally,[1,10,16,31] avoiding intravascular injection, and frequent aspiration[1,10] are important safety measures to decrease the risk of LAST.[7]

Tanawuttiwat et al[32] reported the case of a patient undergoing implantation of a cardioverter defibrillator under local anesthesia. The surgical site at the left infraclavicular area was infiltrated with 20 mL 2% lidocaine followed by another 10 mL to relieve the patient's discomfort. A contrast venogram showed an obstruction in the axillary-subclavian system. The team switched to the right side and infiltrated this site with 30 mL 2% lidocaine. While the surgeon was closing the site, the patient suffered a tonic-clonic seizure followed by pulseless electrical activity. The patient was successfully revived.

The result of the lidocaine level drawn during resuscitation was 8.7 mcg/mL. The normal value at this organization was 1.5 mcg/mL to 5.0 mcg/mL. Contributing factors were the patient's advanced heart failure and age and mixed metabolic and respiratory acidosis. The authors recommended that risk factors for lidocaine toxicity be identified before surgery.[32]

III.a.2. The perioperative RN should document the local anesthetic administered, including the
- medication,
- strength,
- total amount administered,

- route,
- time,
- expiration date,
- lot number,
- response, and
- adverse reactions.[18]

[2: Moderate Evidence]

III.b. The perioperative RN should know the symptoms of LAST, including
- metallic taste,[4,11,16,28]
- numbness of the tongue and lips,[1,4,11,16,20,26,28]
- auditory changes (eg, tinnitus),[4,7,11,16,20,26,28]
- light-headedness,[1,4,7,11,20,26]
- dysarthria (eg, slurred speech),[4,11,26]
- shivering,[5]
- tremors,[5]
- confusion,[11,20,26,28]
- agitation,[11,16,26]
- syncope,[20,26]
- seizures,[1,4,7,11,20,16,26,27]
- coma,[4,7,11,16]
- tachycardia/hypertension (initially),[5,7,16,20,26]
- bradycardia/hypotension (with increased toxicity),[11,16,27,28]
- ventricular arrhythmias,[4,5,16,20,26,28]
- asystole,[4,26,27] and
- respiratory arrest.[4,16,20]

[1: Strong Evidence]

Local anesthetic systemic toxicity is well documented in the literature. The evidence review included a systematic review,[8] a retrospective nonexperimental study,[9] a clinical practice guideline,[16] and 12 literature reviews that describe the signs and symptoms of LAST.[1,7,10,11,20,26,27,30,31,33-35] The collective evidence indicates that the incidence of LAST is rare[8-11] and that LAST occurs as serum levels of the local anesthetic increases, presenting as CNS and CVS complications.[1-7] No randomized controlled trials (RCTs) have studied LAST in humans, and conducting RCTs with human participants raises ethical concerns.[16,36,37]

The CNS signs and symptoms of LAST can be divided into three phases: initial, excitation, and depression. During the initial phase, patients may experience tinnitus, confusion, lightheadedness, dizziness, drowsiness, an abnormal sense of taste (eg, metallic taste), and numbness or tingling of the lips and tongue.[20] During the excitation phase, patients may experience tonic-clonic convulsions. During the depression phase, patients may experience unconsciousness, CNS depression, and respiratory arrest.[20]

The CNS signs and symptoms of LAST also can be divided into three phases. The initial phase includes hypertension and tachycardia during the CNS excitation phase. The intermediate phase includes myocardial depression, decreased cardiac output, and mild to moderate hypertension. The third, terminal phase, includes peripheral vasodilation,[20] hypotension,[7] sinus bradycardia,[20] conduction defects,[20] ventricular dysrhythmias,[20] cardiovascular collapse,[20,7] and death.[7]

Liu et al[8] conducted a systematic review of adverse drug reactions to local anesthetics. Studies included in the review were RCTs, nonrandomized controlled trials, and cross-sectional studies. The 101 articles reviewed contained 1,645 events. Lidocaine was involved in 43.17% of the events and bupivacaine was involved in 16.32% of the events. In 1,645 events, there were seven deaths.

Fuzier et al,[9] in a retrospective review, studied adverse drug reactions to local anesthetics reported to the French Pharmacovigilance System from 1995 to 2006. There were 210,017 reported adverse events. Local anesthetics were suspected in 727 reports, representing 0.3% of the total. The second most common type of adverse event from local anesthetics was neurological (eg, seizures), numbering 161 reports (22.1% of the cases). Cardiovascular events were the fourth most frequently reported at 111 (15.3% of the cases). Ropivacaine was used in 10 of the procedures. The cardiovascular events included chest discomfort, hypotension, cardiac arrest, bradycardia, tachycardia, and circulatory shock. Three of the 22 patients who experienced cardiac arrest died. Respiratory events (eg, dyspnea, bronchoconstriction, respiratory arrest) occurred in 2.8% of the cases.

In the practice advisory of the American Society of Regional Anesthesia and Pain Medicine (ASRA), Neal et al[16] reviewed human and animal experimental studies. In the classic presentation, LAST CNS excitement precedes cardiac toxicity. Examination of published case reports showed variability in the onset, signs, symptoms, and duration of LAST in nearly 40% of the cases. The authors concluded that it is critical for health care practitioners to recognize the early signs of LAST, be aware of the variability, and consider LAST for unexplained agitation, CNS depression or progressive hypotension, or bradycardia or ventricular arrhythmias. Analysis of LAST case reports demonstrated that one-third of the patients with cardiac and CNS toxicity had pre-existing cardiac, neurologic, or metabolic disease (eg, diabetes, renal failure). Symptoms occurred in as little as 56 seconds to more than five minutes after injection.

Di Gregorio et al[26] retrospectively reviewed 93 published reports of LAST during a 30-year period from 1979 to 2009. The cases were analyzed for onset of toxicity and signs and symptoms. The onset of LAST generally occurred after a single injection of a local anesthetic. Onset occurred in less than one minute in more than 50% of the cases and less than five minutes in 75% of the cases. The median time for onset of signs of toxicity was 52.5 seconds. In 25% of the cases, symptoms occurred five minutes or more

LOCAL ANESTHESIA

TABLE 3. TREATMENT FOR LOCAL ANESTHETIC SYSTEMIC TOXICITY

- Suppress seizures (eg, with benzodiazepines)[1,2]
- Avoid vasopressin, calcium channel blockers, beta blockers, or local anesthetics[1]
- Reduce individual epinephrine doses to < 1mcg/kg[1]
- Infuse a 20% lipid emulsion[1,3]
    - Administer an IV bolus 1.5 mL/kg (lean body mass) longer than 1 minute (approximately 100 mL).[1-3]
    - Infuse at 0.25 mL/kg/minute (approximately 18 mL/minute; adjust by roller clamp)[1]
    - Repeat the bolus once or twice for persistent cardiovascular collapse.[1]
    - Double the infusion rate to 0.5 m/kg/minute if blood pressure remains low.[1]
    - Continue infusion for at least 10 minutes after attaining circulatory stability.[1]
    - The recommended upper limit is approximately 10 mL/kg lipid emulsion during the first 30 minutes.[1]
- Avoid propofol in patients showing signs of cardiovascular instability[1,4]
- Alert the nearest facility with cardiopulmonary bypass capability[1]

REFERENCES

1. Neal JM, Bernards CM, Butterworth JF 4th, et al. ASRA practice advisory on local anesthetic systemic toxicity. Reg Anesth Pain Med. 2010;35(2):152-161.
2. AAGBI Safety Guideline: Management of Severe Local Anaesthetic Toxicity. 2010. Association of Anaesthetists of Great Britain & Ireland. http://www.aagbi.org/sites/default/files/la_toxicity_2010_0.pdf. Accessed October 15, 2014.
3. Vanden Hoek TL, Morrison LJ, Shuster M, et al. Part 12: Cardiac arrest in special situations: 2010 American Heart Association guidelines for cardiopulmonary resuscitation and emergency cardiovascular care. Circulation. 2010;122(18 Suppl 3):S829-61.
4. Mercado P, Weinberg GL. Local anesthetic systemic toxicity: prevention and treatment. Anesthesiol Clin. 2011;29(2):233-242.

---

after initial injection. In a single case, the symptoms of LAST occurred at 60 minutes. Central nervous system symptoms were the most common manifestation of LAST, occurring in 44% of the reports; CVS symptoms occurred in 11% of the reports, and a combination of CNS and CVS symptoms occurred in 45% of the reports.

In a review of the mechanisms and toxicity of LAST, Wolfe and Butterworth[38] concluded that short-acting and lower-potency local anesthetics (eg, lidocaine, mepivacaine) depressed cardiac contractility without causing cardiac arrhythmias. The authors further concluded that longer-acting and higher-potency local anesthetics (eg, bupivacaine, levobupivacaine, ropivacaine) produced conduction defects and cardiac arrhythmias with or without reduced contractile function. A lower ratio dose of bupivacaine, levobupivacaine, and ropivacaine can produce cardiovascular toxicity versus CNS toxicity. Treatment of CNS toxicity from local anesthetics is easier and provides better chances for recovery than treatment of cardiovascular toxicity. The outcomes of cardiovascular toxicity from local anesthetics may be serious injury or death.

Byrne and Engelbrecht[20] conducted a review of the toxicity of local anesthetic agents and concluded that no dose of local anesthetic is safe if administered incorrectly (eg, intravascularly, intra-arterially). The authors found that toxicity is dependent on the absolute plasma level and the rate of the rise in the plasma level. Most incidences of toxicity are caused by intravascular injection of local anesthetic, and an intra-arterial injection is more dangerous than an IV injection. Bupivacaine, levobupivacaine, and ropivacaine are more toxic than lidocaine and prilocaine. In 17 of 20 case reports of LAST, the local anesthetic used was ropivacaine or bupivacaine.

III.c. The perioperative RN should receive initial and ongoing education and competency verification of the treatment of LAST. *[2: Moderate Evidence]*

The collective evidence indicates that early recognition of LAST symptoms and treatment are very important.[4,21,39] Initial treatment should focus on airway management.[4] Hypoxemia and acidosis intensify the effects of LAST.[4,36] Four articles describe the importance of early recognition, airway management with oxygenation, and treatment.[4,21,36,39]

III.c.1. If LAST occurs, the perioperative RN should
- call for help (eg, anesthesia professional, code team, 911),[1,10,16,40]
- help maintain the airway,[10,16,40]
- ventilate with 100% oxygen,[1,10,16,40]
- assist with basic or advanced cardiac life support,[6]
- be prepared to establish or assist with IV access,[6,16,40] and
- be prepared to assist with the administration of 20% lipid emulsion therapy.[16]

[1: Strong Evidence]

The "ASRA practice advisory on local anesthetic systemic toxicity,"[16] the Association of Anesthetists of Great Britain and Ireland's *AAGBI Safety Guideline: Management*

LOCAL ANESTHESIA

of Severe Local Anaesthetic Toxicity,[40] and the American Heart Association's guidelines for cardiac arrest in special situations[41] provide guidance for treating LAST (Table 3).

The collective evidence indicates that early recognition and treatment of LAST symptoms with a focus on airway management are important because hypoxemia and acidosis potentiate the effects of LAST.[4,36,39]

The use of lipid emulsion therapy for the treatment of LAST started with animal testing in 1998, and the first clinical use was in 2006.[36] Current recommendations have evolved from the laboratory studies and case reports of lipid emulsion treatment for LAST.[36,42]

Although case reports[43-45] of using lipid emulsion therapy have limitations (eg, reporting only favorable outcomes; underreporting of unfavorable outcomes; variability in dosing and timing), they provide the best evidence available for the treatment of LAST.[3,36,39] Ozcan and Weinberg[39] reviewed 10 case reports in which lipid emulsion was used for bupivacaine-related LAST. The symptoms of all 10 patients resolved after treatment with lipid emulsion. The authors reviewed seven case reports that used lipid emulsion for non-bupivacaine-related LAST. The symptoms of six of the seven patients resolved after treatment. The authors concluded there is mounting clinical evidence that suggests early administration of lipid emulsion with effective cardiopulmonary resuscitation might restore circulation without the use of large doses of vasopressors.

III.c.2. The perioperative RN should monitor the patient with LAST for signs of cardiovascular instability after the patient receives lipid emulsion therapy. *[2: Moderate Evidence]*

The recommended action is supported by a case study. After the successful resuscitation with cardiopulmonary resuscitation and lipid emulsion of a patient who received an accidental intravascular injection of bupivacaine, Marwick et al[44] reported cardiac toxicity 40 minutes after the cessation of lipid emulsion therapy. The authors attributed the cardiovascular instability to a recurrence of LAST after lipid rescue.

III.d. The perioperative RN should receive initial and ongoing education and competency verification on recognition of the signs and symptoms of an allergic reaction to a local anesthetic, including
- anxiety,[13,46]
- bronchospasm,[46,47]
- dizziness,[13,46]
- dyspnea,[46]
- erythema,[13,48]
- edema,[13,46-48]
- heart arrhythmias (ie, tachycardia, bradycardia),[46]
- hypotension,[46-48]
- nausea,[46]
- pallor,[46]
- palpitations,[46,48]
- pruritus,[13,46-48]
- rash,[13,46,47]
- syncope,[13,46,48] and
- urticaria.[13,46-48]

[2: Moderate Evidence]

Allergic reactions to local anesthetics are rare, occurring in less than 1% of all patients who receive a local anesthetic.[12,13] The primary symptoms of an immediate allergic reaction to a local anesthetic are cutaneous and occur within a few minutes of the injection, although symptoms may occur as late as one month after the injection.[47] The evidence review included five retrospective reviews,[13,46-49] nine case reports,[50-58] and a literature review.[12] The retrospective reviews investigated the prevalence of a true local anesthetic allergy among patients who reported a hypersensitivity reaction and sought evaluation.[13,46-49]

Batinac et al[13] retrospectively reviewed and analyzed the medical records of 331 patients who were referred to the dermatology department for evaluation of their local anesthetic hypersensitivity. The aim of the study was to quantify the prevalence of a true local anesthetic allergy among the referred patients. The patients' skin was tested, and three patients (0.91%) had an allergic reaction. Most of the patients' reported adverse reactions to local anesthetics were determined not to be immune related and may have been vasovagal or anxiety reactions. Psychological stress, fear of the procedure, or fear of the injection may cause psychological symptoms that alter blood levels of stress hormones. These symptoms included altered heart rate, generalized weakness, dizziness, fainting, anxiety, and fear. The researchers concluded that allergic reactions to local anesthetics comprise less than 1% of the adverse drug reactions to local anesthetics. The true allergic reactions are type IV immune reactions.

Harboe et al[46] retrospectively reviewed the medical records of 135 patients referred to the allergy department for evaluation of adverse reactions to local anesthetics. Evaluation included a case history review, skin testing, a subcutaneous challenge test, and *in vitro* IgE analysis. Sensitivity tests were also conducted for latex, chlorhexidine, and relevant medications based on the referral information. The researchers found 1.5% of the patients had a hypersensitivity to local anesthetics and concluded that this rate was consistent with the findings of other studies. They also found that 7% of the patients had allergic reactions to the other substances tested. These results indicate that other substances should be investigated as a cause of hypersensitivity reactions to local anesthetics. Psychological reactions were common during the testing.

Saito et al[49] used the leukocyte migration test (LMT) to evaluate 43 patients who had a suspected allergy to amide-type local anesthetic agents (eg, lidocaine, bupivacaine). Twenty patients had a positive LMT for lidocaine hydrochloride. The researchers tested 15 of the positive patients with lidocaine that contained antiseptic agents (eg, parabens, sodium pyrosulfite) and found a 100% positive reaction. When tested with lidocaine hydrochloride alone, only 20% tested positive, indicating that 80% of the reactions were caused by the antiseptic not the lidocaine. Paraben additives are also in cosmetics and hair products, which may lead to sensitization from daily use.

The researchers postulated that there is a risk of a local anesthetic allergy during first-time administration because of the daily paraben sensitization by cosmetic and hair products. Another key finding was the relationship between an amide-type local anesthetic allergy and history of a medication allergy. Patients with a history of a medication allergy had a twentyfold risk of developing an amide-type local anesthetic allergy compared with patients who had no medication allergies. Based on the prevalence of antiseptic allergies, the researchers suggested that using local anesthetic agents with no antiseptics is preferred.[49]

Amado et al[59] patch tested 1,143 patients using the North American Contact Dermatitis Group Standard Allergen Tray. There were 16 cases of allergic contact dermatitis and delayed hypersensitivity to lidocaine. A patient's previous exposure to lidocaine was a factor in determining lidocaine hypersensitivity. The authors concluded that over-the-counter lidocaine products could be the source of exposure and sensitization to lidocaine. Anti-hemorrhoidal products are the most common cause of allergic contact dermatitis. Other commonly used products that contain lidocaine are antiseptics, sunburn relief gels, and pain relief preparations (eg, creams, patches, sprays).

Fuzier et al[47] analyzed documented adverse drug reactions to amide local anesthetics (ie, lidocaine, bupivacaine, ropivacaine, levobupivicaine, mepivacaine) reported to two French databases during a 12-year period. Documentation included a clear and detailed medical history with a positive skin test (eg, patch test, prick test, intradermal injection). The aim of the study was to define the clinical, allergic, and pharmacological components of the adverse drug reactions. The main symptom was skin eruptions (eg, urticaria). The symptoms occurred in as little as a few minutes to as late as one month. Six patients demonstrated cross-reactivity between amide-type local anesthetics.

Bhole et al[12] conducted a review of local allergy reactions that were a type 1 or IgE-mediated immediate hypersensitivity. They identified and analyzed 23 case series involving 2,978 patients. A true IgE-mediated allergy to a local anesthetic was demonstrated in 29 patients, which is a prevalence rate of less than 1%. Seventy-five percent of these patients were allergic to amide local anesthetics. The researchers postulated that the higher rate of allergy to amide agents compared to aminoester agents was a result of the preferred use of amide agents.

There are numerous case reports of local anesthetic allergies confirmed with the patient's medical history and patch testing.[50-58] Reported symptoms include redness,[50-52] swelling,[50,51,54,56] blistering,[50] vesicular dermatitis,[51] eczematous dermatitis,[58] urticaria,[57] itching,[57] conjunctivitis,[56] bronchospasm,[55] lightheadedness,[54] wheezing,[54] and perianal dermatitis.[51,53]

Recommendation IV

The perioperative RN should provide patient education regarding perioperative care of patients undergoing local anesthesia.

One of nursing's primary responsibilities is patient education.[14]

A limitation of the evidence is a lack of studies investigating the benefits of teaching the patient about the local anesthesia care experience.

The benefits of educating the patient outweigh the harms. Benefits include the potential for increased patient cooperation, compliance with postoperative instructions, and anxiety and pain management.

IV.a. Education information for local anesthesia patients should include
- the expected sequence of events before, during,[60] and immediately after the procedure[61];
- instructions on completing a pain level assessment (eg, visual analog scale);
- requesting additional pain relief measures during and after the procedure; and
- postoperative signs and symptoms that should be reported to a designated health care provider.

[2: Moderate Evidence]

Two literature reviews support explaining the intraoperative[60] or postoperative[61] sequence of events to the patient. Mitchell[60] suggested that patient education about the intraoperative experience may reduce anxiety. A literature review by Davis[61] suggests that explaining the sequence of perioperative events may reduce patient anxiety and help the patient establish realistic expectations.

IV.a.1. Teaching strategies should be appropriate to the patient's learning needs, language preference, culture, cognitive ability, and developmental level.[14] *[2: Moderate Evidence]*

IV.a.2. The perioperative RN should assess the patient's comprehension of new information.[17] [2: Moderate Evidence]

Recommendation V

Policies and procedures for the care of the patient receiving local anesthesia should be developed, reviewed periodically, revised as necessary, and readily available in the practice setting.

Policies and procedures assist in the development of patient safety, quality assessment, and performance improvement activities. Policies and procedures establish authority, responsibility, and accountability within the organization. Policies and procedures also serve as operational guidelines that are used to minimize patient risk for injury or complications, standardize practice, direct perioperative personnel, and establish continuous performance improvement programs.

The Centers for Medicare & Medicaid Services (CMS) requires health care organizations that provide care to patients covered by Medicare and Medicaid to establish policies and procedures for patient care.[62,63] The evidence review for this guideline included the CMS regulatory requirements for policies and procedures[62,63] and two literature reviews.[6,28]

V.a. A multidisciplinary team should develop policies and procedures regarding the care of the patient receiving local anesthesia without monitoring by an anesthesia professional. [4: Benefits Balanced with Harms]

The evidence review found no research evidence to support or refute this recommendation. Development of policies and procedures that guide and support patient care, treatment, and services is a regulatory requirement for both hospitals and ambulatory settings.[62,63]

V.a.1. The multidisciplinary team should include representatives from perioperative nursing, surgery, anesthesia, and other health care departments as deemed necessary. [4: Benefits Balanced with Harms]

V.b. Policies and procedures regarding the care of the patient receiving local anesthesia should include
- patient assessment criteria;
- personnel qualifications, competencies, and certifications (eg, certified basic life support, certified advanced cardiovascular life support)[16,40];
- staffing requirements[23];
- monitoring (ie, parameters, frequency);
- risk assessment and criteria for consultation with an anesthesia professional;
- recovery and discharge criteria;
- documentation requirements (eg, vital signs, anxiety level, medication response);
- medication supplies[23] (eg, lipid emulsion, resuscitation medications);
- emergency equipment (eg, supplemental oxygen, suction apparatus, resuscitation)[23,62];
- emergency procedures[16,40]; and
- emergency transfer protocols.[16,62]

[2: Moderate Evidence]

Three clinical practice guidelines[16,23,40] and CMS requirements[62] support portions of the policy and procedure recommendations.

V.b.1. At a minimum, personnel should be competent in basic life support.[16,40] [1: Strong Evidence]

Serious cardiac or respiratory complications can occur abruptly after the administration of local anesthetic medications. If the medication enters the bloodstream directly, seizures, circulatory and respiratory distress, cardiovascular collapse, or even death can result. The initial treatment of LAST is maintaining an airway and basic life support.[16,40]

Glossary

Local anesthetic systemic toxicity (LAST): An uncommon, potentially fatal, toxic reaction that occurs when the threshold blood levels of a local anesthetic are exceeded by an inadvertent, intravascular injection or slow systemic absorption of a large, extravascular volume of local anesthetic.

References

1. Culp WC Jr, Culp WC. Practical application of local anesthetics. *J Vasc Intervent Radiol.* 2011;22(2):111-118. [VA]
2. Bern S, Akpa BS, Kuo I, Weinberg G. Lipid resuscitation: a life-saving antidote for local anesthetic toxicity. *Curr Pharm Biotechnol.* 2011;12(2):313-319. [VA]
3. Ciechanowicz S, Patil V. Lipid emulsion for local anesthetic systemic toxicity. *Anesthesiol Res Pract.* 2012;2012:131784. [VA]
4. Morau D, Ahern S. Management of local anesthetic toxicity. *Int Anesthesiol Clin.* 2010;48(4):117-140. [VB]
5. Khatri KP, Rothschild L, Oswald S, Weinberg G. Current concepts in the management of systemic local anesthetic toxicity. *Adv Anesth.* 2010;28(1):147-159. [VA]
6. Clark MK. Lipid emulsion as rescue for local anesthetic-related cardiotoxicity. *J Perianesth Nurs.* 2008;23(2):111-117. [VB]
7. Bourne E, Wright C, Royse C. A review of local anesthetic cardiotoxicity and treatment with lipid emulsion. *Local Reg Anesth.* 2010;3:11-19. [VA]
8. Liu W, Yang X, Li C, Mo A. Adverse drug reactions to local anesthetics: a systematic review. *Oral Surg, Oral Med, Oral Pathol Oral Radiol.* 2013;115(3):319-327. [IIIB]
9. Fuzier R, Lapeyre-Mestre M, Samii K, Montastruc JL; French Association of Regional Pharmacovigilance Centres. Adverse drug reactions to local anaesthetics: a review of the French pharmacovigilance database. *Drug Saf.* 2009;32(4):345-356. [IIIB]
10. Mercado P, Weinberg GL. Local anesthetic systemic toxicity: prevention and treatment. *Anesthesiol Clin.* 2011;29(2):233-242. [VA]
11. Jackson T, McLure HA. Pharmacology of local anesthetics. *Ophthalmol Clin North Am.* 2006;19(2):155-161. [VB]
12. Bhole MV, Manson AL, Seneviratne SL, Misbah SA. IgE-mediated allergy to local anaesthetics: separating

fact from perception: a UK perspective. *Br J Anaesth.* 2012;108(6):903-911. [VA]

13. Batinac T, Sotosek Tokmadzic V, Peharda V, Brajac I. Adverse reactions and alleged allergy to local anesthetics: analysis of 331 patients. *J Dermatol.* 2013;40(7):522-527. [IIIA]

14. Standards of perioperative nursing. In: *Perioperative Standards and Recommended Practices.* Denver, CO: AORN, Inc; 2014:3-18. [IVB]

15. American Nurses Association. *Nursing: Scope and Standards of Practice.* Silver Spring, MD: American Nurses Association; 2010. [IVB]

16. Neal JM, Bernards CM, Butterworth JF 4th, et al. ASRA practice advisory on local anesthetic systemic toxicity. *Reg Anesth Pain Med.* 2010;35(2):152-161. [IVA]

17. Petersen C. *Perioperative Nursing Data Set: The Perioperative Nursing Vocabulary.* 3rd ed. Denver, CO: AORN, Inc; 2011. [IVB]

18. Guideline for medication safety. In: *Guidelines for Perioperative Practice.* Denver, CO: AORN, Inc; 2015:291-329. [IVB]

19. Treasure T, Bennett J. Office-based anesthesia. *Oral Maxillofac Surg Clin North Am.* 2007;19(1):45-57. [VB]

20. Byrne K, Engelbrecht C. Toxicity of local anaesthetic agents. *Trends Anaesth Crit Care.* 2013;3(1):25-30. [VB]

21. Weinberg GL. Current concepts in resuscitation of patients with local anesthetic cardiac toxicity. *Reg Anesth Pain Med.* 2002;27(6):568-575. [VB]

22. ASA Physical Status Classification System. American Society of Anesthesiologists. http://www.asahq.org/Home/For-Members/Clinical-Information/ASA-Physical-Status-Classification-System. Accessed October 15, 2014. [VA]

23. American Society of Anesthesiologists. Guidelines for Ambulatory Anesthesia and Surgery. American Society of Anesthesiologists. http://www.asahq.org/formembers/~/media/For%20Members/documents/Standards%20Guidelines%20Stmts/Ambulatory%20Anesthesia%20and%20Surgery.ashx. Accessed October 15, 2014. [IVC]

24. Kataria T, Cutter TW, Apfelbaum JL. Patient selection in outpatient surgery. *Clin Plast Surg.* 2013;40(3):371-382. [VB]

25. *AORN Position Statement on One Perioperative Registered Nurse Circulator Dedicated to Every Patient Undergoing an Operative or Other Invasive Procedure.* AORN, In.c http://www.aorn.org/Clinical_Practice/Position_Statements/Position_Statements.aspx. Accessed October 15, 2014.

26. Di Gregorio G, Neal JM, Rosenquist RW, Weinberg GL. Clinical presentation of local anesthetic systemic toxicity: a review of published cases, 1979 to 2009. *Reg Anesth Pain Med.* 2010;35(2):181-187. [VA]

27. Fuzier R, Lapeyre-Mestre M. Safety of amide local anesthetics: new trends. *Expert Opin Drug Saf.* 2010;9(5):759-769. [VA]

28. Kosh MC, Miller AD, Michels JE. Intravenous lipid emulsion for treatment of local anesthetic toxicity. *Ther Clin Risk Manag.* 2010;6:449-451. [VC]

29. Failure to monitor local anesthesia pt. before discharge. Case on point: Messer v. Martin, 2004 WL 1171736 N.W.2d -WI(2004). *Nurs Law Regan Rep.* 2004;45(1):2. [VB]

30. Becker DE, Reed KL. Local anesthetics: review of pharmacological considerations. *Anesth Prog.* 2012;59(2):90-101. [VA]

31. Mulroy MF, Hejtmanek MR. Prevention of local anesthetic systemic toxicity. *Reg Anesth Pain Med.* 2010;35(2):177-180. [VB]

32. Tanawuttiwat T, Thisayakorn P, Viles-Gonzalez JF. LAST (Local Anesthetic Systemic Toxicity) but not least: systemic lidocaine toxicity during cardiac intervention. *J Invasive Cardiol.* 2014;26(1):E13-E15. [VB]

33. Butterworth JF 4th. Models and mechanisms of local anesthetic cardiac toxicity: a review. *Reg Anesth Pain Med.* 2010;35(2):167-176. [VA]

34. Mather LE. The acute toxicity of local anesthetics. *Expert Opin Drug Metab Toxicol.* 2010;6(11):1313-1332. [VA]

35. Conroy PH, O'Rourke J. Tumescent anaesthesia. *Surgeon.* 2013;11(4):210-221. [VA]

36. Weinberg GL. Lipid emulsion infusion: resuscitation for local anesthetic and other drug overdose. *Anesthesiology.* 2012;117(1):180-187. [VB]

37. Manavi MV. Lipid infusion as a treatment for local anesthetic toxicity: a literature review. *AANA J.* 2010;78(1):69-78. [VB]

38. Wolfe JW, Butterworth JF. Local anesthetic systemic toxicity: update on mechanisms and treatment. *Curr Opin Anaesthesiol.* 2011;24(5):561-566. [VB]

39. Ozcan MS, Weinberg G. Update on the use of lipid emulsions in local anesthetic systemic toxicity: a focus on differential efficacy and lipid emulsion as part of advanced cardiac life support. *Int Anesthesiol Clin.* 2011;49(4):91-103. [VA]

40. AAGBI Safety Guideline: Management of Severe Local Anaesthetic Toxicity. 2010. Association of Anaesthetists of Great Britain & Ireland. http://www.aagbi.org/sites/default/files/la_toxicity_2010_0.pdf. Accessed October 15, 2014. [IVC]

41. Vanden Hoek TL, Morrison LJ, Shuster M, et al. Part 12: cardiac arrest in special situations: 2010 American Heart Association Guidelines for Cardiopulmonary Resuscitation and Emergency Cardiovascular Care. *Circulation.* 2010;122(18 Suppl 3): S829-S861. [IVA]

42. Burch MS, McAllister RK, Meyer TA. Treatment of local-anesthetic toxicity with lipid emulsion therapy. *Am J Health Syst Pharm.* 2011;68(2):125-129. [VB]

43. Gallagher C, Tan JM, Foster C-G. Lipid rescue for bupivacaine toxicity during cardiovascular procedures. *Heart Int.* 2010;5(1):20-21. [VB]

44. Marwick PC, Levin AI, Coetzee AR. Recurrence of cardiotoxicity after lipid rescue from bupivacaine-induced cardiac arrest. *Anesth Analg.* 2009;108(4):1344-1346. [VA]

45. Litz RJ. Roessel T, Heller AR, Stehr SN. Reversal of central nervous system and cardiac toxicity after local anesthetic intoxication by lipid emulsion injection. *Anesth Analg.* 2008;106(5):1575-1577. [VB]

46. Harboe T, Guttormsen AB, Aarebrot S, Dybendal T, Irgens A, Florvaag E. Suspected allergy to local anaesthetics: follow-up in 135 cases. *Acta Anaesthesiol Scand.* 2010;54(5):536-542. [IIIB]

47. Fuzier R, Lapeyre-Mestre M, Mertes PM, et al. Immediate- and delayed-type allergic reactions to amide local anesthetics: clinical features and skin testing. *Pharmacoepidemiol Drug Saf.* 2009;18(7):595-601. [IIIC]

48. Grzanka A, Misiolek H, Filipowska A, Miśkiewicz-Orczyk K, Jarzab J. Adverse effects of local anaesthetics—allergy, toxic reactions or hypersensitivity. *Anestezjol Intens Ter.* 2010;42(4):175-178. [IIIB]

49. Saito M, Abe M, Furukawa T, et al. Study on patients who underwent suspected diagnosis of allergy to amide-type local anesthetic agents by the leukocyte migration test. *Allergol Int.* 2014;63(2):267-277. [IIIA]

50. Levy J, Lifshitz T. Lidocaine hypersensitivity after subconjunctival injection. *Can J Ophthalmol.* 2006;41(2):204-206. [VB]

51. Gunson TH, Greig DE. Allergic contact dermatitis to all three classes of local anaesthetic. *Contact Derm.* 2008;59(2):126-127. [VB]

52. Timmermans MW, Bruynzeel DP, Rustemeyer T. Allergic contact dermatitis from EMLA cream: concomitant sensitization to both local anesthetics lidocaine and prilocaine. *J Deutschen Dermatologischen Gesellschaft [Journal of the German Society of Dermatology].* 2009;7(3):237-238. [VA]

53. Yuen WY, Schuttelaar ML, Barkema LW, Coenraads PJ. Bullous allergic contact dermatitis to lidocaine. *Contact Derm.* 2009;61(5):300-301. [VA]

54. Haugen RN, Brown CW. Case reports: type I hypersensitivity to lidocaine. *J Drugs Dermatol.* 2007;6(12):1222-1223. [VA]

55. Caron AB. Allergy to multiple local anesthetics. *Allergy Asthma Proc.* 2007;28(5):600-601. [VC]

56. Fellinger C, Wantke F, Hemmer W, Sesztak-Greinecker G, Wohrl S. The rare case of a probably true ige-mediated allergy to local anaesthetics. *Case Rep Med.* 2013;2013:201586. [VA]

57. Gonzalez-Delgado P, Anton R, Soriano V, Zapater P, Niveiro E. Cross-reactivity among amide-type local anesthetics in a case of allergy to mepivacaine. *J Investig Allergol Clin Immunol.* 2006;16(5):311-313. [VB]

58. Wobser M, Gaigl Z, Trautmann A. The concept of "compartment allergy": prilocaine injected into different skin layers. *Allergy Asthma Clin Immunol.* 2011;7(1):7. [VB]

59. Amado A, Sood A, Taylor JS. Contact allergy to lidocaine: a report of sixteen cases. *Dermatitis.* 2007;18(4):215-220. [VB]

60. Mitchell M. Conscious surgery: influence of the environment on patient anxiety. *J Adv Nurs.* 2008;64(3):261-271. [IIIB]

61. Davis-Evans Chassidy. Alleviating anxiety and preventing panic attacks in the surgical patient. *AORN J.* 2013;97(3): 355-363. [VB]

62. State Operations Manual Appendix L: Guidance for Surveyors: Ambulatory Surgical Centers. Rev 99; 2014. Centers for Medicare & Medicaid Services. http://www.cms.gov/Regulations-and-Guidance/Guidance/Manuals/downloads/som107ap_l_ambulatory.pdf. Accessed October 15, 2014.

63. State Operations Manual Appendix A: Survey Protocol, Regulations and Interpretive Guidelines for Hospitals. Rev 105;2014. Centers for Medicare & Medicaid Services. https://www.cms.gov/Regulations-and-Guidance/Guidance/Transmittals/Downloads/R105SOMA.pdf. Accessed October 15, 2014.

Acknowledgements

Lead Author
Mary J. Ogg, MSN, RN, CNOR
Perioperative Nursing Specialist
AORN Nursing Department
Denver, Colorado

Contributing Author
Ramona L. Conner, MSN, RN, CNOR
Manager, Standards and Guidelines
AORN Nursing Department
Denver, Colorado

The authors and AORN thank Lisa Spruce, DNP, RN, ACNS, ACNP, ANP, CNOR, Director of Evidence-based Perioperative Practice, AORN, Inc, Denver, CO; Elayne Kornblatt Phillips, PhD-BSN, MPH, RN, Clinical Associate Professor, University of Virginia, Charlottesville, VA; Melanie F. Sandoval, PhD, RN, Research Nurse Scientist, Perioperative Services, University of Colorado, Aurora, CO; and Deborah S. Hickman, MS, RN, CNOR, CRNFA, Director, Renue Plastic Surgery, Brunswick, GA, for their assistance in developing this guideline.

Publication History
Originally published May 1984, *AORN Journal.*
    Revised September 1989. Revised August 1993.
    Revised November 1997; published February 1998.
    Reformatted July 2000.
    Revised November 2001; published April 2002, *AORN Journal.*
    Revised 2006; published in *Standards, Recommended Practices, and Guidelines*, 2007 edition.
    Minor editing revisions made to omit *Perioperative Nursing Data Set* codes; reformatted September 2012 for publication in *Perioperative Standards and Recommended Practices*, 2013 edition.
    Revised October 2014; published in *Guidelines for Perioperative Practice*, 2015 edition.

GUIDELINE FOR MINIMALLY INVASIVE SURGERY

The following Guideline for Minimally Invasive Surgery was developed by the AORN Recommended Practices Committee and was approved by the AORN Board of Directors. It was presented as proposed recommendations for comments by members and others. The guideline is effective December 1, 2009. The recommendations in this guideline are intended to be achievable and represent what is believed to be an optimal level of practice. Policies and procedures will reflect variations in practice settings and/or clinical situations that determine the degree to which the guideline can be implemented. AORN recognizes the various settings in which perioperative nurses practice; therefore, this guideline is adaptable to various practice settings. These practice settings include traditional operating rooms (ORs), ambulatory surgery centers, physicians' offices, cardiac catheterization laboratories, endoscopy suites, radiology departments, and all other areas where surgery and other invasive procedures may be performed.

Purpose

This document provides guidance to
- perioperative personnel to reduce risks to patients and the perioperative team during minimally invasive surgery (MIS) and computer-assisted technology procedures;
- perioperative registered nurses (RNs) to assist in managing distention media (eg, gas, fluid) and irrigation fluid; and
- health care administrators to identify considerations, including workplace safety and ergonomics, that need to be addressed when expanding services to accommodate new trends.

Flexible endoscopic gastrointestinal procedures are not addressed in this guideline. For information on the care and cleaning of instruments and related equipment, refer to the AORN "Recommended practices for care and cleaning of instruments and powered surgical equipment"[1] and "Recommended practices for cleaning and processing flexible endoscopes and endoscope accessories."[2] Implementing or expanding MIS and computer-assisted technologies often requires innovative problem solving, state-of-the-art equipment, new relationships between diverse teams, and additional learning requirements for all members of the perioperative team. MIS techniques have evolved from diagnostic techniques to complex operative procedures, primarily because of the documented patient benefits compared to the conventional surgical procedures. Robotic and interventional radiology techniques are examples of computer-assisted trends that continue to evolve and integrate with conventional surgical procedures. Emerging technologies may require construction of new or renovation of existing facilities and also may include audio-visual technology transmission to settings outside the traditional walls of the OR.

Recommendation I

A multidisciplinary planning team should be established to develop the design of new construction or renovation of existing ORs to accommodate MIS, interventional radiology, or other computer-assisted technology equipment. The design considerations should include safety; long-term expansion of services; and compliance with federal, state, and local building regulations.

MIS and computer-assisted procedures are frequently performed in a low-light environment and may involve complex equipment interfaces that include numerous cords, plugs, foot switches, and video equipment. Additional equipment for distention media; fluid management systems; radiologic surveillance; and therapeutic applications (eg, lasers, lithotripsy devices, ultrasound) may contribute to distractions or miscommunications that could compromise safety for both the patient and the perioperative team. An effective OR design accommodates ergonomically safe and efficient use of MIS equipment and supplies, while enabling the perioperative clinical team adequate space to work.[3] Trends for technological expansion in perioperative settings often include complex electronic systems, including web-based information systems and robotic fixtures.[3,4] The goals for technological expansion usually include streamlined communications; better resolution and visualization (eg, augmented reality system, three-dimensional images); increased potential for delineating types of tissue (eg, benign, malignant); and a real-time histological analysis of tissues within the operating field.[5] Progressive nanotechnologies (eg, micro-electrical machinery) and miniaturization of robotic components (eg, intracorporeal mobile devices) open the potential for application of surgical procedures in restricted spaces, including single-cell surgery.[4,5] As design trends and MIS technology evolve toward smaller and more remote equipment, it could result in a reduction in the size of the traditional OR in the future.[6] However, in spite of rapid developments toward miniaturization for diagnostics, expansion to allow for oversized equipment is still a common consideration when planning construction or renovation in perioperative settings. Health care facilities may have a variety of reasons other than financial return for expanding to accommodate new technologies (eg, reputation in the community, growing demand from the public and surgeons to provide state-of-the-art minimally invasive techniques). A cost-benefit analysis for expansion to include robotic services may include the following considerations:

- Procedure times in the OR may increase initially due to the learning curve with robotic technologies, affecting OR utilization.
- Even in an established program, OR productivity may not show increases in efficiency, as robotic procedure times may be the same as conventional techniques.
- The benefits to the patient when a robotic system is used may include reduced blood loss, shortened hospitalization, less postoperative pain, and faster return to normal activities.[4,7,8]
- The benefits to the surgeon when a robotic system is used may include improved ergonomics, improved visualization including three-dimensional imaging, and stabilization of instruments.[9]
- The benefits to the health care organization may include a reduction in length of stay even for patients undergoing more complex procedures with increased patient acuity.

Planning for compliance with local building and zoning codes and state and federal regulations early in the planning stages of a construction or renovation project may prevent costly adjustments later in the project.

I.a. The physical design of the OR, interventional radiology suite, or hybrid OR should allow personnel access to the patient and the surgical field.

I.b. Potential ergonomic hazards specific to MIS and computer-assisted technology should be identified in the design phase of the construction project.[10,11]

Ergonomically positioned monitors help prevent fatigue and musculoskeletal disorders by limiting twisting motions and allowing neck and eye muscles to be relaxed.[12,13] An OR that is too small has restricted walking paths, which increase the risk of slipping, tripping, or falling for members of the perioperative team. An OR that is too large has an increased distance between the supply areas and the surgical field and puts perioperative team members at risk for slipping, tripping, or falling when they have to move quickly across long distances to retrieve supplies or equipment during the procedure.[14-19]

I.b.1. Provisions should be made for preventing slips, trips, and falls.

Floor incongruities of greater than one-fourth of an inch and cords and cables on the floor are factors that increase the risk of slipping, tripping, or falling for members of the perioperative team.[14-19]

I.b.2. Provisions should be made regarding height, hydraulic, or electric mobility and securing ceiling-suspended equipment (eg, booms) to reduce injury risk for the perioperative team.

MIS expansion projects often include physiologic monitors, camera control units, insufflators, and video recording units that are suspended from booms. This allows the premium space around the draped patient to be free of unsterile carts and improves the chances for ergonomic organization of equipment for the sterile surgical team members. Eliminating the need for video carts also allows the unsterile perioperative team members to have fewer obstacles on the floor space and may simplify room cleaning and turnover. The primary disadvantage is the decreased flexibility to move equipment to other rooms.[15,20] Video carts are heavy to move because they have several pieces of equipment on them, increasing the risk of back injury for perioperative team members.[10] Even when ceiling-mounted booms are installed, conventional monitors require heavy-duty booms and substantial physical strength to move.[17] New technologies (eg, flat screen monitors, hydraulic or electric carts and booms) help alleviate the physical strain of moving booms or carts. Securing the monitors to a boom or securing monitors and other equipment to a video cart may prevent injury to patients and personnel as well as damage to equipment.

I.b.3. Provisions should be made for adequate lighting for the unsterile perioperative team to complete their responsibilities without risk of injury despite the low lighting that is required for optimum visualization for the sterile surgical team during MIS procedures.

Ambient blue or green light enhances the MIS screens and allows adequate visibility for other personnel in the room to work safely.[15] However, contrasts in lighting still may have negative consequences for the unsterile perioperative team when they have to adapt their vision between the amplified illumination of the surgical site and the overall dim OR lighting.[14] A wide range of lighting levels can be provided in the OR by using a ring of fluorescent lights around the diffusers and an outer ring of dimmable down-lights. The fluorescent lights can be designed to have two separate switches: one to control a set of white lights, the other to control a set of green lights that are designed to reduce glare.[15] Indirect or diffused lighting in the OR will provide the sterile surgical team with more flexibility in positioning monitors. Voice-activated switching systems also are available.[14]

I.b.4. Video vendors and experts in the field of ergonomic safety should be consulted regarding lighting, optimal procedure table height, and location of booms and monitors.

Five design considerations are associated with non-neutral postures during MIS procedures: position of monitor, use of foot pedals, poorly adjusted table height, the hand-held design of laparoscopic instruments, and static body postures.[12] A study conducted in the Netherlands identified five ergonomically optimal positions and the number of monitors needed for each position when two or three people were scrubbed for the procedure. Each position provided a monitor across from the surgical team member.[17] Ergonomically positioned monitors help prevent fatigue and musculoskeletal disorders by limiting twisting motions and allowing neck and eye muscles to be relaxed.[12,13] Ceiling-suspended monitors that allow monitors to be positioned apart from the rest of the laparoscopic equipment are more versatile when planning ergonomically optimal positions.[21] Research suggests optimal monitor positions include, but are not limited to, the following:

- For the horizontal plane, positioning the monitor straight ahead of the surgical team member, aligned with the forearm-instrument motor axis, will prevent the person from having axial rotation of the spine.
- For the sagittal plane, positioning the monitor lower than eye level, approximately 15 degrees downward, will prevent neck extension.
- For viewing distance, the position of the monitor will depend on the size of the screen. If the monitor is too close, the surgical team member's eyes may undergo extensive accommodation and conversion by the extraocular musculature. If the monitor is too far away, the person may be required to strain and may not be able to see detail.[21]

The amount of glare is another important consideration when positioning monitors. In addition to having high resolution and a high contrast ratio, quality monitors also have a surface material that minimizes the effects of reflected light. Changing the orientation of a monitor (eg, tilt, angle) can create or eliminate glare, which also may be a contributing factor for muscle strain.[14]

I.c. The extent of OR integration and telecommunication technology should be determined and information system interface requirements identified (eg, compatibility between clinical computer-assisted technologies and administrative computer interfaces).

OR integration involves centralized control of audiovisual equipment and information, and is capable of controlling a variety of equipment and activities within the surgical suite.[20] The evolution of software and equipment integration capabilities may require architectural design adjustments or engineering retrofit to accommodate such things as a control desk and housing for the computer and other equipment. Moving the electronics outside the OR room itself frees up space inside the OR, removes a major source of heat from within the OR, and eliminates the need for electronics technicians to enter the sterile environment of an OR to service the equipment.[22] It can save money to install cabling and other infrastructure to accommodate OR integration during construction or renovation, even if a health care facility does not intend to implement OR integration in phase one of the MIS expansion project.[20]

A central database that allows continuous live feeds throughout the health care facility is another important component for ORs that are designed for MIS procedures. The live feed allows data retrieval after the procedure for educational or reporting purposes, including video clips or still images. Full integration of the entire surgical platform can accommodate coordinated scheduling and interfaces with the electronic medical record and monitoring systems.[22] The terms *integrated OR* or *digital OR* may be used for facilities designed with these capabilities.

Picture archiving and communication systems (PACS) monitors, touch-screen, and voice-activated controls are examples of trends that can be incorporated into an MIS expansion project.[15] The term *de-tethering* refers to wireless technology (eg, wireless communications, laptop computers, network portals, e-mail). Privacy, security, and reliability are issues associated with de-tethering.[23]

I.c.1. Planning should include collaboration with vendors to achieve medical device interoperability and upgrade potential.

Consumer electronics with "plug and play" capability have set an expectation that pieces of medical equipment from various manufacturers have the capacity to "talk to each other." The Center for Integration of Medicine and Innovative Technology (CIMIT) is an example of one nonprofit consortium that has established interdisciplinary teams in the Boston area who work toward this goal.[20]

I.c.2. Remote telecommunications technology requirements should be identified to meet the health care organization's strategic plan.

Robotic technology allows an experienced health care provider to gain physical telepresence to interact with patients or other health care providers in remote locations.[24,25] Telemedicine and telesurgery technology have potential for global application for disaster responses (eg, natural disaster, chemical, biological, nuclear attack, battlefields); regional application for providing expertise and access to rural areas to alleviate shortages in medical and surgical specialties; and intraoperative application for allowing anesthesiologists to provide remote support to nurse anesthetists.[25] Current limitations in wireless broadband requirements and the resulting latency in transmission may prevent broad applications of this technology, but the US Army's Telemedicine and Advanced Technology Research Center (TATRC) continues to fund research in this area.[26] Researchers in Canada have found telementoring and telerobotic technologies to be effective tools for providing care to rural areas; however, reimbursement and legal barriers contribute to delays in widespread application and the goal to achieve a uniform standard of care for MIS procedures in rural areas.[24,27]

I.c.3. Considerations to decrease traffic in teaching institutions should be anticipated (eg, integrated camera systems that provide for internal and external web casts).

Audiovisual components are used by OR staff members in providing patient care, but can also be wired to give interns, residents, and visitors a clear view of surgical procedures without requiring them to be in the room. Reducing traffic during patient care decreases the risk for infection and may reduce distraction and noise for the perioperative team.[20,28]

I.d. Work space and architectural and engineering structures should be designed to accommodate progressive technologies and strategic expansion of MIS and computer-assisted services.

Considering expansion (eg, voice-activated technology, centralized command consoles, two-way video and audio connections) and a progression for increased patient acuity and emergencies in the early stages of the design process can potentially increase the long-term value of the construction project and may prevent the necessity for future renovation.[3,20,29,30] Important considerations for MIS expansion projects include, but are not limited to,
- door placement in relation to the sterile field;
- a modular, structural, ceiling system with multiple mounting locations and a center mounting location reserved for a ceiling-mounted robotic arm;
- placement of the equipment boom(s) on the sterile core side of the room away from the OR door;
- placement of a seated workstation facing the procedure bed and adjacent to the door between the OR and the sterile core; and
- adequate expansion space for future robotic systems.[15]

Space planning advisors also may suggest moving the control desk away from the wall and reducing it in scale to accommodate only monitoring screens and keyboards or adding wheels to provide a movable workstation. This creates a peninsula that allows the perioperative RN to sit at one of the monitors on the desk facing the surgical team, providing more direct observation of all activity during the procedure. It also may allow room for another person to sit at a second monitor with touch-screen controls of the integration system or access to video systems.[22]

I.d.1. The perioperative administrator should investigate the feasibility of constructing a dedicated interventional radiology suite versus a hybrid OR.

A hybrid OR may be used for procedures requiring the combined efforts of a surgeon and an interventional radiologist or cardiologist.[31] They also are intended to improve patient care and efficiency by eliminating the need to transfer the patient from radiology or the cardiac catheterization laboratory to the OR when there is an urgent need for a more invasive surgery.[13] The size of a hybrid suite will depend on the required equipment and additional shielding that the equipment may require based on the manufacturer's specifications. Additional square footage will be needed for storage room (eg, perfusion supplies, cardiopulmonary bypass machine); radiology control room; electrical panels; and equipment cooling devices. Sufficient space and anticipated placement of anesthetic equipment may be required to accommodate modern procedure beds that have a movable table top. When the table top is moved longitudinally, away from the broad part of the procedure bed, the surgeon has better ergonomic access to the patient for an open procedure.[13]

I.d.2. A multidisciplinary team should be identified to delineate the procedures (eg, cardiac, neurological) to be performed in the expanded MIS construction project.

Considerations for composition of the team include, but are not limited to, perioperative RNs, physicians, infection preventionists, and staff member representatives from the appropriate service lines.

I.d.3. The multidisciplinary design team should evaluate the benefits of each type of imaging system (ie, portable versus fixed) when choosing a procedure-related imaging system.

A portable system is beneficial because it allows personnel to move the fluoroscopy unit away from the sterile field when the unit is not in use. A fixed system, however, may have better resolution.[13] The imaging system decision will affect all

MINIMALLY INVASIVE SURGERY

other decisions, including the equipment and the square footage required.[19]

I.d.4. Staffing requirements for a hybrid OR should be considered during the design planning phase.

The perioperative team in a hybrid OR may include the following personnel:
- perioperative circulating nurse,
- radiology circulating nurse,
- surgical scrub person,
- radiology scrub person,
- surgeon,
- surgical first assistant,
- anesthesia care provider(s),
- radiology technician,
- interventional radiologist,
- interventional cardiologist, and
- perfusionist.

It may be necessary to have additional personnel present to provide safety and efficiency while interacting with multiple services. The surgeon and the interventional cardiologist or radiologist may work simultaneously; therefore, additional staff members may be necessary.[13,32]

I.e. An infection control risk assessment should be completed before construction or renovation to determine any infection control risks.[33]

An infection control risk assessment before constructing or remodeling existing health care facilities is a regulatory requirement in most states. MIS expansion projects may require specialized equipment that can raise room temperature and increase the risk of infection, and stakeholders may request that traffic patterns be varied from traditional ORs. It is important to continue thorough planning and coordination to minimize the risk for airborne infection both during and after the completion of the expansion project. An ongoing multidisciplinary team may be necessary to assess infection prevention, safety, and personnel implications.[28,30]

I.e.1. The OR or procedure room size should be sufficient to accommodate all equipment and allow ease of movement of personnel without compromising the sterile field.

Large equipment often is needed for MIS and other computer-assisted procedures, which may result in a crowded OR if adequate floor space is not identified in the planning phase of a construction project. The minimum recommended size of a traditional OR is 400 square feet, but this may not be sufficient for MIS rooms. Health care architects currently recommend MIS rooms be at least 600 square feet.[15] Procedures that include computer-assisted or imaging equipment may require an OR in the 750- to 800-square-foot range.[6]

I.e.2. Manufacturers' recommendations for cleaning and disinfection should be considered when selecting equipment for the MIS expansion project.

Liquid crystal diodes (LCD), recording devices, plasma video displays, and other electronic equipment may have specific instructions for cleaning from the manufacturer.

I.f. New and existing air supply, exhaust, and domestic water systems should be assessed for effective adaptation to changing ventilation and fluid management needs in an MIS expansion project.

Imaging systems and computer-assisted technology may require additional cooling systems. Fluid management systems may involve plumbing and additional specifications regarding waste removal.

I.f.1. Electrical panels should be assessed and upgraded, as needed, to provide for the maximum possible concurrent use of advanced technologies.

I.f.2. MIS expansion projects should be built to meet state building code criteria, including, but not limited to,
- air exchanges per hour,
- temperature and humidity control ranges, and
- air flow.

Regulations for outpatient facilities may have different floor-to-floor height requirements when compared to hospital buildings. However, regulations for outpatient imaging centers may require floor-to-floor heights that are similar to hospital buildings. The same may be true for power; heating, ventilation, and air conditioning (HVAC); plumbing; and fire protection systems.[19] The number of air exchanges for interventional radiology suites, cardiac catheterization rooms, and ORs are required to be a minimum rate of 15 total air exchanges per hour with a recommended range of 20 to 25 air exchanges in ORs.[34]

I.f.3. State regulations should be followed regarding radiation protection and building requirements for the walls of the entire suite.

The required radiation protection is based on the selected radiology system's specifications. Radiation protection must be built into the walls between the OR and the control room to protect the personnel working in the control room. If required by state regulations, radiation protection must be built into the walls of the entire suite.[34]

MINIMALLY INVASIVE SURGERY

Recommendation II

Fluids that will be used for irrigation and as distention media at a temperature other than room temperature should be warmed or cooled and stored in a safe manner.

There is an increased risk for patient injury if fluid storage is not systematically monitored and rotated.[35] Solution stability may vary according to composition.[36] The storage container for the fluid also may undergo changes when stored at temperatures higher or lower than room temperature.[37] Intravenous (IV) bags are among the medical devices listed in a safety assessment from the US Food and Drug Administration regarding safe levels of exposure to di-(2-ethylhexyl) phthalate (DEHP), a compound used as a plasticizer to provide flexibility for polyvinyl chloride (PVC). Expert panels have not reached consensus about the toxic and carcinogenic effects of DEHP in humans exposed to devices that contain them. However, the scientific community does agree that DEHP and other phthalate esters produce adverse effects in experiments with animals.[37]

II.a. Sterile water should be segregated from other irrigation solutions during storage.

The purpose of segregating sterile water and irrigation solutions is to reduce the risk for errors. Reports indicate IV bags of sterile water were stored near IV bags of 0.9% sodium chloride resulting in the incorrect administration of sterile water intravenously on a dialysis unit. The use of sterile water for continuous irrigation or as a distention media can cause hemolysis if it is absorbed into the bloodstream.[38]

II.b. Written storage instructions for warming and storing fluids should be obtained from the manufacturer of the fluid and reviewed annually to maintain proper storage protocols.

The manufacturer of the fluid is the best source of information about the duration of time that a fluid can be stored at different temperatures. The expiration date on the solution indicates the duration during which the solution can be used if stored at room temperature. Manufacturers conduct studies to determine how long solutions can be stored at higher temperatures without altering the physical and chemical properties of the solution. The duration for flexible IV bags may be different than the duration for hard plastic pour bottles if DEHP is used in the production process.[37]

II.b.1. Fluids kept in a warming cabinet should be labeled with an expiration date based on the manufacturer's recommendation for storage above room temperature.

Placing the warming expiration date on the fluid container facilitates communication. Adherence to the manufacturer's instructions for safe temperature ranges will provide stability of the solutions being stored.

II.b.2. Fluids kept in a warming cabinet should be rotated on a first-in, first-out basis.

This process helps to facilitate turnover of inventory and increases the probability of using fluid containers before the expiration date.

II.b.3. Unopened fluid containers should be removed from the warming cabinet when the expiration date has been reached.

After removal from the warming cabinet, the irrigation or distention fluid may be used at room temperature until the manufacturer's expiration date has been reached unless information from the manufacturer specifies otherwise.

II.b.4. After the unopened fluid container is removed from the warming cabinet, a "do not re-warm" label should be applied to the fluid container, and the fluid should not be returned to the warming cabinet.

Heat and moisture enhance microbial growth. Temperature fluctuations may contribute to breakdown of the fluid container. Unless information from the manufacturer specifies otherwise, persistent exposure to heat and variations in temperature could increase the risk for contaminants and container breakdown. A "do not re-warm" label on the fluid container increases the probability of compliance among members of the perioperative team.

II.c. A warming cabinet that is designed to warm fluids and has temperature control settings should be used when it is necessary to store fluids for irrigation or distention media at a temperature higher than room temperature.

Using a warming cabinet designed to warm fluids allows for better monitoring of temperatures specific to the safe ranges identified for the fluids. Thermal injuries have occurred as a result of overheating irrigation fluid or IV fluids.[39,40]

II.c.1. Separate warming cabinets or separate compartments with individual temperature control should be designated for blankets and fluids used for irrigation or distention media.

When fluids are placed in warming cabinets with blankets, there is an increased risk that the fluid will be warmed to an unsafe temperature, especially if the blankets can be safely heated to higher temperatures than the fluids.[35]

II.c.2. The temperature in the warming cabinet should be maintained at the temperature range indicated by the fluid manufacturer.

II.c.3. The warming cabinet temperature should be checked at regular intervals per the organization's policy and documented.[41]

MINIMALLY INVASIVE SURGERY

Temperature logs are an indicator that the warming cabinet is functioning properly and is warming fluids within the safe parameters indicated by the fluid manufacturer's specifications. Periodic biomedical inspections and regular preventive maintenance help to keep fluid warming devices in properly functioning condition. Cabinets that are overloaded may not warm fluids uniformly and may not function properly. Follow warming cabinet manufacturers' recommendations for appropriate volume of fluid to be stored.

II.c.4. The warming cabinet should be labeled with the safe temperature range settings for the fluids stored in the warming cabinet as determined by the fluid manufacturer.

Labeling the warming cabinet will help facilitate communication to the perioperative team members about the safe temperature range recommended by the fluid manufacturer.

II.c.5. A microwave or autoclave should not be used to heat irrigation fluids or fluids used for distention media.

Microwaves and autoclaves are uncontrolled methods of warming that could result in an unknown or uneven fluid temperature, increasing the risk of patient injury. Perioperative team members also may be at risk for burns from excessively heating the product or container. The composition of the solution or the container could be at risk when uncontrolled methods of warming are used.

II.d. Fluids used for irrigation should be cooled and stored in a safe manner that prevents contamination and degradation of the solution or container.

The composition of the fluid or container can change with fluctuations in temperature.

II.d.1. Written instructions for storing and cooling fluids should be obtained from the manufacturer of the fluid and reviewed annually.

II.d.2. A systematic rotation and expiration date labeling process should be defined for storing cooled fluids, based on the best available information.

Rotating inventory before the expiration date helps to reduce waste. Expiration dates defining safe duration of time a fluid can be cooled will help to maintain the integrity of the solution and the container and prevent waste.

II.d.3. Fluids that are being cooled below room temperature should be stored in an area that is designated for patient care items and separate from food.[42]

II.e. Fluid containers that have been opened and not completely used should be discarded and should not be returned to a storage area.

Opening a fluid container allows air and potential contaminants to enter the container. The edge of a container is considered contaminated after the contents have been poured; therefore, the sterility of the contents cannot be ensured if the cap is replaced or the seal to the IV bag has been broken.[43]

Recommendation III

During the preoperative nursing patient assessment, the perioperative RN should identify unique patient considerations that require additional precautions or contraindications related to MIS procedures, fluid management, and the medications that may be added to irrigation fluids.

Preoperative nursing assessment of patients for specific risk factors related to MIS patient positioning, fluid management, and medication sensitivities before the invasive procedure will facilitate safe patient care.

III.a. The preoperative patient assessment should include identification of risk factors related to extreme patient positioning that may be required for MIS or computer-assisted procedures.

It is not unusual to have patients in the extreme Trendelenburg or reverse Trendelenburg positions for laparoscopic surgical procedures and procedures involving robotic equipment because the gravitational effect allows organs to move away from the surgical field.[44] The Trendelenburg position increases venous return and increases the risk for cardiac or respiratory congestion. The reverse Trendelenburg position reduces venous return and cardiac output, increases peripheral and pulmonary resistance, and has the potential for misalignment of the patient's extremities.[45]

III.a.1. The preoperative nursing risk assessment related to positioning for MIS procedures should include, but not be limited to, the following:
- age-specific risk factors,
- cardiovascular compromise,
- respiratory compromise,
- pregnancy, and
- increased intraocular or intracranial pressure.

Older adults who have coexisting cardiac or pulmonary disease are at higher risk during laparoscopic procedures that require general anesthetics, pneumoperitoneum, and extreme positions.[46] Premature infants have compromised cardiovascular, respiratory, and thermoregulatory systems that may not tolerate increased intra-abdominal pressure or the Trendelenburg position.[47] Patients who have increased intracranial pressure, severe myopia, and/or retinal detachment are also at high risk during laparoscopic

531

MINIMALLY INVASIVE SURGERY

procedures performed using the Trendelenburg position. Patients who are pregnant, have bullous emphysema, or a history of spontaneous pneumothorax are also at higher risk.[45]

III.a.2. The preoperative nursing risk assessment related to prevention of venous stasis should include, but not be limited to,
- the type of procedure,
- the position required,
- the length of procedure, and
- a patient history that reflects a need for increased surveillance for deep vein thrombosis (DVT).

Laparoscopic surgery patients who will be in the reverse Trendelenburg position and have pneumoperitoneum are at risk for venous stasis. Patients who are undergoing procedures lasting longer than 30 to 45 minutes are at risk for venous stasis, as are patients whose surgery involves the use of a tourniquet (eg, arthroscopy).[48,49] Patients who are scheduled for longer complex laparoscopic procedures (eg, laparoscopic Roux-en-Y gastric bypass patients) are at a higher risk for DVT.[50] Venous thromboembolism prophylaxis is indicated whenever major abdominal operations are performed; however, there are varying opinions about routine prophylaxis if the laparoscopic procedure does not involve stirrups and is expected to be brief, including cholecystectomy and herniorrhaphy.[51-53] Examples of medical history assessment findings that indicate a need for increased surveillance for DVT include, but are not limited to, the following:
- history or family history of thrombosis, coagulopathy blood clots, blood-clotting disorders, DVT, or pulmonary embolism;
- varicosities or leg swelling;
- smoking; or
- sedentary/nonambulatory lifestyle greater than 72 hours.[48]

III.b. The preoperative nursing risk assessment should include safety considerations for intraoperative magnetic resonance imaging (MRI) when applicable.

Physical contraindications for patients in the MRI environment include, but are not limited to, pacemakers, certain cranial aneurysm clips, and certain implants. Manufacturers of the implant can verify whether it is safe or not safe for the intraoperative MRI environment if there is a question.[32]

III.c. The preoperative nursing risk assessment related to fluid management should include, but not be limited to, the following:
- the patient's skin color and turgor,
- weight,
- allergies and sensitivities to medications,
- NPO status,
- patient conditions or diseases that predispose or exacerbate the seriousness of hyponatremia or hypervolemia, and
- medications that predispose or exacerbate the seriousness of hyponatremia or hypervolemia.

The use of improper or excessive amounts of fluid for irrigation or distention media can lead to hypervolemia and hyponatremia. Patients who have congestive heart failure, liver cirrhosis, and renal diseases are more susceptible to hypervolemia and hyponatremia. The main causes of hyponatremia in hypo-osmolar patients are inappropriate antidiuretic hormone secretion, renal disorders, endocrine deficiencies, and certain medications.[54] Medications that predispose or exacerbate the seriousness of hyponatremia and hypervolemia include, but are not limited to, the following:
- diuretics;
- anticonvulsants (eg, carbamazepine); and
- serotonin and norepinephrine reuptake inhibitors.[54]

Medications may be added to irrigation or fluid used for distention media. Identifying allergies and sensitivities in the preoperative phase of care will facilitate communications and decrease the risk of patient complications in the intraoperative and postoperative phases of care.

III.d. The perioperative RN should review preoperative laboratory tests (eg, electrolytes, coagulation studies) and report abnormalities to the surgeon and anesthesia care provider.

Surgeons or anesthesia care providers may order additional laboratory tests for patients who have identified risk factors related to fluid management or DVT. Identifying electrolyte imbalances, coagulopathy, or other unusual laboratory findings preoperatively provides an opportunity to implement corrective measures or postpone the operative or invasive procedure.

III.e. Fluid selection should be based on the individual patient assessment and the intended use.

The selection of fluid to be used for irrigation or distention media depends on the type of procedure being performed, the patient's condition, and the use of electrosurgery. Fluids are divided into electrolyte and nonelectrolyte media. Nonelectrolyte media can lead to hyponatremia when the irrigation or distention fluid is absorbed into the circulatory system.[55]

III.e.1. Nonelectrolyte distention fluids should be used when monopolar electrosurgery is the planned equipment for the MIS procedure.

Electrolyte solutions conduct electricity and dissipate the energy transferred. This can result in ineffective hemostasis or collateral thermal tissue damage. When bipolar electrosurgery is used, electrolyte solutions can be used.[56]

III.e.2. Potential contraindications of fluid distention media should be reported to the surgeon and anesthesia care provider for evaluation of significance and appropriate actions to be taken.

Recommendation IV

Personnel should take additional precautions when using electrosurgery units (ESUs) during MIS and computer-assisted procedures.

MIS procedures using electrosurgery present unique patient safety risks, such as direct coupling of current, insulation failure, and capacitive coupling and tissue damage that may be out of the field of vision.[57]

IV.a. ESUs and accessories should be selected to include technology that minimizes or eliminates the risk of insulation failure and capacitive-coupling injuries.

During MIS procedures, alternate site injuries have resulted from insulation failure and capacitive coupling.[58-63] These injuries are far more serious than skin burns and have increased in number with the increase in MIS procedures.[64] The use of active electrode monitoring has minimized these risks.[61,63,65-68]

IV.b. Personnel should verify the properties of the distention media to minimize risks related to electrosurgery.

Collateral damage secondary to increased temperatures can occur if the distention media conducts current.

IV.b.1. Personnel should verify that the insufflation gas is nonflammable (ie, carbon dioxide).

Carbon dioxide is noncombustible and will not ignite if the active electrosurgical electrode sparks. Gases (eg, oxygen, nitrous oxide, air) are oxidizers that may support combustion. An oxidizer-enriched environment may enhance ignition and combustion.[69,70]

IV.b.2. Nonelectrolyte distention fluids should be used when monopolar electrosurgery is used.

Electrolyte solutions conduct electricity and dissipate the energy transferred. This can result in ineffective hemostasis or burns to internal tissue.

Table 1 presents a comparison of the properties of various fluids used for distention media.

IV.c. Conductive trocar systems should be used.

Conductive trocar cannulas provide a means for the electrosurgical current to flow safely between the cannula and the abdominal wall. This reduces high density current concentration and heating of non-target tissue.[61,62,65,71,72]

IV.c.1. Hybrid trocar (ie, combination plastic and metal) systems should not be used.

Each trocar and cannula can act as an electrical conductor inducing an electrical current from one to the other potentially causing a capacitive-coupling injury.[71]

IV.d. MIS electrodes should be examined for impaired insulation before use.

Insulation failure of electrodes caused by damage during use or reprocessing provides an alternate pathway for the electrical current to leave the active electrode. Some insulation failures are not visible. This has resulted in serious patient injuries.[59,61,62,65-67,71-74]

IV.d.1. Methods should be used to detect insulation failure, including, but not limited to,
- active electrode shielding and monitoring,[65,68]
- using active electrode indicator shafts that have two layers of insulation of different colors,[65]
- using active electrode insulation integrity testers that use high DC voltage to detect full thickness insulation breaks.[65]

Active electrode shielding continuously monitors the endoscopic instruments to minimize the risks of insulation failure or capacitive-coupling injuries.[59,61-63,66-68,71,72] The inner layer of a different color is designed to show through the outer layer if there is an insulation break.[65] Testing the electrode before the procedure identifies damaged electrodes that should be taken out of service. Testing may be done in the sterile processing department, at the sterile field, or with the sterilizable probes and cables that will alert the surgeon of an insulation break during the procedure. The surgical wound can be explored and treated if an alert occurs during the procedure.[65,74]

IV.d.2. The lowest power setting that achieves the desired result should be selected.[72]

Lower power settings for both cut and coagulation reduce the likelihood of insulation failure and capacitive-coupling injuries. Lower power settings also minimize damage from direct coupling when the active electrode is activated while in close proximity to another metal device inserted into an adjacent trocar port.[61,72]

IV.e. The active electrode should not be activated until it is in close proximity to the tissue.[61,62]

Activation only when in close proximity to the tissue minimizes the risk of current arcing and contacting unintended tissue.[61,62] Activating the electrode when it is not in very close proximity to the targeted tissue increases the risk of

MINIMALLY INVASIVE SURGERY

TABLE 1. FLUIDS USED FOR IRRIGATION OR DISTENSION MEDIA

Solution	Electrolyte solution	Uses	Potential contraindications	Adverse reactions
0.9% Sodium chloride[1]	Yes	General irrigation, hysteroscopy, use with laser and bipolar electrosurgery, and urologic procedures[2,3]	Monopolar electrosurgery	Hypervolemia, pulmonary edema, abdominal cramping, nausea and vomiting, diarrhea
Ringer's lactate[4]	Yes	General irrigation	Monopolar electrosurgery	Fluid shift from intracellular to extracellular compartment, hypervolemia
Dextran[1]	No	Hysteroscopy, volume generally limited to 300 mL and not to exceed 500 mL[5]	Allergy to beet sugar;[5] hypersensitivity to dextran or any component of the formulation; hemostatic defects (eg, thrombocytopenia, hypofibrinogenemia); cardiac decompensation; renal disease with severe oliguria or anuria; hepatic impairment	Plasma expander leading to fluid or solute overload; disseminated intravascular coagulation, for every 100 mL absorbed, the plasma volume expands by an additional 860 mL[5]; overdose, marked by pulmonary edema, increased bleeding time, and decreased platelet function
Glycine 1.5%[6]	No	Urologic irrigation, hysteroscopy, and resectoscopy with monopolar electrosurgery[3]	Severe cardiopulmonary or renal dysfunction; decreased liver function; additives may be incompatible, consult with a pharmacist	Aggravated pre-existing hyponatremia caused by shifts from intracellular to extracellular compartment; fluid and electrolyte disturbances (eg, edema, marked diuresis, pulmonary congestion); impaired liver function leading to accumulation of ammonia in the blood; allergic reactions, which are rare
Mannitol 5%[7]	No	Urologic irrigation; hysteroscopy and resectoscopy with monopolar electrosurgery[3]	Severe cardiopulmonary or renal dysfunction	Aggravated pre-existing hyponatremia caused by shifts from intracellular to extracellular compartment; fluid and electrolyte disturbances (eg, edema, marked diuresis, pulmonary congestion); hypernatremia caused by loss of water and excess of electrolytes from continuous administration

continued on next page

capacitive coupling. Capacitance is reduced during closed-circuit activation.

IV.f. Only the user of the active electrode should activate the device whether it is hand- or foot-controlled.[58]

Activation by the user of the active electrode prevents unintentional discharge of the device and minimizes the potential for patient and personnel injury.

IV.g. Bipolar active electrodes (eg, vessel occluding devices) should be used in a manner that minimizes the potential for injuries.

Unlike the monopolar ESU, bipolar technology incorporates an active electrode and a return electrode into a two-poled instrument, such as forceps or scissors.[60,75,76] Current flows only through the tissue contacted between two poles of instruments; thus, the need for a dispersive electrode is eliminated.[76] This also eliminates the chance of stray or alternate pathways for current flow.[76] The bipolar ESU provides precise hemostasis or dissection at the surgical site with less lower voltage and decreased thermal spread to nearby structures.[76]

MINIMALLY INVASIVE SURGERY

Table 1 continued. Fluids Used for Irrigation or Distension Media

Solution	Electrolyte solution	Uses	Potential contraindications	Adverse reactions
Sorbitol 3%[8]	No	Urological irrigation	Severe cardiopulmonary or renal dysfunction, fructose intolerance	Aggravated pre-existing hyponatremia caused by shifts from intracellular to extracellular compartment; hypernatremia caused by loss of water and excess of electrolytes from continuous administration hyperglycemia in patients with diabetes mellitus; allergic reactions (eg, urticaria)
Sorbitol 3%/Mannitol 0.5%[9]	No	Urologic irrigation	Severe cardiopulmonary or renal dysfunction; fructose intolerance	Aggravated pre-existing hyponatremia caused by shifts from intracellular to extracellular compartment; hypernatremia caused by loss of water and excess of electrolytes from continuous administration; hyperglycemia in patients with diabetes mellitus; hyperlactatemia in patients who are metabolically compromised caused by metabolism of sorbitol
Sterile water[10]	No	General irrigation, washing, rinsing, and dilution purposes; transurethral resection of the prostate[11]	Continuous irrigation, as a distention medium; additives may be incompatible, consult with a pharmacist	Hemolysis when absorbed into the bloodstream

Editor's note: This table presents irrigation solutions that are in common use; however, it is not all-inclusive. Use of other irrigation solutions may be indicated in certain patient populations and for certain conditions.

References

1. Lexi-Comp, Inc, AORN. Drug Information Handbook for Perioperative Nursing. Hudson, OH: Lexi-Comp; 2006.
2. Ho HS, Cheng CW. Bipolar transurethral resection of prostate: a new reference standard? *Curr Opin Urol.* 2008;18(1):50-55.
3. ACOG Committee on Practice Bulletins. Endometrial ablation [ACOG Practice Bulletin: Clinical management guidelines for obstetrician-gynecologists, Number 81, May 2007]. *Obstet Gynecol.* 2007;109(5):1233-1248.
4. Lactated Ringer's irrigation [package insert]. Lake Forest, IL: Hospira; 2004.
5. American College of Obstetricians and Gynecologists. Hysteroscopy [ACOG technology assessment in obstetrics and gynecology, Number 4, August 2005]. *Obstet Gynecol.* 2005;106(2):439-442.
6. 1.5% glycine irrigation [package insert]. Lake Forest, IL: Hospira; 1999.
7. 5% mannitol irrigation [package insert]. Irvine, CA: B. Braun Medical, Inc; 2002.
8. 3% sorbitol urologic irrigating solution [package insert]. Deerfield, IL: Baxter Healthcare Corp; 2004.
9. Sorbitol-mannitol irrigation [package insert]. Lake Forest, IL: Hospira; 2004.
10. Sterile water for irrigation [package insert]. Lake Forest, IL: Hospira; 2004.
11. Moharari RS, Khajavi MR, Khademhosseini P, Hosseini SR, Najafi A. Sterile water as an irrigating fluid for transurethral resection of the prostate: anesthetical view of the records of 1600 cases. *South Med J.* 2008;101(4):373-375.

IV.g.1. When bipolar resection devices are used, electrolyte solutions should be used.

Bipolar resection devices need an electrolytic solution to conduct the electrical flow.[77]

IV.h. Argon-enhanced coagulation (AEC) technology poses unique risks to patient and personnel safety and should be used in a manner that minimizes the potential for injury.[57]

Each type of AEC has specific manufacturer's written operating instructions describing safe operation of the unit. The AEC unit uses monopolar alternating current delivered to the tissue through ionized argon gas. The risks of monopolar electrosurgery are present.[78]

IV.h.1. All safety measures for AEC technology outlined in the AORN "Recommended practices for electrosurgery" should be referenced when using AEC technology.[57]

Patient injury and death have occurred as a complication of argon-enhanced technology. There is a significant risk of gas embolism when AEC is used during laparoscopic procedures from abdominal overpressurization and displacement of CO_2 by argon gas.[79-82] (See Recommendation VI.i.)

IV.i. Patients should be instructed to immediately report any postoperative signs or symptoms of electrosurgical injury. Postoperative patient care instructions should include symptoms to look for, including, but not limited to,
- fever,
- inability to void,
- lower gastrointestinal bleeding,
- abdominal pain,
- abdominal distention,
- nausea,
- vomiting, and
- diarrhea.[62]

Symptoms of a minimally invasive electrosurgical injury can occur days after discharge from the perioperative setting and may include infection from an injured intestinal tract. Prompt reporting of electrosurgical injury symptoms ensures timely treatment and minimizes adverse outcomes.[62,73]

IV.j. Potential hazards associated with surgical smoke generated in the practice setting should be identified, and safe practices established.[83]

Surgical smoke (ie, plume) is generated from use of heat-producing instruments such as lasers and electrosurgical devices.[84,85] Analyses of the airborne contaminants produced during electrosurgery have shown that electrosurgery plume contains toxic gas and vapors (eg, benzene, hydrogen cyanide, formaldehyde); bioaerosols; dead and living cell material, including blood fragments; and viruses.[86-91]

Many additional hazardous chemical compounds have been noted in surgical smoke.[89,92-94] These contaminants have been shown to have an unpleasant odor, cause problems with visibility of the surgical site, cause ocular and upper respiratory tract irritation, and demonstrate mutagenic and carcinogenic potential.[86,88,90] Bacterial and/or viral contamination of plume has been highlighted by different studies.[89,91,95,96]

IV.j.1. Surgical smoke should be removed by use of a smoke evacuation system in minimally invasive procedures to prevent patient and health care worker exposure to surgical smoke contaminants.[86]

The National Institute for Occupational Safety and Health (NIOSH) recommends that smoke evacuation systems be used as the primary control to reduce potential acute and chronic health risks to personnel and patients.[94]

Local exhaust ventilation (LEV) is the primary means to protect patients and health care personnel from exposure to airborne contaminants generated by electrosurgery.[86] Potential health and liability risks may be reduced by the evacuation of surgical smoke.[87]

IV.j.2. When surgical smoke is generated, an individual smoke evacuation unit with a 0.1 micron filter (eg, ultra-low particulate air [ULPA] or high efficiency particulate air [HEPA]) should be used to remove surgical smoke.[86,88]

During electrosurgery, cells are heated to a high temperature, which causes the cell membrane to rupture, releasing particles into the cavity. Electrosurgical procedures create particles approximately 0.7 microns in size.[89]

IV.j.3. Surgical smoke should be evacuated and filtered during laparoscopic procedures and at the end of procedures when the pneumoperitoneum is released.

Smoke generated in the pneumoperitoneum may be more concentrated than smoke generated from an open surgical procedure if it accumulates in the closed cavity.[97] The risk to the patient from exposure to this concentrated smoke is not yet identified. Results of studies investigating port site metastasis, also known as the chimney effect, have shown that electrosurgical smoke has the potential to serve as a vehicle for transplanting malignant cells in benign tissue.[85,89,92,97] Surgical smoke contains both large and small particles that negatively affect visibility during laparoscopic procedures.[97,98] At the end of the procedure, if the smoke in the pneumoperitoneum is released directly from a cannula and without a filter, the concentrated smoke can expose the perioperative team members to contaminants.[92,97]

IV.j.4. Used smoke evacuator filters and tubing should be considered potentially infectious waste. These used devices should be handled using standard precautions and disposed of as biohazardous waste.[86-88]

Airborne contaminants produced during laser and electrosurgical procedures have been analyzed and shown to contain gaseous toxic compounds, bioaerosols, and dead and living cell material.[87-89] Bacterial and/or viral contamination of smoke plume also has been identified.[95,96]

Recommendation V

Potential injuries and complications associated with MIS and computer-assisted procedures should be identified and practices should be established to reduce risk.

MIS and computer-assisted procedures often involve use and application of complex technologies that may require unique safety precautions.

V.a. The perioperative team should determine what emergency supplies and equipment should be available before the procedure begins.[99]

MINIMALLY INVASIVE SURGERY

In an analysis of complications from retroperitoneoscopic procedures of the urinary tract, researchers found that the rate of complications was dependent on the complexity of the procedure and the learning curve of the surgeon.[100] The risk of conversion from MIS to an open procedure may not always require a double setup for an open procedure. Conversion rates vary according to specific procedures and complexities, ranging from 4.6% to 7.4%.[7,100,101] Historically, 1.2% of the patients undergoing laparoscopic cholecystectomy required conversion to a laparotomy.[102] Injuries to bowel and major blood vessels in gynecology cases range in frequency from 0.05% to 0.14%.[103]

V.b. Specific positioning devices should be provided to secure the patient and provide safety in accordance with the AORN "Recommended practices for positioning the patient in the perioperative practice setting."[104]

MIS surgery may require exaggerated patient positioning to displace viscera and enhance visibility for the surgical team. More complex procedures are being done with MIS and computer-assisted techniques, consequently the operating procedure time may be prolonged when compared to MIS procedures with lower acuity. Access to the patient may be limited by robotic surgical systems.[105] The patient also may be in extreme positions for extended periods of time, and when a robot is docked to the patient during the procedure, repositioning is improbable, if not impossible.[44,106] Restraints or methods to secure the patient to the procedure bed may be necessary if extreme Trendelenburg or reverse Trendelenburg positions are used.[44] The patient's position may be adjusted to facilitate the surgeon and assistant's view of the monitors and ergonomic access to laparoscopic instruments and accessories. One member of the surgical team may be positioned between the patient's legs when he or she is in the lithotomy position.[21] For surgical reasons, it may be necessary to tuck the patient's arms at his or her sides to make room for other assistants and to avoid moving the armboards to angles of more than 90 degrees.[107] The patient is at risk of injury to the brachial plexus caused by stretching if the arms are positioned in an exaggerated abduction raising them above the head.[108]

V.b.1. The perioperative RN should initiate actions to reduce the risk of pressure on the patient during MIS and computer-assisted procedures.

There is increased risk of adding pressure on the patient when the robotic arms are brought into position and docked. Static positions are often required in MIS procedures, increasing the risk of personnel leaning on the patient during the procedure.

V.b.2. The perioperative RN should ensure the patient is undocked from the robotic system before repositioning is initiated.

If the decision is made to reposition the patient during a long procedure using robotic systems, the patient is at risk for injury if proper procedures for docking and undocking are not followed.

V.c. Electrical cords and plugs should be handled in a manner that minimizes the potential for damage and subsequent patient or staff injuries.

Stress on cords that are too short may cause damage to the cord, posing an electrical hazard. Cords that are too short also increase the risk for tripping members of the perioperative team.[41]

V.c.1. Equipment should be placed near the sterile field, with cords reaching the wall or column outlet without stress on a cord.[41]

It may be necessary to consult with the manufacturer and biomedical personnel to change the cord lengths to avoid the use of extension cords. Cords that do not lie flat or are stretched create a risk for tripping, fraying of the cord, or accidental unplugging of the equipment. Use of extension cords can result in excessive current leakage and/or electrical-system overload.[41]

V.c.2. Cords should be free of kinks, knots, and bends that could damage the cord or cause leakage, current accumulation, and overheating of the cord's insulation.[41]

V.c.3. Cords should be removed from use if they are frayed or char debris is noted.

V.c.4. Cords should be kept away from fluids.

Fluids dripping onto the cord or connections cause electrical hazards.[109]

V.d. Protective measures should be implemented to prevent fire or thermal injury. Measures should include, but not be limited to, the following:
- Turn off light sources when they are not in use.
- Hold fiber-optic light cables away from drapes or place on a moist towel.
- Connect all fiber-optic light cables before activating the source.
- Place the light source on standby when disconnecting fiber-optic light cables.
- Allow all flammable prep solutions to dry fully before placing surgical drapes.[41,110]

The heat from fiber-optic light cables or endoscopes may burn the skin and may cause drapes to burn. Hot fiber-optic light cables increase the risk of fire when in contact with flammable materials. A moist towel can help to cool the light cable.[110]

V.e. Fiber-optic light cables should be inspected regularly for broken light bundles before use.

Broken light bundles will diminish the transmission of light and decrease visibility. Having sterile backup cables readily available decreases surgical delays.

V.e.1. Fiber-optic light cables should be long enough to reach from the surgical field to the equipment without undue stress.

Tension increases the risk that the fiber-optic light cables will become disconnected or break, thereby creating a safety hazard for patients and personnel.

V.e.2. A backup fiber-optic light cable should be available and used if broken light bundles are apparent.

V.f. Considerations to prevent surgical site infection should be implemented with all MIS and computer-assisted procedures.

Specialized cells line the peritoneal cavity and serve as the first line of defense for the immune system in the abdomen. This defense system of the peritoneum may be negatively affected by the pneumoperitoneum used in many MIS procedures. This is important because intra-abdominal infections often begin in the peritoneal cavity.[111] The mechanical distension changes the peritoneal microstructure allowing passage of bacteria. This systemic response coupled with the amount of tissue damage and the duration of the procedure may potentially lead to a higher risk for infection.[112]

Single port access laparoscopy and natural orifice transluminal endoscopic surgery (NOTES) are examples of new approaches for MIS procedures. It is important to clarify access points before the surgery to prepare the skin adequately for the incision and for any expanded incisions that might be necessary.[113-119]

V.f.1. Care should be taken when retrieving specimens to prevent cross contamination and ensure complete extraction.

Infection rates for laparoscopic cholecystectomies has been reported to be as low as 0.38 infections per 100 procedures.[120] However, other procedures may have a higher risk of infection from the extraction of an infected appendix or infected cysts through a small incision. In such procedures, there is a need for careful handling with atraumatic grasping forceps or specimen bags to avoid rupture and contamination into the peritoneal space.[121,122] Morcellators may be used to cut up and remove large specimens.[122,123] There is a potential for retained myomas or dissemination of various cancers when using a morcellator.[123]

V.g. Endoscopic trocars and Veress needles should be selected based on safety criteria established for the practice setting.

Catastrophic patient injuries may occur from excessive use of pressure during trocar insertion. Trocar injuries are grouped into three primary groups: vascular, visceral, or the anterior or posterior abdominal wall.[124] There are three techniques used for trocar insertion: direct or blind insertion, Veress needle technique, and the Hasson technique. Risks of gas embolism or formation of subcutaneous or subfascial emphysema are possible when using a Veress needle before insufflation and trocar insertion. The Hasson technique, also known as a "cut down" or "open" technique, exposes the fascia using a scalpel to make a 2-cm to 3-cm skin incision. Shielded trocars also may help to reduce the risk for trocar injuries.[124,125]

V.h. MIS and computer-assisted equipment and accessories should be used in a manner that minimizes the potential for injuries.

V.h.1. Instructions for MIS and computer-assisted equipment use, warranties, and a manual for maintenance and inspections should be obtained from the manufacturer and be readily available to users.

V.h.2. All MIS and computer-assisted equipment should be checked before use.

White balancing may be required for optimum video image for both traditional laparoscopic and robotic surgery. Appropriate lighting for cameras facilitates surgeon and surgical team visualization for the procedure. Voice-activated systems or other technologies that allow the surgeon to control settings may facilitate efficiency during the procedure.[126]

V.i. Data collected during the procedure should be monitored and retrieved before shutting down the video systems.

V.i.1. Video equipment should have adequate memory and retrieval capabilities throughout the procedure and for documentation.

V.j. Special considerations should be implemented for the intraoperative MRI environment.

V.j.1. Equipment and other items should be labeled as safe for use in the MRI environment or secured to minimize the risk for injury.

Metal objects (eg, oxygen tanks, stretchers, surgical instruments) can become projectiles in the MRI environment. It may be necessary to acquire equipment or other items that are composed of titanium, plastic, ceramic, aluminum, or a high-grade nonmagnetic stainless steel. Metal items that remain in an MRI environment can be tethered to the wall or secured in another way that has been tested to prevent patient or perioperative personnel risk for injury.[32]

V.j.2. When in an MRI environment, electrical cords should not cross each other or loop.

Patient burns may result if there is a coil or antenna placed on the patient over an electrical cord (eg, electrosurgical pad, rectal probe).[32]

Recommendation VI

Potential patient injuries and complications associated with gas distention media used during MIS procedures should be identified, and practices that reduce the risk of injuries and complications should be established.

Although endoscopic procedures are minimally invasive from the surgical perspective, the use of CO_2 to establish pneumoperitoneum increases the risk of hypercarbia, hypoxemia, subcutaneous emphysema, pneumothorax, and other hemodynamic changes depending on the patient's medical history.[45,46,127,128] End tidal CO_2 is closely monitored to detect the onset of hypercarbia, especially for patients with compromised pulmonary function.[129]

Nitrous oxide may be beneficial for patients who have depressed pulmonary function and may be advantageous over other gases if an IV embolization occurs.[45,127] The fear of combustion when using nitrous oxide was a topic studied in 1995. The researchers reported that the risk of combustion is low when using nitrous oxide for the pneumoperitoneum in gastrointestinal laparoscopic procedures because the mixture of methane and hydrogen were not in a high enough concentration for combustion to occur. They concluded nitrous oxide is an option not only for patients with cardiopulmonary and metabolic acidosis, but also for prolonged procedures and for pregnant patients because of the concern for fetal acidosis when using CO_2.[130]

Air and oxygen are not used for insufflations during laparoscopy because of the risk of combustion when electrosurgery or lasers are used. Helium and nitrogen are not used because they are not as soluble as CO_2, which increases the risk for more serious consequences in the event of a gas embolism. There are cost concerns with using helium. Argon has a negative effect on hepatic blood flow.[45]

Carbon dioxide insufflation is one cause of hypothermia because of the exposure of the peritoneal surface to a large volume of CO_2 gas that is insufflated at room temperature.[131] However, the other contributing factors of thermal loss include, but are not limited to,
- irrigation fluids or fluids as distention media,
- OR temperature,
- exposed body surface,
- procedure length, and
- the patient's age and medical condition.

Many studies have been conducted to investigate the potential benefits of heating CO_2 or adding humidity, not only for the prevention of hypothermia but also for the effect on postoperative pain.[131-137] Of the studies reviewed, only one reported a significant decrease in heat loss during the surgery and reduced postoperative shivering, pain, and analgesic requirement.[135] Most researchers report there is no difference in patient outcomes when the temperature or humidity for CO_2 insufflation is changed.[131-134,136,137] Two researchers reported they still prefer to use heated and/or humidified CO_2 for insufflation because it has a positive effect on the total OR time and decreased the amount of time the surgeon spent cleaning the scope and the need for changing the warm saline to prevent fogging.[134,137] Misplacement of the Veress needle directly into a vein or parenchymal organ can lead to a CO_2 gas embolism. Sixty percent (60%) of the symptomatic cases of gas embolism occur during initial insufflation.[127] Gasless laparoscopic techniques rely on an abdominal wall lift to create an intra-abdominal space at atmospheric pressure to eliminate the risk of hypercapnia and CO_2 embolization. This technique or a combination of abdominal wall lifting with low-pressure pneumoperitoneum may be a good alternative for laparoscopic cholecystectomy procedures for elderly patients or those with cardiopulmonary problems.[45] Researchers in Kentucky evaluated five different insufflation techniques from a retrospective analysis of more than 3,000 laparoscopic procedures over a 13-year period. The research findings revealed that certain laparoscopic methods were more appropriate for patients with particular characteristics (eg, previous surgery).[138] There is also a risk for CO_2 embolism during minimally invasive vein harvesting when CO_2 is used to create a closed tunnel to prepare and harvest the greater saphenous vein or radial artery.[139,140]

VI.a. The cylinder should be checked to verify that it contains the appropriate gas and that it is sufficiently full before starting the procedure.

Carbon dioxide is the most commonly used insufflation gas because it is readily absorbed by the body and excreted by the lungs, does not support combustion, and is commonly available.[45,127] Changing the gas tank when it is empty disrupts the gas flow and risks a decrease in the intra-abdominal pressure. In some cases, it also may cause a malfunction in the suction and pumping mechanism. This can lead to a risk of contamination from aspiration of fluids toward the insufflator.[141]

VI.a.1. Before use, gas cylinders should be checked for
- appropriate label,
- appropriate pin-index safety system connector,
- appropriate color coding, and
- volume.[41]

VI.b. The insufflator should be elevated above the level of the surgical cavity.

When the pressure on the patient side is higher than at the insufflator connecting point, body fluid or gas is allowed to flow up the trocar cannula through the insufflation tubing and into the insufflator. This may result in cross contamination or damage to the insufflating device.[141]

VI.c. The insufflator and insufflation tubing should be flushed with gas before personnel connect the tubing to the cannula (eg, Veress needle).

Flushing removes residual air from tubing, reducing the risk of air embolism. It also determines whether residues are present inside the insufflator.[141]

VI.d. Carbon dioxide insufflators should be filtered with a single-use hydrophobic filter that is compatible with the insufflator and impervious to fluids.

A filter helps prevent gas cylinder contaminants from flowing through the insufflator into the surgical cavity, prevents backflow of abdominal fluids and particulates that could contaminate the insufflator, and prevents cross contamination. When the filter is compatible with the insufflator, it does not interfere with flow rate.[141] Cylinders with nonferrous internal surfaces and surfaces incapable of creating residual material that could escape during the gaseous phase of delivery may be helpful in preventing the transfer of particulate matter.[142]

VI.e. Insufflators designed for laparoscopic procedures should not be substituted for insufflators designed for hysteroscopy procedures.

The American College of Obstetricians and Gynecologists recommend that insufflators designed for use with laparoscopic procedures are not to be used for hysteroscopy procedures.[56] Laparoscopic insufflators supply large volumes at low pressures. Hysteroscopic insufflators supply high pressures with low volume.

VI.f. Insufflator pressures should be monitored throughout the procedure.

Maintaining intra-abdominal pressure under 12 mm Hg in adult patients reduces the risk of systemic hemodynamic changes.[127,141,143-145] For heavier or taller patients, an intra-abdominal pressure of 20 mm Hg to 30 mm Hg may be necessary to establish the appropriate pneumoperitoneum.[103] For pediatric patients, the insufflation pressures should be set as low as possible while creating the pneumoperitoneum; however, there are no known studies to define standard ranges.[47] Monitoring intrauterine pressures to less than 100 mm Hg helps minimize the risk of gas embolization.[56]

VI.f.1. A second CO_2 cylinder should be readily available for each procedure.

VI.f.2. The CO_2 cylinder should be replaced before it is empty.

Methods of monitoring the level of remaining gas in the cylinder include, but are not limited to, observing the insufflator gas cylinder gauge level, monitoring the refill history, and tracking cylinder use. The flow of contaminants occurs more readily when the volume of remaining gas in the cylinder is low. Replacing the primary cylinder before the gas level is low helps prevent contamination of the sterile field by particulate matter.[142]

VI.g. The insufflator tubing should be disconnected from the trocar cannula before personnel deactivate the insufflator.

VI.h. Endoscopic CO_2 insufflators should be equipped with alarms that cannot be deactivated.[41]

Alarms alert personnel to equipment malfunction.

VI.i. When using an AEC unit during MIS procedures, personnel should follow all safety measures identified for AEC technology.

AEC acts as a secondary source of pressurized argon gas that can cause the patient's intra-abdominal pressure to rise rapidly and exceed venous pressure, possibly creating argon-enriched gas emboli formation. This has resulted in gas emboli.[79,80]

VI.i.1. The active electrode and argon gas line should be purged according to the manufacturer's recommendations.[79]

VI.i.2. The patient's intra-abdominal cavity should be flushed with several liters of CO_2 between extended activation periods.[79]

Flushing the intra-abdominal cavity with several liters of CO_2 between extended periods of activation reduces the potential for argon gas emboli formation.[79]

VI.i.3. Patient monitoring should include devices that are considered effective for early detection of gas emboli (eg, end-tidal carbon dioxide).[78,79,81]

There is a significant risk of gas embolism when AEC is used during laparoscopic procedures from abdominal overpressurization and displacement of CO_2 by argon gas.[79-82]

Recommendation VII

Potential injuries and complications associated with fluid used for irrigation or as distention media during MIS and computer-assisted procedures should be identified and practices should be established to reduce risk.

Many MIS procedures require irrigation fluid to clear the operative field of blood and debris or fluid used as a distention media to create a broader visual operative field inside a cavity. Patient outcomes may not be optimal, if fluids used for irrigation or as distention media are not managed appropriately. Fluid extravasation, hyponatremia, hypervolemia, cardiovascular and peripheral vascular complications, pulmonary air or fluid emboli, and hypothermia are a few examples of complications resulting from mismanagement of distention media or irrigation fluids.[146,147] Monitoring and early recognition of the complications associated with the intraoperative use of distention media or irrigation fluids are keys to maintaining patient safety and quality control for MIS procedures.

VII.a. Perioperative registered nurses should be aware of uses, contraindications, and risk of fluids used for distention media.

The selection of fluid to be used for irrigation or distention media depends on the type of procedure being performed, the patient's condition, and the use of electrosurgery.

For example, for arthroscopy procedures normal saline (ie, 0.9% sodium chloride) is used unless monopolar electrosurgery is planned.

Normal saline and Lactated Ringer's solution are isotonic, electrolyte fluids. The American College of Obstetricians and Gynecologists considers these solutions to be the media of choice for diagnostic hysteroscopy or intraoperative hysteroscopy when mechanical, laser, or bipolar energy is used.[56] Low viscosity, hyperosmolar, electrolyte-poor fluids (glycine 1.5%, sorbitol 3%, and mannitol 5%) are compatible with monopolar radio-frequency energy but can cause hyponatremia and decreased serum osmolality. Their absorption in excess can result in fatal complications such as cerebral edema and death. Mannitol 5% is iso-osmolar and causes diuresis, which can lead to excessive absorption. Dextran 70 is a high-viscosity fluid and a potent plasma expander. Anaphylaxis and disseminated intravascular coagulopathy have occurred when Dextran 70 has been used for uterine distention. This solution crystallizes on instruments and is very difficult to remove. Dextran 70 is contraindicated for patients who are allergic to beet sugar.[56]

Nonelectrolyte solutions such as glycine, mannitol, or sorbitol often are used in urologic procedures when monopolar electrosurgical devices are used. These solutions do not dissipate the electrical current. Glycine is the fluid medium commonly used with monopolar electrosurgical technology.[148] The complication known as transurethral resection (TUR) syndrome may be observed when glycine is used as irrigating or distention media. Exposed blood vessels from tissue removal and elevated pressure being applied to the distention fluid enables intravasation (ie, distention fluid flows into the vascular system).[149] Monopolar electrosurgical energy can result in temperatures up to 400° C (752° F) because of the resistance with surrounding tissue.[150] Bipolar electrosurgical use has achieved similar clinical efficacy to monopolar procedures, but with shorter catheterization times and shorter hospital stays. For bipolar electrosurgical technology, normal saline, which reduces the occurrence of TUR syndrome, may be used as the fluid medium rather than glycine.[150]

VII.b. Fluids used for irrigation or as distention media should be contained.

Fluid that is not contained cannot be measured. It is important to measure fluids returned from irrigation or distention media to monitor for fluid deficit. Fluid standing on the floor can pose a fall risk to surgical team members. Fluid becomes an electrical hazard when it comes into contact with electrical equipment. Containing the fluid prevents environmental contamination.

VII.b.1. The patient should be draped in a manner that enables as much capture of fluid return as possible.

Drapes designed for collection facilitate the accurate measurement of fluid. Fluid absorption is determined through monitoring the volumetric fluid balance by subtracting the amount of fluid recovered from the amount of fluid instilled. The volumetric calculation does not take into consideration extraneous fluid losses (eg, fluid loss on the floor, on the drape), which cannot be accurately quantified, nor does it consider additives, such as blood.

VII.b.2. Fluid administered to the patient should be collected in a closed container system.

Using a suction canister or fluid collection system prevents the fluid from contaminating the environment and the clothing of personnel. Surgical drapes with fluid collection pouches may assist in preventing fluid from contaminating the floor. Fluid collection mats on the floor may assist with managing fluid that does contact the floor.

VII.b.3. Fluids used for irrigation or as distention media should be prevented from coming into contact with electrical equipment.

Containing fluid used during a procedure prevents contact with electrical outlets, switches, and the internal components of electrical equipment including electrosurgical electrodes. Preventing fluid contact with electrical equipment minimizes the risk of burns, fires, and damage to the equipment.

VII.b.4. Fluid used during a procedure must be handled and discarded as a biohazardous waste in a manner consistent with local, state, and federal regulations.

Fluid that has been used inside a patient's body is considered biohazardous. Management of biohazardous waste is regulated by federal, state, and local agencies.[151]

VII.c. Fluids used for irrigation or as distention media should be monitored for appropriate temperature.

Fluids that are too warm can cause burns.[39] Cool irrigation solutions in body cavities enhance heat transfer from the body core to the solution and increase the risk of heat loss. Perioperative hypothermia is associated with serious cardiac events.[147] Equipment is commercially available to warm irrigation fluid as it is administered.

Warming irrigation fluid to body temperature near 37° C (98.6° F) is an adjunct therapy to decrease heat loss but is insufficient alone to prevent hypothermia.[152] In a study of patients undergoing laparoscopy without forced air warming, patients receiving warmed irrigation solutions maintained higher core body temperatures than those receiving room temperature solutions. However, warmed irrigation fluids alone did not prevent hypothermia.[153] No improvement in body temperature was found when using warmed irrigation during arthroscopic surgery.[154]

The value of warming irrigation solutions during urologic procedures is controversial. The procedure associated with the greatest temperature drop is percutaneous lithotripsy.[155] The combination of warmed irrigation and IV fluids has been found to result in less of a temperature drop in patients undergoing TUR.[156] When active patient surface warming was used during TUR, patients remained normothermic when room temperature irrigation fluids were used. Researchers reported that the temperature of the irrigation fluid did not have as great an effect on the core body temperature as other factors, including ambient temperature of the OR, time spent in the OR, the resection time, and amount of irrigation fluid absorbed.[157]

Using warm distention media for hysteroscopy may dilate the vasculature and lead to intravasation.[158,159]

VII.d. Fluid management systems should be used in a manner that minimizes potential for injury.

Automated fluid management systems calculate the amount of fluid dispensed to the patient and compare this with the amount returned to the system. The deficit is measured and an alarm alerts the user of potential fluid overload. This timely notification of a deficit provides an opportunity to take corrective action before physiologic compromise of the patient.

VII.d.1. The perioperative RN should follow the manufacturer's written instructions for use of fluid management systems.

VII.d.2. The fluid selected for the distention media should be consistent with the fluid management system and the endoscope manufacturer's written instructions.

VII.d.3. Accessories (eg, tubing, collection canisters) should be compatible with the fluid management system.

Fluid management system tubing has a transducer that works with the electronic equipment to measure input and output. Using incompatible tubing results in inaccurate fluid measurements.

VII.d.4. The perioperative RN should calibrate the fluid management system as per the manufacturer's instructions.

Proper calibration of the fluid management system will calculate instillation and total fluid deficit amounts accurately.

VII.d.5. A fluid management system designed for intrauterine distention should be used when distending the uterus with more than 1,000 mL of fluid.

The amount of fluid contained in an IV bag or bottle can be up to 3.3% to 10% more than the amount stated on the label.[160,161] The actual amount of fluid in collection canisters may be 20% more or less than the measured amount. When large volumes of fluid are instilled, this inaccuracy can result in unidentified fluid deficit.[160] This inaccuracy may not be clinically significant when small volumes (ie, less than 1,000 mL) are used.

VII.d.6. The perioperative RN should verify the volume setting for fluid distention with the surgeon before administration.

Volume settings are based on the procedure being done, the size of the patient, and the patient's condition. During operative endoscopic urologic procedures, large volumes of fluid are instilled to enhance visualization and evacuate tissue and blood clots. Irrigation fluid can be absorbed into the intravascular system by instrument perforation during tumor or fibroid resection, or forced into the intraperitoneal or retroperitoneal space. The amount of fluid absorbed increases with the extent of the resection and prolonged exposure.[146] Smoking is the only known risk factor for patients that is associated with an increase in fluid absorption.[162]

VII.e. The perioperative RN should monitor the amount of fluid dispensed and returned during the procedure.

Monitoring irrigation fluid use facilitates calculation of blood loss and determines existing fluid deficit, representing fluid that is being absorbed by the patient (ie, fluid intravasation). Dilutional hyponatremia is associated with intravasation of non-electrolyte solutions. Rapid influx of hypotonic fluid increases circulation of free water and reduces the extracellular sodium concentration.[54,163] During hysteroscopy procedures, fluid is absorbed through the uterine vessels and the bowel if there is a perforation, or the fluid egresses through patent fallopian tubes. This can lead to serious complications. Measuring fluid volume deficit can prevent complications when identified early and the procedure is terminated.[56]

The critical volume of intravasation before symptoms are exhibited is not predictable.[164] The American College of Obstetricians and Gynecologists suggest that 750 mL of fluid absorption implies excessive intravasation. They further advise planning for terminating the procedure for patients who are elderly and

MINIMALLY INVASIVE SURGERY

for those with cardiovascular compromise when this occurs.[56]

The incidence and severity of fluid symptoms from increased amounts of intraoperative or postoperative absorbed fluid have been documented during TUR and endometrial ablation procedures. During TUR procedures where glycine was used as the fluid distention media, patients exhibited symptoms of excessive fluid absorption when 1 L to 2 L of fluid had been absorbed.[146]

VII.e.1. Fluid deficit amount should be reported to the anesthesia care provider and surgeon at regular intervals throughout the procedure.

Fluid absorption increases with increased length of the procedure. Completing procedures in one hour or less may help limit complications from fluid absorption.[146]

VII.e.2. The perioperative RN should initiate corrective action in response to audible alarms from the fluid management system and notify the surgeon and anesthesia care provider if corrective actions do not result in a decrease of fluid volume deficit to a safe level.

VII.e.3. The patient should be monitored for physiologic changes, including core temperature and potential fluid retention.

TUR syndrome, mild to moderately severe absorption of nonelectrolyte solution, occurs in up to 8% of patients undergoing TUR. Absorption of more than 1 L has been reported in 5% to 20% of TURs and results in symptoms.[146] The most serious adverse events occur when more than 3 L of fluid are absorbed.[146] Extravasation can occur during renal stone surgery or when instruments perforate the bladder or prostate capsule.[146] Glycine absorption causes circulatory (ie, chest pain, bradycardia, hypertension) and neurological (ie, blurred vision, nausea and vomiting, apprehension, confusion) symptoms.[146] In a recent study of patients undergoing transurethral resection of the prostate (TURP), glycine absorption was associated with echocardiogram changes and myocardial stress.[149] Physiological responses that can result from excessive fluid absorption include
- cardiac overload,
- cerebral edema,
- dilutional hyponatremia, and
- water intoxication.[146,149,165]

VII.e.4. The patient's neck and facial area should be assessed intraoperatively when volumetric fluid calculations are being performed.

Manual volumetric calculations made intraoperatively provide crude estimates only. Edema of the parotid area is a late sign of interstitial edema that develops as a result of a fluid deficit up to or greater than 1,000 mL. Manual calculation is a simple and inexpensive means to determine fluid deficit over 1,000 mL when accurate volumetric fluid balance calculations are hampered by extraneous fluid losses.[166]

VII.e.5. The nurse should be prepared to coordinate and report laboratory testing of serum electrolytes.

When the patient is at risk of hyponatremia, serum electrolyte or urine electrolyte testing often is performed. Normal serum sodium is 135 mmol/L to 145 mmol/L. Hyponatremia occurs when serum sodium levels fall below 135 mmol/L.[167,168]

VII.f. Patients should be monitored for adverse reactions when medications are added to fluids used for irrigation or distention media.

Antibiotics may be added to irrigation fluid for MIS procedures. For arthroscopy procedures, epinephrine may be added to the irrigation/distention fluid medium resulting in vasoconstriction and hemostasis with an increased visual field for the surgeon.

Recommendation VIII

The patient's physiologic response, including core temperature and potential fluid retention, should be evaluated postoperatively.

Nausea and vomiting are common postoperative complaints after laparoscopic surgery and can cause delays in the patient's discharge.[45] Signs and symptoms related to fluid and medication absorption can occur after the procedure. The most common signs and symptoms reported after a urologic procedure are nausea, hypotension, low urinary output, visual disturbances, and confusion. Abdominal pain accompanied by hypotension and poor urinary output may be an indication of extravasation of fluid.[146] Adverse events related to irrigation and distention fluid may occur postoperatively. Pulmonary edema in the postanesthesia care unit has been reported in healthy, young patients after orthopedic arthroscopy procedures.[169] The potential for complications related to extra-articular fluid migration is likely to increase in relation to the duration and complexity of the arthroscopic procedure. Prolonged use of high irrigation flow rates and pressures (eg, 100 mm Hg for 60 to 90 minutes) may increase the risk of complications.[170,171]

Recommendation IX

Personnel should receive initial and ongoing education and demonstrate competency in the perioperative nursing care of patients who undergo MIS and computer-assisted procedures and in the use of MIS and computer-assisted equipment.

Initial education on the nursing care of MIS patients, procedures, and related equipment provides direction for personnel in providing safe patient care. Additional periodic educational programs provide opportunities

MINIMALLY INVASIVE SURGERY

to reinforce previous learning, introduce new information on changes in technology, its application, compatibility of equipment and accessories, and potential hazards.

IX.a. An introduction and review of policies and procedures for MIS and computer-assisted procedures should be included in orientation and ongoing education of personnel.

Review of policies and procedures assists health care personnel in the development of knowledge, skills, and attitudes that affect patient outcomes.

IX.b. Perioperative RNs should be knowledgeable about new instrumentation; equipment; computer-assisted technology (eg, robotics, voice recognition software); and camera technologies being used in the health care organization.

Technology is continually evolving. Rapid technological advances require continuous learning and skills updating to maintain competency.

IX.b.1. Perioperative personnel should demonstrate competency in the use of MIS and computer-assisted equipment, following manufacturers' written instructions, before use.

Instruction and return demonstration in proper usage minimizes the risk of injury and extends the life of the equipment. Competencies based on the manufacturer's instructions ensure that personnel have the knowledge about the proper use of the fluid management system and other MIS equipment. Incorrect use can result in serious patient complications. Equipment instruction manuals assist in developing operational, safety, and maintenance guidelines and serve as a reference for safe, appropriate use.

IX.b.2. Education and competency validation should include all components of the MIS and computer-assisted equipment including, but not limited to,
- equipment operation and safety considerations,
- computer system use,
- position of equipment for specific surgeries, and
- troubleshooting malfunctioning equipment.[3]

IX.b.3. The perioperative RN should be instructed in the safety considerations and risks of gas insufflation and demonstrate competency in the management of its risks.

IX.b.4. Personnel should be instructed in the safety considerations and risks of electrosurgery and demonstrate competency in the use of electrosurgery equipment and related accessories during MIS and computer-assisted procedures.[57]

IX.b.5. Personnel using AEC should be knowledgeable about signs, symptoms, and treatment of venous emboli.

There is a significant risk of gas embolism when AEC is used during laparoscopic procedures from abdominal overpressurization and displacement of CO_2 by argon gas.[79-82]

IX.c. Personnel should receive education about the selection of fluids used for irrigation and distention media selection, fluid administration equipment and procedures, and fluid storage requirements.

IX.c.1. Education and competency validation should include, but not be limited to,
- fluid storage and fluid warming equipment,
- distention fluid selection,
- proper use of distention fluid management systems,
- patient assessments, and
- response to patient complications.

An understanding of appropriate use, risks, and precautions to minimize these risks provides the foundation for compliance with procedures and the delivery of safe patient care.

IX.d. Team training and team building should be implemented whenever new procedures or new team dynamics are introduced (eg, hybrid/integrated OR).

Creating a hybrid OR requires advanced education of perioperative team members that emphasizes teamwork and the importance of what each member of the team brings to total patient care. Some team members may be resistant to working together in a hybrid OR because of previous departmental borders. Techniques such as those described in the AORN Human Factors in Health Care Tool Kit may be useful for the education process.[172]

Recommendation X

The perioperative RN should document the care of patients undergoing MIS and computer-assisted procedures throughout the continuum of care.

Documentation of all nursing activities performed is legally and professionally important for clear communication and collaboration between health care team members and for continuity of patient care.

X.a. Documentation using the PNDS should include a patient assessment, a plan of care, nursing diagnoses, identification of desired outcomes, interventions, and an evaluation of the patient's response to the care provided.

Documentation provides communication among all care providers involved in planning and implementing patient care. Standardized documentation allows the potential for consistent data retrieval and comparison.

X.b. Documentation should be recorded in a manner consistent with the health care organization's policies and procedures.

X.b.1. Documentation for MIS procedures should include, but not be limited to,
- distention media used;
- equipment used for distention media administration, including the equipment identification number;
- quantity of fluid administered and flow rate;
- quantity of fluid returned, if applicable;
- urinary output;
- medication added to distention fluid; and
- relevant information about equipment used (eg, insufflation, electrosurgery, positioning).

Recommendation XI

Policies and procedures for MIS and computer-assisted procedures should be developed, reviewed periodically, and readily available in the practice setting.

Policies and procedures assist in the development of patient safety, quality assessment, and improvement activities. Policies and procedures establish authority, responsibility, and accountability with the organization. They also serve as operational guidelines that are used to minimize patient risk factors, standardize practice, direct staff members, and establish guidelines for continuous performance improvement activities.

XI.a. The health care organization's policies and procedures for MIS equipment must be in compliance with the *Safe Medical Devices Act (SMDA) of 1990*, as amended in March 2000.[173]

XI.a.1. When patient or personnel injuries or equipment failures occur, the equipment and associated device(s) should be removed from service and the associated devices retained if possible.
Identification and segregation of the complete system allows for a thorough evaluation and identification of the cause of the equipment failure.

XI.a.2. Incidents of patient or personnel injury or equipment failure should be reported as required by regulation to federal, state, and local authorities and to the equipment manufacturer. Device identification, maintenance and service information, and adverse event information should be included in the report from the practice setting.
Documentation of details of the involved equipment and associated devices allows for retrievable information for investigation into an adverse event.

XI.b. Policies and procedures must comply with the *Standards of Privacy and Security of the Health Insurance Portability and Accountability Act of 1996* for the protection of health information.[174]

XI.b.1. MIS patient privacy policies and procedures should include, but not be limited to,
- disclosure of information,
- access to and use of databases,
- access to and use of digital images, and
- data security.

XI.c. Policies should be written and readily available in the practice setting.

XI.c.1. Policies regarding MIS and computer-assisted equipment should include, but not be limited to,
- required qualifications and credentials for operation of specific equipment or devices (eg, radiologic, MRI equipment);
- procedure scheduling related to equipment availability;
- equipment acquisition;
- personnel training and competency validation before use of equipment;
- equipment maintenance and repair;
- types of MIS procedures approved in the practice setting; and
- reporting of adverse events.

Compromised patient safety, delay in care, or cancellation of the procedure may result when required equipment or qualified personnel are not available.[175]

XI.c.2. Policies and procedures regarding the selection, storage, administration, and required monitoring of fluid used for irrigation or distention media and gases used for distention media should include, but not be limited to,
- manufacturers' written instructions for storage, warming, and use of fluid administration or gas insufflation equipment;
- requirements of regulatory and accrediting agencies; and
- evidence from published scientific literature.

Recommendation XII

Quality assurance/performance improvement process should be in place that measures patient; process; and structural (eg, system) outcome indicators.

A fundamental precept of AORN is that it is the responsibility of professional perioperative RNs to ensure safe, high-quality nursing care to patients undergoing operative and other invasive procedures.[176]

XII.a. Structure, process, and clinical outcomes performance measures should be identified.

Performance measures can be used to improve patient care and monitor compliance with facility policy and procedure, national standards, and regulatory requirements.[176]

XII.a.1. Process indicators should be collected, analyzed, and used for performance improvement.[176] Indicators may include, but are not limited to information about adverse patient outcomes and near misses associated with electrosurgery or other MIS or computer-assisted equipment.

XII.b. Quality assurance/performance improvement processes should be in place to evaluate the safety of fluid management in the health care setting.

Quality control programs that enhance personnel performance and monitor fluid management efficacy are established to promote patient and employee safety.

XII.b.1. A quality management program should be in place to evaluate at least the following:
- daily temperature checks of fluid warming storage cabinets,
- temperature of warmed fluids at the point of use,
- bioengineering safety checks for fluid warming and administration equipment, and
- reporting mechanisms for adverse events and near misses related to fluid management.

XII.b.2. Adverse events and near misses related to fluid management or other MIS or computer-assisted equipment should be reported and investigated and corrective action taken.

Reporting adverse events and near misses through an adverse event reporting and investigation system provides a mechanism to determine trends, potential risk factors, and evaluate the effectiveness of corrective actions.

XII.c. Fluid management systems and other MIS and computer-assisted equipment should be evaluated and approved by the health care organization's biomedical personnel before use and assigned an identification or serial number for tracking.[41]

Hazards associated with medical equipment, if not corrected, may result in injury to patients, staff members, or visitors. The identification or serial number facilitates documenting maintenance performed on the individual system and tracking of problems when they occur. Endoscopic equipment manuals provide guidelines for developing operating, safety, and maintenance practices. Proper inspection, testing, use, and processing of equipment reduces the risk of adverse outcomes or damage to equipment. Equipment that functions correctly promotes patient safety and efficiency during the surgical procedure.[175]

XII.c.1. Correct control settings should be labeled on equipment and on a quick reference chart attached to the equipment.

Standardization of equipment allows for interchangeability in the event of equipment malfunction.

XII.c.2. The manufacturer's manual for maintenance and inspections for all MIS-related equipment, written instructions for reprocessing any supplies or accessories, and warranties should be easily retrievable for the clinical perioperative team.

Equipment instruction manuals assist in developing operational, safety, and maintenance guidelines and serve as a reference for safe, appropriate use.

XII.c.3. MIS equipment should have standard safety features including, but not limited to, appropriate alarm and monitoring systems. Clinical alarms should be audible and should not be disabled.[41]

Safety features include, but are not limited to, the following:
- audible alarms for absence of fluid in the dispensing tubing,
- audible alarms to indicate air in the fluid dispensing tubing,
- audible alarms to indicate fluid deficit,
- pressure regulated without fluctuation,
- accurate outflow measure,
- accurate measurement of fluid instilled and returned to the regulator,
- measurement of intrauterine pressure, and
- fluid management systems with accurate calculations of fluid volume deficit.

Glossary

Active electrode: The electrosurgical unit (ESU) accessory that directs current flow to the surgical site (eg, pencils, various pencil tips).

Active electrode indicator shaft: An active electrode composed of two layers of insulated material of different colors. The inner layer is a bright color, the outer layer is black. When the brightly colored inner layer is evident upon visual inspection, a break in the insulation is indicated.

Active-electrode insulation testing devices: Devices designed to test the integrity of the insulation surrounding the conductive shaft of laparoscopic electrosurgical active-electrode instruments. The devices detect full thickness breaks in the insulation layer.

Active electrode monitoring: A dynamic process of searching for insulation failures and capacitive coupling during monopolar surgery. If the monitor detects an unsafe level of stray energy, it signals the generator to deactivate.

MINIMALLY INVASIVE SURGERY

Alternate site injury: Patient injury caused by an electrosurgical device that occurs away from the dispersive electrode site.

Argon-enhanced coagulation (AEC): Radio-frequency coagulation from an electrosurgical generator that is capable of delivering monopolar current through a flow of ionized argon gas.

Automated fluid management system: Mechanical medical devices designed to calculate the amount of fluid dispensed to the patient compared to the amount returned to the system; alarms alert the user to fluid deficit to prompt corrective action.

Bipolar resection devices: Mechanical medical devices that use an electrolytic solution to conduct electrical flow to resect tissue. Often used for hysteroscopy procedures.

Capacitance: Ability of an electrical circuit to transfer an electrical charge from one conductor to another, even when separated by an insulator.

Capacitive coupling: Transfer of electrical current from the active electrode through intact insulation to adjacent conductive items (eg, tissue, trocars).

Capacitors: Two conductors separated by an insulator (eg, insulated active electrode, trocar cannula); instrument for storing electricity.

Computer-assisted technologies: Robotic, interventional radiology, voice-recognition software, or other computer technologies used to enhance minimally invasive surgery.

Dilutional hyponatremia: A decrease in the serum sodium level caused by intravasation of fluids, which dilute the soluble components of the serum.

Digital OR: Technology that includes a centralized database that allows continuous live feeds throughout the health care facility, allowing data retrieval (eg, video clips, still images) after the procedure for educational or reporting purposes. Synonym: Integrated OR.

Direct coupling: The contact of an energized active electrode tip with another metal instrument or object within the surgical field.

Endoscopic surgery: A surgical technique using endoscopic instrumentation inserted through a natural orifice or through one or more small incisions.

Extravasation: To pass by infiltration or effusion from a proper vessel or channel (as a blood vessel) into surrounding tissue.

Fluid deficit: When the amount of fluid infused to the patient is more than the amount returned to suction or fluid management system.

Hybrid OR: An operating room designed with numerous imaging technologies (eg, 3D angiography, computed tomography, magnetic resonance imaging, positron-emission tomography, intravascular ultrasound) to support surgical procedures that require multiple care providers with varied expertise to provide patient care in one location.

Hyponatremia: An abnormally low concentration of sodium ions in circulating blood.

Hydrophobic insufflation filter: An in-line filter that retains a high percentage of particulates greater than a specified size. The hydrophobic media protects against fluid backflow into the insufflation gas.

Hypothermia: A decrease in core body temperature to a level below the normothermic range.

Hypervolemia: An excessive volume of fluid in the vascular space.

Hysteroscopy: Endoscopic visualization of the uterine cavity and tubal orifices.

Insufflate: The introduction of a flow of gas into a body cavity.

Insufflation: The act of blowing gas into a body cavity or the state of being distended with gas for the purpose of visual examination.

Integrated OR: An operating room equipped with technology that centralizes control of audiovideo equipment and information systems and is capable of controlling a variety of equipment and activities within the surgical suite. Synonym: digital OR.

Intracorporeal mobile devices: Miniaturized robotic devices designed to allow access to restricted spaces for surgical or diagnostic purposes.

Intravasation: The entrance of foreign material or solution into a blood vessel.

Light cable: Fiber-optic filaments joined into a cable used to transport light to the surgical field.

Minimally invasive surgery: Surgical procedures performed through one or more small incisions using endoscopic instruments, radiographic and magnetic resonance imaging, computer-assisted devices, robotics, and other emerging technologies.

Nanotechnologies: The science and technology of creating nanoparticles and of manufacturing machines that have sizes within the range of 0.1 to 100 nanometers. An advanced technology involving the fabrication and use of devices so small that the convenient unit of measurement is the nanometer (one billionth of a meter).

NOTES: Natural orifice transluminal endoscopic surgery.

Pneumoperitoneum: The presence of air or gas within the peritoneal cavity of the abdomen often induced for diagnostic purposes.

Single-port access laparoscopy: One incision is used, rather than several incisions, to insert laparoscopic instrumentation.

Telepresence: Robotic and computer technology that allows a health care provider to interact physically with patients or other health care providers in remote locations.

TUR syndrome: A mild to moderately severe absorption of nonelectrolyte solution following transurethral resection.

Water intoxication: An increase in the volume of water in the body, resulting in dilutional hyponatremia.

White balancing: A part of the color balancing process that renders neutral color adjustment to achieve balanced intensities and avoid unrealistic color casts.

References

1. Recommended practices for cleaning and care of surgical instruments and powered equipment. In: *Perioperative Standards and Recommended Practices*. Denver, CO: AORN, Inc; 2009:611-636.

2. Recommended practices for cleaning and processing flexible endoscopes and endoscope accessories.

Perioperative Standards and Recommended Practices. Denver, CO: AORN, Inc; 2009:595-610.

3. Acevedo AL. Construction of an integrated surgical suite in a military treatment facility. *AORN J.* 2009;89(1):151-159.

4. Cepolina F, Michelini RC. Review of robotic fixtures for minimally invasive surgery. *Int J Med Robot.* 2004;1(1):43-63.

5. Taylor GW, Jayne DG. Robotic applications in abdominal surgery: their limitations and future developments. *Int J Med Robot.* 2007;3:3-9.

6. Gordon D. Trends in surgery-suite design. Part I. *Healthcare Design.* 2007;6.

7. Burgess NA, Koo BC, Calvert RC, Hindmarsh A, Donaldson PJ, Rhodes M. Randomized trial of laparoscopic v open nephrectomy. *J Endourol.* 2007;21(6):610-613.

8. Sroga J, Patel S D, Falcone T. Robotics in reproductive medicine. *Front Biosci.* 2008;13:1308-1317.

9. Herron DM, Marohn M; SAGES-MIRA Robotic Surgery Consensus Group. A consensus document on robotic surgery. *Surg Endosc.* 2008;22(2):313-325.

10. Petersen C, ed. AORN Guidance Statement: *Safe Patient Handling and Movement in the Perioperative Setting.* Denver, CO: AORN, Inc; 2007.

11. AORN position statement on ergonomically healthy workplace practices. AORN, Inc. http://www.aorn.org/PracticeResources/AORNPositionStatements/Position_Ergonomics/. Accessed October 13, 2009.

12. van Veelen, Jakimowicz, Kazemier. Improved physical ergonomics of laparoscopic surgery. *Minim Invasive Ther Allied Technol.* 2004;13(3):161-166.

13. Sikkink CJ, Reijnen MM, Zeebregts CJ. The creation of the optimal dedicated endovascular suite. *Eur J Vasc Endovasc Surg.* 2008;35(2):198-204.

14. Brogmus G, Leone W, Butler L, Hernandez E. Best practices in OR suite layout and equipment choices to reduce slips, trips, and falls. *AORN J.* 2007;86(3):384-398.

15. Mathur NS. The next generation of operating rooms. *Acad J.* 2005:8

16. Berguer R. Surgery and ergonomics. *Arch Surg.* 1999;134(9):1011-1016.

17. Albayrak, Kazemier, Meijer, Bonjer. Current state of ergonomics of operating rooms of Dutch hospitals in the endoscopic era. *Minim Invasive Ther Allied Technol.* 2004;13(3):156-160.

18. Sandberg WS, Daily B, Egan M, et al. Deliberate perioperative systems design improves operating room throughput. *Anesthesiology.* 2005;103(2):406-418.

19. Rostenberg B, Horii SC. *The Architecture of Medical Imaging: Designing Healthcare Facilities for Advanced Radiological Diagnostic and Therapeutic Techniques.* Hoboken, NJ: John Wiley & Sons; 2006.

20. ECRI. OR integration: what, why, and how? *Operating Room Risk Management.* 2008;17(4):1-6.

21. van Det MJ, Meijerink WJ, Hoff C, Totté ER, Pierie JP. Optimal ergonomics for laparoscopic surgery in minimally invasive surgery suites: a review and guidelines. *Surg Endosc.* 2009;23(6):1279-1285.

22. Gordon D. Trends in surgery-suite design. Part II. *Healthcare Design.* 2007;7(6):32-40.

23. Catalano K, Fickenscher K. Emerging technologies in the OR and their effect on perioperative professionals. *AORN J.* 2007;86(6):958-969.

24. Latifi R, Peck K, Satava R, Anvari M. Telepresence and telementoring in surgery. *Stud Health Technol Inform.* 2004;104:200-206.

25. Chung KK, Grathwohl KW, Poropatich RK, Wolf SE, Holcomb JB. Robotic telepresence: past, present, and future. *J Cardiothorac Vasc Anesth.* 2007;21(4):593-596.

26. Doarn CR, Hufford K, Low T, Rosen J, Hannaford B. Telesurgery and robotics. *Telemed J E Health.* 2007;13(4):369-380.

27. Sebajang H, Trudeau P, Dougall A, Hegge S, McKinley C, Anvari M. The role of telementoring and telerobotic assistance in the provision of laparoscopic colorectal surgery in rural areas. *Surg Endosc.* 2006;20(9):1389-1393.

28. Recommended practices for traffic patterns in the perioperative practice setting. In: *Perioperative Standards and Recommended Practices.* Denver, CO: AORN, Inc; 2009:327-330.

29. Lindeman WE. Design and construction of an ambulatory surgery center. *AORN J.* 2008;88(3):369-380.

30. Worley DJ, Hohler SE. OR construction project: from planning to execution. *AORN J.* 2008;88(6):917-941.

31. Jacob AL, Regazzoni P, Bilecen D, Rasmus M, Huegli RW, Messmer P. Medical technology integration: CT, angiography, imaging-capable OR-table, navigation and robotics in a multifunctional sterile suite. *Minim Invasive Ther Allied Technol.* 2007;16(4):205-211.

32. Russell L. Intraoperative magnetic resonance imaging safety considerations. *AORN J.* 2003;77(3):590-592.

33. Chapter 1.5: Planning, design, and construction. In: AIA Academy of Architecture for Health, Facilities Guidelines Institute, eds. Guidelines for *Design and Construction of Health Care Facilities.* Washington, DC: American Institute of Architects; 2006:26-30.

34. AIA Academy of Architecture for Health, Facilities Guidelines Institute. *Guidelines for Design and Construction of Health Care Facilities.* Washington, DC: American Institute of Architects; 2006.

35. ECRI Institute upholds recommendations on warming cabinet temperatures. *Risk Management Reporter.* 2007;26(2):9-10.

36. ECRI Institute. Hazard report update: Limiting the temperature of warming cabinets remains a good safety practice. *Health Devices.* 2006;35(12):458-461.

37. US Food and Drug Administration. Safety assessment of Di(2-ethylhexyl)phthalate (DEHP) released from PVC medical devices. 2001.

38. Avoiding mix-ups between sterile water and sodium chloride bags. *ISMP MedicationSafetyAlert.* 2007;12(25).

39. Huang S, Gateley D, Moss AL. Accidental burn injury during knee arthroscopy. *Arthroscopy.* 2007;23(12):1363.e1–1363.e3.

40. Kressin KA. Burn injury in the operating room: a closed claims analysis. *ASA Newsl.* 2004;68(6):9-11.

41. Recommended practices for a safe environment of care. In: *Perioperative Standards and Recommended Practices.* Denver, CO: AORN, Inc; 2009:415-438.

42. Recommended practices for prevention of transmissible infections in the perioperative practice setting. In: *Perioperative Standards and Recommended Practices.* Denver, CO: AORN, Inc; 2009:475-486.

43. Recommended practices for maintaining a sterile field. In: *Perioperative Standards and Recommended Practices.* Denver, CO: AORN, Inc; 2009:317-326.

44. Sullivan MJ, Frost EA, Lew MW. Anesthetic care of the patient for robotic surgery. *Middle East J Anesthesiol.* 2008;19(5):967-982.

45. Gerges FJ, Kanazi GE, Jabbour-Khoury SI. Anesthesia for laparoscopy: a review. *J Clin Anesth.* 2006;18(1):67-78.

46. Henny CP, Hofland J. Laparoscopic surgery: pitfalls due to anesthesia, positioning, and pneumoperitoneum. *Surg Endosc.* 2005;19(9):1163-1171.

47. Harrington S, Simmons K, Thomas C, Scully S. Pediatric laparoscopy. *AORN J.* 2008;88(2):211-236.

48. AORN guideline for prevention of venous stasis. In: *Perioperative Standards and Recommended Practices*. Denver, CO: AORN, Inc; 2009:165-182.

49. Cantrell SW, Ward KS, Van Wickllin SA. Translating research on venous thromboembolism into practice. *AORN J*. 2007;86(4):590-606.

50. Society of American Gastrointestinal and Endoscopic Surgeons (SAGES) Guidelines Committee. Guidelines for deep venous thrombosis prophylaxis during laparoscopic surgery. *Surg Endosc*. 2007;21(6):1007-1009.

51. Rasmussen MS. Is there a need for antithrombotic prophylaxis during laparoscopic surgery? Always. *J Thromb Haemost*. 2005;3(2):210-211.

52. Ljungstrom KG. Is there a need for antithromboembolic prophylaxis during laparoscopic surgery? Not always. *J Thromb Haemost*. 2005;3(2):212-213.

53. Goldfaden A, Birkmeyer JD. Evidence-based practice in laparoscopic surgery: perioperative care. *Surg Innov*. 2005;12(1):51-61.

54. Haskal R. Current issues for nurse practitioners: hyponatremia. *J Am Acad Nurse Pract*. 2007;19(11):563-579.

55. ACOG Committee on Practice Bulletins. Clinical management guidelines for obstetrician-gynecologists [ACOG Practice Bulletin. Number 81, May 2007]. *Obstet Gynecol*. 2007;109(5):1233-1248.

56. American College of Obstetricians and Gynecologists. ACOG technology assessment in obstetrics and gynecology, number 4, August 2005: hysteroscopy. *Obstet Gynecol*. 2005;106(2):439.

57. Recommended practices for electrosurgery. In: *Perioperative Standards and Recommended Practices*. Denver, CO: AORN, Inc; 2010:105-126.

58. ECRI Institute. Electrosurgery. *Healthcare Risk Control*. 2007;4(Surgery and Anesthesia 16).

59. Odell RC. Pearls, pitfalls, and advancements in the delivery of electrosurgical energy during laparoscopy. *Problems in Gen Surg*. 2002;19(2):5-17.

60. ECRI Institute. Operating room risk management: ORRM, Laparoscopic electrosurgery risks. *Operating Room Risk Management*. 1999;2(Surgery 19):1-11.

61. Guidance section: ensuring monopolar electrosurgical safety during laparoscopy. *Health Devices*. 1995;24(1):20-26.

62. Wu MP, Ou CS, Chen SL, Yen EY, Rowbotham R. Complications and recommended practices for electrosurgery in laparoscopy. *Am J Surg*. 2000;179(1):67-73.

63. Vilos GA, Newton DW, Odell RC, Abu-Rafea B, Vilos AG. Characterization and mitigation of stray radiofrequency currents during monopolar resectoscopic electrosurgery. *J Minim Invasive Gynecol*. 2006;13(2):134-140.

64. Physician Insurers Association of America, eds. *Laparoscopic Injury Study*. Rockville, MD: Physician Insurers Association of America; 2000:1-5.

65. ECRI Institute. Safety technologies for laparoscopic monopolar electrosurgery; devices for managing burn risks. *Health Devices*. 2005;34(8):259-272.

66. Evaluation of Electroscope Electroshield System. *Health Devices*. 1995;24(1):11-19.

67. Dennis V. Implementing active electrode monitoring: a perioperative call. *SSM*. 2001;7(2):32-38.

68. Harrell GJ, Kopps DR. Minimizing patient risk during laparoscopic electrosurgery. *AORN J*. 1998;67(6):1194-1196.

69. Surgical fire safety. *Health Devices*. 2006;35(2):45-66.

70. Greilich PE, Greilich NB, Froelich EG. Intraabdominal fire during laparoscopic cholecystectomy. *Anesthesiology*. 1995;83(4):871-874.

71. Tucker RD, Voyles CR, Silvis SE. Capacitive coupled stray currents during laparoscopic and endoscopic electrosurgical procedures. *Biomed Instrum Technol*. 1992;26(4):303-311.

72. Wang K, Advincula AP. "Current thoughts" in electrosurgery. *Int J Gynaecol Obstet*. 2007;97(3):245-250.

73. Shirk GJ, Johns A, Redwine DB. Complications of laparoscopic surgery: How to avoid them and how to repair them. *J Minim Invasive Gynecol*. 2006;13(4):352-359.

74. Yazdani A, Krause H. Laparoscopic instrument insulation failure: the hidden hazard. *J Minim Invasive Gynecol*. 2007;14(2):228-232.

75. Smith TL, Smith JM. Electrosurgery in otolaryngology-head and neck surgery: principles, advances, and complications. *Laryngoscope*. 2001;111(5):769-780.

76. *NFPA 99 Standard for Health Care Facilities*. Quincy, MA: National Fire Protection Association; 2002: Issue D.7.3:203.

77. Garuti G, Luerti M. Hysteroscopic bipolar surgery: a valuable progress or a technique under investigation? *Curr Opin Obstet Gynecol*. 2009;21(4):329-334.

78. Matthews K. Argon beam coagulation. New directions in surgery. *AORN J*. 1992;56(5):885-889.

79. Fatal gas embolism caused by overpressurization during laparoscopic use of argon enhanced coagulation. *Health Devices*. 1994;23(6):257-259.

80. Kizer N, Zighelboim I, Rader JS. Cardiac arrest during laparotomy with argon beam coagulation of metastatic ovarian cancer. *Int J Gynecol Cancer*. 2009;19(2):237-238.

81. Misra S, Kimball WR. Pneumothorax during argon beam-enhanced coagulation in laparoscopy. *J Clin Anesth*. 2006;18(6):446-448.

82. Sezeur A, Partensky C, Chipponi J, Duron JJ. Death during laparoscopy: can 1 gas push out another? Danger of argon electrocoagulation. *Surg Laparosc Endosc Percutan Tech*. 2008;18(4):395-397.

83. Occupational Safety and Health Administration. Sec.5. Duties. OSH Act 1970. http://www.osha.gov/pls/oshaweb/owadisp.show_document?p_table=OSHACT&p_id=3359. Accessed June 7,2012.

84. Brüske-Hohlfeld I, Preissler G, Jauch KW, et al. Surgical smoke and ultrafine particles. *J Occup Med and Toxicol*. 2008;3:31-45.

85. Bigony L. Risks associated with exposure to surgical smoke plume: a review of the literature. *AORN J*. 2007;86(6):1013-1024.

86. *ANSI® Z136.3-2011: American National Standard for Safe Use of Lasers in Health Care*. Washington, DC: American National Standards Institute; 2011.

87. ECRI Institute. Smoke evacuation systems, surgical. Healthcare Product Comparison System. 2007; November.

88. HC11: Control of smoke from laser/electric surgical procedures. http://www.cdc.gov/niosh/hc11.html. Accessed October 13, 2009.

89. Alp E, Bijl D, Bleichrodt RP, Hansson B, Voss A. Surgical smoke and infection control. *J Hosp Infect*. 2006;62(1):1-5.

90. Al Sahaf OS, Vega-Carrascal I, Cunningham FO, McGrath JP, Bloomfield FJ. Chemical composition of smoke produced by high-frequency electrosurgery. *Ir J Med Sci*. 2007;176(3):229-232.

91. Baggish MS, Poiesz BJ, Joret D, Williamson P, Refai A. Presence of human immunodeficiency virus DNA in laser smoke. *Lasers Surg Med*. 1991;11(3):197-203.

92. Ulmer BC. The hazards of surgical smoke. *AORN J*. 2008;87(4):721-738.

93. Hoglan M. Potential hazards from electrosurgery plume—recommendations for surgical smoke evacuation. *Can Oper Room Nurs J.* 1995;13(4):10-16.

94. Safety and health topics: laser/electrosurgery plume. US Department of Labor Occupational Safety and Health Administration. http://www.osha.gov/SLTC/laser electrosurgeryplume/index.html. Accessed October 13, 2009.

95. Garden JM, O'Banion MK, Shelnitz LS, et al. Papillomavirus in the vapor of carbon dioxide laser-treated verrucae. *JAMA.* 1988;259(8):1199-1202.

96. Hallmo P, Naess O. Laryngeal papillomatosis with human papillomavirus DNA contracted by a laser surgeon. *Eur Arch Otorhinolaryngol.* 1991;248(7):425-427.

97. Barrett WL, Garber SM. Surgical smoke: a review of the literature. Is this just a lot of hot air? *Surg Endosc.* 2003;17(6):979-987.

98. Weld KJ, Dryer S, Ames CD, et al. Analysis of surgical smoke produced by various energy-based instruments and effects on laparoscopic visibility. *J Endourol.* 2007;21(3):347-351.

99. Recommended practices for transfer of patient care information. In: *Perioperative Standards and Recommended Practices.* Denver, CO: AORN, Inc; 2010:371-388.

100. Liapis D, de la Taille A, Ploussard G, et al. Analysis of complications from 600 retroperitoneoscopic procedures of the upper urinary tract during the last 10 years. *World J Urol.* 2008;26(6):523-530.

101. Marakis GN, Pavlidis TE, Ballas K, et al. Major complications during laparoscopic cholecystectomy. *Int Surg.* 2007;92(3):142-146.

102. Deziel DJ, Millikan KW, Economou SG, Doolas A, Ko ST, Airan MC. Complications of laparoscopic cholecystectomy: a national survey of 4,292 hospitals and an analysis of 77,604 cases. *Am J Surg.* 1993;165(1):9-14.

103. Abu-Rafea B, Vilos GA, Vilos AG, Hollett-Caines J, Al-Omran M. Effect of body habitus and parity on insufflated CO_2 volume at various intraabdominal pressures during laparoscopic access in women. *J Minim Invasive Gynecol.* 2006;13(3):205-210.

104. Recommended practices for positioning the patient in the perioperative practice setting. In: *Perioperative Standards and Recommended Practices.* Denver, CO: AORN, Inc; 2009:525-548.

105. Underwood S. Reducing positioning changes during robotic lead placement. *AORN J.* 2006;83(2):399-401.

106. Ito F, Gould JC. Robotic foregut surgery. *Int J Med Robot.* 2006;2(4):287-292.

107. Barnett JC, Hurd WW, Rogers RM Jr, Williams NL, Shapiro SA. Laparoscopic positioning and nerve injuries. *J Minim Invasive Gynecol.* 2007;14(5):664-673.

108. Pillai AK, Ferral H, Desai S, Paruchuri S, Asselmeier S, Perez-Gautrin R. Brachial plexus injury related to patient positioning. *J Vasc Interv Radiol.* 2007;18(7):833-834.

109. AORN position statement on fire prevention. AORN, Inc. http://www.aorn.org/PracticeResources/AORNPositionStatements/Position_FirePrevention. Accessed October 14, 2009.

110. Hazard report: Reducing the risk of burns from surgical light sources. *Health Devices.* 2009;38(9):304-305.

111. Whelan RL, Fleshman J, Fowler DL. *The SAGES Manual of Perioperative Care in Minimally Invasive Surgery.* New York, NY: Springer-Verlag; 2006.

112. Strickland AK, Martindale RG. The increased incidence of intraabdominal infections in laparoscopic procedures: potential causes, postoperative management, and prospective innovations. *Surg Endosc.* 2005;19(7):874-881.

113. Shafi BM, Mery CM, Binyamin G, Dutta S. Natural orifice translumenal endoscopic surgery (NOTES). *Semin Pediatr Surg.* 2006;15(4):251-258.

114. Willingham FF, Brugge WR. Taking NOTES: translumenal flexible endoscopy and endoscopic surgery. *Curr Opin Gastroenterol.* 2007;23(5):550-555.

115. Malik A, Mellinger JD, Hazey JW, Dunkin BJ, MacFadyen BV Jr. Endoluminal and transluminal surgery: current status and future possibilities. *Surg Endosc.* 2006;20(8):1179-1192.

116. Kantsevoy SV, Hu B, Jagannath SB, et al. Transgastric endoscopic splenectomy: is it possible? *Surg Endosc.* 2006;20(3):522-525.

117. de la Fuente SG, Demaria EJ, Reynolds JD, Portenier DD, Pryor AD. New developments in surgery: Natural Orifice Transluminal Endoscopic Surgery (NOTES). *Arch Surg.* 2007;142(3):295-297.

118. Robinson TN, Stiegmann GV. Minimally invasive surgery. *Endoscopy.* 2007;39(1):21-23.

119. Jin J, Rosen M, Ponsky J. Minimally invasive surgery 2006-2007. *Endoscopy.* 2008;40(1):61-64.

120. Biscione FM, Couto RC, Pedrosa TM, Neto MC. Factors influencing the risk of surgical site infection following diagnostic exploration of the abdominal cavity. *J Infect.* 2007;55(4):317-323.

121. Gupta R, Sample C, Bamehriz F, Birch DW. Infectious complications following laparoscopic appendectomy. *Can J Surg.* 2006;49(6):397-400.

122. Miller CE. Methods of tissue extraction in advanced laparoscopy. *Curr Opin Obstet Gynecol.* 2001;13(4):399-405.

123. Milad MP, Sokol E. Laparoscopic morcellator-related injuries. *J Am Assoc Gynecol Laparosc.* 2003;10(3):383-385.

124. ECRI Institute. Safe use and selection of trocars in laparoscopy. *Healthcare Risk Control.* 2006;4(Surgery and Anesthesia):25.

125. Vilos GA, Ternamian A, Dempster J, Laberge PY; The Society of Obstetricians and Gynaecologists of Canada. Laparoscopic entry: a review of techniques, technologies, and complications. *J Obstet Gynaecol Can.* 2007;29(5):433-465.

126. Salama IA, Schwaitzberg SD. Utility of a voice-activated system in minimally invasive surgery. *J Laparoendosc Adv Surg Tech A.* 2005;15(5):443-446.

127. Gutt CN, Oniu T, Mehrabi A, et al. Circulatory and respiratory complications of carbon dioxide insufflation. *Dig Surg.* 2004;21(2):95-104.

128. Wadlund DL. Laparoscopy: risks, benefits and complications. *Nurs Clin North Am.* 2006;41(2):219-229.

129. Yoshida H, Kushikata T, Kabara S, Takase H, Ishihara H, Hirota K. Flat electroencephalogram caused by carbon dioxide pneumoperitoneum. *Anesth Analg.* 2007;105(6):1749-1752.

130. Hunter JG, Staheli J, Oddsdottir M, Trus T. Nitrous oxide pneumoperitoneum revisited. Is there a risk of combustion? *Surg Endosc.* 1995;9(5):501-504.

131. Yeh CH, Kwok SY, Chan MK, Tjandra JJ. Prospective, case-matched study of heated and humidified carbon dioxide insufflation in laparoscopic colorectal surgery. *Colorectal Dis.* 2007;9(8):695-700.

132. Jacobs VR, Kiechle M, Morrison JE Jr. Carbon dioxide gas heating inside laparoscopic insufflators has no effect. *JSLS.* 2005;9(2):208-212.

133. Savel RH, Balasubramanya S, Lasheen S, et al. Beneficial effects of humidified, warmed carbon dioxide insufflation during laparoscopic bariatric surgery: a randomized clinical trial. *Obes Surg.* 2005;15(1):64-69.

134. Champion JK, Williams M. Prospective randomized trial of heated humidified versus cold dry carbon dioxide

insufflation during laparoscopic gastric bypass. *Surg Obes Relat Dis.* 2006;2(4):445-450.

135. Hamza MA, Schneider BE, White PF, et al. Heated and humidified insufflation during laparoscopic gastric bypass surgery: effect on temperature, postoperative pain, and recovery outcomes. *J Laparoendosc Adv Surg Tech A.* 2005;15(1):6-12.

136. Farley DR, Greenlee SM, Larson DR, Harrington JR. Double-blind, prospective, randomized study of warmed, humidified carbon dioxide insufflation vs standard carbon dioxide for patients undergoing laparoscopic cholecystectomy. *Arch Surg.* 2004;139(7):739-744.

137. Barragan AB, Frezza EE. Impact of a warm gas insufflation on operating-room ergonometrics during laparoscopic gastric bypass: a pilot study. *Obes Surg.* 2005;15(1):70-72.

138. Pasic RP, Kantardzic M, Templeman C, Levine RL. Insufflation techniques in gynecologic laparoscopy. *Surg Laparosc Endosc Percutan Tech.* 2006;16(1):18-24.

139. Calcaterra D, Salerno TA. Venous gas embolization during endoscopic vein harvesting for coronary artery revascularization: a life-threatening event. *J Card Surg.* 2007;22(6):498-499.

140. Potapov EV, Buz S, Hetzer R. CO(2) embolism during minimally invasive vein harvesting. *Eur J Cardiothorac Surg.* 2007;31(5):944-945.

141. Jacobs VR, Morrison JE Jr, Kiechle M. Twenty-five simple ways to increase insufflation performance and patient safety in laparoscopy. *J Am Assoc Gynecol Laparosc.* 2004;11(3):410-423.

142. Entry of abdominal fluids into laparoscopic insufflators. *Health Devices.* 1992;21(5):180-181.

143. Mertens zur Borg IR, Lim A, Verbrugge SJ, IJzermans JN, Klein J. Effect of intraabdominal pressure elevation and positioning on hemodynamic responses during carbon dioxide pneumoperitoneum for laparoscopic donor nephrectomy: a prospective controlled clinical study. *Surg Endosc.* 2004;18(6):919-923.

144. Meierhenrich R, Gauss A, Vandenesch P, Georgieff M, Poch B, Schutz W. The effects of intraabdominally insufflated carbon dioxide on hepatic blood flow during laparoscopic surgery assessed by transesophageal echocardiography. *Anesth Analg.* 2005;100(2):340-347.

145. Koivusalo AM, Pere P, Valjus M, Scheinin T. Laparoscopic cholecystectomy with carbon dioxide pneumoperitoneum is safe even for high-risk patients. *Surg Endosc.* 2008;22(1):61-67.

146. Hahn RG. Fluid absorption in endoscopic surgery. *Br J Anaesth.* 2006;96(1):8-20.

147. Recommended practices for the prevention of unplanned perioperative hypothermia. In: *Perioperative Standards and Recommended Practices.* Denver, CO: AORN, Inc; 2009:491-504.

148. Moharari RS, Khajavi MR, Khademhosseini P, Hosseini SR, Najafi A. Sterile water as an irrigating fluid for transurethral resection of the prostate: anesthetical view of the records of 1600 cases. *South Med J.* 2008;101(4):373-375.

149. Collins JW, Macdermott S, Bradbrook RA, Drake B, Keeley FX, Timoney AG. The effect of the choice of irrigation fluid on cardiac stress during transurethral resection of the prostate: a comparison between 1.5% glycine and 5% glucose. *J Urol.* 2007;177(4):1369-1373.

150. Ho HS, Cheng CW. Bipolar transurethral resection of prostate: a new reference standard? *Curr Opin Urol.* 2008;18(1):50-55.

151. Recommended practices for environmental cleaning in the perioperative setting. In: *Perioperative Standards and Recommended Practices.* Denver, CO: AORN; 2009:439-453.

152. Sessler DI. Complications and treatment of mild hypothermia. *Anesthesiology.* 2001;95(2):531-543.

153. Moore SS, Green CR, Wang FL, Pandit SK, Hurd WW. The role of irrigation in the development of hypothermia during laparoscopic surgery. *Am J Obstet Gynecol.* 1997;176(3):598-602.

154. Kelly JA, Doughty JK, Hasselbeck AN, Vacchiano CA. The effect of arthroscopic irrigation fluid warming on body temperature. *J Perianesth Nurs.* 2000;15(4):245-252.

155. Mirza S, Panesar S, AuYong KJ, French J, Jones D, Akmal S. The effects of irrigation fluid on core temperature in endoscopic urological surgery. *J Perioper Pract.* 2007;17(10):494-503.

156. Okeke LI. Effect of warm intravenous and irrigating fluids on body temperature during transurethral resection of the prostate gland. *BMC Urol.* 2007;7:15.

157. Jaffe JS, McCullough TC, Harkaway RC, Ginsberg PC. Effects of irrigation fluid temperature on core body temperature during transurethral resection of the prostate. *Urology.* 2001;57(6):1078-1081.

158. Young EC. Hysteroscopy and fluid management. *Perioper Nurs Clin.* 2006;4(1):365-373.

159. de Freitas Fonseca M, Andrade CM Jr, Cardoso MJE, Crispi CP. Temperature of distention fluid and risk of overload in operative hysteroscopy. *J Minim Invasive Gynecol.* 2008;15(6):77S-78S.

160. Boyd HR, Stanley C. Sources of error when tracking irrigation fluids during hysteroscopic procedures. *J Am Assoc Gynecol Laparosc.* 2000;7(4):472-476.

161. Nezhat CH, Fisher DT, Datta S. Investigation of often-reported ten percent hysteroscopy fluid overfill: is this accurate? *J Minim Invasive Gynecol.* 2007;14(4):489-493.

162. Hahn RG. Smoking increases the risk of large scale fluid absorption during transurethral prostatic resection. *J Urol.* 2001;166(1):162-165.

163. Yeates KE, Singer M, Morton AR. Salt and water: a simple approach to hyponatremia. *CMAJ.* 2004;170(3):365-369.

164. Morrison DM. Management of hysteroscopic surgery complications. *AORN J.* 1999;69(1):194-221.

165. Bennett KL, Ohrmundt C, Maloni JA. Preventing intravasation in women undergoing hysteroscopic procedures. *AORN J.* 1996;64(5):792-799.

166. Sinha M, Hegde A, Sinha R, Goel S. Parotid area sign: a clinical test for the diagnosis of fluid overload in hysteroscopic surgery. *J Minim Invasive Gynecol.* 2007;14(2):161-168.

167. Singer GG, Brenner BM. Chapter 46: Fluid and electrolyte disturbances. In: Fauci AS, Braunwald E, Kasper DL, Hauser SL, Longo DL, Jameson JL, Loscalzo J, eds. *Harrison's Principles of Internal Medicine.* 17th ed. New York, NY: McGraw-Hill; 2008.

168. Kaye AD, Riopelle JM. Chapter 54: Intravascular fluid and electrolyte physiology. In: Miller RD, ed. *Miller's Anesthesia.* 7th ed. Edinburgh: Churchill Livingstone; 2009:1705-1737.

169. Ray JM, Conner J, Dillman G, Haynes WB, Lock R. Post-arthroscopic pulmonary edema in two healthy teenage athletes. *J Ky Med Assoc.* 1991;89(2):75-78.

170. Hynson JM, Tung A, Guevara JE, Katz JA, Glick JM, Shapiro WA. Complete airway obstruction during arthroscopic shoulder surgery. *Anesth Analg.* 1993;76(4):875-878.

171. Smith CD, Shah MM. Fluid gain during routine shoulder arthroscopy. *J Shoulder Elbow Surg.* 2008;17(3):415-417.

172. Human Factors in Health Care Tool Kit. AORN, Inc. http://www.aorn.org/PracticeResources/ToolKits/HumanFactorsInHealthCareToolKit. Accessed October 14, 2009.

173. Title 21, Pt. 803: Medical Device Reporting. In: *Code of Federal Regulations.* 2009.

174. HHS Office for Civil Rights. Standards for privacy of individually identifiable health information. Final rule. *Fed Regist.* 2002;67(157):53181-53273.

175. Wiegmann DA, ElBardissi AW, Dearani JA, Daly RC, Sundt TM 3rd. Disruptions in surgical flow and their relationship to surgical errors: an exploratory investigation. *Surgery.* 2007;142(5):658-665.

176. Quality and performance improvement standards for perioperative nursing. In: *Perioperative Standards and Recommended Practices.* Denver, CO: AORN, Inc; 2009:65-74.

Acknowledgments

Lead Author
Bonnie Denholm, RN, MS, CNOR
Perioperative Nursing Specialist
AORN Center for Nursing Practice
Denver, Colorado

Contributing Authors
Sharon Van Wicklin, RN, MSN, CNOR, CRNFA
Educator/Staff Development
Williamson Medical Center
Franklin, Tennessee

Eileen C. Young, RN, CNOR
Senior Clinical Nurse Educator
Gyrus ACMI, an Olympus Company
Kutztown, Pennsylvania

Annette Wasielewski, BSN, RN, CNOR
Administrative Director Minimally Invasive Surgery, Robotics, Bariatrics
Hackensack University Medical Center
Hackensack, New Jersey

Publication History

Originally published as proposed recommended practices February 1994, *AORN Journal.*

Revised November 1998; published February 1999, *AORN Journal.* Reformatted July 2000.

Revised November 2004; published as "Recommended Practices for Endoscopic Minimally Invasive Surgery" in *Standards, Recommended Practices, and Guidelines,* 2005 edition. March 2005, *AORN Journal.*

Revised October 2009 for online publication in *Perioperative Standards and Recommended Practices.*

Editorial revision July 2012. Recommendation IV.j was revised and approved by the Recommended Practices Advisory Board. Reformatted September 2012 for publication in *Perioperative Standards and Recommended Practices,* 2013 edition.

Minor editing revisions made in November 2014 for publication in *Guidelines for Perioperative Practice,* 2015 edition.

GUIDELINE FOR MANAGING THE PATIENT RECEIVING MODERATE SEDATION/ANALGESIA

The Guideline for Managing the Patient Receiving Moderate Sedation/Analgesia was developed by the AORN Recommended Practices Committee and was approved by the AORN Board of Directors. It was presented as proposed recommendations for comments by members and others. The guideline is effective January 1, 2008. The recommendations in the guideline are intended to be achievable and represent what is believed to be an optimal level of practice. Policies and procedures will reflect variations in practice settings and/or clinical situations that determine the degree to which the guideline can be implemented. AORN recognizes the various settings in which perioperative nurses practice; therefore, this guideline is adaptable to various practice settings. These practice settings include traditional operating rooms, ambulatory surgery centers, physician's offices, cardiac catheterization laboratories, endoscopy suites, radiology departments, and all other areas where operative and other invasive procedures may be performed. The reader is referred to the Perioperative Nursing Data Set (PNDS) for an explanation of perioperative nursing diagnoses, interventions, and outcomes.[1]

Purpose

Moderate sedation/analgesia is a drug-induced, mild depression of consciousness achieved by the administration of sedatives or the combination of sedatives and analgesic medications, most often administered intravenously, and titrated to achieve a desired effect. The primary goal of moderate sedation/analgesia is to reduce the patient's anxiety and discomfort. Moderate sedation/analgesia also can facilitate cooperation between the patient and caregivers.[2] Moderate sedation/analgesia produces a condition in which the patient exhibits a mildly depressed level of consciousness and an altered perception of pain, but retains the ability to respond appropriately to verbal and/or tactile stimulation. The patient maintains protective reflexes, may experience some degree of amnesia, and has a rapid return to activities of daily living.[3] The desired effect is a level of sedation with or without analgesia whereby the patient is able to tolerate diagnostic, therapeutic, and invasive procedures through relief of anxiety and pain. The four distinct characteristics of moderate sedation/analgesia are:

- The patient is able to respond purposefully to verbal commands or light tactile stimulation.
- The patient is able to maintain his or her protective reflexes and communicate verbally.
- The patient can maintain adequate, spontaneous ventilation.
- There are minimal variations in vital signs.[2]

Recommendation I

The perioperative registered nurse administering moderate sedation/analgesia must practice within the scope of nursing practice as defined by his or her state and should be compliant with state advisory opinions, declaratory rules, and other regulations that direct the practice of the registered nurse.[4]

The methods of monitoring used with patients who receive moderate sedation/analgesia, the medications selected and administered, and the interventions taken must be within the legal definitions of the scope of practice of the registered nurse.[5]

I.a. In accordance with state and local laws and regulations, a licensed independent practitioner qualified by education, training, and licensure to administer moderate sedation should supervise the administration of moderate sedation.

I.b. The perioperative registered nurse should consult with his or her state board of nursing for any changes or revisions to declaratory rulings and other guidelines that relate to the perioperative registered nurse's role as a provider of moderate sedation/analgesia.[5]

The professional obligation of the perioperative registered nurse to safeguard clients is grounded in the ethical obligation to the patient, the profession, society, the American Nurses Association's (ANA) *Standards of Clinical Nursing Practice*, AORN's "Explications for perioperative nursing," and state nurse practice acts.[4,6]

Recommendation II

Patient selection for moderate sedation/analgesia should be based on established criteria developed through interdisciplinary collaboration by health care professionals.

Certain patients may not be candidates for moderate sedation/analgesia administered by perioperative registered nurses. Such patients may require care provided by an anesthesia provider qualified to administer monitored anesthesia care and to rescue the patient from a deeper level of sedation, or qualified to convert to general anesthesia if needed.[5,7,8]

MODERATE SEDATION/ANALGESIA

TABLE 1. PHYSICAL STATUS CLASSIFICATION

Status	Definition of patient status	Example
P1	A normal healthy patient	No physiologic, psychological, biochemical, or organic disturbance.
P2	A patient with mild systemic disease	Cardiovascular disease, asthma, chronic bronchitis, obesity, or diabetes mellitus.
P3	A patient with severe systemic disease	Cardiovascular or pulmonary disease that limits activity; severe diabetes with systemic complications; history of myocardial infarction, angina pectoris, or poorly controlled hypertension.
P4	A patient with severe systemic disease that is a constant threat to life	Severe cardiac, pulmonary, renal, hepatic, or endocrine dysfunction.
P5	A moribund patient who is not expected to survive without the operation	Surgery is done as a last recourse or resuscitative effort; major multi-system or cerebral trauma, ruptured aneurysm, or large pulmonary embolus.
P6	A declared brain-dead patient whose organs are being removed for donor purposes	

Reproduced with permission from the American Society of Anesthesiologists, Park Ridge, IL.

II.a. The perioperative registered nurse should assess the patient to determine the appropriateness of registered nurse-administered sedation/analgesia based on selection criteria defined by the health care organization.

The American Society of Anesthesiologists (ASA) Physical Status Classification (Table 1) may be used as a means of determining patient appropriateness for registered nurse-administered sedation/analgesia. Patients classified as P1, P2, and a medically stable P3 are normally considered appropriate for registered nurse-administered moderate sedation/analgesia.[5,6]

II.b. Consultation with an anesthesia provider should be obtained if a patient presents with any one of the following:
- known history of respiratory or hemodynamic instability;
- previous difficulties with anesthesia or sedation[2];
- severe sleep apnea or other airway related issues[2];
- one or more significant comorbidities[2];
- pregnancy[2];
- inability to communicate (eg, aphasic);
- inability to cooperate (eg, mentally incapacitated)[2];
- multiple drug allergies;
- multiple medications with potential for drug interaction with sedative analgesics[2,3];
- current substance use (eg, street drugs, herbal supplements, nonprescribed prescription drugs)[5];
- ASA physical classification of an unstable P3[3,5]; and
- ASA physical classification of P4 or above.[3,5]

Recommendation III

The perioperative registered nurse should complete a patient assessment before administering moderate sedation/analgesia.

A presedation assessment determines a patient's suitability for registered nurse-administered moderate sedation/analgesia by identifying the potential for adverse events.

III.a. The presedation assessment should include, but is not limited to,[2,5,7]
- verification of consent explaining the risks, benefits, and alternatives to sedation[2,5];
- review of medical history;
- review of physical examination of the cardiac and pulmonary systems, including vital signs[1];
- review of height and weight[3,5];
- verification of pregnancy test results, when applicable;
- review of present medication regimen (eg, prescribed, over-the-counter, herbals, supplements), medication taken within the last 48 hours including any as needed medications, especially opioids or other narcotics[5];
- review of substance use[1,2,5];
- review of tobacco and alcohol use[1,2,5];
- verification of allergies and sensitivities to medications, latex, chemical agents, foods, and adhesives[1,2,5];
- confirmation of NPO status[2,5];
- determination of patient's ability to tolerate and maintain the required position for the duration of the planned procedure; and
- verification of a responsible adult caregiver to escort the patient home.[5,9]

The fasting guidelines developed by the ASA may be used.[2]

III.b. The perioperative registered nurse should perform an assessment of the patient's airway before administering moderate sedation/analgesia.

Support of the airway and positive-pressure bag-mask ventilation may be necessary if respirations are compromised by the respiratory depressive effects of moderate sedation medications.[2,5]

MODERATE SEDATION/ANALGESIA

III.b.1. The presedation airway assessment should include, but is not limited to, the following risk factors for difficult mask ventilation:
- age > 55 years[10];
- significant obesity (especially of the face, neck, and tongue)[2];
- missing teeth or edentulous[10];
- presence of a beard[10];
- history of snoring or sleep apnea[10]; and
- presence of stridor.[2]

III.c. The perioperative registered nurse should consult with an anesthesia provider if the patient presents with a history of severe obstructive sleep apnea.[2]

Administration of sedatives to the patient with central sleep apnea may inhibit the brain's signal to wake up and breathe.[11]

III.d. Additional precautions should be taken for patients with sleep apnea.

Moderate sedation medications may cause relaxation of the oropharyngeal structures resulting in partial or total airway obstruction.[2,11]

III.d.1. Care of the patient with sleep apnea should include, but is not limited to,
- management by an anesthesia provider if the patient has severe central sleep apnea[2];
- positioning in the lateral or semi-Fowlers position, if at all possible;
- use of continuous positive airway pressure (CPAP) machines during the procedure and recovery periods for patients who routinely use CPAP machines when they sleep[11]; and
- continuous monitoring and positioning to facilitate an open airway.[11]

III.e. The perioperative registered nurse should collaborate with the licensed independent practitioner in developing and documenting the sedation/analgesia plan.[7]

Recommendation IV

The perioperative registered nurse monitoring the patient receiving moderate sedation/analgesia should have no other responsibilities that would require leaving the patient unattended or would compromise continuous monitoring during the procedure.[12]

Continuous monitoring of the patient's physiological and psychological status by the perioperative registered nurse leads to early detection of potential complications.[12]

IV.a. A designated perioperative registered nurse should continually monitor the patient during administration of moderate sedation/analgesia.[1,2,7]

IV.b. An additional perioperative registered nurse should be assigned to the circulating role during the administration of moderate sedation.[7]

IV.c. When moderate sedation is administered, the supervising licensed independent practitioner should remain immediately available during the procedure and recovery period.

Recommendation V

The perioperative registered nurse should know the recommended dose, recommended dilution, onset, duration, effects, potential adverse reactions, drug compatibility, and contraindications for each medication used during moderate sedation/analgesia.

Safe administration of medications for moderate sedation and analgesia requires knowledge of the intended purpose and potential adverse effects of each medication and continuous monitoring of the patient responses to the medications.[2,5]

V.a. When medications are administered by the oral, rectal, intramuscular, or transmucosal routes, sufficient time should be allowed for drug absorption and onset before considering additional medication.[2]

The absorption rate of nonintravenous medications is unpredictable.[2]

V.b. The need for IV access should be assessed and will vary depending on the level of sedation intended; the route of sedative administration (eg, oral); and organizational policy, procedure, and protocol.
- Maintaining IV access throughout the procedure allows for additional sedation as well as resuscitative medications.[2]
- Intravenous administration of both a sedative and an analgesic provides effective moderate sedation/analgesia.[2]
- Sedatives (eg, benzodiazepines) may be prescribed to reduce anxiety.[2,3,5]
- Analgesics (eg, opioid agonists) may be prescribed to manage pain.[2,3,5]

V.c. Each IV agent should be administered separately in incremental doses and titrated to desired effect (ie, moderate sedation/analgesia that enables the patient to maintain his or her protective reflexes, airway patency, spontaneous ventilation).[2,5]

The incremental administration of agents decreases the risk for overdose and respiratory or circulatory depression because the person administrating the agents may better observe the patient's response to the medications given.[2,3,5]

V.d. Opioid antagonists (ie, naloxone) and benzodiazepine antagonists (ie, flumazenil) should be readily available whenever opioids and benzodiazepines are administered.[2,3]

V.e. Only persons trained in administering general anesthesia should administer propofol for moderate sedation/analgesia.

MODERATE SEDATION/ANALGESIA

On April 14, 2004, the American Association of Nurse Anesthetists (AANA) and the ASA in a joint statement said:

> *Because sedation is a continuum, it is not always possible to predict how an individual patient will respond. Due to the potential for rapid, profound changes in sedative/analgesia depth and the lack of antagonistic medications, agents such as propofol require special attention.*
>
> *Whenever propofol is used for sedation/anesthesia, it should be administered only by persons trained in the administration of general anesthesia, who are not simultaneously involved in these surgical or diagnostic procedures. This restriction is concordant with specific language in the propofol insert, and failure to follow these recommendations could put patients at increased risk of significant injury or death.*
>
> *Similar concerns apply when other intravenous induction agents are used for sedation, such as thiopental, methohexital or etomidate.*[2,7,13]

The AORN Board of Directors endorsed this statement on January 14, 2005.

Recommendation VI

The perioperative registered nurse should continuously monitor the patient throughout the procedure.[1,5,7]

Continuous monitoring throughout the procedure enables the perioperative registered nurse to use clinical data to implement or modify the plan of care.[5]

VI.a. The perioperative registered nurse, at a minimum, should continuously monitor the patient's heart rate and function via electrocardiogram (ECG); oxygenation using pulse oximetry; respiratory rate and adequacy of ventilation; blood pressure; level of consciousness (LOC); comfort level; and skin condition at regular intervals.[2,7]

VI.b. The method and the flow rate of administering oxygen should be determined based upon achieving the patient's optimal level of oxygen saturation level as measured with pulse oximetry.

A patient's restlessness resulting from hypercapnia and hypoxia may be misinterpreted as discomfort.

The administration of oxygen does not prevent apnea. Patients manifesting restlessness in the absence of a change in pulse oximetry readings may be overmedicated.[14]

VI.c. Monitoring end-tidal carbon dioxide by capnography should be considered for those patients whose ventilation cannot be directly observed during the procedure.[2]

VI.d. Vital signs should be monitored before the start of the procedure, after administration of sedative or analgesic medications, and at least every five minutes during the procedure based on the patient's condition, type and amount of medication administered, and length of procedure.[2]

VI.e. The patient's LOC and ability to respond to verbal commands should be a routine assessment indicator, except in patients unable to respond (eg, young children, mentally impaired, dental surgery).[2,3]

Assessing the patient's LOC by his or her verbal responses at regular intervals during the procedure can quickly determine if the patient is also breathing well. In addition, verbally reassuring the patient can divert his or her attention and assist in reducing anxiety.[2]

VI.f. Equipment should be present, working properly, and and immediately available in the room where the procedure is performed.[7]

VI.f.1. The following age- and size-appropriate equipment and supplies should be present:
- suction;
- airway management devices (eg, oral, nasal airways; mask ventilation devices);
- noninvasive blood pressure monitoring device;
- pulse oximetry;
- electrocardiograph; and
- sedative and analgesic antagonists.[2,15]

VI.g. An emergency resuscitation cart should be immediately available in every location in which moderate sedation/analgesia is administered.

While careful titration of sedation and analgesics to obtain the desired effect can be very safe when using short-acting agents; respiratory depression, hypotension, or impaired cardiovascular function are common sequelae of sedation and analgesia.[2,5]

VI.g.1. An emergency cart should include
- resuscitation medications;
- intravenous access equipment;
- intravenous fluids; and
- life-support equipment (eg, defibrillator, endotracheal intubation equipment, mechanical positive bag-value mask device).

Recommendation VII

The perioperative registered nurse should monitor the patient who receives moderate sedation/analgesia postoperatively.

Recovery time will depend on the type and amount of sedation/analgesia given, procedure performed, and organizational policy.

MODERATE SEDATION/ANALGESIA

VII.a. The same monitoring parameters used during the procedure should be used during the recovery phase.

VII.a.1. Postoperative patient care and monitoring should be consistent for all patients.

VII.a.2. Postoperative monitoring should include, but is not limited to,
- heart rate and rhythm[5,9];
- LOC[5,7,9];
- blood pressure[5,9];
- cardiac monitoring[5];
- oxygenation monitored by pulse oximetry with an audible pulse rate and alarms[9]; and
- ventilation monitored by direct observation and/or auscultation.[9]

VII.b. All patients should be assessed postoperatively.

VII.b.1. Postoperative patient care assessments should include, but are not limited to:
- wound condition,[5,9]
- dressing condition,[5,9]
- line patency,[5]
- amount of drainage in drains,[5] and
- level of pain.[5,7,9]

Recommendation VIII

The perioperative registered nurse should evaluate the patient for discharge readiness based on specific discharge criteria.[5,7]

Recovery time will depend on the type and amount of sedation/analgesia given, procedure performed, and organizational policy.

VIII.a. Discharge criteria should be developed collaboratively and agreed upon by nursing, surgery, medicine, and anesthesia services.

Establishing discharge criteria may minimize the risk of cardiorespiratory depression after the patient has been released.[16-18]

VIII.b. Patients should remain awake for at least 20 minutes without stimulation before they are considered ready for discharge.[9]

The incorporation of a sedation scale in combination with a modified wakefulness test has been reported as ensuring a more objective criterion as compared to using the caregiver's judgment alone.[9]

VIII.c. Children receiving medication with a long half-life should be monitored post-procedure until able to meet discharge criteria and remain awake for at least 20 minutes without stimulation.[15]

There are numerous reports of deaths of prematurely discharged children that have died in the back seats of cars on the ride home from airway obstruction related to the administration of long-acting agents (eg, chloral hydrate).[9,17]

VIII.d. Discharge criteria should be consistently applied to all patients.

VIII.d.1. Criteria for discharge may include, but are not limited to:
- return to preoperative, baseline LOC;
- stability of vital signs;
- sufficient time interval (eg, two hours) since the last administration of an antagonist (eg, naloxone, flumazenil) to prevent resedation of the patient[2,19];
- use of an objective patient assessment scoring system (eg, Aldrete Recovery Score)[2,20];
- absence of protracted nausea;
- intact protective reflexes;
- adequate pain control; and
- return of motor/sensory control.

VIII.e. Patients and/or their caregivers should receive verbal and written discharge instructions.[5]

Medications used for moderate sedation/analgesia cause retrograde amnesia reducing patient's ability to recall events during the immediate postoperative period.

VIII.e.1. A copy of the written discharge instructions should be given to the patient and a copy should be placed in the patient's medical record.[20]

VIII.e.2. The patient and/or caregiver should be able to verbalize an understanding of the discharge instructions.

Recommendation IX

Competency

The perioperative registered nurse should be clinically competent, possessing the skills necessary to manage the nursing care of the patient receiving moderate sedation/analgesia.

Competency assurance verifies that personnel have an understanding of moderate sedation; the risks of unplanned, deeper sedation; and the safe use of monitoring equipment. This knowledge is essential to minimize the risks of moderate sedation and to provide safe care.[21]

IX.a. The competency of the perioperative registered nurse to administer moderate sedation/analgesia should be assessed, demonstrated, documented, and maintained.[21]

IX.a.1. Competencies related to administration of moderate sedation/analgesia should include, but are not limited to,
- patient selection and assessment criteria;
- selection, function, and proficiency in use of physiological monitoring equipment[1];
- pharmacology of the medications used;
- airway management;
- CPAP use;

MODERATE SEDATION/ANALGESIA

- basic dysrhythmia recognition and management;
- emergency response and management;
- advanced cardiac life support (ACLS) and pediatric advanced life support (PALS) according to patients served[18];
- recognition of complications associated with sedation/analgesia; and
- knowledge of anatomy and physiology.[12]

IX.b. The perioperative registered nurse administering moderate sedation/analgesia should be able to rescue patients whose level of sedation progresses to deep sedation.

Sedation occurs on a continuum from fully conscious to deep sedation[2,7] (Table 2).

IX.c. The perioperative registered nurse should, at a minimum, have the ability to manage a compromised airway and to provide adequate oxygenation and ventilation.

Patients receiving moderate sedation/analgesia may unexpectedly slip to the next level (ie, deep sedation or general anesthesia). A provider with bag-, valve-, mask-ventilation; advance life support; and resuscitation skills should be immediately available (eg, within one to five minutes).[2,7]

IX.d. Administrators should ensure that initial and ongoing educational opportunities are provided to meet the needs of personnel who perform moderate sedation/analgesia.

Initial education provides a baseline to support a beginning level of competency to assist in the development of knowledge, skills, and attitudes that positively affect patient outcomes. Ongoing education offers personnel an opportunity to enhance skills and learn about changes in practice, regulations, and standards.[21]

IX.d.1. An introduction and review of moderate sedation/analgesia policies and procedures should be included in the orientation and ongoing education of personnel.

IX.e. Administrators should ensure that perioperative registered nurses who administer moderate sedation/analgesia for procedures are competent to perform these skills.[21]

IX.f. Competencies should reflect current regulations, nurse practice acts, standards, recommended practices, and guidelines affecting the administration of moderate sedation/analgesia.

Regulations, nurse practice acts, standards, recommended practices, and guidelines affecting the administration of moderate sedation/analgesia are evolving and may change over time.

IX.g. The perioperative registered nurse should have the additional knowledge and skills necessary to provide care to the pediatric patient populations they serve.[15]

Recommendation X

Documentation

The perioperative registered nurse should document the care of the patient and their physiological responses throughout the continuum of care.[7]

Documentation of all nursing activities performed is legally and professionally important for clear communication and collaboration between health care team members, and for continuity of patient care.

X.a. Documentation using the PNDS, should include a patient assessment, a plan of care, nursing diagnoses, identification of desired outcomes, interventions, and an evaluation of the patient's response to the care provided.

X.b. Documentation should be recorded in a manner consistent with health care organization policies and procedures and should include, but is not limited to,
  - name, dose, route, time, and effects of all medications;
  - patient's LOC;
  - ventilation and oxygenation status;

TABLE 2. Continuum of Depth of Sedation				
Levels of sedation/analgesia	Minimal sedation (ie, anxiolysis)	Moderate sedation/analgesia (ie, conscious sedation)	Deep sedation/analgesia	General anesthesia
Responsiveness	Normal response to verbal stimulation	Purposeful response to verbal or tactile stimulation	Purposeful response following repeated or painful stimulation	Unarousable even with painful stimulation
Airway	Unaffected	No intervention required	Intervention may be required	Intervention often required
Ventilations	Unaffected	Adequate	May be adequate	Frequently inadequate
Cardiovascular function	Unaffected	Usually maintained	Usually maintained	May be impaired

Reproduced with permission from the American Society of Anesthesiologists, Park Ridge, IL.

- vital signs documented at intervals dependent on the type and quantity of medication administered;
- procedure start and end times; and
- condition of the patient.[1]

Recommendation XI

Policies and Procedures

Policies and procedures for managing patients who receive moderate sedation/analgesia should be written, reviewed periodically, and readily available within the practice setting.

Policies and procedures are operational guidelines that are used to minimize patient risk factors, standardize practice, direct staff members, and establish guidelines for continuous performance improvement activities.

XI.a. Policies and procedures should establish authority, responsibility, and accountability.

XI.b. Policies and procedures for managing patients receiving moderate sedation/analgesia should include, but are not limited to,
- patient selection criteria;
- personnel requirements;
- staffing requirements;
- monitoring;
- risk assessment and criteria for consultation (eg, anesthesia);
- moderate sedation/analgesia medication administration and dosage guidelines;
- recovery and discharge criteria;
- documentation;
- emergency procedures[3,7]; and
- alternative care arrangements when the patient's acuity and or level of care required is outside the capabilities and scope of practice of the perioperative registered nurse.[22]

Recommendation XII

Quality

A quality assurance/performance improvement process should be in place that measures patient, process, and structural (eg, system) outcome indicators.

A fundamental precept of AORN is that it is the responsibility of professional perioperative registered nurses to ensure safe, high-quality nursing care to patients undergoing operative and invasive procedures.[24]

XII.a. Structure, process, and clinical outcomes performance measures should be identified that can be used to improve patient care and that also monitor compliance with facility policy and procedure, national standards and regulatory requirements.[23,25]

XII.a.1. The measures should have universality across the continuum and relevance to all providers of sedation for procedures.[25]

XII.a.2. Process indicators may include, but are not limited to,
- consent for sedation and procedure;
- NPO status confirmed;
- history and physical completed;
- airway assessment conducted;
- factors requiring anesthesia consultation are noted;
- ASA classification;
- anesthesia intervention required (eg, loss of protective reflexes, bag mask ventilation required);
- reversal agents used;
- providers credentialed for procedure/sedation and practice in compliance with facility policy and procedure; and
- adherence to required physiological monitoring.

XII.b. Adverse events should be reported and investigated through the health care organization's quality review process (eg, root cause analysis).[25]

XII.b.1. Any of the following adverse events should be reviewed, and some may require reporting to the appropriate regulatory agency or accrediting organization:[25]
- death;
- aspiration;
- use of antagonists (eg, reversal agents);
- unplanned transfer to a higher level of care;
- cardiac or respiratory arrest;
- sedation using nonapproved agents (eg, anesthetic agent by nonanesthesia provider); and
- emergency procedure without a licensed, independent practitioner in attendance.

Glossary

Anxiolytic: Pharmacologic agent used to treat anxiety. Synonym for anti-anxiety agent.[21]

Benzodiazepine: Pharmacological agent that has sedative, anxiolytic, amnesic, muscle relaxant, and anticonvulsant properties.[24]

Deep sedation/analgesia: A medication-induced depression of consciousness that allows patients to respond purposefully only after repeated or painful stimulation. The patient cannot be aroused easily, and the ability to independently maintain a patent airway may be impaired with spontaneous ventilation possibly inadequate. Cardiovascular function usually is adequate and maintained.[21]

General anesthesia: Patients cannot be aroused, even by painful stimulation, during this medication-induced loss of consciousness. Patients usually require assistance in airway maintenance and often require positive pressure ventilation due to depressed spontaneous ventilation or depression of neuromuscular function. Cardiovascular function also may be impaired.

Immediately available: Defined by the ASA practice guidelines as having a health care provider trained in ACLS and resuscitation skills available to assist with patient care within one to five minutes.[2]

Licensed independent practitioner: Any individual who is permitted by law and the health care organization to provide care and services, without supervision or direction. The care and services should be within the scope of the individual's license and granted clinical privileges.

Moderate sedation/analgesia: A minimally depressed level of consciousness that allows a surgical patient to retain the ability to independently and continuously maintain a patent airway and respond appropriately to verbal commands and physical stimulation. Often referred to as *conscious sedation.*

Opioid: Pharmacologic agent that produces varying degrees of analgesia and sedation, and relieves pain. Fentanyl, morphine, and hydromorphone are opiod analgesic medications that may be used for moderate sedation/analgesia.[3]

Sedative: Pharmacologic agent that reduces anxiety and may induce some degree of short-term amnesia. Diazapam and midazolam are two benzodiazepines commonly used for sedation.

References

1. Beyea SC, ed. *Perioperative Nursing Data Set.* Rev 2nd ed. Denver CO: AORN, Inc; 2007.
2. American Society of Anesthesiologists Task Force on Sedation and Analgesia by Non-Anesthesiologists. Practice guidelines for sedation and analgesia by non-anesthesiologists. *Anesthesiology.* 2002; 96:1004-1017.
3. King CA. *Moderate Sedation/Analgesia Competency Assessment Module.* 2nd ed. Denver CO: Competency & Credentialing Institute; 2005:9, 13-16, 19-21, 23, 25-26, 29, 37-38.
4. AORN explications for perioperative nursing. In: *Standards, Recommended Practices, and Guidelines.* Denver CO: AORN, Inc; 2007:171-201.
5. Odom-Forren J, Watson D. *Practical Guide to Moderate Sedation/Analgesia.* St. Louis MO: Elsevier Mosby; 2005:4-5;242-257.
6. American Nurses Association. *Nursing: Scope and Standards of Practice.* Washington DC: Nursebooks.org; American Nurses Association; 2004:36;39;42.
7. Operative and other high-risk procedures and/or the administration of moderate or deep sedation or anesthesia. In: *Comprehensive Accreditation Manual for Hospitals: The Official Handbook.* Oakbrook Terrace IL: Joint Commission on Accreditation of Healthcare Organizations; 2007 PC-41 to PC-43.
8. American Society of Anesthesiologists. Distinguishing monitored anesthesia care ("MAC") from moderate sedation/analgesia (conscious sedation) (Oct 27, 2004). http://www.asahq.org/publicationsAndServices/standards/35.pdf. Accessed July 23, 2007.
9. Malviya S, Voepel-Lewis T, Ludomirsky A, Marshall J, Tait AR. Can we improve the assessment of discharge readiness? a comparative study of observational and objective measures of depth of sedation in children. [Comment]. *Anesthesiology.* 2004; 100:218-224.
10. Langeron O, Masso E, Huraux C, et al. Prediction of difficult mask ventilation. *Anesthesiology.* 2000; 92:1229-1236.
11. Gross JB, Bachenberg KL, Benumof JL, et al. Practice guidelines for the perioperative management of patients with obstructive sleep apnea: a report by the American Society of Anesthesiologists task force on perioperative management of patients with obstructive sleep apnea. *Anesthesiology.* 2006; 104:1081-1093.
12. American Nurses Association. The role of the registered nurse (RN) in the management of patients receiving IV conscious sedation for short-term therapeutic, diagnostic, or surgical procedures. In: *Compendium of American Nurses Association Position Statements.* Washington, DC: American Nurses Pub; 1996; 148-150.
13. American Association of Nurse Anesthetists, American Society of Anesthesiologists. *AANA-ASA Joint Statement Regarding Propofol Administration.* Available at: http://www.asahq.org/news/propofolstatement.htm. Accessed September13, 2007.
14. Harkness GA, Dincher JR. *Medical-Surgical Nursing: Total Patient Care.* 10th ed. St Louis, MO: Mosby; 1999:502.
15. Committee on Drugs American Academy of Pediatrics. Guidelines for monitoring and management of pediatric patients during and after sedation for diagnostic and therapeutic procedures: addendum. *Pediatrics.* 2002; 110:836-838.
16. Newman DH, Azer MM, Pitetti RD, Singh S. When is a patient safe for discharge after procedural sedation? The timing of adverse effects events in 1367 pediatric procedural sedations. *Ann Emerg Med.* 2003; 42:627-635.
17. Cote CJ, Karl HW, Notterman DA, Weinberg JA, McCloskey C. Adverse sedation events in pediatrics: analysis of medications used for sedation. *Pediatrics.* 2000; 106:633-644.
18. Cote CJ, Notterman DA, Karl HW, Weinberg JA, McCloskey C. Adverse sedation events in pediatrics: a critical incident analysis of contributing factors. *Pediatrics.* 2000; 105:805-814.
19. *Drug Information Handbook for Perioperative Nursing.* Hudson OH: Lexi-Comp; 2006: 739, 1220.
20. American Society of PeriAnesthesia Nurses. *Standards of Perianesthesia Nursing Practice.* Thorofare NJ: American Society of Perianesthesia Nurses; 2004:63-67.
21. Management of human resources. In: *Comprehensive Accreditation Manual for Hospitals: The Official Handbook.* Oakbrook Terrace IL: Joint Commission on Accreditation of Healthcare Organizations; 2007: HR-2.
22. America Nurses Association. The right to accept or reject an assignment. Available at: http://nursingworld.org/MainMenuCategories/HealthcareandPolicyIssues/ANA PositionStatements/workplac/wkassign14540.aspx. Accessed September 18, 2007.
23. AORN. Quality and performance improvement standards for perioperative nursing. In: *Standards, Recommended Practices, and Guidelines.* Denver, CO: AORN, Inc; 2007:437-446.
24. Lee A, Fan LT, Gin T, Karmakar MK, Ngan Kee WD. A systemic review (meta-analysis) of the accuracy of the Mallampati tests to predict the difficult airway. *Anesth & Analg.* 2006;102:1867-1878.
25. Improving organization performance. In: *Comprehensive Accreditation Manual for Hospitals: The Official Handbook.* Oakbrook Terrace IL: Joint Commission on Accreditation of Healthcare Organizations; 2007:PI-8 to PI-9.

MODERATE SEDATION/ANALGESIA

PUBLICATION HISTORY

Originally published April 1993, *AORN Journal*, as "Recommended practices for monitoring the patient receiving intravenous conscious sedation."

Revised; published in January 1997, *AORN Journal*, as "Recommended practices for managing the patient receiving conscious sedation/analgesia." Reformatted July 2000.

Revised November 2001; published March 2002, *AORN Journal*, as "Recommended practices for managing the patient receiving moderate sedation/analgesia."

Revised 2007; published in *Perioperative Standards and Recommended Practices*, 2008 edition.

Minor editing revisions made to omit PNDS codes; reformatted September 2012 for publication in *Perioperative Standards and Recommended Practices*, 2013 edition.

Minor editing revisions made in November 2014 for publication in *Guidelines for Perioperative Practice*, 2015 edition.

MODERATE SEDATION/ANALGESIA

GUIDELINE FOR POSITIONING THE PATIENT

The Guideline for Positioning the Patient was developed by the AORN Recommended Practices Committee and was approved by the AORN Board of Directors. It was presented as proposed recommendations for comments by members and others. The guideline is effective January 1, 2008. The recommendations in this guideline are intended to be achievable and represent what is believed to be an optimal level of practice. Policies and procedures will reflect variations in practice settings and/or clinical situations that determine the degree to which the guideline can be implemented. AORN recognizes the various settings in which perioperative registered nurses practice; therefore, this guideline is adaptable to various practice settings. These practice settings include traditional operating rooms, ambulatory surgery centers, physicians' offices, cardiac catheterization laboratories, endoscopy suites, radiology departments, and all other areas where surgery may be performed. The reader is referred to the Perioperative Nursing Data Set (PNDS) for an explanation of nursing diagnoses, interventions, and outcomes.[1]

Purpose

This document provides guidance for positioning the patient in the perioperative setting. It is not intended to cover aspects of perioperative patient care addressed in other AORN guidelines. Prevention of positioning injury requires anticipation of the positioning equipment necessary based on the patient's identified needs and the planned operative or invasive procedure, application of the principles of body mechanics and ergonomics, ongoing assessment throughout the perioperative period, and coordination with the entire perioperative team.[1] Attention should be given to patient comfort and safety, as well as to assessing circulatory, respiratory, integumentary, musculoskeletal, and neurological structures. Working as a member of the team, the perioperative registered nurse can minimize the risk of perioperative complications related to positioning.

Recommendation I

Personnel who purchase positioning equipment should make decisions based on the health care organization's patient population, current research findings, and the equipment design safety features required to minimize risks to patients and personnel.

The technology used to create mattresses, padding, and other positioning equipment continues to evolve, and it is important for perioperative registered nurses to be aware of products and current research to support their product selection.

The primary safety feature consideration for positioning equipment is that it redistribute pressure, especially at bony prominences on the patient's body. The National Pressure Ulcer Advisory Panel Support Surface Standards Initiative defines a support surface as "a specialized device for pressure redistribution designed for management of tissue loads, micro-climate, and/or other therapeutic functions (ie, any mattresses, integrated bed system, mattress replacement, overlay, or seat cushion, or seat cushion overlay)."[2]

Although physiologic blood and lymphatic flow rates vary among individuals, capillary pressures may increase to as much as 150 mm Hg during prolonged, unrelieved pressure without position change.[3]

The traditional procedure bed mattress usually is constructed of one to two inches of foam covered with a vinyl or nylon fabric. Research studies have found that foam overlays or replacement pads, which represent most OR and procedure bed mattresses, do not have effective pressure-reduction capabilities.[4] Studies comparing the pressure-reducing abilities of standard foam procedure bed mattresses to gel mattresses (ie, viscoelastic polymer) have found gel mattresses to be more effective.[4,5] One research study reported that polyether mattresses generate a lower capillary interface pressure when the patient was in the supine position than gel mattresses or foam mattresses.[6] Another study found that foam and gel mattresses are effective for preventing skin changes, but visco-elastic overlays are effective for preventing both skin changes and pressure sore formation.[7]

Clinical support surfaces (ie, padding) function differently for persons of different height and weight.[8] A performance improvement study reported that supplemental padding on the procedure bed mattress or the use of other positioning devices may not reduce capillary interface pressure for all body types or for all areas of bony prominences even in patients with the same body type.[9]

Postoperative use of alternating pressure mattresses has been found to minimize the incidence of pressure ulcers. Intraoperative use of this technology may be limited due to concerns about patient movement, electrical safety, and asepsis.[3]

There are studies reporting a reduction in the postoperative incidence of pressure ulcers when pressure-relieving overlays are used on procedure bed mattresses and in the postoperative period; however, use of mattress overlays intraoperatively may not minimize this risk.[10] It is difficult, therefore, to draw firm conclusions about the most effective means of intraoperative pressure relief. Future studies of pressure-relieving surfaces are needed and

must address methodological deficiencies associated with many of the available studies. Examples of current study limitations include the following:
- Trials that do not clearly reflect whether a reduction in risk for skin changes is due to intraoperative or postoperative pressure relief or whether application of the trial is necessary in both settings to achieve a risk reduction.[10]
- Studies that do not include information gathered on the postoperative skin care of the patient make it difficult to assess the clinical significance of the studies' findings.[10]
- Cross comparisons of study results often are not effective because of variations of selection criteria. In addition, limited sample sizes, interrater reliability, and contradictory findings further contribute to weak scientific support for recommendations on how to predict and prevent pressure ulcers resulting from intraoperative procedure bed mattresses.[11]
- Studies that measure only interface pressure (ie, the pressure on different parts of the patient's body that are in contact with the support surface) have serious limitations. The process that leads to the development of a pressure ulcer involves the complex interplay of several factors.[10]

The most frequent predictors of perioperative pressure ulcers have been found to be
- increasing age of the patient,
- a patient diagnosed with diabetes or vascular disease, and
- vascular procedures.[11]

I.a. Personnel selecting procedure bed mattresses and positioning equipment for purchase and use should make decisions based on criteria that include, but are not limited to,
  o ability to hold the patient in the desired position;
  o available in a variety of sizes and shapes;
  o suitable for the patient population and anticipated position requirements;
  o ability to support maximum weight requirements;
  o durable material and design (eg, maintains resilience under constant use);
  o evidence that it is able to disperse skin interface pressure;
  o resistance to moisture;
  o low risk for moisture retention;
  o radiolucent, if necessary;
  o fire retardant;
  o nonallergenic;
  o promotes air circulation;
  o low risk of harboring bacteria (eg, replacements may be needed when soiled);
  o easy to use and store; and
  o cost effective.[3,4,7,12]

One study found the viscoelastic mattress overlay appears to offer the most benefit for older patient populations; patients who have more serious or chronic health problems, where there is a prevalence of vascular disease; or in situations where surgical procedures extend beyond two-and-one-half hours.[7]

I.a.1. Positioning equipment for obese patients should include, but is not limited to,
- lateral transfer devices or patient lifts to move obese patients from stretcher procedure bed to the OR procedure bed;[13] and
- stretchers and beds in the postanesthesia care unit (PACU) that are able to accommodate at least a 30-degree elevation of the patient's upper body and head to avoid respiratory distress.

Whether or not a facility has a bariatric surgery program, it is necessary to accommodate the unique needs of the obese patient population. Patient demographics, baseline utilization requirements, and peak census requirements may help to determine whether caseloads justify purchasing rather than leasing special bariatric equipment. Upgrading existing equipment with bariatric accessories may be a viable option rather than replacing equipment in its entirety.[14]

I.a.2. The manufacturer should be consulted for both weight capacity and articulation abilities of the procedure bed.

Many procedure beds are designed to safely support a 500-pound patient, but maximum weight for special functioning capabilities is an important consideration. Heavy-duty procedure beds are available that lift, articulate, and support patients weighing 800 to 1,000 lb.[15]

I.b. Procedure bed mattresses and positioning equipment should be evaluated according AORN's "Recommended practices for product selection in the perioperative practice setting."[16]

Recommendation II

During the planning phase of patient care, the perioperative registered nurse should anticipate the positioning equipment needed for the specific operative or invasive procedure.

The patient's position should provide optimum exposure for the procedure while providing access to IV lines and monitoring devices. The nurse determines the equipment to be used based on the planned procedure, surgeon's preference, and patient condition. Assessment of surgical case characteristics (eg, procedure length, surgical approach, use of radiological equipment) helps determine positioning equipment and modifications in positioning needed to safely accommodate a patient's physical needs.

II.a. The perioperative registered nurse should review the surgery schedule before the patient's arrival, preferably before the day of surgery, to identify potential conflicts in availability of positioning equipment.

Compromises in patient safety may result when proper equipment is not available.

II.a.1. When a procedure is scheduled, the availability of special equipment should be verified.

II.b. The perioperative registered nurse should confirm that the room is set up appropriately for the planned procedure before the patient arrives.

Compromises in patient safety may result when the room arrangement is not specific to the planned procedure and its laterality.[17]

II.b.1. The correct patient position and related equipment should be verified during the time out period.[18]

Recommendation III

Positioning and transporting equipment should be periodically inspected and maintained in properly functioning condition.

Properly functioning equipment contributes to patient safety and assists in providing adequate exposure of the surgical site. Patients and health care workers are at risk for injury if equipment is not used according to manufacturers' specifications.

III.a. Scheduled preventive maintenance and repair should be performed on all equipment used for patient transport.

Preventive maintenance and repair promote proper functioning and decrease the risk for injury to patients and personnel.

III.b. Surfaces of positioning and transporting equipment should be smooth and intact.

Loss of equipment surface integrity can result in bacterial growth. Surfaces that hold moisture or wrinkle contribute to skin breakdown.

III.c. Proper working condition of positioning and transporting equipment should be verified before use.

Creating a culture of safety includes designing a work environment that minimizes factors that contribute to errors or injuries.[19]

III.d. Potential hazards associated with the use of positioning and transporting equipment should be identified, and safe practices should be established in accordance with AORN's "Recommended practices for a safe environment of care."[20]

Recommendation IV

During the preoperative assessment, the perioperative registered nurse should identify unique patient considerations that require additional precautions for procedure-specific positioning.

Assessing patients for pressure ulcer development risk factors serves as a key step to preventing them. Patients who are immobile, as is required during operative procedures, are at increased risk.[3]

Additional precautions may be necessary when positioning special patient populations (eg, neonatal, elderly, malnourished, morbidly obese patients; patients with chronic diseases; patients with existing pressure ulcers) to reduce the risk for integumentary, respiratory, or cardiovascular compromises, and nerve impairment.[12,21] For example:

- Obesity adversely affects most body systems.[22] Routine skin condition assessments may be difficult because of the patient's size, lack of landmarks, and chronic conditions.[23] Traditional foam positioning products may prove ineffective, due to compression resulting from the patient's weight.[15,23]
- Patients with vascular disease may have existing tissue ischemia and often have additional risk factors (eg, age, nutritional deficits, obesity, diabetes). Patients with vascular disease who are hypertensive may react unexpectedly to a reduction in blood pressure that is considered normotensive for many patients, but which results in loss of blood flow through stenotic vessels.[24]
- Patients who smoke often experience vasoconstriction, another mechanism that contributes to pressure ulcer formation.[24]

IV.a. Patient needs should be assessed by a registered nurse before transport to determine the required equipment and the skill level and number of transport personnel needed.

Advance preparation for transport may be required for obese patients or other patients with special needs.[21]

IV.b. The preoperative nursing assessment should include questions to determine patient tolerance to the planned operative position.

IV.b.1. The perioperative registered nurse should take additional precautions to decrease the risk for pressure ulcers in patients who
- are more than 70 years of age;
- require vascular procedures or any procedure lasting longer than four hours;
- are thin, small in stature, or who have poor preoperative nutritional status;
- are diabetic or have vascular disease; and
- have a preoperative Braden Scale score that is less than 20.[11]

Studies report that the duration of a procedure is a significant predictor of pressure ulcer development. One study reported that intraoperative pressure ulcers increased when the procedure time extended beyond three hours. Cardiac, general, thoracic, orthopedic, and vascular procedures were reported to be the most common types of procedures associated with pressure ulcer formation.[25]

IV.b.2. Preoperative assessment should include evaluation of both patient and intraoperative factors.
- Patient assessment should include, but is not limited to,
  ○ age;
  ○ height;

POSITIONING THE PATIENT

- weight;
- body mass index (BMI);
- skin condition;
- presence of jewelry;
- nutritional status;
- allergies (eg, latex);
- preexisting conditions (eg, vascular, respiratory, circulatory, neurological, immune system suppression);
- laboratory results;
- physical or mobility limitation (eg, range of motion);
- presence of prosthetics or corrective devices;
- presence of implanted devices (eg, pacemakers, orthopedic implants);
- presence of external devices (eg, catheters, drains, orthopedic immobilizers);
- presence of peripheral pulses;
- perception of pain;
- level of consciousness; and
- psychosocial and cultural considerations.[1,12]
- Intraoperative assessment factors should include, but are not limited to,
  - anesthesia care provider's access to patient;
  - estimated length of procedure; and
  - desired procedural position.

IV.c. Special procedure beds and accessories designed to meet unique patient needs should be used.

When assessing a patient's body weight and condition it is important to assess more than just their BMI. Patients of the same BMI (a relative ratio of height and weight) can have significantly different body composition that affects positioning needs and their risk for pressure ulcer development; therefore, procedure bed and positioning device requirements may be quite different.

The perioperative nursing assessment should include the length and weight capacity of the procedure bed.

IV.d. Perioperative registered nurses should participate in their health care organization's fall-reduction program by including an assessment of the patient's risk for falling.

Patients may be prone to falls before they enter the operating room, during transfer to the procedure bed, and when attempting to sit up or transfer to a recliner in the PACU.[26] Patients may be at a higher risk for falling if the following conditions are present:
- history of a fall during the past three months;
- use of certain medications (eg, psychotropics, antidepressants, benzodiazepines, cardiovascular agents, antihypertensives, diuretics, anticoagulants, antihistamines, bowel preparation medications, medications related to treating nocturia);[27]
- confusion or depression;
- function or mobility problems (ie, gait),
- age, and
- dizziness.[27,28]

The top three risk factors for predicting falls include a previous fall, medications used, and gait.[27] Age ranks fourth as a risk factor, however, it is not a good predictor of falls because studies show a wide range of age groups experience falls. One study reported a high percentage of injuries due to falls occurring in the 20- to 24-year-old age group.[28]

IV.d.1. Regardless of age, patients who have poor vision, postural hypotension, or an altered mental status should be considered to be at a high risk for falling.[27]

Recommendation V

Perioperative personnel should use proper body mechanics when transporting, moving, lifting, or positioning patients.

The incidence of work-related back injuries in nursing is among the highest of any profession worldwide.[29] Manual lifting and other patient-handling tasks are high-risk activities that can result in musculoskeletal disorders.[13] Most injuries are due to overexertion when lifting patients; tasks that require staff members to twist or bend forward; and high-risk tasks performed on a horizontal plane (eg, lateral transfer from bed to stretcher, repositioning patient in bed).[29,30]

Biomechanical studies have demonstrated that health care personnel are at risk for injury, despite the use of proper body mechanics, if patient-handling tasks are beyond reasonable limits and the caregiver's capabilities.[29] The combination of frequency, duration, and the stress of performing high-risk tasks that push the limits of human capabilities (eg, heavy loads; sustained, awkward positions; bending and twisting; reaching fatigue or stress; force; standing for long periods of time) predisposes nurses to musculoskeletal disorders.[13]

V.a. An adequate number of personnel should be available to ensure patient and personnel safety when transporting the patient.

Procedure beds can be very heavy and difficult to move, even without the presence of a patient. When a procedure bed is moved with a patient on it, the risk of injury is increased for both the worker and the patient.[13]

V.b. The perioperative registered nurse should identify high-risk tasks and implement ergonomic solutions to eliminate or reduce occupational risks for injury.

Transferring, lifting, and handling patients have been identified as the most frequent precipitating trigger of back and shoulder problems for nurses.[13] Nurses are often required to use the weaker muscles of the arms and shoulders as the primary lifting muscles, rather than the stronger muscles of the legs, because lifting, turning, or repositioning patients is often performed on a horizontal plane, such as a bed or stretcher.[29]

Experts do not always agree on the safest methods for lifting or assisting dependent patients. One research center recommends the use of a roller or mechanical lifting equipment to reduce the risk of strain when moving a patient who is unable to move independently. The same center studied nurses' behaviors regarding use of lifting equipment and identified the following reasons for continued manual lifting:
- devices were purchased in insufficient quantities,
- lifts were stored in inconvenient locations, and
- equipment was not maintained adequately.[29]

V.c. All perioperative personnel should be educated in the principles of body mechanics and ergonomics.

The majority of musculoskeletal disorders reported by nurses working in the private sector are back injuries that require time away from work. Several studies report that nurses complain of chronic back pain, are unable to do their work because of injuries to shoulder and neck, or are planning to leave the profession because of their concern for personal safety in the health care environment.[13]

Recommendation VI

Potential hazards associated with patient transport and transfer activities should be identified, and safe practices should be established.

Preoperative patient observation and assessment by a perioperative registered nurse allows for identification of potential problems during transport and transfer activities that can be prevented by the implementation of appropriate precautions.

VI.a. When selecting the appropriate transport vehicle, design features to be considered should include, but are not limited to,
- locking devices on wheels;
- protective devices (eg, safety straps, side rails, cribs rails high enough to prevent a standing child from falling out);
- stable, adjustable IV poles or stands;
- holding devices for oxygen tanks;
- positioning capabilities;
- controls that are easy to operate and within reach of the operator;
- maneuverability;
- sufficient size;
- removable head and foot boards;
- mattress-stabilizing devices;
- easily cleanable surfaces; and
- a rack or shelf to hold monitoring equipment.

Equipment safety design features help reduce the risk of injury to patients and personnel during transport.

VI.b. The patient should be attended during transport and transfer by personnel deemed appropriate by the perioperative registered nurse or as determined by the anesthesia care provider or surgeon.

VI.c. Safety measures to be implemented during transport and transfer activities should include, but are not limited to,
- presence of locking wheels on the transport vehicle and the patient's bed during transfer activities;
- side rails that can be elevated;
- use of safety straps;
- hanging and securing IV containers away from the patient's head;
- ensuring that the patient's head, arms, and legs are protected;
- ensuring that one staff member remains at the head of the patient transport vehicle;
- pushing the transport vehicle with the patient's feet first and avoiding rapid movement through hallways or when turning corners;
- maintaining the integrity and function of IV infusions, indwelling catheters, tubes, drainage systems, and monitoring equipment; and
- obtaining appropriately skilled assistance personnel and specific instructions for the patient with special needs.

Locking wheels, raising side rails, and securing safety straps reduce the risk of patient falls. Maintaining proximity to the patient's head provides access to the patient's airway in the event of respiratory distress or vomiting. Rapid movements can cause patient disorientation, nausea and vomiting, and dizziness.

Recommendation VII

Positioning equipment should be used in a safe manner and according to manufacturers' written instructions.

To reduce the risk of injury, it is important to follow manufacturers' written instructions regarding weight limits in flat, articulated, and reverse orientation positions for each type of procedure bed. One researcher reviewed 16 perioperative incident reports and found that 63% involved patients who were above the specified weight limit for the positioning equipment used for back surgery. In all of the reports, it was noted that a staff member notified the surgeon of the problem before the beginning of the surgery, but the equipment was used anyway because alternative equipment was not available.[31]

VII.a. The perioperative registered nurse should verify that the positioning equipment to be used has been designed specifically for surgical procedure positioning.

The goal of using positioning equipment is to use equipment that is designed to redistribute pressure and that decreases the risk for positioning injuries.

POSITIONING THE PATIENT

The number of pads, blankets, and warming blankets beneath the patient has been implicated as a risk factor for pressure ulcer development.[4,11,26,32,33]

- Foam pads may not be effective as padding devices because they quickly compress under heavy body areas.[33-35] In some situations, however, foam can be an effective pressure-reducing material equal to that of gel or visco-elastic.
- Convoluted foam mattress overlays (eg, egg crate mattresses) may be more effective in redistributing pressure if they are made of thick, dense foam that resists compression. The effectiveness of this type of mattress overlay depends on the weight of the patient and may not provide adequate pressure reduction in obese patients.
- Pillows, blankets, and molded-foam devices may produce only a minimum amount of pressure redistribution and are less effective during long procedures.
- Towels and sheet rolls do not reduce pressure and may contribute to friction injuries.[3]

VII.b. The perioperative registered nurse should select a surface that is able to reduce excessive pressure on the patient's bony prominences.

Pressure against the skin above 32 mm Hg interferes with tissue perfusion.[36,37] Firm, stable devices may help hold the patient in position but may not help redistribute pressure. If care is not taken to minimize pressure points caused by positioning equipment, the positioning equipment may not adequately decrease the potential for injury and may actually increase the potential for pressure injury.

VII.b.1. Rolled sheets and towels should not be used beneath the procedure bed mattress or an overlay. When using positioning equipment such as a uterine displacing wedge or chest rolls, the positioning devices should be placed underneath the patient and not beneath the mattress or overlay.

When rolled towels, sheets, or other positioning equipment are placed beneath the mattress or the overlay, they may negate the pressure-reducing effect of the mattress or overlay.[11]

VII.c. Patients should not be transported in procedure beds unless the manufacturer's written instructions state that the bed is safe to use as a transportation device.

Procedure bed designs vary. Unlocking the bed may make it unstable. Moving an occupied procedure bed is not recommended because the risk of injury increases for both the worker and the patient.[13] There are some procedure beds, however, that are designed for patient transport. It is important to consult the manufacturers' written instructions to determine if unlocking and moving a patient-occupied procedure bed is recommended.

Recommendation VIII

The perioperative registered nurse should actively participate in safely positioning the patient under the direction of and in collaboration with the surgeon and anesthesia provider.

The physiologic effects of anesthesia increase the patient's vulnerability to the effects of pressure. Patients may have preexisting conditions that limit the positions they can assume and may influence the positions they can tolerate.[37]

VIII.a. The perioperative registered nurse should provide for patient dignity and privacy during transport, transfer, and positioning.

Maintaining patient privacy is essential to preserving the trust developed in the nurse-patient relationship. The perioperative registered nurse is responsible for developing a caring environment that promotes the well-being of patients. Perioperative registered nurses should provide care that recognizes the importance of each patient's values, beliefs, and health practices and is culturally relevant to a diverse patient population.[38]

VIII.a.1. The perioperative registered nurse should implement actions that include, but are not limited to, the following:
- Restrict OR patient care area access to designated authorized personnel only.
- Keep doors to patient care areas closed.
- Limit traffic coming into OR procedure rooms.
- Expose only the areas of the patient's body needed to provide care or access to the surgical site during the planned procedure.
- Provide auditory privacy for patient and staff member conversations during transport and transfer.
- Provide care without prejudicial behavior.[38]

VIII.b. Patient jewelry and body piercing accessories should be removed before positioning or transferring to the procedure bed if it will cause potential injury or interfere with the surgical site.

Patients positioned on jewelry may be subject to pressure injuries.[39] Patient jewelry can become entangled in bedding or caught on equipment while moving the patient and cause injuries due to accidental removal.

VIII.c. Movement or positioning of the patient should be coordinated with the surgical team.

Sliding or pulling the patient can result in shearing forces and/or friction on the patient's skin. Shearing can occur when the patient's skin remains stationary and underlying tissues shift or move, as might occur when the patient is

POSITIONING THE PATIENT

pulled or dragged without support to the skeletal system or while using a draw sheet. Friction occurs when skin surfaces rub over a rough stationary surface.[3,40]

VIII.c.1. Specific patient needs should be communicated to the perioperative team before initiating transfer or positioning the patient.

VIII.c.2. Attention should be given to protecting the patient's airway at all times during patient transfer and positioning.

VIII.c.3. Before and during transfer or positioning, perioperative team members should communicate with each other regarding securing tubes, drains, and catheters; take actions to support these devices and prevent dislodging; and confirm that the devices have maintained patency after transfer, positioning, or repositioning.

Indwelling catheters, tubes, or cannulas may be dislodged without proper support.

VIII.c.4. The perioperative registered nurse should actively participate in monitoring the patient's body alignment and confirming that the patient's legs are not crossed during transfer and positioning.

Maintaining the patient's correct body alignment and supporting his or her extremities and joints decreases the potential for injury during transfer and positioning.[12]

VIII.c.5. When on the procedure bed, the patient should be attended by surgical team members at all times.

A lack of clear communication about who should be watching the patient after the safety straps are removed or before the patient is transferred has been reported as a contributing factor for patient falls in the operating room.[28]

VIII.d. The number of personnel and required equipment should be adequate to safely position the patient.

Inadequate numbers of personnel and/or equipment can result in patient or personnel injury.

VIII.e. The perioperative registered nurse should actively participate in monitoring the patient's tissue integrity based on sound physiologic principles.

VIII.f. The perioperative registered nurse should implement general positioning safety measures including, but not limited to, the following:
- Positioning equipment should be used to protect, support, and maintain the patient's position.
- Padding should be used to protect the patient's bony prominences.
- The patient's arms should be positioned to protect them from nerve injury.[37,41]
- The location of the patient's fingers should be confirmed to ensure they are in a position that is clear of procedure bed breaks or other hazards.
- Safety restraints should be applied carefully to avoid nerve compression injury and compromised blood flow.[42]
- The patient's body should be protected from coming in contact with metal portions of the procedure bed.
- The patient's heels should be elevated off the underlying surface when possible.[43]
- The patient's head and upper body should be in alignment with the hips. The patient's legs should be parallel and the ankles uncrossed to reduce pressure to occiput, scapulae, thoracic vertebrae, olecranon processes (ie, elbows), sacrum/coccyx, calcaneae (ie, heel),[12,44] and ischial tuberosities.[9,45]
- The patient's head should be in a neutral position and placed on a headrest.
- A pillow may be placed under the back of the patient's knees to relieve pressure on the lower back.[12]
- If the patient is pregnant, a wedge should be inserted under the patient's right side to displace the uterus to the left and prevent supine hypotensive syndrome, caused by the gravid uterus compressing the aorta and vena cava.[46]
- If patient is attached to a robot, caution should be used before moving either the patient or the robot.

VIII.f.1. Unless necessary for surgical reasons, the patient's arms should not be tucked at his or her sides when in the supine position. If there are surgical reasons to secure the patient's arms at his or her side with the use of a draw sheet, the draw sheet should extend above the elbows and should be tucked between the patient and the procedure bed's mattress.[37,44]

When a patient's arms are tucked tightly at his or her side with sheets, it may add unnecessary pressure on the tucked arms and may lead to tissue injury and ischemia. It may also cause interference with physiologic monitoring (eg, blood pressure monitoring, arterial catheter monitoring) and result in an inability to resuscitate during an emergency due to unrecognized IV infiltration in the tucked arm. There is also an increased risk for the patient to develop compartment syndrome in the upper extremity.[47]

VIII.f.2. Direct pressure on the eye should be avoided to reduce the risk of central retinal artery occlusion and other ocular damage, including corneal abrasion.

Patients who are at increased risk for development of postoperative visual loss

POSITIONING THE PATIENT

are those that are undergoing procedures that are prolonged (ie, > 6.5 hrs), have substantial blood loss (ie, > 44.7% of estimated blood volume), or who are in a prone position.[48]

- Patients at risk for ocular injury should be positioned so that their heads are level with or higher than their hearts, when possible. In addition, their heads should be maintained in a neutral forward position without significant neck flexion, extension, lateral flexion, or rotation, when possible. The use of a horseshoe headrest may increase the risk of ocular compression.
- The eyes of patients in the prone position should be assessed regularly.
- The surgeon may consider using a series of staged spine procedures for high-risk patients.

VIII.g. Perioperative team members should implement measures to reduce the risk of nerve injuries when positioning the patient's extremities.

○ Patients who undergo general anesthesia are at an increased risk for nerve injury resulting from patient positioning.[42]
○ Trauma may result from compression or stretching of nerves, with the most frequent injuries involving the ulnar nerve and brachial plexus. Why some of these injuries occur is unknown.[12,41,42,49,50,51]
○ The saphenous, sciatic, and peroneal nerves are vulnerable when the patient is in the lithotomy position. The peroneal nerve is also at risk with the patient in the lateral position.[50]
○ Injury to the pudendal nerve may result from inadequate padding or incorrect placement of the positioning post, when using a fracture table.[37,52,53]

VIII.g.1. To minimize the risk of nerve injury, safety measures should include, but are not limited to, the following:

- Padded arm boards should be attached to the procedure bed at less than a 90-degree angle for supine patients.[37,41,44,50]
- The patient's palms should be facing up and the fingers should be extended when his or her arms are placed on arm boards.[37,41,50]
- When the patient's arms are placed at the side of the body, they should be in a neutral position (ie, elbows slightly flexed, wrist in neutral position, palms facing inward).[37,41,50]
- Patient shoulder abduction and lateral rotation should kept be to a minimum.[42]
- Patient extremities should be prevented from dropping below procedure bed level.
- The patient's head should be placed in a neutral position, if not contraindicated by the surgical procedure or the patient's physical limitations.[50]
- Adequate padding is required for the saphenous, sciatic, and peroneal nerves, especially when the patient is in a lithotomy or lateral position.[50]
- A well-padded perineal post should be placed against the perineum between the genitalia and the uninjured leg when a patient is positioned on a fracture table.[37,52,53]

VIII.h. Perioperative team members should implement measures to reduce the risk of injuries when positioning the patient in the supine position.

The supine position may be modified into a sitting or semi-sitting position for access to the shoulder, posterior cervical spine, or posterior or lateral head. While there is better lung excursion and diaphragmatic activity in these positions, there is increased risk for poor venous return from the lower extremities and pooling of blood in the patient's pelvis.[12]

○ When using only a draw sheet without a lateral transfer device for a lateral patient transfer in the supine position, the care provider exerts a pull force up to 72.6% of the patient's weight.[54]
○ When one care provider (eg, anesthesia care provider) supports the patient's head and neck, the remaining mass of the patient's body equals 91.6% of his or her total body mass.[55] To accommodate this body mass, each caregiver can safely contribute a pull force required to transfer up to 48 lb.[13]
○ When moving the patient into and out of a sitting or modified sitting position, the mass of a patient's body from the waist up, including the head, neck, and upper extremities, equals almost 69% of the patient's total body weight.[55]

VIII.h.1. A lateral transfer device (eg, friction-reducing sheets, slider board, air-assisted transfer device) should be used for supine-to-supine patient transfer. One caregiver and one anesthesia care provider (who is managing the airway, head, and neck) should be assigned to safely transfer a patient who weighs 52 lb. Two caregivers plus the anesthesia care provider should be assigned to safely transfer a patient up to 104 lb. Three caregivers plus the anesthesia care provider should be assigned to safely transfer a patient up to 157 lb. For patients who weigh more than 157 lb, an appropriate mechanical lifting device (ie, mechanical lift with supine sling, mechanical lateral transfer device, or air-assisted lateral transfer device) should be used and a minimum of three to four caregivers should be assigned.[13]

VIII.h.2. When moving the patient into and out of a sitting or modified sitting position, three

POSITIONING THE PATIENT

caregivers should be assigned to work together to lift up to 67 lb (30 kg). It is preferable to use mechanical devices and a minimum of three caregivers if the patient weighs more than 68 lb.[13]

VIII.i. The perioperative team should implement measures to reduce the risk of injuries when positioning the patient in the prone position.

The prone position may be modified into the jackknife position to provide exposure to sacral, rectal, and perineal areas, or modified into the knee-chest position to provide exposure for spinal procedures.[11,36]

Respiratory function may be affected by the ultimate positioning of the patient and is mitigated by many factors, including the angle of incline, external pressure on the rib cage, and whether the diaphragm is free to move.

Respiratory function may be decreased as a result of mechanical restriction of the rib cage and diaphragm when the patient is in a prone position.[12,37]

Ophthalmic complications, including vision loss, have been reported in association with patients undergoing spinal surgery in a prone position.[56] There is an increased risk for direct compression to the orbit and corneal abrasion when the patient is in a prone position. During spinal surgeries, the patient may be turned to a prone position using a frame that causes the head to be lower than the rest of the body. This cerebral-dependent position may lead to a decreased venous return from the head, which can lead to capillary bed stasis and decreased perfusion to the optic nerve and result in blindness.[57]

When transferring a patient from a supine position to a prone position, the most common physiologic changes are related to hypotension.[37]

VIII.i.1. General safety considerations for the prone position should include, but are not limited to, the following.
- The patient's cervical neck alignment should be maintained.
- Protection for the patient's forehead, eyes, and chin should be provided.
- A padded headrest should be used to provide airway access.
- Chest rolls (ie, from clavicle to iliac crest) should be used to allow chest movement and decrease abdominal pressure.
- Breasts and male genitalia should be positioned in a way that frees them from torsion or pressure.
- The patient's toes should be positioned to allow them to hang over the end of the bed or to be elevated off the bed by placing padding under the patient's shins so the shins are high enough to avoid pressure on the tips of the toes.[11]

VIII.i.2. When in the prone position, direct pressure on the patient's eyes and face should be avoided.[58]

Although ocular injuries have been reported with and without the use of a headrest (eg, the head held with pins), the use of a horseshoe headrest may increase the risk of ocular compression and perioperative central retinal artery occlusion.[57]

VIII.i.3. Ideally, the patient's arms should be placed down by his or her sides in the prone position. If this is not possible, each arm should be placed on an arm board with the arms abducted to less than 90 degrees, the elbows flexed, and the palms facing downwards. To safely secure the patient's arms at his or her sides, the palms of the hands should be facing in toward the thighs, the elbows and hands should be protected with padding, and the hands and wrists should be kept in anatomical alignment.[37]

Positioning the arms above the patient's head can cause a stretch injury to the lower trunks of the brachial plexus.[50]

VIII.i.4. Four caregivers should be available for a supine-to-prone patient transfer. One anesthesia care provider should maintain the airway and support the patient's head, while other members of the team are responsible for the patient's trunk and extremities.

Two caregivers, plus the anesthesia care provider, can safely transfer a patient weighing up to 48.5 lb (22.0 kg) from the supine to the prone position. Three caregivers, plus an anesthesia care provider, can safely transfer a patient weighing up to 72.7 lb (33.0 kg). If the patient's weight is greater than 73 lb, it is necessary to use assistive technology and a minimum of three to four caregivers.[13]

VIII.j. The perioperative team should implement measures to reduce the risk of injuries when positioning the patient in the Trendelenburg and reverse Trendelenburg positions.

When the patient is in Trendelenburg position, excessive pressure on the clavicle can compress the brachial plexus as it exits the thorax between the clavicle and the first rib. Morrell closed claims files revealed that brachial plexus injuries were related to the use of shoulder braces and the head-down position.[51]

Positioning a patient with a history of heart failure secondary to increased venous return and increased pulmonary blood flow in a steep, head-down tilt may adversely affect heart function. Trendelenburg position causes redistribution of the blood supply due to increased venous return

POSITIONING THE PATIENT

from the lower extremities. To ventilate the patient's lungs while in this position, the diaphragm must push against the displaced abdominal contents, which increases the risk for the alveoli to collapse resulting in atelectasis.[12,44]

Circulatory response changes can be rapid and dramatic when moving the patient into or out of Trendelenburg position. During surgery, there is gravitational flow of blood away from the surgical field, which can mask significant blood loss. The patient may be hypotensive as a result of hypovolemia when returned from Trendelenburg position to the supine position. Cerebral blood flow may fall as venous and intracranial pressure rises; therefore, patients with known or suspected intracranial pathology should not be placed in Trendelenburg position if it can be avoided.[12,44] Trendelenburg position can lead to visual loss related to decreased venous return from the head.[57]

VIII.j.1. Measures should be taken to prevent patient from sliding on the procedure bed.
Risk for shear injuries increase when changing the patient's position from supine to Trendelenburg or reverse Trendelenburg.[59]

VIII.j.2. To prevent injury to the shoulders, brachial plexus, or feet in Trendelenburg or reverse Trendelenburg positions,[41,42,49,60]
- shoulder braces should be avoided, and
- a padded footboard should be used for reverse Trendelenburg position.

VIII.k. The perioperative team should implement measures to reduce the risk of injury to patients and caregivers associated with the lithotomy position.
- Some type of leg holder is used in all lithotomy positions. Modifications of the position include low, standard, high, and exaggerated positions depending on how high the legs and pelvis need to be elevated for the procedure.[37,61]
- The length of time that a patient may remain in the lithotomy position without risk of injury is unknown and is related to patient condition.
- In the lithotomy position the patient's heels are at risk for pressure ulcers at the heel support sites, particularly when the legs are supported by the heel in the standard, high, or exaggerated lithotomy position for prolonged procedures.[61]
- Injury to the peroneal nerve on the lateral aspect of the knee is common and results from the fibular neck resting against the vertical post of the stirrup when the patient is in the lithotomy position. This injury can result in foot drop and lateral, lower-extremity paresthesia.[12,37,50,60]
- Compartment syndrome, although infrequent, has been reported as a complication of surgical positioning, especially the lithotomy position.[37,62-64]

There is increased risk for poor venous return from the lower extremities and pooling of blood in the patient's pelvis when the patient is in a lithotomy position. At the end of the procedure, the patient's overall circulating blood volume may be depleted when the patient's legs are lowered to the procedure bed due to the blood returning quickly into the patient's peripheral circulation. Respiratory compromises may occur due to pulmonary congestion. There is increased risk for deep vein thrombus formation due to the increased risk of blood pooling in the calf muscles.[12]

When positioning the patient into and out of the lithotomy position, the maximum load for a two-handed lift is 22.2 lb (10.1kg). Each complete lower patient extremity (including thigh, calf, and foot) weighs almost 16% of the patient's total body mass.[13]

VIII.k.1. General positioning considerations for patients in the lithotomy position include, but are not limited to, the following:
- Stirrups should be placed at an even height.
- The patient's buttocks should be even with the lower break of the procedure bed and positioned in a manner that securely supports the sacrum on the bed surface. Confirm proper positioning of the patient buttocks before surgery is initiated.[12]
- The patient's legs should be moved slowly and simultaneously into the leg holders to prevent lumbosacral strain.
- The patient's legs should be removed from stirrups slowly and brought together simultaneously before lowering the legs to the bed surface when removing the patient from leg holders, to prevent lumbosacral strain. To maintain the patient's hemodynamic status, his or her legs should be slowly returned to the bed, one at a time if possible.[37]
- The patient's arms should be placed on padded arm boards, extended less than 90 degrees from the long axis of the procedure bed, with the patient's palms up and gently secured.[37,60] The arms should be tucked at the patient's sides only if surgically necessary. When it is necessary to tuck the arms at the patient's side, the elbows should be padded and the palms should be facing in toward the patient's body. The hands should be enclosed and secured within a foam protector.[37]
- The patient's fingers should be protected from injury when the foot of the procedure bed is repositioned.[37]
- The patient's heels should be placed in the lowest position possible.[61]

POSITIONING THE PATIENT

- Support should be provided over the largest surface area of the leg possible.[61]
- The patient's legs should not rest against the stirrup posts.[60]
- Scrubbed personnel should not lean against the patient's thighs.[60,62]
- The patient should be in the lithotomy position for the shortest time possible.[61]
- Care should be exercised to avoid shearing when moving the patient to the break in the procedure bed during repositioning.

VIII.k.2. In prolonged procedures (ie, longer than four hours), the perioperative team should consider repositioning the patient in the lithotomy position as a strategy to reduce the risk of pressure injury (eg, skin damage, nerve injury, compartment syndrome).[60,62]

One research review suggests that perioperative team members remove the patient's legs from support structures every two hours, if the procedure is anticipated to last four hours or more.[63] Research does not identify how long the patient's legs should be out of the stirrups before repositioning.

VIII.k.3. The perioperative registered nurse should monitor the patient at all times, especially when the safety strap is removed.

Proper placement of the safety strap is difficult in the lithotomy position. The perioperative registered nurse may not be able to place the safety strap low across the patient's pelvis without restricting access to the surgical site. Use of a safety strap that is placed high or too tight across the abdomen increases the risk of restricting respiration or causing pressure injuries. The patient's legs may seem to be secure in leg holders with his or her arms tucked at the side. It is important to remember that there is still a risk for the patient to shift on the procedure bed, especially when moving into or out of Trendelenburg position, which is often used in conjunction with the lithotomy position.

VIII.k.4. When positioning the patient into and out of the lithotomy position, a minimum of two caregivers is needed to lift the legs. Mechanical devices such as support slings can be used to lift the legs to and from the lithotomy position.[13]

VIII.l. The perioperative team should implement measures to reduce the risk of injury to patient and caregivers associated with the lateral position.

The patient in the lateral position is at risk of injury due to spinal misalignment and vulnerable pressure points on the dependent side, specifically the ear, acromion process, iliac crest, greater trochanter, lateral knee, and malleolus.[9]

In a lateral position, the patient is positioned on the nonoperative side. This dependent side is the reference point for documentation. For example, when documenting a right lateral position, the patient is lying on his or her right side. This position provides exposure for a left-sided procedure (eg, upper chest or kidney procedure). When documenting the left lateral position, the patient is lying on the left side. The left lateral position provides exposure for a surgical or invasive procedure on the patient's right side.

One research study on interface pressures found that the highest pressures occurred in the lateral position and that there was an increased risk for the procedure bed mattress to become fully compressed under the weight of the patient's body and cause a "bottoming out" effect.[6] Another study found an increased risk for ulceration when a solid object or positioning device (eg, "bean bag" product) is used to maintain patients in a specific position. The firm pressure of the positioning device may compromise the circulatory system due to the tight restraint and because of the overall effect of gravity on the horizontal body posture.[25]

The lateral position increases the risk of damage to the common peroneal nerve if there is not padding to protect the nerve on the dependent leg from being compressed between the fibula and the procedure bed.[50]

VIII.l.1. Safety considerations for the lateral position should include, but are not limited to, the following:
- The patient's spinal alignment should be maintained during turning.
- The patient's dependent leg should be flexed for support.[37]
- The patient's straight upper leg should be padded and supported with pillows between the legs.
- Padding should be used under the patient's dependent knee, ankle, and foot.
- A headrest or pillow should be placed under the patient's head to keep the cervical and thoracic vertebrae aligned.
- The patient's dependent ear should assessed to ensure that it is not folded, and the ear should be well padded.[37]
- The patient's arm should be secured to prevent movement during the procedure.

VIII.l.2. To safely position a patient weighing up to 76 lb (ie, 34.5 kg) into and out of the lateral position, three caregivers should be assigned; one caregiver (eg, the anesthesia care provider) should be assigned specifically to support the patient's head and neck and maintain the patient's airway during the lateral transfer.

When positioning or repositioning the anesthetized patient into and out of the lateral

573

position, pushing and pulling forces can occur rather than lifting forces. Three caregivers plus an anesthesia care provider can safely position a patient weighing up to 115 lb (ie, 52.2 kg). If the patient's weight exceeds 115 lb (ie, 52.2 kg), it is important to use lateral positioning devices.[13]

VIII.m. The perioperative team members should implement measures to reduce the risk of injury to patient and caregivers associated with the morbidly obese patient.

Morbid obesity is associated with patients who have a BMI of greater than 40 or who weigh 100 lb or more over their recommended weight. Patients who are morbidly obese tend to have other health conditions, such as type II diabetes, hypertension, atherosclerosis, arthritis of weight bearing joints, sleep apnea, alveolar hypoventilation, urinary stress incontinence, and gastroesophageal reflux disease. Morbidly obese patients are at increased risk for stroke and sudden death.[65]

It is essential for perioperative team members to understand the pathophysiology of obesity and the effects that various positions have on the obese patient's cardiopulmonary function.[66]

- Respiratory issues include
  - airway compromise due to a patient's short, thick neck;
  - risk of difficult intubation;
  - increased risk for hypoxia;
  - increased risk for intra-abdominal pressure on diaphragm; and
  - increased risk of aspiration.
- Circulatory issues include
  - increased cardiac output,
  - increased pulmonary artery pressure, and
  - risk of inferior vena cava compression.

VIII.m.1. Safety considerations for positioning the morbidly obese patient should include, but are not limited to, the following:

- The procedure bed should be capable of articulating and supporting patients weighing 800 to 1000 lb (363.2 kg to 454 kg).[15] Specialized hydraulics should be capable of lifting patients weighing 800 to 1000 lb (363.2 kg to 454 kg).[67]
- Mattresses should provide sufficient support and padding and should not "bottom out."[23]
- The width of the patient's legs determines whether the lower legs will remain on the procedure bed or must be supported by stirrups. Side attachments may be available on more recent procedure bed models.
- The patient's size may cause difficulty in determining if arms are positioned at less than a 90-degree angle. Padded sleds/toboggans may be used to contain the patient's arms at the side of the body if necessary, provided they can be used without causing excessive pressure on the arms.
- An extra wide, extra long safety strap should be used for patients who exceed the length limits for a regular size safety strap. Sheets should not be substituted for inadequately sized safety straps. Two separate safety straps may be necessary to decrease the risk for the patient falling off the procedure bed due to instability and weight load shifts. One safety strap should be placed across the patient's thighs and one over the patient's lower legs.[22]
- When in the supine position, a roll or wedge should be placed under the patient's right flank to relieve compression of vena cava.
- Patients may not be able to tolerate the supine position due to respiratory or circulatory compromises; it may be necessary to reposition the patient into a sitting or lateral position.[66]
- When in the prone position, the patient's upper chest and pelvis should be adequately supported to free the abdominal viscera to reduce pressure on the diaphragm and inferior vena cava.[66]
- Trendelenburg position should be avoided because the added weight of the abdominal contents press against the diaphragm causing respiratory compromise, and the increased blood flowing from the lower extremities into central and pulmonary circulation causes vascular congestion.
- In reverse Trendelenburg position, care should be taken when placing the patient's feet against a padded footboard to ensure that his or her feet are aligned and flat against the board. This prevents rotation and increased pressure on the ankle.
- The lithotomy position should be avoided, if possible, due to the weight of the patient's thighs pressing on his or her abdomen and raising intra-abdominal pressure, thus increasing the risk of circulatory complications.
- If the patient is placed in the lithotomy position, heavy-duty stirrups should be used, and the perioperative nurse should be aware of and institute measures to reduce risks for respiratory, circulatory, and neurological complications.
- The lateral position may be preferred over the prone position as the bulk of the patient's panniculus can be displaced off the abdomen. The perioperative nurse

should be aware, however, that a shift of the patient's panniculus may increase the risk of falling or other injury due to unintentional change in position.[15]

Recommendation IX

After positioning the patient, the perioperative registered nurse should assess the patient's body alignment, tissue perfusion, and skin integrity.

Respiratory function may be compromised after positioning the surgical patient depending on individual factors and patient position.[12,37]

Circulatory function is influenced by anesthetic agents and surgical techniques that may result in vasodilatation, hypertension, decreased cardiac output, and inhibition of normal compensatory mechanisms.[37]

Intraoperative skin injury occurs because of a combination of events:
- unrelieved pressure,
- duration of the pressure, and
- the individual patient's ability to withstand the insult.

Several studies indicate that procedures over two-and-one-half to three hours significantly increase the patient's risk for pressure ulcer formation.[37,68] External skin pressure exceeding normal capillary interface pressure (ie, 23 to 32 mm Hg) can cause capillary occlusion that will restrict or block blood flow. The resulting tissue ischemia leads to tissue breakdown. Both high pressure for a short duration and low pressure for extended duration are pressure injury risk factors. Other extrinsic factors for skin injury include shear forces and friction.[3,4,7,34,64,68]

IX.a. After the desired patient position is attained, the perioperative registered nurse should reassess the patient to include, but not be limited to, the following systems:
- respiratory,
- circulatory,
- neurological, and
- musculoskeletal/integumentary.[1,11]

Positions such as lithotomy and Trendelenburg can cause redistribution and congestion of the patient's blood supply.[12,43]

Circulatory responses to certain positions or position changes can be rapid and dramatic.[12,43]

IX.b. The perioperative registered nurse should monitor the patient for external pressure from surgical team members leaning against the patient's body.

Retractors, equipment, or instruments resting on the patient and members of the perioperative team resting or leaning on the patient add to the risk of pressure injuries that cause nerve or tissue damage.[37,60]

IX.b.1. The perioperative registered nurse should communicate with the surgical team about the position of surgical instruments, retractor frames, Mayo stands, or other items placed on or over the patient throughout the procedure.[12,60]

IX.c. The perioperative registered nurse should reassess the patient's body alignment, placement of the safety strap, and the placement of all padding after repositioning or any movement of the patient, procedure bed, or any equipment that attaches to the procedure bed.[12]

Changing the patient's position may expose or damage otherwise protected body tissue. The safety strap may shift and apply increased pressure when repositioning the patient or adding extra padding.

Patient repositioning may increase the risk of pressure ulcer development due to shearing of tissue.[24,40]

An injury may result from adding or deleting positioning equipment, adjusting the procedure bed, or moving the patient on the procedure bed.[12]

In nonsurgical settings, patients who are identified as being at risk for developing pressure injuries are turned or repositioned at least once every two hours. If a patient is chair-bound preoperatively, it is optimal to reposition the patient once every hour.[3] When patients receive anesthesia, they are even more vulnerable to the effects of pressure due to physiological changes.[67] One study found that the incidence of occipital alopecia was significantly reduced when the patient's head was repositioned at regular intervals during prolonged procedures (ie, longer than four hours).[69]

When a prolonged surgical procedure is expected, a patient who is in the lithotomy position may need to be repositioned every two hours to reduce the risk of pressure injury and compartment syndrome.[60,62,63]

Patients who have a radial intra-arterial catheter in place throughout the procedure may have their wrists in a hyperextended position for the duration of the surgical procedure. One study suggests that patients' wrists should be returned to the neutral position following arterial catheter placement as a strategy to decrease the risk of injury to the median nerve.[70]

Literature searches demonstrate that it is difficult to determine the effect of patient repositioning during a surgical procedure because, while position changes are documented, these changes are not normally identified as a strategy to prevent pressure injuries.[71,72]

IX.c.1. The perioperative registered nurse should communicate with anesthesia personnel and the surgeon when assessing the need for repositioning the patient every two hours for prolonged procedures.

IX.c.2. The perioperative registered nurse should place his or her hand between the safety strap and the patient to ensure the strap is

POSITIONING THE PATIENT

IX.c.3. not applying excessive pressure to the patient's tissue.[12]

IX.c.3. The perioperative registered nurse should assess the patient for adequate padding by positioning a hand, palm up, below the part of the body at risk to be sure there is more than an inch of support material between the body part and any hard surface.[3]

IX.c.4. The perioperative registered nurse should confirm that prep solutions have not pooled beneath the patient and check for excessive moisture (eg, urine from incontinence) between the patient and positioning devices before the start of the surgical procedure.

A patient's skin may be more susceptible to pressure and friction due to prep solutions that change the pH of the skin and remove protective oils. When prep solutions pool beneath a patient, there is increased risk for skin maceration.[4,24]

Recommendation X

The perioperative registered nurse should collaborate with the postoperative patient caregiver to identify patient injury due to intraoperative positioning.

The incidence of pressure ulcers occurring as a result of surgery may be as high as 66%. Pressure ulcers that originate in surgery may be assessed and documented as burns and may not appear until one to four days postoperatively. Operating room-acquired pressure injuries have a unique purple appearance initially. They tend to progress outwardly with origination at the muscle overlying bony prominences, which explains why they may not be detected when the initial skin assessment is done in the operating room. Pressure injuries in nonsurgical patients progress inward, getting deeper as the tissue injury advances[3] (Table 1).

Epithelialization may be delayed in patients who are obese, which may cause poor postoperative wound healing and increased risk of infection.[21]

X.a. Perioperative registered nurses should evaluate the patient for signs and symptoms of physical injury related to intraoperative positioning.

Pressure ulcers are staged according to the degree of tissue damage.[4,73,74] Refer to Table 1 for assessment descriptors.

X.a.1. Perioperative registered nurses should identify patients who are high risk for postoperative injuries due to positioning and communicate areas of concern with postoperative care provider.

X.a.2. When the patient has been in the lateral position for an extended amount of time in the OR, the perioperative nurse should alert the nurses caring for the patient postoperatively to carefully inspect the areas that are at high risk for pressure injuries. It is important to change the patient's positions postoperatively to avoid recurring pressure on those high risk areas.[6]

X.a.3. Patients who have been identified to be at-risk for development of postoperative vision loss should be assessed when the patient becomes alert postoperatively.

The patient who has anemia preoperatively, who undergoes a prolonged procedure, and who experiences substantial blood loss is identified as a high-risk patient for perioperative vision loss. Patient assessment, position modification, and staged procedures are strategies identified to minimize the risk of this rare complication.[56,58]

The incidence of postoperative eye injury in nonocular surgery is relatively uncommon, but the risk may be greater in patients whose surgery involves the face, head, or neck, and in patients whose surgery requires use of the lateral position. The patient's age and length of procedure are also factors for ocular injury.[75]

X.b. Perioperative registered nurses should establish open communications with postoperative care providers to obtain feedback about postoperative injuries due to positioning.

X.b.1. When patients are discharged the same day as the surgery, perioperative registered nurses should include an evaluation for signs and symptoms of injury due to positioning in the postoperative phone call.

Recommendation XI

Competency

Perioperative personnel should receive initial education, competency validation, and updated information on patient positioning, new positioning equipment and procedures, and ergonomic safety.

Competency verification serves as an indicator that personnel have a basic understanding of patient positioning, the risks of injury to patient and to staff members, and understand what may be implemented as appropriate corrective action when a process failure occurs.

XI.a. The perioperative registered nurse should be educated in, and demonstrate knowledge about, the physiologic effects and implications of positioning in relation to the patient's assessed status and limitations.[3,12]

Knowledge of anatomy and physiology enhances the perioperative registered nurse's appreciation of injury mechanisms associated with common intraoperative patient positions.[12]

POSITIONING THE PATIENT

XI.b. Perioperative personnel should be familiar with the proper function and use of positioning equipment.

Ongoing education of perioperative personnel will assist them in developing skills that will decrease the risk of patient injury due to positioning.

XI.c. Perioperative personnel should receive education and competency validation in new positioning equipment as they are introduced into the perioperative setting.

XI.d. Members of the perioperative team who transport patients should demonstrate competency in operating transport equipment.

XI.e. Administrative personnel should periodically assess and document the competency of personnel in safe patient positioning and use of positioning equipment according to facility and department policy.

Recommendation XII

Documentation

Patient care and use of positioning devices should be documented on the intraoperative record by the registered nurse circulator.

Documenting nursing activities provides a description of the perioperative nursing care administered, status of patient outcomes upon transfer, and provides information for continuity of patient care.[76]

XII.a. Documentation should include, but not be limited to,
- preoperative assessment including a description of the patient's overall skin condition on arrival and discharge from the perioperative suite;
- type and location of positioning equipment;
- name and titles of persons participating in positioning the patient;
- patient position and new position, if repositioning becomes necessary; and

TABLE 1. PRESSURE ULCER STAGES

Suspected deep tissue injury
Purple or maroon localized area of discolored intact skin or blood-filled blister due to damage of underlying soft tissue from pressure and/or shear. The area may be preceded by tissue that is painful, firm, mushy, boggy, warmer, or cooler as compared to adjacent tissue.

Further description: Deep tissue injury may be difficult to detect in individuals with dark skin tones. Evolution of the injury may include a thin blister over a dark wound bed. The wound may further evolve and become covered by thin eschar. Evolution may be rapid, exposing additional layers of tissue even with optimal treatment.

Stage I
Intact skin with nonblanchable redness of a localized area usually over a bony prominence. Darkly pigmented skin may not have a visible blanching; its color may differ from the surrounding area.

Further description: The area may be painful, firm, or soft, and warmer or cooler than adjacent tissue. Stage I may be difficult to detect in individuals with dark skin tones.

Stage II
Partial-thickness loss of dermis presenting as a shallow, open ulcer with a red-pink wound bed, without slough. May also present as an intact or open/ruptured serum-filled blister.

Further description: Presents as a shiny or dry shallow ulcer without slough or bruising.* This stage should not be used to describe skin tears, tape burns, perineal dermatitis, maceration, or excoriation.

Stage III
Full-thickness tissue loss. Subcutaneous fat may be visible, but bone, tendon, or muscles are not exposed. Slough may be present but does not obscure the depth of tissue loss. May include undermining and tunneling.

Further description: The depth of a stage III pressure ulcer varies by anatomical location. The bridge of the nose, ear, occiput, and malleolus do not have subcutaneous tissue, and stage III ulcers can be shallow. In contrast, areas of significant adiposity can develop extremely deep stage III pressure ulcers. Bone/tendon is not visible or directly palpable.

Stage IV
Full-thickness tissue loss with exposed bone, tendon, or muscle. Slough or eschar may be present on some parts of the wound bed. Often include undermining and tunneling.

Further description: The depth of a stage IV pressure ulcer varies by anatomical location. The bridge of the nose, ear, occiput, and malleolus do not have subcutaneous tissue, and these ulcers can be shallow. Stage IV ulcers can extend into muscle and/or supporting structures (eg, fascia, tendon, joint capsule), making osteomyelitis possible. Exposed bone/tendons are visible or directly palpable.

Unstageable
Full-thickness tissue loss in which the base of the ulcer is covered by a yellow, tan, gray, green, or brown slough and/or tan, brown, or black eschar in the wound bed.

Further description: Until enough slough and/or eschar are removed to expose the base of the wound, the true depth, and therefore stage, cannot be determined. Stable wounds are dry, adherent, and intact without erythema or fluctuance. Eschar on the heels serves as "the body's natural (ie, biological) cover" and should not be removed.

*Bruising indicates suspected deep tissue injury.
Adapted with permission from The National Pressure Ulcer Advisory Panel, Washington, DC.

POSITIONING THE PATIENT

- postoperative assessment for injury related to position.[1,76]

XII.b. Photography used to document injuries due to positioning should be consistent with health care organizations' policies regarding medical photography and videotaping.

Although the American Medical Directors Association's guidelines for pressure-ulcer prevention and treatment suggest photographs as a means to monitor the progress of wound care, risk management experts and health care attorneys may advise against photographs being included in the patient's chart. If photography is used, high-definition grid film may be recommended for accuracy. Digital images can be modified, resulting in questions about the accuracy and integrity of the image.[3]

Recommendation XIII

Policies and Procedures

Policies and procedures related to positioning should be developed, reviewed annually, revised as necessary, and readily available in the practice setting.

Policies and procedures establish authority, responsibility, and accountability. Policies also assist in the development of performance improvement activities. These recommendations should be used to guide the development of policies and procedures within the individual perioperative practice setting.

XIII.a. Policies and procedures for positioning should include, but not be limited to,
- assessment and evaluation criteria,
- required documentation,
- safety interventions,
- positioning equipment care and maintenance, and
- ergonomic safety.

XIII.b. Perioperative policies on positioning should be consistent with the health care organization's risk-control plan for pressure ulcer prevention and management.

Recommendation XIV

Quality

A quality management program should be in place to evaluate the outcomes of patient positioning practices and to improve patient safety.

To evaluate the quality of patient care and formulate plans for corrective action, it is necessary to maintain a system of evaluation.[77,78]

XIV.a. Perioperative administration members should participate in developing and monitoring an organization-wide risk control plan for pressure ulcer prevention and management.

XIV.a.1. Pressure ulcer prevention and management risk-control plans should include, but not be limited to, the following:
- a method for identifying patients at risk for pressure ulcers;
- a documentation system to follow the progress of a wound;
- prevention protocols that protect the patient's skin integrity; and
- education programs for caregivers, patients, and family members.[3,79]

XIV.b. Information about adverse patient outcomes and "near-miss incidents" associated with positioning should be collected, analyzed, and used for performance improvement as part of the institution-wide performance improvement program.

To demonstrate that all reasonable efforts were made to protect the patient's safety, it is considered a sound professional practice to document information according to organizational policy when an event occurs.[80]

XIV.b.1. Following organizational policy, documentation of an event related to positioning should include, but not be limited to,
- a description of what happened,
- the date and time of the incident,
- location of the incident,
- witnesses,
- corrective action to be implemented, and
- communications made regarding the outcome.

XIV.b.2. Data on health care personnel injuries related to positioning activities should be collected, analyzed, and used for performance improvement.

Glossary

Body mass index (BMI): The measure of a person's body fat based on height and weight that applies to both adult men and women.

Braden scale: A widely used assessment tool for predicting the development of pressure sores.

Capillary interface pressure: The amount of pressure placed on the skin's resting surface over a bony prominence.

Compartment syndrome: A pathologic condition caused by the progressive development of arterial compression and consequent reduction of blood supply. Clinical manifestations include swelling, restriction of movement, vascular compromise, and severe pain or lack of sensation.

Ergonomics: The science of fitting the demands of work to the anatomical, physiological, and psychological capabilities of the worker to enhance efficiency and well-being.

Friction: The act of rubbing one object (or tissue surface) against another.

Morbid obesity: A person whose body mass index (BMI) is more than 40.

Procedure bed: A type of bed used in ORs or procedure rooms that allow the surgical team access to the patient and the ability to position the patient for a surgical procedure through the use of the bed, its positions, and its attachments.

Positioning equipment/devices: Any device or piece of equipment used for positioning the patient and/or providing maximum anatomic exposure. Devices include, but are not limited to,
- support devices for head, arms, chest, iliac crests, and lumbar areas;
- pads in a variety of sizes and shapes for pressure points (eg, head, elbows, knees, ankles, heels, sacral areas);
- securing devices (eg, safety belts, tapes, kidney rests, vacuum-pack positioning devices);
- procedure beds equipment (eg, headrest/holders, overhead arm supports, stirrups, footboard); and
- specialty surgical beds (eg, fracture table, ophthalmology carts/stretchers, chairs).[16]

Shearing: A sliding movement of skin and subcutaneous tissue that leaves the underlying muscle stationary.

REFERENCES

1. Petersen C, ed. *Perioperative Nursing Data Set.* Rev 2nd ed. Denver, CO: AORN, Inc; 2007:43-44, 64-66.
2. National Pressure Ulcer Advisory Panel Support Surface Standards Initiative. Terms and definitions related to support surfaces. Ver. 01/29/07. http://invisiblecaregiver.com/docs/NPUAP_Standards.pdf. Accessed December 7, 2007.
3. ECRI. Pressure ulcers. *HRC Risk Analysis.* 2006;3(Nursing 4):1-37.
4. Armstrong D, Bortz P. An integrative review of pressure relief in surgical patients. *AORN J.* 2001;73:645, 647-648, 650-653.
5. Nixon J, McElvenny D, Mason S, Brown J, Bond S. A sequential randomised controlled trial comparing a dry visco-elastic polymer pad and standard operating procedure bed mattress in the prevention of postoperative pressure sores. *Int J Nurs Stud.* 1998;35:193-203.
6. Defloor T, De Schuijmer JD. Preventing pressure ulcers: an evaluation of four operating-table bed mattresses. *Applied Nursing Research.* 2000;13:134-141.
7. Hoshowsky VM, Schramm CA. Intraoperative pressure sore prevention: an analysis of bedding materials. *Res Nurs Health.* 1994;17:333-339.
8. Shelton F, Lott JW. Conducting and interpreting interface pressure evaluations of clinical support surfaces. *Geriatr Nurs.* 2003;24:222-227.
9. King CA. Comparison of pressure relief properties of operating room surfaces. *Perioperative Nursing Clinics.* 2006;1:261-265.
10. Cullum N, McInnes E, BellSyer SEM, Legood R. Support surfaces for pressure ulcer prevention. *Cochrane Database Syst Rev.* 2007;(1):ID10300075320-100000000-01074.
11. Schultz A. Predicting and preventing pressure ulcers in surgical patients. *AORN J.* 2005;81:986-1006.
12. McEwen DR. Intraoperative positioning of surgical patients. *AORN J.* 1996;63:1058-1063, 1066-1075, 1077-1082.
13. Petersen C, ed. *AORN Guidance Statement: Safe Patient Handling and Movement in the Perioperative Setting.* Denver, CO: AORN, Inc; 2007:1-32.
14. Facility design, equipment, and supplies. In: *Bariatric Services: Safety, Quality, and Technology Guide.* Plymouth Meeting, PA: ECRI; 2004:77-110.
15. Dybec RB. Intraoperative positioning and care of the obese patient. *Plastic Surgical Nursing.* 2004;24:118-122.
16. Recommended practices for product selection in perioperative practice settings. In: *Standards, Recommended Practices, and Guidelines.* Denver, CO: AORN, Inc; 2007:637-640.
17. AORN position statement on correct site surgery. In: *Standards, Recommended Practices, and Guidelines.* Denver, CO: AORN, Inc; 2007:371-374.
18. Joint Commission. Implementation expectations for the universal protocol for preventing wrong site, wrong procedure, and wrong person surgery, 2003. http://www.jointcommission.org/NR/rdonlyres/DEC4A816-ED52-4C04-AF8C-FEBA74A732EA/0/up_guidelines.pdf. Accessed May 3, 2007.
19. AORN guidance statement: creating a patient safety culture. In: *Standards, Recommended Practices, and Guidelines.* Denver, CO: AORN, Inc; 2007:305-310.
20. Recommended practices for a safe environment of care. In: *Standards, Recommended Practices, and Guidelines.* Denver, CO: AORN, Inc; 2008:351-373.
21. Keller C. The obese patient as a surgical risk. *Semin Perioper Nurs.* 1999;8:109-117.
22. Graling P, Elariny, H. Perioperative care of the patient with morbid obesity. *AORN J.* 2003;77:801-819.
23. Bushard S. Trauma in patients who are morbidly obese. *AORN J.* 2002;76:585-589.
24. Sieggreen M. OR-acquired pressure ulcers in vascular surgery patients. *Adv Wound Care.* 1998;11:12.
25. Aronovitch SA. Intraoperatively acquired pressure ulcer prevalence: a national study. *Journal of WOCN.* 1999/5;26:130-136.
26. Catalano, K. Update on the national patient safety goals—changes for 2005. *AORN J.* 2005;81:336-341.
27. Robey-Williams C, Rush KL, Bendyk H, Patton LM, Chamberlain D, Sparks T. Spartanburg Fall Risk Assessment Tool: a simple three-step process. *Applied Nursing Research.* 2007;20:86-93.
28. Beyea S. Preventing patient falls in perioperative settings. [Patient Safety First]. *AORN J.* 2005; 81:393-395.
29. Nelson A, Fragala G, Menzel N. Myths and facts about back injuries in nursing. *Am J Nurs.* 2003;103:32-40.
30. Stetler CB, Burns M, Sander-Buscemi K, Morsi D, Grunwald E. Use of evidence for prevention of work-related musculoskeletal injuries. *Orthop Nurs.* 2003; 22:32-41.
31. Chappy, S. Perioperative patient safety: a multisite qualitative analysis. *AORN J.* 2006; 83:871-897.
32. Sewchuk D, Padula C, Osborne E. Prevention and early detection of pressure ulcers in patients undergoing cardiac surgery. *AORN J.* 2006; 84:75-96.
33. Feuchtinger J, de Bie R, Dassen T, Halfens R. A 4-cm thermoactive viscoelastic foam pad on the operating room procedure bed to prevent pressure ulcer during cardiac surgery. *J Clin Nurs.* 2006;15:162-167.
34. Ramsay J. Pressure ulcer risk factors in the operating room. *Advances in Wound Care.* 1998;11:5-6.
35. Reddy M, Gill SS, Rochon PA. Preventing pressure ulcers: a systematic review. *JAMA.* 2006; 296: 974-984.
36. Landis EM. Micro-injection studies of capillary blood pressure in human skin. *Heart.* 1930;15:209-228.
37. O'Connell MP. Positioning impact on the surgical patient. *Nurs Clin North Am.* 2006;41:173-192.
38. AORN explications for perioperative nursing. In: *Standards, Recommended Practices, and Guidelines.* Denver, CO: AORN, Inc; 2007:171-201.

39. Larkin BG. The ins and outs of body piercing. *AORN J.* 2004;79:333-342.
40. Aronovitch SA, Wilber M, Slezak S, Martin T, Utter D. A comparative study of an alternating air mattress for the prevention of pressure ulcers in surgical patients. *Ostomy Wound Management.* 1999;45:34-40.
41. Practice advisory for the prevention of perioperative peripheral neuropathies: a report by the American Society of Anesthesiologists Task Force on Prevention of Perioperative Peripheral Neuropathies. *Anesthesiology.* 2000;92:1168-1182.
42. Fritzlen T, Kremer M, Biddle C. The AANA Foundation Closed Malpractice Claims Study on nerve injuries during anesthesia care. *AANA J.* 2003;71:347-352.
43. Ayello EA. Preventing pressure ulcers and skin tears. In: Mezey M, Fulmer T, Abraham I, Zwicker DA, eds. *Geriatric Nursing Protocols for Best Practice.* 2nd. ed. New York, NY: Springer Publishing Company, Inc; 2003:165-184.
44. Walsh J. *AANA Journal* course: update for nurse anesthetists—patient positioning. *AANA J.* 1994;62:289-298.
45. Lindgren M, Unosson M, Krantz AM, Ek AC. Pressure ulcer risk factors in patients undergoing surgery. *J Adv Nurs.* 2005;50:605-612.
46. **Birnbach DJ, Browne IM. Anesthesia for obstetrics.** In: *Miller's Anesthesia, Volume Two.* Miller RD, ed. 6th ed. Philadelphia, PA: Elsevier; 2006: 2309.
47. Liau, DW. **Injuries and liability related to peripheral catheters: a closed claims analysis. *ASA Newsletter.* June 2006.** http://www.asahq.org/newsletter/2006/06/liau06_06.html. **Accessed December 12, 2007.**
48. **Faust RJ, Cucchiara RF, Bechtel PS. Patient positioning.** In: *Miller's Anesthesia,* **Volume One.** Miller RD, ed. 6th ed. Philadelphia, PA: Elsevier; 2006:**1155-1158.**
49. Coppieters MW, Van de Velde M, Stappaerts KH. Positioning in anesthesiology: toward a better understanding of stretch-induced perioperative neuropathies. [Comment]. *Anesthesiology.* 2002;97:75-81.
50. Sawyer RJ, Richmond MN, Hickey JD, Jarrratt JA. Peripheral nerve injuries associated with anaesthesia. [Comment]. *Anaesthesia.* 2000;55:980-991.
51. Cheney FW, Domino KB, Caplan RA, Posner KL. Nerve injury associated with anesthesia: a closed claims analysis. *Anesthesiology.* 1999;90:1062-1069.
52. France MP, Aurori BF. Pudendal nerve palsy following fracture procedure bed traction. *Clinical Orthopaedics & Related Research.* 1992;276:272-276.
53. Toolan BC, Koval KJ, Kummer FJ, Goldsmith ME, Zuckerman JD. Effects of supine positioning and fracture post placement on the perineal countertraction force in awake volunteers. *J Orthop Trauma.* 1995;9:164-170.
54. Lloyd JD, Baptiste A. Friction-reducing devices for lateral patient transfers: a biomechanical evaluation. *American Association of Occupational Health Nurses.* 2006;54:113-119.
55. Chaffin DB, Andersson G, Martin BJ. *Occupational Biomechanics.* 3rd ed. New York: J Wiley & Sons; 1999:73.
56. American Society of Anesthesiologists Task Force on Perioperative Blindness. Practice advisory for perioperative visual loss associated with spine surgery: a report by the American Society of Anesthesiologists Task Force on Perioperative Blindness. *Anesthesiology.* 2006; 104:1319-1328.
57. Rupp-Montpetit K, Moody, ML. Visual loss as a complication of non-ophthalmologic surgery: a review of the literature. *AANA Journal.* 2004;72:285-292.
58. Giarrizzo-Wilson S. Postoperative vision loss; cellular telephones; medical gas handling; roller latches. [Clinical Issues]. *AORN J.* 2006;84:107-108, 111-114.
59. Biddle C, Cannaday MJ. Surgical positions. their effects on cardiovascular, respiratory systems. *AORN J.* 1990;52:350-359.
60. Irvin W, Andersen W, Taylor P, Rice L. Minimizing the risk of neurologic injury in gynecologic surgery. *Obstet Gynecol.* 2004;103:374-382.
61. Roeder RA, Geddes LA, Corson N, Pell C, Otlewski M, Kemeny A. Heel and calf capillary-support: pressure in lithotomy positions. *AORN J.* 2005;81:821-830.
62. Wilde S. Compartment syndrome. the silent danger related to patient positioning and surgery. *Br J Perioper Nurs.* 2004;14:546-550.
63. Raza A, Byrne D, Townell N. Lower limb (well leg) compartment syndrome after urological pelvic surgery. *J Urol.* 2004;171:5-11.
64. Pfeffer SD, Halliwill JR, Warner MA. Effects of lithotomy position and external compression on lower leg muscle compartment pressure. [Comment]. *Anesthesiology.* 2001;95:632-636.
65. Recommendations for facilities performing bariatric surgery. *Bull Am Coll Surg.* 2000;85:20-23.
66. Brodsky JB. Positioning the morbidly obese patient for anesthesia. *Obesity Surg.* 2002;12:751-758.
67. ECRI. Bariatric surgery. *Operating Room Risk Management.* May 2005:14-17.
68. Schouchoff B. Pressure ulcer development in the operating room. *Crit Care Nurs Q.* 2002;25:76-82.
69. Lawson N, Mills NL, Oschner JL. Occipital alopecia following cardiovascular bypass. *J Thorac Cardiovasc Surg.* 1976;71:342-347.
70. Chowet AL, Lopez JR, Brock-Utne JG, Jaffe RA. Wrist hyperextension leads to median nerve conduction block: Implications for intra-arterial catheter placement. *Anesthesiology.* 2004;100:287-291.
71. Stotts, NA. Risk assessment of pressure ulcer development in surgical patients. *Adv Skin Wound Care.* 1998;11(suppl 3):7.
72. Price MC, Whitney JD, King CA. Wound care. development of a risk assessment tool for intraoperative pressure ulcers. *J WOCN.* 2005;32:19-32.
73. Schoonhoven L, Defloor T, Grypdonck MH. Incidence of pressure ulcers due to surgery. *J Clin Nurs.* 2002;11:479-487.
74. National Pressure Ulcer Advisory Panel. Pressure ulcer definition and stages. February 2007. http://www.npuap.org/pr2.htm. Accessed November 6, 2007.
75. Roth S, Thisted RA, Erickson JP, Black S, Schreider BD. Eye injuries after nonocular surgery. A study of 60,965 anesthetics from 1988 to 1992. *Anesthesiology.* 1996;85:1020-1027.
76. Recommended practices for documentation of perioperative nursing care. In: *Standards, Recommended Practices, and Guidelines.* Denver, CO: AORN, Inc; 2007:511-514.
77. Dunn D. Incident reports: their purpose and scope. First in a two-part series. [Home Study Program]. *AORN J.* 2003;78:45-46, 49-61, 65-70.
78. Quality and performance improvement standards for perioperative nursing. In: *Standards, Recommended Practices, and Guidelines.* Denver, CO: AORN, Inc; 2007:437-446.
79. Agency for Healthcare Research and Quality. Pressure Ulcers in Adults: Prediction and Prevention. *Clinical Practice Guideline Number 3.* Pub No 92-0047 (May 1992). http://www.ncbi.nlm.nih.gov/books/bv.fcgi?rid=hstat2.chapter.4409. Accessed November 6, 2007.
80. Liang BA. The adverse event of unaddressed medical error: Identifying and filling the holes in the health-care and legal systems. *J Law Med Ethics.* 2001;29:346-368.

POSITIONING THE PATIENT

PUBLICATION HISTORY

Originally published November 1990, *AORN Journal*. Revised November 1995; published August 1996, *AORN Journal*.

Revised and reformatted; published January 2001, *AORN Journal*.

Revised 2007; published in *Perioperative Standards and Recommended Practices*, 2008 edition.

Minor editing revisions made to omit PNDS codes; reformatted September 2012 for publication in *Perioperative Standards and Recommended Practices*, 2013 edition.

Minor editing revisions made in November 2014 for publication in *Guidelines for Perioperative Practice*, 2015 edition.

POSITIONING THE PATIENT

PATIENT CARE

GUIDELINE FOR TRANSFER OF PATIENT CARE INFORMATION

The Guideline for Transfer of Patient Care Information was developed by the AORN Recommended Practices Committee and was approved by the AORN Board of Directors. It was presented as proposed recommendations for comments by members and others. The guideline is effective December 1, 2009. The recommendations in the guideline are intended to be achievable recommendations representing what is believed to be an optimal level of practice. Policies and procedures will reflect variations in practice settings and/or clinical situations that determine the degree to which the guideline can be implemented. AORN recognizes the various settings in which perioperative nurses practice; therefore, this guideline is adaptable to various practice settings. These practice settings include traditional operating rooms (ORs), ambulatory surgery centers, physicians' offices, cardiac catheterization laboratories, endoscopy suites, radiology departments, and all other areas where operative and other invasive procedures may be performed.

Purpose

This document provides guidance to perioperative nurses for safe transfer of patient information to subsequent health care providers. In order to be proactive in addressing patient safety concerns, transfer of patient information processes should be incorporated into the overall perioperative plan of care. The recommendations are aimed toward establishing consistent and reliable methods for improved communication across the continuum of care that are evidence-based and should be realistically transferred into everyday practice. AORN's Patient Hand Off Tool Kit is a companion resource for this guideline.

Recommendation I

A transfer of patient information process should be developed, standardized, and based upon the best available and most current evidence.

Standardization of transfer of patient information processes improves the accuracy, reliability, and quality of information. A model that is based upon standardization of the process and content, and tailored to individual organizations and disciplines may improve patient safety.[1] Standardized hand offs and transfer protocols were identified as methods to prevent communication breakdowns.[2]

I.a. A multidisciplinary team, composed of caregivers who participate in the transfer of patient information, should be assembled to develop a structure and process for transfer of patient information processes. All members of the multidisciplinary team, regardless of title or stature, should be encouraged to participate. Team members may include, but are not limited to
- registered nurse (eg, perioperative, perianesthesia, critical care, emergency department, registered nurse first assistant);
- physician (eg, surgeon, anesthesiologist, proceduralist, resident);
- allied health personnel (eg, certified surgical technologist, perfusionist, radiology technician);
- anesthesia care provider (eg, certified registered nurse anesthetist, anesthesiologist assistant);
- other licensed independent practitioners (eg, advanced practice registered nurse, physician assistant); and
- support personnel (eg, patient care assistant, transporter).

A multidisciplinary team's planning and coordination of the process ensures that the needs and perspectives of the patient and all caregivers are included, which can decrease risk and promote the safe transfer of patient information. (The team should be representative of the disciplines that care for the particular patient population.[3])

I.b. The process for transferring patient information should include verbal components and written components in a standardized documentation format. If possible, interaction should occur using a face-to-face format.

A standardized documentation format will assist the practitioner in ensuring the continuity of information flow. In a review of more than 14,000 medical records from 28 hospitals, it was found that 6,200 patients incurred some type of adverse event during their hospital stay.[4] Forty-nine percent of the adverse events occurred in the OR. In all clinical categories, 27% of adverse events were rule-based errors that could possibly have been prevented by the implementation of some type of standardized documentation format such as a checklist.[4] Additional study results indicated that data loss was minimal when nurses used both verbal communication and a pre-printed form during the process to transfer patient information.[5] Aside from the written portion, an effective communication exchange between the giver and receiver of patient information provides time for the opportunity to dialogue and ask questions.[6] Direct communication reduces the

TRANSFER OF PATIENT CARE INFORMATION

number of assumptions made by the practitioners regarding patient status, allows for a more effective exchange of information, and provides an opportunity to ask questions. In face-to-face exchanges, all communication channels are available including body language, facial expression, and eye contact.[7] Results from an observational study of hand-off strategies showed that a face-to-face exchange of information improved the effectiveness of the hand off.[8]

I.b.1. Only individuals involved with the patient's care should be allowed to view or hear protected information. Examples include, but are not limited to,
- appropriate members of the health care team,
- family members, and
- designated support person(s).

Confidentiality ensures compliance with Health Insurance Portability and Accountability Act (HIPAA) regulations[9] and protects the patient's right to privacy.[10,11]

I.c. All phases of patient care should be addressed in the process for transferring patient information. Phases of care should include, but not be limited to, the
- surgeon's office;
- scheduling department;
- preanesthesia testing unit;
- preoperative holding unit;
- OR;
- postanesthesia care unit (PACU); and
- other areas where postoperative care is provided (eg, intensive care unit, ambulatory care discharge unit).

Research results have indicated that information loss and degradation has occurred across the major phases of patient care.[12,13]

I.d. Contents of the transfer-of-patient-information process for each perioperative phase should include, but not be limited to, the following:

Preoperative phase:
- verification of correct patient (ie, two identifiers), site, and procedure;
- evidence of site marking, if applicable;
- diagnosis, surgeon, anesthesia type;
- required legal documents (eg, complete and signed consent form, durable power of attorney);
- required clinical documentation (eg, complete and signed history and physical by attending physician, informed consent statement);
- laboratory/diagnostic/radiologic test results;
- required blood products, implants, devices, and/or special equipment or instrumentation;
- precautions (eg, isolation, respiratory);
- presence of prostheses and implants (eg, sensory aids, hardware, pacemaker, implanted electronic device [IED]);
- NPO status, allergies, vital signs (eg, temperature, pulse, respiration, blood pressure, pain assessment), as well as pulse oximetry, height, and weight);
- advanced directives documents;
- medication profile including preoperative medications;
- relevant cultural, generational, spiritual, and/or educational patient needs;
- primary language;
- family/significant other information;
- risk for hypothermia, deep vein thrombosis (DVT), difficult airway, and surgical site infection;
- performance measures (eg, antibiotic prophylaxis, beta-blocker administration);
- patient seen by surgeon and anesthesia care provider; and
- patient ready for transfer.

Intraoperative phase:
- verification of correct patient (ie, two identifiers), site, position, and procedure;
- allergies;
- diagnosis, surgeon, and anesthesia type;
- current or pending laboratory or other test results;
- precautions (eg, isolation, respiratory);
- advanced directives;
- special equipment, instrumentation, and implants;
- surgical count status;
- family communication;
- available blood products and blood loss;
- catheter and/or invasive lines present;
- medications (including dose and time);
- IV and irrigation fluids;
- specimens;
- thermal interventions;
- DVT prophylaxis; and
- patient family and/or significant other information.

Postoperative phase:
- verification of correct patient (ie, two identifiers), site, position, and procedure;
- anesthesia type;
- anesthesia care provider's orders related to oxygenation/ventilation, and IV medications;
- surgeon's orders for drains, diet, and medications;
- administered medications including dose and time;
- administered IV fluids and irrigation;
- advanced directives;
- estimated blood loss;
- related information about the surgical site (eg, dressings, tubes, drains, packing);
- vital signs;
- hemodynamic status;
- airway and oxygenation status;
- thermal status;
- urine output;
- presence or absence of surgical complications;

TRANSFER OF PATIENT CARE INFORMATION

- precautions (eg, isolation, respiratory);
- any significant events; and
- patient family and/or significant other information.

Patient needs vary among phases of perioperative care. Key elements for inclusion may depend on different circumstances (eg, clinical environment, health care provider involved in the transfer process, patient acuity, identified safety risks).[14,15]

I.e. The timing of the transfer of patient information during a change in personnel (eg, breaks, permanent shift relief) or during periods of high activity (eg, conducting counts) should be addressed.

Communicating case status and critical information in the transfer of patient information during a change in personnel (eg, breaks, permanent shift relief) or during periods of high activity (eg, counting protocol) has been identified as a point of vulnerability to information loss, which may have a negative effect on patient safety.[12,13,16]

I.f. Standardized documentation formats (eg, checklists, electronic records, scripts, briefings) should be adopted in processes for the transfer of patient information. Practitioners should ensure that the format for the safe transfer of patient information allows for a smooth and efficient exchange of information.

Standardized documentation formats provide adequate and purposeful information to ensure safe patient care transitions.[17] Standardized transfers and hand-off protocols have the potential to reduce communication breakdowns.[2] Examples of standardized documentation formats include
- SBAR: situation, background, assessment, recommendation[18];
- I PASS the BATON: introduction, patient, assessment, situation, safety concerns, (the) background, actions, timing, ownership, next[19];
- SURgical PAtient Safety System (SUR-PASS)[15]; and
- SHARED: situation, history, assessment, request, evaluate, document.[20]

I.g. Interruptions and distractions (eg, cellular telephones, pagers, music) during the transfer of patient information should be minimized and eliminated, if possible.

Interruptions and distractions during verbal and/or written patient information exchanges can lead to errors, forgetfulness on the part of the practitioner, and decreased attention. An interruption-driven environment can cause failures in a person's working memory, which is described as the memory that actively processes information.[21] In an analysis of observational data for evidence of use of 21 hand-off strategies in non-health care formats, limiting interruptions was found to be a useful strategy for improving the effectiveness of the hand-off process.[8]

I.h. Transfer of patient information should be delayed until members of the patient care team have had an opportunity to ask and respond to patient care questions or concerns. Questions may include but not be limited to
- the process,
- the readiness of the incoming provider, and
- staffing or bed availability.[22,23]

I.i. Health care organization leaders should support the implementation of a process for the transfer of patient information.

Support at all levels of the organization, including clinical, is needed to implement safe patient practices.[24-26] Encouragement on the part of health care organization leaders creates a familiar environment in which all team members feel safe to speak and participate.[24] It was found in a prospective study that OR leaders and managers were supportive if shown how the use of a preoperative checklist could improve communication and promote safer teamwork.[27]

Recommendation II

Patients, families, and significant others should have an active role in transfer of patient information processes whenever possible.

It was found that a structured, individualized method of transfer that engaged the patient and family members reduced family members' anxiety. The intervention provided family members with details regarding what to expect after the patient and relevant information were transferred.[28]

II.a. Patients, families, and significant others should be informed as soon as possible if the patient's transfer plan changes (eg, patient is transferred directly to a unit instead of the PACU).

It was concluded from an extensive review of the literature that patients' families incur transfer anxiety that can be reduced through nursing interventions.[29] Patient and family anxiety, related to changes in care providers and the physical environment, was reduced after they received written information. Anxiety was decreased in patients and their relatives when they received individualized education on transfers.[30,31]

Recommendation III

Personnel should receive education, training, and competency validation on effective communication skills and processes for the transfer of patient information.

Communication is central in maintaining the continuity of patient care.[32] Communication was cited as the root cause of the nearly 3,000 sentinel events, such as unexpected deaths and catastrophic injuries, reported to the Joint Commission between 1995 and 2005.[33] A relationship exists between effective communication skills and positive patient outcomes.[34,35]

III.a. The health care organization leaders should determine the type and frequency of competency assessment (eg, upon hire and periodically thereafter) for processes for the transfer of patient information. Team members accompanying the patient should be selected according to their training and validated competency and the patient's ongoing or anticipated needs during transport.[36]

Competency assessment validates the clinician's knowledge acquisition to implement processes for the transfer of patient information.

III.b. Training sessions, using different teaching modalities (eg, simulation, role-playing, case studies), should be conducted to educate personnel.

Simulation is a valuable tool in aiding effective communication and teamwork during the transfer of patient information.[24] Data has shown that simulation improves communication and teamwork skills.[37-39]

Recommendation IV

The perioperative registered nurse should document the process for the transfer of patient information using a standardized documentation format, and the document should be recorded and retained in a manner consistent with the health care organization's policies and procedures.

Documentation of the process for the transfer of patient information provides a record of patient care. A standardized documentation format allows clear and timely communication of patient information affecting patient safety. The Perioperative Nursing Data Set (PNDS) contains specific data elements related to the continuity of care and communication of patient information.[40]

Recommendation V

Policies and procedures for standardized transfer of patient information processes should be developed, reviewed periodically, readily available in the practice setting, and reflect the rules and recommendations from regulatory and accreditation bodies.

Policies and procedures are operational guidelines that are used to minimize patient risk factors, standardize practice, direct staff members, and establish guidelines for continuous performance improvement activities.

V.a. The policy and procedure for the transfer of patient information should be developed by a multidisciplinary team and written according to the established guidelines and format of the health care organization. Components of the policy should include the documentation and communication methods as well as tools and what information and equipment (eg, electrocardiogram monitor, portable oxygen, lifting devices) are needed in various patient information transfer situations.

V.b. The policy and procedure should outline a contingency plan should a patient's status change.

A contingency plan has been shown to improve the effectiveness of the transfer of information in settings with high consequences for failure.[8]

Recommendation VI

A quality management program should be implemented to evaluate and monitor the processes for the transfer of patient information. Components should include patient; process; and structural (eg, format) outcome indicators. A fundamental precept of AORN is that it is the responsibility of professional perioperative registered nurses to provide safe, high-quality nursing care to patients undergoing operative and invasive procedures.[11]

Feedback should be solicited from practitioners to validate the implementation of the standardized documentation format, its ease of use, and the required training process.[20] Regularly evaluating and monitoring processes for the transfer of patient information may assist in identifying areas for improvement.[22]

VI.a. Barriers to effective communication that interfere with processes for the transfer of patient information should be identified and corrected through quality review activities. The areas that should be evaluated include but are not limited to
- physical setting;
- social setting (eg, status, hierarchy);
- language; and
- communication.[7]

Barriers to effective communication resulting in poorly executed patient care processes can result in delays in surgical intervention, delays in obtaining consents, and delays and/or duplications of tests or treatments thereby placing the patient at risk.[41] Methods to reduce information loss include confirming and repeating verbal orders; using standardized and accepted abbreviations, symbols, acronyms, and dose designations; and avoiding colloquialisms.[6,42] A combination of verbal and written communication provides multiple pathways for the exchange of information.[7]

VI.b. An evaluation period should occur to assess the efficacy of the standardized documentation format. Data on past transfer of patient information processes that were deemed deficient and compromised patient safety should be reviewed. Ongoing evaluation efforts may include focus groups, surveys, and direct observations.

During the evaluation period following the implementation of a preoperative team checklist, team members indicated that the most valuable functions of the checklist were providing detailed case-related information and team-building.[43] Results from a follow-up study using the same checklist showed that communication failures were reduced after the checklist was implemented.[27] Improved accuracy and completeness of transfer-of-patient information may result from evaluation efforts by team members.[44]

VI.c. An evaluation tool for measuring the effectiveness of the standardized documentation process should be considered, and if desired, completed anonymously by health care personnel.[45]

Through the use of an evaluation tool, particular transfer of patient information situations can be evaluated for efficiency, including determining risks that could cause miscommunication. Areas to assess include adequate time, likelihood of interruptions, accessible information, and how many personnel are required.[16] Data results should be shared with the team members to solicit suggestions or comments on identified deficiencies.[1] Review of data may provide insight into the success of the transfer of patient information process.[46]

References

1. Arora V, Johnson J. A model for building a standardized hand-off protocol. *Jt Comm J Qual Patient Saf.* 2006;32(11):646-655.
2. Greenberg CC, Regenbogen SE, Studdert DM, et al. Patterns of communication breakdowns resulting in injury to surgical patients. *J Am Coll Surg.* 2007;204(4):533-540.
3. Manning ML. Improving clinical communication through structured conversation. *Nurs Econ.* 2006;24(5):268-271.
4. Wilson RM, Runciman WB, Gibberd RW, Harrison BT, Newby L, Hamilton JD. The Quality in Australian Health Care Study. *Med J Aust.* 1995;163(9):458-471.
5. Pothier D, Monteiro P, Mooktiar M, Shaw A. Pilot study to show the loss of important data in nursing handover. *Br J Nurs.* 2005;14(20):1090-1093.
6. National Patient Safety Goals. In: *Comprehensive Accreditation Manual for Hospitals: The Official Handbook.* Oakbrook Terrace, IL: The Joint Commission; 2009: NPSG-1–NPSG-24.
7. Solet DJ, Norvell JM, Rutan GH, Frankel RM. Lost in translation: challenges and opportunities in physician-to-physician communication during patient handoffs. *Acad Med.* 2005;80(12):1094-1099.
8. Patterson ES, Roth EM, Woods DD, Chow R, Gomes JO. Handoff strategies in settings with high consequences for failure: lessons for health care operations. *Int J Qual Health Care.* 2004;16(2):125-132.
9. *Summary of the HIPAA Privacy Rule.* Washington, DC: US Department of Health and Human Services; 2003.
10. Code of Ethics for Nurses With Interpretive Statements. American Nurses Association. http://nursingworld.org/ethics/code/protected_nwcoe813.htm. Accessed October 6, 2009.
11. Standards of perioperative nursing. In: *Perioperative Standards and Recommended Practices.* Denver, CO: AORN, Inc; 2010. In press.
12. Christian CK, Gustafson ML, Roth EM, et al. A prospective study of patient safety in the operating room. *Surgery.* 2006;139(2):159-173.
13. Roth EM, Christian CK, Gustafson M, et al. Using field observations as a tool for discovery: analysing cognitive and collaborative demands in the operating room. *Cogn Tech Work.* 2004;6(3):148-157.
14. Committee on Patient Safety and Quality Improvement. Communication strategies for patient handoffs [ACOG committee opinion, Number 367]. *Obstet Gynecol.* 2007;109(6):1503-1505.
15. de Vries EN, Hollmann MW, Smorenburg SM, Gouma DJ, Boermeester MA. Development and validation of the SURgical PAtient Safety System (SURPASS) checklist. *Qual Saf Health Care.* 2009;18(2):121-126.
16. Gregory BS. Patient safety first. Standardizing hand-off processes. *AORN J.* 2006;84(6):1059-1061.
17. Vidyarthi AR, Arora V, Schnipper JL, Wall SD, Wachter RM. Managing discontinuity in academic medical centers: strategies for a safe and effective resident sign-out. *J Hosp Med.* 2006;1(4):257-266.
18. SBAR checklist can cut risk at patient handoff. *Healthc Risk Manage.* 2006;28(9):102-104.
19. *Strategies and Tools to Improve Healthcare Handoffs and Transitions.* Washington, DC: US Department of Defense; 2005.
20. Sharing information at transfers: proven technique to aid handoff communications. *Joint Comm Perspect Patient Saf.* 2005;5(12):9-10.
21. Parker J, Coiera E. Improving clinical communication: a view from psychology. *J Am Med Inform Assoc.* 2000;7(5):453-461.
22. Simpson KR. Handling handoffs safely. *MCN Am J Matern Child Nurs.* 2005;30(2):152.
23. 2010 National Patient Safety Goals. The Joint Commission. http://www.jointcommission.org/PatientSafety/NationalPatientSafetyGoals. Accessed October 6, 2009.
24. Leonard M, Graham S, Bonacum D. The human factor: the critical importance of effective teamwork and communication in providing safe care. *Qual Saf Health Care.* 2004;13(Suppl 1):85-90.
25. Pronovost PJ, Goeschel CA, Marsteller JA, Sexton JB, Pham JC, Berenholtz SM. Framework for patient safety research and improvement. *Circulation.* 2009;119(2):330-337.
26. Pronovost PJ, Rosenstein BJ, Paine L, et al. Paying the piper: investing in infrastructure for patient safety. *Jt Comm J Qual Patient Saf.* 2008;34(6):342-348.
27. Lingard L, Regehr G, Orser B, et al. Evaluation of a preoperative checklist and team briefing among surgeons, nurses, and anesthesiologists to reduce failures in communication. *Arch Surg.* 2008;143(1):12-17.
28. Mitchell ML, Courtney M. Reducing family members' anxiety and uncertainty in illness around transfer from intensive care: an intervention study. *Int J Qual Health Care.* 2004;20(4):223-231.
29. Mitchell ML, Courtney M, Coyer F. Understanding uncertainty and minimizing families' anxiety at the time of transfer from intensive care. *Nurs Health Sci.* 2003;5(3):207-217.
30. Paul F, Hendry C, Cabrelli L. Meeting patient and relatives' information needs upon transfer from an intensive care unit: the development and evaluation of an information booklet. *J Clin Nurs.* 2004;13(3):396-405.
31. Tel H, Tel H. The effect of individualized education on the transfer anxiety of patients with myocardial infarction and their families. *Heart Lung.* 2006;35(2):101-107.

32. Kerr MP. A qualitative study of shift handover practice and function from a socio-technical perspective. *J Adv Nurs.* 2002;37(2):125-134.

33. *Front Line of Defense: the Role of Nurses in Preventing Sentinel Events.* Oakbrook Terrace, IL: Joint Commission Resources; 2007.

34. Mazzocco K, Petitti DB, Fong KT, et al. Surgical team behaviors and patient outcomes. *Am J Surg.* 2009;197(5):678-685.

35. McKeon LM, Cunningham PD, Oswaks JS. Improving patient safety: patient-focused, high-reliability team training. *J Nurs Care Qual.* 2009;24(1):76-82.

36. Warren J, Fromm RE Jr, Orr RA, Rotello LC, Horst HM; American College of Critical Care Medicine. Guidelines for the inter- and intrahospital transport of critically ill patients. *Crit Care Med.* 2004;32(1):256-262.

37. Gettman MT, Pereira CW, Lipsky K, et al. Use of high fidelity operating room simulation to assess and teach communication, teamwork and laparoscopic skills: initial experience. *J Urol.* 2009;181(3):1289-1296.

38. Paige JT, Kozmenko V, Yang T, et al. High-fidelity, simulation-based, interdisciplinary operating room team training at the point of care. *Surgery.* 2009;145(2):138-146.

39. Powers KA, Rehrig ST, Irias N, et al. Simulated laparoscopic operating room crisis: an approach to enhance the surgical team performance. *Surg Endosc.* 2008;22(4):885-900.

40. Petersen C, ed. *Perioperative Nursing Data Set.* 2nd ed Rev. Denver, CO: AORN, Inc; 2007.

41. Carr DD. Case managers optimize patient safety by facilitating effective care transitions. *Prof Case Manag.* 2007;12(2):70-80.

42. Sutcliffe KM, Lewton E, Rosenthal MM. Communication failures: an insidious contributor to medical mishaps. *Acad Med.* 2004;79(2):186-194.

43. Lingard L, Espin S, Rubin B, et al. Getting teams to talk: development and pilot implementation of a checklist to promote interprofessional communication in the OR. *Qual Saf Health Care.* 2005;14(5):340-346.

44. Wayne JD, Tyagi R, Reinhardt G, et al. Simple standardized patient handoff system that increases accuracy and completeness. *J Surg Educ.* 2008;65(6):476-485.

45. Measure understanding during handoffs: a naval hospital uses an evaluation tool to determine whether information is understood. *Brief Patient Saf.* 2006;7(7):4-5.

46. SBAR initiative to improve staff communication. *Healthcare Benchmarks Qual Improv.* 2005;12(4):40-41.

Acknowledgments

Lead Author
Robin Chard, PhD, RN, CNOR
Perioperative Nursing Specialist
AORN Center for Nursing Practice
Denver, Colorado

Contributing Authors
Jane Kuhn, MSN, RN, CNOR, CNAA
Health Care Consultant
Carson, California

Maria C. Arcilla, BSN, RN, CNOR
Education Coordinator
Texas Children's Hospital
Houston, Texas

Terri Goodman, PhD, RN
Health Care Consultant
Dallas, Texas

Thomas Hilbert, MS, CRNA
American Association of Nurse Anesthetists Liaison
Marshfield Clinic Ambulatory Surgery Center
Marshfield, Wisconsin

Publication History
Originally published December 2009 online in *Perioperative Standards and Recommended Practices.*

Minor editing revisions made in November 2010 for publication in *Perioperative Standards and Recommended Practices*, 2011 edition.

Reformatted September 2012 for publication in *Perioperative Standards and Recommended Practices*, 2013 edition.

Minor editing revisions made in November 2014 for publication in *Guidelines for Perioperative Practice*, 2015 edition.

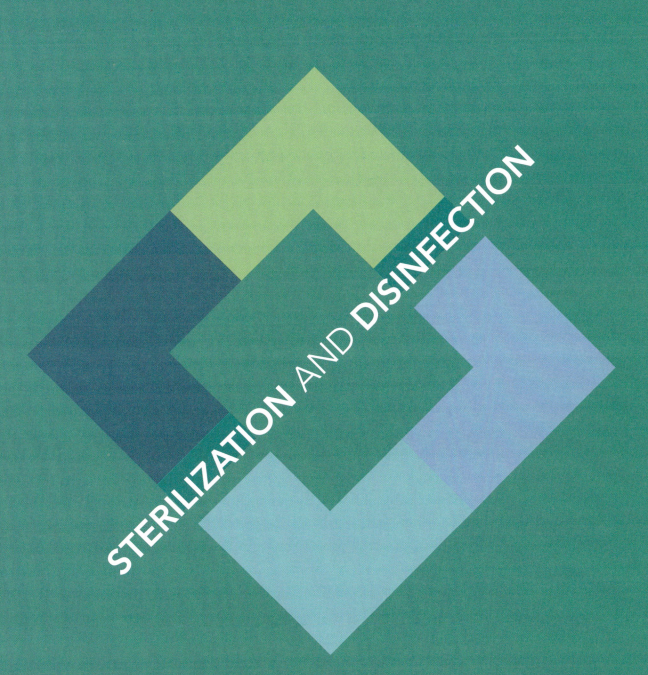

GUIDELINE FOR CLEANING AND PROCESSING FLEXIBLE ENDOSCOPES AND ENDOSCOPE ACCESSORIES

The Guideline for Cleaning and Processing Flexible Endoscopes and Endoscope Accessories was developed by the AORN Recommended Practices Committee and was approved by the AORN Board of Directors. It was presented as proposed recommendations for comments by members and others. The guideline is effective January 1, 2009. The recommendations in the guideline are intended to be achievable and represent what is believed to be an optimal level of practice. Policies and procedures will reflect variations in practice settings and/or clinical situations that determine the degree to which the guideline can be implemented. AORN recognizes the various settings in which perioperative nurses practice; therefore, this guideline is adaptable to various practice settings. These practice settings include traditional operating rooms, ambulatory surgery centers, physician's offices, cardiac catheterization laboratories, endoscopy suites, radiology departments, and all other areas where operative and other invasive procedures may be performed.

Purpose

This document provides guidance to assist personnel in the care, cleaning, decontamination, maintenance, handling, storage, sterilization, and/or disinfection of flexible endoscopes and related accessories. Use of this guideline will assist personnel in providing a safe environment for patients and health care workers.

The guideline is based on the most current evidence available at the time of development. It should be used to develop policies and procedures for the care of flexible endoscopes and accessories in the practice setting. As new information becomes available, perioperative nurses should consult with infection preventionists and epidemiologists to review and revise procedures as appropriate. This guideline pertains only to flexible endoscopes and is divided into the following sections:

- following manufacturer's instructions,
- precleaning,
- transport to decontamination,
- leak testing,
- cleaning,
- high-level disinfection,
- alcohol treatment,
- drying,
- inspection,
- storage,
- handling damaged flexible endoscopes,
- care of accessories, and
- personal protective equipment (PPE).

Competencies, documentation, policies and procedures, and quality management suggestions also are discussed. For more information on the care and cleaning of rigid endoscopes and related equipment, refer to the AORN "Recommended practices for cleaning and care of surgical instruments and powered equipment."[1]

Recommendation I

Flexible endoscopes should be cleaned and stored in accordance with the manufacturer's written instructions.

Failure to follow the manufacturer's written instructions could result in ineffective cleaning that interferes with high-level disinfection or sterilization, creating a risk of infection for the patient. The manufacturer's warranty may be void if the written instructions for care and use of the device are not followed.

I.a. The manufacturer's written instructions for flexible endoscopes and all accessories should be followed regarding
   o cleaning processes,
   o selection of cleaning product,
   o selection of disinfectant/sterilization products,
   o use of alcohol, and
   o compatibility with automatic endoscope reprocessors.

   Flexible endoscopes manufactured by different companies require different cleaning processes as described in the manufacturer's written instructions. The flexible endoscope manufacturer is required to demonstrate to the US Food and Drug Administration in the premarket clearance application that the cleaning /disinfecting instructions are adequate and that the results are reproducible.[2] All flexible endoscopes and accessories cannot be processed successfully in all automatic endoscopic reprocessors.[3]

I.b. High-level disinfectant and chemical cleaner manufacturers' written instructions should be followed regarding
   o compatibility with the flexible endoscope and accessories,
   o water quality,
   o dilution,

FLEXIBLE ENDOSCOPES

- temperature of solution,
- testing for minimum effective concentration,
- time of exposure, and
- rinsing.[4]

Following the manufacturer's written instructions will deliver the recommended concentration of cleaning solution, disinfectant, or sterilant required for adequate cleaning and to create effective high-level disinfection or sterilization.[5,6] Improper dilution may result in ineffective high-level disinfection or sterilization if the solution is too weak. If the solution is too strong, it may become abrasive or corrosive, possibly contributing to corrosion and degradation of the surfaces of the flexible endoscope.[7] The high-level disinfectant and chemical cleaner may remain on the scope if the manufacturer's written instructions for rinsing are not followed. For more information on high-level disinfection, refer to the AORN "Recommended practices for high-level disinfection."[8]

I.c. New, repaired, or refurbished flexible endoscopes and accessories should be leak tested, cleaned, and high-level disinfected or sterilized before use in a health care organization.

Cleaning and high-level disinfection of newly acquired or repaired flexible endoscopes removes any soil related to manufacturing, repairing, refurbishing, or shipping. Leak tests determine if perforations in either the outer covering or the lining of the internal channels may have occurred during manufacturing, shipping, repairing, or refurbishing.[9]

Recommendation II

Precleaning of flexible endoscopes and accessories should occur at the point of use, before organic material has dried on the surface or in the channels of the endoscope, and before transport to the decontamination area.

Flexible endoscopes, by virtue of the body cavities in which they are used, acquire high levels of microbial contamination during each use. Failure to completely follow the defined cleaning process, beginning with precleaning, has been shown to cause inadequate decontamination leading to patients being exposed to infectious agents.[10] Precleaning of endoscopes and related equipment at the point of use before transport to the decontamination area helps prevent drying of the organic material on the flexible endoscope surfaces.

The presence of dried organic material makes decontamination/disinfection more difficult. Organic materials (eg, blood and body fluids) that have dried on the flexible endoscope surfaces are difficult to remove and can inhibit sterilization and high-level disinfection.[11] Precleaning reduces the likelihood of the formation of biofilms, which contain viable and nonviable microorganisms that become trapped within a matrix of organic matter (eg, proteins, glycoproteins, carbohydrates) and adhere to the surfaces of flexible endoscopes. Biofilms are difficult to remove, and it is difficult for sterilizing/disinfecting agents to penetrate and kill the microorganisms within the biofilms. The biofilm formation process can begin within minutes after completion of a procedure.[7,12]

II.a. Precleaning measures include the following:
(1) External surfaces of the flexible endoscope insertion tube should be washed with an enzymatic detergent solution using a soft cloth or sponge.
(2) Internal suction/biopsy channels should be cleaned by suctioning copious amounts of enzymatic solution (ie, enzymatic detergent mixed with tap water) and air.
(3) Air and water channels should be flushed with an enzymatic solution, then flushed using low-pressure compressed air (ie, pressure should not exceed maximum channel pressure specified by manufacturer), if available. If low-pressure compressed air is not available, a syringe may be used for flushing with air.
(4) Additional complex design components or channels (eg, forward water jet channel, exposed elevator wire channels, balloon channels) should be flushed or purged with water and/or enzymatic detergent solution as described in the manufacturer's written instructions.
(5) The tip of the endoscope should be visually inspected for damage to any surface and any working part and for cleanliness.
(6) The video protective cap, if available, should be attached after removing the flexible endoscope from the light source and suction.
(7) All detachable parts (eg, hoods, valves, water bottle) should be removed and immersed in an enzymatic detergent solution until transport to the decontamination room. When flexible endoscopes and accessories are used on a sterile field,
- the external surfaces should be wiped with a lint-free cloth saturated with sterile water;
- sterile water and air should be alternately suctioned through the channels; and
- the endoscope and accessories should be handed to the circulator as soon as possible, enabling steps 1–7 to be accomplished.
(8) The enzymatic detergent solution should be discarded after a single use.

Washing the external surfaces of the endoscope and flushing the internal channels with enzymatic solution helps to soften, moisten, dilute, and remove organic soils (eg, blood, feces, respiratory secretions).[13]

Alternating cleaning solution with air may help to soften, moisten, dilute, and remove organic soils (eg, blood, feces, respiratory secretions). It is more effective to alternate the use of air and water when cleaning rather than to prolong the use of either.[13]

Flushing with low-pressure compressed air helps to dry the channel. Low-pressure compressed air should be used because it is possible to damage the channel linings with uncontrolled or high-flow air.[7]

Depending upon design and intended use, endoscopes vary in complexity. Certain flexible endoscopes may have more channels than the standard air, water, and suction. Therefore, whenever scopes have additional channels or complex components, each should also be flushed or purged by following the original scope manufacturer's recommendations.

A visual inspection after precleaning should be done to verify that no obvious organic debris remains.

The video protective cap protects video connections from moisture during decontamination and disinfection.[13]

Soaking the detachable parts of the endoscope in enzymatic detergent solution assists in degrading and preventing biofilms.[7] Wiping the flexible endoscope and accessories with lint-free cloth saturated with sterile water and alternately suctioning sterile water and air while the endoscope remains on the sterile field will prevent drying of proteins on the endoscope surfaces until the cleaning process may be accomplished.

The enzymatic detergent cleaning solution should be discarded after each use because it does not possess bactericidal activity and may support growth of organisms if stored. There are no tests to verify the strength of the solution prior to use.

Recommendation III

After precleaning, contaminated flexible endoscopes and accessories should be transported to the decontamination area before remaining organic material dries on the surface or in the channels of the endoscope.

Transport to the decontamination area before remaining organic material is able to dry on the surface or in the channels of the flexible endoscope facilitates cleaning which helps to reduce the formation of biofilms.[7,12]

III.a. During transport to the decontamination area, soiled flexible endoscopes must be contained (eg, enclosed by a plastic bag, container with a lid) in a manner to prevent exposure of environmental surfaces, patients, and personnel to bloodborne pathogens and other potentially infectious organisms. If the decontamination area is adjacent to the procedure room, the contaminated items may be transported in an open container by personnel wearing appropriate PPE.[14]

Contaminated flexible endoscopes and accessories present a risk of contaminating the environment and can expose health care workers to blood and other potentially infectious materials during transport to the decontamination area.[14]

III.b. The transport container must be labeled to indicate biohazardous contents. The types of label may include, but are not limited to, magnetic signs, stickers, or plastic placards.[14]

Labeling the transport container communicates to others that the items are potentially infectious.[14]

Recommendation IV

In the decontamination area and before cleaning, pressure (ie, leak) tests should be performed on flexible endoscopes with leak testing capabilities.[9]

Leak tests determine if there are any openings in the external surfaces and internal channels that would permit fluid to enter the internal body of the endoscope.[9]

IV.a. During leak testing, the flexible endoscope control knobs should be manipulated in all directions.

Manipulating the flexible endoscope control knobs in all directions exposes the surfaces to the maximum extension, thereby revealing small perforations, if present.[9]

IV.b. When using a leak test system requiring water, the leak test system should be attached to the flexible endoscope, followed by submersion of the entire endoscope in water that does not contain cleaning agents, to check for the presence of bubbling.[9]

Leakage in either the covering or one or more of the internal channels can be determined by the presence of air bubbles when air pressure is applied to the inside of the insertion tube. Discoloration and foam caused by the detergent agent may prevent small bubbles from being visible.[9]

IV.b.1. When a leak is detected, the leak testing device should remain attached to the flexible endoscope and under pressure until the endoscope is removed from the water.[9]

Continuous air pressure helps to prevent water from entering the internal (ie, working) portions of the flexible endoscope, which may cause more extensive damage to the internal parts.[15]

FLEXIBLE ENDOSCOPES

IV.c. When using a leak test system that does not require water, the leak test should be completed before submersion in water or cleaning solution.[9]

Leaks in either the covering or one or more of the inside channels can be determined by a drop in pressure after inflation or by the inability to inflate the inside of the insertion tube.[9]

Recommendation V

Following leak testing and before high-level disinfection using a manual process or an automatic endoscope reprocessor, flexible endoscopes and their accessories should be manually cleaned before any remaining organic material dries on the surface or in the channels of the endoscope.[16]

Immediate cleaning reduces the amount of microbial contamination and the formation of biofilms. For the high-level disinfectant to be effective, the solution must reach all surfaces of the flexible endoscope. If the microbial contamination and biofilm are not removed, the surface under the bioburden will not be disinfected.[7]

V.a. When manually cleaning flexible endoscopes:
(1) The flexible endoscope should be submerged in an enzymatic detergent solution.
(2) The insertion tube of the flexible endoscope should be washed using a soft, lint-free cloth or sponge.[17]
(3) All internal channels should be flushed thoroughly with an enzymatic detergent using manufacturer-provided channel cleaning adapters.
(4) All endoscope components (eg, shroud, valves) should be flushed thoroughly with an enzymatic detergent.
(5) Brushes should be inspected prior to insertion to confirm that they are sized appropriately to the channel(s), not kinked, not missing bristles, and that a protective tip is present to prevent damage to the channel.[17]
(6) The brush should be inserted through the channel with the entire endoscope submerged to prevent aerosolization. The bristles should be wiped to remove excess moisture prior to retracting the brush back through the channel.[17] All channels should be flushed thoroughly and all exterior surfaces of the flexible endoscope and accessories rinsed with potable tap water.[4]
(7) The flexible endoscope should be dried using low-pressure forced air through the internal channels and the exterior surfaces wiped with a soft cloth before placing the endoscope in high-level disinfecting solution or an automatic endoscope reprocessor.

Submersion of the flexible endoscope in enzymatic detergent solution helps ensure contact between the solution and all surfaces of the endoscope and decreases the potential for the cleaning solution to splash.[17]

Washing the exterior of the insertion tube with an enzymatic detergent and a soft cloth removes organic material remaining after precleaning.

Flushing all internal channels with detergent solution exposes these surfaces to the enzymatic detergent solution. Using the manufacturer-provided channel cleaning adapters facilitates opening of the ports.

Brushing accessible channels removes particulate matter. Using the appropriate size brush will maximize the amount of soil removed without damaging the inside of the channel. Using a brush that is kinked or missing bristles or without its protective tip may cause damage to the flexible endoscope.[12,17]

The tip of the flexible endoscope and the lens may be abraded by vigorous brushing and wiping. Brushing and wiping the tip of the flexible endoscope removes any debris or tissue that might be lodged around the air-water outlet.[17] Thorough flushing of the channels and rinsing of the flexible endoscope and accessories with potable tap water removes residual debris and cleaning agents. Potable tap water may be used at this point if it does not cause corrosion or tarnishing or leave salt deposits on the flexible endoscope or its accessories. If corrosion, tarnishing, or salt deposits are found on the flexible endoscope, the water filtration process should be examined.[4]

Moisture remaining on the surface and in the flexible endoscope's lumens may dilute the high-level disinfecting solution, potentially reducing its effectiveness.

Recommendation VI

After cleaning, flexible endoscopes and accessories should be high-level disinfected or sterilized.[8,18]

Flexible endoscopes and accessories contact mucous membranes and/or nonintact skin during use and require a minimum of high-level disinfection. Some flexible endoscopes are heat-labile and cannot be steam sterilized. Sterilization is only required if the flexible endoscope is to be used on a sterile field.[11]

VI.a. When using a manual process for high-level disinfection:
(1) The flexible endoscope and its accessories should be manually cleaned, as described in Recommendation V, before beginning the manual high-level disinfection process.
(2) The flexible endoscope and its accessories should be completely immersed in the disinfecting solution.

(3) All channels should be flushed with disinfecting solution after immersion.[19]

For the high-level disinfectant to be effective, the solution must reach all surfaces of the item. If the microbial contamination and biofilm are not removed, the surface under the bioburden will not be disinfected.[7,16] Complete immersion is required to ensure complete coverage of all surfaces of the flexible endoscope.[20] Flushing helps to ensure that the high-level disinfectant has contact with all surfaces, including internal channels, which is necessary for complete disinfection.[19,20]

VI.b. When using an automatic endoscope reprocessor for high-level disinfection:
(1) Manual cleaning should be accomplished as described in Recommendation V.
(2) The flexible endoscope and components should be inserted into the automatic endoscope reprocessor.
(3) All the flexible endoscope channels should be attached to the unit using compatible connectors.[19]

For the high-level disinfectant to be effective, the solution must reach all surfaces of the flexible endoscope. If the microbial contamination and biofilm are not removed, the surface under the bioburden will not be disinfected.[7,16] Failure to use approved connectors may result in disinfection failure because the disinfectant/sterilant may not reach all surfaces of the flexible endoscope. The use of incompatible connectors have lead to the transmission of infections.[7,21]

VI.b.1. When the compatible connectors of the automatic endoscope reprocessor cannot be connected to a specific channel (ie, the wire elevator channel of a duodenoscope), the steps for manual high-level disinfection should be followed for this channel or for the entire flexible endoscope.[7,22]

Manual high-level disinfection is the only method by which the high-level disinfectant will reach the entire inner surface of the channel.[3,7,21,22]

Recommendation VII

After high-level disinfection, flexible endoscopes should be rinsed and the internal channels flushed with water (eg, sterile water, filtered or unfiltered tap water) followed by a 70% to 90% ethyl or isopropyl alcohol rinse and flush, unless contraindicated by the manufacturer's written instructions.[4,19]

The water rinse and flush removes the residual disinfecting solution. Use of filtered tap water or sterile water reduces the potential for recontamination by waterborne microorganisms. Filtered tap water is created at the point of use, using a filter with 0.2 or 0.1 micron pores.[4,7,19] Rinsing with alcohol assists with removing the water because the alcohol binds with the water remaining in the channel, facilitating the drying process and killing any microorganisms contained in the water.[7,19,23]

VII.a. After rinsing with 70% to 90% ethyl or isopropyl alcohol, the channels should be dried using low pressure forced air.

Using forced air assists with removal of moisture remaining in the channels. Dry air channels do not support microbial growth.[7]

Recommendation VIII

Flexible endoscopes, accessories, and associated equipment should be inspected for integrity, function, and cleanliness:
- **before use,**
- **during the procedure,**
- **after the procedure,**
- **immediately after decontamination, and**
- **before disinfection or sterilization.[24]**

Visual inspection helps to identify structural damage, when and where the damage occurred, what caused the damage, and how to prevent further damage. Loss of function and gross soil that may affect further processing and patient outcomes can also be identified during visual inspection.[16]

VIII.a. Damaged flexible endoscopes and accessories should be removed from use, and the manufacturer should be consulted for directions regarding actions to be taken prior to shipping for repair, such as reprocessing or not reprocessing the damaged flexible endoscope.

Immediate removal from use will prevent further damage to the internal mechanisms of the flexible endoscope that may be caused by water entering the mechanism and will prevent the damaged endoscope from being inadvertently used. The manufacturer will determine the correct method of shipping and whether the endoscope should be cleaned before shipping based on the nature of the damage.[9]

VIII.a.1. Unless otherwise specified in the manufacturer's instructions, a damaged flexible endoscope should not be submerged.[9]

Submersion may lead to additional damage related to water entering the interior of the flexible endoscope.[9]

VIII.a.2. Before shipping a contaminated flexible endoscope or its accessories, the item must be packaged in impervious material in compliance with Department of Transportation shipping regulations.[14]

Flexible endoscopes and accessories returned to the manufacturer for repair are considered a biohazard and precautions must be taken to protect anyone who may come in contact with the device.[14]

FLEXIBLE ENDOSCOPES

VIII.a.3. Flexible endoscopes and accessories returned to the manufacturer for repair must be labeled with a biohazardous label visible during shipping.

Contaminated flexible endoscopes and accessories returned to the manufacturer for repair are considered a biohazard. The biohazard label will act as a warning of potentially infectious material for anyone who handles the package.[14]

Recommendation IX

Flexible endoscopes should be stored in a manner that protects the device from damage and minimizes microbial contamination.

IX.a. Flexible endoscopes should be stored
- in a closed cabinet with
  - venting that allows air circulation around the flexible endoscopes,
  - internal surfaces composed of cleanable materials,
  - adequate height to allow flexible endoscopes to hang without touching the bottom of the cabinet, and
  - sufficient space for storage of multiple endoscopes without touching;
- hanging in a secure vertical position;
- with all removable endoscope components (eg, valve mechanisms, biopsy valve covers, irrigation tubes) detached;
- with all accessories removed; and
- with scope protectors applied if the protector does not interfere with the flexible endoscope hanging straight or restrict the air movement around channel openings.[25-28]

When flexible endoscopes are hung in the vertical position, coiling or kinking is prevented, allowing any remaining moisture to drain out of the endoscope and decreasing the potential development of an environment conducive to microbial growth in the endoscope. Proper storage facilitates drying and decreases potential for contamination. Opening all valves and removing all accessories facilitates drying. The scope protector may create an environment favorable for microbial growth if the flexible endoscope is not dry and cannot hang straight.[28-30]

IX.a.1. Flexible endoscopes should not be stored in the original shipment cases.

The cases are difficult to clean, may be contaminated, and are designed for shipping only.

IX.b. Flexible endoscopes should be reprocessed before use if unused for more than five days.[25-27,31]

In research studies, flexible endoscopes cleaned and processed as recommended and stored by hanging in closed cabinets have been shown to grow organisms after five days of no use. In a prospective observational study, flexible endoscopes in active service during the three-week study period were microbiologically sampled prior to reprocessing before the first case of the day. The contamination rate was 15.5%, with a pathogenic contamination rate of 0.5%. Mean shelf life (ie, time between the last reprocessing one day and reprocessing before the first case on the following day) was 37.62 hours (standard deviation [SD] 36.47). Median shelf life was 18.8 hours (range 5.27 to 165.35 hours). The most frequently identified organism was coagulase-negative *Staphylococcus*, an environmental nonpathogenic organism.[31]

One study evaluated the contamination of high-level disinfection of upper endoscopes, duodenoscopes, and colonoscopes endoscopes stored in a dust-proof cabinet for five days. After completion of the endoscopic procedure, the endoscopes were subjected to an initial decontamination, followed by manual cleaning with the endoscope immersed in detergent. The endoscopes then were placed in an automatic reprocessor that provides high-level disinfection. They then were stored by hanging in a dust-proof cabinet. Bacteriologic samples were obtained from the surface of the endoscopes, the openings for the piston valves, and the accessory channels daily for five days and by flush-through (combined with brushing) from the accessory channels after five days of storage. Samples were cultured for all types of aerobic and anaerobic bacteria, including bacterial spores, and for *Candida* species. For all assays, all endoscopes were bacteria-free immediately after high-level disinfection. Only four assays (of 135) were positive (for skin bacteria cultured from endoscope surfaces) during the subsequent five-day assessment. All flush-through samples were sterile. The study concluded that when endoscope reprocessing guidelines are strictly observed and endoscopes are stored in appropriate cabinets for up to five days, reprocessing before use may not be necessary.[25]

In a multiphase study, four endoscopic retrograde cholangiopancreatography (ERCP) scopes and three colonoscopes were evaluated. In phase 1, endoscopes were assayed after initial high-level disinfection and daily for a period of two weeks. In phase 2, this procedure was repeated to confirm phase 1 results. In phase 3, endoscopes were assayed after high-level disinfection and again following a seven-day storage period. In phase 1, 6 of 70 (8.6%) assays were positive. This involved two colonoscopes and two ERCP scopes out of the seven total scopes (57%) and was limited to the first five days of the study. No cultures were positive in phase 2. In phase 3, one endoscope had a positive culture. Positive cultures grew only *Staphylococcus epidermidis*, a low-virulence skin organism.[27]

One study conducted in the clinical environment to determine shelf life for flexible colonoscopes, which were processed using peracetic acid, suggests that colonoscopes with all channels thoroughly reprocessed and dried may be stored for up to one week before needing to be reprocessed. This study was limited by the small sample size, completion at a single site with a single processing method, and artificial contamination of a single colonoscope without a control measure to measure the level of contamination following inoculation.[26]

IX.c. Flexible endoscopes should be reprocessed before use if evidence of improper drying exists (eg, evidence of discoloration, wet spots, or stains, or soil in the storage cabinet) when the scope is removed from storage.[25-27,31]

Evidence of improper drying may include wet spots or stains on the bottom of the cabinet where the flexible endoscopes have been hanging. Improper drying creates an environment conducive to growth of microorganisms.[31]

IX.d. Storage cabinets should be cleaned and disinfected with an Environmental Protection Agency (EPA)-registered disinfectant when visibly soiled and on a weekly or monthly schedule.[32]

Cleaning and disinfecting storage cabinets periodically will decrease dust and soil buildup.[32]

Recommendation X

Flexible endoscope accessories (eg, water bottle, cap, water tubing, biopsy forceps, cytology brushes, cleaning brushes) should be decontaminated after use and inspected for damage.

Flexible endoscope accessories have been found to be a source of contamination.[30,33]

X.a. Endoscopic accessories (eg, biopsy forceps, cytology brushes) that enter sterile tissue or the vascular system should be cleaned and sterilized between use as described in the AORN "Recommended practices for cleaning and care of surgical instruments and powered equipment" and the AORN "Recommended practices for sterilization in the perioperative practice setting."[1]

These devices enter sterile tissue and, if contaminated, increase the risk of patient infection.[11]

X.a.1. All surfaces of accessories should be brushed using brushes of the appropriate size and style.

Brushing all surfaces of accessories, some of which may be irregular, assists with removing all organic debris.[17]

X.a.2. Insulated electrosurgical instruments should be handled as described in the AORN "Recommended practices for cleaning and care of surgical instruments and powered equipment" and the AORN "Recommended practices for electrosurgery."[1,34]

X.a.3. Reusable cleaning brushes should be thoroughly cleaned using an ultrasonic cleaner, inspected for integrity, and sterilized or high-level disinfected after each use.[17]

Damaged reusable brushes can cause perforations in any flexible endoscope surface. Reusable brushes may be a cause for cross-contamination. Ultrasonic cleaning of reusable endoscopic accessories removes soil and organic material from hard to clean places. Disposable cleaning brushes are available commercially and may be safer, more efficient, and more economic to use.[17]

Recommendation XI

Flexible endoscopes should be decontaminated in an area physically separated from locations where clean items are handled and patient care activities are performed.[35]

Physical separation of decontamination areas from areas where clean items are handled minimizes the risk of cross-contamination. Cross-contamination can result when soiled items are placed in close proximity to clean items or placed on surfaces upon which clean items are later placed. Aerosols created during cleaning can also cause cross-contamination.[7]

XI.a. The decontamination area should be physically separated from clean patient care areas and include a door.[35] This area should contain, but not be limited to,
- sinks to manually clean flexible endoscopes,
- hand-washing facilities,[14]
- eyewash station,[36]
- automated equipment consistent with the types of flexible endoscopes to be decontaminated,
- adapters and accessories to connect the flexible endoscopes with cleaning equipment and utilities,
- leak testing equipment,
- low-pressure air,
- closed storage facilities, and
- proper ventilation.

The design of the decontamination area facilitates the safe and effective decontamination of flexible endoscopes and accessories. Appropriate equipment and utilities facilitate desired infection control practices. Keeping the door closed supports the functioning of the building ventilation system which is designed to vent potentially contaminated room air out of the building, minimizing contamination of adjacent areas.

Sinks are required to manually clean or remove gross bioburden from flexible endoscopes before high-level disinfection via manual or automatic endoscope reprocessor methods.

Hand washing facilities are required to decontaminate hands after removal of PPE.[14]

FLEXIBLE ENDOSCOPES

An eyewash station is required to flush eyes when cleaning and disinfecting chemicals are accidentally splashed into the health care worker's face.[37]

Automated cleaning and decontamination of flexible endoscopes and accessories provides a high level of cleaning that is difficult to consistently replicate using manual methods.

Compressed air is needed to dry lumens after cleaning.[7]

Closed storage facilities help to prevent contamination of stored supplies.[1]

Adequate ventilation is required to protect personnel from the high-level disinfecting fumes.[35]

XI.b. The decontamination area should be supplied at a minimum with
- enzymatic detergent,
- soft-bristle brushes,
- cleaning cloths,
- alcohol, and
- personal protective equipment (PPE).

Enzymatic cleaner is used for manual and automated cleaning of flexible endoscopes. Soft-bristle brushes, designed for flexible endoscope cleaning, can effectively clean scopes and accessories without damaging surfaces. Cleaning cloths are used for external surfaces. Alcohol is used to irrigate after the final rinse to assist with drying. When cleaning flexible endoscopes with water, it can be reasonably anticipated that there is a potential for exposure to chemicals and bloodborne pathogens.[14]

XI.c. Flexible endoscopes and accessories should not be decontaminated in scrub or hand sinks.

Cleaning soiled instruments in a scrub or hand sink can contaminate the sink and faucet, which also may be used for clean activities (eg, hand washing, surgical hand antisepsis).

Recommendation XII

Personnel handling contaminated endoscopic equipment must wear appropriate PPE.[14]

Personal protective equipment (PPE) helps to protect the employee from exposure to bloodborne pathogens and other potentially infectious materials.

XII.a. Personal protective equipment consistent with the anticipated exposure must be worn.[11,37] The appropriate PPE for these types of exposures include, but is not limited to,
- a fluid-resistant gown,
- disposable chemical resistant glove,
- a mask, and
- face protection.

Splashes, splatters, and skin contact can be reasonably anticipated when handling contaminated flexible endoscopes. Glutaraldehyde may be absorbed through neoprene and PVC gloves; use gloves made of butyl rubber, nitrile, and Viton®. Latex surgical exam or polyethylene gloves may be used for short-term, or incidental contact only.[8,38]

XII.a.1. Hands must be washed after removing PPE.[14]

Perforations can occur in gloves, and hands can become contaminated when removing PPE.[14]

XII.a.2. Reusable protective attire must be decontaminated and the integrity of the attire confirmed between uses.[14]

Reusable gloves, gowns, aprons, and face shields become contaminated and their integrity can be compromised during use. Decontamination and confirmation of integrity helps to protect the wearer from exposure.[37]

Recommendation XIII

Personnel should demonstrate competency in the use, care, and processing of flexible endoscopes and related equipment periodically and before new endoscopic equipment and/or accessories are introduced into the practice setting.[11]

Ongoing competency validation and education of personnel facilitates the development of knowledge, skills, and attitudes that affect patient and health care worker safety.

XIII.a. Personnel working with flexible endoscopes and accessories should demonstrate competency commensurate with their responsibilities, including but not limited to,
- cleaning/decontamination methods;
- preparation of flexible endoscopes and related accessories for sterilization/high-level disinfection;
- selection of cleaning agents and methods;
- proper use of cleaning agents, including an understanding of specific applications, appropriate dilution, and special precautions;
- decontamination of specialized flexible endoscopes and related accessories used within the practice setting;
- personal protection required during instrument processing;
- exposure risk associated with chemical cleaning agents; and
- location of material safety data sheets.[11,37]

Workers have the right to know the hazards that exist in the workplace.[37] An understanding of procedures involved in cleaning each type of flexible endoscope is necessary to provide the foundation for compliance with procedures. Failure to follow decontamination practices has been shown to be the leading cause of flexible endoscope contamination.[10] Knowing the location of the material safety data sheets assists in obtaining information in the event of an emergency.

- XIII.a.1. Education programs should be specific to the type and design of flexible endoscopes used and the procedures performed in the facility.[11]
- XIII.a.2. Orientation and ongoing education activities for personnel should include an introduction to and/or review of policies and procedures to be applied in the practice setting.
- XIII.b. Personnel should receive education before new flexible endoscopes, accessories, cleaning agents, cleaning methods, and procedures are introduced.
- XIII.c. Designated administrative personnel should validate the competencies of personnel participating in decontamination of flexible endoscopes and accessories. The validation of competencies should include all types of flexible endoscopes and accessories the individual is authorized to reprocess.

  Validation of competencies provides an indication that personnel are able to appropriately perform inspection, decontamination, cleaning, and sterilization or high-level disinfection procedures.

Recommendation XIV

Cleaning and processing of flexible endoscopes, accessories, and related equipment should be documented to enable the identification of trends and demonstrate compliance with regulatory and accrediting agency requirements.

Documentation provides a source of data to review processes and evaluate corrective actions.

- XIV.a. Records of flexible endoscope cleaning and processing should include, but not be limited to,
  - date,
  - time,
  - flexible endoscope identification,
  - method of cleaning,
  - number or identifier of automatic endoscope reprocessor,
  - name of person performing the cleaning,
  - dilution testing results on high-level disinfectants if used multiple times,
  - routine and unscheduled maintenance or repairs, and
  - disposition of defective equipment.

  Most high-level disinfection and sterilization failures result from inadequate cleaning. Some automatic endoscope reprocessors have digital readouts or printers that facilitate recordkeeping. Records of testing of the dilution of the high-level disinfectant provide a source of evidence for review when investigating clinical issues.[7]

- XIV.b. High-level disinfection and sterilization records should be maintained for a time period specified by the health care organization and in compliance with local, state, and federal regulations.

Recommendation XV

Policies and procedures for cleaning and processing flexible endoscopes, accessories, and related equipment should be developed, reviewed regularly, revised as necessary, and readily available in the practice setting.

Policies and procedures serve as operational guidelines to develop/reinforce knowledge, skills, and attitudes and establish authority, responsibility, and accountability within the organization. Policies and procedures also assist in the development of patient safety guidelines and quality assessment and improvement activities.

- XV.a. Policies and procedures should establish authority, responsibility, and accountability for flexible endoscope care, cleaning, and processing; should be developed by a multidisciplinary team; and should be based on current literature and manufacturer's written instructions.

  Multidisciplinary team participation in policy and procedure development and review provides varied input and improves compliance. Involving surgeons, infection preventionists, and health care workers in review of policies educates them on the requirements of flexible endoscope reprocessing and facilitates safe patient care.

- XV.b. Policies should include, but not be limited to,
  - review of manufacturers' written instructions before purchase,
  - cleaning of flexible endoscopes and accessories before initial use,
  - precautions to be taken when handling contaminated items,
  - precautions to be taken when handling chemical agents,
  - frequency and method of evaluation of mechanical washers,
  - frequency and method of evaluation of manual cleaning,
  - frequency of checking insulated electrosurgery instruments for leakage current,
  - documentation of cleaning,
  - initial education and annual competency,
  - maintenance of material safety data sheets,
  - reporting exposures to bloodborne pathogens, and
  - reporting adverse events.

- XV.c. A procedure should be developed in the event of a potential disinfection or sterilization failure and should include, but not be limited to,
  - assessment to confirm failure;
  - assessment of patient risk;

FLEXIBLE ENDOSCOPES

- removal of all improperly disinfected equipment;
- removal of defective cleaning equipment from use;
- notification of departments and physicians involved;
- root cause analysis;
- corrective action plan;
- identification of potentially involved patients;
- determination if patients require notification;
- identification of regulatory, accrediting, and governing agencies requiring notification;
- notification of all medical device manufacturers potentially related to the disinfection or sterilization failure; and
- development of an action plan for disinfection/sterilization failure prevention.[11]

A procedure provides an outline of the steps to follow after a potential disinfection or sterilization failure has occurred.

Recommendation XVI

The health care organization's quality management program should evaluate the cleaning and processing of flexible endoscopes and accessories.

Evaluation of cleaning and processing of flexible endoscopes and accessories improves patient safety.

XVI.a. A quality management program should be in place to test mechanical and manual cleaning processes when new types of flexible endoscopes and accessories are purchased and at intervals determined by the health care organization.[39]

Testing of mechanical cleaners assures proper functioning to the equipment because malfunctioning automatic endoscope reprocessors have been shown to cause contamination of flexible endoscopes.[10] Periodic testing of cleaning methods provides an opportunity to evaluate the performance of personnel and equipment. Manual cleaning is a learned skill and subject to human error.[23,39] New instruments can pose unique challenges when cleaning.

XVI.a.1. Automatic endoscope reprocessors should be tested for proper functioning before initial use, annually during service, and after major repair.[40]

Testing automatic endoscope reprocessors on a regular basis verifies that the equipment is functioning properly or identifies an opportunity for corrective action. Washer testing products (eg, protein indicators) are commercially available to assist with this evaluation.[39]

XVI.a.2. Adverse events and near misses related to flexible endoscope and accessory cleaning should be reported in the health care organization's adverse event reporting system and reviewed for potential opportunities for improvement.

Reporting mechanisms assist in the discovery of opportunities for improvement and prevention of repeat adverse events.

XVI.b. Water quality should be tested periodically for bacterial contamination and purity (eg, hardness, mineral content, pH).[4]

Contaminated water has been shown to cause contamination of flexible endoscopes after the decontamination process has been completed.[4,10]

XVI.c. Perioperative nurses should collaborate with infection preventionists to monitor and validate flexible endoscope cleaning, disinfection, and storage processes.

XVI.d. A program should be developed to monitor appropriate storage conditions, including but not limited to,
- length of storage time, and
- lack of evidence of the presence of moisture in or on the flexible endoscope after hanging.

Improper storage conditions may cause bacterial growth.

XVI.d.1. The length of storage time after high-level disinfection and before next use should be measured and monitored using a system to determine the date for removal of the flexible endoscope from use for reprocessing (eg, expiration date label on endoscope, log of serial numbers and the date of processing).

Recording the date the flexible endoscope was last processed will reduce the risk of a flexible endoscope being used more than five days after processing.

Glossary

Automated endoscope reprocessor: A unit for mechanical cleaning, disinfecting, and rinsing of flexible endoscopes.

Bioburden: The degree of microbial load; the number of viable organisms contaminating an object.

Biofilms: "A thin coating containing biologically active organisms, that have the ability to grow in water, water solutions, or in vivo, which coat the surface of structures (eg, teeth, inner surfaces of catheters, tubes, implanted or indwelling devices, instruments, other medical devices). Biofilms contain viable and nonviable microorganisms that adhere to surfaces and become trapped within a matrix of organic matter (eg, proteins, glycoproteins, carbohydrates), which prevents antimicrobial agents from reaching the cells." (Source: Favero MS, Bond WW. Chemical disinfection of medical and surgical materials. In: *Disinfection, Sterilization, and Preservation.* 5th ed. Block SS, ed. Philadelphia, PA: Lippincott Williams & Wilkins; 2001:910-911.)

Chemical disinfectant/germicide: A generic term for a government-registered agent that destroys microorganisms. Germicides are classified as sporicides, general disinfectants, sanitizers, and others.

Cleaning: A process using friction, detergent, and water to remove organic debris; the process by which any type of soil, including organic debris, is removed. Cleaning removes rather than kills microorganisms.

Contaminated: The presence of potentially infectious, pathogenic organisms (eg, blood, other potentially infectious material) on or in animate or inanimate objects.

Critical item: An item that has contact with the vascular system or enters sterile tissue, or body cavities and thus poses the highest risk of transmission of infection.

Decontamination: A process that removes contaminating infectious agents and renders reusable medical products safe for handling.

Disinfection: A process that kills most forms of microorganisms on inanimate surfaces. Disinfection destroys pathogenic organisms (excluding bacterial spores) or their toxins or vectors by direct exposure to chemical or physical means.

Electrosurgical accessories: Electrosurgical accessories are defined as the active electrode with tip(s), dispersive electrode, adapters, and connectors to attach these devices to the generator.

Enzymatic cleaner: A cleaner that uses enzymes to remove protein from surgical instruments.

High-level disinfection: A process that kills all microorganisms with the exception of high numbers of bacterial spores and prions. High-level disinfectants have the capability to inactivate the hepatitis B and C viruses, HIV, and *Mycobacterium tuberculosis*, but do not inactivate the virus-like prion that causes Creutzfeld-Jakob disease. Government-registered high-level disinfection agents kill vegetative bacteria, tubercle bacilli, some spores and fungi, and lipid and nonlipid viruses, given appropriate concentration, submersion, and contact time.

Minimum effective concentration: The minimum concentration of a liquid chemical germicide that achieves the claimed microbicidal activity as determined by dose-response testing.

Personal protective equipment (PPE): Specialized equipment or clothing for eyes, face, head, body, and extremities; protective clothing; respiratory devices; and protective shields and barriers designed to protect the worker from injury or exposure to a patient's blood, tissue, or body fluids. Used by health care workers and others whenever necessary to protect themselves from the hazards of processes or environments, chemical hazards, or mechanical irritants encountered in a manner capable of causing injury or impairment in the function of any part of the body through absorption, inhalation, or physical contact.

Potable water: Water that is of sufficient quality to be considered appropriate for drinking.

Semicritical item: An item that comes in contact with mucous membranes or with skin that is not intact.

Sterile: The absence of all living microorganisms.

Sterilization: Processes by which all microbial life, including pathogenic and nonpathogenic microorganisms, and spores, are killed.

Tap water: High-quality potable water that meets federal clean water standards at the point of use.

References

1. Recommended practices for cleaning and care of surgical instruments and powered equipment. In: *Perioperative Standards and Recommended Practices.* Denver, CO: AORN; 2008:421-446.

2. *ANSI/AAMI ST81:2004—Sterilization of Medical Devices: Information to Be Provided by the Manufacturer for the Processing of Resterilizable Medical Devices.* Arlington, VA: Association for the Advancement of Medical Instrumentation; 2004.

3. The Steris Reliance EPS endoscope processing system: A new automated endoscope reprocessing technology. *Health Devices* 2007;36(1):22.

4. *AAMI TIR34:2007—Water for the Reprocessing of Medical Devices.* Arlington, VA: Association for the Advancement of Medical Instrumentation; 2007.

5. Zuhlsdorf B, Emmrich M, Floss H, Martiny H. Cleaning efficacy of nine different cleaners in a washer-disinfector designed for flexible endoscopes. *J Hosp Infect* 2002;52(3):206.

6. Zuhlsdorf B, Winkler A, Dietze B, Floss H, Martiny H. Gastroscope processing in washer-disinfectors at three different temperatures. *J Hosp Infect* 2003;55(4):276.

7. Rutala WA, Weber DJ. Reprocessing endoscopes: United States perspective. In: Proceedings of the 7th International BODE Hygiene Days, May 2003. *J Hosp Infect* 2004 (April); 56 Supplement 2:S27-S39.

8. Recommended practices for high-level disinfection. In: *Perioperative Standards and Recommended Practices.* Denver, CO: AORN; 2008:303-310.

9. Thomas L A. Essentials for endoscopic equipment: Leak testing. *Gastroenterol Nurs* 2005;28(5):430.

10. Seoane-Vazquez E, Rodriguez-Monguio R, Visaria J, Carlson A. Endoscopy-related infections and toxic reactions: An international comparison. *Endoscopy* 2007;39(8):742.

11. Rutala WA, Weber DJ. How to assess risk of disease transmission to patients when there is a failure to follow recommended disinfection and sterilization guidelines. *Infect Control Hosp Epidemiol* 2007;28(2):146.

12. Martiny H, Floss H, Zuhlsdorf B. The importance of cleaning for the overall results of processing endoscopes. In: Proceedings of the 7th International BODE Hygiene Days, May 2003. *J Hosp Infect* 2004 (April); 56 Supplement 2:S16.

13. Standards of infection control in reprocessing of flexible gastrointestinal endoscopes. *Gastroenterol Nurs* 2006;29(2):142.

14. Bloodborne Pathogens. (29 CFR §1910.1030.) Occupational Safety and Health Administration. http://www.osha.gov/pls/oshaweb/owadisp.show_document?p_table=STANDARDS&p_id=10051. Accessed December 15, 2008.

15. Thomas LA. Essentials for endoscopic equipment: Endoscope staging. *Gastroenterol Nurs* 2005;28(3):243.

16. Garces E. Endoscope repair prevention: It takes a team. *Healthc Purchasing News* 2006;30(11):50, 55.

17. Thomas L A. Essentials for endoscopic equipment:

Manual cleaning. *Gastroenterol Nurs* 2005;28(6):512.

18. Recommended practices for sterilization in the perioperative practice setting. In: *Perioperative Standards and Recommended Practices*. Denver, CO: AORN; 2008:575.

19. Pang J, Perry P, Ross A, Forbes GM. Bacteria-free rinse water for endoscope disinfection. *Gastrointest Endosc* 2002;56(3):402.

20. *ANSI/AAMI ST58:2005—Chemical Sterilization and High-Level Disinfection in Health Care Facilities*. Arlington, VA: Association for the Advancement of Medical Instrumentation; 2005.

21. Thomas LA. Essentials for endoscopic equipment: Care of the specialty scope. *Gastroenterol Nurs* 2006;29(1):68.

22. Nelson DB, Jarvis WR, Rutala WA, et al; Society for Healthcare Epidemiology of America. Multi-society guideline for reprocessing flexible gastrointestinal endoscopes. *Infect Control Hosp Epidemiol* 2003;24(7):532.

23. Alfa MJ, Olson N, Degagne P, Jackson M. A survey of reprocessing methods, residual viable bioburden, and soil levels in patient-ready endoscopic retrograde choliangiopancreatography duodenoscopes used in Canadian centers. *Infect Control Hosp Epidemiol* 2002;23(4):198.

24. Fisher C. The blame game: Don't play it. *Surg Technol* 2007;39(3):121.

25. Rejchrt S, Cermak P, Pavlatova L, McKova E, Bures J. Bacteriologic testing of endoscopes after high-level disinfection. *Gastrointest Endosc* 2004;60(1):76.

26. Riley R, Beanland C, Bos H. Establishing the shelf life of flexible colonoscopes. *Gastroenterol Nurs* 2002; 25(3):114.

27. Vergis AS, Thomson D, Pieroni P, Dhalla S. Reprocessing flexible gastrointestinal endoscopes after a period of disuse: Is it necessary? *Endoscopy* 2007; 39(8):737.

28. Thomas L A. Essentials for endoscopic equipment. Recommended care and handling of flexible endoscopes: Endoscope storage. *Gastroenterol Nurs* 2005; 28(1):45.

29. Goldstine S. Endoscopy storage: Preventing distal tip protector contamination. *Gastroenterol Nurs* 28(1), 45-46.

30. Bisset L, Cossart YE, Selby W, West R, Catterson D, O'Hara K, Vickery K. A prospective study of the efficacy of routine decontamination for gastrointestinal endoscopes and the risk factors for failure. *Am J Infect Control* 2006; 34(5):274.

31. Osborne S, Reynolds S, George N, Lindemayer F, Gill A, Chalmers M. Challenging endoscopy reprocessing guidelines: a prospective study investigating the safe shelf life of flexible endoscopes in a tertiary gastroenterology unit. *Endoscopy* 2007; 39(9):825.

32. Recommended practices for environmental cleaning in the perioperative setting. In: *Perioperative Standards and Recommended Practices*. Denver, CO: AORN; 2008:375-382.

33. Reprocessing of endoscopic accessories and valves. *Gastroenterol Nurs* 2006; 29(5):394.

34. Recommended practices for electrosurgery. In: *Perioperative Standards and Recommended Practices*. Denver, CO: AORN; 2008:315-330.

35. AIA Health Facilities Guidelines Institute. *Guidelines for Design and Construction of Health Care Facilities*. Washington, DC: American Institute of Architects; 2006.

36. *OSH Act of 1970*. Public Law 91-596 84; STAT. 1590; 91st Congress, S.2193 (December 29, 1970). http://www.osha.gov/pls/oshaweb/owadisp.show_document?p_id=2743&p_table=OSHACT. Accessed December 15, 2008.

37. *Hazard Communication*. (29 CFR §1910.) Occupational Safety and Health Administration. Washington, DC: US Government Printing Office; 2007. Available at http://www.osha.gov/SLTC/hazardcommunications/standards.html. Accessed December 5, 2008.

38. Hospital eTool: Healthcare wide hazards module—Glutaraldehyde. Occupational Safety and Health Administration. http://www.osha.gov/SLTC/etools/hospital/hazards/glutaraldehyde/glut.html. Accessed December 5, 2008.

39. *ANSI/AAMI ST79:2006—Comprehensive Guide to Steam Sterilization and Sterility Assurance in Health Care Facilities*. Arlington, VA: Association for the Advancement of Medical Instrumentation; 2008.

40. Gillespie EE, Kotsanas D, Stuart RL. Microbiological monitoring of endoscopes: 5-year review. *J Gastroenterol Hepatol* 2008 (July); 23(7 Pt 1):1069-1074.

Acknowledgments

Lead Authors

Byron Burlingame, RN, BSN, MS, CNOR
Perioperative Nursing Specialist
AORN Center for Nursing Practice
Denver, Colorado

Maria Arcilla, RN, BSN, CNOR
Perioperative Coordinator
Texas Children's Hospital
Houston, Texas

Contributing Author

Carla McDermott, RN, CNOR
Educator, Staff Development
South Florida Baptist Hospital
Plant City, Florida

Publication History

Originally published February 1993, *AORN Journal*. Revised November 1997; published January 1998. Reformatted July 2000.

Revised November 2002; published in *Standards, Recommended Practices, and Guidelines*, 2003 edition. Reprinted February 2003, *AORN Journal*.

Revised November 2008; published in *Perioperative Standards and Recommended Practices*, 2009 edition.

Reformatted September 2012 for publication in *Perioperative Standards and Recommended Practices*, 2013 edition.

Minor editing revisions made in November 2014 for publication in *Guidelines for Perioperative Practice*, 2015 edition.

GUIDELINE FOR HIGH-LEVEL DISINFECTION

The Guideline for High-Level Disinfection was developed by the AORN Recommended Practices Committee and was approved by the AORN Board of Directors. It was presented as proposed recommendations for comments by members and others. The guideline is effective January 1, 2009. The recommendations in the guideline are intended to be achievable and represent what is believed to be an optimal level of practice. Policies and procedures will reflect variations in practice settings and/or clinical situations that determine the degree to which the guideline can be implemented. AORN recognizes the various settings in which perioperative nurses practice; therefore, this guideline is adaptable to various practice settings. These practice settings include traditional operating rooms, ambulatory surgery centers, physician's offices, cardiac catheterization laboratories, endoscopy suites, radiology departments, and all other areas where operative and other invasive procedures may be performed.

Purpose

This document provides guidance for achieving safe and effective high-level disinfection (HLD) of reusable instruments and equipment. Care and cleaning of flexible endoscopes is outside the scope of this guideline. Refer to the AORN "Recommended practices for cleaning and processing endoscopes and endoscope accessories."

Recommendation I

Items to be reprocessed should be categorized as critical, semicritical, and noncritical.

The Spaulding classification system, developed by Earle Spaulding in 1968, has withstood the passage of time and continues to be used today by infection preventionists and others to determine the correct processing methods for preparing instruments and other items for patient use. According to the Spaulding system, the level of processing required is based on the nature of the item requiring processing and the manner in which it is to be used (Table 1).[1-5]

I.a. Items that enter sterile tissue or the vascular system are categorized as critical and should be sterile when used. Sterility may be achieved by physical or chemical processes.[1,5-9]

ABsence When critical items are contaminated with microorganisms, including bacterial spores, the risk of infection is substantial.[2,10-12] Examples of critical items include, but are not limited to,
- surgical instruments;
- cutting endoscopic accessories that break the mucosal barrier;
- endoscopes used in sterile body cavities;
- cardiac, vascular, and urinary catheters;
- implants;
- needles; and
- ultrasound probes used in sterile body cavities.

I.b. Items that come in contact with nonintact skin or mucous membranes are considered semicritical and should receive a minimum of high-level disinfection.[1,5-9,13]

Intact mucous membranes generally provide a barrier to common bacterial spores but not to organisms such as tubercle bacilli and viruses.[2,11] Examples of semicritical items include, but are not limited to,
- vaginal and rectal probes, even when sheaths are used;
- respiratory therapy equipment;
- anesthesia equipment;
- bronchoscopes; and
- gastrointestinal endoscopes and accessories.

I.b.1. Semicritical devices contaminated or potentially contaminated with hepatitis B virus (HBV), hepatitis C virus (HCV), HIV, multi-drug resistant bacteria, or *Mycobacterium tuberculosis* (TB) should receive a minimum of high-level disinfection.[2]

Literature has supported and research has demonstrated that high-level disinfectants inactivate these and other pathogens that may contaminate semicritical devices.[3,6,10,14-22] The practice of using HLD is consistent with standard precautions, which presume that all patients potentially are infected.[2]

I.c. Items that contact only intact skin are categorized as noncritical items and should receive intermediate-level disinfection, low-level disinfection, or cleaning.[1,5-9]

Intact skin acts as an effective barrier to most organisms.[2] Examples of noncritical items include, but are not limited to,
- tourniquets and blood pressure cuffs,
- linens,
- Mayo stands, and
- other OR furnishings.

Recommendation II

Items should be thoroughly cleaned and decontaminated before high-level disinfection.[10]

HIGH-LEVEL DISINFECTION

TABLE 1. Spaulding Classification System[1-7]

Device category/classification	Level of disinfection	Effectiveness of method	Examples
Critical Items that come in contact with the bloodstream or sterile body tissues	**Sterilization** *Examples:* saturated steam, ethylene oxide, dry heat, ozone, low-temperature hydrogen peroxide gas plasma, glutaraldehyde-based formulations, peracetic acid, stabilized hydrogen peroxide 6% **Chemical sterilants** *Examples:* glutaraldehyde-based formulations, peracetic acid, stabilized hydrogen peroxide 6%, wet pasteurization, sodium hypochlorite	Sterilization kills all microbial life, including pathogenic and nonpathogenic microorganisms and spores.	• surgical instruments • acupuncture needles • foot care instruments • implants • cardiac and urinary catheters • endoscope accessories that penetrate the mucosal barrier
Semicritical Items that come in contact with mucous membranes or non-intact skin	**High-level disinfection** Use when sterilization is not possible. *Examples:* glutaraldehyde-based formulations, peracetic acid, stabilized hydrogen peroxide 6%, wet pasteurization, sodium hypochlorite	High-level disinfection kills all microorganisms but not necessarily a large number of bacterial spores.	• scopes (eg, bronchoscopes, colonoscopes, and similar scopes) • laryngoscope handles and blades, • reusable peak flow meters • vaginal and rectal probes • cryosurgical instruments • thermometers
Noncritical Items that come in contact with intact skin and those exposed to blood or other potentially infectious material	**Intermediate-level disinfection** Use an EPA-registered hospital disinfectant with label claim for tuberculocidal activity. *Examples:* chlorine-based products, phenolics	Intermediate-level disinfection kills viruses, mycobacteria, fungi, and vegetative bacteria but not bacterial spores.	• skin probes • blood pressure cuffs • pneumatic tourniquet cuffs • hydrotherapy tanks • examination tables
Items that do not come in contact with the patient's skin and have not been exposed to blood or other potentially infectious material	**Low-level disinfection** Use an EPA-registered hospital disinfectant without label claim for tuberculocidal activity. *Examples:* chlorine-based products, phenolics, quaternary ammonium compounds, hydrogen peroxide (approximately 3%), iodophors, 70% to 90% alcohol	Low-level disinfection kills vegetative forms of bacteria, some fungi, and lipid viruses but cannot be relied on to destroy mycobacteria, bacterial endospores, or nonlipid viruses.	• stethoscopes • dishes • scales • furniture • bed pans

References

1. Spaulding EH. Clinical disinfection and antisepsis in the hospital. J Hosp Res. 1972:95.

2. Appendix B: Decontamination and disinfection. In: Biosafety in Microbiological and Biomedical Laboratories (BMBL). 5th ed. Centers for Disease Control and Prevention; National Institutes of Health, eds. Washington, DC: US Government Printing Office; 2007:328-336. Available at http://www.cdc.gov/od/ohs/biosfty/bmbl5/bmbl5toc.htm. Accessed December 5, 2008.

3. Alvarado CJ, Reichelderfer M. APIC guideline for infection prevention and control in flexible endoscopy. Association for Professionals in Infection Control. Am J Infect Control 2000;28(2):138.

4. AAMI TIR12:2004—Designing, Testing and Labeling Reusable Medical Devices for Reprocessing in Health Care Facilities: A Guide for Medical Device Manufacturers. Arlington, VA: Association for the Advancement of Medical Instrumentation; 2005.

5. Rutala WA, Weber DJ. How to assess risk of disease transmission to patients when there is a failure to follow recommended disinfection and sterilization guidelines. Infect Control Hosp Epidemiol. 2007;28(2):146.

6. Multi-society guideline for reprocessing flexible gastrointestinal endoscopes. Am J Infect Control. 2003; 31(5):309.

7. Rutala WA, Weber DJ. Cleaning, disinfection, and sterilization in healthcare facilities. In: APIC Text of Infection Control and Epidemiology. Washington, DC: Association for Professionals in Infection Control and Epidemiology; 2005:21-31.

HIGH-LEVEL DISINFECTION

Cleaning and decontamination are the initial and most critical steps in breaking the chain of disease transmission. Debris, blood, mucous, fat, tissue, and organic matter will interfere with the action of the disinfectant. Microbial biofilms (ie, collections of bacteria and fungi existing in a multicellular matrix) adhere to each other or to medical devices, particularly those with lumens, where they affect tissues adjacent to virtually any medical device. Biofilms are difficult to remove and may serve as sources of bacterial toxin that can affect remote locations in the body. Friction and oxidizing chemicals must be used to remove biofilms. Initiating cleaning immediately after use reduces or eliminates the growth of biofilm-forming microorganisms.[10,23-43]

II.a. Appropriate personal protective equipment (PPE) should be worn during cleaning and decontamination.[6,22,44]

Personal protective equipment protects the worker from hazardous chemicals and exposure to blood and other potentially infectious materials.

II.a.1. Personnel should wear PPE that may include, but is not limited to,
- 100% nitrile rubber or 100% butyl rubber gloves when handling glutaraldehyde (polyvinyl chloride [PVC] gloves are not recommended because they absorb glutaraldehyde)[18];
- less than 100% nitrile or butyl rubber gloves for handling all other HLD solutions except glutaraldehyde;
- protective eyewear (eg, goggles, face shields);
- masks (ie, to prevent contact with skin and not inhalation of fumes); and
- moisture-repellent or splash-proof skin protection (eg, gowns, jumpsuits, aprons).[45]

Chemical disinfectants can irritate or stain skin and mucous membranes.[46,47] Use of protective apparel decreases the potential for exposure to the chemical agent.[48]

II.b. Soiled instruments and devices should be handled using PPE and transported in a contained, covered, and secure manner to the point of decontamination and processing.[22]

These practices prevent environmental contamination and protect employees from blood-borne pathogen exposure.

II.c. Meticulous cleaning and decontamination should precede high-level disinfection.

Adherence to a written cleaning protocol results in consistency of practice and facilitates the disinfection process.[6,12,22,44,49,50] According to the US Food and Drug Administration (FDA), manufacturers are obliged to provide users with adequate instructions for the safe and effective use of an instrument or device, including methods to clean and disinfect or sterilize the item if it is marked as reusable.[51,52]

II.c.1. Particular attention should be given to complex medical devices with multiple pieces (eg, endoscopes, robotic devices) that have crevices, joints, lumens, ports, and channels because they are difficult to clean.[12]

II.d. Instruments to be disinfected should be cleaned according to AORN's "Recommended practices for cleaning and care of surgical instruments and powered equipment"[49] and "Recommended practices for cleaning and processing flexible endoscopes and endoscope accessories."[53]

Adherence to a written cleaning protocol results in consistency of practice and facilitates the disinfection process.[12,22,49]

II.e. High-level disinfection should not be used for items exposed to prions. Refer to the AORN "Recommended practices for sterilization in the perioperative practice setting."[15,49,53-55]

Prions present unique infection prevention and control challenges. Prions are proteinaceous, infectious agents containing no DNA or RNA and may be transmitted iatrogenically by direct inoculation. Prions cause transmissible spongiform encephalopathies (TSE), including Creutzfeldt-Jakob disease (CJD) and variant Creutzfeldt-Jakob disease (vCJD). Prions are resistant to traditional chemical and physical decontamination methods. High-level disinfection does not inactivate prions. Critical and semicritical items or surfaces contaminated with the CJD agent require unique decontamination procedures because of an extremely resistant subpopulation of prions.[36,49] Although some discrepancies exist among studies, all studies show that these prions resist normal inactivation methods.[33,54,56]

II.e.1. Critical and semicritical devices that come into contact with internal tissues of patients with known or suspected TSE should be processed using the highest level and method of decontamination that can be tolerated by the instrument.[54]

Many complex and expensive instruments such as intracardiac monitoring devices, fiber-optic endoscopes, and microscopes cannot be decontaminated by the harsh procedures recommended for the decontamination of critical items exposed to high-infectivity tissue.

II.e.2. Extended steam sterilization cycles are the preferred method of inactivating resistant prions on critical and semicritical devices. Effective exposure inactivation parameters for gravity displacement are 30 minutes at 131° C (268° F) and 18 minutes at 134° C to 138° C (273° F to 280° F) for dynamic-air removal.[2] Critical and noncritical items used in low-infectivity tissue (eg, intestines) do not have to be incinerated.[54]

II.e.3. Disposable endoscopic accessories should be used whenever possible when there is a

HIGH-LEVEL DISINFECTION

patient with known or suspected TSE infectivity.

Prions are highly resistant to chemical and physical processes that normally inactivate microorganisms. The risk of transferring prion protein is greatest in cases that manipulate high-risk tissue (ie, brain, dura matter, cornea). Few reports have revealed transmission of spongiform encephalopathy from endoscopic procedures; however, iatrogenic transmission of the disease has catastrophic consequences that warrants conservative treatment of accessories.[39,57]

II.e.4. Disposable cover sheets should be used whenever possible to avoid environmental contamination of noncritical items.[54]

Transmissible spongiform encephalopathy infectivity persists for long periods on work surfaces, although they have not been implicated in iatrogenic transmission.

II.e.5. Noncritical patient care items and surfaces should be disinfected with double-strength sodium hydroxide solution (2N NaOH) or undiluted sodium hypochlorite for one hour and rinsed with water. Sodium hypochlorite may be corrosive to some surfaces.[57]

Noncritical patient care items and surfaces have not been implicated in disease transmission.[2]

Recommendation III

Pasteurization may be used to achieve thermal high-level disinfection.

Pasteurization is a heat-automated high-level disinfection process that employs time and heat (ie, 160° F to 170° F [71° C to 77° C] for 30 minutes) for HLD of heat-sensitive semicritical patient care items. Pasteurization destroys all microorganisms except high numbers of bacterial spores.[15] The process originally developed by Louis Pasteur consists of heating milk, wine, or other liquids to between 140° F and 212° F (60° C to 100° C) for approximately 30 minutes to kill or significantly reduce the number of pathogenic and spoilage organisms.

III.a. Items to be high-level disinfected using pasteurization should be placed inside the washer/pasteurizer chamber according to the manufacturer's written instructions.

Medical washer/pasteurizers have wash, rinse, and pasteurization cycles. The wash cycle is accomplished either through a horizontal agitation method or a vertical rotational method, depending on the manufacturer's specifications, using warm water and detergent cleaning solution. The length of this cycle is determined by the manufacturer's written instructions. At the conclusion of the wash and rinse cycles, the tank automatically drains in preparation for the pasteurization cycle. Pasteurization is achieved by immersing all devices in a hot water bath heated to 140° F to 212° F (60° C to 100° C) and held for 30 minutes.[58] Medical washer/pasteurizers may offer quality assurance data recorders that document the temperature of the pasteurizing bath and cycle time.

Recommendation IV

An FDA-cleared agent should be used to achieve chemical high-level disinfection of medical devices.

The FDA has primary responsibility for premarket review of safety and efficacy requirements for liquid chemical germicides intended for use on critical and semicritical devices.[59] A list of products that have been cleared for marketing by the FDA can be found on the web site of the FDA Center for Devices and Radiological Health (CDRH).[17]

IV.a. Products selected for chemical disinfection should be efficacious and compatible with the materials or items to be disinfected. Many disinfectants are used in the practice setting (eg, glutaraldehyde, stabilized hydrogen peroxide, peracetic acid, ortho-phthalaldehyde [OPA]). These agents are not interchangeable.[48]

Devices may be damaged by these chemicals. The use of incompatible chemicals can damage the surfaces of the instrument, causing corrosion, scratches, and other surface irregularities. This damage can create a challenge for cleaning and high-level disinfection, interfere with the proper function, and reduce the life and cosmetic appearance of the device.

IV.a.1. Factors that influence the efficacy of a chemical agent include, but may not be limited to,
- organic load present on the items to be disinfected;
- type and level of microbial contamination;
- precleaning, rinsing, and drying of the items;
- active ingredients of the chemical agent;
- concentration of the chemical agent;
- exposure time to the chemical agent;
- physical configuration of the item;
- temperature and pH of the chemical agent;
- inorganic matter present;
- water hardness; and
- presence of surfactants.

IV.a.2. An ideal high-level disinfectant should
- possess a broad spectrum of antimicrobial effectiveness,
- demonstrate rapid activity,
- possess material compatibility,
- be nontoxic,
- be odorless,
- have no disposal restrictions,
- possess prolonged reuse and shelf life,

HIGH-LEVEL DISINFECTION

- be easy to use,
- demonstrate resistance to organic material,
- be able to be monitored for concentration, and
- be cost effective.[17]

Emerging pathogens such as *Cryptosporidium parvum,* human papilloma virus, rotavirus, Norwalk virus, *Helicobacter pylori, Escherichia coli 0157:H7,* multidrug-resistant bacteria, nontuberculous mycobacteria *(M chelonae),* and prions are a growing concern for members of the public and infection preventionists. The susceptibility of each of these pathogens has been studied, and with the exception of *C parvum* and prions, all are susceptible to available chemical disinfectants and chemical sterilants.[21,46] Glutaraldehyde-resistant strains of *M chelonae* have been isolated in some automated endoscope reprocessors but have been found to be sensitive to other high-level disinfectants such as ortho-phthalaldehyde.[38,47]

IV.a.3. FDA-approved high-level disinfectant liquid chemical agents should be used according to workload requirements, instrumentation characteristics, and workplace design (Table 2). *Note:* A full and comprehensive list of high-level disinfectant solutions and contact conditions is available from the FDA.

IV.a.4. High-level disinfection should occur at appropriate temperature, contact time, and length of use following solution activation. Table 2 provides FDA-approved chemicals for HLD with recommended conditions for use.[2,16,17,27,46,51,56,60,61]

Improper use of cleaners and disinfectants can cause contamination and lead to outbreaks.[62]

IV.b. Chemical high-level disinfection should be achieved by immersing an item for specified contact conditions (ie, period of time, temperature, concentration) in a chemical agent (also called a chemical germicide) that has been cleared by the FDA as a high-level disinfectant.

Disease transmission can result from improper selection and/or use of disinfecting agents.

IV.c. Manufacturers' written instructions should be followed when preparing disinfectant solutions, calculating expiration dates, and labeling solution soaking containers.

The appropriate conditions for use are provided on solution container labels. Labels indicate clearly the appropriate time for discarding solutions that may no longer be effective. Most chemical disinfectants are effective for only a specific period of time.[36]

IV.c.1. Manufacturers' written instructions about the type of container used should be followed.

The correct container ensures that no interaction occurs between the container and the active ingredients of the disinfectant.[36]

IV.c.2. A test strip or other FDA-cleared testing device specific for the disinfectant and minimum effective concentration of the active ingredient should be used for monitoring solution potency prior to each use.[36,51]

The test strip expiration date should be checked before use.

IV.c.3. If a solution falls below its minimum effective concentration, it should be discarded, even if the designated expiration date has not been reached.

High-level disinfection solution potency cannot be guaranteed when the solution falls below the minimum effective concentration.

IV.d. Items to be chemically disinfected should be cleaned and completely immersed in the disinfectant solution according to device and HLD solution manufacturers' written instructions and consistent with established infection control practice.

Total immersion permits contact of all surfaces. Perfusion of the disinfectant into all channels eliminates air pockets and ensures contact with internal channels.

IV.e. Lumens and ports should be flushed and filled with the disinfectant and the entire item completely immersed for the designated exposure time.

Disinfection of all surfaces can be achieved only if all surfaces of the items are clean and in constant contact with the disinfecting solution. Flushing lumens and ports eliminates air pockets and facilitates contact of the disinfectant with internal channels.[2,12,21]

IV.f. The automated endoscopic reprocessor (AER) manufacturer's written instructions should be congruent with the endoscope manufacturer's written instructions when an AER is used for high-level disinfection, or the endoscope should not be processed in the AER.

Device-specific instructions ensure adequate function of the reprocessing equipment and prevent damage to the scope.[6]

IV.g. After being exposed to the disinfectant solution for the required exposure time, critical and semicritical items should be thoroughly rinsed with water according to the manufacturer's written instructions.

Rinsing removes toxic and irritating residues that can result in tissue damage or staining.[7,63] Rinsing critical and semicritical items with sterile water prevents potential recontamination that could result from tap water.[2,6,9,15,25]

605

HIGH-LEVEL DISINFECTION

TABLE 2. USE OF FDA-APPROVED CHEMICAL AGENTS FOR HIGH-LEVEL DISINFECTION (HLD)[1-5]

NOTE: This is not intended to be a comprehensive list of all HLD products. Manufacturers' directions for use should be followed.

HLD chemical	Advantages	Disadvantages	Concentration	Contact time/Conditions
Peracetic acid (PA) and hydrogen peroxide solutions	No activation required. Odor or irritation not significant.	Concerns regarding compatibility with materials (eg, lead, brass, copper, zinc) and both cosmetic and functional damage. Limited clinical use. Potential for eye and skin damage.	0.08% PA and 1.0% hydrogen peroxide 0.23% PA and 7.35% hydrogen peroxide	25 min contact time at 20° C (68° F); 14 days maximum reuse 15 min contact time at 20° C (68° F); 14 days maximum reuse
Glutaraldehyde solutions	Numerous published studies of use. Relatively inexpensive. Excellent compatibility with materials.	Respiratory irritation from glutaraldehyde vapor. Pungent and irritating odor. Relatively slow mycobactericidal activity. Coagulates blood and fixes tissue to surfaces. Allergic contact dermatitis.	2.5% glutaraldehyde automated endoscopic reprocessor (AER) 1.12% glutaraldehyde and 1.93% phenol	5.0 min at 35° C (95° F); 28 days maximum reuse 20 min contact time at 25° C (77° F); 14 days maximum reuse
Hydrogen peroxide	No activation required. May enhance removal of organic material and organisms. No disposal issues. No odor or irritation issues. Does not coagulate blood or fix tissues to surfaces. Inactivates *Cryptosporidium*. Published studies of use.	Concerns regarding compatibility with materials (eg, brass, zinc, copper, nickel/silver plating) and both cosmetic and functional damage. Serious eye damage with contact.	7.5% hydrogen peroxide	30 min contact time at 20° C (68° F); 21 days maximum reuse
Ortho-phthalaldehyde	Fast-acting high-level disinfectant. No activation required. Odor not significant. Claim of excellent compatibility with materials. Claim of not coagulating blood or fixing tissues to surfaces.	Stains protein gray (eg, skin, mucous membranes, clothing, environmental surfaces). More expensive than glutaraldehyde. Eye irritation with contact. Slow sporicidal activity. Repeated exposure may result in hypersensitivity in some patients with bladder cancer.	5.75% ortho-phthalaldehyde 0.55% ortho-phthalaldehyde manual processing AER	5 min at 50° C (122° F); single use 12 min at 20° C (68° F); 14 days maximum reuse 5 min at 25° C (77° F); 14 days maximum reuse
Peracetic acid *Indication for sterilization only*	Environmentally friendly by-products (ie, acetic acid, oxygen, and water). Fully automated. Single-use system eliminates need for concentration testing. Standardized cycle. May enhance removal of organic material and endotoxins. No adverse health effects to operators under normal operating conditions.	Potential incompatibility with materials (eg, aluminum anodized coating becomes dull). Used for immersible instruments only. Biological indicator may not be suitable for routine monitoring. Only one endoscope or a small number of instruments can be processed in a cycle. More expensive (eg, endoscope repairs, operating costs, purchase costs) than high-level disinfection. Serious eye and skin damage after contact with concentrated solution. Point-of-use system; cannot save sterilized items for later use or storage.	0.2% peracetic acid	rapid sterilization cycle time (30 to 45 min) low-temperature (50° C to 55° C [122° F to 131° F]) liquid-immersion sterilization; single use

REFERENCES

1. Appendix B: Decontamination and disinfection. In: Biosafety in Microbiological and Biomedical Laboratories (BMBL). 5th ed. Centers for Disease Control and Prevention; National Institutes of Health, eds. Washington, DC: US Government Printing Office; 2007:328-336. Available at http://www.cdc.gov/od/ohs/biosfty/bmbl5/bmbl5toc.htm. Accessed December 5, 2008.

2. Alvarado C J, Reichelderfer M. APIC guideline for infection prevention and control in flexible endoscopy. Association for Professionals in Infection Control. Am J Infect Control 2000;28(2):138.

3. Favero MS, Bond WW. Chemical disinfection of medical and surgical materials. In: Block SS, ed. Disinfection, Sterilization, and Preservation. 5th ed. Philadelphia, PA: Lippincott Williams & Wilkins; 2001:881.

4. FDA-cleared sterilants and high-level disinfectants with general claims for processing reusable medical and dental devices; September 28, 2006. US Food and Drug Administration. http://www.fda.gov/cdrh/ode/germlab.html. Accessed December 5, 2008.

5. Association for the Advancement of Medical Instrumentation. ANSI/AAMI ST58:2005—Chemical Sterilization and High-Level Disinfection in Health Care Facilities. Arlington, VA: Association for the Advancement of Medical Instrumentation; 2005.

Recommendation V

HLD items should be protected from contamination until the item is delivered to the point of use.

Use of aseptic technique will protect the items from being contaminated before patient use.[2,6,36,59]

V.a. High-level disinfected items should be transported to the point of use using a technique that does not result in recontamination of the instrument (eg, aseptic technique).

Performance of hand hygiene, donning gloves to handle HLD items, and transferring immediately to point of use following processing are examples of practices that minimize recontamination.

V.b. High-level disinfected items should be processed immediately before use. Flexible endoscopes should be cleaned, high-level disinfected, and stored according to the "Recommended practices for cleaning and processing flexible endoscopes and endoscope accessories.[36,53]

HLD devices that cannot be placed in appropriate barrier materials are prone to recontamination when stored.

Recommendation VI

Health care organizations should provide a safe environment for personnel who are using chemical disinfectants.

Health care organizations are responsible for providing a safe work and patient care environment. Patients, visitors, and health care workers should be protected from injuries and illnesses caused by hazardous chemicals used in the facility.

VI.a. When handling chemical disinfectants, personnel should wear protective apparel that may include, but is not limited to,
- 100% nitrile rubber or 100% butyl rubber gloves when handling glutaraldehyde (polyvinyl chloride [PVC] gloves are not recommended because they absorb glutaraldehyde)[18];
- less than 100% nitrile or butyl rubber gloves for handling all other HLD solutions except glutaraldehyde;
- protective eyewear (eg, goggles, face shields);
- masks (ie, to prevent contact with skin and not inhalation of fumes); and
- moisture-repellent or splash-proof skin protection (eg, gowns, jumpsuits, aprons).[45]

Chemical disinfectants can irritate or stain skin and mucous membranes, cause allergic reactions, and may pose other health risks.[46,47] Use of protective apparel decreases the potential for exposure to the chemical agent.[36]

VI.b. Chemical disinfectants should be contained and used in well-ventilated areas.

Vapor generated from glutaraldehyde can be irritating to the respiratory tract and may aggravate preexisting respiratory conditions. Glutaraldehyde should be used in well-ventilated areas or in freestanding or vented chemical fume hoods. The American Conference of Governmental Industrial Hygienists (ACGIH) recommends a ceiling limit of 0.05 parts per million (ppm) for occupational exposure to glutaraldehyde vapors. The Occupational Safety and Health Administration (OSHA) has established occupational exposure limits for several agents. No exposure limits have been established by OSHA for glutaraldehyde; however, OSHA can regulate exposure to glutaraldehyde and has recommended that the ACGIH limits be followed.[22]

VI.b.1. Chemical disinfectants should be kept in covered containers with tight-fitting lids and clearly labeled with contents and expiration date.

VI.b.2. Methods (eg, transfer pumps) should be used to limit worker exposure during loading of chemical disinfectants into automated endoscopic reprocessors.

VI.b.3. Chemical disinfectants should be used according to manufacturers' written instructions and federal, state, and local regulations.

Recommendation VII

Chemical disinfectants should be disposed of according to federal, state, and local regulations.[64,65]

The most stringent regulations should be followed. State and local regulations may be more stringent than those imposed at the federal level.[36,66]

VII.a. Personnel should know their obligations under state laws and local ordinances and use appropriate PPE when disposing of high-level disinfectants.

Recommendation VIII

Personnel should receive initial education and competency validation on procedures, chemicals used, and personal protection and should receive additional training when new equipment, instruments, supplies, or procedures are introduced.

Ongoing education and competency validation of perioperative personnel facilitates the development of knowledge, skills, and attitudes that affect patient and worker safety.[8,67]

VIII.a. Personnel should receive initial education on
- decontamination methods;
- preparation of instruments and equipment for high-level disinfection;
- selection of cleaning agents and methods;
- proper use of cleaning agents, including an understanding of specific applications, appropriate dilution, and special precautions;
- decontamination of specific instruments and equipment used within the practice setting;

HIGH-LEVEL DISINFECTION

- procedures for decontamination of instruments contaminated with prions and the effectiveness of various methods of deactivation;
- personal protection required during instrument processing; and
- exposure risk associated with chemical cleaning agents.[22]

Workers have the right to know the about the safe use of disinfectants and about the hazards in the workplace. The OSHA requires that employers provide hazardous material safety information to employees.[22]

VIII.b. Personnel should receive education on new instruments and equipment, new cleaning agents and methods, and new procedures.[9,67-69]

VIII.c. Personnel responsible for HLD should maintain the technical skills needed to establish and maintain a safe practice environment for patients and other staff members.

Adverse effects resulting from the exposure to HLD is well documented in patients and health care workers.[70-74] Adverse effects include, but are not limited to,
- OPA-related anaphylaxis in patients with carcinoma of the urinary bladder,[32,56]
- OPA-related bronchial asthma in health care workers,[75]
- glutaraldehyde-related asthma and contact dermatitis,[76]
- glutaraldehyde-induced bowel injury after laparoscopy,[77] and
- toxic anterior segment syndrome with glutaraldehyde.[78]

VIII.d. Administrative personnel should ensure competency validation of personnel participating in decontamination and high-level disinfection of invasive instruments.[67,79]

Competency validation is an essential component to providing safe and effective patient care.

VIII.e. The validation of competencies should include all types of instruments that the individual is authorized to reprocess.

Validation of competency supports demonstration of mastery level knowledge and skill required to correctly perform decontamination procedures.

VIII.f. Employers must provide employees with the information and training needed to protect themselves from chemical hazards in the workplace according to federal standards.[22]

Employers must provide a written hazard communication program, hazard evaluation, hazardous materials inventory, materials safety data sheets (MSDS), labels on all containers of hazardous chemicals, and employee training.

VIII.f.1. Employee training includes an explanation of the standard, identification of hazards and health effects, location of the written hazard communication program and MSDS, procedures to detect and measure contaminants, safe work practices, appropriate PPE, an explanation of labeling, and locations of spill kits and eyewash stations in accordance with employees' right to know about hazards in the workplace.[6,22]

VIII.f.2. The latest version of the MSDS must be maintained on site and be readily accessible to personnel when they are in their work areas. Material may be available in hard copy and/or electronic format.[22]

The MSDS provides users with valuable information about toxicity, reactivity, required protective equipment and apparel, storage, and disposal of the material.[36]

Recommendation IX

Documentation should be completed to enable the identification of trends and demonstrate compliance with regulatory and accrediting agency requirements.

Documentation policies and procedures establish authority, responsibility, and accountability and serve as operational guidelines.[80]

IX.a. HLD processing records should be kept and include, but not be limited to,
- the patient identifier, when applicable;
- the procedure and physician;
- load contents (item description, serial number if applicable);
- name of the individual performing cleaning, disinfection, rinsing, and transport;
- method of cleaning;
- number or identifier of the mechanical decontaminator;
- date and time disinfection was performed;
- type of disinfectant used and lot number;
- test results before each load, indicating the solution used was at the proper concentration (ie, MEC) and within the expiration date;
- temperature of the disinfectant;
- submersion time;
- verification of rinsing of the disinfected item;
- use of device-specific biological and chemical indicators (BI, CI) for automated peracetic acid processors;
- testing results of insulated electrical instruments; and
- disposition of defective equipment.[2,36,81]

Some washer decontaminators have digital readouts or printers that facilitate recordkeeping. Records of washer testing provide a source of evidence for review when investigating clinical issues, including surgical site infections.

IX.b. Records should be maintained for a time period specified by the health care organization and in compliance with local, state, and federal regulations.[22]

HIGH-LEVEL DISINFECTION

Employers are required to maintain hazardous communication training to ensure that employees are aware and knowledgeable of hazardous chemical exposure and exposure consequences.[22]

Recommendation X

Policies and procedures for high-level disinfection should be developed using the validated instructions provided by the medical device manufacturers, reviewed at regular intervals, revised as necessary, and readily available in the practice setting.

Policies and procedures establish authority, responsibility, and accountability and serve as operational guidelines. Policies and procedures also assist in the development of patient safety, quality assessment, and improvement activities. Policies and procedures are subject to change with the advent of new technologies.

X.a. Policies regarding high-level disinfection should be developed by a multidisciplinary team to include perioperative nurses, sterile processing personnel, surgeons, and infection preventionists.

Using a multidisciplinary team provides varied input and improved ownership of policies and procedures. Involving surgeons in review of policies educates them on the expectations for high-level disinfection and facilitates planning for instrument use. The expertise of infection preventionists facilitates establishment of minimum standards of infection control.

X.b. Policies should include, but not be limited to
- review of validated manufacturers' written instructions before purchase or consignment,
- cleaning of instruments before initial use,
- precautions to be taken when handling contaminated items,
- precautions to be taken when handling chemical agents,
- frequency of AER checks,
- frequency and method of evaluation of manual cleaning,
- criteria for identification and precautions taken for instruments used on patients with known or suspected prion disease,
- documentation of high-level disinfection,
- initial education and annual competency,
- maintenance of material safety data sheets,
- reporting exposures to bloodborne pathogens, and
- reporting adverse events.

X.c. Introduction to and review of policies and procedures should be included in the orientation and ongoing education of personnel to help develop knowledge, skills, and attitudes that affect patient care and occupational safety.

Policies and procedures may guide performance improvement activities.

X.d. Written policies and procedures should be in place to designate how critical and semicritical items are transported from the area where disinfection takes place to the point of use in patient areas.[44,48,82]

Recommendation XI

A quality-control program should be established for the health care organization in all areas where high-level disinfection is used.

The health care organization's quality management program should evaluate high-level disinfection to improve patient and worker safety.[52,67,79,83-85]

XI.a. Quality-control programs should be documented and should include, but not be limited to,
- orientation programs;
- competency assurance;
- continuing education;
- quality-control checks;
- investigation of adverse events, including outbreaks and exposures; and
- monitoring of solution replacement intervals.

Quality and performance improvement functions ensure that organizations design processes well and systematically monitor, analyze, and improve their outcomes.

XI.a.1. The HLD solution should be tested prior to each use.[9,86]

XI.a.2. The solution should be discarded even if it is within its use life if the test strip indicates the solution is below the minimum effective concentration.[36]

The test strip is the only indicator that the solution is effective.

XI.a.3. In the event of test strip failure, items processed with HLD solution below the minimum effective concentration should be considered inadequately processed and should not be used until reprocessed in an acceptable minimum effective concentration of high-level disinfection solution.[36]

XI.b. A comprehensive quality management program should include ongoing monitoring including scheduled testing of mechanical cleaning and AER equipment with supportive documentation.

Adequate cleaning and processing of endoscopes are essential to removing or destroying microorganisms and eliminating endotoxins.

XI.b.1. Mechanical instrument washers and AERs should be tested for proper functioning according to AORN "Recommended practices for cleaning and processing flexible endoscopes and endoscope accessories."[53]

Testing washer decontaminators and AERs on a regular basis verifies that the

609

HIGH-LEVEL DISINFECTION

equipment is functioning properly or identifies an opportunity for corrective action. Washer-testing products are commercially available.

XI.b.2. Manual cleaning processes and skills should be evaluated when new types of instruments are reprocessed and at periodic intervals determined by the health care organization.

Periodic testing provides an opportunity to evaluate the health care worker's understanding of principles and validate performance. Manual cleaning is a learned skill and subject to human error. New instruments can pose unique challenges when cleaning.

XI.b.3. Personnel should identify and respond to opportunities for improvement.

XI.c. Reporting mechanisms for adverse events and near misses related to HLD should be in place.

Systematic performance measures (ie, indicators) and/or priority areas are identified as opportunities for improvement based on the functions and processes of the perioperative episode.[87]

XI.c.1. Adverse events should be reported in the adverse event reporting system and reviewed for potential opportunities for improvement.[36]

Continuous quality improvement opportunities arise from documented and structured quality processes and measures that can define and resolve problems.

XI.c.2. Near misses should be investigated and corrective action taken to prevent serious adverse events.

XI.d. When investigating surgical infections, documentation of the decontamination and HLD processes should be reviewed.[6,8,9,32,39]

Pathogen transmission from endoscopy has been associated with failure to follow cleaning and disinfection protocols.[6,9,15]

Glossary

Automated endoscope reprocessor: A unit for mechanical cleaning, disinfecting, and rinsing of flexible endoscopes.

Bioburden: The degree of microbial load; the number of viable organisms contaminating an object.

Biofilms: "A thin coating containing biologically active organisms, that have the ability to grow in water, water solutions, or in vivo, which coat the surface of structures (eg, teeth, inner surfaces of catheters, tubes, implanted or indwelling devices, instruments, other medical devices). Biofilms contain viable and nonviable microorganisms that adhere to surfaces and become trapped within a matrix of organic matter (eg, proteins, glycoproteins, carbohydrates), which prevents antimicrobial agents from reaching the cells." (Source: Favero MS, Bond WW. Chemical disinfection of medical and surgical materials. In: *Disinfection, Sterilization, and Preservation.* 5th ed. Block SS, ed. Philadelphia, PA: Lippincott Williams & Wilkins; 2001:910-911.)

Cavitation: "A process by which high-frequency sound wave energy is produced in an ultrasonic cleaner causing microscopic bubbles to form, become unstable, and implode, thus creating minute vacuum areas that draw particles of debris off of instrument surfaces and from crevices in instruments." (Source: Topical antimicrobial drug products for over-the-counter human use; tentative final monograph for health-care antiseptic drug products. In: *Code of Federal Regulations (CFR) 21: Food and Drugs, Parts 333 and 369.* Washington, DC: US Government Printing Office; 1994:31402-31453.)

Chemical disinfectant/germicide: A generic term for a government-registered agent that destroys microorganisms. Germicides are classified as sporicides, general disinfectants, sanitizers, and others.

Critical item: An item that has contact with the vascular system or enters sterile tissue, or body cavities and thus poses the highest risk of transmission of infection.

Decontamination: A process that removes contaminating infectious agents and renders reusable medical products safe for handling.

Disinfection: A process that kills most forms of microorganisms on inanimate surfaces. Disinfection destroys pathogenic organisms (excluding bacterial spores) or their toxins or vectors by direct exposure to chemical or physical means.

Free-rinsing: Ability to be removed without leaving residue.

High-level disinfection: A process that kills all microorganisms with the exception of high numbers of bacterial spores and prions. High-level disinfectants have the capability to inactivate the hepatitis B and C viruses, HIV, and *Mycobacterium tuberculosis,* but do not inactivate the virus-like prion that causes Creutzfeldt-Jakob disease. Government-registered high-level disinfection agents kill vegetative bacteria, tubercle bacilli, some spores and fungi, and lipid and nonlipid viruses, given appropriate concentration, submersion, and contact time.

Hospital disinfectant: A chemical germicide with label claims for effectiveness against *Salmonella, Staphylococcus,* and *Pseudomonas.* Hospital disinfectants may be low-, intermediate-, or high-level disinfectants.

Iatrogenic: A response to a medical or surgical treatment, usually denoting an unfavorable response.

In vitro: Outside the living body and in an artificial environment.

Intermediate-level disinfection: A process that kills *Mycobacterium tuberculosis,* vegetative bacteria, most viruses, and most fungi, but does not necessarily kill bacterial spores.

Low-level disinfection: A process by which most bacteria, some viruses, and some fungi are killed. This process cannot be relied on to kill resistant microorganisms such as *Mycobacterium tuberculosis* or bacterial spores.

Minimum effective concentration: The minimum concentration of a liquid chemical germicide that achieves the claimed microbicidal activity as determined by dose-response testing.

Nidus; (pl) *nidi:* A focus of infection; or the coalescence of small particles that is the beginning of a solid deposit.

Pasteurization: "A process originally developed by Louis Pasteur of heating milk, wine, or other liquids to between 140° F and 212° F (60° C to 100° C) for approximately 30 minutes to kill or significantly reduce the number of pathogenic and spoilage organisms" (Source: Block SS. Definition of terms. In: *Disinfection, Sterilization, and Preservation.* 5th ed. Block SS, ed. Philadelphia, PA: Lippincott Williams & Wilkins; 2001:19-28.) A process that employs time and heat (ie, 160° F to 170° F [71.1° C to 76.7° C] for 30 minutes) for high-level disinfection. The intensity of heat and duration of exposure must be determined by the manufacturer of the pasteurization unit and the manufacturer of the product or device to be cleaned.

Personal protective equipment (PPE): Specialized equipment or clothing for eyes, face, head, body, and extremities; protective clothing; respiratory devices; and protective shields and barriers designed to protect the worker from injury or exposure to a patient's blood, tissue, or body fluids. Used by health care workers and others whenever necessary to protect themselves from the hazards of processes or environments, chemical hazards, or mechanical irritants encountered in a manner capable of causing injury or impairment in the function of any part of the body through absorption, inhalation, or physical contact.

Sterilization: Processes by which all microbial life, including pathogenic and nonpathogenic microorganisms, and spores, is killed.

References

1. Spaulding EH. Clinical disinfection and antisepsis in the hospital. *J Hosp Res* 1972;95.
2. Rutala WA. APIC guideline for selection and use of disinfectants. 1994, 1995, and 1996 APIC Guidelines Committee. Association for Professionals in Infection Control and Epidemiology, Inc. *Am J Infect Control* 1996; 24(4):313.
3. Tablan OC, Anderson LJ, Besser R, Bridges C, Hajjeh R, et al. Guidelines for preventing health care-associated pneumonia, 2003: Recommendations of CDC and the Healthcare Infection Control Practices Advisory Committee. *MMWR Recomm Rep* 2004;53(RR-3):1.
4. Class II special controls guidance document: Medical washers and medical washer-disinfectors; guidance for the medical device industry and FDA review staff. US Food and Drug Administration. http://www.fda.gov/cdrh/ode/guidance/1252.html. Accessed December 5, 2008.
5. Appendix B: Decontamination and disinfection. In: *Biosafety in Microbiological and Biomedical Laboratories (BMBL).* 5th ed. Centers for Disease Control and Prevention; National Institutes of Health, eds. Washington, DC: US Government Printing Office; 2007:328-336. Available at http://www.cdc.gov/od/ohs/biosfty/bmbl5/bmbl5toc.htm. Accessed December 5, 2008.
6. Alvarado CJ, Reichelderfer M. APIC guideline for infection prevention and control in flexible endoscopy. Association for Professionals in Infection Control. *Am J Infect Control* 2000;28(2):138.
7. *AAMI TIR12:2004—Designing, Testing and Labeling Reusable Medical Devices for Reprocessing in Health Care Facilities: A Guide for Medical Device Manufacturers.* Arlington, VA: Association for the Advancement of Medical Instrumentation; 2005.
8. Rutala WA, Weber DJ. How to assess risk of disease transmission to patients when there is a failure to follow recommended disinfection and sterilization guidelines. *Infect Control Hosp Epidemiol* 2007;28(2):146.
9. Multi-society guideline for reprocessing flexible gastrointestinal endoscopes. *Am J Infect Control* 2003;31(5):309.
10. Rutala WA, Gergen MF, Weber DJ. Disinfection of a probe used in ultrasound-guided prostate biopsy. *Infect Control Hosp Epidemiol* 2007;28(8):916.
11. Perkins JJ. *Principles and methods of sterilization in health sciences.* 2nd ed. Springfield, Ill.: Thomas; 1969.
12. Favero MS, Bond WW. Chemical disinfection of medical and surgical materials. In: Block SS, ed. *Disinfection, Sterilization, and Preservation.* 5th ed. Philadelphia, PA: Lippincott Williams & Wilkins; 2001:881.
13. Thomas LA. Essentials for endoscopic equipment. High-level disinfection. *Gastroenterol Nurs* 2006;29(2):179.
14. Camp S, Dawson C. Best practice forum: Standard high-level disinfection protocol development. *ORL Head Neck Nurs* 2003; 21(2):18-21.
15. Rutala WA, Weber DJ. Disinfection and sterilization in health care facilities: what clinicians need to know. *Clin Infect Dis.* 2004;39(5):702-709.
16. Bolding B. Choosing a reprocessing method. *Can Oper Room Nurs J.* 2004;22(2):24.
17. FDA-cleared sterilants and high-level disinfectants with general claims for processing reusable medical and dental devices; September 28, 2006. US Food and Drug Administration. http://www.fda.gov/cdrh/ode/germlab.html. Accessed December 5, 2008.
18. Society of Gastroenterology Nurses and Associates Inc. Guidelines for the use of high-level disinfectants and sterilants for reprocessing of flexible gastrointestinal endoscopes. *Gastroenterol Nurs* 2004;27(4):198.
19. Lee JH, Rhee PL, Kim JH, Kim JJ, Paik SW, Rhee JC, Song JH, Yeom JS, Lee NY. Efficacy of electrolyzed acid water in reprocessing patient-used flexible upper endoscopes: Comparison with 2% alkaline glutaraldehyde. *J Gastroenterol Hepatol* 2004;19(8):897-903.
20. Bhattacharyya N, Kepnes LJ. The effectiveness of immersion disinfection for flexible fiberoptic laryngoscopes. *Otolaryngol Head Neck Surg* 2004;130(6):681.
21. Rutala WA, Weber DJ. Disinfection of endoscopes: Review of new chemical sterilants used for high-level disinfection. *Infect Control Hosp Epidemiol* 1999; 20(1):69.
22. *Hazard Communication.* (29 CFR §1910.) Occupational Safety and Health Administration. Washington, DC: US Government Printing Office; 2007. Available at http://www.osha.gov/SLTC/hazardcommunications/ standards.html. Accessed December 5, 2008.
23. Rutala WA, Weber DJ. Cleaning, disinfection, and sterilization in healthcare facilities. In: *APIC Text of*

Infection Control and Epidemiology. Washington, DC: Association for Professionals in Infection Control and Epidemiology; 2005:21-31.

24. Cantrell S. High-level disinfection vs sterilization: Six of one, half dozen of the other? *Healthc Purchasing News* 2005;29(4):38, 40, 42.

25. Rutala WA, Weber DJ. Reprocessing endoscopes: United States perspective. In: Proceedings of the 7th International BODE Hygiene Days, May 2003. *J Hosp Infect* 2004 (April); 56 Supplement 2:S27-S39.

26. Alfa MJ. Can biofilm prevent high-level disinfection? *J Genca* 2006;16(1):23.

27. Raffo P, Salliez AC, Collignon C, Clementi M. Antimicrobial activity of a formulation for the low temperature disinfection of critical and semicritical medical equipment and surfaces. *New Microbiol* 2007;30(4):463.

28. Marion K, Freney J, James G, Bergeron E, Renaud FN, Costerton JW. Using an efficient biofilm detaching agent: An essential step for the improvement of endoscope reprocessing protocols. *J Hosp Infect* 2006;64(2):136.

29. Murdoch H, Taylor D, Dickinson J, Walker JT, Perrett D, Raven ND, Sutton JM. Surface decontamination of surgical instruments: An ongoing dilemma. *J Hosp Infect* 2006;63(4):432.

30. Rerknimitr R, Eakthunyasakul S, Nunthapisud P, Kongkam P. Results of gastroscope bacterial decontamination by enzymatic detergent compared to chlorhexidine. *World J Gastroenterol* 2006;12(26):4199.

31. Thomas LA. Manual cleaning. *Gastroenterol Nurs* 2005;28(6):512.

32. Dettenkofer M, Block C. Hospital disinfection: Efficacy and safety issues. *Curr Opin Infect Dis* 2005; 18(4):320.

33. Kampf G, Bloss R, Martiny H. Surface fixation of dried blood by glutaraldehyde and peracetic acid. *J Hosp Infect* 2004;57(2):139.

34. Vickery K, Pajkos A, Cossart Y. Removal of biofilm from endoscopes: Evaluation of detergent efficiency. *Am J Infect Control* 2004;32(3):170.

35. Cowen AE. The clinical risks of infection associated with endoscopy. *Can J Gastroenterol* 2001;15(5):321.

36. Association for the Advancement of Medical Instrumentation. *ANSI/AAMI ST58:2005—Chemical Sterilization and High-Level Disinfection in Health Care Facilities.* Arlington, VA: Association for the Advancement of Medical Instrumentation; 2005.

37. Morck DW, Olson ME, Ceri H. Microbial biofilms: Prevention, control, and removal. In: Block SS, ed. *Disinfection, Sterilization, and Preservation.* 5th ed. Philadelphia, PA: Lippincott Williams & Wilkins; 2001:675.

38. McDonnell G, Pretzer D. New and developing antimicrobials. In: Block SS, ed. *Disinfection, Sterilization, and Preservation.* 5th ed. Philadelphia, PA: Lippincott Williams & Wilkins; 2001:431.

39. Cowen A, Jones D, Wardle E. *Guidelines: Infection Control in Endoscopy.* 2nd ed. Sydney, Australia: Gastroenterological Society of Australia; 2003.

40. Spach DH, Silverstein FE, Stamm WE. Transmission of infection by gastrointestinal endoscopy and bronchoscopy. *Ann Intern Med* 1993;118(2):117.

41. Weber DJ, Rutala WA, DiMarino AJ. The prevention of infection following gastrointestinal endoscopy: The importance of prophylaxis and reprocessing. In: DiMarino AJ, Benjamin SB, eds. *Gastrointestinal Disease: An Endoscopic Approach.* Thorofare, NJ: Slack; 2002:87.

42. Miner N, Harris V, Ebron T, Cao T. Sporicidal activity of disinfectants as one possible cause for bacteria in patient-ready endoscopes. *Gastroenterol Nurs* 2007; 30(4):285.

43. Cheetham NWH. Comparative efficacy of medical instrument cleaning products in digesting some blood proteins [corrected]. *Aust Infect Control* 2005;10(3):103; erratum *Aust Infect Control* 2005;10(4):142.

44. Nelson DB, Jarvis WR, Rutala WA, et al; Society for Healthcare Epidemiology of America. Multi-society guideline for reprocessing flexible gastrointestinal endoscopes. *Infect Control Hosp Epidemiol* 2003;24(7):532.

45. Hospital eTool: Healthcare-wide hazards module—Glutaraldehyde. Occupational Safety and Health Administration. http://www.osha.gov/SLTC/etools/hospital/hazards/glutaraldehyde/glut.html. Accessed December 5, 2008.

46. Fraud S, Maillard J Y, Russell AD. Comparison of the mycobactericidal activity of ortho-phthalaldehyde, glutaraldehyde, and other dialdehydes by a quantitative suspension test. *J Hosp Infect* 2001;48(3):214.

47. Rutala W A, Weber D J. New disinfection and sterilization methods. *Emerg Infect Dis* 2001;7(2):348.

48. *ANSI/AAMI ST58:2005—Chemical Sterilization and High-Level Disinfection in Health Care Facilities.* Arlington, VA: Association for the Advancement of Medical Instrumentation; 2005.

49. Recommended practices for cleaning and care of surgical instruments and powered equipment. In: *Perioperative Standards and Recommended Practices.* Denver, CO: AORN; 2008:421-446.

50. Banerjee S, Nelson DB, Dominitz JA, et al. Reprocessing failure. *Gastrointest Endosc* 2007; 66(5):869.

51. Lin CS, Fuller J, Mayhall ES. Federal regulation of liquid chemical germicides by the US Food and Drug Administration. In: Block SS, ed. *Disinfection, Sterilization, and Preservation.* 5th ed. Philadelphia, PA: Lippincott Williams & Wilkins; 2001:1293.

52. Procedures for performance standards development. (21 CFR §861.) US Food and Drug Administration. Washington, DC: US Government Printing Office; 2008. Available at http://www.accessdata.fda.gov/scripts/cdrh/cfdocs/cfcfr/CFRSearch.cfm?CFRPart=861. Accessed December 5, 2008.

53. Recommended practices for cleaning and processing flexible endoscopes and endoscope accessories. In: *Perioperative Standards and Recommended Practices.* Denver, CO: AORN; 2009:595-610.

54. WHO infection control guidelines for transmissible spongiform encephalopathies. Report of a WHO consultation, Geneva, Switzerland, 23-26 March 1999. World Health Organization. http://www.who.int/csr/resources/publications/bse/WHO_CDS_CSR_APH_2000_3/en. Accessed December 5, 2008.

55. Rutala WA, Weber DJ. Creutzfeldt-Jakob disease: Recommendations for disinfection and sterilization. *Clin Infect Dis* 2001;32(9):1348.

56. Gray J. How safe is your endoscope disinfectant? *Br J Perioper Nurs* 2005;15(3):134.

57. NINDS Creutzfeldt-Jakob disease information page. National Institute of Neurological Disorders and Stroke. http://www.ninds.nih.gov/disorders/cjd/cjd.htm. Accessed December 5, 2008.

58. Definition of terms. In: Block SS, ed. *Disinfection, Sterilization, and Preservation.* 5th ed. Philadelphia, PA: Lippincott Williams & Wilkins; 2001:19.

59. Nelson DB, Jarvis WR, Rutala WA, et al. Multi-society guideline for reprocessing flexible gastrointestinal endoscopes. *Dis Colon Rectum* 2004;47(4):413.

60. Acosta-Gío AE, Rueda-Patiño JL, Sánchez-Pérez L. Sporicidal activity in liquid chemical products to sterilize or high-level disinfect medical and dental instruments. *Am J Infect Control* 2005;33(5):307-309.

61. Omidbakhsh N. A new peroxide-based flexible endoscope-compatible high-level disinfectant. *Am J Infect Control* 2006;34(9):571.

62. Weber DJ, Rutala WA, Sickbert-Bennett EE. Outbreaks associated with contaminated antiseptics and disinfectants. *Antimicrob Agents Chemother* 2007; 51(12):4217.

63. *AAMI TIR34:2007—Water for the Reprocessing of Medical Devices.* Arlington, VA: Association for the Advancement of Medical Instrumentation; 2007.

64. Guidelines for protecting the safety and health of health care workers, chapter 6: Hazardous waste disposal. National Institute for Occupational Safety and Health. http://www.cdc.gov/niosh/hcwold6.html. Accessed December 5, 2008.

65. *Code of Federal Regulations.* Title 40: Protection of Environment. http://ecfr.gpoaccess.gov/cgi/t/text/text-idx?c=ecfr;sid=4990e762d7b81851bef18f82dc851826;rgn=div5;view=text;node=40:25.0.1.1.2;idno=40;cc=ecfr#40:25.0.1.1.2.3.1.4. Accessed December 5, 2008.

66. Public health notification from FDA, CDC, EPA and OSHA: Avoiding hazards with using cleaners and disinfectants on electronic medical equipment. US Food and Drug Administration. http://www.fda.gov/cdrh/safety/103107-cleaners.html. Accessed December 5, 2008.

67. AORN explications for perioperative nursing. In: *Perioperative Standards and Recommended Practices.* Denver, CO: AORN; 2008:633-660.

68. Newsome C. Education in product safety: glutaraldehyde in high-level disinfection applications. *Occup Health Rev* 2005;118:18-20.

69. Rideout K, Teschke K, DimichWard H, Kennedy S M. Considering risks to healthcare workers from glutaraldehyde alternatives in high-level disinfection. *J Hosp Infect* 2005;59(1):4-11.

70. Suzukawa M, Yamaguchi M, Komiya A, Kimura M, Nito T, Yamamoto K. Ortho-phthalaldehyde-induced anaphylaxis after laryngoscopy. *J Allergy Clin Immunol* 2006; 117(6):1500.

71. Cohen NL, Patton CM. Worker safety and glutaraldehyde in the gastrointestinal lab environment. *Gastroenterol Nurs* 2006;29(2):100.

72. Ghasemkhani M, Jahanpeyma F, Azam K. Formaldehyde exposure in some educational hospitals of Tehran. *Ind Health* 2005;43(4):703.

73. Cogliano V, Grosse Y, Baan R, Straif K, Secretan B, El Ghissassi F; WHO International Agency for Research on Cancer. Advice on formaldehyde and glycol ethers. *Lancet Oncol* 2004; 5(9):528.

74. Sokol WN. Nine episodes of anaphylaxis following cystoscopy caused by Cidex OPA (ortho-phthalaldehyde) high-level disinfectant in 4 patients after cytoscopy. *J Allergy Clin Immunol* 2004; 114(2):392.

75. Fujita H, Ogawa M, Endo Y. A case of occupational bronchial asthma and contact dermatitis caused by ortho-phthalaldehyde exposure in a medical worker. *J Occup Health* 2006; 48(6):413.

76. Best practices for the safe use of glutaraldehyde in health care. OSHA document number 3258-08N-2006. Occupational Safety and Health Administration. http://www.osha.gov/Publications/3258-08N-2006-English.html. Accessed December 5, 2008.

77. Karpelowsky JS, Maske CP, Sinclair-Smith C, Rode H. Glutaraldehyde-induced bowel injury after laparoscopy. *J Pediatr Surg* 2006; 41(6):e23.

78. Unal M, Yücel I, Akar Y, Oner A, Altin M. Outbreak of toxic anterior segment syndrome associated with glutaraldehyde after cataract surgery. *J Cataract Refract Surg* 2006 Oct;32(10):1696-1701.

79. Standards of perioperative administrative practice. In: *Perioperative Standards and Recommended Practices.* Denver, CO: AORN; 2008:15.

80. Recommended practices for documentation of perioperative nursing care. In: *Perioperative Standards and Recommended Practices.* Denver, CO: AORN; 2008:311-314.

81. American Society for Healthcare Central Service Professionals. *Training Manual for Health Care Central Service Technicians.* 5th ed. San Francisco, CA: Jossey-Bass; 2006.

82. Thomas LA. Essentials for endoscopic equipment. Recommended care and handling of flexible endoscopes: Endoscope storage. *Gastroenterol Nurs* 2005; 28(1):45.

83. Perioperative patient care quality. In: *Perioperative Standards and Recommended Practices.* Denver, CO: AORN; 2008:11-12.

84. Standards of perioperative professional practice. In: *Perioperative Standards and Recommended Practices.* Denver, CO: AORN; 2008:23-26.

85. Sciortino CV Jr, Xia EL, Mozee A. Assessment of a novel approach to evaluate the outcome of endoscope reprocessing. *Infect Control Hosp Epidemiol* 2004; 25(4):284.

86. Standards of infection control in reprocessing of flexible gastrointestinal endoscopes. Society of Gastroenterology Nurses and Associates. http://www.sgna.org/Resources/standards.cfm. Accessed December 5, 2008.

87. Quality and performance improvement standards for perioperative nursing. In: *Perioperative Standards and Recommended Practices.* Denver, CO: AORN; 2008:27-36.

Acknowledgments

Lead Authors

Sheila Mitchell, RN, BSN, MS, CNOR
Perioperative Nursing Specialist
AORN Center for Nursing Practice
Denver, Colorado

Judith Goldberg, RN, MSN, CNOR
Clinical Director
Backus Hospital
Norwich, Connecticut

Contributing Author
Ardene Nichols, RN, MSN, CNS, CNOR, PAHM
Health Care Consultant
Conroe, Texas

Publication History

Originally published August 1980, *AORN Journal*, as AORN "Recommended practices for sterilization and disinfection."

Format revision July 1982; revised February 1987.

Revised October 1992 as "Recommended practices for disinfection"; published as proposed recommended practices September 1994 as "Recommended practices for chemical disinfection."

Revised November 1998 as "Recommended practices for high-level disinfection"; published March 1999, *AORN Journal*.

HIGH-LEVEL DISINFECTION

Revised November 2004; published in *Standards, Recommended Practices, and Guidelines*, 2005 edition. Reprinted February 2005, *AORN Journal*.

Revised November 2008; published in *Perioperative Standards and Recommended Practices*, 2009 edition.

Minor editing revisions made in November 2009 for publication in *Perioperative Standards and Recommended Practices*, 2010 edition

Reformatted September 2012 for publication in *Perioperative Standards and Recommended Practices*, 2013 edition.

Minor editing revisions made in November 2014 for publication in *Guidelines for Perioperative Practice*, 2015 edition.

GUIDELINE FOR CLEANING AND CARE OF SURGICAL INSTRUMENTS

The Guideline for Cleaning and Care of Surgical Instruments has been approved by the AORN Guidelines Advisory Board. It was presented as a proposed guideline for comments by members and others. The guideline is effective November 15, 2014. The recommendations in the guidelines are intended to be achievable and represent what is believed to be an optimal level of practice. Policies and procedures will reflect variations in practice settings and/or clinical situations that determine the degree to which the guideline can be implemented. AORN recognizes the many diverse settings in which perioperative nurses practice; therefore, this guideline is adaptable to all areas where operative and other invasive procedures may be performed.

Purpose

This document provides guidance for cleaning surgical instruments, including point-of-use cleaning, selecting cleaning chemicals, and determining water quality. Guidance is also provided for decontaminating, transporting, inspecting, and care of surgical instruments. Processing of laryngoscope blades and handles and ophthalmic instruments, special precautions necessary to minimize the risk for transmitting prion diseases from contaminated instruments, and the use of personal protective equipment (PPE) that must be worn during cleaning and care of instruments are also addressed. The recommendations are general recommendations, as it is not possible to make a separate recommendation for every instrument used.

Sterilization, packaging for terminal sterilization, high-level disinfection, and processing of flexible endoscopes are outside the scope of this document. Guidance for these topics is provided in the AORN Guideline for Sterilization,[1] Guideline for High-Level Disinfection,[2] Guideline for Selection and Use of Packaging Systems for Sterilization,[3] and Guideline for Cleaning and Processing Flexible Endoscopes and Endoscope Accessories.[4]

Evidence Review

On August 2, 2013, a medical librarian conducted a systematic search of the databases MEDLINE®, CINAHL®, and the Cochrane Database of Systematic Reviews for meta-analyses, systematic reviews, randomized controlled and non-randomized trials and studies, case reports, letters, reviews, and guidelines. The search was limited to literature published in English from January 2008 through June 2013.

Search terms included *surgical instruments, equipment reuse, surgical procedures, instrument reprocessing, cross infection, infection control, surgical wound infection, surgical site infection, equipment contamination, washing system, washer-disinfector, medical device washer, presoak, soak, disinfection, decontamination, sterilization, detergents, sterile water, water purification, water microbiology enzymatic detergents, non-enzymatic detergents, ultrasonic, impingement, maintenance, storage, transport, case cart, inspection, magnification, staining, corrosion, adenosine triphosphate, photobacterium, luciferases, luminescent measurements, microbial sensitivity tests, ninhydrin, antineoplastic agents, toxic anterior segment syndrome, toxic endothelial cell deconstruction, prion diseases, Creutzfeldt-Jakob syndrome, fatal familial insomnia,* and *Gerstmann-Straussler-Scheinker.* Surgical instruments as a broad search term was augmented by the inclusion of terms related to specific instruments, such as *laryngoscopes, blades, forceps, scalpels, dilators, lumens, drills,* and *retractors.*

At the time of the initial search, the librarian established weekly alerts on the search topics and until June 2014, presented relevant results to the lead author. During the development of this guideline, the author requested supplementary literature searches and additional literature that either did not fit the original search criteria or was discovered during the evidence-appraisal process; this additional literature included book chapters and manufacturers' materials. The librarian and author also identified relevant guidelines from government agencies and standards-setting bodies.

Articles were excluded if they addressed the use of a device or the care of patients rather than the practices associated with instrument processing. Articles related to processing single-use devices were excluded as outside the scope of this document. Articles that were clearly biased or written as product promotion for marketing purposes also were excluded.

Articles identified in the search were provided to the lead author and assigned evidence reviewer for review and critical appraisal using the AORN Research or Non-Research Evidence Appraisal Tools as appropriate. The literature was independently evaluated and appraised by the lead author and evidence reviewer according to the strength and quality of the evidence. Each article was then assigned an appraisal score determined by consensus. The appraisal score is noted in brackets after each reference as applicable.

The evidence supporting each activity and intervention statement within a specific recommendation was summarized, and the AORN Evidence-Rating Model was used to rate the strength of the collective evidence. Factors considered in the review of the collective body of evidence were the quality of similar evidence on a given topic, the consistency of the evidence supporting a recommendation, and the

INSTRUMENT CLEANING

potential benefits and harms. The assigned evidence rating is noted in brackets after each intervention and activity statement.

Editor's note: *MEDLINE is a registered trademark of the US National Library of Medicine's Medical Literature Analysis and Retrieval System, Bethesda, MD. CINAHL, Cumulative Index to Nursing and Allied Health Literature, is a registered trademark of EBSCO Industries, Birmingham, AL.*

Recommendation I

All instruments and devices used in surgery should be cleared by the US Food and Drug Administration (FDA) for use in surgery and have written, manufacturer-validated cleaning and decontamination instructions for use (IFU).

Manufacturers of reusable instruments and devices cleared by the FDA provide validated cleaning and decontamination instructions and instructions on how to process devices between uses. Items cannot be assumed to be clean, decontaminated, or sterile unless the manufacturer's IFU are derived from validation testing and the user has followed those instructions. Instructions for use provide users with validated techniques for processing instruments.[5,6]

I.a. A multidisciplinary team consisting of sterile processing personnel, perioperative registered nurses (RNs), physicians, infection preventionists, and other stakeholders should develop a mechanism for evaluating and selecting the products that require cleaning and decontamination and the associated cleaning products that will be used at the health care facility.[7] *[2: Moderate Evidence]*

Involvement of a multidisciplinary team in the product selection process allows input from personnel with expertise beyond that of the clinical end users. Facility areas in which personnel are responsible for cleaning, decontamination, and care of instruments may include operating rooms (ORs), sterile processing areas, procedure areas, physician offices, and clinics where processing is performed. Personnel working in these areas have information concerning equipment and resource capabilities that will help determine the facility's ability to follow the manufacturer's written IFU.

A standardized product evaluation and selection process that includes input from key personnel may assist in the selection of functional and reliable products that are safe, cost-effective, and environmentally friendly; promote quality care; and prevent duplication or rapid obsolescence.[7]

I.b. Before the purchase of surgical instruments and other devices used for surgical or other procedures performed in the facility, a designated person responsible for processing surgical instruments should obtain and evaluate the applicable manufacturer's written IFU, including
- instructions for precleaning at the point of use,
- transport of the soiled device,
- cleaning,
- decontamination,
- inspection,
- functionality testing,
- packaging,
- high-level disinfection, and
- sterilization,

to determine whether the facility has the capability to comply with the manufacturer's instructions. *[2: Moderate Evidence]*

Cleaning, decontamination, and handling instructions recommended by device manufacturers vary widely. Some instruments may require special cleaning, packaging, sterilization, or maintenance procedures that cannot be provided by the facility.[6,8-12]

I.b.1. A designated person responsible for processing surgical instruments should review the instrument manufacturer's written IFU to determine the requirements for replicating the validated cleaning and processing methods. *[4: Benefits Balanced with Harms]*

I.b.2. The manufacturer's written IFU should be reviewed for requirements related to
- utilities (eg, water, compressed air);
- cleaning equipment;
- device disassembly required for cleaning;
- accessories (eg, adaptors for creating a correct connection between the device and equipment, utilities, and cleaning equipment);
- accessories for cleaning lumens, ports, and internal parts;
- cleaning agents;
- lubricants; and
- procedures for handling, cleaning, disinfecting, testing, packaging, and sterilizing.[5,6,13,14]

[3: Limited Evidence]

I.b.3. Prepurchase evaluation of the health care facility's capability to comply with the instrument manufacturer's instructions for care and cleaning should include determining requirements for cleaning and decontaminating equipment (eg, washer/decontaminators, ultrasonic cleaners, forced-air dryers, sinks, detergents, brushes, adaptors, lubricants) and whether
- the instructions are clear and understandable to personnel who will be handling the instrument or device,
- a water supply of the specified quality is available, and
- utilities (eg, electrical, ventilation, steam supply) are in place.

[3: Limited Evidence]

The instrument manufacturers' IFU provide instructions for cleaning and processing that are required to achieve the validated results.[6]

Recommendation II

Before use, all new, repaired, refurbished, and loaned instruments and devices should be cleaned and decontaminated, inspected, and sterilized or high-level disinfected according to the instrument or device manufacturer's written IFU.

It is not possible to verify how all new, repaired, refurbished, and loaned instruments and devices have been handled, cleaned, inspected, or processed before receipt in the facility. Failure to clean, inspect, disinfect, or sterilize an item may lead to transmission of pathogenic microorganisms from a contaminated device and create a risk for patient injury, including surgical site infection (SSI).[15-25]

Inspecting instruments and devices upon receipt and before processing in accordance with the manufacturer's written IFU can help verify that there are no obvious defects and may prevent damaged or incorrectly functioning devices from being used in patient care.[26]

Cleaning and decontamination remove soil that may interfere with subsequent processing and reduce or eliminate viable microorganisms, thereby rendering devices safe to handle.[2,10]

II.a. The manufacturer's written IFU should be readily available to the personnel responsible for processing instruments and devices used for surgical or other procedures performed in the facility.[27] *[1: Strong Evidence]*

Instructions for use identify the processes necessary to achieve effective decontamination and sterility.[10]

II.a.1. Manufacturer's IFU should be reviewed periodically, and processing practices should comply with the most current IFU. *[2: Moderate Evidence]*

Manufacturers may make modifications to their IFU when new technology becomes available, when regulatory requirements change, or when modifications are made to a device.[28]

II.b. Accessories specified by the device manufacturer for cleaning and processing should be obtained at the time of the device purchase and used in accordance with the IFU. *[3: Limited Evidence]*

Using accessories that are designed and manufactured to the device manufacturer's specifications facilitates performance of the required cleaning and processing procedures.[6]

II.c. Instruments and related accessories should be removed from external shipping containers and web-edged or corrugated cardboard boxes before transfer into the decontamination area. *[2: Moderate Evidence]*

External shipping containers and web-edged cardboard boxes may collect dust, debris, and insects during transport and may carry contaminants into the facility.[1,10]

II.d. Instruments should be inspected for defects and correct function upon receipt.[29,30] Instrument inspection should include verifying
- tip integrity and alignment,
- security of screws,
- ability of ratchets to hold,
- sharpness of cutting edges,
- integrity of box locks,
- freedom of moveable parts, and
- insulation integrity (for instruments used for electrosurgery).

[2: Moderate Evidence]

Inspection of instruments before processing may minimize the risk of damaged, nonfunctioning, or incorrectly functioning instruments being used in patient care.

II.e. A multidisciplinary team appointed by the health care facility should establish policies and procedures for managing loaned items (eg, instruments). The policies and procedures should include
- a process for requesting and communicating the need for loaned instrument sets;
- time requirements for preprocedure delivery, product testing, and processing (ie, cleaning, decontaminating, inspecting, packaging, sterilizing) and for postprocedure processing and pick-up;
- requirements for education and competency verification of personnel before new or loaned instrumentation is used;
- a process for obtaining and reviewing manufacturers' written IFU;
- delivery requirements (eg, location, documentation);
- a process for returning the item(s) to the lender;
- time requirements for vendor retrieval;
- inventory requirements and a process for taking inventory;
- processes for care, cleaning, decontaminating, inspecting, packaging, and sterilizing before use;
- responsibility for ensuring each instrument set weighs no more than 25 lb (11.3 kg);
- method of transport;
- processes for point-of-use and postprocedure cleaning and decontamination; and
- documentation of processes and transactions related to loaned instruments.[31,32]

[3: Limited Evidence]

A successful loaned instrument management program begins with clear and detailed policies and procedures developed in collaboration with all stakeholders.[29]

II.e.1. Loaned instruments should be cleaned, decontaminated, inspected, and sterilized

INSTRUMENT CLEANING

by the receiving health care organization before use. *[3: Limited Evidence]*

Conditions of transport vary, and an event could occur during transport that could compromise sterility or cause damage to the instruments before they are received at the facility. Inspection verifies that the instruments have no visible defects or damage. Parameters of inhouse sterilization can be verified immediately after a cycle is complete. Even if the instruments have been sterilized in another health care facility, the user will have no record of the sterilization process in the event of a recall.[29,30]

II.e.2. Before processing and preferably before receipt of loaned instruments, a designated person responsible for processing surgical instruments should obtain and review the manufacturers' written IFU for cleaning. *[3: Limited Evidence]*

When instructions are received in advance, preparations can be made for cleaning and sterilization before the arrival of the instruments. Advance preparation can prevent potential delays in patient care and help ensure correct cleaning and sterilization procedures are followed. Review of processing instructions before receipt of the instruments may improve the efficiency of processing.[33]

II.e.3. The accessories needed to process loaned instruments according to the manufacturer's written IFU should be received before processing.[5] *[3: Limited Evidence]*

Accessories specified in the manufacturer's written IFU are those the manufacturer has determined are needed to perform required cleaning procedures.[6]

II.e.4. Loaned instruments should be requested when the surgery is scheduled and delivered to the health care facility in sufficient time to allow inhouse inventorying, inspection, disassembly, cleaning, packaging, and terminal sterilization in accordance with the manufacturer's written IFU.[29,32] *[3: Limited Evidence]*

When there is insufficient time to process instruments according to the manufacturers' written IFU, patient safety may be at risk.[29,32,34] Management of loaned instruments requires planning. Requesting the instruments well in advance of the surgical procedure allows adequate time for the vendor to deliver the instruments and for facility personnel to perform the required cleaning; decontamination; inspection; sterilization; and if needed, product quality assurance testing procedures.

II.e.5. Loaned instruments and accessories should be removed from external shipping containers and web-edged or corrugated cardboard boxes before transfer into the decontamination area. *[2: Moderate Evidence]*

External shipping containers and web-edged cardboard boxes may collect dust, debris, and insects during transport and may carry contaminants into the facility.[1,10]

II.e.6. The recipient should inventory and document the type and quantity of loaned instruments and confirm receipt with the lender upon delivery.[29] *[3: Limited Evidence]*

Inventory lists of instruments help provide verification that the instrument set is complete upon receipt. Taking inventory is critical to verifying that all required instruments have been received and are available for use during the procedure. When an inventory is not performed, it is not possible to determine whether the instruments that were intended to be delivered were actually received and that all instruments are returned to the lender. If an instrument critical to the procedure is not available when needed, the surgeon may not be able to perform the procedure as planned and patient care may be compromised or delayed.[16,35]

II.e.7. Loaned instruments should be inspected for defects and correct function upon receipt.[29,30] Instrument inspection should include verifying
- tip integrity and alignment,
- security of screws,
- ability of ratchets to hold,
- sharpness of cutting edges,
- integrity of box locks,
- freedom of moveable parts, and
- insulation integrity (for instruments used for electrosurgery).

[3: Limited Evidence]

Inspection of instruments before processing may minimize the risk of damaged, nonfunctioning, or incorrectly functioning instruments being used in patient care.

II.e.8. Loaned instruments, regardless of whether they were processed in another health care facility, should be considered contaminated and should be delivered directly to a sterile processing area and decontaminated as soon as possible after delivery.[10,29] *[3: Limited Evidence]*

It is not possible to know under what conditions instruments were processed at another facility or for the receiving facility to monitor or control events that may contaminate items during transport. The receiving facility is responsible for providing the surgical patient with sterile products and is therefore responsible for monitoring the cleaning and sterilization process.[19,29,30]

The evidence review for this guideline found only one published article related to the condition of loaned instruments. This limited, single-facility, quality assurance project evaluated the cleanliness of loaned instruments upon receipt. A total of 139 sets were visually inspected and tested for blood residue during a two-month period. Six sets (4.3%) were visibly contaminated. Twenty-three sets (16.5%) tested positive for blood residue. The authors recommended that that all loaned instruments be enclosed in biohazard containers, that some method of documentation of the decontamination and quality assurance processes used by the lending institution be included with each shipment, that designated receiving areas be established, that institutions establish standard procedures for loaned instrumentation, and that the procedure be communicated not only to sterile processing personnel and the hospital infection prevention committee, but also to perioperative personnel.[33]

II.e.9. Loaned instruments should be disassembled, cleaned, decontaminated, and inspected before they are returned to the vendor or lending facility.[1,30] *[2:Moderate Evidence]*

Instruments used in surgery may be contaminated with blood, body fluids, or other potentially infectious materials and may pose a safety risk to health care and other personnel if they are not handled or decontaminated correctly.[10]

II.e.10. Loaned instruments should be inventoried and documentation should be provided to the lender and receiver regarding the processing and disposition of items after decontamination.[29,30] *[3: Limited Evidence]*

Documentation makes it possible to determine where an instrument may have been lost or damaged and provides a description of the steps taken to help ensure the return of items that are safe to handle.

Recommendation III

Instruments should be cleaned and decontaminated as soon as possible after use.

Cleaning instruments as soon as possible after use can help prevent formation of biofilm and dried blood. When blood or other bioburden is allowed to dry on instruments, it can become more difficult to remove. The effectiveness of disinfection or sterilization can be compromised when thorough cleaning is not accomplished.[6,10,19,28]

III.a. Preparation for decontamination of instruments should begin at the point of use.[10,12,28] *[2: Moderate Evidence]*

Moistening and removing gross soil at the point of use can help prevent organic material and debris from drying on instruments. Organic material and debris are more difficult to remove from surgical instruments when they are allowed to dry. Removal of organic material and debris at the point of use can improve the efficacy and effectiveness of cleaning and decontamination.[2,6,10]

III.b. Instruments should be kept free of gross soil during the procedure. *[2: Moderate Evidence]*

Gross soil left to dry on instruments can affect the efficacy of subsequent disinfection and sterilization processes.[2,10,22,36-38]

III.b.1. During the procedure, the scrub person should remove gross soil from instruments by wiping the surfaces with a sterile surgical sponge moistened with sterile water. Saline should not be used to wipe instrument surfaces. *[3: Limited Evidence]*

Blood, organic material, debris, and saline are highly corrosive to instrument surfaces and can cause corrosion, rusting, and pitting when allowed to dry on surgical instruments. These materials can be difficult to remove from all surfaces during the cleaning and decontamination process, reducing the efficacy of the subsequent sterilization process.[6,10,12,36]

III.b.2. Periodically during the procedure, the scrub person should use sterile water to irrigate instruments with lumens. *[1: Strong Evidence]*

Irrigating instrument lumens periodically throughout a procedure removes gross soil and may reduce the risk of biofilm formation. Biofilm can form on many surfaces but is particularly problematic when it forms in lumens because it is difficult to see and remove. After a biofilm forms, mechanical action is required to remove it.[38]

In an experimental longitudinal study, Vickery et al[38] grew a mature biofilm of *Pseudomonas aeruginosa* on 20 Teflon® endoscope tubings and subjected them to 20 decontamination and recontamination cycles. Decontamination consisted of a manual wash followed by a 2% glutaraldehyde disinfection in an automated endoscope reprocessor. This process was repeated 20 times. At the 20th cycle, 90% of the tubing was biofilm free. The researchers concluded that washing endoscopes under high flow rates with some detergents removed established biofilms. Although the researchers examined endoscopes, the results of this study may be applicable to decontamination of other lumened instruments.

If not removed, a biofilm can reduce the efficacy of subsequent disinfection or sterilization processes.[2,10,28,38]

INSTRUMENT CLEANING

III.c. All instruments opened onto the sterile field in the operating or procedure room should be cleaned and decontaminated whether or not they have been used.[10,28] *[2: Moderate Evidence]*

Scrubbed persons may touch and contaminate instruments without being aware of it. Instruments that were used may come in contact with unused items. Airborne microorganisms may come in contact with instruments that have not been used. Contamination of unused instruments on the sterile field can occur without the occurrence being noticed.[12]

III.d. In preparation for transport to a decontamination area, sharp instruments must be segregated from other instruments and confined in a puncture-resistant container. *[1: Regulatory Requirement]*

Segregation of sharps from other instruments minimizes the risk of injury to personnel handling instruments during cleaning and decontamination. The Occupational Safety and Health Administration (OSHA) prohibits processes that require employees to place their hands into basins of sharp instruments because of the risk for percutaneous exposure to bloodborne pathogens.[39] The reader should refer to the Guideline for Sharps Safety[40] for guidance related to preventing sharps injuries.

III.d.1. Disposable sharps (eg, scalpel blades, suture needles) must be removed and discarded into a closeable, puncture-resistant container that is leak-proof on its sides and bottom and is labeled or color-coded as biohazardous.[39,40] *[1: Regulatory Requirement]*

III.e. When an instrument is composed of more than one piece, it should be opened and disassembled according to the manufacturer's written IFU and arranged in a manner that will permit contact of cleaning solutions with all surfaces of the instruments. *[1: Strong Evidence]*

When surfaces cannot be contacted by cleaning solutions, thorough cleaning cannot be achieved; thus, these surfaces can retain organic material and debris. These retained materials can prevent contact of cleaning solutions and disinfecting or sterilizing agents with instrument surfaces, reduce the effectiveness of subsequent disinfection or sterilization processes,[2,10,12] and cause patient injury if they are not removed before sterilization.[17,21,23,41] Further research is warranted to determine the clinical significance of retained organic material and debris on instruments during disinfection and sterilization processes.

In a case series investigation, Parada et al[23] characterized the relationship between sterilization failure and SSIs. During a 14-week period, the investigators collected laboratory data on five patients who sustained SSIs after anterior cruciate ligament reconstruction and determined the infection rate was 12.2%. Before this period, the infection rate for anterior cruciate ligament reconstruction was 0.3%. The investigators found gross organic material inside an instrument common to all the surgical procedures. The inadequate removal of debris had occurred because there was no brush available with a diameter small enough to clean the cannula on the device.

III.f. Delicate instruments should be protected from damage during transport to a decontamination area. Delicate and other easily damaged instruments, such as fiberoptic cords, rigid endoscopes, and microsurgical instruments, should be placed on top of heavier instruments or segregated into separate containers.[10,12] *[3: Limited Evidence]*

Instruments may shift during transport, causing heavy instruments to damage more-delicate instruments.

III.g. Instruments should be kept moist until they are cleaned. A towel moistened with water placed over the instruments may be used. Saline should not be used. *[3: Limited Evidence]*

Keeping instruments moist helps prevent blood, organic materials, and debris from drying and adhering to the instruments. Dried organic materials and debris can make instruments more difficult to clean and potentially lead to the formation of biofilm. Prolonged exposure of instruments to saline can cause pitting.[10,12]

III.g.1. Instruments that cannot be cleaned immediately should be treated with an instrument cleaner according to the device and the instrument cleaner manufacturers' written IFU.[8,10,12] *[2: Moderate Evidence]*

Treating instruments with an instrument cleaner at the point of use can help prevent rusting and corrosion; prevent blood, organic materials, and debris from drying on the instruments; and inhibit biofilm formation.[8,10]

III.g.2. Liquids used to soak contaminated items at the point of use should be discarded before transport. When disposal of the solution is not feasible, it must be transported in a leak-proof container to the decontamination area for disposal.[39] *[1: Regulatory Requirement]*

Contaminated liquids may be spilled during transport, presenting a risk of contaminating the environment and exposing personnel to blood, body fluids, and other potentially infectious materials.[10,12,39]

Recommendation IV

Contaminated instruments must be contained during transport to a decontamination area.[10,39]

Containment of contaminated instruments decreases the potential for injury to personnel or their exposure to blood, body fluids, or other potentially infectious materials and helps prevent damage to the instruments during transport.

IV.a. Contaminated instruments should be transported to the decontamination area as soon as possible after completion of the procedure. *[1: Strong Evidence]*

Removal of blood, organic materials, and debris from instruments becomes more difficult after they have dried.[2,10,37,42]

IV.b. Soiled instruments must be transported to the decontamination area in a closed container or enclosed transport cart. The container or cart must be
- leak proof,[39]
- puncture resistant,[39]
- large enough to contain all contents, and
- labeled with a fluorescent orange or orange-red label containing a biohazard legend.[39]

[1: Regulatory Requirement]

Transporting soiled instruments in a manner that prevents exposing personnel to bloodborne pathogens and other potentially infectious materials is an OSHA requirement.[39]

Labeling the transport containment device communicates to others that the contents are potentially infectious.

IV.b.1. Biohazard labels should be affixed so as to prevent separation from the contents. When appropriate to the configuration of the contents, a red bag or red container may be used instead of a label to indicate contaminated waste.[39] *[1: Regulatory Requirement]*

IV.b.2. If the instrument containment device has been contaminated, it must be either cleaned at the point of use or placed inside another containment device and labeled as biohazardous.[39,43] *[1: Regulatory Requirement]*

Contact with contaminated surfaces can transmit potentially infectious microorganisms.[39,43] The reader should refer to the AORN Guideline for Prevention of Transmissible Infections[44] for guidance.

IV.b.3. Contaminated instruments and other items should be separated from clean and sterile supplies before transport to the processing area. *[3: Limited Evidence]*

Separation of soiled instruments from clean supplies minimizes the risk of cross-contamination.[10]

Recommendation V

Instruments should be cleaned and decontaminated in an area separate from locations where clean items are handled.[10,45,46]

Physical separation of decontamination areas from areas where clean items are handled minimizes the risk of cross-contamination. Cross-contamination can result when soiled items are placed in close proximity to clean items or are placed on surfaces upon which clean items are later placed. Droplets and aerosols created during cleaning of soiled instruments can cause cross-contamination of any nearby clean items or surfaces.

V.a. The sterile processing area should have
- separate clean and decontamination spaces, which may be rooms or areas;
- decontamination and clean spaces that are separated by one of three methods:
  - a wall with a door or pass-through,
  - a partial wall or partition that is at least 4 ft high and at least the width of the counter, or
  - a distance of 4 ft between the instrument washing sink and the area where the instruments are prepared for sterilization;
- separate sinks for washing instruments and for hand hygiene;
- decontaminating equipment (eg, automated washer, ultrasonic cleaner); and
- storage space for PPE and cleaning supplies in the decontamination area.

[3: Limited Evidence]

The requirements for processing reusable medical devices do not vary by location. Equivalent procedures, supplies, and equipment are needed in all locations where sterile processing is performed.[45,46]

V.b. Instruments should not be cleaned or decontaminated in scrub or hand sinks. *[4: Benefits Balanced with Harms]*

Cleaning soiled instruments in a scrub or hand sink can contaminate the sink and faucet, which are intended to be used for clean activities (eg, hand washing, surgical hand antisepsis).

V.c. The decontamination area must contain
- an eyewash station[10,47,48] and
- a hand-washing sink.[39]

[1: Regulatory Requirement]

The Occupational Safety and Health Administration requires that an eyewash station be provided where chemicals that are hazardous to the eyes are located.[47] Hand hygiene facilities are required by OSHA for use after removal of PPE.[39]

V.c.1. Eyewash stations, either plumbed or self contained, must be provided within the immediate area where chemicals such as instrument cleaning solutions or disinfectants that are hazardous to the eyes are located.[47,49]

Eyewash stations should be located so that travel time is no greater than 10 seconds from the location of chemical use or storage, or should be immediately available if the chemical is caustic or is a strong acid.[49] Eyewash stations should be located on the same level as the hazard, with the path of travel free of obstructions (eg, doors) that may inhibit immediate use of the eyewash station.[49]

Eyewash stations should
- be identified with a highly visible sign[49];
- deliver warm water (ie, 60° F to 100° F [15.6° C to 37.8° C]) at a rate of 1.5 L/minute for 15 minutes[49];
- be designed to flush both eyes simultaneously using a hands-free, stay-open feature[49];
- be flushed weekly to remove stagnant water, which may contain microbial contamination, from thoe system[49]; and
- be tested regularly and maintained in accordance with the manufacturer's written IFU.[49]

V.d. The decontamination area should contain
- automated equipment consistent with the types of instruments to be cleaned and decontaminated,
- adaptors and accessories to connect instruments with cleaning equipment and utilities,
- a filtered medical-grade compressed air supply,[10] and
- access to water of appropriate quality for rinsing instruments (eg, deionized or reverse-osmosis water).

[2: Moderate Evidence]

Automated cleaning and decontamination provides an effective level of cleaning that is difficult to replicate consistently using manual methods.[50-52] Compressed air is used to clear lumens of detergent and rinse water after cleaning.

V.e. The decontamination area should be stocked with the accessories and supplies needed to clean and decontaminate instruments in accordance with the manufacturers' written IFU.[10] Supplies should include
- brushes or other devices intended to remove organic material and debris from lumens, with a diameter and length appropriate to the lumen to be cleaned;
- enzymatic and nonenzymatic detergent;
- soft, low-linting cleaning cloths;
- testing equipment;
- a source of treated water (eg deionized, reverse osmosis, filtered);
- 70% to 90% alcohol;
- a thermometer; and
- a measuring device.

[3: Limited Evidence]

Brushes or devices of the correct size used in accordance with the brush or device manufacturer's IFU can facilitate cleaning of lumens. The instrument manufacturer's IFU may recommend either an enzymatic or a nonenzymatic detergent for cleaning. Soft, low-linting cleaning cloths may prevent scratches to the surface of instruments and prevent lint from adhering to the surfaces of the instruments.

Treated water is used for final rinsing. Impurities in untreated water can leave residues on instruments that may lead to corrosion, pitting, or staining.[10,51,53] A thermometer is used to measure that the detergent solution is within the recommended temperature range as specified by the detergent manufacturer's written IFU. Measuring devices are used to mix detergents at the concentration specified by the detergent manufacturer's written IFU.

V.f. The decontamination area heating, ventilation, and air conditioning (HVAC) system should be maintained within the HVAC design parameters at the rate that was applicable according to regulatory and professional guidelines at the time of design or most recent renovation of the HVAC system.[46]

The HVAC system controls the air quality, temperature, humidity, and pressure of the room in comparison with the surrounding areas. The HVAC system is designed in accordance with the American Society of Heating, Refrigerating and Air-Conditioning Engineers (ASHRAE)[54] and local regulatory requirements to reduce the amount of environmental contaminants and to provide a comfortable environment for occupants in the area.[46] [2: Moderate Evidence]

V.f.1. A multidisciplinary team that includes infection preventionists, perioperative RNs, sterile processing personnel, representatives from facility maintenance, and other stakeholders representing the health care organization should develop and implement a systematic process for monitoring HVAC performance parameters in the decontamination area and a mechanism for resolving variances.[46] [3: Limited Evidence]

The HVAC parameters recommended by ASHRAE and the Facilities Guidelines Institute for decontamination areas are
- 2 outdoor air changes per hour,[45,54]
- 6 total air changes per hour,[45,54]
- negative air pressure,[45,54] and
- temperature between 72° F and 78° F (22° C and 26° C).[45,54]

Room temperature may be intentionally adjusted to accommodate the individual comfort needs of the occupants.[45] Negative pressure helps prevent contaminated air from entering into positive-pressure, clean areas. The evidence on the effect of relative humidity on bacterial, fungal, and viral growth is inconclusive. Further research is warranted to determine optimal relative humidity levels to control environmental contamination.

In a descriptive study, Panagopoulou et al[55] examined air and surface fungal levels of two buildings in a Greek tertiary care hospital during a 12-month period. Each room in building A had a separate air-conditioning unit. Building B had a central air-conditioning unit. The researchers determined that, independent of the method of air-conditioning, the fungal levels were higher during the months in which the temperature and humidity levels were higher.

In a literature review on the effects of humidity on bacterial survival, Tang[56] found that various levels of humidity created differing responses in different strains of bacteria. The responses included structural changes and death. The bacterial survival rates were dependent on the species. The author was unable to find a link between humidity and bacterial survival.

In a laboratory setting, Thompson et al[57] found that aerosolized *Staphylococcus epidermidis*, used as a surrogate for *Staphylococcus aureus*, survived at relative humidity levels of < 20%, 40% to 60%, 70% to 80%, and > 90%. The researchers concluded that *S epidermidis* was not affected by the level of relative humidity.

In a literature review of the effect of temperature and humidity on viruses, Memarzadeh[58] reviewed 120 articles and found no conclusive evidence supporting a maximum or minimum relative humidity level to decrease the survival rate of viruses and the ability of viruses to cause diseases.

The ASHRAE guidelines related to room temperature ranges for the decontamination area are the accepted professional guidelines for HVAC systems in the United States.[54] Personnel working in the decontamination area and wearing PPE may become uncomfortable at room temperatures above 72° F (22° C). Lower room temperatures may contribute to the comfort of personnel wearing PPE.

V.f.2. Designated personnel should perform a risk assessment of the decontamination area if a variance in the parameters of the HVAC system occurs. Based on the risk assessment, measures should be taken to restore the area to full functionality after the HVAC system variance has been corrected.[46] *[5: No Evidence]*

The evidence review did not reveal any evidence of clinical significance related to the degree of variance in the HVAC system design parameters. The effect of the HVAC system parameters falling out of range is variable. A small variance for a short period of time may not be of clinical concern, whereas a large variance for a longer period may have clinical significance. Further research on this topic is warranted.

V.f.3. Personnel who identify an unintentional variance (ie, variances other than intentional temperature adjustments) in the predetermined HVAC system parameters should report the variance according to the health care organization's policy and procedure.[46] *[5: No Evidence]*

Rapid communication between affected and responsible personnel may help facilitate resolution of the variance.

Recommendation VI

Personnel working in the decontamination area and handling contaminated instruments must wear PPE.[39]

Contaminated instruments are a potential source of transmissible pathogens. Personnel in the decontamination area are at risk for exposure to blood, body fluids, and other potentially infectious materials. Personal protective equipment helps to protect the individual from exposure to infectious materials.

VI.a. Personal protective equipment consistent with exposure risks in the decontamination area must be worn,[39] including
- a fluid-resistant gown with sleeves,
- gloves (ie, general purpose utility gloves with a cuff that extends beyond the cuff of the gown),
- a mask and eye protection or a full face shield, and
- shoe covers or boots designed for use as PPE.[39]

[1: Regulatory Requirement]

Splashes, splatters, and skin contact can be reasonably anticipated by personnel handling contaminated instruments. Fluid-resistant gowns can prevent transfer of microorganisms from contaminated items to skin.[10] General purpose utility gloves can minimize the potential for punctures, cuts, and nicks and exposure of the hands to blood, body fluids, and other potentially infectious materials.[10] Utility glove cuffs that extend beyond the cuff of the gown help to provide adequate fluid protection during instrument cleaning in a sink. A mask and eye protection or a full face shield can protect the face and eyes from contact with contaminated aerosols and chemicals used for cleaning purposes.[10] Fluid-resistant shoe covers can protect shoes from contaminants and splashes, splatters, and spills.

VI.a.1. Personal protective equipment should be placed where it is readily available to personnel entering an area in which there is a risk of exposure to transmissible pathogens.[27] *[1: Regulatory Requirement]*

There is potential for exposure to transmissible pathogens in the decontamination area, and OSHA requires the employer to provide PPE.[39] Placing PPE in an area readily available to decontamination area personnel can facilitate compliance with OSHA requirements for wearing PPE when there is

INSTRUMENT CLEANING

danger of exposure to blood, body fluids, or other potentially infectious materials.

VI.b. Hand hygiene must be performed after PPE is removed.[39] *[1: Regulatory Requirement]*

Perforations can occur in gloves, and hands can become contaminated during removal of PPE; OSHA requires hand hygiene after removal of PPE.[39]

VI.c. Reusable PPE must be cleaned and decontaminated and its integrity confirmed between uses. *[1: Regulatory Requirement]*

Personal protective equipment is appropriate only if it does not permit potentially infectious materials to pass through and contact the individual.[39] Reusable gloves, gowns, aprons, face shields, and eye wear can become contaminated and their integrity compromised during use. Decontamination and confirmation of integrity helps to protect the wearer from exposure.

Recommendation VII

The type of water used for cleaning should be consistent with the manufacturers' written IFU and the intended use of the equipment and cleaning product.[6,10,28,53]

Water quality is affected by the presence of dissolved minerals, solids, chlorides, and other impurities and by its acidity and alkalinity (ie, pH).[53,59] Minerals can cause deposits, scale, or water spots to form on instruments.[53,59] Excessive chlorides can cause pitting.[53,59] The pH level affects the performance of enzymatic and detergent agents.[6,53,59] Untreated water quality fluctuates over time, varies with geographic location and season, and can affect the outcome of cleaning actions.[51,53,60]

VII.a. The final rinse should be performed with treated (eg, distilled, reverse osmosis, filtered) water of a quality that will not stain or cause damage to instruments or contribute to recontamination of the instrument.[10] *[2: Moderate Evidence]*

Untreated water can contain contaminants, including endotoxins, which can be deposited on instruments during the final rinse. Rinsing with treated water can prevent deposits of impurities or contaminants on instruments.[10,51]

Endotoxins are heat stable and may not be destroyed by subsequent steam sterilization. Tissue contaminated with endotoxins can cause severe inflammation.[53]

Treated water can prevent spotting, stains, deposits, and corrosion on the surfaces of instruments.[53,59]

VII.b. Device-processing personnel, in collaboration with clinical engineering personnel, should perform a water-quality assessment periodically[53] and after major maintenance to the water supply system to determine water quality relative to the requirements for cleaning as specified in the detergent and cleaning equipment manufacturers' written IFU. *[3: Limited Evidence]*

Water quality varies seasonally and after water-source maintenance. Periodic testing can indicate whether the chemical combination used to condition the cleaning and decontamination water requires adjusting. Water-quality checks determine the hardness (ie, mineral content) of the water and any impurities present.

Water quality that does not meet the requirements specified in the detergent or the cleaning equipment manufacturers' IFU can adversely affect the efficacy of cleaning chemistries.[6,53] The need for repairs or modifications to the treatment system can be identified from a water-quality check.[53]

A nonexperimental study by Harnroongroj et al[60] compared 32 first-burst water samples with 29 running tap samples of water supplied to an OR and found the bacterial count in first-burst water was three times higher than in running tap water. This research was performed in Thailand and may not be generalizable to the United States.

In a nonexperimental study to determine the effectiveness of a commercially available test for determining the presence of organic soil on instruments after cleaning in automated washers, Alfa et al[51] found that surgical instruments cleaned in automated washers may have visually undetected high post-cleaning residuals of carbohydrate and endotoxin. An objective of the researchers was to determine the level of protein, hemoglobin, carbohydrate, and endotoxin before and after cleaning in an automated washer. The researchers evaluated five types of surgical instruments from plastic surgery trays for residuals both before and after cleaning. Of a total of 25 instruments tested, 21 (84%) had substantially higher carbohydrate levels and 15 (60%) had higher endotoxin levels after cleaning than before cleaning. The results of the study suggest that endotoxins remaining on surgical instruments after cleaning in automated washers may be related to water quality. The researchers recommended monitoring of water quality.

Recommendation VIII

Surgical instrument, cleaning product, and cleaning equipment manufacturers' validated, written IFU should be reviewed for compatibility during selection and followed during use of cleaning products and equipment for cleaning and decontaminating surgical instruments.[10]

The intended use of cleaning products and cleaning equipment varies. Following the manufacturers' written IFU decreases the possibility of selecting and using cleaning products and equipment that may damage instruments.[6]

INSTRUMENT CLEANING

VIII.a. A multidisciplinary team that includes infection preventionists, perioperative RNs, sterile processing personnel, and other stakeholders representing the health care organization should develop a mechanism for evaluating and selecting products for cleaning surgical instruments. *[3: Limited Evidence]*

The chemical actions of cleaning products vary, and products are intended for different applications. Some cleaning products target specific types of bioburden (eg, protein, lipids, other organic material); others are intended for general purpose cleaning.

Some cleaning products contain one or more enzymes to break up soil and facilitate its removal.[6,61] Enzymes are specific in terms of the soils they remove.[6,61] Some enzymatic detergents contain more than one enzyme and are intended to be used as all-purpose detergents; others are intended for a specific type of soil.[6,61] Protease enzymes target blood and body salts.[6] Amylases target carbohydrates, starches, and sugars.[6,61] Lipases break down fats and oils.[6,61] The pH and the rinsability of cleaning products vary.

Cleaning equipment manufacturers' requirements for selection and use of cleaning products also vary. Some instrument manufacturers' written IFU specifically recommend against using some cleaning agent formulations.

VIII.a.1. Neutral detergents with a pH of 7 that are low foaming and easy to remove during rinsing should be used for manual or mechanical cleaning unless contraindicated by the device or cleaning equipment manufacturer's IFU. *[2: Moderate Evidence]*

Detergents help to dislodge solids from the surface of instruments. Neutral pH or slightly alkaline detergents are compatible with most instruments and work well with enzymes that may be added to detergents to help break down and facilitate removal of organic materials.[2] Detergents that are low foaming facilitate observation of the cleaning process.[5]

VIII.a.2. Cleaning products should
- be nonabrasive,
- be low foaming,
- be easy to remove during rinsing,
- be biodegradable,
- provide for soil dispersion,
- be nontoxic in the specific-use dilution,
- be effective for clinically relevant soils under specified conditions,
- have a long shelf life,
- be cost-effective, and
- be able to be tested for effective concentration.[6]

[3: Limited Evidence]

Cleaning products that are nonabrasive can help protect the surface of instruments from damage. Cleaning products that are low foaming are less likely to interfere with the action of mechanical cleaning equipment. Cleaning products that are easy to remove facilitate removal of detergent during rinsing.[6] Cleaning products that are nontoxic contribute to personnel safety. Use of cleaning products that are effective on clinically relevant soils may increase the efficacy of the cleaning process.

VIII.b. Cleaning products must be handled according to the safety data sheets (SDSs) and the manufacturers' written IFU. The SDSs must be readily accessible to employees within the workplace.[62] *[1: Regulatory Requirement]*

Highly acidic or alkaline cleaning agents are corrosive and can cause injury to skin or mucus membranes.[6] Exposure to enzymatic detergents can cause asthma.[2] Access to the cleaning product IFU and SDS provides opportunities for personnel to use the product correctly and obtain information useful for implementing processes that prevent injury.[48]

VIII.c. The cleaning product manufacturer's written IFU should be followed for[2,10]
- water quality, hardness, and pH;
- concentration and dilution;
- water temperature;
- contact time;
- conditions of storage; and
- shelf life and use life.

[2: Moderate Evidence]

Water quality, including hardness and pH, can affect the effectiveness of cleaning products.[53] Using the product in the concentration recommended by the manufacturer's written IFU helps to ensure consistent and accurate cleaning chemistry.[10] The manufacturer has determined the correct temperature and contact time to facilitate cleaning with the specific product. Shelf life and use life indicate the time span or use after which the cleaning product's effectiveness cannot be assured. Using the product after expiration or at a temperature other than specified in the IFU can render the product ineffective.[6]

VIII.c.1. An automated titration unit may be used to efficiently concentrate chemicals at a consistent ratio. *[4: Benefits Balanced with Harms]*

The concentration of the solution can vary when it is mixed manually. Use of a titration unit can aid in accurate measurement of the chemical during preparation of the cleaning solution and help personnel to consistently obtain the recommended concentration of the cleaning product.

VIII.d. Abrasive devices and products should not be used to clean instruments unless their use is

INSTRUMENT CLEANING

specified in the device manufacturer's written IFU.[10] *[3: Limited Evidence]*

Abrasive devices and products, such as metal scouring pads, scouring powders, and bleach can cause permanent damage to instrument surfaces and can result in pitting, providing a place that can harbor microorganisms and debris. In some circumstances, the device manufacturer may recommend using a metal brush.[10] In circumstances in which instruments were used on prion-contaminated tissue, the guidelines for processing may recommend use of a corrosive chemical[63,64] (see Recommendation XIII).

VIII.d.1. Brushes or other items used to clean crevices and lumens should have a diameter and length appropriate for the area within or on the instrument or device being cleaned and be made of a material specified as compatible by the instrument or device manufacturer.[10] *[3: Limited Evidence]*

Tissue and debris can become lodged in crevices, box locks, lumens, and other areas of instruments. Use of a brush intended for these difficult-to-clean areas may be required to effectively remove organic material and debris.[10,23]

VIII.d.2. Brushes used to clean lumens should
- meet the requirement for cleaning as specified in the instrument or device manufacturer's written IFU,[10]
- be long enough to clean the entire length of the lumen and exit at the distal end,
- contact the inner surface of the lumen without collapsing,
- have bristles soft enough to prevent damage to the internal lumen surface, and
- be either designed for single use and discarded after each use or be reusable and decontaminated at least daily or more frequently as needed.[10]

[3: Limited Evidence]

Brushes that are too short to exit the distal length of a lumen can push debris to a point in the lumen but fail to remove it. Brushes with bristles that are too small or too large in diameter can prevent thorough cleaning. Bristles that are abrasive can damage instruments.

Reusable brushes that are not decontaminated can cause contaminants to be transferred from one device to another. Use of single-use disposable brushes helps ensure that a clean brush is used each time.

Recommendation IX

Surgical instruments and equipment should be cleaned and decontaminated according to the manufacturer's validated, written IFU.[10]

Cleaning of instruments (ie, removal of organic and inorganic soil) is the first step in decontamination and can be accomplished through manual or mechanical processes. The instrument and equipment manufacturers have determined the manual or mechanical steps and processes necessary to effectively clean a device.[6,10] Decontamination (ie, rendering instruments safe to handle) may require a microbiocidal process after cleaning (eg, wiping with 70% to 90% alcohol). Factors that determine whether a microbiocidal process is required after cleaning include device materials and design (see Recommendation XIII).

IX.a. Manual cleaning as specified in the instrument manufacturer's written IFU should be used for instruments that cannot tolerate mechanical cleaning.[12] *[3: Limited Evidence]*

Manual cleaning is often recommended for devices that cannot tolerate the action of mechanical cleaning or cannot be immersed (eg, power drills, delicate microsurgical instruments, flexible endoscopes, cameras). Seals on lensed instruments can be damaged when processed through ultrasonic equipment.[10] Mechanical cleaning of devices when the manufacturer's written IFU recommend against it can result in damage to instruments and can limit the associated warranty.

IX.a.1. In preparation for manual cleaning, instruments should be disassembled and ports, valves, stop cocks, ratchets, and joints should be opened.[10,12] *[3: Limited Evidence]*

Opening and disassembling instruments facilitates contact of the cleaning solution with all surfaces of the instruments.

IX.a.2. Instruments should be rinsed in cool water before washing.[6,10] *[2: Moderate Evidence]*

Hot water can denature blood proteins, which makes them more difficult to remove.[10] Cool water can help to prevent coagulation of blood on instruments and can help remove gross soil from lumens, joints, and crevices.[2,6,10] Rinsing with cool water can wash away water-soluble blood proteins and prevent denaturing.[10]

IX.a.3. Unless contraindicated in the device manufacturer's written IFU, the instrument should be submerged for cleaning in a solution of water and detergent intended for cleaning surgical instruments. The detergent should be compatible with the device to be cleaned and used at the concentration and temperature specified in the detergent manufacturer's IFU.[10] *[3: Limited Evidence]*

Full submersion of the instrument in the cleaning solution reduces the risk of splashing potentially contaminated cleaning solution onto personnel and into the environment. The concentration and temperature of the cleaning solution specified in the detergent IFU have been validated by the detergent manufacturer as necessary for the detergent to be effective.[6]

INSTRUMENT CLEANING

IX.a.4. Lumens should be flushed with cleaning solution and brushed with a brush of the length, diameter, type, and material specified in the device manufacturer's IFU.[6] *[3: Limited Evidence]*

Brushing is necessary to ensure detergent contact of the cleaning solution within lumens. Brushes that are too short cannot contact the entire lumen. Brushes with a diameter that is too small will not contact all surfaces within the lumen.[65]

IX.a.5. Devices with lumens should be immersed in the cleaning solution in a vertical position.[10] *[3: Limited Evidence]*

Air may become trapped within lumens when the device is soaked in a horizontal position. Entrapped air may prevent contact of the cleaning solution with the surfaces within the lumen.

IX.b. Cleaning solutions should be changed before they become heavily soiled, when the temperature of the solution does not meet the temperature specified in the manufacturer's written IFU, and as needed.[10] *[3: Limited Evidence]*

Bioburden is deposited in the cleaning solution during the cleaning process. Frequent changes of the cleaning solution can help to minimize bioburden. Following the manufacturer's written IFU helps facilitate effective cleaning.

IX.c. Instruments that require lubrication should be lubricated with a type of lubricant that is recommended by the instrument manufacturer and is compatible with the subsequent sterilization method. *[3: Limited Evidence]*

Instruments require different types of lubricant depending on the design of the device or the sterilization method. Oil-based lubricants may be recommended for the internal mechanisms of powered devices. Water-soluble lubricants are compatible with steam sterilization.[12] Following the device manufacturer's instructions for lubrication can facilitate selection and use of the correct lubricant.

IX.d. Mechanical methods (eg, ultrasonic cleaner, washer disinfector/decontaminator) should be used for cleaning surgical instruments unless otherwise specified by the instrument manufacturer.[5,6,50] *[1: Strong Evidence]*

Mechanical cleaning is preferred over manual cleaning because it is reproducible and provides consistent detergent concentration, temperature control, and washing and rinsing processes, whereas manual cleaning is subject to variation among personnel.[5,50-52] Mechanical cleaning reduces the risk to personnel of exposure to blood, body fluids, other potentially infectious materials, and other hazards.[5,6] Mechanical cleaning is more easily monitored for quality than manual cleaning.[6]

IX.d.1. When mechanical equipment incorporates cleaning accessories specifically intended for use with specific types of instruments (eg, robotic or laparoscopic instruments), these accessories should be used according to the equipment and device manufacturers' written IFU.[6] *[3: Limited Evidence]*

IX.e. Ultrasonic cleaners may be used to remove soil from hard-to-access areas of instruments.[10] *[3: Limited Evidence]*

Ultrasonic cleaners can provide an effective means of removing soil from hard-to-reach areas, such as joints and crevices.[6] Ultrasonic cleaners vary by design, intended use, operation, and maintenance. Some ultrasonic cleaners are designed and intended for use on specific instruments. Instructions for use will vary accordingly.[66]

IX.e.1. Cleaning products compatible with the ultrasonic cleaner should be used.[6] *[3: Limited Evidence]*

Ultrasonic cleaners remove debris through a process of cavitation. Cleaning chemistries that are not compatible with the ultrasonic cleaner can interfere with the cavitation process and result in inadequate cleaning.[67]

IX.e.2. Ultrasonic cleaning device manufacturers' written IFU should be followed regarding degassing the cleaning solution before instrument processing. *[3: Limited Evidence]*

Water contains air bubbles that can interfere with the cavitation process if not removed.[67]

IX.e.3. Gross soil should be removed from instruments before they are placed in the ultrasonic cleaner. *[3: Limited Evidence]*

Ultrasonic cleaners are not designed to remove gross soil. They are designed to remove debris from joints, crevices, lumens, and hard-to-reach areas.[10]

IX.e.4. Only instruments made of similar metals should be combined in the ultrasonic cleaner unless otherwise specified in the instrument manufacturer's written IFU.[10] Instruments composed of brass, copper, aluminum, or chrome should not be mixed with instruments made of stainless steel in an ultrasonic cleaner.[6] *[3: Limited Evidence]*

Placing instruments made of dissimilar metals in the ultrasonic cleaner can cause the transfer of ions from one instrument to another (ie, electroplating), which can result in etching and pitting of the instrument. Damage to the finish of the instrument can create surface imperfections that can harbor microorganisms and debris.[6]

IX.e.5. Only instruments compatible with the ultrasonic cleaning process should be subjected to ultrasonic cleaning. *[3: Limited Evidence]*

INSTRUMENT CLEANING

Some instruments, such as lensed instruments, air-powered drills, flexible endoscopes, and chrome-plated instruments, will sustain damage if cleaned in an ultrasonic cleaner.[67] Lenses may loosen, internal components of air-powered drills may sustain damage if immersed, and chrome plating can loosen.[68]

IX.e.6. Instruments with lumens should be thoroughly submerged and filled with cleaning solution.[6] If the ultrasonic cleaner includes adaptors or connections for internal lumen flushing, these should be attached to lumens that are intended to be cleaned. *[3: Limited Evidence]*

The presence of air prevents the cleaning solution from contacting the inner lumen of instruments and affects the cavitation process[10,67]

IX.e.7. Instruments should be thoroughly rinsed after ultrasonic cleaning.[8] The rinse should be performed with treated (eg, distilled, reverse osmosis, filtered) water of a quality that will not stain or cause damage to the instruments or contribute to recontamination of the instruments.[10] *[2: Moderate Evidence]*

Rinsing removes the cleaning solution. Solution in the cleaner may contain debris that can be deposited on the instruments as they are removed.[8]

IX.e.8. The lid should be closed when the ultrasonic cleaner is in use. *[3: Limited Evidence]*

A closed lid prevents aerosolization of contaminants.[66]

IX.e.9. The cleaning solution in the ultrasonic cleaner should be changed before it becomes visibly soiled, when the temperature of the solution does not meet the temperature specified in the manufacturer's written IFU, and as needed.[10,67] *[3: Limited Evidence]*

Organic material and debris that is lifted from instruments during the ultrasonic processing is deposited in the solution and can become a growth medium for bacteria and other microorganisms. The effectiveness of the cleaning can be reduced when the cleaning solution is heavily soiled. Some manufacturer's written IFU specify using a fresh cleaning solution each time an ultrasonic cycle is run. Following the manufacturer's written IFU helps facilitate effective cleaning.

IX.e.10. Ultrasonic cleaners should be emptied, cleaned, disinfected, rinsed, and dried at least daily or, preferably, after each use.[10] If not contraindicated by the ultrasonic cleaner manufacturer's written IFU, the chamber should be wiped with 70% to 90% alcohol and dried with a lint-free cloth.[8,69] *[2: Moderate Evidence]*

Inadequately cleaned ultrasonic cleaners and endotoxins have been associated with toxic anterior segment syndrome (TASS).[70] Fluid in the ultrasonic cleaner can harbor gram-negative bacteria.[8,69,71,72] Growth of these bacteria can result in the production of endotoxins, which are heat resistant, can survive steam sterilization, and can cause serious consequences for patients.[8,71,72] Alcohol promotes drying, inhibits microbial growth, and can prevent biofilm formation.[67,69]

IX.f. Mechanical washer disinfectors/decontaminators should be used according to the manufacturer's written IFU.[10] *[3: Limited Evidence]*

Washer disinfector equipment designs vary among manufacturers and models. Following the manufacturer's written IFU will help ensure that the equipment is used correctly and functions as intended.

IX.f.1. Surgical instruments and their containment devices and accessories should be positioned in the washer disinfector in a manner that ensures contact of the cleaning solution with all surfaces of the items.[10]
- Items composed of more than one part should be disassembled according to the manufacturer's IFU. Small parts should be contained.
- Instruments should be placed in open mesh-bottom pans.
- Ports and stopcocks should be opened.
- Stylets should be removed from lumened instruments.
- Instrument ratchets should be in the open position.
- Items with surfaces that will retain water should be placed on edge.
- Electrical cords and insulated instruments should be segregated from sharp instruments.

[3: Limited Evidence]

Preparing and positioning items as described above helps ensure contact of the cleaning solution with all surfaces of the instrument. Contact with the cleaning solution is critical to effective cleaning and decontamination.[10] Containing small parts helps to prevent loss. Placing on edge the items with surfaces that will retain water helps prevent water retention. Sharp items can damage the softer material of cords and cables and can damage insulation coverings.

IX.f.2. The instrument manufacturer's written IFU should be followed during use of automated washing equipment, including placement of the instrument within mechanical washers, cycle parameters, and any other specific cleaning requirements. *[3: Limited Evidence]*

The variety of equipment available and the complexity of devices make it essential to consult and follow the manufacturer's IFU to achieve optimal cleaning effectiveness.[10]

IX.f.3. The operator of the mechanical washer should consult with the mechanical washer manufacturer's written IFU to determine
- the level of decontamination that is achieved (eg, low-level, intermediate) and
- how to monitor the cycle to determine that the parameters necessary to render the processed items safe to handle are met (see Recommendation XVII).

[4: Benefits Balanced with Harms]

Recommendation X

Surgical instruments should be inspected and evaluated for cleanliness and correct working order after decontamination and if soiled or defective, should be removed from service until they are cleaned or repaired.[10]

Items that are not clean or do not function correctly can put a patient at risk for injury or SSI.[17,20,22,23,69] Inspection and evaluation provide an opportunity to identify soiled or damaged instruments and to remove these items from service until they are cleaned or repaired.

X.a. Items should be inspected and evaluated for
- cleanliness;
- correct alignment;
- corrosion, pitting, burrs, nicks, cracks;
- sharpness of cutting edges;
- wear and chipping of inserts and plated surfaces;
- missing parts;
- integrity of insulation on insulated devices;
- integrity of cords and cables;
- clarity of lenses;
- integrity of seals and gaskets;
- presence of moisture;
- correct functioning; and
- other defects.

[2: Moderate Evidence]

Use of instruments that are not thoroughly cleaned, are damaged, or do not function correctly poses a risk to patient safety.[17,20,23,24,26,73,74]

X.a.1. Powered equipment should be checked before use to verify that power ceases when the device is turned off and that the device is functioning as intended. Instruments that require power to operate should be attached to the power source for testing as specified in the manufacturer's written IFU. *[3: Limited Evidence]*

Power that does not cease when a powered device is turned off can cause harm to personnel or patients.[6] Verifying that instruments requiring a power source are functioning as intended may help to prevent injury to patients and personnel.

X.a.2. Instruments that require assembly or that work with an accessory instrument should be assembled to confirm correct fit and that locking mechanisms work as intended. After inspection, these instruments should be disassembled before packaging for sterilization.[75] *[3: Limited Evidence]*

Attachments and accessory items not designed to the instrument manufacturer's specifications may not fit or seal correctly and may be ejected with force and pose a risk to patients and personnel. Disassembling items before sterilization helps ensure that the sterilant contacts all surfaces of the item being sterilized.

X.a.3. Lighted magnification should be used to inspect hard-to-clean areas of devices for cleanliness. *[2: Moderate Evidence]*

An instrument that appears clean to the naked eye may harbor debris that cannot be seen without magnification.[76]

Lipscomb et al[77] compared the results of 202 cleaned and decontaminated instruments by first visually examining them and then examining them using microscopic analysis (ie, episcopic differential interference contrast microscopy). Visual inspection by the researchers showed that 37% of the instruments (75 of 202) had a low level of contamination, and 4% (eight of 202) had a high level of contamination. The microscopic assessment showed 66% (133 of 202) were severely contaminated and 27% (55 of 202) were moderately contaminated.

X.a.4. The internal channels of reusable arthroscopic shavers should be inspected using an endoscopic camera or borescope.[78] *[2: Moderate Evidence]*

It is not possible to visually inspect lumens without a device that can penetrate the lumen. Retained organic material or debris in lumens can lead to patient injury.[22,23]

In a 2007 case-control study, Tosh et al[22] reported on an outbreak of *Pseudomonas aeruginosa* SSI in seven patients on whom the same arthroscopic shaver was used. Upon investigation, the researchers found debris in a lumen of the shaver although the shaver had undergone repeated decontamination and sterilization procedures. The researchers concluded that the retained surgical debris allowed the bacteria to survive the sterilization process, and the subsequent use of the shaver was likely related to the SSI outbreak.

The FDA recommends that the inside of the device be inspected and that consideration be given to using a 3-mm videoscope

INSTRUMENT CLEANING

to inspect the channels of the shaver hand piece.[78]

X.a.5. Insulated devices should be visually examined and tested using equipment designed to detect insulation failure. *[2: Moderate Evidence]*

Electrode insulation damage caused during use or processing may create an alternate pathway for the electrical current to leave the active electrode and cause patient injury. Some insulation failures are not visible. Damage to insulation may not be seen during visual inspection.[20]

In a two-part study, Espada et al[26] tested 78 robotic and 298 insulated laparoscopic instruments for insulation failure using a porosity detector. The researchers found that 25 of 78 robotic instruments (32%) had an insulation defect, but only seven of 25 defects (28%) were visible to the naked eye. Thirty-nine of the 298 laparoscopic instruments (13%) had an insulation defect, but only 27 of the 39 defects (69%) were visible to the naked eye.

In a nonexperimental study that examined insulated instruments from four hospitals, Montero et al[20] used a porosity detector to detect insulation failure. The researchers found that 33 of 226 insulated instruments (15%) had an insulation failure. There was no significant difference in insulation failure between hospitals that routinely checked for failure and those that did not.

Serious patient injury, such as thermal bowel injury, can occur when instruments with insulation defects are used.[26]

X.b. Defective instruments should be identified, removed from service, and repaired or discarded.[10] *[3: Limited Evidence]*

Identification of defective instruments and removal from service facilitates segregation of these instruments from instruments to be used when assembling sets. Removing defective instruments from service reduces the risk that defective instruments will be used.[10]

X.c. Instruments should be thoroughly dried before they are assembled in packaging systems in preparation for sterilization.[10] *[3: Limited Evidence]*

Moisture can interfere with sterilization processes.[10] Excess moisture on instrument surfaces can alter the content of steam and can pose a challenge for effective heating of the instrument during steam sterilization.[10] Hydrogen peroxide vapor and hydrogen peroxide gas plasma sterilization cycles may abort in the presence of excess moisture.[79] Ethylene oxide combines with water to form ethylene glycol (ie, antifreeze), which is toxic and is not removed during aeration.[80]

Recommendation XI

Special precautions should be taken during processing of intraocular ophthalmic instruments.[8]

Prevention of toxic anterior segment syndrome (TASS), an acute inflammation of the anterior segment of the eye, requires thorough cleaning and rinsing of intraocular instruments and strict adherence to the manufacturer's written IFU and to professional guidelines.[81-83] Toxic anterior segment syndrome is a complication of anterior segment eye surgery and is most commonly associated with cataract surgery.[84] According to the FDA, hundreds of surgical centers in North America reported outbreaks of TASS between 2000 and 2011.[84]

Most instances of TASS appear to be related to instrument processing.[69,70,81-83,85-90] Factors associated with TASS include

- contaminated instruments,
- contaminated ultrasonic cleaners,
- detergent residues (eg, soaps, enzymatic cleaners) remaining on instruments,
- insufficient rinsing of instruments,
- endotoxin residues on instruments,
- steam impurities during steam sterilization,[91]
- use of glutaraldehyde during processing,[92]
- dried debris and residues of ophthalmic viscoelastic (OV) material remaining on instruments,
- use of reusable cannulated instruments, and
- insufficiently dried lumens.[83]

Further research is warranted to determine the multifactorial risk factors for TASS.[83]

In response to a number of TASS outbreaks, the American Society of Cataract and Refractive Surgery (ASCRS) and the American Society of Ophthalmic Registered Nurses issued recommended practices for processing ophthalmic instruments.[8] The ASCRS formed a task force composed of members of industry and the ASCRS to educate surgeons who perform anterior segment eye surgery on the causes, symptoms, and treatment of TASS, and to help investigate outbreaks of TASS.[69] The task force posted a questionnaire on the ASCRS web site to allow surgeons to self-report cases of TASS and provide information about instrument cleaning and processing practices; surgical protocols; substances and techniques used for cleaning phacoemulsification and irrigation/aspiration hand pieces; and products used during the perioperative period, including medications, irrigation fluids, cannulas, and instrument tips.[69,85] The questionnaire has been maintained on the ASCRS web site since June 2007.[85] In addition, members of the TASS task force made site visits at the request of personnel from the facilities reporting TASS cases.[69]

Cutler Peck et al[69] conducted a retrospective analysis of 77 questionnaires submitted to the ASCRS web site from June 1, 2007, through May 31, 2009, and evaluated the findings from 54 TASS task force site visits conducted between October 1, 2005, and May 31, 2009. The researchers found there were common practices associated with TASS that included

- inadequately flushing phacoemulsification and irrigation/aspiration hand pieces,

INSTRUMENT CLEANING

- using enzymatic cleaners,
- using detergents at the wrong concentration,
- using contaminated fluids in ultrasonic cleaners,
- adding antibiotics to balanced salt solutions,
- using epinephrine with preservatives,
- using preoperative skin antiseptics incorrectly,
- using powdered gloves,
- reusing single-use products, and
- failing to maintain instruments correctly.

The researchers concluded that changing these practices could help prevent TASS.

Bodnar et al[85] conducted a retrospective analysis of 130 questionnaires submitted to the ASCRS web site from June 1, 2007, through March 1, 2012, and of information from 71 site visits conducted by the TASS task force between October 1, 2005, and December 31, 2011. The researchers noted several trends when comparing their data with the data previously analyzed by Cutler Peck et al.[69] When analyzing data obtained from the questionnaires, the researchers found a 26% reduction in sites reporting inadequate flushing of hand pieces and a 27% increase in sites reporting the use of deionized or distilled water for the final rinse. When analyzing data from the site visits, the researchers found a 36% reduction in the use of epinephrine with preservatives and a 36% reduction in the use of enzymatic detergents; however, they found a 21% increase in the handling of intraocular lenses and instrument tips with gloved hands, a 47% increase in poor instrument maintenance, and a 34% increase in use of contaminated fluids in ultrasonic cleaners. The researchers concluded that education had improved some practices but had not improved others.

The findings from these studies indicate a need to improve education of personnel who use or process ophthalmic instruments regarding best practices for care and processing of ophthalmic instruments to prevent TASS.

XI.a. Immediately after use during the procedure, ophthalmic instruments should be wiped clean with sterile water and a lint-free sponge and flushed or immersed in sterile water according to the manufacturer's written IFU.[8,10] *[1: Strong Evidence]*

Ophthalmic viscoelastic material can harden and dry within minutes, making subsequent removal difficult.[8,10,82,85,88] Keeping OV or other organic material moist can prevent drying and hardening of such material on ophthalmic devices.[8]

Biofilm adheres to the surfaces of instruments and is very difficult to remove. Keeping the OV and organic material moist helps facilitate removal and prevent biofilm formation.

XI.b. The instrument manufacturer's written instructions for cleaning should be reviewed and followed.[8,10] *[2: Moderate Evidence]*

The method of cleaning and the compatibility of cleaning products may vary among instrument manufacturers. Instructions for cannulated instruments indicate the type and volume of solution to be used for rinsing and cleaning and the number of times and for how long the cannula should be flushed.[8,82]

XI.c. Adequate time, an adequate number of personnel, and sufficient instrument inventory should be provided to permit thorough instrument cleaning and sterilization.[8,10] *[2: Moderate Evidence]*

Time constraints may create a disincentive for personnel to adhere to recommended cleaning and disinfection procedures.[69]

In a retrospective analysis of 77 questionnaires and 54 site visits to identify risk factors associated with TASS, an ASCRS task force reported that 23 of the sites (43%) were noted to have an insufficient number of instrument sets or of personnel to provide adequate time to process ophthalmic instruments. Personnel at six sites (11%) did not follow the manufacturer's written IFU, and four individuals were observed to perform inadequate flushing of phacoemulsification and irrigation/aspiration hand pieces.[69]

XI.c.1. An inventory of ophthalmic instruments sufficient to meet the anticipated demand should be maintained.[8,10] *[2: Moderate Evidence]*

An adequate instrument inventory provides sufficient time for personnel to follow correct cleaning, decontamination, and terminal sterilization procedures and helps eliminate or reduce the need for immediate-use steam sterilization (IUSS).[8,10,83]

XI.d. Intraocular instruments should be cleaned in a designated cleaning area. Intraocular instruments should be cleaned separately from general surgical instruments.[10] *[2: Moderate Evidence]*

Procedures for processing ophthalmic instruments differ from those for general surgery instruments.[85] Cleaning intraocular instruments separately from general surgery instruments can help prevent cross-contamination with bioburden from heavily soiled nonophthalmic surgical instruments.[8,10]

XI.e. Single-use disposable cannulae should be used whenever possible.[8] *[1: Strong Evidence]*

Thorough cleaning of these devices is difficult because the lumens are exceptionally small.[8] Use of reusable cannulae has been associated with TASS.[82,87]

In a 2006 review of the literature to identify possible causes of TASS, Mamalis et al[86] identified detergent residues and denatured OV material on reusable intraocular instruments as possible causes.

XI.f. The scrub person should flush the irrigation and aspiration ports of phacoemulsification and irrigation/aspiration hand pieces and accessory reusable tips and tubing with sterile water according to the manufacturer's written IFU

INSTRUMENT CLEANING

before disconnecting the hand piece from the unit.[8] *[2: Moderate Evidence]*

Inadequate flushing of phacoemulsification hand pieces has been associated with TASS.[69] When OV material is allowed to dry on phacoemulsification hand pieces, it is difficult to remove. Flushing immediately after the procedure can help prevent OV material from drying. Flushing the hand piece prevents buildup of OV material inside the hand piece, which is difficult to remove during cleaning.[93]

XI.g. Cleaning products used to clean intraocular instruments should be selected and used in accordance with the instrument manufacturer's written IFU.[8,10] *[2: Moderate Evidence]*

Some IFU for ophthalmic instruments recommend against the use of enzymatic detergents.[69]

In a retrospective analysis of questionnaires and site visits to examine instrument cleaning and processing of extraocular and intraocular products used during cataract surgery, Culter-Peck et al[69] identified common practices associated with TASS. They analyzed 77 questionnaires and 54 site visits; 909 cases of TASS were reported. Use of enzymatic cleaners was reported in 36 questionnaires (47%) and observed at 48 sites (89%). The researchers concluded that the benefit of using enzymatic cleaners to clean ophthalmic instruments had not been established and, in fact, was prohibited in some manufacturers' instructions for specific-use products.

In a randomized controlled trial (RCT) to determine whether enzymatic detergents used to clean ophthalmic instruments could cause TASS, Leder et al[94] randomly assigned rabbits into seven treatment groups to receive intracameral injection of three different doses of enzymatic detergent. Although the enzymatic detergent caused a severe inflammatory response, the response did not include TASS. The researchers concluded that given that patient exposure to an enzymatic detergent would be significantly less than the lowest dose used in the experiment, enzymatic detergent on ophthalmic instruments was not a cause of TASS.

Mamalis and Edelhauser raised concerns about the validity and generalizability of the study conducted by Leder et al[94] in a letter to the editor and stated "there are significant differences in the inflammatory reaction of the rabbit, as well as their response to toxic insults, that make it difficult to extrapolate findings from the rabbit to the human."[93(p651)] They noted that the conclusions of the researchers were inconsistent with the results presented in the study and contended that the results of the study actually provided additional support for the role of enzymatic detergents as a potential cause of TASS.

Following the instrument manufacturer's IFU helps ensure compatibility of the cleaning product with the device. Incorrect selection and incorrect detergent dilution has been associated with TASS.[69]

XI.g.1. After cleaning, ophthalmic instruments should be rinsed with a copious amount of water.[8] *[2: Moderate Evidence]*

Thorough rinsing helps remove residual cleaning product. Detergent residue has been identified as a possible cause of TASS, although studies performed on rabbits have not supported enzymatic detergent residues alone as a cause of TASS.[83,94]

In a review of the literature, Ozcelik et al[83] identified detergent residues/soaps, enzymatic cleaners, inappropriate rinsing, and dried debris and OV material residues as potential causes or risk factors for TASS. However, in an RCT to investigate whether enzymatic detergents used to clean ophthalmic instruments could cause TASS, Leder et al[94] concluded that enzymatic detergent residues alone did not cause TASS. The researchers randomly assigned 35 rabbits into seven treatment groups (ie, low, medium, and high detergent concentration of three detergents, plus a control group of untreated rabbits) and injected their eyes with detergent accordingly. The enzymatic detergents caused a severe but unusual response; however, this response has not been reported in humans.

When the instructions for cleaning are strictly followed, it is possible to remove all detergent.[82,87]

XI.g.2. A final rinse should be performed with sterile distilled or sterile deionized water.[8,69,86] *[2: Moderate Evidence]*

Untreated water may contain endotoxins, which are heat stable and as such will remain biologically active after sterilization and which have been implicated in occurrences of TASS.[70,83,85,86]

Residual enzymes and detergents not rinsed from instruments have been associated with TASS.[8,70,85,86]

XI.g.3. After cleaning, lumens should be rinsed with sterile deionized or distilled water. The rinse fluid should be expelled from the lumen into a drain and not back into the rinse water. Lumens should be dried with medical-grade compressed air.[8,83] *[2: Moderate Evidence]*

Rinsing removes detergent and other residue from the lumens. Expelling the lumen rinse into a drain prevents reuse of the rinse water and prevents recontamination of the lumen with debris that has been rinsed out of the lumen. Compressed air forced through the lumen eliminates moisture that can serve as a medium for microbial growth.

XI.g.4. After manual cleaning, unless contraindicated in the manufacturer's written IFU, instruments should be disinfected by wiping and by rinsing lumens with 70% to 90% alcohol and should be dried before they are packaged for sterilization. *[2: Moderate Evidence]*

Wiping with alcohol disinfects the instruments and renders them safe to handle. Endotoxins are removable with alcohol.[88] Rinsing lumens with alcohol facilitates drying.

XI.h. If an ultrasonic cleaner is used, it should be emptied, cleaned, disinfected, rinsed, and dried at least daily or, preferably, after each use.[10] If not contraindicated by the ultrasonic cleaner manufacturer's written IFU, the chamber should be wiped with 70% to 90% alcohol and dried with a lint-free cloth.[8,69] *[2: Moderate Evidence]*

Inadequately cleaned ultrasonic cleaners and endotoxins have been associated with TASS.[70] Fluid in the ultrasonic cleaner can harbor gram-negative bacteria.[8,69,71,72] Growth of these bacteria can result in the production of endotoxins, which are heat resistant, can survive steam sterilization, and can cause serious consequences for patients.[8,71,72] Alcohol promotes drying, inhibits microbial growth, and can prevent biofilm formation.[67,69]

XI.h.1. Ophthalmic instruments should be thoroughly rinsed after ultrasonic cleaning.[8] A final rinse should be performed with treated water before drying, inspecting, and packaging in preparation for sterilization. *[1: Strong Evidence]*

Adequate rinsing removes the cleaning solution. Residual cleaning products have been implicated in the occurrence of TASS.[69,82]

In an RCT, Tamashiro et al[82] filled 30 reusable 25-gauge injection cannulas with OV material and allowed them to dry for 50 minutes. Cannulas were then presoaked, washed using a high-pressure water jet, backwashed with enzymatic detergent in an ultrasonic cleaner, rinsed with tap water, rinsed with sterile distilled water, dried with compressed filtered air, wrapped in surgical-grade paper, and steam sterilized. After sterilization, the cannulas were tested for cytotoxicity. The results showed that all extracts were noncytotoxic. Six of the cannulas were then immersed in enzymatic detergent and rinsed, and the extracts from these were tested for cytotoxicity. The researchers found that the extracts were not cytotoxic; however, they observed changes in cell morphology and a reduction in cell growth. The researchers concluded that the cleaning protocol had the potential to minimize the occurrence of TASS associated with residues of OV material and enzymatic detergents remaining on ophthalmic instruments.

XI.i. After cleaning and decontamination, instruments that have been in contact with OV material should be inspected for residual OV material under magnification.[8] *[1: Strong Evidence]*

Retained OV material has been associated with TASS.[8,69]

Viscoelastic material is difficult to remove during cleaning, especially if it has been allowed to dry. Inspection under magnification can facilitate detection of residual OV material. Although studies conducted on rabbits showed that OV material alone, even if denatured by steam sterilization, did not cause ocular inflammation, the presence of endotoxin in OV material can cause severe ocular reaction.[95]

Buchen et al[96] conducted an RCT to determine the ocular reactivity of rabbits to bacterial endotoxin contained in an aqueous medium and in a cohesive and dispersive OV material. The researchers found that inflammation occurred after injection of as little as 0.02 endotoxin units in OV material and 0.08 endotoxin units in a phosphate buffered saline.

XI.j. Records should be maintained of all cleaning methods, cleaning solutions, and lot numbers of cleaning solutions used with ophthalmic instruments. *[2: Moderate Evidence]*

Records of cleaning methods and solutions can assist in surveillance efforts[84] and be used to facilitate investigation of any suspected or confirmed cases of TASS.

Recommendation XII

Laryngoscope blades and their handles should be cleaned, decontaminated, dried, and stored in a manner that reduces the risk of exposing patients and personnel to potentially pathogenic microorganisms.

Laryngoscope blades and handles may be a potential source of contamination.[97,98] In a comprehensive integrative review, Negri de Sousa et al[97] identified 77 articles that addressed the laryngoscope blade or handle as a potential source of contamination.[97] Based on the quality of the research, the authors selected 20 articles for further review. In five of the studies, blood was found on the laryngoscope blade. None of the studies that investigated the handles found blood.

In a descriptive study of laryngoscope blades and handles, Phillips and Monaghan[99] found that although none of the blades or handles had visible blood, 13 of 65 blades (20%), and 26 of 65 handles (40%) tested positive for occult blood.

XII.a. After each use, laryngoscope blades should be cleaned and high-level disinfected or sterilized according to the manufacturer's written IFU.[2] *[1: Strong Evidence]*

633

INSTRUMENT CLEANING

Cleaning and disinfection minimizes the risk of pathogen transmission.[2] Semicritical items are those that contact mucus membranes or nonintact skin.[2] Laryngoscope blades are considered semicritical items that require a minimum of high-level disinfection.[2,100]

Jones et al[101] conducted an investigation of an outbreak of *Serratia marcescens* that involved two geographically distinct neonatal intensive care units during a nine-week period. They found that 17 infants were colonized and three developed septicemia, two of whom died. The investigators found that during the outbreak, two infants had been transferred between the two units and two employees worked in both units. Because of a shortage of laryngoscope blades, the blades had been shared without being sterilized between uses. At one of the facilities, *S marcescens* was isolated from a laryngoscope blade and a sample of breast milk. The outbreak isolates were of the identical serotype and phage type as those identified in the outbreak. The investigators concluded that infection prevention measures, including disinfection of laryngoscope blades, were insufficient at these facilities.

Foweraker[102] reported four cases of *Pseudomonas aeruginosa* infection in a pediatric cardiac intensive care unit. They infections were believed to have been transmitted by a single laryngoscope blade disinfected between uses by wiping with alcohol. Sampling of the laryngoscope blade in question revealed *P aeruginosa* of the identical type as a blood culture from one child who died from the infection. The author recommended thorough cleaning and disinfection of blades and handles to reduce the potential for infection.

XII.b. Laryngoscope handles should be cleaned and low-level disinfected after each use and may be high-level disinfected or sterilized according to the manufacturer's written IFU. *[2: Moderate Evidence]*

Laryngoscope handles are classified as noncritical items according to the Spaulding Classification.[2] Noncritical items are those that contact intact skin.[2] According to the Centers for Disease Control and Prevention (CDC), low-level disinfectants are used for noncritical items.[2] Although the laryngoscope handle by itself is a noncritical device, the laryngoscope consists of two parts that are handled concurrently. In a comprehensive, integrative review, Negri de Sousa et al[97] recommended that both parts of the laryngoscope be classified as semicritical.

Laryngoscope handles have a knurled surface (ie, a series of small ridges cut into the metal) to facilitate grip; the rough surface can accumulate bioburden.[97,103] When the laryngoscope blade is folded closed, the tip of the blade is in contact with the handle. Studies have demonstrated the presence of microorganisms on laryngoscope handles.[97,103-105] To date, no studies have demonstrated patient infection as a result of contaminated laryngoscope handles[97]; however, studies have demonstrated the potential for pathogen transmission from the laryngoscope handle to the patient.[103,104]

In a nonexperimental study to identify the extent and nature of contamination of laryngoscope handles considered to be clean and ready for use in the OR, Williams et al[103] cultured 192 laryngoscope handles. The researchers found 99 positive cultures that yielded a total of 128 different microorganisms on the handles.

In a quasi-experimental study, Call et al[104] sampled 60 laryngoscope handles considered to be clean and ready for use in the OR. Samples from 40 handles were sent to the laboratory for aerobic bacterial culture; samples from 20 handles were examined for viral contamination. The researchers found that 30 of the 40 samples sent for bacterial culture (75%) were positive for bacterial contamination, and all 20 of the other handles were negative for viral contamination. The researchers recommended a minimum of low-level disinfection of laryngoscope handles after each use.

Some manufacturer's IFU recommend low-level surface disinfection while others recommend high-level disinfection or sterilization between uses.[106,107]

Recommendations for processing vary within the published literature;[97] however, the Association of Anaesthetists of Great Britain and Ireland suggests that laryngoscope handles do become contaminated with bacteria and blood during use and as such they should be cleaned, disinfected, and sterilized after every use.[100]

Further research is warranted regarding processing protocols and the risk of infection associated with laryngoscope handles.

XII.c. Cleaned and disinfected laryngoscope blades and handles should be packaged and stored in a manner that prevents contamination.[100,107] *[1: Strong Evidence]*

Packaging assists in preventing recontamination of items that have been high-level disinfected. Packaging of laryngoscope blades to prevent recontamination is a CDC recommendation.[2]

XII.c.1. Laryngoscope blades should be stored in individual packages.[107] *[2: Moderate Evidence]*

Storing blades individually minimizes the potential for contaminating multiple blades, which could occur if a contaminated blade is placed back into a package of uncontaminated blades. Individual storage eliminates the need to process multiple blades.[107]

Recommendation XIII

Special precautions should be taken to minimize the risk of transmission of prion diseases from contaminated instruments.

Prions are a unique class of infectious proteins that cause fatal neurological diseases known as transmissible spongiform encephalopathies (TSEs).[63] Examples of prion diseases are Gertsmann-Straussler-Scheinker syndrome, fatal familial insomnia syndrome, and Creutzfeldt-Jakob disease (CJD).[63] Variant Creutzfeldt-Jakob Disease (vCJD) is acquired from cattle with bovine spongiform encephalopathy or "mad cow disease."[63] Transmissible spongiform encephalopathies have been described in a number of animal species.[64] To date, with the exception of cattle, there is no evidence of transmission of TSEs to humans from animals.[63]

Creutzfeldt-Jakob disease has been transmitted iatrogenically through direct inoculation (ie, with contaminated cadaveric human growth hormone), use of contaminated cadaveric dura mater, and use of contaminated medical equipment.[63] Human cadaveric growth hormone has been replaced with growth hormone produced using recombinant DNA technology, and cadaveric dura mater is no longer used in neurosurgeries.[63]

Iatrogenic CJD resulting from use of contaminated medical equipment has been reported in two circumstances: two cases from contaminated electroencephalography electrodes and four suspected cases from contaminated neurosurgical devices[63]; all occurred in Europe during the period from 1952 through 1976.[63] No other cases have been reported of transmission from instruments used in other types of surgeries or since that time.[109]

Prions are resistant to conventional physical and chemical sterilization.[63] Special precautions and protocols are required to inactivate prions.[63,109-112] Instrumentation used for neurosurgery procedures performed on a patient suspected or known to have a prion disease is of particular concern because of the high concentrations of prions in the brain and spinal cord.[110]

XIII.a. A multidisciplinary team that includes infection preventionists, perioperative RNs, sterile processing personnel, surgeons, representatives from the clinical pathology laboratory, and other stakeholders should establish, document, and implement evidence-based policies and procedures to minimize the risk of prion disease transmission.[110] *[2: Moderate Evidence]*

These processes should be based on
- the patient's risk of having a prion disease;
- the level of infectivity of the tissue involved, as defined by the World Health Organization (WHO) *Tables on Infectivity Distribution in Transmissible Spongiform Encephalopathies*[110,113]; and
- the intended use of the medical device.

A defined protocol based on available evidence provides guidance to protect patients and health care workers from prion transmission. Anesthesia professionals, infection preventionists, perioperative team members, risk management personnel, neurosurgeons, and sterile processing personnel are involved when surgery is performed on a patient known or suspected to have a prion disease. A coordinated effort among disciplines is important and may increase the likelihood of developing effective strategies to protect patients and personnel.[110]

Common laboratory methodologies are ineffective in diagnosing prion disease. Diagnosis can be confirmed through neuropathological examinations of brain tissue, usually performed at autopsy. Research to develop additional laboratory techniques for diagnosis is ongoing.[109,114]

The WHO has published clinical diagnostic criteria for CJD.[112] These criteria are used to identify patients at risk of having or developing CJD. Patients at high risk of having or developing prion disease include those with
- progressive dementia consistent with CJD in whom a diagnosis has not been confirmed or ruled out,
- a familial history of a prion disease,
- a history of dura mater transplants, or
- a history of receiving cadaveric-derived pituitary hormone.[63]

Although all prion diseases are infectious, the risk of infection is not the same for all tissue. Based on successful experimental transmission, the risk of infection from tissue types is categorized as high, low, or no risk.[113]
- Tissue from the posterior eye retina or optic nerve, brain, pituitary gland, and spinal cord are categorized as high risk.[113]
- Liver, lung, spleen, kidney, and lymph nodes are categorized as low risk, as are body fluids, blood, and urine.[113,114]

Prions are found in other tissue, and studies to determine whether they can transmit prion disease are ongoing.[111] The definition of high- and low-risk tissue has continued to change.[111] Infectivity in similar tissue can vary according to the type of prion.[111]

Research directed toward understanding tissue infectivity is ongoing.[111] In particular, blood has been studied to determine whether transfusion is a risk factor.[114-119] Four potential cases of vCJD from blood transfusion have been reported.[110,114] The risks associated with having received blood or blood components from a donor with CJD have been studied.[114-119] Although there is no direct evidence of a causal relationship, the long incubation of CJD, as long as 20 years, is a limitation of these studies.[114-119] The risk associated with receipt of blood or blood products from a donor with vCJD is significantly higher than that associated with receipt of blood or blood components from a donor with CJD.[117-119]

INSTRUMENT CLEANING

There are no known cases of prion disease transmission attributable to the reuse of devices contaminated with blood.[115] Because of the long incubation period of CJD and the discovery of prion protein in tonsils, gut, and muscle, the risk of prion contamination may extend to surgeries on tissue not currently listed as high risk, and categories of high-risk tissue may continue to change.[110,111]

XIII.b. Patients should be screened for the risk of prion disease before surgery, and information about patients identified to be at risk should be communicated to personnel who are directly or indirectly involved in the patient's care (eg, anesthesia professional, surgeon, nurses, infection preventionist, clinical pathology laboratory representatives, sterile processing personnel, risk manager, surgery scheduler).[63] *[1: Strong Evidence]*

Preoperative screening provides a mechanism to identify patients at high risk of having a prion disease. Early communication provides an opportunity to plan for the provision of instruments that can be discarded or taken out of service (ie, quarantined) until a definitive diagnosis is made or to identify alternatives to the use of complex instruments.

Early communication is crucial as it provides an opportunity for review of policies and procedures related to sterilization, disinfection, and environmental cleaning. Early communication may allow time to track the instruments used in surgery, and prevent them from being discarded or returned to service without undergoing special disinfection and sterilization procedures.

XIII.c. Single-use surgical drapes, gowns, and supplies should be used whenever possible and discarded after use.[63,112] *[1: Strong Evidence]*

The use and disposal of single-use gowns and supplies eliminates the need to institute special protocols for laundering and may reduce the risk of exposing personnel to prion-contaminated materials.

Although there is no known correlation between contact with work surfaces and attire worn in surgery with transmission of prion diseases, use of single-use gowns and drapes eliminates the need to determine protocols for reusable drapes and gowns potentially contaminated with prions.

Use and incineration of single-use gowns and drapes is recommended in the 1999 *WHO Infection Control Guidelines for Transmissible Spongiform Encephalopathies*.[112] The more current 2010 Society for Healthcare Epidemiology of America (SHEA) "Guideline for disinfection and sterilization of prion-contaminated medical instruments"[63] recommends that masks, gowns, and protective eyewear be worn if mucus membrane or skin exposure to blood, body fluids, or other potentially infectious materials is anticipated and that laundry be managed according to the OSHA bloodborne pathogens standard.[39,63]

XIII.c.1. Noncritical work surfaces should be covered with fluid-resistant drapes, and if contaminated with high-risk tissue, the drape should be discarded as nonregulated medical waste. Regulated waste, (eg, bulk blood, pathologic waste, sharp devices) should be managed according to state regulations.[63] *[1: Strong Evidence]*

Minimizing contamination of surfaces reduces the need for special precautions or protocols for environmental cleaning.

There are no known studies that correlate prion disease transmission with the disposal of waste contaminated with high-risk tissue from a patient known or suspected to have a prion disease. Previous WHO guidelines[63] recommended incineration of potentially prion-contaminated medical waste; however, current guidelines[112] recommend disposal as nonregulated waste.

XIII.d. If the need for an implant is anticipated, only the implant essential for the specific patient should be delivered to the sterile field. Implants opened and handled by scrubbed personnel after the surgery has started should be discarded and not processed for subsequent use. *[4: Benefits Balanced with Harms]*

Discarding potentially contaminated implants eliminates the risk of implanting a prion-contaminated implant into a patient. Implants, such as screws, are often supplied in racks that hold multiple implants. When sets containing multiple implants are open, there is a risk of cross-contamination of implants that are not used. Removing implants that will not be needed for the patient before sterilizing the tray decreases the amount of implant inventory that will need to be discarded.

XIII.e. Reusable instruments used on high-risk tissue of patients suspected of having prion disease should be easy to clean and should tolerate exposure to an extended steam sterilization cycle. *[1: Strong Evidence]*

Depending on the cleaning management before sterilization (eg, cleaning process, cleaning product), extended steam sterilization cycles may not be necessary. However, at the time of this publication and on the basis of current knowledge, an extended cycle steam sterilization is still recommended as the option for sterilization that provides the greatest margin of safety.[63,111]

XIII.f. Instruments used on high-risk tissue of patients at high risk for prion disease should be designed for single use.[63] If single-use instruments are not available, reusable instruments

INSTRUMENT CLEANING

should be limited to those that are easy to clean. The number of instruments used should be kept to a minimum. *[1: Strong Evidence]*

Use of single-use instruments eliminates the need to implement special processing protocols and eliminates the risk of instruments contaminated with prions being used on another patient. Use of single-use instruments also eliminates the risk of exposure of personnel who process instruments.

Successful cleaning is a critical step in processing instruments exposed to high-risk tissue. When instruments are difficult to clean thoroughly, the potential for incomplete cleaning is increased. The challenge to cleaning is reduced when easy-to-clean devices are used.

XIII.f.1. Single-use brain biopsy sets should be used on all patients undergoing brain biopsy. *[2: Moderate Evidence]*

Creutzfeldt-Jakob disease is often definitively diagnosed by brain biopsy, and whether the patient has a prion disease may not be known at the time of surgery.

Until the later stages of CJD, most patients developing a prion disease cannot be identified.[120] Patients undergoing surgery for a brain biopsy are considered to be at high risk for prion disease.[109] Commercial single-use brain biopsy sets are available, or sets can be assembled using instruments at the end of their useful life and discarding them after use.

XIII.f.2. Rigid, as opposed to flexible, neuroendoscopes should be used for patients with known or suspected prion disease. *[4: Benefits Balanced with Harms]*

Flexible neuroendoscopes contain narrow lumens. Narrow lumens are difficult to clean. Neuroendoscopes may not be compatible with the cleaning procedures and extended steam sterilization cycles recommended for items contaminated with prions.

XIII.f.3. Power drills and saws should not be used for patients with known or suspected prion disease. *[1: Strong Evidence]*

Power drills and saws create aerosols and may splatter potentially infectious material. Although there are no reported cases of occupational transmission of prion disease through exposure to aerosols, much about prions and their infectivity is unknown.[63,109,121]

Stitz and Aguzzi[122] reviewed the literature related to prion-containing aerosols and concluded that although not identified as a source of prion transmission in humans, the high rate of prion transmission by way of aerosols in mice suggested that it was advisable to avoid inhaling aerosols from prion-containing materials.

In a series of experiments that tested the cellular and molecular characteristics of prion propagation after aerosol intranasal exposure in mice, Haybaeck et al[123] demonstrated that prions could be transmitted to mice through aerosols. They exposed both immunocompetent and immunodeficient mice to prion aerosols that were produced by using a nebulizing device with prion-contaminated brain homogenates of concentrations ranging from 0.1% to 20%. All mice exposed to infectious aerosols developed clinical mouse scrapie (a form of TSE) or displayed brain tissue indicative of subclinical prion infection. The longer the exposure time, the shorter the incubation time; notably, exposure of only one minute resulted in infection. The researchers concluded that although there have been no reports of prion transmission to humans by aerosols under normal conditions, it remains prudent to minimize exposure to aerosols that may contain prions. They recommended that prion-containing aerosols be considered a potential vector for prion infection.

Power drills are difficult to clean, and the cleaning and sterilization methods recommended to eliminate prion infectivity may damage these instruments.

XIII.f.4. Single-use instruments that have come in contact with high-risk tissue from patients known or suspected to have a prion disease should be discarded.[63] *[1: Strong Evidence]*

Prions are highly resistant to conventional disinfection and sterilization processes.[10,63,111] Discarding these devices eliminates the risk of inadequate prion inactivation.

XIII.g. Reusable instruments that have come in contact with high-risk tissue from patients known or suspected to have a prion disease should be treated in accordance with the most current infection prevention guidelines.[63] *[1: Strong Evidence]*

Reducing infectivity is crucial to providing instruments that are safe to use on patients. When a potentially contaminated device can be cleaned and prion tissue removed, the risk of prion disease transmission is minimized. There is currently no consensus on the best method of managing instruments that are likely to be contaminated with prions. Until recently, the most referenced guidelines for managing prevention of TSEs were the WHO *Infection Control Guidelines for Transmissible Spongiform Encephalopathies*.[112] These were published in 1999 and were based on studies that

- did not incorporate conventional cleaning procedures that reduce protein contamination,
- investigated inactivation using tissue homogenates dried onto carriers, and

INSTRUMENT CLEANING

- investigated inactivation using various strains and concentrations of prions and a variety of tissue.[10,109]

Although they are effective, the WHO guidelines for managing instruments contaminated with prions[112] are impractical and are corrosive to instruments. The more current SHEA "Guideline for disinfection and sterilization of prion-contaminated medical instruments,"[63] published in 2010, reflect research conducted after the WHO publication. These guidelines identify practices that can eliminate prion infectivity with a wide margin of safety.[63]

XIII.g.1. Instruments that cannot be cleaned or require sterilization using low-temperature technologies should not be used or should be discarded.[63] *[1: Strong Evidence]*

Steam sterilization for an extended cycle time is the only sterilization method recommended in national guidelines at this time.[63] Low-temperature sterilization technologies have not been incorporated into recognized guidelines for inactivating prions.

Research into the effectiveness of gaseous hydrogen peroxide for inactivating prions is ongoing. Several studies have demonstrated that hydrogen peroxide vapor and some hydrogen peroxide gas plasma technologies in combination with specific cleaning agents are effective in inactivating prions, and researchers have suggested that sterilization with gaseous hydrogen peroxide protocols will be practical and widely used in the future.[63,124]

In a quasi-experimental study designed to test the effectiveness of a gaseous hydrogen peroxide sterilization process to inactivate prions, Fichet et al[124] contaminated stainless steel wires with prion-infected brain homogenates and then exposed them to gaseous hydrogen peroxide sterilization. Sterilization parameters included a vacuum process at 86° F (30° C) for three or six pulses. The researchers concluded that exposure under these conditions demonstrated that gaseous hydrogen peroxide was effective in inactivating prions.

In a quasi-experimental study to test effectiveness of decontamination methods to inactivate prions, Yan et al[125] contaminated stainless steel wires with prion-infected brain homogenate material and subjected them to a variety of decontamination and sterilization procedures including exposure to gaseous hydrogen peroxide, steam sterilization, sodium hydroxide, enzymatic detergent, enzymatic detergent plus gaseous hydrogen peroxide, peracetic acid, alkaline detergent, alkaline detergent plus orthophthalaldehyde, alkaline detergent plus steam sterilization, and alkaline detergent plus gaseous hydrogen peroxide. The researchers injected the wires into the brains of living hamsters. Successful processing was defined as a total group survival time of 18 months after implantation. After 18 months, only those hamsters incubated with wires reprocessed with an alkaline detergent followed by sterilization with a four injection gaseous hydrogen peroxide cycle showed no clinical signs of prion disease.

In a quasi-experimental study to determine the effectiveness of hydrogen peroxide gas plasma for inactivating animal and human prions, Rogez-Kreuz et al[126] decontaminated prion-contaminated steel wires with combinations of enzymatic or alkaline detergents and gaseous hydrogen peroxide. The researchers found that gaseous hydrogen peroxide decreased the infectivity of the prions; however, its efficacy was dependent on the concentration of the hydrogen peroxide and the systems used to deliver it. Only one specific model of a hydrogen peroxide gas plasma sterilizer was 100% effective in inactivating prions.

XIII.g.2. Instruments should be kept moist until they are cleaned and decontaminated.[63] Instruments may be kept moist by immersion in water, a wet cloth draped over the instruments, or use of a transport gel or foam.[63] *[1: Strong Evidence]*

When prions are allowed to dry on instruments, they become highly resistant to removal.[127-129] Dried films of tissue are more resistant to prion inactivation by steam sterilization than tissue that is kept moist.[63]

Prions are hydrophobic and in the absence of moisture can strongly attach to surfaces, particularly stainless steel.[128] Keeping instruments moist until cleaning and decontamination can help reduce the tenacity of prions to adhere to surfaces.

XIII.g.3. Instruments should be decontaminated in a mechanical washer as soon as possible after use.[63] *[1: Strong Evidence]*

Mechanical washing is preferred because process consistency is more likely than with manual washing, and the mechanical process is more easily monitored. Automation of cleaning helps ensure reproducibility.[74] Mechanical washers employ a validated cycle that is not possible with manual cleaning.

Stainless steel has a high affinity for prion adsorption. The longer prion-contaminated instruments are permitted to dry, the greater the adsorption and the more difficult the prion removal.[128]

XIII.g.4. Cleaning chemicals that have evidence of prionicidal activity and that are compatible with the instruments to be cleaned should be used.[63] *[1: Strong Evidence]*

It is important that product selection decisions take into consideration the combined effect of precleaning, cleaning, disinfection, and sterilization and effectiveness against other infectious diseases and not just the ability to inactivate prions.

The WHO recommendation to soak instruments in 1 N sodium hydroxide (NaOH)[112] is effective at eliminating prion infectivity but, because of incompatibility with most instruments, is impractical. A number of alkaline and enzymatic cleaning agents in combination with steam sterilization have been shown to be effective as well and are compatible with instruments.[63,111]

Some cleaning formulas have a demonstrated ability to remove and inactivate prions.[111,130] However, it has also been shown that some cleaning agents may increase the resistance of prions to subsequent steam sterilization.[111,130] In an investigative study of the effectiveness of innovative physical and chemical methods of prion inactivation, Fichet et al[130] subjected prion-contaminated stainless steel wires to a variety of cleaning chemistries and sterilization technologies. The researchers found that one phenolic formulation increased the resistance of prions to inactivation.

In a quasi-experimental study, McDonnell et al[111] found that cleaning with certain chemical formulations, alkaline formulations in particular, in combination with steam sterilization was an effective prion-decontamination process. The researchers found that low-temperature gaseous hydrogen peroxide sterilization reduced infectivity in both the presence and absence of cleaning.

In an RCT to determine effectiveness of prion inactivation, Schmitt et al[131] subjected prion-contaminated stainless steel wires to either an automated decontamination procedure developed for prion decontamination, or a routine automated alkaline disinfection process used for sterile processing in Germany. The routine procedure included an alkaline wash and thermal disinfection. The specially designed prion decontamination process included an alkaline wash, thermal disinfection, and an oxidizing process using hydrogen peroxide combined with an alkaline detergent. After processing, the researchers implanted the wires into the brains of eight hamsters. The researchers found that the specially designed process was more effective than conventional alkaline cleaning, was as effective as exposure to a steam sterilization process at 273° F (134° C) for two hours, and left no detectable prion infectivity. The researchers also found that although the alkaline cleaning resulted in significant reduction of prion infectivity, it did not eliminate prion infectivity in six of eight animals in which the stainless steel wires were implanted.

XIII.g.5. After decontamination, one of the following three methods recommended by SHEA should be used to steam sterilize instruments exposed to high-risk tissue:
- prevacuum sterilization at 273° F (134° C) for 18 minutes[63,111];
- gravity displacement sterilization at 270° F (132° C) for 60 minutes[63,111]; or
- immersion in 1 N NaOH for 60 minutes, then removal, rinsing with water, and sterilization using one of the cycles noted above (1 N NaOH is a solution of 40 g NaOH in 1 L water).[63,111]

[1: Strong Evidence]

These measures have demonstrated safety and efficacy.[63,111]

The SHEA guidelines state "it is unclear from the published literature which of these options is best for complete inactivation of prions because some studies have revealed excellent but not complete inactivation of the test prions with autoclaving only . . . and the same result for use of NaOH and autoclaving. . . ."[63(p111)]

A fourth option described in the SHEA guidelines is to immerse the contaminated instruments in 1 N NaOH for 60 minutes and heat them in a gravity displacement sterilizer at 250° F (121° C) for 30 minutes, then clean and subject the instruments to routine sterilization.[63] This option is effective for prion inactivation; however, it can damage many devices, especially anodized aluminum-containing devices (depending on the quality and finish of the materials used) and therefore is not recommended by many device manufacturers.[111]

XIII.h. Instruments exposed to high-risk tissue should not be subjected to IUSS.[10,63] *[1: Strong Evidence]*

Steam sterilization cycles for IUSS of surgical instruments are different from those recommended by SHEA for prion inactivation.[63] The steam sterilization cycles recommended by SHEA for instruments exposed to high-risk tissue are supported by prion investigational studies and have been shown to inactivate prions.[63]

XIII.i. Semicritical and critical devices contaminated with low-risk tissue from high-risk patients should be processed using conventional processing procedures.[63] *[1: Strong Evidence]*

INSTRUMENT CLEANING

Instruments contaminated with low-risk tissue are unlikely to transmit infection after processing using conventional protocols because those instruments would not be used in the central nervous system.[63]

The SHEA guidelines make no recommendation regarding processing of devices exposed to low-risk tissue.[63] Studies to determine the risk associated with low-risk tissues are ongoing, and until evidence indicates that special processing protocols are required to prevent transmission of infection, SHEA makes no recommendation. Transmission of infection from low-risk tissue has only been demonstrated in animal studies of direct inoculation into the brain.[63]

XIII.j. Instruments that require special prion processing procedures should be identified in a manner that alerts personnel who handle and process instruments that the instruments are contaminated or potentially contaminated with prions.[10] *[3: Limited Evidence]*

Awareness that instruments are contaminated or potentially contaminated with prions reduces the risk of these instruments being ineffectively processed and subsequently used on other patients.

XIII.j.1. An instrument-tracking process should be used that provides for tracking of surgical instruments used on high-risk tissue (eg, spinal and brain tissue). *[4: Benefits Balanced with Harms]*

Instrument tracking systems identify items used during the procedure and also identify the patient for whom the items were used.

XIII.k. Noncritical environmental surfaces contaminated with high-risk tissue from a patient known or suspected to have a prion disease should be cleaned and then spot decontaminated with a 1:5 or 1:10 dilution of hypochlorite for a contact time of 15 minutes or with 1 N NaOH.[63,132] *[1: Strong Evidence]*

Because there is no Environmental Protection Agency-registered antimicrobial product specifically for prion-contaminated environmental surfaces, a solution of diluted hypochloride or 1 N NaOH is recommended.[63]

No transmission of prion diseases from environmental surfaces, other than devices used in surgery, has been reported. However, current evidence on prion diseases suggests the need for continued research to better explain transmission. It remains prudent to eliminate highly infectious material from OR surfaces that patients and personnel will be in contact with during subsequent surgeries.

XIII.l. Noncritical environmental surfaces contaminated with low-risk tissue should be cleaned using standard disinfection processes.[63] *[1: Strong Evidence]*

Transmission of prion disease from surfaces contaminated with low-risk tissue has not been reported.

XIII.m. When a patient is identified postoperatively as having had a prion disease at the time of surgery, special precautions should be taken. Devices determined to be potentially contaminated with high-risk tissue from the patient should be removed from service and decontaminated according to the most current professional guidelines for prion inactivation.[63] *[1: Strong Evidence]*

Inadequately decontaminated instruments may pose a risk to subsequent patients who have contact with the instruments. The current SHEA Guidelines[63] describe six cases of CJD transmitted by neurosurgical instruments in Europe between 1952 through 1976, demonstrating prion survival of several years. Two of these cases occurred in 1967. These patients developed CJD 15 and 18 months after stereotactic electroencephalographic explorations using electrodes that had been implanted earlier in a patient with CJD and sterilized with 70% alcohol and formaldehyde vapor. Two years later, the electrodes were retrieved and implanted into the brain of a chimpanzee who then developed CJD.[63,64] These classic cases are frequently cited in prion-related articles.[110,116,133,134]

XIII.n. Perioperative personnel who may be exposed to prions should review current research on methods of detecting prion infectivity and decontamination methods and incorporate new evidence into practice.[111] *[2: Moderate Evidence]*

Research related to prion disease, tissue infectivity, potential risks of transmission, and effectiveness of cleaning chemistries and sterilization technologies and cycles is ongoing. Incorporating current, evidence-based knowledge into practice may help minimize risks associated with prions.

Recommendation XIV

Documentation of instrument cleaning and disinfection processes should be maintained.

Documentation provides data for the identification of trends and demonstration of compliance with regulatory requirements and accreditation agency standards.

Effective management and collection of health care information that accurately reflects the patient's care, treatment, and services is a regulatory requirement and accreditation agency standard for both hospitals and ambulatory settings.[135-140]

XIV.a. Cleaning and decontamination documentation should include the
- date,

- time,
- identification of instruments,
- method and verification of cleaning and results of cleaning audits,
- number or identifier of the mechanical instrument washer and results of washer efficacy testing,
- name of the person performing the cleaning and decontamination,
- lot numbers of cleaning agents,
- testing results for insulated instruments,
- disposition of defective equipment, and
- maintenance of cleaning equipment.

[3: Limited Evidence]

Documentation enables traceability in the event of a failure.[10] Records of washer testing provide a source of evidence for review during investigation of clinical issues, including SSIs. Documentation of equipment maintenance provides evidence that equipment has been maintained.

XIV.b. Records should be maintained for a time period specified by the health care organization and in compliance with local, state, and federal regulations.[1,10] *[2: Moderate Evidence]*

Recommendation XV

Perioperative team members with responsibilities for cleaning and care of instruments used in surgery should receive initial and ongoing education and complete competency verification activities related to cleaning and care of surgical instruments.

It is the responsibility of the health care organization to provide initial and ongoing education and to verify the competency of perioperative team members.[141] Initial and ongoing education of perioperative personnel about cleaning and care of instruments facilitates the development of knowledge, skills, and attitudes that affect safe patient care.

Competency verification activities measure individual performance, provide a mechanism for documentation, and help verify that perioperative personnel have an understanding of the principles and processes related to recommended practices for cleaning and care of surgical instruments.

XV.a. Perioperative team members should receive education and complete competency verification activities that address specific knowledge and skills related to cleaning and care of surgical instruments. *[1: Regulatory Requirement]*

Ongoing development of knowledge and skills and documentation of personnel participation is a regulatory requirement and accreditation agency standard for both hospital and ambulatory settings.[135,136,142-144]

XV.a.1. Education regarding cleaning and care of surgical instruments should include
- adherence to manufacturers' IFU,
- methods of cleaning and verification of cleaning,
- types of contamination of medical devices,
- methods of decontamination,
- selection of cleaning chemistries,
- safe use of cleaning chemistries,
- safe use of cleaning equipment,
- how to verify washer cleaning efficacy,
- use of PPE during instrument processing,
- risks and hazards associated with contaminated instruments,
- prions and risks associated with prion-contaminated instruments,
- procedures for decontaminating instruments that are potentially contaminated or known to be contaminated with prions,
- measures to minimize risks of exposure to transmissible pathogens,
- TASS and measures to prevent its occurrence,
- corrective actions to employ in the event of a cleaning failure,
- corrective actions to employ in the event of an equipment or instrument failure,
- new instruments and equipment, and
- evidence-based information about changes in cleaning chemistries and technologies.

[4: Benefits Balanced with Harms]

Recommendation XVI

Policies and procedures for cleaning and care of instruments used in surgery should be developed, reviewed periodically, revised as necessary, and readily available in the practice setting in which they are used.

Policies and procedures assist in the development of patient safety, quality assessment, and performance improvement activities. Policies and procedures also serve as operational guidelines used to minimize patients' risk for injury or complications, standardize practice, direct perioperative personnel, and establish continuous performance improvement programs. Policies and procedures establish authority, responsibility, and accountability within the practice setting.

XVI.a. Policies and procedures regarding cleaning and care of surgical instruments used in surgery should be developed using professional guidelines and validated, written manufacturers' IFU. *[1: Regulatory Requirement]*

Having policies and procedures that guide and support patient care, treatment, and services is a regulatory requirement and an accreditation agency standard for both hospital and ambulatory settings.[135,136,145-148]

XVI.a.1. Policies and procedures related to cleaning and care of surgical instruments should include
- prepurchase evaluation;
- a review of the manufacturer's IFU before purchase or consignment;
- management of loaned instruments, including advance notification, time frame

INSTRUMENT CLEANING

- for delivery and pickup, requirements for and delineation of responsibilities for inventory, and processes for care and handling, cleaning, decontamination, packaging, and sterilization of instruments;
- point-of-use cleaning of instruments;
- transport of contaminated instruments;
- precautions to be taken when handling contaminated instruments;
- precautions to be taken when handling cleaning chemistries;
- processes for cleaning and decontaminating instruments after use in surgery;
- care and handling of accessories and supplies necessary for cleaning and decontaminating contaminated instruments;
- processes for manual and automated cleaning;
- use and care of cleaning equipment and cleaning chemistries;
- requirements for water quality used for cleaning instruments;
- methods for processing ophthalmic instruments;
- design of decontamination areas to accommodate efficient workflow;
- requirements for ventilation, temperature, and humidity of decontamination areas;
- use of PPE in relation to cleaning and decontaminating instruments;
- methods for monitoring cleaning processes and cleaning equipment;
- inspection and testing of instruments to determine cleanliness, integrity, and function;
- preparation of instruments for packaging;
- procedures for managing laryngoscope blades and handles;
- criteria for identification and precautions taken for instruments used on patients with known or suspected prion disease;
- documentation of cleaning;
- education and competency verification;
- maintenance of SDSs;
- procedures for reporting exposure to bloodborne pathogens; and
- procedures for reporting adverse events.

[4: Benefits Balanced with Harms]

Recommendation XVII

The health care organization's quality management program should evaluate the cleaning, decontamination, and care of instruments.

Quality assurance and performance improvement programs can facilitate the identification of problem areas and assist personnel in evaluating and improving the quality of patient care and formulating plans for corrective actions. These programs provide data that may be used to determine whether an individual organization is within benchmark goals and, if not, to identify areas that may require corrective actions. A quality management program provides a mechanism to evaluate effectiveness of processes, compliance with manufacturers' written IFU, sterile processing policies and procedures, and function of equipment.

Collecting data to monitor and improve patient care, treatment, and services is a regulatory requirement and an accreditation agency standard for both hospital and ambulatory settings.[135,136,149-152]

XVII.a. A quality management program should include monitoring of manual and mechanical cleaning. *[2: Moderate Evidence]*

Cleaning is a critical component of instrument processing and can affect the efficacy of a subsequent sterilization processes. Items that have been sterilized after inadequate cleaning processes have caused patient injury.[21-23,153]

XVII.a.1. Mechanical cleaners (eg, washer disinfectors/decontaminators) should be tested for correct function on installation, at least weekly (preferably daily) during routine use, after major repairs, and after significant changes in cleaning parameters (eg, changing cleaning solutions).[10] *[3: Limited Evidence]*

Monitoring washer function provides information about whether the equipment is functioning correctly. Thorough cleaning is dependent on how the equipment is used, how instruments are placed in the machine, and whether the equipment is functioning correctly.

Adequate cleaning is essential to remove or destroy microorganisms and eliminate endotoxins. Testing washer disinfectors/decontaminators on a regular basis verifies that the equipment is functioning correctly or identifies an opportunity for corrective action. Commercial tests to monitor cleaning efficacy of mechanical washer disinfector/decontaminators are available.

XVII.a.2. Manual cleaning should be evaluated using objective measures (eg, chemical reagent tests for detecting clinically relevant soils [eg, protein]) when new types of instruments requiring manual cleaning are processed and periodically at intervals determined by the health care facility. *[4: Benefits Balanced with Harms]*

Manual cleaning is a learned skill and is subject to human error.

XVII.a.3. When verifying the effectiveness of manual cleaning, the instruments most difficult to clean should be used. *[5: No Evidence]*

Using the most difficult instruments to clean provides a robust measure of cleaning effectiveness.

XVII.a.4. Testing should be performed to assess efficacy of cleaning of medical devices. *[1: Strong Evidence]*

INSTRUMENT CLEANING

Currently, there is no single standard of clean, nor is there a standard test soil. Agreement as to what level of residual soil is acceptable after cleaning and what level of residual soil is clinically significant is also lacking.[5,51]

Efficacy of cleaning has traditionally been evaluated visually. Several studies comparing visual analysis with microscopic analysis have demonstrated that visual inspection alone is not sufficient to determine levels of cleanliness.[21,51,77,154] Visual inspection is subjective. In addition, infectious microorganisms and residues are not visible to the naked eye. It is also not possible to visually inspect most lumens. Even under ideal cleaning conditions, instruments may retain debris.[42]

There are, however, a number of tests that can be used to assess cleaning efficiency.[155-158] Qualitative tests usually involve swabbing a device, immersing it in a reagent, and observing for a color change that indicates the presence of organic markers, such as protein or blood.[5,10,82,158] Quantitative tests provide a measure or action limit against which test results are measured. Adenosine tri-phosphate (ATP) bioluminescence is an example of a quantitative test.[155-157] The item to be tested is swabbed to collect ATP, the swab is inserted into a reaction tube, and the ATP on the swab is released using chemicals in the reaction tube. The reaction tube is then inserted into a hand-held luminometer that converts the ATP released from microorganisms or human cells into a light signal, which is measured in relative light units (ie, RLUs). Manufacturers may establish "benchmark cutoffs" for manual cleaning of instruments (eg, flexible endoscopes) that users can employ so that any instrument failing this quantitative cutoff after cleaning is re-cleaned before disinfection/sterilization.[158]

Quantitative testing can be used in a quality monitoring program to observe for trends and to monitor performance of a washer disinfector/decontaminator or of manual processes.[37,154,159] Readings that trend lower indicate improved cleaning, whereas readings that trend higher can indicate a need for improvement.

XVII.b. Instruments and equipment should be maintained and serviced in accordance with the device manufacturer's written IFU. *[2: Moderate Evidence]*

Preventive maintenance requirements or recommendations are what the device manufacturer has determined are necessary to keep instruments and equipment in optimal working order. Providing instruments and equipment in optimal working order is critical to patient safety.[23]

XVII.b.1. Cleaning equipment should be maintained and serviced in accordance with the equipment manufacturer's written IFU, and maintenance and service should be documented. *[4: Benefits Balanced with Harms]*

The manufacturer has determined that the maintenance requirements specified in the manufacturer's written IFU are necessary for optimal performance.

Documentation of maintenance provides a record that can be used to determine compliance with the IFU. Documentation of service can provide information useful in determining whether equipment needs to be replaced.

XVII.b.2. Instruments and cleaning equipment should be serviced by personnel who are qualified to repair the instruments and equipment in need of service. Instrument or equipment service should be documented. *[4: Benefits Balanced with Harms]*

Instruments and cleaning equipment used in surgery are complex. Having qualified personnel service instruments and equipment increases the probability that repair and service will be performed correctly.

Documentation of instrument repairs may help to identify trends in instrument and cleaning equipment damage and define practices that may reduce damage.

XVII.c. Insulated equipment should be tested for current leakage before use and after decontamination. *[4: Benefits Balanced with Harms]*

Testing before use and after decontamination allows a defective device to be replaced before use or sterilization and provides an opportunity for corrective action in advance of the surgical procedure.[25]

XVII.d. Adverse events should be reported and documented according to the health care organization's policy and procedure and should be reviewed for potential opportunities for improvement. *[4: Benefits Balanced with Harms]*
- During investigation of SSIs, the cleaning process and its documentation should be reviewed by infection preventionists, perioperative RNs, and designated sterile processing personnel.
- Near misses (ie, unplanned events that do not result in injury, such as organic or inorganic material discovered in a processed instrument tray) should be investigated and corrective action taken to prevent serious adverse events. Surgical site infection has been documented as a result of inadequate cleaning of surgical instruments.[22,23] Reports of near misses can be used to identify actions that should be taken to

INSTRUMENT CLEANING

prevent actual adverse events and can reveal opportunities for improvement.

Editor's note: *Teflon is a registered trademark of DuPont, Wilmington, DE.*

Glossary

Adsorption: The adhesion of extremely thin layers of molecules to the solid surfaces they contact.

Aerosol: A suspension of fine solid or liquid particles in air.

Borescope: A device used to inspect the inside of an instrument through a small opening or lumen of the instrument.

Cavitation: A process that uses high-frequency sound waves to form microscopic bubbles that become unstable and implode, creating tiny vacuums capable of removing debris from instrument surfaces and crevices.

Cleaning: A process that uses friction, detergent, and water to remove organic debris; the process by which any type of soil, including organic debris, is removed to the extent necessary for further processing or for the intended use. Cleaning removes rather than kills microorganisms.

Creutzfeldt-Jakob disease: A fatal degenerative neurological disease caused by a prion.

Decontamination: Any physical or chemical process that removes or reduces the number of microorganisms or infectious agents and renders reusable medical products safe for handling or disposal. The process by which contaminants are removed, either by hand cleaning or mechanical means, using specific solutions capable of rendering blood and debris harmless and removing them from the surface of an object or instrument.

Distilled water: Water that has been boiled, vaporized, cooled, and condensed to remove impurities.

Electroplating: A process whereby electrical current reduces dissolved metal cations that then form a coating on an electrode, causing a change in the surface properties of a device.

Gross soil: Organic material (eg, blood, tissue, bone) and debris (eg, bone cement) that accumulates on surgical instruments during operative or other invasive procedures.

Homogenate: A tissue that is or has been made homogenous, as by grinding cells into a creamy consistency for laboratory studies. A homogenate usually lacks cell structure.

Hydrophobic: Absence of affinity to water.

Loaned items: Medical devices used in health care facilities that are not owned by the facility.

Lumen: A channel or path through a tubular structure.

Medical-grade compressed air: Air supplied from cylinders, bulk containers, or medical air compressors or reconstituted from oxygen USP and oil-free dry nitrogen NF.

Porosity detector: A high-voltage device designed to find pinholes and flaws in nonconductive coatings. Porosity detectors can only be used to find flaws in coatings when the layer beneath the coating is made of a conductive material.

Product quality assurance testing: A quality assurance process used to verify that a device manufacturer's instructions for sterile processing can be achieved in the health care setting.

Reverse osmosis: A water purifying process whereby water under pressure is passed through a semi-permeable membrane to eliminate impurities.

Toxic anterior segment syndrome (TASS): A complication of ophthalmic surgery involving a severe, noninfectious inflammation of the anterior segment of the eye, caused by various contaminants in solutions, medications, steam, and residue on surgical instruments and supplies.

Transmissible spongiform encephalopathies (TSEs): A fatal prion disease that effects the brain and nervous system. The development of tiny holes in the brain cause it to appear like a sponge, hence the term "spongiform."

Treated water: Water that has been filtered, deionized, distilled, or subjected to reverse osmosis to reduce impurities.

Ultrasonic cleaner: A processing unit that transmits ultrasonic waves through the cleaning solution in a mechanical process known as cavitation. Ultrasonic cleaning is particularly effective in removing soil deposits from hard-to-reach areas.

Validating: A documented procedure performed by manufacturers for obtaining, recording, and interpreting the results required to establish that a process will consistently yield product that complies with predetermined specifications.

Variant Creutzfeldt-Jakob disease (vCJD): A fatal degenerative neurological disease caused by a prion. The human form of bovine spongiform encephalopathy (ie, mad cow disease).

Viscoelastic: A gel injected into the anterior chamber during ophthalmic surgery to maintain the depth of the chamber, protect the corneal endothelium, and stabilize the vitreous.

Washer/decontaminator: A processing unit that, either by use of single or multiple chambers, automatically decontaminates surgical instruments. It employs a cool water rinse, hot water wash, rinse, and drying. An ultrasonic cleaning feature and lubricant rinse may be added.

References

1. Guideline for sterilization. In: *Guidelines for Perioperative Practice*. Denver, CO: AORN, Inc; 2015:665-692. [IVA]

2. *Guideline for Disinfection and Sterilization in Healthcare Facilities*, 2008. Atlanta, GA: Centers for Disease Control and Prevention; 2008. [IVA]

3. Guideline for selection and use of packaging systems for sterilization. In: *Guidelines for Perioperative Practice*. Denver, CO: AORN, Inc; 2015:651-664. [IVA]

4. Guideline for cleaning and processing flexible endoscopes and endoscope accessories. In: *Guidelines for Perioperative Practice*. Denver, CO: AORN, Inc; 2015:589-600. [IVB]

5. *ANSI/AAMI TIR30:2011 A Compendium of Processes, Materials, Test Methods, and Acceptance Criteria for Cleaning Reusable Medical Devices.* Arlington, VA: Association for the Advancement of Medical Instrumentation; 2011. [IVC]

6. *AAMI TIR12: 2010 Designing, Testing, and Labeling Reusable Medical Devices for Reprocessing in Health Care Facilities: a Guide for Medical Device Manufacturers.* Arlington, VA: Association for the Advancement of Medical Instrumentation; 2010. [IVC]

7. Guideline for product selection. In: *Guidelines for Perioperative Practice.* Denver, CO: AORN, Inc; 2015:179-186. [IVB]

8. American Society of Cataract and Refractive Surgery, American Society of Ophthalmic Registered Nurses. Recommended practices for cleaning and sterilizing intraocular surgical instruments. *J Cataract Refract Surg.* 2007;33(6):1095-1100. [IVB]

9. Hensell MG. Instrumentation for robotic surgery. *Perioper Nurs Clin.* 2010;5(1):69-81. [VA]

10. *ANSI/AAMI ST79: Comprehensive Guide to Steam Sterilization and Sterility Assurance In Health Care Facilities.* Arlington, VA: Association for the Advancement of Medical Instrumentation; 2013. [IVC]

11. Meredith SJ, Sjorgen G. Decontamination: back to basics. *J Periop Pract.* 2008;18(7):285-288. [VA]

12. Spry CC, Brooks Tighe SM. Care and handling of surgical instruments. In: Brooks Tighe S, ed. *Instrumentation for the Operating Room: a Photographic Manual.* 8th ed. St Louis, MO: Elsevier/Mosby; 2012:1-2. [VB]

13. Howlin RP, Harrison J, Secker T, Keevil CW. Acquisition of proteinaceous contamination through the handling of surgical instruments by hospital staff in sterile service departments [corrected]. 2009;10(3):106-111. [IA]

14. Seavey R. Reprocessing in the ambulatory surgery setting. *Healthc Purch News.* 2012;36(12):38-41. [VA]

15. Rutala WA, Weber DJ. Disinfection and sterilization: an overview. *Am J Infect Control.* 2013;41(5):S2-S5. [VA]

16. Hercules PA. Instrument readiness: a patient safety issue. *Perioper Nurs Clin.* 2010;5(1):15-25. [VA]

17. Dancer SJ, Stewart M, Coulombe C, Gregori A, Virdi M. Surgical site infections linked to contaminated surgical instruments. *J Hosp Infect.* 2012;81(4):231-238. [VB]

18. Cordero I. Sharpening and tightening surgical scissors. *Comm Eye Health J.* 2011;24(76):44-45. [VB]

19. Goldberg JL. What the perioperative nurse needs to know about cleaning, disinfection, and sterilization. *Perioper Nurs Clin.* 2010;5(3):263-272. [VB]

20. Montero PN, Robinson TN, Weaver JS, Stiegmann GV. Insulation failure in laparoscopic instruments. *Surg Endosc.* 2010;24(2):462-465. [IIIA]

21. Shimono N, Takuma T, Tsuchimochi N, et al. An outbreak of Pseudomonas aeruginosa infections following thoracic surgeries occurring via the contamination of bronchoscopes and an automatic endoscope reprocessor. *J Infect Chemother.* 2008;14(6):418-423. [VA]

22. Tosh PK, Disbot M, Duffy JM, et al. Outbreak of Pseudomonas aeruginosa surgical site infections after arthroscopic procedures: Texas, 2009. *Infect Control Hosp Epidemiol.* 2011;32(12):1179-1186. [IIIA]

23. Parada SA, Grassbaugh JA, Devine JG, Arrington ED. Instrumentation-specific infection after anterior cruciate ligament reconstruction. *Sports Health.* 2009;1(6):481-485. [VA]

24. Yasuhara H, Fukatsu K, Komatsu T, Obayashi T, Saito Y, Uetera Y. Prevention of medical accidents caused by defective surgical instruments. *Surgery.* 2012;151(2):153-161. [IIIA]

25. Saito Y, Kobayashi H, Uetera Y, Yasuhara H, Kajiura T, Okubo T. Microbial contamination of surgical instruments used for laparotomy. *Am J Infect Control.* 2014;42(1):43-47. [IIIC]

26. Espada M, Munoz R, Noble BN, Magrina JF. Insulation failure in robotic and laparoscopic instrumentation: a prospective evaluation. *Am J Obstetr Gynecol.* 2011;205(2):121.e1-121.e5. [IIIA]

27. *Guide to Infection Prevention for Outpatient Settings: Minimum Expectations for Safe Care.* Atlanta, GA: Centers for Disease Control and Prevention; 2011. [IVA]

28. Spry CC. Care and handling of basic surgical instruments. *AORN J.* 2007;86(Suppl 1):S77-S81. [VA]

29. Seavey R. Reducing the risks associated with loaner instrumentation and implants. *AORN J.* 2010;92(3):322-334. [VA]

30. Huter-Kunish GG. Processing loaner instruments in an ambulatory surgery center. *AORN J.* 2009;89(5):861-866. [VA]

31. Duro M. New IAHCSMM loaner instrumentation position paper and policy template. *AORN J.* 2011;94(3):287-289. [VA]

32. IAHCSMM Position Paper on the Management of Loaner Instrumentation. IAHCSMM. http://www.iahcsmm.org/137-resources/news/association-news/association-archives/767-iahcsmm-releases-loaner-instrumentation-position-paper,-sample-policy.html?highlight=WyJsb2FuZXIiLCJpbnN0cnVtZW50YXRpb24iLCJsb2FuZXIgaW5zdHJ1bWVudGF0aW9uIl0=. Accessed September 29, 2014. [IVC]

33. Winthrop TG, Sion BA, Gaines C. Loaner instrumentation: processing the unknown. *AORN J.* 2007;85(3):566-573. [VB]

34. Seavey R. High-level disinfection, sterilization, and antisepsis: current issues in reprocessing medical and surgical instruments. *Am J Infect Control.* 2013;41(5):S111-S117. [VA]

35. McNamara SA. Instrument readiness: an important link to patient safety. [Patient Safety First]. *AORN J.* 2011;93(1):160-164. [VA]

36. Root CW, Kaiser N, Antonucci C. What, how and why: enzymatic instrument cleaning products in healthcare environments. *Healthc Purchasing News.* 2008;32(11):50. [VA]

37. Azizi J, Anderson SG, Murphy S, Pryce S. Uphill grime: process improvement in surgical instrument cleaning. *AORN J.* 2012;96(2):152-162. [IIA]

38. Vickery K, Ngo Q, Zou J, Cossart YE. The effect of multiple cycles of contamination, detergent washing, and disinfection on the development of biofilm in endoscope tubing. *Am J Infect Control.* 2009;37(6):470-475. [IA]

39. Toxic and Hazardous Substances: Bloodborne Pathogens, 29 CFR §1910.1030 (2012). Occupational Safety and Health Administration. http://www.osha.gov/pls/oshaweb/owadisp.show_document?p_table=STANDARDS&pid=10051. Accessed September 23, 2014.

40. Guideline for sharps safety. In: *Guidelines for Perioperative Practice.* Denver, CO: AORN, Inc; 2015:365-388. [IVA]

41. Bruins MJ, Wijshake D, de Vries-van Rossum SV, Klein Overmeen RG, Ruijs GJ. Otitis externa following aural irrigation linked to instruments contaminated with *Pseudomonas aeruginosa.* *J Hosp Infect.* 2013;84(3):222-226. [IIIB]

INSTRUMENT CLEANING

42. Azizi J, Basile RJ. Doubt and proof: the need to verify the cleaning process. *Biomed Instrum Technol.* 2012;Spring(Suppl):49-54. [IIIA]

43. Weber DJ, Rutala WA, Miller MB, Huslage K, Sickbert-Bennett E. Role of hospital surfaces in the transmission of emerging health care-associated pathogens: norovirus, *Clostridium difficile* and Acinetobacter species. *Am J Infect Control.* 2010;38(Suppl 1):S25-S33. [VA]

44. Guideline for prevention of transmissible infections. In: *Guidelines for Perioperative Practice.* Denver, CO: AORN, Inc; 2015:419-451. [IVA]

45. Facility Guidelines Institute, American Society for Healthcare Engineering. *Guidelines for Design and Construction of Hospitals and Outpatient Facilities.* Chicago, IL: American Society for Healthcare Engineering; 2014. [IVC]

46. Guideline for a safe environment of care, part 2. In: *Guidelines for Perioperative Practice.* Denver, CO: AORN, Inc; 2015:265-290. [IVA]

47. Medical services and first aid, 29 CFR §1910.151. Occupational Safety and Health Administration. http://www.gpo.gov/fdsys/granule/CFR-2013-title29-vol5/CFR-2013-title29-vol5-sec1910-151. Accessed September 23, 2014.

48. Guideline for a safe environment of care, part 1. In: *Guidelines for Perioperative Practice.* Denver, CO: AORN, Inc; 2015:239-263. [IVA]

49. *ANSI/ISEA Z358.1-2009: American National Standard for Emergency Eyewash and Shower Equipment.* New York, NY: American National Standards Institute; 2009. [IVC]

50. Alfa MJ, Nemes R. Manual versus automated methods for cleaning reusable accessory devices used for minimally invasive surgical procedures. *J Hosp Infect.* 2004;58(1):50-58. [IA]

51. Alfa MJ, Olson N, Al-Fadhaly A. Cleaning efficacy of medical device washers in North American healthcare facilities. *J Hosp Infect.* 2010;74(2):168-177. [IIIA]

52. Ofstead CL, Wetzler HP, Snyder AK, Horton RA. Endoscope reprocessing methods: a prospective study on the impact of human factors and automation. *Gastroenterol Nurs.* 2010;33(4):304-311. [IIIA]

53. *AAMI TIR34:2007: Water for the Reprocessing of Medical Devices.* Arlington, VA: Association for the Advancement of Medical Instrumentation; 2007. [IVC]

54. American Society of Heating, Refrigerating and Air-Conditioning Engineers. Room design. In: *HVAC Design Manual for Hospitals and Clinics.* 2nd ed. Atlanta, GA: ASHRAE; 2013:151-202. [IVC]

55. Panagopoulou P, Filioti J, Farmaki E, Maloukou A, Roilides E. Filamentous fungi in a tertiary care hospital: environmental surveillance and susceptibility to antifungal drugs. *Infect Control Hosp Epidemiol.* 2007;28(1):60-67. [IIIB]

56. Tang JW. The effect of environmental parameters on the survival of airborne infectious agents. *J R Soc Interface.* 2009;6(Suppl 6):S737-S746. [VB]

57. Thompson KA, Bennett AM, Walker JT. Aerosol survival of Staphylococcus epidermidis. *J Hosp Infect.* 2011;78(3):216-220. [IIIB]

58. Memarzadeh F. Literature review of the effect of temperature and humidity on viruses. *ASHRAE Transactions.* 2012;18(Part I):1049-1060. [VB]

59. *Proper Maintenance of Instruments.* 8th ed. Morfelden-Walldorf, Germany: Arbeitskreis Instrumenten-Aufbereitung [Instrument Working Group]; 2004. [IVC]

60. Harnroongroj T, Leelaporn A, Limsrivanichayakorn S, Kaewdaeng S, Harnroongroj T. Comparison of bacterial count in tap water between first burst and running tap water. *J Med Assoc Thailand.* 2012;95(5):712-715. [IIIC]

61. Enzymatic detergents and contamination control: a guide for instrument reprocessing. Infection Control Today. http://www.infectioncontroltoday.com/articles/2010/06/enzymatic-detergents-and-contamination-control-a.aspx. Accessed September 23, 2014. [VB]

62. Hazard Communication Standard Final Regulatory Text 2012. Occupational Safety and Health Administration. https://www.osha.gov/dsg/hazcom/ghs-final-rule.html. Accessed September 23, 2014.

63. Rutala WA, Weber DJ. Guideline for disinfection and sterilization of prion-contaminated medical instruments. *Infect Control Hosp Epidemiol.* 2010;31(2):107-117. [IVA]

64. Rutala WA, Weber DJ. Creutzfeldt-Jakob disease: recommendations for disinfection and sterilization. *Clin Infect Dis.* 2001;32(9):1348-1356. [IVA]

65. Williamson JE. Brushing up on brush basics. *Healthc Purchasing News.* 2009;33(5):28. [VB]

66. Czyrko C. Ultrasonic cleaners in dental decontamination. *Dent Nurs.* 2012;8(4):210-213. [VB]

67. Kauffman M, Joseph C. Ultrasonic cleaning in the healthcare setting. *Healthc Purchasing News.* 2011;35(1):30-33. [VA]

68. Kohn Rachel. Ultra-sound reasons to use an ultrasonic cleaner for surgical instruments. *Healthc Purchasing News.* 2011;35(5):54-54. [VB]

69. Cutler Peck CM, Brubaker J, Clouser S, Danford C, Edelhauser HE, Mamalis N. Toxic anterior segment syndrome: common causes. *J Cataract Refract Surg.* 2010;36(7):1073-1080. [IIIA]

70. Mamalis N. Toxic anterior segment syndrome update. *J Cataract Refract Surg.* 2010;36(7):1067-1068. [VA]

71. Richburg FA, Reidy JJ, Apple DJ, Olson RJ. Sterile hypopyon secondary to ultrasonic cleaning solution. *J Cataract Refract Surg.* 1986;12(3):248-251. [VA]

72. Kreisler KR, Martin SS, Young CW, Anderson CW, Mamalis N. Postoperative inflammation following cataract extraction caused by bacterial contamination of the cleaning bath detergent. *J Cataract Refract Surg.* 1992;18(1):106-110. [VA]

73. Gilmour D. Instrument integrity and sterility: the perioperative practitioner's responsibilities. *J Perioper Pract.* 2008;18(7):292-296. [VC]

74. Alfa MJ. Monitoring and improving the effectiveness of cleaning medical and surgical devices. *Am J Infect Control.* 2013;41(5 Suppl):S56-S59. [VA]

75. Instrument inspections lead to detections. *Healthc Purchasing News.* 2012;36(11):38-40. [VB]

76. Alfa MJ. The "Pandora's Box" dilemma: reprocessing of implantable screws and plates in orthopedic tray sets. *Biomed Instrum Technol.* 2012;Spring(Suppl):55-59. [VA]

77. Lipscomb IP, Sihota AK, Keevil CW. Comparison between visual analysis and microscope assessment of surgical instrument cleanliness from sterile service departments. *J Hosp Infect.* 2008;68(1):52-58. [IIIB]

78. Ongoing Safety Review of Arthroscopic Shavers. US Food and Drug Administration. http://www.fda.gov/MedicalDevices/Safety/AlertsandNotices/ucm170639.htm. Accessed on Feb 21, 2014.

79. *ANSI/AAMI ST58:2013: 2010 Chemical Sterilization and High-level Disinfection in Health Care Facilities.* Arlington, VA: Association for the Advancement of Medical Instrumentation; 2013. [IVC]

80. *ANSI/AAMI ST41:2008/(R)2012: Ethylene Oxide Sterilization in Health Care Facilities: Safety and*

81. Shunmugam M, Hugkulstone CE, Wong R, Williamson TH. Consecutive toxic anterior segment syndrome in combined phaco-vitrectomy. *Int Ophthalmol.* 2013;33(3):289-290. [VA]

82. Tamashiro NS, Souza RQ, Goncalves CR, et al. Cytotoxicity of cannulas for ophthalmic surgery after cleaning and sterilization: evaluation of the use of enzymatic detergent to remove residual ophthalmic viscosurgical device material. *J Cataract Refract Surg.* 2013;39(6):937-941. [IA]

83. Ozcelik ND, Eltutar K, Bilgin B. Toxic anterior segment syndrome after uncomplicated cataract surgery. *Eur J Ophthalmol.* 2010;20(1):106-114. [VB]

84. FDA collaboration to monitor rare eye condition associated with cataract surgery [FDA News Release]. US Food and Drug Administration. http://www.fda.gov/NewsEvents/Newsroom/PressAnnouncements/ucm284239.htm. Accessed on September 23, 2014. [VB]

85. Bodnar Z, Clouser S, Mamalis N. Toxic anterior segment syndrome: update on the most common causes. *J Cataract Refract Surg.* 2012;38(11):1902-1910. [IIIA]

86. Mamalis N, Edelhauser HF, Dawson DG, Chew J, LeBoyer RM, Werner L. Toxic anterior segment syndrome. *J Cataract Refract Surg.* 2006;32(2):324-333. [VA]

87. McCormick PJ, Kaiser JJ, Schoene MJ, et al. Ophthalmic viscoelastic devices as a cleaning challenge. *Biomed Instrum Technol.* 2013;47(4):347-355. [IIA]

88. Maier P, Birnbaum F, Bohringer D, Reinhard T. Toxic anterior segment syndrome following penetrating keratoplasty. *Arch Ophthalmol.* 2008;126(12):1677-1681. [VA]

89. Mathys KC, Cohen KL, Bagnell CR. Identification of unknown intraocular material after cataract surgery: evaluation of a potential cause of toxic anterior segment syndrome. *J Cataract Refract Surg.* 2008;34(3):465-469. [VB]

90. Providing safe surgical instruments: factors to consider. Infection Control Today. http://www.infectioncontroltoday.com/articles/2008/04/providing-safe-surgical-instruments-factors-to-co.aspx. Accessed September 23, 2014. [VB]

91. Hellinger WC, Hasan SA, Bacalis LP, et al. Outbreak of toxic anterior segment syndrome following cataract surgery associated with impurities in autoclave steam moisture. *Infect Control Hosp Epidemiol.* 2006;27(3):294-298. [VA]

92. Ayaki M, Shimada K, Yaguchi S, Koide R, Iwasawa A. Corneal and conjunctival toxicity of disinfectants—assessing safety for use with ophthalmic surgical instruments. *Regul Toxicol Pharmacol.* 2007;48(3):292-295. [IB]

93. Mamalis N, Edelhauser HF. Enzymatic detergents and toxic anterior segment syndrome. *Ophthalmology.* 2013;120(3):651-652. [VA]

94. Leder HA, Goodkin M, Buchen SY, et al. An investigation of enzymatic detergents as a potential cause of toxic anterior segment syndrome. *Ophthalmology.* 2012;119(7):e30-e35. [IB]

95. Buchen SY, Calogero D, Tarver ME, Hilmantel G, Tang X, Eydelman MB. Evaluation of intraocular reactivity to organic contaminants of ophthalmic devices in a rabbit model. *Ophthalmology.* 2012;119(7):e24-e29. [IB]

96. Buchen SY, Calogero D, Hilmantel G, Eydelman MB. Rabbit ocular reactivity to bacterial endotoxin contained in aqueous solution and ophthalmic viscosurgical devices. *Ophthalmology.* 2012;119(7):e4-e10. [IA]

97. Negri de Sousa AC, Levy CE, Freitas MI. Laryngoscope blades and handles as sources of cross-infection: an integrative review. *J Hosp Infect.* 2013;83(4):269-275. [VA]

98. Simmons SA. Laryngoscope handles: a potential for infection. *AANA J.* 2000;68(3):233-236. [IIA]

99. Phillips RA, Monaghan WP. Incidence of visible and occult blood on laryngoscope blades and handles. *AANA J.* 1997;65(3):241-246. [IIIC]

100. Tablan OC, Anderson LJ, Besser R, et al. Guidelines for preventing health-care–associated pneumonia, 2003: recommendations of CDC and the Healthcare Infection Control Practices Advisory Committee. *MMWR Recomm Rep.* 2004;53(RR-3):1-36. [IVA]

101. Jones BL, Gorman LJ, Simpson J, et al. An outbreak of Serratia marcescens in two neonatal intensive care units. *J Hosp Infect.* 2000;46(4):314-319. [VB]

102. Foweraker JE. The laryngoscope as a potential source of cross-infection. *J Hosp Infect.* 1995;29(4):315-316. [VC]

103. Williams D, Dingley J, Jones C, Berry N. Contamination of laryngoscope handles. *J Hosp Infect.* 2010;74(2):123-128. [IIIB]

104. Call TR, Auerbach FJ, Riddell SW, et al. Nosocomial contamination of laryngoscope handles: challenging current guidelines. *Anesth Analg.* 2009;109(2):479-483. [IIA]

105. Howell V, Thoppil A, Young H, Sharma S, Blunt M, Young P. Chlorhexidine to maintain cleanliness of laryngoscope handles: an audit and laboratory study. *Eur J Anaesthesiol.* 2013;30(5):216-221. [IIIB]

106. Rosing J. What's needed for reprocessing, storage of laryngoscope blades? *OR Manager.* 2011;27(12):15. [VC]

107. Standards FAQs details: laryngoscopes—blades and handles—how to clean, disinfect and store these devices. The Joint Commission. http://www.jointcommission.org/mobile/standards_information/jcfaqdetails.aspx?StandardsFAQId=508&StandardsFAQChapterId=69. Accessed September 23, 2014. [VB]

108. Association of Anaesthetists of Great Britain and Ireland. Infection control in anaesthesia. *Anaesthesia.* 2008;63(9):1027-1036. [IVA]

109. Thomas JG, Chenoweth CE, Sullivan SE. Iatrogenic Creutzfeldt-Jakob disease via surgical instruments. *J Clin Neurosci.* 2013;20(9):1207-1212. [VA]

110. McDonnell G. Prion disease transmission: can we apply standard precautions to prevent or reduce risks? *J Perioper Pract.* 2008;18(7):98-304. [VA]

111. McDonnell G, Dehen C, Perrin A, et al. Cleaning, disinfection and sterilization of surface prion contamination. *J Hosp Infect.* 2013;85(4):268-273. [IIA]

112. *WHO Infection Control Guidelines for Transmissible Spongiform Encephalopathies.* Report of a WHO consultation, Geneva, Switzerland, 23-26 March 1999. World Health Organization. http://www.who.int/csr/resources/publications/bse/WHO_CDS_CSR_APH_2000_3/en/. Accessed September 23, 2014. [IVB]

113. *WHO Tables on Tissue Infectivity Distribution in Transmissible Spongiform Encephalopathies.* Geneva, Switzerland: WHO Press; 2010. [IVA]

114. Barrenetxea G. Iatrogenic prion diseases in humans: an update. *Eur J Obstetr Gynecol Reproduct Biol.* 2012;165(2):165-169. [VB]

115. Henson M, Ireton M, Mortensen JE. Prions: a brief overview. *Amt Events.* 2013;30(2):72-84. [VA]

116. Blattler T. Implications of prion diseases for neurosurgery. *Neurosurg Rev.* 2002;25(4):195-203. [VA]

117. Dorsey K, Zou S, Schonberger LB, et al. Lack of evidence of transfusion transmission of Creutzfeldt-Jakob

disease in a US surveillance study. *Transfusion.* 2009;49(5):977-984. [IIIA]

118. Puopolo M, Ladogana A, Vetrugno V, Pocchiari M. Transmission of sporadic Creutzfeldt-Jakob disease by blood transfusion: risk factor or possible biases. *Transfusion.* 2011;51(7):1556-1566. [IIIC]

119. Molesworth AM, Mackenzie J, Everington D, Knight RS, Will RG. Sporadic Creutzfeldt-Jakob disease and risk of blood transfusion in the United Kingdom. *Transfusion.* 2011;51(8):1872-1873. [IIIC]

120. McDonnell Gerald. Prion diseases and device reprocessing: a time gone or a time bomb? *Br J Neurosci Nurs.* 2013;9(5):229-233. [VA]

121. Alcalde-Cabero E, Almazan-Isla J, Brandel J-P, et al. Health professions and risk of sporadic Creutzfeldt-Jakob disease, 1965 to 2010. *Euro Surveill.* 2012;17(15):pii-20144. http://www.eurosurveillance.org/ViewArticle.aspx?ArticleId=20144. Accessed October 1, 2014. [VA]

122. Stitz L, Aguzzi A. Aerosols: an underestimated vehicle for transmission of prion diseases? *Prion.* 2011;5(3):138-141. [VA]

123. Haybaeck J, Heikenwalder M, Klevenz B, et al. Aerosols transmit prions to immunocompetent and immunodeficient mice. *PLoS Pathog.* 2011;7(1):e1001257. [IIB]

124. Fichet G, Antloga K, Comoy E, Deslys JP, McDonnell G. Prion inactivation using a new gaseous hydrogen peroxide sterilisation process. *J Hosp Infect.* 2007;67(3):278-286. [IIB]

125. Yan ZX, Stitz L, Heeg P, Pfaff E, Roth K. Infectivity of prion protein bound to stainless steel wires: a model for testing decontamination procedures for transmissible spongiform encephalopathies. *Infect Control Hosp Epidemiol.* 2004;25(4):280-283. [IIB]

126. Rogez-Kreuz C, Yousfi R, Soufflet C, et al. Inactivation of animal and human prions by hydrogen peroxide gas plasma sterilization. *Infect Control Hosp Epidemiol.* 2009;30(8):769-777. [IIB]

127. Hesp JR, Poolman TM, Budge C, et al. Thermostable adenylate kinase technology: a new process indicator and its use as a validation tool for the reprocessing of surgical instruments. *J Hosp Infect.* 2010;74(2):137-143. [IA]

128. Secker TJ, Hervé R, Keevil CW. Adsorption of prion and tissue proteins to surgical stainless steel surfaces and the efficacy of decontamination following dry and wet storage conditions. *J Hosp Infect.* 2011;78(4):251-255. [IIB]

129. Lipscomb IP, Pinchin H, Collin R, Keevil CW. Effect of drying time, ambient temperature and pre-soaks on prion-infected tissue contamination levels on surgical stainless steel: concerns over prolonged transportation of instruments from theatre to central sterile service departments. *J Hosp Infect.* 2007;65(1):72-77. [IA]

130. Fichet G, Comoy E, Duval C, et al. Novel methods for disinfection of prion-contaminated medical devices. *Lancet.* 2004;364(9433):521-526. [IIB]

131. Schmitt A, Westner IM, Reznicek L, Michels W, Mitteregger G, Kretzschmar HA. Automated decontamination of surface-adherent prions. *J Hosp Infect.* 2010;76(1):74-79. [IA]

132. Lehmann S, Pastore M, Rogez-Kreuz C, et al. New hospital disinfection processes for both conventional and prion infectious agents compatible with thermosensitive medical equipment. *J Hosp Infect.* 2009;72(4):342-350. [IA]

133. Belay ED, Blase JM, Sehulster LA, Maddox RB, Schonberger L. Management of neurosurgical instruments and patients exposed to Creutzfeldt-Jakob disease. *Infect Control Hosp Epidemiol.* 2013;34(12):1272-1280. [VA]

134. Bernoulli C, Siegfried J, Baumgartner G, et al. Danger of accidental person-to-person transmission of Creutzfeldt-Jakob disease by surgery. *Lancet.* 1977;209(8009):478-479. [VB]

135. *State Operations Manual Appendix A—Survey Protocol, Regulations and Interpretive Guidelines for Hospitals. Rev. 105; 3/21/14.* Washington, DC: Department of Health and Human Services, Centers for Medicare & Medicaid; 2014.

136. *State Operations Manual Appendix L: Guidance for Surveyors: Ambulatory Surgical Centers. Rev. 99; 1/31/14.* Washington, DC: Department of Health and Human Services, Centers for Medicare & Medicaid; 2014.

137. RC.01.01.01: The hospital maintains complete and accurate medical records for each individual patient. In: *Hospital Accreditation Standards 2014.* 2014 ed. Oakbrook Terrace, IL: Joint Commission Resources; 2014.

138. RC.01.01.01: The organization maintains complete and accurate clinical records. In: *Standards for Ambulatory Care 2014: Standards, Elements of Performance, Scoring, Accreditation Polices.* Oakbrook Terrace, IL: Joint Commission Resources; 2014.

139. MS.16: Medical record maintenance. In: *NIAHO Interpretive Guidelines and Surveyor Guidance. 10.1* ed. Milford, OH: DNV Healthcare Inc; 2012: 2029.

140. Clinical records and health information. In: *2014 Accreditation Handbook for Ambulatory Health Care.* Skokie, IL: Accreditation Association for Ambulatory Health Care; 2014:37-39.

141. Standards of perioperative nursing practice. In: *Perioperative Standards and Recommended Practices.* Denver, CO: AORN, Inc; 2014:3-42. [IVB]

142. HR.01.05.03: Staff participate in ongoing education and training. In: *Comprehensive Accreditation Manual: CAMH for Hospitals.* 2014 ed. Oakbrook Terrace, IL: Joint Commission Resources; 2014.

143. HR.01.05.03: Staff participate in ongoing education and training. In: *Comprehensive Accreditation Manual: CAMAC for Ambulatory Care.* 2014 ed. Oakbrook Terrace, IL: Joint Commission Resources; 2014.

144. MS.10: Continuing education. In: *NIAHO Interpretive Guidelines and Surveyor Guidance. 10.1 ed.* Milford, OH: DNV Healthcare Inc; 2012:24.

145. LD.04.01.07: The hospital has policies and procedures that guide and support patient care, treatment, and services. In: *Hospital Accreditation Standards 2014.* 2014 ed. Oakbrook Terrace, IL: Joint Commission Resources; 2014.

146. LD.04.01.07: The organization has policies and procedures that guide and support patient care, treatment, or services. In: *Standards for Ambulatory Care 2014: Standards, Elements of Performance, Scoring, Accreditation Polices.* Oakbrook Terrace, IL: Joint Commission Resources; 2014.

147. SS.1: Organization. In: *NIAHO Interpretive Guidelines and Surveyor Guidance. 10.1 ed.* Milford, OH: DNV Healthcare Inc; 2012:70-71.

148. Governance. In: *2014 Accreditation Handbook for Ambulatory Health Care.* Skokie, IL: Accreditation Association for Ambulatory Health Care; 2014:19-26.

149. PI.03.01.01: The hospital improves performance on an ongoing basis. In: *Hospital Accreditation Standards 2014.* 2014 ed. Oakbrook Terrace, IL: Joint Commission Resources; 2014.

150. PI.03.01.01: The organization improves performance. In: *Standards for Ambulatory Care 2014: Standards, Elements of Performance, Scoring, Accreditation*

Polices. Oakbrook Terrace, IL: Joint Commission Resources; 2014.

151. Quality management and improvement. In: *2014 Accreditation Handbook for Ambulatory Health Care*. Skokie, IL: Accreditation Association for Ambulatory Health Care; 2014:32-36.

152. Quality management system. In: *NIAHO Interpretive Guidelines and Surveyor Guidance. 10.1 ed.* Milford, OH: DNV Healthcare Inc; 2012:10-16.

153. Xia Y, Lu C, Zhao J, et al. A bronchofiberoscopy-associated outbreak of multidrug-resistant *Acinetobacter baumannii* in an intensive care unit in Beijing, China. *BMC Infect Dis.* 2012;Dec12:335. [VB]

154. Heathcote R, Stadelmann B. Measuring of ATP bioluminescence as a means of assessing washer disinfector performance and potentially as a means of validating the decontamination process. *Healthc Infect.* 2009;14(4):147-151. [IIIB]

155. Alfa MJ, Fatima I, Olson N. The adenosine triphosphate test is a rapid and reliable audit tool to assess manual cleaning adequacy of flexible endoscope channels. *Am J Infect Control.* 2013;41(3):249-253. [IIIA]

156. Shama G, Malik DJ. The uses and abuses of rapid bioluminescence-based ATP assays. *Int J Hyg Environ Health.* 2013;216(2):115-125. [VA]

157. Anderson RE, Young V, Stewart M, Robertson C, Dancer SJ. Cleanliness audit of clinical surfaces and equipment: who cleans what? *J Hosp Infect.* 2011;78(3):178-181. [IIIB]

158. Alfa MJ, Olson N, DeGagné P, Simner PJ. Development and validation of rapid use scope test strips to determine the efficacy of manual cleaning for flexible endoscope channels. *Am J Infect Control.* 2012;40(9):860-865. [IA]

159. Jagrosse D, Bommarito M, Stahl JB. Monitoring the cleaning of surgical instruments with an ATP detection system. *Am J Infect Control.* 2012;40(5):e90-e91. [IIIC]

Acknowledgements

Lead Author
Cynthia Spry, MA, MS, RN, CNOR(E), CBSPDT
Independent Consultant
New York, New York

Contributing Author
Ramona L. Conner, MSN, RN, CNOR
Manager, Standards and Guidelines
AORN Nursing Department
Denver, Colorado

The authors and AORN thank Michelle Alfa, PhD, FCCM, Winnipeg, MB, Canada; Jane Rothrock, PhD, RN, CNOR, FAAN, Professor and Director, Perioperative Programs, Delaware County Community College, Media, PA; Paula Berrett, BS, CRCST, Intermountain Healthcare Urban South Region CP Manager, Utah Valley Regional Medical Center, Provo, Utah; Antonia Hughes, MA, BSN, RN, CNOR, Perioperative Education Specialist, Baltimore Washington Medical Center, Glen Burnie, MD; George D. Allen, PhD, RN, CNOR, CIC, Director of Infection Control, Downstate Medical Center, Fresh Meadows, NY, for their assistance in developing this guideline.

Publication History

Originally published February 1988, *AORN Journal*. Revised March 1992.

Revised November 1996; published January 1997, *AORN Journal*.

Reformatted July 2000.

Revised November 2001; published March 2002, *AORN Journal*.

Revised 2007; published in *Perioperative Standards and Recommended Practices*, 2008 edition.

Minor editing revisions made to omit PNDS codes; reformatted September 2012 for publication in *Perioperative Standards and Recommended Practices*, 2013 edition.

Revised September 2014 for online publication in *Perioperative Standards and Recommended Practices*.

Minor editing revisions made in November 2014 for publication in *Guidelines for Perioperative Practice*, 2015 edition.

INSTRUMENT CLEANING

STERILIZATION AND DISINFECTION

GUIDELINE FOR SELECTION AND USE OF PACKAGING SYSTEMS FOR STERILIZATION

The Guideline for Selection and Use of Packaging Systems for Sterilization has been approved by the AORN Recommended Practices Advisory Board. It was presented as proposed recommendations for comments by members and others. The guideline is effective November 15, 2013. The recommendations in the guideline are intended to be achievable and represent what is believed to be an optimal level of practice. Policies and procedures will reflect variations in practice settings and/or clinical situations that determine the degree to which the guideline can be implemented. AORN recognizes the many diverse settings in which perioperative nurses practice; therefore, this guideline is adaptable to all areas where operative and other invasive procedures may be performed.

Purpose

This document provides guidance to perioperative personnel for evaluating, selecting, and using packaging systems and for packaging the items to be sterilized and subsequently used in the perioperative setting. Packaging systems should permit sterilization of the contents within the package, protect the integrity of the sterilized contents, prevent contamination of the contents until the package is opened for use, and permit the aseptic delivery of the contents to the sterile field. Packaging systems include woven fabrics, nonwoven materials, paper-plastic pouches, Tyvek®-plastic pouches, plastic-plastic pouches, and containment devices (eg, sterilization containers, instrument cases, cassettes, organizing trays) composed of a variety of materials. This guideline does not include recommendations for cleaning contaminated instruments, loading a sterilizer, or sterilization. The reader should refer to the AORN Guideline for Cleaning and Care of Surgical Instruments[1] and Guideline for Sterilization.[2]

Evidence Review

A medical librarian conducted a systematic literature search of the databases MEDLINE®, CINAHL®, Scopus®, and Cochrane Database of Systematic Reviews for meta-analyses, randomized and nonrandomized trials and studies, systematic and nonsystematic reviews, and opinion documents and letters. Search terms included *surgical equipment, surgical instruments, dental instruments, organizing tray, instrument set, loaner instrument, medical packaging, product packaging, device packaging, product labeling, packaging material, sterilization container, rigid container, instrument case, instrument cassette, packaging system, reusable pack, pouch, heat sealer, sequential wrapping, plastics, textiles, fabrics, Mylar, Tyvek, Kraft, olefin, paper, polypropylene, polypropene, barrier integrity, barrier system, barrier properties, sterility maintenance cover, sterilization, flash sterilization, immediate use sterilization, infection control, microbial colony count, cross infection, equipment contamination, humidity, steam, condensation, equipment reuse, single-use, event-related, time-related, time-dependent, event-dependent, outdating, monitoring, quality control, materials testing, indicators and reagents, package integrity, equipment failure, safety management, hospital central supply, sterile processing,* and *hospital purchasing.*

The lead author and the medical librarian identified and obtained relevant guidelines from government agencies, other professional organizations, and standards-setting bodies. The lead author assessed additional professional literature, including some that was cited in other articles provided to the author. The initial search was confined to the years 2005 to 2012 and limited to English-language articles. The time restriction was not applied in subsequent searches. The librarian also established continuing alerts on the topics included in this guideline and provided relevant results to the lead author. The majority of research regarding packaging was related to shelf life and was conducted more than 10 years ago when facilities were transitioning from time-related shelf life to event-related shelf life. Articles addressing other aspects of packaging were quite limited. It is evident from the literature search that there is a need for additional research on all aspects of packaging for sterilization.

Articles identified by the search were provided to a doctorally prepared evidence appraiser and to the lead author for evaluation. Articles were critically appraised using the Johns Hopkins Evidence-Based Practice Model and the Research or Non-Research Evidence-Appraisal Tools as appropriate. The articles were independently evaluated and appraised according to the strength and quality of the evidence. Each article was then assigned an appraisal score as agreed upon by the researcher and the lead author. The appraisal score is noted in brackets after each reference citation, as applicable.

The collective evidence supporting each intervention within a specific recommendation was summarized and used to rate the strength of the evidence using the AORN Evidence Rating Model. Factors considered in review of the collective evidence were the quality of the research, quantity of similar studies on a given topic, and consistency of results supporting a recommendation. The evidence rating is noted in brackets after each intervention.

Editor's note: MEDLINE is a registered trademark of the US National Library of Medicine's Medical

PACKAGING SYSTEMS

Literature Analysis and Retrieval System, Bethesda, MD. CINAHL, Cumulative Index to Nursing and Allied Health Literature, is a registered trademark of EBSCO Industries, Birmingham, AL. Scopus is a registered trademark of Elsevier B.V., Amsterdam, Netherlands. Tyvek is a registered trademark of DuPont, Wilmington, DE. Mylar is a registered trademark of DuPont Tejin Films, Chester, VA.

Recommendation I

Packaging systems and packaging materials should be evaluated before purchase and use.[3]

When packaging systems are compatible with the sterilization method and equipment, the probability is increased that sterility can be achieved and maintained until use of the packaged items.[4-6]

I.a. Packaging systems should
- have US Food and Drug Administration (FDA) clearance for performance claims for intended use;
- be suitable for the items being sterilized;
- include a manufacturer's instructions for use (IFU);
- be free of toxic ingredients;
- be odor free;
- be low linting;
- be large enough to permit equal distribution of the contents;
- be easy to use for personnel who prepare, transport, and/or open the package;
- permit secure and complete closure of items;
- permit sealing that is tamper-evident;
- permit identification of the contents before opening;
- allow adequate air removal;
- allow sterilant penetration and direct contact with the item(s) and surfaces;
- allow removal of the sterilant;
- be resistant to tears and punctures;
- protect contents from physical damage;
- maintain sterility of the contents until opened;
- permit aseptic delivery of the contents to the sterile field (eg, minimal wrap memory, easy removal of lids from rigid sterilization containers);
- have a favorable cost-benefit ratio; and
- be free of restrictive waste-disposal regulatory requirements.[3,7,8]

[3: Limited Evidence]

I.a.1. Prepurchase evaluation of packaging systems should include consideration of the environmental impact of the product throughout its life cycle.[5,9-12]

Estimates of the amount of waste generated by health care facilities vary, with some estimates as high as 4 billion pounds annually. Much of that waste is generated in the operating room and consists of packaging and disposable supplies.[13,14] Some experts suggest that use of environmentally responsible packaging results in cost savings.[13,15]

I.b. Before selecting a packaging system, purchasers should evaluate and verify the performance of the packaging system and materials in the environment in which they will be used to determine whether conditions for sterilization, shelf life, transport, storage, and handling can be met.[3] *[3: Limited Evidence]*

I.b.1. Prepurchase evaluation of packaging materials should determine
- FDA clearance for performance claims for intended use;
- ability to verify the manufacturer's IFU through facility product testing;
- barrier effectiveness;
- compatibility with the intended sterilization method(s) and cycles used within the facility;
- biocompatibility;
- availability of an external chemical indicator (CI);
- durability;
- useful product life (including all components);
- requirements for tracking use;
- method for tracking use;
- method for labeling;
- ability of the seal to maintain package integrity;
- requirements for disassembly, laundering, or cleaning requirements;
- maintenance requirements;
- storage requirements;
- ease of use;
- weight;
- available sizes;
- ease of transport;
- ease of aseptic presentation;
- environmental impact; and
- cost-effectiveness.

I.c. Manufacturers' IFU should be evaluated to verify that the packaging system and packaging material are intended for use with both the method(s) of sterilization and the specific equipment to be used.[3] *[3: Limited Evidence]*

Packaging manufacturers' IFU provide information that identifies correct use with the intended sterilization method(s) and equipment.

I.c.1. The manufacturer's validation information should be reviewed and evaluated before purchase.

Validation information may include items such as sterilant penetration, resistance to tears and punctures, barrier performance, use with extended steam sterilization cycles, sterility maintenance, and shelf life.[3,7,16,17]

I.d. Prepurchase product testing should be performed if the packaging represents a major change in packaging type (eg, a change from using woven to using nonwoven materials, a change from using nonwoven materials to using rigid sterilization containers).[3] *[3: Limited Evidence]*

Product testing is used to verify that adherence to the device manufacturer's instructions for sterilization is achievable in the health care setting.

I.d.1. Product testing should include
- evaluation of sterilization efficacy by placing biological indicators (BIs) and CIs inside a variety of sets and packages to be processed (eg, basin sets, instrument sets);
- placement of BIs and CIs within the package in the areas that present the greatest challenge to sterilant contact (medical device and packaging manufacturers may be able to assist in identifying challenging areas);
- moisture assessment;
- documentation of product testing activities to include the date of the test, a description of the package and contents, the location of BIs and CIs within the test package, and test results; and
- reprocessing of the product before use.[3]

Recommendation II

Packaging systems should be compatible with the specific sterilization method for which they will be used.

The interaction among packaging systems, medical devices, and sterilizer technologies is complex. Not all packaging systems are suitable for all methods of sterilization.

II.a. Packaging systems for steam sterilization should permit steam penetration and adequate drying.[3] *[3: Limited Evidence]*

Attention to steam penetration and drying decreases the possibility that steam sterilization efficacy will be adversely affected by humidity; elevation; packaging material; package contents; load; position of items within the sterilizer; size, weight, and density of the pack or rigid sterilization container; and other parameters of the sterilization cycle.[3]

II.b. Packaging systems for ethylene oxide (EO) should
- be permeable to EO and moisture;
- permit aeration;
- include recommendations for aeration time and parameters; and
- be specified by the packaging manufacturer as for use in EO sterilization.[18]

[3: Limited Evidence]

Woven, nonwoven, and peel-pouch packages and some rigid sterilization container systems can be permeated by EO and do not impede rapid aeration of the contents. However, some packaging materials can retain EO residuals, making them difficult to aerate. Woven materials may absorb a large amount of relative humidity that is needed for EO sterilization.[18]

Sufficient humidity helps maintain adequate hydration of microorganisms, thereby increasing their susceptibility to destruction by EO.[18]

II.c. Packaging systems used for low-temperature hydrogen peroxide gas plasma sterilization and low-temperature hydrogen peroxide vapor sterilization systems should
- allow hydrogen peroxide sterilants to penetrate packaging materials,
- be compatible (ie, nondegradable, nonabsorbable) with the designated sterilization process, and
- be constructed of a material recommended by the sterilizer manufacturer.

[3: Limited Evidence]

Sterilization methods that use low-temperature hydrogen peroxide gas plasma or low-temperature hydrogen peroxide vapor are affected by absorbable packaging materials (eg, cellulose-based packaging material, textile wrappers, paper-plastic pouches, porous wrap). Absorption of the sterilant (ie, hydrogen peroxide) by paper-plastic pouches or porous wrap has been shown to adversely affect the sterilization process.[19]

II.c.1. Written documentation of the acceptability of use of low-temperature hydrogen peroxide gas plasma sterilization or low-temperature hydrogen peroxide vapor sterilization systems with specific containment devices should be obtained from the device and sterilizer manufacturers. Only containment devices validated for use in hydrogen peroxide gas plasma or hydrogen peroxide vapor should be used.

II.c.2. If a rigid sterilization container that requires a filter is used, the filter should be made of noncellulose material.

Not all rigid sterilization containers and their accessories are compatible with low-temperature hydrogen peroxide gas plasma or low-temperature hydrogen peroxide vapor.

II.d. Packaging systems for ozone sterilization should
- allow ozone to penetrate packaging materials,
- be compatible (ie, nondegradable, nonabsorbable) with the designated sterilization process, and
- be constructed of a material recommended by the sterilizer manufacturer.[19]

[3: Limited Evidence]

Use of packaging systems that are intended for use in ozone sterilizers facilitates compatibility with the ozone sterilization process.[19]

PACKAGING SYSTEMS

Recommendation III

Packaging materials should be processed and stored in a way that maintains the qualities required for sterilization.

Some manufacturers of packaging materials may specify environmental storage condition requirements for their product. Temperature and humidity equilibrium may be necessary to permit adequate sterilant penetration and to avoid superheating. Wrap material that is too dry and stored in areas of low humidity may lead to superheating and sterilization failure.[3,20]

III.a. Reusable woven textiles should be laundered after every use to maintain hydration. *[3: Limited Evidence]*

Resterilization without relaundering may lead to superheating and could create a deterrent to sterilization. Overdrying, heat pressing (eg, ironing), and storage in areas of low humidity may lead to superheating and sterilization failure. In addition, when woven textiles are not rehydrated after sterilization and/or if repeated sterilization is attempted, the textiles may absorb the available moisture present in the steam, thereby possibly creating a dry or superheated steam effect.[3]

III.b. Packaging materials should be stored at room temperature and at a relative humidity that is in accordance with the packaging manufacturer's IFU.[3] *[3: Limited Evidence]*

III.c. Wrapping materials labeled for single-use should be discarded after one sterilization cycle.[21] *[1: Strong Evidence]*

Products labeled as single-use or disposable are intended for one use and are not intended to be reprocessed.[22]

III.c.1. Single-use packaging materials can be recycled if the product is suitable for recycling.[10-14]

III.d. The shelf life of a packaged sterile item should be considered event-related.[2,3] *[1: Strong Evidence]*

The sterility of an item does not change with the passage of time, but may be affected by particular events (eg, amount of handling) or environmental conditions (eg, humidity).[2,3,21]

In a randomized controlled trial, researchers assessed the sterility of 700 porcelain cylinders sterilized in four different packaging materials (125 each of cotton serge fabric, crepe paper, nonwoven wrap, and peel pouches) and then stored for up to six months. The external package was deliberately contaminated with *Serratia marcescens*. No growth of the test microorganisms was identified inside the packages in any of the storage intervals (ie, seven, 14, 28, 90, and 180 days).[23]

In another randomized controlled trial that examined the effect of time on the sterile integrity of single-sealed peel pouches, double-sealed pouches, linen-wrapped devices, and double-linen wrapped trays, a total of 600 sterile packages were studied. A control group of 60 packages was sent for analysis of microbial contamination immediately after sterilization. The remaining 540 sterilized packages were stored at randomly selected storage sites. Samples were tested for microbial contamination at one, three, six, and 12 months. Results showed a nonstatistically significant effect of time on the odds of a nonsterility event.[24]

Recommendation IV

Items to be sterilized should be packaged in a manner that facilitates sterilization and provides for an aseptic presentation of the package contents. Packaging should be used according to the packaging manufacturer's and sterilizer manufacturer's written IFU.

Incorrect packaging may prevent sterilization from occurring. Inappropriate handling can lead to loss of package integrity. Incorrect packaging can make aseptic delivery of the contents to the sterile field difficult or impossible.

IV.a. Packaging materials, including filters for rigid sterilization container systems, should be inspected for defects and extraneous matter before use.[3] Packaging materials with defects should not be used.[4] *[1: Strong Evidence]*

Defective packaging materials can permit migration of pathogens into the package. In an observational study to determine susceptibility of packaging materials to bacterial transmission, nails ranging in size from 1.1 mm to 10.0 mm that were contaminated with three colonies of skin flora were used to make holes in 90 samples of a polypropylene wrap. Results showed bacterial transmission occurred through the entire range of holes.[25]

IV.b. The size of the wrapping material should be selected to achieve adequate coverage of the item(s) being packaged. The item(s) should be wrapped securely to prevent gapping, billowing, or formation of air pockets.[3] *[3: Limited Evidence]*

Gapping, billowing, or air pockets may prevent sterilant contact with the surface of the device or allow penetration of contaminants into the package.[3]

IV.c. Items to be sterilized should be positioned within packages to allow sterilant contact with all surfaces.[3] *[3: Limited Evidence]*

Sterilant contact is necessary for sterilization to be achieved.

IV.d. The total weight of instrument containment devices, including the contents, should not exceed 25 lb.[3,26,27] *[2: Moderate Evidence]*

Instrument sets weighing more than 25 lb are known to be difficult to dry without lengthy drying times and present an increased risk of ergonomic injury to health care personnel.[3,27]

IV.e. Instruments composed of more than one part that can be disassembled should be disassembled unless the manufacturer's written and validated IFU specifies that disassembly is not required.[3] *[3: Limited Evidence]*

Sterilization of assembled instruments can prevent exposure of some areas of the device to the sterilant.[3]

IV.f. Items to be sterilized that have concave or convex surfaces that create potential for water retention should be positioned within packages in a manner that prevents those surfaces from retaining water.[3,4] *[1: Strong Evidence]*

Preventing water retention can help avoid the occurrence of wet packs and sterilization failure.

IV.g. Towels placed within instrument sets should be lint-free, freshly laundered, and thoroughly rinsed by a health care-accredited laundry facility. *[3: Limited Evidence]*

Adequate rinsing reduces the risk of leaving chemical residues that could be transferred from the towels to instruments.[28] Lint left on sterile instruments may be transferred to the surgical wound and may cause a foreign-body reaction.

IV.h. Items to be sterilized should be placed in the package or tray in an open or unlocked position. *[3: Limited Evidence]*

The open or unlocked position facilitates sterilant contact of all surfaces of the item.[3]

IV.h.1. Racks or stringers designed and intended for sterilization can be used to maintain instruments in their open position.[3]

IV.i. Packaging should be performed in a manner that facilitates maintenance of sterility and aseptic presentation of the contents. Sequential wrapping with two single wraps or single wrapping with a doubled-bonded wrap may be used. *[2: Moderate Evidence]*

Sequential wrapping using two nonwoven, disposable, barrier-type wrappers provides a tortuous pathway to impede microbial migration and permits ease of presentation to the sterile field without compromising sterility.

A fused or double-bonded, disposable, nonwoven single wrapper used according to the manufacturer's IFU provides a bacterial barrier comparable to the sequential double wrap.[7] In one study conducted during a five-month period, 200 packs wrapped in two FDA-cleared and manufacturer-validated barrier-type wrappers were compared with 200 packs wrapped in a single FDA-cleared and manufacturer-validated double-bonded, nonwoven wrapper to determine whether the risk of contamination was greater with either method. Results indicated that use of a single double-bonded wrapper was not associated with a greater risk of contamination. A statistically significant reduction in time required to wrap was identified with use of the single double-bonded, disposable, nonwoven wrapper.[12]

IV.j. The health care organization should weigh the risks and benefits of placing a nonvalidated product (ie, count sheet) in instrument trays against the need for inventory control and instrument count procedures. *[4: Benefits Balanced with Harms]*

Although there are no known reports of adverse events related to sterilized count sheets, there is limited research regarding the safety of toners or various papers subjected to any sterilization method. Chemicals used in the manufacturing of paper and toner inks pose a theoretical risk of reaction in some sensitized individuals.

A literature search related to cytotoxicity of count sheets yielded only one study. This limited controlled study, employing commonly used inks and paper under extremely exaggerated conditions, found that label and toner inks transferred to instruments during sterilization were not cytotoxic.[29] Results from this study are not generalizable and definitive conclusions regarding the safety of all count papers and all inks used in count sheets placed within sterilized instrument sets is not possible.

Recommendation V

Chemical indicators specific to the sterilization method selected should be used with each package.[2]

Chemical indicators are used to verify that one or more of the conditions necessary for sterilization have been achieved within each package. External and internal CIs do not verify sterility of the contents.[3,4]

V.a. A CI should be placed on the outside and inside of every package to be processed unless the internal indicator is readable through the package material.[3,4] *[1: Strong Evidence]*

External CIs are used to verify that the package has been exposed to the sterilization process. External indicators are intended to differentiate processed packages from unprocessed packages.

Internal CIs are used to verify that the sterilant has reached the contents of the package and that critical variables of the sterilization process have been met. The number of critical process variables that are monitored with an internal indicator is dependent on the specific type of internal indicator that is used.

V.a.1. A class I CI (ie, process indicator) should be placed externally. Examples of process indicators are indicator tape and indicator labels.

PACKAGING SYSTEMS

V.a.2. A class III CI (ie, single-parameter indicator), class IV CI (ie, multiparameter indicator), class V CI (ie, integrating indicator), or class VI CI (ie, emulating indicator) should be placed internally.

V.a.3. More than one CI may be required for multi-layered trays and should be placed according to the tray manufacturer's IFU.

V.a.4. The CI manufacturer's written instructions for storage, use, and expiration date should be followed.[3]

V.b. Chemical indicators should be placed in an area within the package that presents a challenge for air removal and sterilant contact. When there is a question concerning the appropriate number and placement of internal CIs, the CI manufacturer, the device manufacturer, and the containment device manufacturer should be consulted for additional information.[2,3] *[3: Limited Evidence]*

The number and placement of internal CIs may be affected by the contents of the package, the configuration of the items within the set, and the packaging or containment device.

Recommendation VI

Reusable woven packaging materials should be inspected and monitored throughout the life of the product.

Multiple launderings and processings will eventually diminish the protective barrier of the material.

VI.a. Textiles should be inspected on a light table for defects (eg, holes, tears, worn spots). Small defects can be repaired using a vulcanized patch; the number of repairs should be kept to a minimum.[3] *[3: Limited Evidence]*

Vulcanized patches do not permit penetration of most sterilants. Keeping the quantity and concentration of patches to a minimum may decrease the risk of compromised penetration of the sterilant.

A search for published literature on the patching of textiles intended for use as a sterilization wrap did not result in any articles that identified the number or placement of patches that could prevent or compromise sterilization of the package contents.

VI.a.1. All woven reusable textiles should be de-linted after washing and before packaging.

VI.a.2. When there is a question about the suitability of a woven wrap, it should be discarded. Defects should not be sewn.

Sewing increases the number of holes in the textile into which microbes can enter.

VI.b. A method should be established to monitor, control, and determine the useful life of reprocessed woven materials. This should include the number of sterilization processes and washing cycles that may occur while maintaining the acceptable barrier quality of the material.[30] *[3: Limited Evidence]*

The barrier qualities of woven materials are diminished by repeated laundering and sterilization cycles. Processes to evaluate material quality after each use are needed to determine suitability for continued use.

VI.b.1. If a printed area (eg, grid system) for marking the number of uses is available on the woven textile, the printed area should be marked each time the item is used. When the grid is full, the item should be removed from service.[30]

VI.b.2. The manufacturer's IFU should be followed for the suggested number of reprocessings.[30]

Recommendation VII

Peel pouches (ie, paper-plastic, Tyvek, Mylar) should be used according to manufacturers' written IFU.[3]

Manufacturers' IFU provide steps that the manufacturers have determined should be followed to achieve and maintain sterility of the package contents.

VII.a. Peel pouches should be used only for small, lightweight, low-profile items (eg, one or two clamps, scissors). Heavy devices, such as drills and weighted vaginal speculums, should not be packaged in peel pouches.[3] *[3: Limited Evidence]*

Heavy or sharp items may compromise the package seal.

VII.b. Peel pouches should not be used within wrapped sets or containment devices unless the pouch manufacturer can supply documented validation for this practice.[3] *[3: Limited Evidence]*

The impervious plastic side of a peel pouch in contact with devices within sets may prevent sterilant from contacting the devices.[3]

VII.c. Double pouching (ie, placing the item within one pouch and then placing this pouch inside another) should not be performed without written instructions from the pouch manufacturer indicating that this practice has been validated and the pouch in question has been cleared by the FDA for this purpose.[3] *[3: Limited Evidence]*

Sterilization validation studies performed by the manufacturer provide confirmation that the pouch will perform as intended when two pouches are used in a single package.

VII.d. Unless otherwise specified in the manufacturer's IFU, when double pouching is used,
- the inner pouch should fit within the outer pouch without folding,[3] and
- the inner pouch should face in the same direction as the outer pouch (ie, plastic or

Mylar faces plastic or Mylar, and paper or Tyvek faces paper or Tyvek).[3]
[3: Limited Evidence]

Folding the inner pouch may entrap air and inhibit sterilant contact.[18]

The plastic side of the pouch is impervious to sterilant penetration. The paper side of the pouch permits sterilant penetration. Facing the inner pouch in the same direction as the outer pouch results in paper-to-paper contact through which the sterilant can penetrate. If the paper side of the inner pouch is in contact with the plastic side of the outer pouch, penetration of the sterilant through the paper side of the inner pouch is prevented.[3]

VII.e. When loading the sterilizer, peel pouches should be placed on edge and spaced to permit sterilant contact and drying.[3] *[3: Limited Evidence]*

Separation of pouch packages facilitates sterilant contact with all surfaces of each package.

VII.e.1. Racks designed and intended for sterilization that separate and hold all the pouches in a vertical position can be used to position peel pouches.

VII.f. Peel pouches should be labeled according to the pouch manufacturer's IFU. Labels should be placed on the plastic side of the pouch.[3] *[3: Limited Evidence]*

Writing or placing a label on the paper side of the pouch may compromise the barrier properties by causing damage to the package.[3]

VII.f.1. A marker with nontoxic ink may be used for writing on the plastic side of the pouch.

Use of a nontoxic ink will prevent toxins from being deposited on the package contents. The force of writing with a ballpoint pen or a pencil may cause perforation of the pouch.[3]

Recommendation VIII

A rigid sterilization container should be used, cleaned, inspected, repaired, and maintained according to the manufacturer's written IFU.

Rigid sterilization container design and materials may affect compatibility with the sterilization process (eg, penetration of the sterilant, release of the sterilant and moisture). Directions related to the method of sterilization may vary by manufacturer.

VIII.a. The recommended sterilization method and cycle exposure times for each rigid sterilization container system should be provided by and obtained from the manufacturer.[3] *[3: Limited Evidence]*

Manufacturers of rigid sterilization containers with FDA clearance have validated that their containers will permit sterilization using specific sterilization methods and cycle exposure times.

VIII.a.1. Sterilization efficacy and drying effectiveness of rigid sterilization containers should be evaluated before initial use as well as periodically, according to the manufacturer's written IFU.[3]

Rigid sterilization container systems vary widely in design, mechanics, and construction. Such variables affect the performance of the containers and their compatibility with sterilization methods.

Health care personnel are responsible for ensuring that rigid sterilization container systems are suitable for proposed sterilization uses and are compatible with existing sterilizers.

VIII.b. Before placing cassettes or organizing trays within rigid sterilization containers, users should refer to the containment device or organizing tray manufacturer's IFU to determine whether this practice is acceptable and/or consult with the rigid sterilization container manufacturer and the device manufacturer to determine whether this practice is acceptable.[3] *[3: Limited Evidence]*

Some device manufacturers provide specifications that should be met to ensure sterilization efficacy when cassettes or organizing trays are used within rigid sterilization containers.

VIII.c. The integrity of the rigid container should be inspected after each use. Inspections should include that
- the mating surfaces and edges of the container and lid are free of dents and chips;
- the lid and container fit together properly and securely;
- the filter retention mechanisms and fasteners are secure and not distorted or burred;
- the latching mechanisms are functioning as they should;
- the handles are in working order;
- the integrity of the filter media is not compromised;
- the gaskets are pliable, securely fastened, and without breaks or cuts; and
- the valves are in working order.

[3: Limited Evidence]

Improperly maintained valves, worn gaskets, dents, or other damage may compromise both the integrity of the container and the ability of the container to maintain sterility.[3]

VIII.c.1. Single-use or reusable filters and valve systems should be secured and in proper working order before sterilization. Filter plates should be examined for integrity before and after the sterilization process. Only intact filters should be used. If the filter is damp, dislodged, or has holes, tears, or punctures, the contents should be considered unsterile.

PACKAGING SYSTEMS

VIII.c.2. Damaged items should be removed from service and repaired or replaced.

VIII.d. Rigid sterilization containers should be cleaned after each use.[3] For proper cleaning, all components (eg, filter retention plates) should be disassembled unless otherwise specified in the manufacturer's IFU. *[3: Limited Evidence]*

Retained debris on container surfaces and components can inhibit sterilant contact.

VIII.e. Additional materials (eg, silicone mats, towels) should not be placed within rigid sterilization containers unless the container manufacturer has provided directions for their use.[3] *[3: Limited Evidence]*

Adding materials to the container in a manner that is not in accordance with the manufacturer's IFU may inhibit sterilization and the performance of the container.

VIII.f. Before devices are placed within rigid sterilization containers, the manufacturer's IFU should be consulted to determine limitations related to density of materials, weight, and distribution of contents.[3] *[3: Limited Evidence]*

Following the manufacturer's requirements for density of materials and weight and distribution of contents will facilitate sterilization and optimize the performance of the container.

Recommendation IX

Packages to be sterilized should be labeled.

Accurate labeling provides identification of the package contents as well as information that enables tracking of the sterilizer, sterilization cycle, personnel involved in the sterilization process, and the patient for whom the items were used.[2]

IX.a. Packages should be labeled before sterilization. Package labels should include
- the sterilizer number or unique identifier if more than one sterilizer is in use;
- the cycle or load number[2,3];
- the date of sterilization[2];
- a description of the package contents (eg, major abdominal set, Kerrison rongeur, Kleppinger bipolar forceps); and
- identification of the assembler.

[2: Moderate Evidence]

Package label information allows items to be identified or retrieved in the event of a sterilization processing error or equipment malfunction.[3]

IX.b. Package labels should be visible and remain securely fixed to the package throughout processing, storage, and distribution to the point of use.[3] *[3: Limited Evidence]*

Visible and secure packaging labels are necessary for verification of package contents and tracking of sterilization cycles and personnel involved in the sterilization process.

IX.c. When a marker is used to enter label information, the ink should be nontoxic, nonbleeding, and indelible.[3] *[3: Limited Evidence]*

Using nontoxic, nonbleeding ink may help to prevent toxic deposits on or in sterile packages. Using indelible ink may help to prevent loss of labeling information.[3]

IX.c.1. Writing should be entered on the indicator tape or affixed label of wrapped packages or on the plastic side of peel pouches, and not on the packaging material.[3]

Writing on the wrapper or on the paper side of peel pouches may damage the package and compromise its barrier function.[3]

Recommendation X

Perioperative team members with responsibilities for selection and/or use of packaging systems should receive initial and ongoing education and competency verification on their understanding of selection and use of packaging systems.

It is the responsibility of the health care organization to provide initial and ongoing education and to verify the competency of perioperative team members.[5]

Initial and ongoing education of perioperative personnel about selection and use of packaging systems facilitates the development of knowledge, skills, and attitudes that affect safe patient care.

Periodic education programs provide the opportunity to reinforce principles of packaging and packaging systems evaluation and may be used to introduce relevant new equipment and practices.

Competency verification measures individual performance, provides a mechanism for documentation, and may verify that perioperative personnel have an understanding of the principles and processes related to selection and use of packaging systems.[31-35]

X.a. Perioperative team members should receive education and complete competency verification activities that address specific knowledge and skills related to selection and use of packaging systems. *[1: Regulatory Requirement]*

Ongoing development of knowledge and skills and documentation of personnel participation are regulatory and accreditation requirements for both hospital and ambulatory settings.[36-46]

X.a.1. Education regarding selection and use of packaging systems should include
- adhering to manufacturers' IFU,
- safe use of packaging systems,
- risks and potential hazards associated with packaging,
- measures to minimize risk,
- product testing,
- corrective actions to employ in the event of a failure of the packaging system, and
- new information about changes in packaging technology and its compatibility

with sterilization equipment and processes.

X.b. Relative to the selection and use of packaging systems, the perioperative registered nurse (RN) should
- participate in ongoing educational activities[5];
- identify personal learning needs[5];
- seek experiences to acquire, maintain, and augment personal knowledge and skills proficiency[5];
- share knowledge and skills[5];
- communicate pertinent information to perioperative team members[5];
- contribute to a healthy work environment by using appropriate and courteous verbal and nonverbal communication techniques[5]; and
- develop and implement conflict resolution skills to manage difficult behavior, promote positive working relationships, and advocate for patient safety.[5]

[2: Moderate Evidence]

Education, collegiality, and collaboration are standards of perioperative nursing and a primary responsibility of the RN who practices in the perioperative setting.[5,47]

Recommendation XI

Policies and procedures for selection and use of packaging systems should be developed, reviewed periodically, revised as necessary, and readily available in the practice setting in which they are used.

Policies and procedures assist in the development of patient safety, quality assessment, and performance activities. Policies and procedures also serve as operational guidelines used to minimize patient risk of injury or complications, standardize practice, direct perioperative personnel, and establish continuous performance improvement programs. Policies and procedures establish authority, responsibility, and accountability within the practice setting.

XI.a. Policies and procedures regarding the selection and use of packaging systems should be developed. *[1: Regulatory Requirement]*

Having policies and procedures that guide and support patient care, treatment, and services is a regulatory and accrediting agency requirement for both hospital and ambulatory settings.[36,37,41,42,48-50]

XI.a.1. Policies and procedures regarding selection and use of packaging systems should include
- prepurchase evaluation;
- assembly of devices within packaging systems;
- weight limitations;
- product testing;
- labeling;
- placement and positioning of packages within the sterilizer;
- storage requirements pre- and post-sterilization;
- shelf life;
- use of internal and external sterilization monitors;
- wrapping requirements and technique;
- use of peel pouches; and
- maintenance of packaging materials, peel pouches, rigid container systems, and heat sealers.

Recommendation XII

Perioperative personnel should participate in a variety of quality assurance and performance improvement activities that are consistent with the health care organization's plan to improve understanding of and compliance with the principles and processes of selection and use of packaging systems.

Quality assurance and performance improvement programs assist in evaluating and improving the quality of packaging items to be sterilized for operative and other invasive procedures. Quality assurance programs provide information used to determine whether packaging practices are in compliance with recognized standards and to identify areas that may require corrective action.

XII.a. The health care organization should establish quality assurance and performance improvement programs to monitor the workplace environment and practices associated with selection and use of packaging systems.[2,3] *[3: Limited Evidence]*

Monitoring the packaging processes allows results to be compared against a predetermined level of quality. Reviewing the findings provides information for identifying problems and trends that can be used to improve practice.[2]

XII.b. Performance improvement activities for selection and use of packaging systems should include monitoring personnel for understanding of the principles and processes of selection and use of packaging systems. *[1: Regulatory Requirement]*

Collecting data to monitor and improve patient care, treatment, and services is a regulatory and accrediting agency requirement for both hospital and ambulatory settings.[36,37,40,51-55]

XII.b.1. Process monitoring for activities related to selection and use of packaging systems should include monitoring compliance with policies and procedures for the following:
- using packaging systems and their IFU;
- verifying the compatibility of packaging systems with sterilization processes;
- storing packaging materials;
- assembling, handling, and packaging wrapped, pouched, and containerized items;
- labeling packages for sterilization;
- determining event-related sterility;
- product testing; and

659

PACKAGING SYSTEMS

- investigating wet packs.

XII.b.2. The quality assurance and performance improvement program for selection and use of packaging systems should include
- periodically reviewing and evaluating activities to verify compliance or to identify the need for improvement,
- identifying corrective actions directed toward improvement priorities, and
- taking additional actions when improvement is not achieved or sustained.

Reviewing and evaluating quality assurance and performance improvement activities helps to identify failure points that contribute to errors in the use of packaging systems and helps define actions for improvement and increased competency.

Taking corrective actions may improve patient safety by enhancing understanding of the principles of and compliance with the processes for selection and use of packaging systems.

XII.c. Quality assurance testing of packaging systems and related equipment (eg, heat sealers) should be performed before initial use as well as periodically, according to the manufacturers' written IFU.[3] *[3: Limited Evidence]*

Packaging systems and related equipment vary in design, mechanics, and construction. These variables affect the performance and compatibility of packaging systems with sterilization methods.[2,3]

XII.c.1. The packaging system manufacturer should be consulted to determine the areas within the package that present the greatest challenge.[2]

XII.c.2. Testing and monitoring of heat seal equipment should be performed in accordance with the manufacturer's IFU.

XII.c.3. During periodic product quality assurance testing of packaging systems, sterilization efficacy and drying effectiveness should be evaluated for each sterilizer and cycle used.[2]

Health care organizations are responsible for obtaining and maintaining manufacturers' documentation of methodology and performance testing for packaging systems.[2]

Health care personnel are responsible for ensuring that packaging systems are suitable for proposed sterilization uses and compatible with existing sterilizers.[2]

XII.d. Product testing should be performed whenever there is a major change in packaging systems, such as a change from using wrapping materials to using rigid sterilization containers, or when there are changes to materials, tray configuration, or content density.[2,3]

Two types of tests should be performed:

- Biological indicators and CIs/integrators/emulating indicators should be placed inside a set, tray, or pack being tested. The set should be run in a full load and the indicators evaluated for pass or fail results.[3]
- After steam sterilization, the package should be inspected for any moisture on the outside and/or on its contents (ie, a wet pack).[3]

[3: Limited Evidence]

Product testing verifies the ability to achieve a sterile, dry package and contents in the health care facility.[3]

XII.e. The occurrence of wet packs should be investigated and resolved.

Internal or external moisture has the potential to compromise the integrity of the barrier material and the sterility of the contents. Moisture present inside the package after steam sterilization is indicative of problems with the packaging or the sterilization process.[3] *[3: Limited Evidence]*

XII.e.1. Measures to resolve wet packs should include an evaluation of the
- package weight, density, and configuration;
- packaging materials and methods used;
- load contents and configuration;
- placement of the package on the sterilizer cart;
- compliance with the manufacturer's recommendations for containers, instruments, and wrappers;
- process of removal of the load from the sterilizer after sterilization;
- conditions (eg, temperature, humidity) in the cooldown area;
- location of air-conditioning vents in the cooldown area; and
- water and steam quality.[3,21,56]

Sterilizer performance, utility supply, and steam quality issues may require evaluation by engineering personnel or the sterilizer manufacturer representative.[56]

XII.f. Perioperative RNs should participate in ongoing quality assurance and performance improvement activities related to selection and use of packaging systems by
- identifying processes that are important for quality monitoring (eg, weight of containment devices not exceeding 25 lb),
- developing strategies for compliance,
- establishing benchmarks to evaluate quality indicators,
- collecting data related to levels of performance and quality indicators,
- evaluating practice based on the cumulative data collected,
- taking action to improve compliance, and
- assessing the effectiveness of the actions taken.

[2: Moderate Evidence]

Participating in ongoing quality assurance and performance improvement activities is a standard of perioperative nursing and a primary responsibility of the RN who is engaged in practice in the perioperative setting.[5]

Glossary

Chemical indicators: Devices used to monitor exposure to one or more sterilization parameters.
- *Class I:* Process indicator that demonstrates that the package has been exposed to the sterilization process to distinguish between processed and unprocessed packages.
- *Class II:* Process indicator that is used for a specific purpose, such as the dynamic air removal test (Bowie-Dick test).
- *Class III:* A single-parameter indicator that reacts to one of the critical parameters of sterilization.
- *Class IV:* A multi-parameter indicator that reacts to one, two, or more of the critical parameters of sterilization.
- *Class V* (integrating indicator): An indicator that reacts to all critical parameters of sterilization.
- *Class VI* (emulating indicator): An indicator that reacts to all critical parameters of a specified sterilization cycle.

Containment device: Reusable rigid sterilization container, instrument case, cassette, or organizing tray intended for the purpose of containing reusable devices for sterilization.

Hydrogen peroxide gas plasma sterilization: A sterilization process that involves the combined use of hydrogen peroxide and low-temperature gas plasma. Gas plasmas are highly ionized gases composed of ions, electrons, and neutral particles.

Hydrogen peroxide vapor sterilization: A sterilization process in which vaporized hydrogen peroxide acts as a sterilant.

Instrument case/cassette: A container with a lid and a base to sterilize devices that permits air removal and sterilant penetration/removal. The devices require wrapping in packaging material if sterility of the contents is to be maintained.

Nonwoven material: Fabric made by bonding fibers together as opposed to weaving threads.

Organizing tray: A reusable metal or plastic tray that permits organization and protection of the contents. Some organizing trays have diagrams for the representative instruments etched onto the surface of the tray to facilitate their identificaton and location within the tray.

Package integrity: Unimpaired physical condition of a final package.

Paper-plastic pouch (peel pouch): A type of packaging made of Mylar® (a polyester film manufactured by DuPont) and paper that is suitable for packaging items to be sterilized in steam or a type of packaging made of Mylar® and Tyvek® (a polyethelene material manufactured by DuPont) that is suitable for packaging items to be sterilized in EO, low-temperature hydrogen gas plasma, or hydrogen peroxide vapor.

Rigid sterilization container system: Specifically designed heat-resistant, metal, plastic, or anodized aluminum receptacles used to package items, usually surgical instruments, for sterilization. The lids and/or bottom surfaces contain steam- or gas-permeable, high-efficiency microbial filters.

Sequential wrapping: A double-wrapping procedure that creates a package within a package.

Shelf life: When this term is used in conjunction with a sterile device, shelf life is considered to be the length of time a device is safe to use.

Sterility maintenance cover (dust cover): A plastic bag, usually 2 to 3 thousandths of an inch (ie, mils) in thickness, applied to a cooled, sterilized item to provide extra protection from dust, moisture, and other environmental contaminates. These covers can be heat-sealed or self-sealed closed.

Sterilization validation studies: Tests performed by a device manufacturer that demonstrate that a sterilization process will consistently yield sterile product under defined parameters.

Superheating: A condition in which dehydrated textiles are subjected to steam sterilization. The superheated package or product becomes too dry, which causes destructive effects on the strength of the cloth fibers. When woven textiles are not re-hydrated after sterilization, and/or if repeated sterilization is attempted, the textiles could absorb the available moisture present in the steam, thereby creating a dry or superheated steam effect and adversely affecting the steam sterilization process.

Useful life: The length of time, as determined by the manufacturer, for which a product maintains acceptable safety and performance characteristics. The manufacturer should provide data to support the useful life of the product.

Wet packs: Packs are considered wet when there is moisture in the form of dampness, droplets, or puddles of water found on or within a textile pack, instrument, basin set, rigid sterilization container, or other containment device after a completed sterilization cycle and after a cool-down period. Wet packs are associated with steam sterilization; however, they can occur with EO sterilization.

Woven textile: A reusable fabric constructed from yarns made of natural and/or synthetic fibers or filaments that are woven or knitted together to form a web in a repeated interlocking pattern.

References

1. Guideline for cleaning and care of surgical instruments. In: *Guidelines for Perioperative Practice.* Denver, CO: AORN, Inc; 2015:615-650.

2. Guideline for sterilization. In: *Guidelines for Perioperative Practice.* Denver, CO: AORN, Inc; 2015:665-692.

3. *ANSI/AAMI ST79:2010 & A1:2010, & A2:2011, & A3:2012: Comprehensive Guide to Steam Sterilization and Sterility Assurance in Health Care Facilities.* Arlington, VA: Association for the Advancement of Medical Instrumentation; 2012. [IVC]

4. *Guideline for Disinfection and Sterilization in Healthcare Facilities, 2008.* Centers for Disease Control and Prevention. http://www.cdc.gov/hicpac/

disinfection_sterilization/13_0sterilization.html. Accessed on November 8, 2013. [IVA]

5. Standards of perioperative nursing. In: *Perioperative Standards and Recommended Practices*. Denver, CO: AORN, Inc; 2013:3-20. [IVB]

6. Diab-Elschahawi M, Blacky A, Bachhofner N, Koller W. Challenging the Sterrad 100NX sterilizer with different carrier materials and wrappings under experimental "clean" and "dirty" conditions. *Am J Infect Control*. 2010;38(10):806-810. [IIIB]

7. Rutala WA, Weber DJ. Choosing a sterilization wrap for surgical packs. *Infect Control Today*. May 1, 2000. http://www.infectioncontroltoday.com/articles/2000/05/choosing-a-sterilization-wrap-for-surgicalpacks.aspx. Accessed September 20, 2013. [VC]

8. *ANSI/AAMI/ISO 11607-1:2006/(R)2010: Packaging for terminally sterilized medical devices—Part 1: Requirements for materials, sterile barrier systems and packaging*. Arlington, VA: Association for the Advancement of Medical Instrumentation; 2010. [IVC]

9. Brusco J, Ogg M. Health care waste management and environmentally preferable purchasing. *AORN J*. 2010;92(6 Suppl):S62-S66. [VB]

10. *EPA's Final Guidance on Environmentally Preferable Purchasing*. August 20, 1999. Environmental Protection Agency. http://www.epa.gov/epp/pubs/guidance/finalguidance.htm. Accessed September 20, 2013. [IVA]

11. *AORN Position Statement: Environmental Responsibility*. http://www.aorn.org/Clinical_Practice/Position_Statements/Position_Statements.aspx. AORN, Inc. Accessed September 20, 2013. [IVB]

12. Laustsen G. Reduce-recycle-reuse: guidelines for promoting perioperative waste management. *AORN J*. 2007;85(4):717-728. [VA]

13. Lee RJ, Mears SC. Greening of orthopedic surgery. *Orthopedics*. 2012;35(6):e940-e944. [VB]

14. Belkin NL. Green nursing: the environment and economics. *AORN J*. 2007;86(1):15-16. [VC]

15. Conrardy J, Hillanbrand M, Myers S, Nussbaum GF. Reducing medical waste. *AORN J*. 2010;91(6):711-721. [IIIB]

16. Herman P, Larsen C. Measuring porous microbial barriers, part 1. Medical Device and Diagnostic Industry. http://www.mddionline.com/article/measuring-porous-microbial-barriers-part-1. Accessed September 20, 2013. [IVA]

17. Herman P, Larsen C. Measuring porous microbial barriers, part 2. Medical Device and Diagnostic Industry. http://www.mddionline.com/article/measuring-porous-microbial-barriers-part-2. Accessed September 20, 2013. [IVA]

18. *ANSI/AAMI ST41:2008: Ethylene Oxide Sterilization in Health Care Facilities: Safety and Effectiveness*. Arlington, VA: Association for the Advancement of Medical Instrumentation; 2008. [IVC]

19. *ANSI/AAMI ST58:2005/(R)2010: Chemical Sterilization and High-level Disinfection in Health Care Facilities*. Arlington, VA: Association for the Advancement of Medical Instrumentation; 2006. [IVC]

20. Kimberly-Clarke. KimGuard Sterilization Wrap. KimGuard One-Step Sterilization Wrap. Directions for use. http://www.njcl.us/images/KIMBERLY_CLARK_WRAP_DIRECTIONS_FOR_USE.PDF. Accessed September 20, 2013.

21. Rutala WA, Weber DJ; Healthcare Infection Control Practices Advisory Committee. *Guideline for Disinfection and Sterilization in Healthcare Facilities, 2008*. Atlanta, GA: Centers for Disease Control and Prevention; 2008. [IVA]

22. *Guidance Documents (Medical Devices and Radiation-Emitting Products) > Labeling Recommendations for Single-Use Devices Reprocessed by Third Parties and Hospitals; Final Guidance for Industry and FDA*. US Food and Drug Administration. http://www.fda.gov/MedicalDevices/DeviceRegulationandGuidance/GuidanceDocuments/ucm071058.htm. Accessed September 20, 2013.

23. Moriya GA, Souza RQ, Pinto FM, Graziano KU. Periodic sterility assessment of materials stored for up to 6 months at continuous microbial contamination risk: laboratory study. *Am J Infect Control*. 2012;40(10):1013-1015. [IA]

24. Joan LSP, Norhashimawati Khor S. Time versus event-related sterility: linen & pouch packaging remain sterile over a year of storage and handling. *Singapore Nurs J*. 2010;37(1):34-42. [IB]

25. Waked WR, Simpson AK, Miller CP, Magit DP, Grauer JN. Sterilization wrap inspections do not adequately evaluate instrument sterility. *Clin Orthop Relat Res*. 2007;462:207-211. [IA]

26. *ANSI/AAMI ST77: Containment Devices for Reusable Medical Device Sterilization*. Arlington, VA: Association for the Advancement of Medical Instrumentation; 2013. [IVC]

27. AORN guidance statement: safe patient handling and movement in the perioperative setting. In: *Perioperative Standards and Recommended Practices*. Denver, CO: AORN; 2013:553-572. [IVB]

28. American Society of Cataract and Refractive Surgery, American Society of Ophthalmic Registered Nurses. Recommended practices for cleaning and sterilizing intraocular surgical instruments. *J Cataract Refract Surg*. 2007;33(6):1095-1100. [IVB]

29. Lucas AD, Chobin N, Conner R, et al. Steam sterilization and internal count sheets: assessing the potential for cytotoxicity. *AORN J*. 2009;89(3):521-531. [IIB]

30. *ANSI/AAMI ST65:2008: Processing of Reusable Surgical Textiles for Use in Health Care Facilities*. Arlington, VA: Association for the Advancement of Medical Instrumentation; 2008. [IVC]

31. Nicholson P, Gillis S, Dunning AM. The use of scoring rubrics to determine clinical performance in the operating suite. *Nurse Educ Today*. 2009;29(1):73-82. [IIIB]

32. Ringerman E, Flint LJ, Hughes DE. An innovative education program: the peer competency validator model. *J Nurses Staff Dev*. 2006;22(3):114-123. [VB]

33. Sportsman S. Competency education and validation in the United States: what should nurses know? *Nurs Forum*. 2010;45(3):140-149. [VA]

34. Stobinski JX. Perioperative nursing competency. *AORN J*. 2008;88(3):417-436. [VB]

35. Whittaker S, Carson W, Smolenski MC. Assuring continued competence—policy questions and approaches: how should the profession respond? *Online J Issues Nurs*. 2000;5(3). http://www.nursingworld.org/MainMenuCategories/ANAMarketplace/ANAPeriodicals/OJIN/TableofContents/Volume52000/No3Sept00/ArticlePreviousTopic/ContinuedCompetence.aspx. Accessed September 20, 2013. [VA]

36. Centers for Medicare & Medicaid Services. *State Operations Manual Appendix A: Survey Protocol, Regulations and Interpretive Guidelines for Hospitals*. Rev.78; 2011.

37. Centers for Medicare & Medicaid Services. *State Operations Manual Appendix L: Guidance for Surveyors: Ambulatory Surgical Centers*. Rev. 76; 2011.

38. HR.01.05.03: Staff participate in ongoing education and training. In: *Comprehensive Accreditation Manual:*

CAMH for Hospitals. Oakbrook Terrace, IL: Joint Commission Accreditation; 2013.

39. HR.01.05.03: Staff participate in ongoing education and training. In: *Comprehensive Accreditation Manual for Ambulatory Care*. Oakbrook Terrace, IL: The Joint Commission; 2013.

40. Quality management and improvement. In: 2013 *Accreditation Handbook for Ambulatory Health Care*. Skokic, IL: Accreditation Association for Ambulatory Health Care; 2013:30-34.

41. Personnel: personnel records. In: *Procedural Standards and Checklist for Accreditation of Ambulatory Surgery Facilities*. Version 3 ed. Gurnee, IL: American Association for Accreditation of Ambulatory Surgery Facilities; 2011:77-79.

42. Personnel: personnel records; resumes. In: *Regular Standards and Checklist for Accreditation of Ambulatory Surgery Facilities*. Version 13 ed. Gurnee, IL: American Association for Accreditation of Ambulatory Surgery Facilities; 2011:77-78.

43. Personnel: knowledge, skill & CME training. In: *Regular Standards and Checklist for Accreditation of Ambulatory Surgery Facilities*. Version 13 ed. Gurnee, IL: American Association for Accreditation of Ambulatory Surgery Facilities; 2011:78-79.

44. Personnel: personnel safety. In: *Regular Standards and Checklist for Accreditation of Ambulatory Surgery Facilities*. Version 13 ed. Gurnee, IL: American Association for Accreditation of Ambulatory Surgery Facilities; 2011:80.

45. Personnel: knowledge, skill & CME training. In: *Procedural Standards and Checklist for Accreditation of Ambulatory Surgery Facilities*. Version 3 ed. Gurnee, IL: American Association for Accreditation of Ambulatory Surgery Facilities; 2011:79.

46. Personnel: personnel safety. In: *Procedural Standards and Checklist for Accreditation of Ambulatory Surgery Facilities*. Version 3 ed. Gurnee, IL: American Association for Accreditation of Ambulatory Surgery Facilities; 2011:79-80.

47. Jordan C, Thomas MB, Evans ML, Green A. Public policy on competency: how will nursing address this complex issue? *J Contin Educ Nurs*. 2008;39(2):86-91. [VA]

48. LD.04.01.07: The hospital has policies and procedures that guide and support patient care, treatment, and services. In: *Hospital Accreditation Standards* 2013. 2013 ed. Oakbrook Terrace, IL: Joint Commission Resources; 2013.

49. LD.04.01.07: The organization has policies and procedures that guide and support patient care, treatment, or services. In: *Standards for Ambulatory Care 2013: Standards, Elements of Performance Scoring Accreditation Polices*. Oakbrook Terrace, IL: The Joint Commission; 2013.

50. Governance. In: *2013 Accreditation Handbook for Ambulatory Health Care*. Skokie, IL: Accreditation Association for Ambulatory Health Care; 2013:17-24.

51. PI.03.01.01: The hospital improves performance on an ongoing basis. In: *Hospital Accreditation Standards 2013*. 2013 ed. Oakbrook Terrace, IL: Joint Commission Resources; 2013.

52. PI.03.01.01: The organization improves performance. In: *Standards for Ambulatory Care 2012: Standards, Elements of Performance Scoring Accreditation Polices*. Oakbrook Terrace, IL: The Joint Commission; 2013.

53. Quality improvement/quality assessment: quality improvement. In: *Procedural Standards and Checklist for Accreditation of Ambulatory Surgery Facilities*. Version 3 ed. Gurnee, IL: American Association for Accreditation of Ambulatory Surgery Facilities; 2011:67.

54. Quality assessment/quality improvement: quality improvement. In: *Regular Standards and Checklist for Accreditation of Ambulatory Surgery Facilities*. Version 13 ed. Gurnee, IL: American Association for Accreditation of Ambulatory Surgery Facilities; 2011:67.

55. Quality assessment/quality improvement: unanticipated operative sequelae. In: *Regular Standards and Checklist for Accreditation of Ambulatory Surgery Facilities*. Version 13 ed. Gurnee, IL: American Association for Accreditation of Ambulatory Surgery Facilities; 2011:69-71.

56. Brown JM, Bliley J. How to solve wet packs, and evaluate water issues. *Mater Manag Health Care*. 2008;17(7):50-52. [VB]

Acknowledgements

Lead Author
Cynthia Spry, MA, MS, RN, CNOR, CBSPDT
Independent Consultant
New York, New York

Contributing Author
Ramona Conner, MSN, RN, CNOR
Manager, Standards and Guidelines
AORN Nursing Department
Denver, Colorado

The authors and AORN thank Paula Berrett, BS, CRCST, Intermountain Healthcare Urban South Region CP Manager, Utah Valley Regional Medical Center, Provo, Utah; Paula Morton, MS, RN, CNOR, Director of Perioperative Services, Sherman Health, Elgin, Illinois; Judith Goldberg, DBA, MSN, RN, CNOR, CRCST; Nurse Manager, Pequot Surgical Center, Groton, Connecticut; and Jane Rothrock, PhD, RN, CNOR, FAAN, Professor, Delaware Community College, Media, Pennsylvania, for their assistance in developing this guideline.

Publication History
Originally published February 1983, *AORN Journal*.

Revised November 1988, February 1992.

Revised November 1995; published May 1996, *AORN Journal*.

Revised and reformatted; published December 2000, *AORN Journal*.

Revised 2006; published in *Standards, Recommended Practices, and Guidelines*, 2007 edition.

Minor editing revisions made to omit PNDS codes; reformatted September 2012 for publication in *Perioperative Standards and Recommended Practices*, 2013 edition.

Revised September 2013 for online publication in *Perioperative Standards and Recommended Practices*.

Minor editing revisions made in November 2014 for publication in *Guidelines for Perioperative Practice*, 2015 edition.

GUIDELINE FOR STERILIZATION

The Guideline for Sterilization has been approved by the AORN Recommended Practices Advisory Board. It was presented as proposed recommendations for comments by members and others. The guideline is effective June 15, 2012. The recommendations in the guideline are intended to be achievable and represent what is believed to be an optimal level of practice. Policies and procedures will reflect variations in practice settings and/or clinical situations that determine the degree to which the guideline can be implemented. AORN recognizes the various settings in which perioperative nurses practice; therefore, this guideline is adaptable to various practice settings. These practice settings include traditional operating rooms (ORs), ambulatory surgery centers, physicians' offices, cardiac catheterization laboratories, endoscopy suites, radiology departments, and all other areas where operative and other invasive procedures may be performed.

Purpose

This document provides guidance for sterilizing items to be used in the perioperative setting. The creation and maintenance of an aseptic environment has direct influence on patient outcomes. A major responsibility of the perioperative registered nurse (RN) is to minimize patient risk for surgical site infections (SSIs). One of the measures for preventing SSIs is to provide reusable surgical items that are free of contamination at the time of use. This can be accomplished by subjecting them to cleaning and decontamination, followed by a disinfection or sterilization process.

The Spaulding classification system is commonly used to classify patient care items to determine the appropriate level of processing.[1] The Spaulding classification system, developed by Earl Spaulding in 1968, classifies items as noncritical, semicritical, or critical and identifies the appropriate processing method for each category. Infection preventionists and others use this system to determine the correct processing methods for preparing instruments and other items for patient use. According to the Spaulding classification system, the level of processing required is based on the nature of the item that requires processing and the manner in which the item is to be used.

The guideline addresses processing of critical medical devices. Processing of noncritical and semicritical devices is outside the scope of this document. The difference between noncritical and semicritical devices is as follows.

Noncritical devices are devices that contact only intact skin. Noncritical devices require low-level disinfection or cleaning. Examples of noncritical devices include

- tourniquets and blood pressure cuffs,
- stethoscopes, and
- Mayo stands.

Semicritical devices are devices that come in contact with nonintact skin or with mucous membranes and require a minimum of high-level disinfection. Examples of semicritical devices include

- vaginal and rectal probes,
- respiratory therapy equipment,
- bronchoscopes, and
- laryngoscope blades.[2,3]

Sterilization provides the highest level of assurance that surgical items are free of viable microbes.[1] Although these recommendations include several references to cleaning, decontamination, disinfection, and packaging, the major focus is on sterilization.

The guideline includes recommendations for high-temperature sterilization (ie, sterilization by steam), low-temperature sterilization (ie, ethylene oxide, low-temperature hydrogen peroxide gas plasma, low-temperature hydrogen peroxide vapor, dry heat, ozone), and processing using a liquid chemical sterilant system using peracetic acid.

Cleaning, decontamination, disinfection, and packaging of sterile medical devices are outside the scope of this document. The reader should refer to the AORN Guideline for Cleaning and Care of Surgical Instruments[4] and Guideline for High-Level Disinfection[5] for additional guidance.

Evidence Review

A medical librarian conducted a systematic literature search of the databases MEDLINE®, CINAHL®, Scopus®, and Cochrane Database of Systematic Reviews for meta-analyses, randomized and nonrandomized trials and studies, systematic and nonsystematic reviews, and opinion documents and letters. Search terms included *sterilization, ethylene oxide, steam, peracetic acid, dry heat, hydrogen peroxide gas, ozone, hospital equipment and supplies, prostheses and implants, surgical equipment, infusion pumps, disposable equipment, diagnostic equipment, flash sterilization, immediate use, surgical equipment and supplies, equipment contamination, microbial contamination, indicators and reagents, fungi, bacterial contamination, ethylene oxide toxicity,* and *biofilms,* as applicable.

The search was limited to articles published in English between 2005 and 2011. Older articles were included where there were no articles within this time period. Additional articles not identified in the original literature search were obtained by reviewing the reference lists of the original articles. The librarian also established continuing alerts on the sterilization topics. The lead author and medical librarian identified relevant documents from government agencies, standards-setting bodies, and equipment manufacturers, with the lead author requesting other guidelines, professional literature, and book chapters as necessary.

Articles identified by the search were provided to the project team for evaluation. The team consisted of the lead author, two members of the Recommended Practices Advisory Board, two members of the Research Committee, and an ad hoc member of the Evidence Rating Task Force. The lead author divided the search results into topics and assigned members of the team to review and critically appraise each article using the Johns Hopkins Evidence-Based Practice Model and the Research or Non-Research Evidence Appraisal Tools as appropriate. The literature was independently evaluated and appraised according to the strength and quality of the evidence. Each article was then assigned an appraisal score as agreed upon by consensus of the team. The appraisal score is noted in brackets after each reference citation, as applicable.

The collective evidence supporting each intervention within a specific recommendation was summarized and used to rate the strength of the evidence using the AORN Evidence Rating Model. Factors considered in review of the collective evidence were the quality of research, quantity of similar studies on a given topic, and consistency of results supporting a recommendation. The evidence rating is noted in brackets after each intervention.

Editor's note: *MEDLINE is a registered trademark of the US National Library of Medicine's Medical Literature Analysis and Retrieval System, Bethesda, MD. CINAHL, Cumulative Index to Nursing and Allied Health Literature, is a registered trademark of EBSCO Industries, Birmingham, AL. Scopus is a registered trademark of Elsevier B.V., Amsterdam, Netherlands.*

Recommendation I

Patient care items should be processed for reuse based on the intended use of the item.

I.a. Items that enter sterile tissue or the vascular system are categorized as critical and should be sterile when used.[1,6] Sterilization may be accomplished using a variety of sterilization methods and technologies (eg, steam, ethylene oxide, hydrogen peroxide). *[1: Strong Evidence]*

    Examples of critical items include
- surgical instruments,
- cutting endoscopic accessories that break the mucosal barrier, and
- implants.

I.a.1. If it is determined that in-house reprocessing of single-use devices is feasible, a program for reprocessing of single-use devices that meets US Food and Drug Administration (FDA) requirements and includes policies, procedures, competencies, and educational requirements should be developed. Reprocessing of single-use medical devices is outside the scope of this document.

I.a.2. If it is determined that in-house reprocessing of single-use items is not feasible and it is still the intention of the facility to target some single-use devices for reprocessing, the facility should investigate the feasibility of using the services of a third-party reprocessing company. Criteria for evaluating the services of a third-party reprocessor and identifying single-use items for reprocessing are outside the scope of this document.

Recommendation II

Devices labeled as single-use should not be reprocessed unless the FDA guidelines for reprocessing of single-use devices can be met.

In 2000 the FDA issued a guidance document for reprocessing of single-use devices.[7] This document details the requirements that a reprocessor must meet. These requirements are the same requirements that the original device manufacturer must meet. They include
- registering as a reprocessing firm and listing all products that are reprocessed;
- submitting reports of associated adverse events to the FDA;
- tracking devices that, in the event of failure, could have serious outcomes;
- correcting or removing from the market unsafe devices; and
- meeting manufacturing and labeling requirements.

An in-depth explanation of these guidelines can be accessed on the FDA web site.[7,8] Meeting these requirements is beyond the capabilities of most health care facilities.

II.a. Health care facilities considering reprocessing single-use devices should identify devices labeled as single-use that they would like to reprocess, review the FDA guidance document, and, based on the requirements within the document, make a determination as to the feasibility of reprocessing those devices within the facility.[7] *[1: Regulatory Requirement]*

Recommendation III

Items to be sterilized should be cleaned, decontaminated, inspected, packaged, sterilized, and stored in a controlled environment and in accordance with the AORN Guideline for Cleaning and Care of Surgical Instruments[4] and the device manufacturer's validated and written instructions for use.

A controlled environment is intended to facilitate effective decontamination, assembly, sterilization, and storage and to minimize environmental contamination and maintain sterility of sterilized items.

Effective sterilization cannot take place without effective cleaning. The process of sterilization is negatively affected by the amount of bioburden and the number, type, and inherent resistance of microorganisms, including biofilms, on the items to be sterilized.

STERILIZATION

TABLE 1. ATTIRE AND PERSONAL PROTECTIVE EQUIPMENT REQUIREMENTS[1]

Work area	Scrubs	Head covers	Gloves*	Gowns#	Eye protection+	Masks or face shields±
Decontamination	X	X	X	X	X	X
Preparation and packaging	X	X				
Sterilization processing	X	X				
Sterile storage	X	X				

*Gloves should be waterproof, general-purpose utility, or heavy duty.
#Gowns must be liquid-resistant with sleeves.
+Eye protection includes goggles/eye glasses with side shields or chin-length face shields.
± Masks should be fluid-resistant.
Other protective equipment (such as shoe covers) may be worn as needed. The type and characteristics will depend on the task and degree of anticipated exposure.

REFERENCE
1. Occupational Safety & Health Administration. US Department of Labor. Toxic and hazardous substances. Appendix A: bloodborne pathogens. 29 CFR §1910.1030. Fed Regist. 1991;56(235):64004-64182. Effective December 6, 1991. http://www.osha.gov/pls/oshaweb/owadisp.show_document?p_table=standards&p_id=10051. Accessed April 25, 2012.

Soils, oils, and other materials may shield microorganisms on items from contact with the sterilant or combine with and inactivate the sterilant.[1,6,9]

III.a. Items sterilized outside of the facility in which they will be used, unless they are processed in a commercial FDA-regulated instrument sterilization facility, should be removed from their container or wrapper and cleaned, decontaminated, and sterilized according to the manufacturer's validated and written instructions for use within the organization in which they will be used. *[3: Limited Evidence]*

Controlled conditions reduce the risk of contamination.[6] It is not possible to know the conditions under which items were cleaned, packaged, and sterilized at another facility or to know the conditions of transport.

III.a.1. Facilities in which instruments are routinely processed at a satellite facility or at a campus site that requires transportation of the sterilized items from one building to another should develop policies and procedures to ensure standardized processing procedures, controlled conditions of transport, and oversight of all aspects of processing and transport. Criteria for such a practice are outside the scope of this document.

III.b. Functional workflow patterns should be established to create and maintain physical separation between the decontamination and sterilization areas.[6,10] *[3: Limited Evidence]*

Physical separation aids in achieving environmental and microbial control. During manual cleaning of instruments, particulates, aerosolized matter, dust, and microbial counts are elevated. Physical separation and vented airflow to the outside minimizes potential contamination of processed items.[10]

III.b.1. Attire, use of personal protective equipment (PPE), and limitations in personnel access and movement should be based on expected contamination levels (Table 1).

III.b.2. Functional workflow patterns should be established in the following order, from potentially high contamination areas to clean areas:
1. decontamination area,
2. preparation and packaging,
3. sterilization processing,
4. sterile storage, and
5. clean distribution.

A workflow pattern that begins in the decontamination area (ie, dirty) and flows to the clean distribution area can help to prevent clean or sterile items from reentering a contaminated area where they may be recontaminated.

III.b.3. Traffic patterns should be established to protect personnel, equipment, supplies, and instrumentation from sources of potential contamination. Traffic patterns should define access restrictions, movement of personnel, and appropriate attire according to AORN guidelines.[10]

III.c. Room temperature, humidity, and ventilation must be controlled and monitored in accordance with local, state, and federal policy and regulation. Table 2 provides parameters for the controlled environment.[6] *[3: Limited Evidence]*

Bacteria and fungi thrive at warm temperatures, whereas cooler temperatures may impede bacterial and fungal growth in the decontamination area. Regulated environmental controls in work areas are essential for the comfort of personnel wearing appropriate attire and PPE.[6]

STERILIZATION

III.d. Monitoring results should be readily retrievable.[6] *[2: Moderate Evidence]*

Monitoring and recording environmental controls in each area will assist in verification that minimum recommended parameters are met and maintained and will identify when corrective action needs to be taken.

A mechanism with memory for history of temperature and humidity can alert personnel if there was a deviation during unmanned times.

III.e. Items to be sterilized should be decontaminated before inspection, packaging, and sterilization.[4,6] *[1: Strong Evidence]*

III.e.1. Health care personnel should use standard precautions when performing decontamination activities.

Standard precautions are designed to protect patients and health care workers from contact with recognized and unrecognized sources of infectious diseases.[11,12]

Recommendation IV

Items to be sterilized should be inspected for cleanliness and proper function in accordance with AORN's Guideline for Cleaning and Care of Surgical Instruments.[4]

Debris remaining on a device may compromise the subsequent sterilization process.[1]

IV.a. Instruments should be inspected for cleanliness and function before packaging and sterilization. *[3: Limited Evidence]*

Although commercially available tests can be used to verify the cleaning process,[1] there is no universally accepted standard for clean. Visual inspection is a subjective assessment that depends on the operator. It has limited efficacy but is commonly used to determine cleanliness. Inspection under magnification and ancillary lighting can assist in viewing residual soil and determining cleanliness.[13]

In one study, investigators rated 91% of cleaned instruments as visually clean. However, upon examination under a microscope, they determined that 84% of the instruments that looked clean contained residual debris.[14]

IV.b. The device manufacturer should be consulted for the appropriate methods for testing function.[6] *[3: Limited Evidence]*

Instruments that malfunction or are not intact when used in surgery have the potential to cause patient harm.

TABLE 2. Parameters for Controlled Environments During Sterilization[1,2]

Functional area	Airflow	Minimum number of air exchanges per hour	All air exhausted directly to the outdoors	Temperature	Relative humidity
Soiled/decontaminated	Negative (in)	10 *(6)	Yes	60° F to 65° F (16° C to 18° C)	20% to 60%
Sterilizer equipment access	Negative (in)	10	Yes	75° F to 85° F (24° C to 29° C)	20% to 60%
Sterilizer loading/unloading	Positive (out)	10	Yes	68° F to 73° F (20° C to 23° C)	20% to 60%
Restrooms/housekeeping	Negative (in)	10	Yes	68° F to 73° F (20° C to 23° C)	20% to 60%
Preparation and packaging	Positive (out)	10 (downdraft type)	No	68° F to 73° F (20° C to 23° C)	20% to 60%
Textile packaging room	Positive (out)	10 (downdraft type)	No	68° C to 73° F (20° C to 23° C)	20% to 60%
Clean/sterile storage	Positive (out)	4 (downdraft type)	No	≤ 75° F (≤ 24° C)	≤ 70%

* The Facilities Guideline Institute recommends a minimum of 6 air exchanges an hour in decontamination. AAMI recommends 10 exchanges.

Regulatory agencies may enforce the American Society for Healthcare Engineering (ASHE) or AAMI recommendations listed in Table 2. They also may enforce other recommendations, such as the 2000 NFPA 101, which states the relative humidity should be at 35%. As stated in the ASHE document, these parameters are intended to be used for the design of the heating, ventilation, and air conditioning systems and there may be daily fluctuations based on the environmental conditions.

References

1. Association for the Advancement of Medical Instrumentation. ANSI/AAMI ST79:2010, A1:2010 & A2:2011, Comprehensive guide to steam sterilization and sterility assurance in health care facilities. Arlington, VA: Association for the Advancement of Medical Instrumentation; 2010 & 2011. Adapted and reprinted with permission. Further reproduction or distribution prohibited.

2. ANSI/ASHRAE/ASHE Addendum D to ANSI/ASHRAE/ASHE Standard 170-2008. Atlanta, GA: American Society of Heating, Refrigerating and Air-Conditioning Engineers; 2010.

Recommendation V

Items to be sterilized should be packaged in a manner that promotes successful sterilization. Items should be packaged in accordance with AORN's Guideline for Selection and Use of Packaging Systems for Sterilization.[15]

Appropriate packaging increases the probability that sterility can be achieved and maintained to the point of use.[1,16]

V.a. Manufacturers of packaging systems should be consulted for package preparation, configuration, and sterilization. *[3: Limited Evidence]*

V.b. The total weight of an instrument set should not exceed 25 lb.[6,17] *[2: Moderate Evidence]*

Instrument sets weighing more than 25 lb are known to be difficult to dry without lengthy drying times and present an increased risk of ergonomic injury.[6,15,18,19]

V.c. Combination paper-plastic peel pouches should not be placed in a container or wrapped set unless the pouch or container manufacturer has validated this process.[6] Medical-grade, all-paper pouches or other containment devices validated for use within instrument sets may be used to segregate small items within a set. *[3: Limited Evidence]*

When placing paper-plastic peel pouches within a wrapped set or rigid sterilization container, it may not be possible to position them in a manner that allows adequate air removal, steam contact, or drying.[6]

Recommendation VI

Saturated steam under pressure should be used to sterilize heat- and moisture-stable items unless otherwise indicated by the device manufacturer.[1]

Saturated steam under pressure is a preferred sterilization method. It has a large margin of safety because of its reliability, consistency, and lethality. It is an effective, inexpensive, and relatively rapid sterilization method for most porous and nonporous materials.[1]

VI.a. Manufacturers' written instructions for operating steam sterilizers should be followed. *[2: Moderate Evidence]*

Steam sterilizers vary in size, design, and performance characteristics. Steam sterilizers may be large capacity—greater than 2 cubic feet—or small table-top models and may differ in how they generate steam.

Types of steam sterilizers include gravity-displacement sterilizers that permit only gravity-displacement cycles, dynamic air-removal sterilizers (eg, prevacuum, high vacuum, steam-flush pressure-pulse) that permit only dynamic air-removal cycles, and sterilizers that permit either gravity-displacement or dynamic air-removal cycles.[1]

Health care organizations may use both gravity-displacement cycles and dynamic air-removal cycles. Immediate use steam sterilization (IUSS), formerly referred to as flash sterilization, can be performed in either a gravity-displacement or a dynamic air-removal cycle.[20,21]

Air removal is critical to successful steam sterilization. Medical device manufacturers may validate a specific method of air removal and therefore recommend a specific type of steam sterilization cycle or specify the achievement of certain cycle parameters in their written instructions for use.

Steam sterilizers may be used for both terminal sterilization, which permits storage of items after sterilization, and IUSS.[20]

Cycle parameters vary according to sterilizer and device manufacturers' instructions for use, and whether terminal or IUSS is desired.

Table 3 and Table 4 provide typical minimum sterilization times for gravity-displacement and dynamic air-removal steam sterilization cycles, respectively.

It is critical to refer to the device and container manufacturers' instructions to determine the required cycle. Many devices require extended exposure times and some rigid sterilization containers, such as those intended for IUSS, may require exposure times greater than those identified in the tables (Table 3 and Table 4).

VI.b. Cycle parameters recommended by the device manufacturer should be reconciled with the sterilizer manufacturer's written instructions for the specific sterilization cycle and load configuration.[6,21] *[2: Moderate Evidence]*

Certain types of devices (eg, some pneumatically powered instruments; specialty orthopedic, neurosurgery, trauma instruments) and implants may require prolonged exposure times or drying times. These cycle times may not have been validated by the sterilizer manufacturer.

VI.b.1. When the sterilizer and the device manufacturers' instructions cannot be reconciled, the device manufacturers' instructions should be followed.[20]

The device manufacturer has validated the cycle, identified in the instructions for use, that must be used to ensure sterility.

VI.c. A quality monitoring program that includes physical monitors (eg, printouts, digital readings, graphs, gauges), chemical indicators, and biological indicators should be used to verify that conditions necessary for steam sterilization have been met.[6] *[1: Strong Evidence]*

Attention to sterility monitoring to ensure compliance with recommended guidelines is a critical component of quality assurance. Deviation from recommended practices and recommendations can compromise the quality of sterilization processes.

STERILIZATION

TABLE 3. TYPICAL MINIMUM CYCLE TIMES FOR GRAVITY-DISPLACEMENT STEAM STERILIZATION[1]

Item	Exposure time at 250° F (121° C)	Exposure time at 270° F (132° C)	Exposure time at 275° F (135° C)	Drying time
Packaged instruments	30 minutes	15 minutes		15 to 30 minutes
Textile packs	30 minutes	25 minutes		15 minutes
			10 minutes	30 minutes
Nonporous items subject to immediate use steam sterilization (IUSS)		See device and container manufacturer instructions for use	See device and container manufacturer instructions for use	See IUSS container manufacturer instructions for use
Nonporous and porous items in mixed load subject to IUSS		See device and container manufacturer instructions for use	See device and container manufacturer instructions for use	See IUSS container manufacturer instructions for use

REFERENCE
1. Association for the Advancement of Medical Instrumentation. ANSI/AAMI ST79:2010, A1:2010 & A2:2011, Comprehensive guide to steam sterilization and sterility assurance in health care facilities. Arlington, VA: Association for the Advancement of Medical Instrumentation; 2010 & 2011. Adapted and reprinted with permission. Further reproduction or distribution is prohibited.

VI.c.1. Each sterilization cycle should be monitored to verify that parameters required for sterilization have been met.[1,6]

VI.c.2. The sterilizer operator should review physical monitors to verify cycle parameters for every load.[6]

Physical monitors can provide a rapid means of identification of sterilizer failure. Physical monitors record cycle parameters (eg, time for each phase of the cycle, temperature during each phase of the cycle).

VI.c.3. External and internal chemical indicators should be used with each package.
- A class 1 chemical indicator (ie, process indicator) should be placed on the outside of every package unless the internal indicator is visible through the package material.[6] Examples of process indicators are indicator tape and indicator labels.
- A class 5 chemical indicator (ie, integrating indicator) or class 6 chemical indicator (ie, emulating indicator) should be placed inside every package.[6]
- A class 3 or 4 chemical indicator may be used within a package to meet requirements for internal monitoring.[6]

Chemical indicators are used to verify that one or more of the conditions necessary for sterilization have been achieved within each package.[6]

VI.c.4. Chemical indicators should be placed in an area within the package that presents a challenge for air removal and steam contact. When there is a question concerning the appropriate number and placement of internal chemical indicators, the user should consult with the chemical indicator manufacturer, the device manufacturer, and the container manufacturer for additional information.

The number and the placement of internal chemical indicators may be affected by the contents of the package, the configuration of the items within the set, and the packaging or container.[6]

VI.c.5. Biological indicators should be used to monitor sterilizer efficacy. Efficacy monitoring should be performed at least weekly and preferably daily.

Frequent sterilizer efficacy monitoring reduces the possibility that items will be processed under suboptimal conditions and for load release.[6] (See Recommendation XX for further recommendations concerning a quality monitoring program and application of monitors.)

VI.c.6. Biological indicators should be used for load release purposes. For example, loads containing an implant should be monitored with a biological indicator and not released for use until the result of the test is available.

VI.d. After steam sterilization, the contents of the sterilizer should be removed from the chamber and left untouched until they are cool enough to handle without concern that retained moisture may act as a wick for bacteria that is on the hands of personnel who touch the package. *[3: Limited Evidence]*

A period of 30 minutes to two hours may be necessary for the cooldown, but there is a lack of scientific evidence to support an exact amount of time needed for cooling. Cooling time will vary according to how hot items are at the end of the cycle, the density and composition of the materials contained within the load, the packaging material, and the temperature and

STERILIZATION

TABLE 4. TYPICAL MINIMUM CYCLE TIMES FOR DYNAMIC AIR-REMOVAL STEAM STERILIZATION[1]

Item	Exposure time at 270° F (132° C)	Exposure time at 275° F (135° C)	Drying times
Packaged instruments	4 minutes		20 to 30 minutes
		3 minutes	16 minutes
Textile packs	4 minutes		5 to 20 minutes
		3 minutes	3 minutes
Nonporous items subject to IUSS	See device and container manufacturer instructions for use	See device and container manufacturer instructions for use	See IUSS container manufacturer instructions for use
Nonporous and porous items in mixed load subject to IUSS	See device and container manufacturer instructions for use	See device and container manufacturer instructions for use	See IUSS container manufacturer instructions for use

REFERENCE
1. Association for the Advancement of Medical Instrumentation. ANSI/AAMI ST79:2010, A1:2010 & A2:2011, Comprehensive guide to steam sterilization and sterility assurance in health care facilities. Arlington, VA: Association for the Advancement of Medical Instrumentation; 2010 & 2011. Adapted and reprinted with permission. Further reproduction or distribution is prohibited.

humidity of the ambient environment.[6] Containers made from plastic may require an extended cooling period to ensure moisture is removed from the container. High-density items retain heat and may require extended cooling times.

At the end of a steam sterilization cycle, packages may contain moisture that migrates out of the package as a gas or water vapor during the drying and cooling period. Depending on the type of packaging, a moist area may be created that can act as a wick and draw bacteria from hands before appropriate cooling and drying.

The potential for the formation of condensation is decreased by allowing the contents of the sterilizer to remain untouched until the equalization of the temperature differential between the chamber and outside environment has occurred.[6]

There is a lack of definitive studies to support cracking the sterilizer door to facilitate drying. However, some sterilizer manufacturers' instructions for use may recommend cracking the sterilizer door.[22]

VI.d.1. Warm or hot items should not be placed on cool or cold surfaces. Items should be allowed to cool on the sterilization rack.

When hot and cold surfaces are brought together, moisture may condense from both inside and outside the package.[6]

VI.d.2. Sterilized packages or containers that have formed condensate should be considered unsterile, and the contents should not be used.[6]

Moisture can compromise the integrity of barrier material and the sterility of the contents. Moisture may indicate problems with the packaging and/or sterilization process.

Recommendation VII

Immediate use steam sterilization (IUSS) should be kept to a minimum and should be used only in selected clinical situations and in a controlled manner.[20,23]

Immediate use steam sterilization may be associated with increased risk of infection to patients.[1] Time constraints may result in pressure on personnel to eliminate or modify one or more steps in the cleaning and sterilization process.

The term *flash sterilization* has historically been used to describe steam sterilization of unwrapped items intended to be used immediately. Flash sterilization cycles have traditionally been either 3 or 10 minutes of exposure, depending on the nature of the device being sterilized or the type of cycle indicated, minimal or no dry time, and no cooldown, thereby making the entire cycle time shorter than the cycle times for wrapped or terminally sterilized items. However, current manufacturers' instructions for use may require a variety of cycle times and the use of single wrappers or flash containers as opposed to sterilizing unwrapped items. The term "flash sterilization" no longer serves to describe the various steam sterilization cycles and processes that are used to process items that are not intended to be stored for later use. For this reason, the more appropriate term is *IUSS*.

Immediate use is considered the shortest time possible between a sterilized item's removal from the sterilizer and its aseptic transfer to the sterile field. The term IUSS has been endorsed by AORN, the Association for Professionals in Infection Control and Epidemiology (APIC), the International Association of Healthcare Central Service Materiel Management (IAHCSMM), the Accreditation Association of Ambulatory Healthcare (AAAHC), and the Association of Surgical Technologists (AST), as well as the ASC Quality Collaboration, which represents the ambulatory surgery center industry.[20]

STERILIZATION

VII.a. Immediate use steam sterilization should be used only when there is insufficient time to process by the preferred wrapped or container method intended for terminal sterilization. Immediate use steam sterilization should not be used as a substitute for sufficient instrument inventory.[6,23] *[1: Strong Evidence]*

VII.a.1. Items to be steam sterilized for immediate use should be subjected to the same decontamination processes as described in AORN's Guideline for Cleaning and Care of Surgical Instruments.[4] Decontamination should be performed in an area intended, designed, and equipped for decontamination activities.

As with terminal sterilization, proper decontamination is essential for removing bioburden and preparing an item for IUSS. Failures in instrument cleaning have resulted in transmission of infectious agents.[24]

VII.a.2. Immediate use steam sterilization should be performed only if all of the following conditions are met:
- The device manufacturer's written instructions include instructions for IUSS.
- The device manufacturer's written instructions for cleaning, cycle type, exposure times, temperature settings, and drying times (if recommended) are available and followed.
- Items are placed in a containment device that has been validated for IUSS and cleared by the FDA for this purpose and in a manner that allows steam to contact all instrument surfaces.
- The containment device manufacturer's written instructions for use are followed.
- Measures are taken to prevent contamination during transfer to the sterile field.
- Items subjected to IUSS are used immediately and not stored for later use or held from one procedure to another.[6]

VII.b. Packaging and wrapping (eg, textiles, paper-plastic pouches, nonwoven wrappers) should not be used in IUSS cycles unless the sterilizer and the packaging are specifically intended and labeled for this use.[6] *[3: Limited Evidence]*

Cycle parameters vary according to sterilizer design.[21]

VII.b.1. Sterilizer manufacturers' written instructions should be followed and reconciled with packaging and device manufacturers' instructions for sterilization.[6]

VII.c. Each sterilization cycle should be monitored to verify that parameters required for sterilization have been met.[6] *[1: Strong Evidence]*

VII.c.1. The sterilizer operator should use physical monitors to verify cycle parameters for each load.[6]

Physical monitors (eg, printouts, digital reading, graphs, gauges) can indicate immediate sterilizer failure. Physical monitors record cycle parameters (eg, time, temperature) for each cycle.

VII.c.2. Biological and chemical indicators should be used to monitor sterilizer efficacy and to assess whether conditions of sterilization have been achieved.

Although products used to monitor sterilizer efficacy and achievement of required parameters vary according to type of cycle or type of sterilizer, monitoring requirements are the same for all types of steam sterilization. (See Recommendation XX for more detailed recommendations for a quality monitoring program and application of monitors.)

VII.c.3. A class 5 chemical integrating indicator or a class 6 indicator should be used within each sterilization container or tray used for IUSS.[6] Class 6 indicators are cycle-specific and should be used only in the specific cycles for which they are labeled.

VII.d. Devices processed using IUSS should be transported to the point of use in a manner that minimizes the risk of contamination of the item and injury to personnel handling the hot, wet, and possibly heavy trays. *[3: Limited Evidence]*

Immediate use steam sterilized items may be vulnerable to contamination by exposure to the environment and handling by personnel while transporting the sterile device to the point of use. It is important that sterilization processing be carried out in a clean environment and that IUSS devices are transferred to the point of use in a manner that prevents contamination.[20,25]

Because drying time is not usually part of a preprogrammed IUSS cycle, the items processed are assumed to be wet at the conclusion of the cycle and will be hot when removed from the sterilizer chamber immediately after the cycle.

VII.e. Rigid sterilization containers designed and intended for IUSS cycles should be used. *[3: Limited Evidence]*

Rigid IUSS containers protect items so as to reduce the risk of contamination during transport of items to the point of use and facilitate ease of presentation to the sterile field.[6,25]

VII.e.1. After each use, IUSS containers should be cleaned, inspected (eg, for wear of gaskets and other critical components), and maintained according to the manufacturer's written instructions.[6]

VII.e.2. Immediate use steam sterilization containers should be opened and the contents used immediately. Instruments processed in IUSS containers should not be stored for later use or held from one procedure to the next.[20]

VII.e.3. Items processed using IUSS should be differentiated from items processed using terminal sterilization.

VII.f. Immediate use steam sterilization should not be used for implantable devices except in cases of defined emergency when no other option is available.[1,6] *[1: Strong Evidence]*

Implants are foreign bodies and they increase the risk of SSI.[23] Careful planning, appropriate packaging, and inventory management in cooperation with suppliers can minimize the need for IUSS of implantable medical devices.

VII.f.1. When IUSS of an implant is unavoidable, cycle selection should be determined by the manufacturer's written instructions for use, and a biological indicator and a class 5 chemical integrating indicator should be run with the load.[6,21] When an implant is used before the biological indicator results are known and the biological indicator is later determined to have a positive result, the surgeon and infection preventionists should be notified as soon as the results are known. If the implant is not used, it should not be saved as sterile for future use. If, after inspection, it is determined that the implant is suitable for future use, resterilization of the implant is required.[6]

VII.f.2. Every implant should be fully traceable to the patient in whom it was implanted.[6]

VII.g Documentation of cycle information and monitoring results should be maintained in a log (ie, electronic or manual).[6] *[3: Limited Evidence]*

Documentation of cycle information provides a means for tracking items that are processed using IUSS to individual patients and for quality monitoring.

VII.g.1. Immediate use steam sterilization records should include information on each load, including
- the items processed,
- the patient on whom the items were used,
- the type of cycle (eg, gravity-displacement, dynamic air-removal),
- the cycle parameters used (eg, temperature, duration of cycle),
- monitoring results,
- the date and time the cycle was run,
- the operator information (ie, person who initiated the cycle, person who retrieved the item from the sterilizer), and
- the reason for IUSS.[6]

VII.g.2. A record describing what could have been done to prevent IUSS of the implant should be completed and used as part of a quality monitoring system.

A record of IUSS of implants can be helpful in determining problems, trends, or circumstances that can be addressed to prevent IUSS of implants in the future.

Recommendation VIII

Ethylene oxide sterilization is a low-temperature process that may be used for moisture- and heat-sensitive surgical items and when indicated by the device manufacturer.

At sterilizing temperatures, ethylene oxide kills microbes in hard-to-reach areas, and it does so with no damage to devices. Ethylene oxide is an alkylating agent that results in microbial death when used under controlled parameters. Ethylene oxide substitutes for hydrogen atoms on molecules needed to sustain life and, by attaching to these molecules, ethylene oxide stops these molecules' normal life-supporting functions. Some of the key molecules that ethylene oxide disrupts are proteins and DNA. Under low-temperature sterilizing conditions, so much ethylene oxide is used that this disruption proves lethal to microbial life.[26]

VIII.a. Ethylene oxide may be used if alternate methods of sterilization are not available or compatible with the medical devices being processed.[26,27] *[1: Strong Evidence]*

Health care organizations use 100% concentrations of ethylene oxide or ethylene oxide in mixtures with inert diluent gases (eg, carbon dioxide, hydrochlorofluorocarbons [HCFCs]) for ethylene oxide sterilization procedures. Until the 1990s, chlorofluorocarbons (CFCs) were used as diluents for ethylene oxide. Chlorofluorocarbons cause depletion of the ozone layer and are no longer produced in the United States. Hydrochlorofluorocarbons deplete the ozone layer, but to a lesser degree than CFCs.[27]

In 2015 the Environmental Protection Agency (EPA) will begin regulation of HCFCs, and production will terminate.[28] One hundred percent concentrations of ethylene oxide will continue to be available.

VIII.a.1. Users of HCFCs should be aware of and comply with federal, state, and local regulations regarding HCFC use in ethylene oxide sterilizers.

VIII.b. The manufacturer's written instructions should be reviewed to determine whether a heat- or moisture-sensitive item is compatible with ethylene oxide. *[3: Limited Evidence]*

VIII.c. Items, including all lumens, should be clean and dry before being packaged for ethylene oxide sterilization.[26] *[3: Limited Evidence]*

Soil inhibits sterilization, and moisture may produce toxic by-products. The combination of water and ethylene oxide results in the formation of ethylene glycol (a form of antifreeze).

STERILIZATION

VIII.d. Sterilizer manufacturers' written instructions should be followed for ethylene oxide-sterilization parameters and placement of items within the sterilizer.[26] *[3: Limited Evidence]*

Ethylene oxide sterilizers differ in design and operating characteristics.

VIII.d.1. Items should be placed in ethylene oxide sterilizers in baskets or on loading carts in a manner that allows free circulation and penetration of the ethylene oxide and moisture vapor.[26]

VIII.d.2. Full loads of items with common aeration times should be run unless the sterilizer is equipped with an air pollution control device.[29]

A full load is not the same as a full chamber. What constitutes a full load will vary among facilities.

VIII.e. A quality monitoring program that includes physical, chemical, and biological monitors should be used to verify that conditions necessary for sterilization have been met.[26] *[1: Strong Evidence]*

VIII.e.1. Each sterilization cycle should be monitored to verify that parameters required for sterilization have been met.[26]

VIII.e.2. The sterilizer operator should use physical monitors to verify cycle parameters for every load.

Physical monitors (eg, printouts, digital readings, graphs, gauges) can indicate immediate sterilizer failure. Physical monitors record cycle parameters (eg, time, temperature, humidity, gas concentration).

VIII.e.3. Chemical indicators designed for ethylene oxide monitoring should be used to verify that one or more of the conditions for sterilization have been met. A class 1 chemical indicator should be placed on the outside of every package unless the internal indicator is visible.[6,26] A chemical indicator validated for use in ethylene oxide should be placed inside every package.

VIII.e.4. Biological indicators should be used to monitor sterilizer efficacy and for load release. Every load should be monitored with a biological indicator.[26]

VIII.f. Ethylene oxide penetrates packaging materials. Items sterilized in ethylene oxide sterilizers should be properly aerated in a mechanical aerator to remove ethylene oxide. *[1: Regulatory Requirement]*

Ethylene oxide is a known human carcinogen and a chemical that has the potential to cause adverse reproductive effects in humans. The Occupational Safety and Health Administration (OSHA) has established exposure limits for ethylene oxide in the workplace.[30] If not removed, ethylene oxide residue absorbed into sterilized items represents a hazard to patients and personnel. Items that are not sufficiently aerated may cause patient or personnel injury (eg, chemical burns). Aeration is the only safe and effective way to remove residual ethylene oxide.[26,31]

Adequate aeration times reduce ethylene oxide vapors and residue to a level safe for exposure of both patients and health care personnel.

Rinsing an inadequately aerated item does not remove ethylene oxide and can create hazardous by-products.

VIII.f.1. Items should be sterilized and properly aerated in a single chamber.[32]

The EPA does not permit transfer of ethylene oxide-sterilized loads to a separate aerator.

VIII.f.2. Health care personnel should wear butyl rubber, nitrile, or neoprene gloves that provide protection to the skin when a situation arises in which it is necessary to handle unaerated ethylene oxide-sterilized items.[26]

Safety measures are necessary to prevent health care personnel from coming in contact with ethylene oxide residues.

VIII.f.3. Required aeration times are validated by the medical device manufacturer and should be established based on
- item composition and size,
- item preparation and packaging,
- density of the load,
- type of ethylene oxide sterilizer/aerator used,
- the device and sterilizer manufactures' written instructions for use, and
- temperature penetration pattern of the aerator's chamber.[26]

VIII.f.4. All ethylene oxide-sterilized items must be completely aerated before they can be used safely.
- Aeration cycles should not be interrupted to remove items for use.
- Items should remain in aerators until the aeration time has been completed.
- Aeration requirements for the most difficult-to-aerate products may require increased aeration time.

Ethylene oxide vapors and residues diffuse from sterilized items over time. This aeration or degassing process can be expedited by raising the temperature and by increasing the flow of air around the item.

VIII.f.5. Device manufacturers' written instructions should be followed for specific aeration requirements.

VIII.f.6. All aeration cycle parameters should be documented and the correct aeration time and temperature verified.

VIII.f.7. A program for monitoring occupational exposure to ethylene oxide must be established to document that worker exposure to ethylene oxide is below permissible exposure limits established by OSHA.

Compliance with regulations promotes a safe work environment that is within federal and state mandated limits.[30,33]

VIII.g. Personnel who have the potential for exposure should wear ethylene oxide-monitoring badges that meet the National Institute for Occupational Safety and Health standards for accuracy.[26,30,34] *[1: Regulatory Requirement]*

VIII.g.1. The ethylene oxide monitoring program in each organization must comply with OSHA regulations.

General environmental monitoring is not required, although it may provide an indicator of problems with the ventilation or ethylene oxide system. Monitoring of short-term exposures during a 15-minute period also is required while sterilization and aeration activities are being performed.

Permissible limits, as established by OSHA, for exposure to ethylene oxide are 1 part per million (ppm) of airborne ethylene oxide expressed as a time weighted average for an eight-hour work shift in a 40-hour work week, or 5 ppm for short-term exposure.[1,26,30]

VIII.h. Health and safety procedures should be developed for health care personnel who are at risk for exposure to ethylene oxide.[26] *[1: Regulatory Requirement]*

Established procedures help to identify, eliminate, or minimize risk from exposure to hazards as well as facilitate timely responses to accidental exposure and emergencies.

VIII.h.1. Personnel must be informed about the health effects and potential hazards associated with exposure to ethylene oxide.[30]

VIII.h.2. Information on ethylene oxide health effects and potential hazards must be provided at the time of assignment to an area where ethylene oxide is used and at least annually thereafter.[30]

VIII.h.3. Periodic employee and environmental physical assessment and testing should be carried out and documented according to current OSHA regulations.[26,30]

VIII.h.4. Personnel should be familiar with the organization's emergency spill plan.[30]

VIII.h.5. Personnel should be aware of safety procedures that should be implemented following exposure to ethylene oxide. The material safety data sheet (MSDS) for the type of ethylene oxide used should be consulted for specific first-aid measures after exposure. People who have inhaled concentrated ethylene oxide gas
- should seek fresh air immediately,
- may require the administration of oxygen, and
- may require cardiopulmonary resuscitation if respiratory or cardiac collapse occurs.[26,30,31]

VIII.i. Documentation of employee monitoring must be maintained in compliance with federal regulations. *[1: Regulatory Requirement]*

Regulations from OSHA require that documentation of employee breathing zone monitoring must be maintained in employees' health records for the duration of employment plus 30 years after termination of employment.[26,30]

Documentation establishes a continuous history of the work environment.

Recommendation IX

Low-temperature hydrogen peroxide gas plasma sterilization methods should be used to sterilize moisture- and heat-sensitive items and when indicated by the device manufacturer.[35]

Low-temperature hydrogen peroxide gas plasma sterilization uses a combination of hydrogen peroxide vapor and low-temperature hydrogen peroxide gas plasma. In this process, hydrogen peroxide, a strong oxidizing agent, kills microorganisms via the hydroxyl free radical. The hydroxyl free radical, being highly reactive, can attack membrane lipids, DNA, and other essential cell components. The plasma breaks down the hydrogen peroxide into a "cloud" of highly energized species that recombine, converting the hydrogen peroxide into water and oxygen.

Items processed using low-temperature hydrogen peroxide gas plasma do not require aeration because the residuals and by-products are oxygen and water in the form of humidity, and these by-products are nontoxic.[35,36] Items are dry at the end of the cycle.
Hydrogen peroxide is an irritant of the eyes, mucous membranes, and skin.[37] It is considered nonmutagenic and noncarcenogenic.[38,39]

IX.a. The sterilizer manufacturer's written instructions for use, monitoring, and maintenance should be followed when using a low-temperature hydrogen peroxide gas plasma sterilization system.[35] *[3: Limited Evidence]*

IX.a.1. Written documentation of the acceptability of low-temperature hydrogen peroxide gas plasma sterilization for specific devices should be obtained from the device and sterilizer manufacturers.

IX.a.2. Devices with lumens should be evaluated to determine whether the lumen diameter and length are within the sterilizer manufacturer's acceptable dimensions as specified in

STERILIZATION

the sterilizer manufacturer's instructions for use.[35,40]

IX.a.3. The placement of items within the chamber should comply with the sterilizer manufacturer's instructions for use.

Correct placement and configuration of items within the chamber facilitates contact of the sterilant with the items to be sterilized. Sterilant contact is essential for sterilization.[6]

IX.b. Items to be sterilized using low-temperature hydrogen peroxide gas plasma sterilization should be clean, thoroughly dry, and packaged in sterilization wraps, pouches, trays, or containers cleared by the FDA for use in hydrogen peroxide gas plasma. *[1: Strong Evidence]*

Liquids and cellulose-based (ie, paper-based) packaging materials or products are not suitable for low-temperature hydrogen peroxide gas plasma sterilization.[1]

IX.b.1. Trays, mats, containers, and other accessories designed and validated for use with low-temperature hydrogen peroxide gas plasma should be used.

IX.c. A quality monitoring program that includes physical monitors (eg, printouts, digital readings, graphs, gauges), chemical indicators, and biological indicators should be used. *[1: Strong Evidence]*

These monitors and indicators verify that conditions necessary for sterilization have been met.[6]

IX.c.1. Each sterilization cycle should be monitored to verify that parameters required for sterilization have been met.[6]

IX.c.2. The sterilizer operator should use physical monitors to verify cycle parameters for every load.

Physical monitors can indicate immediate sterilizer failure. Physical monitors record cycle parameters (eg, pressure, time) for each cycle.

IX.c.3. Chemical and biological indicators should be used to monitor sterilizer efficacy and to assess whether parameters of sterilization have been achieved.[6]

IX.c.4. A class 1 chemical indicator should be placed on the outside of every package unless the internal indicator is visible.[6]

IX.c.5. An FDA-cleared chemical indicator recommended by the manufacturer of the selected sterilization system should be placed within each package to be sterilized.[6,41]

IX.c.6. Biological monitors should be used to assess sterilizer efficacy.[6] Routine sterilizer efficacy monitoring should be performed daily, preferably with every load.[35]

Recommendation X

Low-temperature hydrogen peroxide vapor sterilization methods should be used for moisture- and heat-sensitive items and when indicated by the device manufacturer.

Low-temperature hydrogen peroxide vapor sterilization uses vaporized hydrogen peroxide as the sterilant. For this process, hydrogen peroxide sterilant is introduced into the chamber through a vaporizer under low pressure, creating a vapor that fills the sterilization chamber. As the hydrogen peroxide vapor diffuses and contacts surfaces, an oxidative process inactivates microorganisms. Devices sterilized using this process do not require aeration because the by-products are oxygen and water vapor, which are nontoxic.[1,42]

X.a. The sterilizer manufacturer's written instructions for use, monitoring, and maintenance should be followed when using a low-temperature hydrogen peroxide vapor sterilization system.[35] *[3: Limited Evidence]*

X.a.1. Written documentation of the acceptability of low-temperature hydrogen peroxide vapor should be obtained from the device manufacturer or the sterilizer manufacturer's list of validated devices.

X.a.2. Devices with lumens should be evaluated to determine whether the lumen diameter and length are within the sterilizer manufacturer's acceptable dimensions as specified in the instructions for use.[42]

X.a.3. Items should be placed within the chamber in compliance with the sterilizer manufacturer's instructions for use.

Correct placement and configuration of items within the chamber facilitates contact of the sterilant with the items to be sterilized. Sterilant contact is essential for sterilization.[6]

X.b. Items to be sterilized using low-temperature hydrogen peroxide vapor should be clean, thoroughly dry, and packaged in sterilization wraps, pouches, trays, or containers cleared by the FDA for use in the specific low-temperature hydrogen peroxide vapor system. *[1: Strong Evidence]*

Liquids and cellulose-based (eg, paper-based) packaging materials or products and liquids are not suitable for low-temperature hydrogen peroxide vapor sterilization.[1]

X.b.1. Trays, mats, containers, and other accessories designed and validated for use with low-temperature hydrogen peroxide vapor sterilization should be used.

X.c. A quality monitoring program that includes physical monitors (eg, printouts, digital readings, graphs, gauges), chemical indicators, and biological indicators should be used to verify that conditions necessary for sterilization have been met.[6] *[1: Strong Evidence]*

X.c.1. Each sterilization cycle should be monitored to verify that parameters required for sterilization have been met.[6]

X.c.2. The sterilizer operator should use physical monitors to verify that required sterilization parameters are met for every load.[6]

Physical monitors can indicate immediate sterilizer failure. Physical monitors record cycle parameters (eg, time, pressure) for each cycle.

X.c.3. Chemical and biological indicators should be used to monitor sterilizer efficacy and to assess whether parameters of sterilization have been achieved.[6] Efficacy testing should be performed in accordance with manufacturers' instructions.

X.c.4. A class 1 chemical indicator should be placed on the outside of every package unless the internal indicator is visible.[6]

X.c.5. An FDA-cleared chemical indicator recommended by the manufacturer of the selected sterilization system should be placed within each package to be sterilized.[6,41]

Recommendation XI

Sterilization systems using ozone should be used for moisture- and heat-sensitive items when indicated by the device manufacturer.

Ozone has been cleared by the FDA for use in the sterilization of metal and plastic surgical instruments, including some instruments with lumens.[43] Ozone is a strong oxidizer, which makes ozone sterilization an effective low-temperature sterilization process. Ozone is generated within the sterilizer using only oxygen and water. On completion of the sterilization cycle, ozone is exhausted through a catalytic converter, where it is converted back into the raw materials of oxygen and water. No aeration of sterilized items is necessary because these by-products are nontoxic.[35,36,44]

XI.a. Manufacturers' written instruction for operating, monitoring, and maintaining ozone sterilizers should be followed. *[3: Limited Evidence]*

XI.a.1. Written documentation of the acceptability of ozone sterilization should be obtained from the device manufacturer or the sterilizer manufacturer's list of validated devices.

XI.a.2. Devices with lumens should be evaluated to determine whether lumen diameter and length are within the sterilizer manufacturer's acceptable dimensions as specified in the instructions for use.

XI.b. Items to be sterilized using ozone should be packaged in nonwoven pouches or reusable rigid sterilization containers cleared by the FDA for use in ozone sterilizers.[35,44] *[2: Moderate Evidence]*

Cellulose-based (eg, paper-based) packaging materials or products are not suitable for ozone sterilization.[43]

XI.c. Items should be placed in the sterilizer chamber in compliance with the sterilizer manufacturer's instructions for use. *[3: Limited Evidence]*

Correct placement and configuration of items in the chamber facilitates contact of the sterilant with the items to be sterilized. Sterilant contact is essential for sterilization.[6]

XI.d. A quality monitoring program that includes physical monitors (eg, printouts, digital readings, graphs, gauges), chemical indicators, and biological indicators should be used to verify that conditions necessary for sterilization have been met.[6] *[1: Strong Evidence]*

XI.d.1. Each sterilization cycle should be monitored to verify that parameters required for sterilization have been met.[6]

XI.d.2. The sterilizer operator should use physical monitors to verify parameters for every load.[6]

Physical monitors can indicate immediate sterilizer failure. Physical monitors record cycle parameters (eg, time, pressure) for each cycle.

XI.d.3. Chemical and biological indicators should be used to monitor sterilizer efficacy and to assess whether parameters of sterilization have been achieved.[6] Efficacy testing should be performed in accordance with manufacturers' instructions.

XI.d.4. A class 1 chemical indicator should be located on the outside of every package unless the internal indicator is visible.[6]

XI.d.5. An FDA-cleared chemical indicator recommended by the manufacturer of the selected sterilization system should be placed within each package to be sterilized.[6,41]

Recommendation XII

Dry-heat sterilization should be used only for materials that are impenetrable to moist heat.[1] Dry heat may be used to sterilize anhydrous (ie, waterless) items that can withstand high temperatures and when indicated by the device manufacturer.

Sharp instruments that would be damaged by the moisture of steam may be sterilized by dry heat.[45] Dental instruments, burrs, reusable needles, glassware, and heat-stable powders and oils are examples of items that can withstand the high temperatures generated by dry-heat sterilization. Dry heat is an oxidation or slow-burning process that coagulates protein in microbial cells. Sterilization is accomplished through the transfer of heat energy to objects on contact. There is no moisture present in a dry-heat process, so

STERILIZATION

microorganisms are destroyed by a very slow process of heat absorption.[46]

Presterilized oils and powders are commercially available and may eliminate the need for a dry heat sterilizer.

XII.a. Dry-heat sterilizers should be used, monitored, and maintained according to the manufacturer's written instructions.[46] *[3: Limited Evidence]*

Dry-heat sterilizers may vary in design and performance characteristics.

XII.b. Only packaging and container materials designed and validated by the packaging manufacturer to withstand the high temperature of dry-heat sterilization should be used.[46] *[3: Limited Evidence]*

If packaging is not formulated for dry-heat sterilization, pouches may char, compromising the package integrity of sterilized items.

XII.b.1. Closed containers or cassettes should be used based on the manufacturer's instructions and biological indicator monitoring results. Closed containers or cassettes may extend the time needed to achieve sterilization.

XII.b.2. Packaging manufacturers should be consulted to confirm the compatibility of the packaging material with sterilizer temperatures before packaging materials are selected for dry-heat sterilization.[46]

Most types of tape are not designed to withstand the high temperatures of dry-heat sterilization. Tape adhesive melts when subjected to dry-heat sterilization and may leave a sticky residue on sterilized packages that degrades, leaving baked-on tape residue on the items, or can result in loss of tape adhesion.[46]

XII.b.3. When possible, small containers should be used for items to be dry-heat sterilized, and package density should be as low as possible.[46]

XII.c. Items should be placed within the sterilizer chamber according to the sterilizer manufacturer's instructions for use. *[3: Limited Evidence]*

Correct placement and configuration of items within the chamber facilitates contact of the sterilant with the items to be sterilized. Sterilant contact is essential for sterilization.[46]

XII.d. The operator should be aware of the hazards associated with dry-heat sterilization and use the appropriate PPE (eg, insulated gloves, transfer handles).[46] *[3: Limited Evidence]*

Burns are the most common safety hazard associated with dry-heat sterilization.[46]

XII.d.1. On completion of a dry-heat sterilization cycle, both the sterilizer chamber and the items in the chamber are very hot and should not be touched.

XII.d.2. Packages should be cooled before being handled or removed from the dry-heat sterilizer.

XII.e. A quality monitoring program that includes physical monitors (eg, printouts, digital readings, graphs, gauges), chemical indicators, and biological indicators should be used to verify that conditions necessary for sterilization have been met.[46] *[1: Strong Evidence]*

XII.e.1. Each sterilization cycle should be monitored to verify that parameters for sterilization have been met.[46]

XII.e.2. The sterilizer operator should use physical monitors to verify parameters for every load.[6]

Physical monitors can indicate immediate sterilizer failure. Physical monitors record cycle parameters (eg, time, pressure) for each cycle.

XII.e.3. A class 1 chemical indicator should be located on the outside of every package unless the internal indicator is visible.[6]

XII.e.4. An FDA-cleared chemical indicator recommended by the manufacturer of the selected sterilization system should be placed within each package to be sterilized.[6,41]

Recommendation XIII

Liquid chemical sterilant instrument processing systems that use peracetic acid as a low-temperature sterilant should be used for devices that are heat-sensitive, can be immersed, are approved for this process by the device manufacturer, and cannot be sterilized using terminal sterilization methods.[47,48]

Peracetic acid is an oxidizing agent that is an effective biocide at low temperatures and is effective in the presence of organic matter.[1] It has a chemical formula of acetic acid plus an extra oxygen atom. This extra oxygen atom is highly reactive, reacts with most cellular components, and causes cellular death. The ability of peracetic acid to inactivate many different critical cell systems is responsible for its broad spectrum antimicrobial activity. As peracetic acid returns to acetic acid (ie, vinegar) and the oxygen decomposes, it is rendered nontoxic and environmentally safe. Following liquid chemical sterilant processing, devices are rinsed with potable tap water that has been passed through pre-filters, subjected to an ultraviolet light treatment, and then passed through two 0.1-micron filter membranes.[47]

XIII.a. Liquid chemical sterilant systems using peracetic acid should be used only to process items validated for processing in liquid peracetic acid.[1,48] *[1: Strong Evidence]*

Items processed in liquid chemical sterilant systems that are not validated for these systems may not be compatible with the sterilant or the

STERILIZATION

process, which could result in damage or an ineffective process.

XIII.a.1. The ability to successfully process devices intended for use with a liquid chemical sterilant system that uses peracetic acid should be validated by the device manufacturer and comply with the liquid chemical sterilant processing system manufacturer's written instructions.[35]

Processing devices that are incompatible with liquid chemical sterilant processing systems can shorten the life of the devices.

XIII.a.2. Documentation of devices that can and cannot be processed in liquid chemical sterilant systems using peracetic acid should be obtained from the device and the liquid chemical sterilant system manufacturers.

XIII.b. Critical items processed in liquid chemical sterilant systems should be used immediately and not stored for later use or held from one procedure to another.[47] *[1: Strong Evidence]*

Processing trays used in liquid chemical sterilant systems are not intended for storage of processed items.

XIII.c. Systems using liquid peracetic acid should be used, monitored, and maintained according to the manufacturer's written instructions. *[3: Limited Evidence]*

Peracetic acid is an effective sterilizing agent that does not leave toxic residues on sterilized items when items are rinsed properly. Serious injuries (eg, burns) may result if the chemical is not handled, neutralized, and rinsed properly. Peracetic acid is corrosive to the skin at concentrations of 3.4% or higher and corrosive to the eyes at concentrations of 0.35% or higher.[49]

XIII.d. When using liquid chemical sterilant processing systems, health care personnel should verify proper selection of adapters and connect the device to the appropriate adapters as recommended by the manufacturer of both the device and the liquid chemical sterilant processing system.[50] *[2: Moderate Evidence]*

Failure to do so may result in failure of the liquid chemical sterilant to contact the lumen of the item.

XIII.e. Items processed in a liquid chemical sterilant system using peracetic acid should be transported to the point of use and used immediately.[1] *[1: Strong Evidence]*

Items processed with peracetic acid are wet and the cassette or container in which they are processed is not sealed to prevent contamination, thereby increasing the risk of contamination if the items are not used immediately.

XIII.f. A quality monitoring program that includes physical monitors (eg, printouts, digital readings, graphs, gauges) and chemical indicators should be used to verify that conditions necessary for processing have been met.[1,6] *[1: Strong Evidence]*

XIII.f.1. Each sterilization cycle should be monitored to verify that parameters required for processing have been met.[6]

XIII.f.2. The liquid chemical sterilant processing system operator should use physical monitors to verify that parameters required for processing have been met.[35]

Physical monitors can indicate immediate failure to achieve required parameters.

XIII.f.3. Each cycle should be monitored with a chemical indicator validated for use in the liquid chemical sterilant system according to the manufacturer's instructions for use.[35] Biological indicators have not been cleared by the FDA for use with liquid peracetic acid systems.

Recommendation XIV

A formalized program between the health care organization and health care industry representatives should be established for the receipt and use of loaned instrumentation.[51]

Implementation of tracking and quality controls and procedures is necessary to manage instrumentation and implants that are brought in from outside organizations and companies.[52]

XIV.a. Interdisciplinary collaboration between health care organizations' sterile processing and surgical services personnel and commercial health care industry representatives should be established.[6] *[3: Limited Evidence]*

The systematic management of loaned instrumentation reduces loss and ensures proper decontamination and sterilization through increased collaboration, communication, and accountability.

XIV.b. The loaned instrumentation program should include processes to
- request loaned instrumentation or implants;
- receive loaned items, including a detailed inventory list;
- obtain manufacturers' written instructions for instrument care, cleaning, assembly, and sterilization;
- determine responsibility for ensuring sets weigh no more than 25 lb;
- clean, decontaminate, and sterilize loaned instrumentation at the receiving facility in accordance with AORN's Guideline for Cleaning and Care of Surgical Instruments[4];
- transport processed loaned instrumentation to the point of use;
- return items to the sterile processing department after the procedure for decontamination, processing, inventory, and return to the health care industry representative; and

STERILIZATION

- maintain records of transactions.
  [3: Limited Evidence]

XIV.c. The manufacturer's instructions for cleaning, packaging, and sterilizing should be obtained before loaned items are received.[52] *[3: Limited Evidence]*

Advanced delivery of instructions for cleaning, packaging, and sterilizing is useful in determining whether a facility has the required equipment and resources to process loaned instruments according to the device manufacturer's written instructions.

XIV.d. Personnel should coordinate requests for loaned instrumentation in sufficient time for loaned items to be processed by conventional terminal sterilization methods.[52] *[3: Limited Evidence]*

Advanced delivery of loaned items to the receiving health care organization ensures sufficient time to permit inhouse disassembly, cleaning, packaging, quality assurance testing, and sterilization of the instruments before scheduled procedures.

XIV.d.1. Personnel requesting loaned items should specify quantities, estimated time of use and return, and restocking requirements to circumvent the need for IUSS.

XIV.d.2. Late receipt of loaned instruments should not be used to justify IUSS.[23,53]

XIV.e. Sterility assurance related to loaned instruments should begin at the point at which the health care organization assumes responsibility for the items.[6] *[3: Limited Evidence]*

Failures in instrument cleaning have resulted in transmission of infectious agents.[24,53]

XIV.e.1. All loaned instruments, regardless of whether they were processed in another health care facility, should be considered contaminated and delivered directly to the sterile processing department for decontamination.[51] Instruments should be thoroughly cleaned and dried in a manner consistent with AORN's Guideline for Cleaning and Care of Surgical Instruments[4] and the guidelines of the Association for the Advancement of Medical Instrumentation (AAMI)[51] before sterilization.

It is not possible to know under what conditions instruments were processed at another facility. Sterilized instruments may become contaminated during transport.

XIV.e.2. Newly manufactured loaned items should be properly decontaminated before sterilization to remove bioburden and substances (eg, oil, grease) that may remain on the item from the manufacturing process.[6]

XIV.e.3. Loaned instruments should be removed from external shipping containers before transport to the sterile processing area.[6]

External shipping containers may have potentially high microbial contamination because of environmental exposure during transport.

XIV.e.4. Rigid sterilization containers should be thoroughly inspected upon receipt and cleaned and decontaminated according to the container manufacturer's instructions.

XIV.e.5. The type and quantity of loaned items should be inventoried and documented.

XIV.e.6. Implants and instruments should be visually inspected for damage.

XIV.e.7. Manufacturers' instructions for processing and sterilizing loaned items should be followed.

XIV.e.8. Implantable devices should be sterilized with a biological indicator and a class 5 integrating indicator and documented in accordance with regulatory requirements and AORN guidelines.

XIV.e.9. After use, loaned items should be decontaminated and returned to the lender in accordance with the health care organization's policy.

Recommendation XV

Sterilized materials should be labeled and stored in a manner to ensure sterility, and each item should be marked with the sterilization date.[6]

Limiting exposure to moisture, dust, excessive light or handling, and temperature and humidity extremes decreases potential contamination of sterilized items.[6] Factors that contribute to contamination include air movement, humidity, temperature, location of storage, presence of vermin, whether shelving is open or closed, and properties of the packaging material.[1]

XV.a. The shelf life of a packaged sterile item should be considered event-related. *[2: Moderate Evidence]*

Shelf life is dependent on packaging material, storage conditions, transport, and handling. An event must occur to compromise package content sterility. Events that may compromise the sterility of a package include

- multiple instances of handling that leads to seal breakage or loss of package integrity,
- moisture penetration, and
- exposure to airborne contaminants.[6,26,46]

Several studies have resulted in data that support event-related shelf life. One study examined the effect of time on the sterility of peel pouches, paper envelopes, and nylon sleeves and showed no increased rate of contamination over time when packages were placed in covered storage.[54] Another study showed that items covered with 3 mil (3/1,000

STERILIZATION

inch) polyethylene overwrap were sterile nine months after sterilization.[1] Another microbiological study examined items after two years of storage and showed no contamination.[55] The prospective study, which was conducted over a two-year period, evaluated the effectiveness of event-related shelf life and included placing 152 items that were terminally sterilized on shelves in various wards. Every three months, several items were tested for microbial contamination and all were found to be sterile.

XV.b. Sterile packages should be stored under environmentally controlled conditions.[6] *[3: Limited Evidence]*

Controlled conditions reduce the risk of contamination of sterile items.

XV.b.1. Room temperature, humidity, and ventilation should be controlled in accordance with local, state, and federal policies and regulations.

Regulatory agencies may enforce American Society for Healthcare Engineering (ASHE)[56] or AAMI[6] recommendations or they may enforce other guidelines. As stated in the ASHE document, these parameters are intended to be used for the design of the heating, ventilation, and air-conditioning (HVAC) systems and there may be daily fluctuations based on the environmental conditions.

Recommendations from AAMI include that temperature in sterile storage areas not exceed 75° F (24° C), that there be a minimum of 4 air exchanges per hour, and that relative humidity is between 20% and 60% and not higher than 70%.[6] The ASHE recommends temperatures in the sterile storage area of between 72° F to 78° F (22° C to 26° C) and that humidity not exceed 60%.[56]

Research on the relationship between temperature, humidity, air exchange, and maintenance of sterility is lacking.

XV.b.2. When selecting a temperature and humidity level or range, the perioperative team should collaborate with infection preventionists and facility engineers and consider the pathogens that pose risk to patients and personnel and the effect of temperature and humidity on those organisms.

Other considerations when determining temperature and humidity levels include personnel comfort and the fact that high temperature and humidity levels may lead to the development of condensate on walls and surfaces, which could serve as a wicking agent for the transmission of microorganisms and result in contamination of sterile items.

XV.b.3. Access to sterile supply areas should be limited to personnel who are trained in handling sterile supplies.

XV.b.4. Sterile storage areas, including racks, shelves, bins, and containers, should be kept clean and dry.[57]

XV.b.5. Supplies should be stored in a manner that allows adequate air circulation and ease of cleaning in compliance with local fire codes and in a manner that reduces the risk of contamination.

Recommendations for supply storage are generally 8 to 10 inches from the floor and 2 inches from outside walls. Fire code regulations specify the minimum clearance between sprinkler heads and stored items, with the typical minimum distance being 18 inches, to allow the sprinkler system to be effective.[58]

XV.b.6. Sterile items should not be stored under sinks or in other locations where they can become wet.[1]

XV.b.7. Sterile items should be stored in closed cabinets or covered carts. Open shelving may be used if it is located in a secure, environmentally controlled, clean area.[1]

XV.b.8. Supplies and equipment should be removed from external shipping containers and web-edged or corrugated cardboard boxes before transfer into the sterile storage area.

External shipping containers and web-edged cardboard boxes may collect dust, debris, and insects during shipment and may carry contaminants into the surgical suite.[6,26,46]

Recommendation XVI

Transportation of sterile items should be controlled.

Sterility is event-related and is dependent on the amount of handling, the conditions during transportation and storage, and the quality of the packaging material.[1]

XVI.a. Sterile items should be transported in covered or enclosed carts with solid-bottom shelves.[6] *[3: Limited Evidence]*

Covered or enclosed carts protect sterile items from exposure to environmental contaminants during transportation.

XVI.b. Carts and reusable covers should be cleaned after each use. *[3: Limited Evidence]*

Contaminants may be picked up from the environment during transport.[6]

STERILIZATION

Recommendation XVII

Personnel should receive initial and ongoing education and competency validation for sterilization practices.

Initial and ongoing education of perioperative personnel on sterilization practices facilitates the development of knowledge, skills, and attitudes that affect safe patient care.

Periodic educational programs provide the opportunity to reinforce the principles of sterilization, the compatibility of equipment and accessories, and the potential hazards to patients and personnel; and to introduce new information on technology changes and new applications.

Competency validation measures individual performance and provides a mechanism for documentation. Competency assessment verifies that perioperative personnel have an understanding of sterilization and sterilization practices.

XVII.a. An introduction to and review of policies and procedures should be included in personnel orientation to sterile processing of surgical instruments in the perioperative setting. Continuing education should be provided for employees when new equipment, instruments, and processes are introduced. *[5: No Evidence]*

Operator and processing errors may be minimized with regularly scheduled education, training, and competency demonstration.

XVII.b. Sterilization-specific education and competency assessment should encompass all sterilization methodologies that are in use in the organization, including
- operation and maintenance of sterilization equipment;
- selection and monitoring of sterilization cycles;
- use of chemical, biological, and physical monitors; and
- documentation requirements.

[5: No Evidence]

XVII.c. Education should address topics that include
- orientation to equipment and work areas;
- infection control policies and procedures, including exposure plans;
- potential hazards in the environment and methods of hazard protection;
- safe ergonomic practices;
- use and location of MSDSs; and
- standards, guidelines, recommended practices, and regulations related to instrument processing.

[5: No Evidence]

Recommendation XVIII

Documentation should reflect activities related to sterilization.[6]

Documentation demonstrates compliance with regulatory and accrediting agency requirements and identifies trends and quality improvement opportunities.

XVIII.a. Sterilization records should be maintained for the amount of time specified in the health care organization's policies and should be in compliance with professional standards and local, state, and federal regulations.[1,6,26,46] *[2: Moderate Evidence]*

Accurate and complete records are required for process verification and are used in sterilizer function analysis.

XVIII.b. Every sterilization cycle and modality, including steam (eg, gravity-displacement, dynamic air-removal), ethylene oxide, hydrogen peroxide gas plasma, hydrogen peroxide vapor, ozone, and dry heat should be documented. Documentation should include
- contents of each load;
- load identification;
- exposure parameters;
- the operator's name or initials; and
- results of physical, chemical, and biological monitors.[1]

[1: Strong Evidence]

Recommendation XIX

Policies and procedures for sterilization and sterilization-related processes and practices should be developed, reviewed periodically, revised as necessary, and readily available in the practice setting.

Policies and procedures assist in the development of patient safety, quality assessment, and performance improvement activities. Policies and procedures establish authority, responsibility, and accountability within the facility. They also serve as operational guidelines that are used to minimize patient risk factors for complications, standardize practice, direct perioperative personnel, and establish continual performance improvement programs.

XIX.a. The recommendations for sterilization should be used to guide the development of policies and procedures within individual perioperative practice settings. *[5: No Evidence]*

XIX.b. Policies and procedures should be developed and implemented for processes including
- routine cleaning of sterilizer chambers, carts, and exterior surfaces;
- transport of contaminated devices and equipment to the decontamination area;
- selection of sterilization modality and cycle;
- evaluation and selection of sterilization equipment and accessories[59];
- release of implants that are not terminally sterilized;
- care and handling of loaned instruments;
- orientation of and competency review for personnel who are responsible for sterilizing items;

- sterilization of items intended for immediate use;
- documentation of sterilization processes, environmental conditions, load contents, and load numbers;
- sterilization process monitoring;
- sterilization equipment maintenance;
- storage of sterile items;
- transport and distribution of sterile items; and
- product testing.

[5: No Evidence]

Capital equipment and medical device procurement are collaborative processes that require clinical, business, financial, and legal acumen. Goals of product standardization and value analysis processes are to select functional and reliable products that are safe, cost-effective, and environmentally friendly and that promote quality care and avoid duplication or rapid obsolescence.

XIX.c. The sterilizer manufacturer's written instructions for cleaning, operation, and maintenance should be reviewed and reflected in instrument processing policies and procedures. *[5: No Evidence]*

XIX.c.1. User manuals for all sterilization equipment should be readily available to the sterilizer operators.

As new sterilization technologies are introduced for use in perioperative practice settings, it is imperative that health care personnel strictly follow manufacturers' written instructions for the operation and maintenance of sterilization equipment and be aware of the occupational hazards that different sterilants may pose to patients, health care personnel, and the environment.

XIX.c.2. Equipment and device manuals that provide instructions for use should be retained for the life of the device and sterilizer.

Recommendation XX

A quality assurance and performance improvement process should be in place to measure patient, process, and system outcome indicators.

Quality assurance and performance improvement programs assist in evaluating the quality of patient care and the formulation of plans for corrective actions. These programs provide data that may be used to determine whether an individual organization is within benchmark goals and, if not, identify areas that may require corrective actions.

XX.a. The health care organization should establish quality control and improvement programs to monitor the workplace environment and practices associated with cleaning, disinfection, and sterilization of surgical instruments.[6] *[3: Limited Evidence]*

Monitoring the sterilization process allows results to be compared to a predetermined level of quality. Reviewing the findings provides information identifying problems and trends, which can be used to improve practice.

XX.a.1. Physical, chemical, and biological monitors should be used to monitor sterilization processes. They should be used for routine load release, routine sterilizer efficacy testing, and sterilizer qualification testing (eg, after installation, relocation, malfunction, major repair, sterilization process failure). Table 5 and Table 6 illustrate recommendations for process monitoring and types of monitors, respectively.

XX.b. All sterilizer failures and corrective actions should be documented and reported to the infection preventionist, quality assurance or risk management committee, and to administrators.[6] *[3: Limited Evidence]*

XX.c. All physical, chemical, and biological monitoring results, including results from controls, should be interpreted by qualified personnel in the time frame specified by the manufacturer of the monitor and should be included in the sterilization records. *[3: Limited Evidence]*

Accurate interpretation and reporting of results promotes safe patient care.[6]

XX.d. Immediate investigation and corrective action should be taken in the event of a physical, chemical, or biological monitor failure.[6] *[3: Limited Evidence]*

XX.d.1. The sterilizer printout should be checked first to determine whether cycle parameters were met. If parameters were not met, the sterilizer should be removed from service, the load should be quarantined, and the cause of the failure should be investigated.[6]

XX.d.2. If the cause of the failure is immediately identified (eg, operator error) or the failure is confined to a single item within the load, the cause should be corrected, the sterilizer returned to service, and the load reprocessed.[6]

XX.d.3. If the cause of the failure is not immediately identified, the load should be quarantined and the sterilizer taken out of service. The cause should be investigated and the sterilizer only returned to service when the cause is identified and rectified.[6]

XX.d.4. If they are retrievable, items that were processed in the suspect sterilizer (ie, back to the last known negative biological indicator test) should be recalled and reprocessed before use.[6] When a tracking system is present, it can be used to identify items and the patient or patients on whom the items may have been used before it was known that

STERILIZATION

Table 5. Steam Sterilization Process Monitoring Recommendations[1]

Routine load release		Routine sterilizer efficacy monitoring	Sterilizer qualification testing (after installation, relocation, malfunction, major repair, sterilization process failure)	Periodic product quality assurance testing
Nonimplants	**Implants**			
Physical monitoring of cycle	Physical monitoring of cycle	Physical monitoring of cycle	Physical monitoring of cycle	Physical monitoring of cycle
External and internal chemical indicator (CI) monitoring of packages	External and internal CI monitoring of packages	External and internal CI monitoring of packages	External and internal CI monitoring of packages	Placement of BIs and CIs within product test sample
Optional monitoring of the load with a process challenge device (PCD) containing one of the following: • a biological indicator (BI) • a BI and a class 5 integrating indicator • a class 5 integrating indicator • a class 6 emulating indicator	Monitoring of every load with a PCD containing a BI and a class 5 integrating indicator	Weekly, preferably daily (ie, each day the sterilizer is used), monitoring with a PCD containing a BI; the PCD also may contain a CI	For sterilizers larger than 2 cubic feet and for IUSS cycles, monitoring of three consecutive cycles in an empty chamber with a PCD containing a BI; the PCD also may contain a CI	
		For sterilizers larger than 2 cubic feet and for table-top sterilizers, monitoring performed in a fully loaded chamber	For table-top sterilizers, monitoring of three consecutive cycles in a fully loaded chamber with a PCD containing a BI; the PCD also may contain a CI	
		In immediate use steam sterilization (IUSS) cycles, monitoring performed in an empty chamber	For dynamic air-removal sterilizers, monitoring of three consecutive cycles in an empty chamber with a Bowie-Dick test pack	
		For dynamic air-removal sterilizers, daily Bowie-Dick testing in an empty chamber		

Reference
1. Association for the Advancement of Medical Instrumentation. ANSI/AAMI ST79:2010, A1:2010 & A2:2011, *Comprehensive guide to steam sterilization and sterility assurance in health care facilities*. Arlington, VA: Association for the Advancement of Medical Instrumentation; 2010 & 2011. Adapted and reprinted with permission. Further reproduction or distribution prohibited.

---

the items should be retrieved. This information can be used to determine further patient care.
- The positive biological indicator vial should be sent to the laboratory for subculturing for bacilli. The recall should not be delayed during this testing.
- All actions taken in response to a positive biological indicator should be documented.

A positive control should be placed in each incubator each day a test vial is run and incubated. The control and the test vials should be from the same lot.[6]

XX.d.5. Positive biological indicator results should be reported immediately so that appropriate action can be taken.

XX.e. Processed items should be labeled with load control numbers to identify the sterilizer used, the cycle or load number, and the date of sterilization. Where tracking systems exist, documentation should be used to track instruments to the patient on whom they were used. *[3: Limited Evidence]*

Load control numbers allow items to be identified or retrieved in the event of a sterilizer failure or malfunction.[6,26,46]

XX.e.1. Information should be recorded from each sterilization cycle and should include the
- identification of the sterilizer (eg, "sterilizer #1"),
- type of sterilizer and cycle used,
- load control number,
- load contents (eg, major set, Kelly clamps),
- critical parameters for the specific sterilization methodology (eg, exposure time, temperature for steam sterilization),
- operator's name, and
- results of sterilization process monitoring (ie, biological, chemical, physical).[1]

Documentation is an important component of a quality control program.

STERILIZATION

XX.f. Physical monitors should be used to verify that parameters (eg, time, temperature, pressure, humidity, gas concentration) for sterilization have been met. *[3: Limited Evidence]*

Physical monitoring provides real-time assessments of cycle conditions as well as historic records by means of printouts, digital readings, graphs, or gauges. Reviewing data from physical monitoring can readily identify sterilizer malfunctions to expedite corrective actions.[6]

XX.f.1. Recordings of physical data should be used, when available, for all sterilization methods to ascertain that sterilization systems function within manufacturers' specifications.[6,26]

XX.f.2. The printout should be reviewed at the end of each cycle and signed by the sterilizer operator, verifying that all sterilization parameters were met.

XX.g. A sterilization chemical indicator should be used inside and outside of each package that is sterilized.[1,6,26] *[1: Strong Evidence]*
- An external indicator should be used on the outside of each package unless the internal indicator is visible.[6]
- Chemical indicators should be reviewed for a proper end point response (eg, color, migration, other change).
- An FDA-cleared chemical indicator recommended by the manufacturer of the selected sterilization system should be placed within each package to be sterilized.[6]

The purpose of the external chemical indicator is to differentiate between processed and unprocessed items.[41] Chemical indicators do not establish whether the item is sterile, but they do demonstrate that the contents were exposed to the sterilant.[41] Although chemical indicators do not verify sterility, they help detect procedural errors and equipment malfunctions.

XX.g.1. If the interpretation of the external or internal process monitors suggests inadequate processing, the item should not be used.[26,41]

XX.g.2. The internal chemical indicator should be reviewed for a proper end point response (eg, color, migration, other change) before placing the items or tray on the sterile field. If the proper end point is not achieved, items or trays should not be placed on the sterile field.

XX.h. Biological monitors should be used routinely to test for sterilizer efficacy, for sterilizer qualification testing (eg, after installation, relocation, malfunction, major repair, sterilization process failure), for routine load release, for implant load release, and for periodic product quality assurance testing for all sterilization processes.[6] *[3: Limited Evidence]*

XX.h.1. **Steam sterilizers:** *Geobacillus stearothermophilus* biological indicators should be used for routine load release, routine sterilizer efficacy monitoring, sterilizer qualification testing, and periodic product quality assurance testing as follows:
- Routine sterilizer efficacy monitoring should be performed weekly, but preferably daily. A process challenge device (PCD) containing a biological indicator should be used to test sterilizer efficacy.
- If a steam sterilizer is intended to be used for multiple types of cycles (eg, gravity-displacement, dynamic air-removal, IUSS), each sterilization cycle type should be tested.
- If one temperature is used but with different exposure times, only the cycle with the shortest exposure time needs to be tested.[6] The shortest time is the most challenging cycle.
- For table-top sterilizers and for sterilizers larger than 2 cubic feet, efficacy testing should be conducted in a fully loaded chamber.
- Efficacy testing of IUSS cycles should be conducted in an empty chamber unless an IUSS container is used.
- The biological monitor should be placed in the most challenging location within the sterilizer chamber and within the IUSS container as indicated by the sterilizer and container manufacturers.
- Each load containing an implantable device should be monitored with a PCD containing a biological indicator and a class 5 indicator and quarantined until the results of the biological indicator testing are available.
- One biological indicator PCD should be run in three consecutive empty cycles for sterilizer qualification testing.
- Qualification testing for sterilizers larger than 2 cubic feet and for IUSS cycles should be conducted in an empty chamber.
- Qualification testing of table-top sterilizers should be conducted in a fully loaded chamber.

XX.h.2. **Dynamic air-removal steam sterilizers:** A Bowie-Dick air-removal test should be performed daily in an empty chamber as follows:
- A Bowie-Dick air-removal test should be performed each day that the sterilizer is used and should be performed before the first load of the day but after a warm-up cycle is run.
- A warm-up cycle should be run so that Bowie-Dick testing is performed under the conditions in which the sterilizer will be used.

STERILIZATION

TABLE 6. TYPES AND APPLICATIONS FOR USE OF STEAM STERILIZATION MONITORING DEVICES[1]

Monitor	Frequency of use	Application (release of sterilizer, package, load)
Physical monitors		
Time, temperature, and pressure recorders; displays; digital printouts; and gauges	Should be used in every load of every sterilizer	Part of load release criteria
Chemical indicators (CIs)		
External CIs Class 1 (process indicators)	Should be used on the outside of every package unless the internal CI is visible	Part of routine load and package release criteria
Bowie-Dick-type indicators Class 2 (Bowie-Dick)	For routine sterilizer testing (dynamic air-removal sterilizers only), should be run within a test pack each day in an empty sterilizer before the first processed load	Test of sterilizer for efficacy of air removal and steam penetration; part of release criteria for using the sterilizer for the day
	For sterilizer qualification testing (dynamic air-removal sterilizers only), should be run within a test pack after sterilizer installation, relocation, malfunction, major repair or sterilization process failure; test should be run three times consecutively in an empty chamber after biological indicator (BI) tests	Part of release criteria for placing the sterilizer into service after qualification testing
Internal CIs	Should be used inside each package	Part of routine package release criteria at the use site
	Should be used in periodic product quality assurance testing	Part of release criteria for changes made to routinely sterilized items, load configuration, and/or packaging
		Release criteria should include BI results
Class 3 (single-variable indicator) Class 4 (multi-variable indicator)	May be used to meet internal CI recommendation	Part of routine package release criteria at the use site; not to be used for release of loads
Class 5 (integrating indicator)	May be used to meet internal CI recommendation	Part of routine package release criteria at the use site
	Within a process challenge device (PCD), may be used to monitor non-implant sterilizer loads	Part of load release criteria for nonimplant loads
	Within a PCD, should be used to monitor each sterilizer load containing implants; the PCD also should contain a BI	Part of release criteria for loads containing implants
		Except in emergencies, implants should be quarantined until BI results are known

continued on next page

- The test should be run in accordance with the test manufacturer's instructions before the routine biological indicator testing.
- Whenever a dynamic air-removal sterilizer is installed or relocated, malfunctions, undergoes a major repair, or has a sterilization process failure, three consecutive cycles in an empty chamber should be tested with a biological indicator PCD followed by three consecutive cycles in an empty chamber with a Bowie-Dick air-removal test.[6]
- The air-removal test is designed to detect residual air in the sterilizer chamber.

XX.h.3. **Ethylene oxide sterilizers:** *Bacillus atrophaeus* biological indicators should be used to test sterilizer efficacy. Sterilizer efficacy testing should be performed with every load.[26] Qualification testing should be performed after installation, relocation, malfunction, major repair, or sterilization process failure. Qualification testing should be performed in accordance with AAMI guidelines[26] and in consultation with the sterilizer manufacturer.

STERILIZATION

TABLE 6 CONTINUED. TYPES AND APPLICATIONS FOR USE OF STEAM STERILIZATION MONITORING DEVICES[1]

Monitor	Frequency of use	Application (release of sterilizer, package, load)
Class 6 (emulating indicator)	May be used to meet internal CI recommendation	Part of routine package release criteria at the use site
	Within a PCD, may be used to monitor sterilizer loads	Part of load release criteria for non-implant loads
		Part of release criteria for loads containing implants
		Implants should be quarantined until BI results are known, except in emergency situations
BIs	Within a PCD, may be used to monitor nonimplant loads	Part of routine load release criteria
	Within a PCD, should be used in every load containing implants; the PCD also should contain a class 5 integrating indicator	Part of release criteria for loads containing implants
		Implants should be quarantined until BI results are known, except in emergency situations
	Within a PCD, should be used for weekly, but preferably daily (ie, each day the sterilizer is used), routine sterilizer efficacy testing; the PCD also may contain a CI	Except in emergencies, implants should be quarantined until BI results are known
		Part of sterilizer/load release and recall criteria
	Should be run in a full load for wrapped items; for table-top sterilization, should be run in a fully loaded chamber; for immediate use steam sterilization, should be run in an empty chamber	Part of routine release criteria for placing the sterilizer into service after qualification testing
	Within a PCD, should be used for sterilizer qualification testing (after sterilizer installation, relocation, malfunction, major repair, sterilization process failure); the PCD also may contain a CI	Part of release criteria for changes made to routinely sterilized items, load configuration, and/or packaging
	Test should be run three times consecutively in an empty chamber, except for table-top sterilizers, for which the test should be run three times consecutively in a full load	
	Should be used for periodic product quality assurance testing	

REFERENCE
1. Association for the Advancement of Medical Instrumentation. ANSI/AAMI ST79:2010, A1:2010 & A2:2011, Comprehensive guide to steam sterilization and sterility assurance in health care facilities. Arlington, VA: Association for the Advancement of Medical Instrumentation; 2010 & 2011. Adapted and reprinted with permission. Further reproduction or distribution is prohibited.

XX.h.4. **Low-temperature hydrogen peroxide gas plasma sterilizers:** *Geobacillus stearothermophilus* biological indicators should be used for routine load release, routine sterilizer efficacy monitoring, sterilizer qualification testing, and periodic product quality assurance testing.[35] Routine sterilizer efficacy monitoring should be performed at least daily on each cycle type, preferably with each load, as follows:

- The sterilizer manufacturer should be consulted for the specific monitoring product to use and the appropriate placement of the product within the sterilizer.
- For each cycle type enabled on low-temperature hydrogen peroxide gas plasma sterilizers (eg, standard, advanced), one biological indicator PCD should be run in three consecutive empty cycles for sterilizer qualification testing.

STERILIZATION

XX.h.5. **Hydrogen peroxide vapor sterilizer:** *Geobacillus stearothermophilus* biological indicators should be used for routine load release, routine sterilizer efficacy monitoring, sterilizer qualification testing, and periodic product quality assurance testing.[35] Routine sterilizer efficacy monitoring should be performed at least daily on each cycle type, preferably with each load, as follows:
- The sterilizer manufacturer should be consulted for the specific monitoring product to use and the appropriate placement of the product within the sterilizer.
- For each cycle offered (eg, lumen, nonlumen), one biological indicator PCD should be run in three consecutive empty cycles for sterilizer qualification testing.[35]

XX.h.6. **Ozone sterilizers:** *Geobacillus stearothermophilus* biological indicators should be used for routine load release, routine sterilizer efficacy monitoring, sterilizer qualification testing, and periodic product quality assurance testing.[35] Routine sterilizer efficacy monitoring should be performed at least daily, preferably with each load, as follows:
- One biological indicator PCD should be run in three consecutive empty cycles for sterilizer qualification testing.
- The sterilizer manufacturer should be consulted for the specific monitoring product(s) to use and the appropriate placement of the product(s) within the sterilizer.[35]

XX.h.7. **Liquid peracetic acid sterilant systems:** A diagnostic cycle to verify the system is operating according to specification should be run every 24 hours according to the manufacturer's instructions for use.[60] Routine efficacy monitoring considerations include the following:
- Biological indicator monitoring is not required for liquid peracetic acid sterilant systems. A microprocessor monitors use dilution, temperature, and sterilant contact time.[47]
- Chemical indicators may be used according to the equipment manufacturer's instructions for use.

XX.h.8. **Dry-heat sterilizers:** *Bacillus atrophaeus* biological indicators should be used for routine load release, routine sterilizer efficacy monitoring, sterilizer qualification testing, and periodic product quality assurance testing. Routine sterilizer efficacy monitoring should be performed at least weekly, but preferably daily, as follows:
- Each load containing an implantable device should be monitored with a biological indicator and quarantined until the results of the biological indicator testing are available.
- Sterilizer qualification testing biological indicator PCDs should be run in three consecutive empty cycles.
- Mechanical convection (ie, forced-air) dry-heat sterilizers should be monitored according to the manufacturer's recommendations. Additional monitoring of three consecutive sterilization cycles should be performed after sterilizer installation, relocation, malfunction, major repair, or sterilization process failure.
- Testing should be performed in an empty sterilizer.[46]

XX.i. Preventive maintenance on sterilizers should be performed by qualified personnel on a scheduled basis. *[3: Limited Evidence]*

Periodic inspections, maintenance, and replacement of components that are subject to wear (eg, recording devices, steam traps, filters, valves, drain pipes, gaskets) help maintain proper functioning of sterilizers.[6]

XX.i.1. Inspection and cleaning should be performed as outlined in the manufacturer's written instructions.[46]

Proper inspection and cleaning minimizes sterilizer downtime and helps prevent sterilizer malfunctions.

XX.i.2. Preventive maintenance and repairs should be performed by qualified personnel as specified in the manufacturer's written instructions.

XX.i.3. Maintenance records should be kept for each sterilizer. Information noted in the sterilizer maintenance records should include the
- date of service;
- sterilizer model and serial number;
- sterilizer location;
- description of any malfunction;
- name of the person who is performing the maintenance and the name of his or her company;
- description of the type of service and any parts that are replaced;
- results of biological indicator testing, if performed;
- results of Bowie-Dick testing, if performed;
- name of the person requesting the service, where appropriate; and
- signature and title of the person acknowledging the completed work.

Accurate and complete records are required for sterilization process verification.

XX.j. Quality assurance testing of packaging systems including rigid containers is part of a quality assurance program and should be performed before initial use, as well as periodically, according to the manufacturer's written instructions.[6] *[3: Limited Evidence]*

Rigid sterilization container systems vary widely in design, mechanics, and construction. These variables can affect the performance and compatibility of containers with sterilization methods.

XX.j.1. Sterilization efficacy and drying effectiveness should be evaluated when conducting periodic product quality assurance testing of packaging systems, including sterilization containers for each sterilizer used.

Health care organizations are responsible for obtaining and maintaining manufacturers' documentation of methodology and performance testing for packaging systems.

Health care personnel are responsible for ensuring that container systems are suitable for proposed sterilization uses and are compatible with existing sterilizers.

XX.k. Periodic product testing of routinely processed items representing a product family should be performed on a continual basis.[6] *[3: Limited Evidence]*

Criteria that may be used to identify product families include
- design configuration,
- number of components,
- size or surface area,
- materials of construction,
- surface finish or texture,
- mated surfaces,
- presence of cannulations or lumens,
- the need for disassembly, and
- written processing instructions provided by manufacturers.

Product testing is used to verify that the device manufacturer's instructions for sterilization can be achieved in the health care setting.

Information related to product testing is evolving. Users are advised to review current literature for additional information as it becomes available.

XX.k.1. Product testing should be performed when major changes are made, before first use of loaned instruments, before use of newly purchased sets (eg, new specialty), or when there is no preexisting product family. Examples of major changes include
- significant changes in packaging (eg, changing from wrap to containerized systems),
- weight changes, and
- package configuration changes.

XX.k.2. During product testing of sterilization, conditions such as exposure time should be evaluated with physical, biological, and chemical monitors by strategically placing monitors alongside each other at locations that present the greatest challenge to air evacuation and sterilant penetration and contact.

XX.k.3. The container manufacturer should be consulted to determine the areas within the container that present the greatest challenge.

Glossary

Aeration: Method by which absorbed ethylene oxide (EO) is removed from EO-sterilized items by circulating warm air in an enclosed cabinet specifically designed for this purpose.

Anyhdrous: Items that are free of water.

Bioburden: The degree of microbial load; the number of viable organisms contaminating an object.

Biological indicator: A sterilization process-monitoring device commercially prepared with a known population of highly resistant spores that tests the effectiveness of the method of sterilization being used. The indicator is used to demonstrate that conditions necessary to achieve sterilization were met during the sterilizer cycle being monitored.

Bowie-Dick test (Class 2 chemical indicator): A test designed to detect air leaks, ineffective air removal, and presence of noncondensable gases in dynamic air-removal steam sterilizers. This test is not a test for sterilization efficacy. It is not used in gravity-displacement sterilizers.

Chemical indicator: A sterilization process-monitoring device used to monitor the attainment of one or more critical parameters required for sterilization. A characteristic color or other visual change indicates a defined level of exposure based on the classification of the chemical indicator used.
- *Class 1:* Process indicator that demonstrates that the package has been exposed to the sterilization process to distinguish between processed and unprocessed packages.
- *Class 2 (Bowie-Dick):* Process indicator that is used to detect air leaks, ineffective air removal, and presence of noncondensable gases. Used in dynamic air-removal sterilizers.
- *Class 3:* Process indicator that reacts to a single parameter of the sterilization process.
- *Class 4:* Process indicator that reacts to two or more of the critical parameters of sterilization.
- *Class 5 (integrating indicator):* Process indicator designed to react to all critical parameters over a specified range of sterilization cycles; performance has been correlated to the performance of the stated test organism under the labeled conditions of use.
- *Class 6 (emulating indicator):* Process indicator designed to react to all of the critical parameters of a specific cycle.

Decontamination area: Area designated for collection, retention, and cleaning of soiled and/or contaminated items.

Downtime: A period of time when an item or device is not operational.

STERILIZATION

Dynamic air removal: Mechanically assisted air removal from the sterilization chamber. Includes prevacuum and steam-flush pressure-pulse steam sterilizers.

Emergency spill plan: A plan of action for any unanticipated release of ethylene oxide or other hazardous chemicals into the workplace.

Gravity displacement: Type of sterilization cycle in which incoming air displaces residual air through a port or drain near the bottom of the sterilizer chamber.

Immediate use steam sterilization (IUSS): Steam sterilization of patient care items intended for immediate use. Formerly known as "flash sterilization."

Physical monitor: Automated devices (eg, printouts, digital readings, graphs, gauges) that monitor sterilization parameters for the sterilization method in use.

Prevacuum: A steam sterilization cycle in which air is removed from the chamber and load via a series of pressure and vacuum excursions.

Process challenge device (PCD): A device designed to represent a defined challenge or resistance to a sterilization process. A commercially prepared PCD may contain a biological indicator, a chemical indicator, or a biological indicator and a chemical indicator. A PCD is used to test the efficacy of the sterilization process.

Qualification testing: Sterilizer testing performed after installation, relocation, malfunction, major repair, or sterilizer process failure to verify that the sterilizer equipment performs within predetermined limits when used in accordance with the manufacturer's instructions for use.

Short-term exposure limits: Durations of exposure to a potentially toxic or harmful substance lasting for less than 15 minutes that cannot be repeated more than four times per day.

Sterilization: Processes by which all microbial life, including pathogenic and nonpathogenic microorganisms and spores, are killed.

Sterilization process monitoring device: A device used to monitor sterilization processes. Sterilization monitoring devices can be biological, chemical, or mechanical.

Terminal sterilization: A process by which the product is sterilized within a sterile barrier that permits storage for use at a later time.

References

1. Rutala WA, Weber DJ; Healthcare Infection Control Practices Advisory Committee. *Guideline for Disinfection and Sterilization in Healthcare Facilities*, 2008. Atlanta, GA: Centers for Disease Control and Prevention; 2008. [IVA]

2. Tablan OC, Anderson LJ, Besser R, et al. Guidelines for preventing health-care–associated pneumonia, 2003: recommendations of CDC and the Healthcare Infection Control Practices Advisory Committee. *MMWR Recomm Rep.* 2004;53(RR-3):1-36. [IVA]

3. Standards FAQ details: how should we process and store laryngoscope blades? The Joint Commission. October 24, 2011. http://www.jointcommission.org/standards_information/jcfaqdetails.aspx?StandardsFAQChapterId=69&StandardsFAQId=386. Accessed April 25, 2012.

4. Guideline for Cleaning and Care of Surgical Instruments. In: *Guidelines for Perioperative Practice.* Denver, CO: AORN, Inc; 2015:615-650.

5. Guideline for high-level disinfection. In: *Guidelines for Perioperative Practice.* Denver, CO: AORN, Inc; 2015:601-614.

6. Association for the Advancement of Medical Instrumentation (AAMI). ANSI/AAMI ST79:2010/A2:2011: Comprehensive guide to steam sterilization and sterility assurance in health care facilities. Arlington, VA: AAMI; 2011. [IVC]

7. Enforcement priorities for single-use devices reprocessed by third parties and hospitals. Food and Drug Administration. Center for Devices and Radiological Health. August 14, 2000. http://www.fda.gov/MedicalDevices/DeviceRegulationandGuidance/GuidanceDocuments/ucm107164.htm. Accessed April 26, 2012.

8. Medical devices; reprocessed single-use devices; termination of exemptions from premarket notification; requirement for submission of validation data. *Fed Regist.* 2005;70(188):56911-56925. https://federalregister.gov/a/05-19510. Accessed April 25, 2012.

9. Diab-Elschahawi M, Blacky A, Bachhofner N, Koller W. Challenging the Sterrad 100NX sterilizer with different carrier materials and wrappings under experimental "clean" and "dirty" conditions. *Am J Infect Control.* 2010;38(10):806-810. doi:10.1016/j.ajic.2010.05.023. [IB]

10. Recommended practices for traffic patterns in the perioperative practice setting. In: *Perioperative Standards and Recommended Practices.* Denver, CO: AORN, Inc; 2011:95-98. [IVB]

11. Occupational Safety & Health Administration. US Department of Labor. Toxic and hazardous substances. Appendix A: bloodborne pathogens. 29 CFR §1910.1030. *Fed Regist.* 1991;56(235):64004-64182. Effective December 6, 1991. http://www.osha.gov/pls/oshaweb/owadisp.show_document?p_table=standards&p_id=10051. Accessed April 25, 2012.

12. Siegel JD, Rhinehart E, Jackson M, Chiarello L; Healthcare Infection Control Practices Advisory Committee. *2007 Guideline for Isolation Precautions: Preventing Transmission of Infectious Agents in Healthcare Settings.* Atlanta, GA: Centers for Disease Control and Prevention; 2007. http://www.cdc.gov/hicpac/pdf/isolation/Isolation2007.pdf. Accessed April 25, 2012. [IVA]

13. Lipscomb IP, Sihota AK, Keevil CW. Comparison between visual analysis and microscope assessment of surgical instrument cleanliness from sterile service departments. *J Hosp Infect.* 2008;68(1):52-58. [IIC]

14. DesCoteaux JG, Poulin EC, Julien M, Guidoin R. Residual organic debris on processed surgical instruments. *AORN J.* 1995;62(1):23-30. [IIIC]

15. Guideline for selection and use of packaging systems for sterilization. In: *Guidelines for Perioperative Practice.* Denver, CO: AORN, Inc; 2015:651-664.

16. Association for the Advancement of Medical Instrumentation. ANSI/AAMI/ISO 11607-1:2006/(R)2010: Packaging for terminally sterilized medical devices—Part 1: Requirements for materials, sterile barrier systems, and packaging systems. Arlington, VA: AAMI; 2010. [IVB]

17. Association for the Advancement of Medical Instrumentation (AAMI). ANSI/AAMI ST77:2006/(R)2010: Containment devices for reusable medical device sterilization. Arlington, VA: AAMI; 2010. [IVC]

18. AORN position statement on ergonomically healthy workplace practices. AORN, Inc. http://www.aorn.org/WorkArea/DownloadAsset.aspx?id=21921. Accessed on April 24, 2012. [IVB]

19. AORN guidance statement: safe patient handling and movement in the perioperative setting. In: *Perioperative Standards and Recommended Practices*. Denver, CO: AORN, Inc; 2011:617-638. [IVB]

20. AAMI, Accreditation Association for Ambulatory Health Care, Inc, AORN, et al. Immediate-use steam sterilization statement. http://www.aami.org/publications/standards/ST79_Immediate_Use_Statement.pdf. Accessed April 25, 2012. [IVC]

21. Association for the Advancement of Medical Instrumentation (AAMI). *ANSI/AAMI ST8: Hospital Steam Sterilizers*. Arlington, VA: AAMI; 2008. [IVC]

22. Clement L, Bliley J. Cracking the steam sterilizer door: dispelling the myth. *Healthc Purchasing News*. 2007:40-42. [VC]

23. Mangram AJ, Horan TC, Pearson ML, Silver LC, Jarvis WR. Guideline for prevention of surgical site infection, 1999. Hospital Infection Control Practices Advisory Committee. *Infect Control Hosp Epidemiol*. 1999;20(4):250-78. doi:10.1086/501620. [IVA]

24. Centers for Disease Control and Prevention (CDC). Bronchoscopy-related infections and pseudoinfections—New York, 1996 and 1998. *MMWR Morb Mortal Wkly Rep*. 1999;48(26):557-560. [IVA]

25. Update: The Joint Commission position on steam sterilization. *Jt Comm Perspect*. 2009;29(7):8, 11.

26. Association for the Advancement of Medical Instrumentation (AAMI). ANSI/AAMI ST41: Ethylene oxide sterilization in health care facilities: safety and effectiveness. Arlington, VA: AAMI; 2008. [IVC]

27. Identification and listing of hazardous waste. 40 CFR §261. *Fed Regist*. 2011;76:74709-74717. Effective December 1, 2011. https://federalregister.gov/a/2011-30152. Accessed April 25, 2012.

28. Ozone layer protection – regulatory programs. Phaseout of HCFCs (class II ozone-depleting substances). US Environmental Protection Agency. http://www.epa.gov/ozone/title6/phaseout/classtwo.html. Accessed April 25, 2012.

29. National emission standards for hospital ethylene oxide sterilizers—EPA. Final rule. *Fed Regist*. 2007;63(248):73611-73625.

30. Ethylene oxide. 29 CFR §1910.1047. July 1, 2010. http://www.osha.gov/pls/oshaweb/owastand.display_standard_group?p_toc_level=1&p_part_number=1910. Accessed April 25, 2012.

31. Steris. Envirosystems ethylene oxide sterilant. [VB]

32. Pesticides: reregistration. Ethylene oxide (ETO): hospitals and healthcare facilities must use a single chamber when sterilizing medical equipment with ETO. US Environmental Protection Agency. http://www.epa.gov/oppsrrd1/reregistration/ethylene_oxide/ethylene_oxide_fs.html. Accessed April 25, 2012.

33. Hazard communication in the 21st century workplace. Occupational Safety & Health Administration. http://www.osha.gov/dsg/hazcom/finalmsdsreport.html. Updated March 2004. Accessed April 25, 2012.

34. Ethylene oxide: Evidence of carcinogenicity. Appendix I: Guidelines for minimizing worker exposure to ethylene oxide. http://www.cdc.gov/niosh/81130_35.html#Appendix I ed. 1981.

35. Association for the Advancement of Medical Instrumentation (AAMI). ANSI/AAMI ST58: Chemical sterilization and high-level disinfection in health care facilities. Arlington, VA: AAMI; 2005. [IVC]

36. Joslyn LJ, Block SS. Gaseous chemical sterilization. In: Block SS, ed. *Disinfection, Sterilization, and Preservation*. 5th ed. Philadelphia, PA: Lippincott Williams & Wilkins; 2001:337-359. [IVA]

37. Occupational safety and health guideline for hydrogen peroxide. Occupational Safety & Health Administration. http://www.osha.gov/SLTC/healthguidelines/hydrogenperoxide/recognition.html. Accessed April 25, 2012.

38. *Material Safety Data Sheet MS 52013: Hydrogen Peroxide Cassette*. Irvine, CA: Advanced Sterilization Products; 2008. [VB]

39. *Material Safety Data Sheet MSDS 09461-0-001: Hydrogen Peroxide Solution*. Irvine, CA: Advanced Sterilization Products; 2008.

40. Rutala WA, Weber DJ, Rutala WA. An overview of disinfection and sterilization in health care facilities. In: Rutala WA, ed. *Disinfection, Sterilization, and Antisepsis: Principles, Practices, Current Issues, and New Research*. Washington, DC: Association for Professionals in Infection Control and Epidemiology; 2007:12-48. [IVA]

41. ANSI/AAMI/ISO 15882: Chemical indicators—guidance for selection, use, and interpretation of results. Arlington, VA: Association for the Advancement of Medical Instrumentation; 2008. [IVC]

42. *510(k) Summary for Amsco V-PRO™ 1 Low Temperature Sterilization System*. STERIS Corp. Aug. 4, 2006. http://www.accessdata.fda.gov/cdrh_docs/pdf6/K062297.pdf. Accessed April 24, 2012.

43. TSO3 125L Ozone Sterilizer 510(k) summary. TSO3 Inc. March 15, 2002. http://www.accessdata.fda.gov/cdrh_docs/pdf2/K020875.pdf. Accessed April 24, 2012.

44. Weavers LK, Wickramanayake GB, Block SS. Disinfection and sterilization using ozone. In: Block SS, ed. *Disinfection, Sterilization, and Preservation*. 5th ed. Philadelphia, PA: Lippincott Williams & Wilkins; 2001:205-214. [IVA]

45. Joslyn LJ, Block SS. Sterilization by heat. In: Block SS, ed. *Disinfection, Sterilization, and Preservation*. 5th ed. Philadelphia, PA: Lippincott Williams & Wilkins; 2001:695-728. [IVA]

46. ANSI/AAMI ST40: Table-top dry heat (heated air) sterilization and sterility assurance in health care facilities. Arlington, VA: Association for the Advancement of Medical Instrumentation; 2004. [IVC]

47. *Revised 510(k) Summary for SYSTEM 1E Liquid Chemical Sterilant Processing System*. Mentor, OH: STERIS Corp; 2010. [VB]

48. STERIS System 1E (SS1E) liquid chemical sterilant - K090036. US Food and Drug Administration. http://www.fda.gov/MedicalDevices/ProductsandMedicalProcedures/DeviceApprovalsandClearances/RecentlyApprovedDevices/ucm207489.htm. Updated June 30, 2011. Accessed April 25, 2012.

49. Malchesky PS, Block SS. Medical applications of peracetic acid. In: Block SS, ed. *Disinfection, Sterilization, and Preservation*. 5th ed. Philadelphia, PA: Lippincott Williams & Wilkins; 2001:979-996. [IVA]

50. Petersen BT, Chennat J, Cohen J, et al. Multisociety guideline on reprocessing flexible GI endoscopes: 2011. *Infect Control Hosp Epidemiol*. 2011;32(6):527-537. doi:10.1086/660676. [IVB]

51. Winthrop TG, Sion BA, Gaines C. Loaner instrumentation: processing the unknown. *AORN J*. 2007;85(3):566-573. doi:10.1016/S0001-2092(07)60128-8.

52. ASHCSP/IAHCSMM Position Paper on Loaner Instrumentation. http://www.iahcsmm.org/pdfs/ASHCSP-IAHCSMMLoanerPaper.pdf. [IVC]

53. Villarrubia A, Palacin E, Gomez del Rio M, Martinez P. Description, etiology, and prevention of an outbreak of diffuse lamellar keratitis after LASIK. *J Refract Surg*. 2007;23(5):482-486. [IIIC]

STERILIZATION

54. Butt WE, Bradley DV Jr, Mayhew RB, Schwartz RS. Evaluation of the shelf life of sterile instrument packs. *Oral Surg Oral Med Oral Pathol.* 1991;72(6):650-654. [IA]

55. Webster J, Lloyd W, Ho P, Burridge C, George N. Rethinking sterilization practices: evidence for event-related outdating. *Infect Control Hosp Epidemiol.* 2003;24(8):622-624. doi:10.1086/502264. [IIB]

56. *ASHRAE/ASHE Standard: Ventilation of Health Care Facilities.* Atlanta, GA: American Society of Heating, Refrigerating, and Air-Conditioning Engineers; 2008. [IVB]

57. Guideline for environmental cleaning. In: *Guidelines for Perioperative Practice.* Denver, CO: AORN, Inc; 2015:9-30.

58. Standard pendent and upright spray sprinklers. In: *NFPA 13: Standard for the Installation of Sprinkler Systems.* 2010 ed. Quincy, MA: National Fire Protection Association; 2010: 51-58. [IVA]

59. Guideline for product selection. In: *Guidelines for Perioperative Practice.* Denver, CO: AORN, Inc; 2015: 179-186.

60. Medical device reporting: manufacturer reporting, importer reporting, user facility reporting, distributor reporting. 65(17) *Fed Regist.* (January 26, 2000) 4112-4121 (codified at 21 CFR §803-804).

Acknowledgments

LEAD AUTHOR
Cynthia Spry, MA, MS, RN, CNOR, CSIT
Independent Consultant
New York, New York

CONTRIBUTING AUTHOR
Ramona Conner, MSN, RN, CNOR
Manager, Standards and Guidelines
AORN Nursing Department
Denver, Colorado

The authors and AORN thank Paula Berrett, BS, CRCST, Intermountain Healthcare Urban South Region CP Manager, Utah Valley Regional Medical Center, Provo, Utah; Patricia A. Graybill-D'Ercole, MSN, RN, CNOR, CRCST, CHL, Consultant, Soyring Consulting, York, Pennsylvania; James X. Stobinski, PhD, RN, CNOR, Director of Education and Credentialing, Competency and Credentialing Institute, Denver, Colorado; and Julia A. Thompson, PhD, RN, APRN, CNOR, Administrative Director, Harris County Hospital District, Houston, Texas, for their assistance in developing this guideline.

PUBLICATION HISTORY

Originally published August 1980, *AORN Journal.* Format revision July 1982.

Revised February 1987, October 1992. Published as proposed recommended practices in July 1994.

Revised; published August 1999, *AORN Journal.* Reformatted July 2000.

Revised November 2005; published March 2006, *AORN Journal.*

Revised 2007; published in *Perioperative Standards and Recommended Practices*, 2008 edition.

Minor editing revisions made in November 2010 for publication in *Perioperative Standards and Recommended Practices*, 2011 edition.

Revised June 2012 for online publication in *Perioperative Standards and Recommended Practices.*

Reformatted September 2012 for publication in *Perioperative Standards and Recommended Practices*, 2013 edition.

Evidence ratings revised 2013 to conform to the AORN Evidence Rating Model.

Minor editing revisions made in November 2014 for publication in *Guidelines for Perioperative Practice*, 2015 edition.

STANDARDS
OF PERIOPERATIVE NURSING PRACTICE

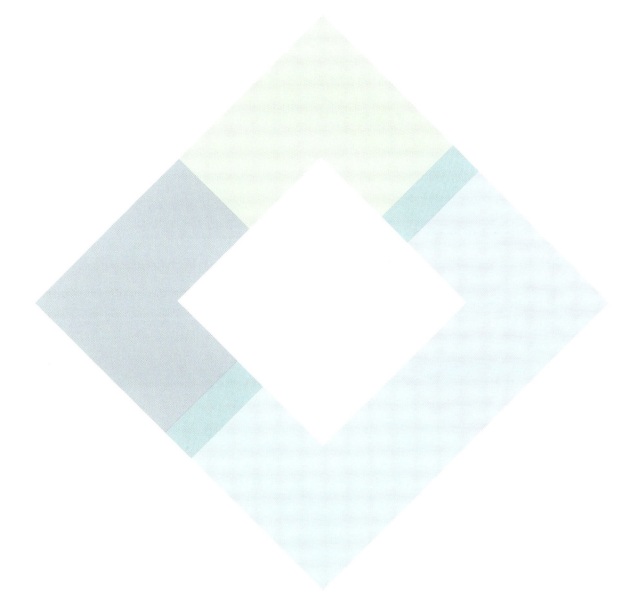

SECTION II

STANDARDS OF PERIOPERATIVE NURSING

Introduction

AORN is dedicated to enhancing the professionalism of perioperative registered nurses (RNs), promoting standards of perioperative nursing practice to better serve the needs of society, and providing a forum for interaction and exchange of ideas related to perioperative health care. Standards are authoritative statements that describe the responsibilities for which RNs are accountable and that reflect the values and priorities of the profession. The history of the Standards of Perioperative Nursing is detailed in Exhibit A.

As recipients of care, patients are entitled to privacy, confidentiality, personal dignity, and quality health services. The delivery of patient-focused care is guided by ethical, legal, and moral principles. These inherent principles serve as a foundation for perioperative nursing practice and are paramount in achieving optimal patient outcomes.

The standards of perioperative nursing focus on the process of providing nursing care and performing professional role activities. These standards apply to all nurses in the perioperative setting and were developed by AORN using the American Nurses Association's (ANA) scope and standards of practice for nursing and nursing administration as the foundation.[1,2]

It is the perioperative RN's responsibility to meet these standards, assuming that adequate environmental working conditions and necessary resources are available to support and facilitate the nurse's attainment of these standards. It is the responsibility of health care employers to provide an appropriate environment for nursing practice. It is important to recognize the link between working conditions and the nurse's ability to deliver care.

Several related themes underlie the standards of perioperative nursing. Nursing care must be individualized to meet a patient's unique needs and situation. This care should be provided in the context of disease or injury prevention, health promotion, health restoration, health maintenance, or palliative care. The cultural, racial, and ethnic diversity of the patient always must be taken into account while providing nursing care.

The perioperative RN must respect the patient's goals and preferences in developing and implementing a plan of care. One of nursing's primary responsibilities is patient education; therefore, nurses should provide patients with appropriate information to make informed decisions regarding their care and treatment. It is recognized, however, that some state regulations or institutional policies or procedures may prohibit full disclosure of information to patients.

The perioperative RN's partnership with the patient and other health care providers is recognized in the standards. It is assumed that the nurse will work with other health care providers in a coordinated manner throughout the process of caring for patients undergoing operative or other invasive procedures. The involvement of the patient and designated support person(s) is paramount. The appropriate degree of participation that is expected of the patient, designated support person(s), and other health care providers is determined by the clinical environment and the patient's unique situation.

It is beyond the scope of documents such as these to account for all possible scenarios that the perioperative RN may encounter in practice. The nurse will need to exercise judgment based on education and experience to determine what is appropriate, pertinent, or realistic. Further direction also may be available from documents such as recommended practices, guidelines for care, agency standards, policies, procedures, protocols, and current research findings.

The standards of perioperative nursing provide a mechanism to delineate the responsibilities of RNs engaged in practice in the perioperative setting. These standards serve as the basis for quality monitoring and evaluation systems; databases; regulatory systems; the development and evaluation of nursing service delivery systems and organizational structures; certification activities; job descriptions and performance appraisals; agency policies, procedures, and protocols; and educational offerings. The standards of perioperative nursing are generic and apply to all RNs engaged in perioperative practice, regardless of clinical setting, practice setting, or educational preparation.

A. Perioperative Patient Focused Model

A.1. Conceptual Framework

The Perioperative Patient Focused Model (Figure 1) is the conceptual framework for perioperative nursing practice and the Perioperative Nursing Data Set (PNDS).[3] At the core of the Model, the patient and his or her designated support person(s) provide the focus of perioperative nursing care. Concentric circles expand beyond the patient and designated support person(s) representing the perioperative nursing domains and elements. The Model illustrates the relationship between the patient, designated support person(s), and care provided by the perioperative RN.

STANDARDS OF PERIOPERATIVE NURSING

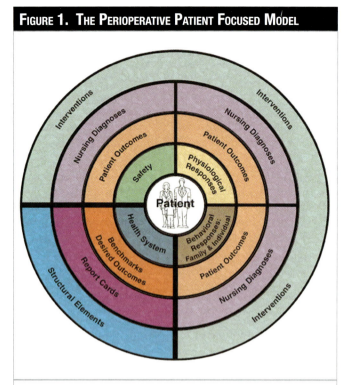

FIGURE 1. THE PERIOPERATIVE PATIENT FOCUSED MODEL

Petersen C, ed. Perioperative Nursing Data Set. *3rd ed. Denver, CO: AORN, Inc; 2011. Reprinted with permission.*

A.2. Patient Centered

The patient is at the center of the Model, which clearly represents the true focus of perioperative patient care. Regardless of practice setting, geographic location, or nature of the patient population, there is nothing more important to the perioperative RN than the patient.

A.3. Four Domains

The Model is divided into four quadrants, three representing patient-centered domains:
- patient safety,
- patient physiologic responses to operative and other invasive procedures, and
- patient and designated support person(s) behavioral responses to operative and other invasive procedures.

The fourth quadrant represents the health system in which the perioperative care is delivered. The health system domain designates administrative concerns and structure elements essential to successful perioperative outcomes.

A.4. Outcome Focused

The Model focuses on patient outcomes. This is important, because nursing theories and models should embrace and represent all elements of the nursing process. AORN's Model represents the outcomes focus of perioperative RNs by placing outcomes immediately adjacent to the patient care domains. Perioperative RNs have a unique knowledge base that supports high-quality patient outcomes. An individualized patient assessment guides the identification of nursing diagnoses and selection of nursing interventions for each patient.

B. Goal for Perioperative Nursing Practice

The goal of perioperative nursing practice is to assist patients and their designated support person(s) with achieving a level of wellness equal to or greater than that which they had before their operative or other invasive procedures.

C. Scope of Perioperative Nursing Practice

C.1. Definition of Perioperative RN

C.1.1. Perioperative RNs use the nursing process to develop individualized plans of care and to coordinate and deliver care to patients undergoing operative or other invasive procedures. Perioperative RNs identify patient needs, set goals with patients, and implement nursing interventions and activities to achieve optimal patient outcomes.

C.1.2. Perioperative RNs address the physiological, psychological, socio-cultural, and spiritual responses of patients.

C.1.3. Perioperative RNs use standards, knowledge, judgment, and skills based on scientific principles.

C.1.4. Perioperative RNs are ethical, responsible, and accountable for quality patient care.

C.1.5. Perioperative RNs use evidence as the foundation for practice.

C.1.6. Perioperative RNs assume responsibility for lifelong learning.

C.2. Definition of Perioperative Nursing Practice

C.2.1. Perioperative nursing practice is consistent with the ANA's definition of nursing, which states,

> *Nursing is the protection, promotion, and optimization of health and abilities, prevention of illness and injury, alleviation of suffering through the diagnosis and treatment of human response, and advocacy in the care of individuals, families, communities, and populations.*[4(p6)]

C.2.2. Perioperative nursing practice is based on holistic caring relationships that facilitate health and healing within the range of human experiences.

C.2.3. Perioperative nursing practice is enhanced by interdisciplinary collaboration and appropriate resource utilization.

STANDARDS OF PERIOPERATIVE NURSING

C.2.4. Perioperative RNs use AORN guidelines as a foundation for practice and specialized educational preparation.

C.3. Span of Perioperative Nursing Practice

C.3.1. Perioperative RNs provide care across the surgical continuum, beginning when patients are first informed that they need an operative or invasive procedure and ending when they return to their usual roles and responsibilities.

C.3.2. Perioperative RNs focus on patients and their designated support person(s).

C.4. Settings of Perioperative Nursing Practice

Perioperative RNs provide care in a variety of clinical settings. These settings include traditional ORs, ambulatory surgery centers, physicians' offices, cardiac catheterization suites, endoscopy suites, radiology departments, and all other areas where operative and other invasive procedures may be performed.

Perioperative RNs influence community, regulatory, and legislative activities through employment or voluntary participation at the local, state, national, or international level.

C.5. Role Functions

Perioperative RNs function in a variety of roles that are dynamic and continually evolving through increased education and experience to meet the changing needs of society. These may include, but are not limited to, staff RN, RN first assistant, advanced practice RN, manager, administrator, educator, informatics nurse specialist, and researcher.

Perioperative RNs act in the public interest when providing the unique service society has entrusted to them. Accountability is accomplished through self-regulation, professional regulation, and legal regulation. Perioperative RNs positively influence health care services and delivery by promoting a safe environment.

D. Standards of Perioperative Nursing

D.1. Standard 1: Assessment

The perioperative RN collects patient health data that are relevant to the operative or invasive procedure.

Measurement

D.1.1. **Perioperative RN:**
D.1.1.1. Determines data collection priorities based on the patient's condition or needs, and the relationship to the proposed intervention.
D.1.1.2. Collects pertinent data using systematic, comprehensive, and evidence-based techniques.
D.1.1.3. Conducts a systematic and ongoing process for data collection.
D.1.1.4. Involves the patient, designated support person(s), and health care providers in the data-collection process.
D.1.1.5. Reviews the results of diagnostic studies relevant to the patient's current status and planned operative or invasive procedure.
D.1.1.6. Documents relevant data in a retrievable format.

Additional measurement

D.1.2. **Advanced practice RN:**
D.1.2.1. Uses advanced assessment techniques, independently or collaboratively, to gather appropriate data pertinent to patients and populations.
D.1.2.2. Recognizes complex physiologic responses.
D.1.2.3. Initiates diagnostic studies relevant to the patient's current status and planned operative or invasive procedure.
D.1.2.4. Interprets results of diagnostic studies relevant to the patient's current status and planned operative or invasive procedure.
D.1.2.5. Synthesizes assessment data to identify trends and improve perioperative outcomes.
D.1.2.6. Assigns American Society of Anesthesiologists (ASA) physical status classification.

D.2. Standard 2: Diagnosis

The perioperative RN analyzes the assessment data to determine nursing diagnoses.

Measurement

D.2.1. **Perioperative RN:**
D.2.1.1. Identifies nursing diagnoses that are consistent with the assessment data.
D.2.1.2. Sets priorities using nursing diagnoses based on assessment data.
D.2.1.3. Validates nursing diagnoses with the patient, designated support person(s), and health care providers when possible.
D.2.1.4. Documents nursing diagnoses using standardized nursing language in a retrievable format.

Additional measurement

D.2.2. **Advanced practice RN:**
D.2.2.1. Synthesizes assessment data using advanced knowledge and clinical judgment to formulate differential diagnoses for risk reduction and clinical problems.
D.2.2.2. Sets priorities using differential diagnoses.

STANDARDS OF PERIOPERATIVE NURSING

D.3. Standard 3: Outcome Identification

The perioperative RN identifies expected outcomes that are unique to the patient.

Measurement

D.3.1. Perioperative RN:

D.3.1.1. Uses ethical principles to determine expected outcomes that are mutually formulated with the patient, designated support person(s), and health care providers when appropriate.

D.3.1.2. Develops culturally and age-appropriate expected outcomes based on the patient's present and potential physical capabilities and behavioral patterns.

D.3.1.3. Defines expected outcomes that are attainable with considerations to the human and material resources available to the patient.

D.3.1.4. Identifies measurable criteria to determine outcome attainment.

D.3.1.5. Sets priorities including a time estimate for attaining expected outcomes.

D.3.1.6. Modifies expected outcomes based on patient status.

D.3.1.7. Communicates expected and attained outcomes to health care providers to provide direction for continuity of care.

D.3.1.8. Documents outcomes in a retrievable format.

Additional measurement

D.3.2. Advanced practice RN:

D.3.2.1. Develops peer education that emphasizes identification and use of culturally appropriate patient outcome measures.

D.3.2.2. Acts as a resource to determine an outcome-driven plan for individual patients and patient populations.

D.3.2.3. Synthesizes evidence to determine optimal outcomes for individual patients and patient populations.

D.4. Standard 4: Planning

The perioperative RN develops an individualized plan of care to attain expected outcomes.

Measurement

D.4.1. Perioperative RN:

D.4.1.1. Uses nursing diagnoses to identify nursing interventions.

D.4.1.2. Uses current trends and scientific evidence in the planning process.

D.4.1.3. Designs a plan of care that includes strategies for health promotion and restoration.

D.4.1.4. Collaborates with the patient and designated support person(s), as appropriate, while planning care.

D.4.1.5. Creates a plan of care that supports continuity among providers.

D.4.1.6. Specifies a logical sequence of interventions to attain expected outcomes.

D.4.1.7. Identifies human and material resources necessary to implement the plan of care.

D.4.1.8. Communicates the plan of care to the patient, designated support person(s), and health care providers.

D.4.1.9. Documents the plan of care using standardized language in a retrievable format.

Additional measurement

D.4.2. Advanced practice RN:

D.4.2.1. Synthesizes research findings and applies expert clinical knowledge to expand the plan of care for individuals and patient populations.

D.4.2.2. Develops priorities for care reflecting the signs, symptoms, and behavioral responses within the realm of care for the advanced practice nurse.

D.5. Standard 5: Implementation

The perioperative RN implements the identified plan of care.

Measurement

D.5.1. Perioperative RN:

D.5.1.1. Determines that the nursing interventions are consistent with the plan of care.

D.5.1.2. Verifies that nursing interventions reflect the rights and desires of the patient and designated support person(s).

D.5.1.3. Implements nursing interventions safely and efficiently.

D.5.1.4. Implements the ongoing plan of care in collaboration with the patient, designated support person(s), and health care providers based on the patient's responses.

D.5.1.5. Anticipates and responds to situational changes.

D.5.1.6. Modifies the plan of care based on the patient's responses.

D.5.1.7. Incorporates new knowledge and strategies to initiate change in nursing care practices if desired outcomes are not achieved.

D.5.1.8. Documents interventions using standardized language in a retrievable format to promote continuity of care.

STANDARDS OF PERIOPERATIVE NURSING

Additional measurement

D.5.2. Advanced practice RN:
D.5.2.1. Integrates advanced knowledge and skills to implement the plan of care.
D.5.2.2. Performs ongoing physical examinations, selecting, ordering, and interpreting diagnostic tests.
D.5.2.3. Provides advanced interpretation of conditions and gives rationale for the procedure.
D.5.2.4. Performs interventions that apply advanced nursing therapies and include medication management and clinical procedures.

D.5.a. Standard 5a: Coordination of Care

The perioperative RN coordinates patient care continually throughout the patient's perioperative experience.

Measurement

D.5.a.1. Perioperative RN:
D.5.a.1.1. Delegates tasks and functions according to applicable laws, regulations, and standards, taking into consideration the competency of the assignee.
D.5.a.1.2. Assists the patient and designated support person(s) with identifying alternative options for care.

Additional measurement

D.5.a.2. Advanced practice RN:
D.5.a.2.1. Uses advanced knowledge to initiate new treatments or change existing treatment based on changing trends or scientific evidence.
D.5.a.2.2. Makes referrals to other health care professionals and community agencies.
D.5.a.2.3. Initiates interdisciplinary team meetings or other communication to improve the health of individual patients and patient populations.

D.5.b. Standard 5b: Health Teaching— Health Promotion

The perioperative RN promotes holistic wellness and a safe environment.

Measurement

D.5.b.1. Perioperative RN:
D.5.b.1.1. Teaches modifications for activities of daily living.
D.5.b.1.2. Provides information to patients to reduce high-risk behaviors.
D.5.b.1.3. Advocates for healthy lifestyle choices.
D.5.b.1.4. Uses teaching strategies that are appropriate to the situation and the patient's developmental level, cognitive ability, learning needs, readiness, language preference, culture, and beliefs.
D.5.b.1.5. Alters teaching strategies based on feedback.
D.5.b.1.6. Reports information to the appropriate source regarding local, state, and national health issues that affect safety according to policy, guidelines, or regulations.

Additional measurement

D.5.b.2. Advanced practice RN:
D.5.b.2.1. Uses advanced theoretical knowledge to organize and deliver educational programs for patients, designated support person(s), health care professionals, and the community.
D.5.b.2.2. Initiates referrals promoting health or risk reduction.
D.5.b.2.3. Analyzes and disseminates information regarding local, state, and national health issues that affect safety.

D.5.c. Standard 5c: Consultation

The perioperative RN seeks specialized dialogue appropriate to the patient.

Measurement

D.5.c.1. Perioperative RN:
D.5.c.1.1. Facilitates communication between health care professionals to enhance patient outcomes.

Additional measurement

D.5.c.2. Advanced practice RN:
D.5.c.2.1. Provides independent consultation services based on expertise using advanced knowledge within the scope of practice.
D.5.c.2.2. Collaborates and coordinates with medical, nursing, and other disciplines to plan and implement monitoring of physiologic responses for individuals or patient populations.
D.5.c.2.3. Consults with the appropriate health care providers to determine a need for new treatments or a change in existing treatments.

STANDARDS OF PERIOPERATIVE NURSING

D.5.c.2.4. Initiates new treatment based on consultation.

D.5.d. Standard 5d: Prescriptive Authority

The advanced practice RN prescribes medications, treatments, and therapies in compliance with state and federal laws and regulations.

Measurement

D.5.d.1. Prescriptive authority does not apply to the perioperative RN.

Additional measurement

D.5.d.2. Advanced practice RN:
D.5.d.2.1. Uses prescriptive authority within the scope of practice.
D.5.d.2.2. Uses scientific evidence to order, prescribe, or initiate diagnostic, therapeutic, or pharmacologic interventions based on patient status.
D.5.d.2.3. Monitors the patient for therapeutic and potential adverse effects in response to diagnostic or pharmacologic interventions.
D.5.d.2.4. Modifies diagnostic, therapeutic, or pharmacologic interventions based on the patient's status and responses.
D.5.d.2.5. Educates patients and designated support person(s) about intended and potential adverse effects of proposed prescribed therapies.
D.5.d.2.6. Informs patients and designated support person(s) about potential costs, alternative treatment options, and procedures as appropriate.

D.6. Standard 6: Evaluation

The perioperative RN evaluates the patient's progress toward attaining outcomes.

Measurement Criteria

D.6.1. Perioperative RN:
D.6.1.1. Conducts a systematic and ongoing evaluation measuring the effectiveness of the interventions in relation to achieving identified outcomes.
D.6.1.2. Monitors the patient's progress toward achieving outcomes in the time frame identified in the plan.
D.6.1.3. Documents the patient's progress toward achieving outcomes accurately and consistently using standardized language in a retrievable format.
D.6.1.4. Revises diagnoses, outcomes, and the plan of care, based on ongoing assessment and evaluation.
D.6.1.5. Documents revisions in diagnoses, outcomes, and the plan of care using standardized language in a retrievable format.
D.6.1.6. Involves the patient, designated support person(s), and health care providers in the evaluation process whenever possible.
D.6.1.7. Disseminates evaluation results as appropriate to the patient and others according to state and federal laws and regulations.
D.6.1.8. Recommends policy, procedure, protocol, process, or structural changes, as appropriate, based on evaluation data.

Additional measurement

D.6.2. Advanced practice RN:
D.6.2.1. Evaluates responses to interventions systematically and revises differential diagnoses as needed in relation to the patient's progress toward attaining outcomes.
D.6.2.2. Uses advanced knowledge of learning and change theories, human behavior, stress and coping mechanisms, crisis management, growth, and development to evaluate patient responses to care.
D.6.2.3. Modifies the patient's plan of care, recommending additional diagnostic testing and treatments if necessary to attain outcomes.
D.6.2.4. Synthesizes knowledge of diagnostic tests, therapeutic regimens, and the patient's responses as they relate to progress toward attaining expected outcomes.
D.6.2.5. Uses advanced knowledge to synthesize evaluation data that have a potential effect on current and future health care practices for individual patients and patient populations.

Standards of Perioperative Professional Practice

D.7. Standard 7: Quality of Practice

The perioperative RN systematically evaluates the quality and appropriateness of nursing practice.

Measurement

D.7.1. Perioperative RN:
D.7.1.1. Demonstrates the quality of perioperative nursing care by documenting use of the nursing process using standardized language in a retrievable format.
D.7.1.2. Participates in ongoing quality improvement activities as appropriate to the individual's position, education, and practice environment. Such activities may include, but are not limited to, the following:

STANDARDS OF PERIOPERATIVE NURSING

- Identifying aspects of the perioperative nursing practice that are important for quality monitoring.
- Assigning responsibility for quality monitoring and evaluation activities.
- Identifying dimensions of performance related to perioperative nursing practice.
- Developing quality indicators for each identified dimension of performance.
- Establishing benchmarks to evaluate the quality indicators.
- Collecting data related to the dimensions of performance and quality indicators.
- Evaluating perioperative nursing practice and care based on the cumulative data collected.
- Identifying strategies to improve perioperative nursing care or services based on quality indicators as necessary.
- Taking action to improve perioperative nursing care or services.
- Assessing the effectiveness of the action(s) taken.
- Communicating the data collected organization-wide to other agencies, regulatory bodies, or data repositories while maintaining confidentiality.

D.7.1.3. Initiates changes in perioperative nursing practice through knowledge gained and shared via the quality and performance improvement process.

D.7.1.4. Improves perioperative nursing practice, services, and care through the quality improvement process.

D.7.1.5. Monitors perioperative nursing practice and compares it to national guidelines, standards, or existing research.

D.7.1.6. Uses internal and external data to create innovative quality indicators.

Additional measurement

D.7.2. **Advanced practice RN:**

D.7.2.1. Applies advanced theoretical knowledge, research findings, and assessment data to design and implement ongoing quality monitoring activities to evaluate perioperative nursing practice.

D.7.2.2. Works with multidisciplinary groups to design or implement advanced practices and alternative solutions to patient care issues based on quality monitoring data.

D.7.2.3. Synthesizes data from clinical investigations and scientific research to improve the safety, efficiency, and effectiveness of perioperative patient care.

D.7.2.4. Publishes or presents results of quality monitoring and evaluation activities to influence and improve perioperative nursing practice.

D.7.2.5. Maintains certification in advanced nursing practice.

D.8. Standard 8: Education

The perioperative RN acquires and maintains specialized knowledge and skills in nursing practice.

Measurement

D.8.1. **Perioperative RN:**

D.8.1.1. Completes an individualized orientation based on identified learning needs.

D.8.1.2. Demonstrates skill proficiency relevant to perioperative nursing practice.

D.8.1.3. Seeks experiences to maintain skills and competency necessary to practice perioperative nursing.

D.8.1.4. Participates in ongoing educational activities relevant to professional issues and trends in perioperative nursing.

D.8.1.5. Maintains records and documents to support competence in perioperative nursing.

D.8.1.6. Strives to achieve certification in perioperative nursing.

Additional measurement

D.8.2. **Advanced practice RN:**

D.8.2.1. Incorporates current research, national guidelines, standards, and evidence-based practices to develop advanced clinical knowledge and augment performance in perioperative nursing.

D.8.2.2. Develops, coordinates, implements, and evaluates educational programs for individual patients, designated support person(s), patient populations, and local, regional, or state communities based on identified needs.

D.8.2.3. Maintains educational requirements necessary for advanced certification and licensure to practice.

D.9. Standard 9: Professional Practice Evaluation

The perioperative RN evaluates his or her practice in context with current professional practice standards, rules, and regulations.

Measurement

D.9.1. **Perioperative RN:**

D.9.1.1. Provides care consistent with the institution's policies and procedures.

D.9.1.2. Practices nursing in accordance with the state board of nursing statutes, as well as the standards and guidelines of accrediting and regulatory bodies.

D.9.1.3. Maintains current knowledge of and adheres to ANA standards, practice guidelines, and position statements.

STANDARDS OF PERIOPERATIVE NURSING

D.9.1.4. Maintains current knowledge of and adheres to AORN standards, recommended practices, guidelines, and position statements.

D.9.1.5. Maintains current knowledge of and adheres to standards, recommended practices, guidelines, and position statements from other nursing organizations as relevant to practice.

D.9.1.6. Participates in an ongoing evaluation process to ensure practice is current, legal, ethical, culturally competent, and age-appropriate.

D.9.1.7. Seeks evaluative input from peers, colleagues, patients, and patients' designated support person(s) regarding nursing practice.

D.9.1.8. Participates in peer review to evaluate nursing practice of fellow RN colleagues.

D.9.1.9. Identifies goals and develops an action plan for professional development as part of an ongoing evaluation process.

D.9.1.10. Interprets and facilitates staff member and agency compliance with current local, state, and federal regulations and standards.

D.9.1.11. Participates in legislative and policy-making activities that influence health services and nursing practice.

D.9.1.12. Respects diversity in all interactions.

Additional measurement

D.9.2. **Advanced practice RN:**

D.9.2.1. Devises innovative, evidence-based evaluation strategies to ensure that care is being delivered in a legal, ethical, culturally competent and age-appropriate manner.

D.9.2.2. Applies advanced theoretical knowledge, research findings, and assessment data to design, implement, and evaluate perioperative nursing practice.

D.9.2.3. Works with multidisciplinary groups to design or implement advanced practices and alternative solutions to patient care issues based on quality monitoring data.

D.9.2.4. Synthesizes data from clinical investigations and scientific research to improve the safety, efficiency, and effectiveness of perioperative patient care.

D.9.2.5. Publishes or presents results of quality monitoring and evaluation activities to influence and improve perioperative nursing practice.

D.10. Standard 10: Collegiality

The perioperative RN interacts with and contributes to the professional growth of peers, colleagues, and others.

Measurement

D.10.1. **Perioperative RN:**

D.10.1.1. Shares knowledge and skills through a variety of methods including, but not limited to,
- providing inservice education, programs, seminars, and workshops;
- precepting;
- mentoring;
- role modeling;
- participating in peer evaluation;
- publishing; and
- participating in professional associations.

D.10.1.2. Contributes to a supportive and healthy work environment by using appropriate verbal and nonverbal communication techniques.

D.10.1.3. Builds trust by being approachable, honest, and accountable.

D.10.1.4. Acts as a role model for professional behavior.

D.10.1.5. Supports colleagues' professional development.

D.10.1.6. Interacts with team members and others in a respectful and courteous manner.

D.10.1.7. Uses conflict resolution skills to manage difficult behavior, promote positive working relationships, and advocate for patient safety.

Additional measurement

D.10.2. **Advanced practice RN:**

D.10.2.1. Shares knowledge and skills as a role model and mentor.

D.10.2.2. Uses advanced knowledge to assist staff members with applying the nursing process to complex patient situations in the perioperative setting.

D.10.2.3. Develops evidence-based guidelines to influence policy, change practice, and support professional development of colleagues.

D.10.2.4. Acts as a preceptor for advanced practice nurses.

D.11. Standard 11: Collaboration

The perioperative RN collaborates with the patient and designated support person(s) when practicing professional nursing.

Measurement

D.11.1. **Perioperative RN:**

D.11.1.1. Communicates pertinent information relating to patient care to internal and external stakeholders as appropriate.

STANDARDS OF PERIOPERATIVE NURSING

D.11.1.2. Demonstrates accountability and flexibility when interacting with others.

D.11.1.3. Includes the patient and designated support person(s) and health care team members, as appropriate, in decision making when providing perioperative nursing care.

D.11.1.4. Provides continuity of care when implementing referrals.

D.11.1.5. Supervises allied health care providers and support personnel with appropriate authority.

D.11.1.6. Delegates tasks and functions according to applicable law, regulation, and standards, taking into consideration the competency of the assignee.

Additional measurement

D.11.2. **Advanced practice RN:**

D.11.2.1. Participates with the interdisciplinary team to promote the use of nationally accepted clinical practice guidelines and standards in advanced nursing practice.

D.11.2.2. Serves as a resource for perioperative staff members, surgeons, ancillary departments, and community groups requiring advanced nursing expertise.

D.11.2.3. Fosters a collaborative environment and recognizes the value of each provider's contribution to comprehensive health care.

D.11.2.4. Acts in partnership with appropriate health care providers to initiate new treatments or change existing treatments to promote positive outcomes.

D.12. Standard 12: Ethics

The perioperative RN uses ethical principles to determine decisions and actions.

Measurement

D.12.1. **Perioperative RN:**

D.12.1.1. Practices nursing according to the ANA *Code of Ethics for Nurses with Interpretive Statements* (Exhibit B).

D.12.1.2. Acts as a patient advocate.

D.12.1.3. Encourages patient self-advocacy.

D.12.1.4. Maintains patient confidentiality within legal and regulatory guidelines.

D.12.1.5. Delivers care in a nonjudgmental and nondiscriminatory manner that is sensitive to cultural, racial, and ethnic diversity.

D.12.1.6. Delivers care in a way that preserves and protects patient autonomy, dignity, and human rights.

D.12.1.7. Upholds the professional and therapeutic boundaries of the nurse-patient relationship.

D.12.1.8. Formulates ethical decisions by using available resources.

D.12.1.9. Reports illegal, incompetent, or impaired practices.

D.12.1.10. Recognizes own physical and psychological limitations to provide safe, competent patient care.

D.12.1.11. Participates on ethics committees as appropriate.

Additional measurement

D.12.2. **Advanced practice RN:**

D.12.2.1. Develops treatment plans while instructing the patient and designated support person(s) about the risks, benefits, and possible outcomes of the plan.

D.12.2.2. Contributes to the development of consistent policies and services that are comparable in all settings and that are within the legal and ethical scope of advanced practice.

D.12.2.3. Provides independent or collaborative care that is nondiscriminatory and nonprejudicial regardless of the setting.

D.12.2.4. Initiates treatments in a nonjudgmental and nondiscriminatory manner that is sensitive to the patient's cultural, racial, socioeconomic, and ethnic diversity.

D.12.2.5. Considers ethical implications of scientific advances, cost, and clinical effectiveness, as well as patient and designated support person(s)' acceptance or satisfaction.

D.13. Standard 13: Research

The perioperative RN incorporates research findings into practice.

Measurement

D.13.1. **Perioperative RN:**

D.13.1.1. Uses the best available research evidence to guide practice.

D.13.1.2. Initiates change using scientific evidence to develop policies and procedures or influence perioperative nursing practice.

D.13.1.3. Supports nursing practice changes based on research evidence.

D.13.1.4. Seeks new knowledge that is evidence-based through print, web-based, and other sources.

D.13.1.5. Participates in research activities by involvement in one or more of the following:
- identifying clinical problems pertinent to perioperative nursing practice;
- participating in data collection;
- reading, analyzing, critiquing, and interpreting research findings to determine applicability to practice;

- sharing research activities and findings with others;
- participating on a research committee;
- participating in a research study; or
- joining a journal club.

Additional measurement

D.13.2. Advanced practice RN:
D.13.2.1. Collects and aggregates data to analyze care decisions, patient responses, and health outcomes for potential research projects.
D.13.2.2. Synthesizes current and emerging research findings that contribute to positive patient outcomes and incorporates them into advanced practice decisions.
D.13.2.3. Performs a literature review and critically appraises findings to advocate for analysis or review of system-wide clinical practices.
D.13.2.4. Conducts research to contribute to nursing knowledge and evidence-based practice.
D.13.2.5. Disseminates research findings through writing, publishing, and presenting to influence general and advanced nursing practice.
D.13.2.6. Pursues funding for perioperative nursing research.

D.14. Standard 14: Resource Utilization

The perioperative RN considers factors related to safety, effectiveness, efficiency, and the environment, as well as the cost in planning, delivering, and evaluating patient care.

Measurement

D.14.1. Perioperative RN:
D.14.1.1. Assigns tasks or delegates care based on knowledge and skills of perioperative team members to meet the needs of the patient and keep him or her free from harm.
D.14.1.2. Assists the patient and designated support person(s) with identifying human and material resources that are available to address perioperative patient needs.
D.14.1.3. Advocates for technical advances in clinical care to increase efficiency or improve outcomes.
D.14.1.4. Promotes the use of electronic information systems to provide perioperative patient care efficiently and safely.
D.14.1.5. Advocates for reusing, recycling, and renewing supplies whenever appropriate in the perioperative setting.
D.14.1.6. Conserves supplies to minimize waste and decrease costs without compromising safety or negatively affecting outcomes.

Additional measurement

D.14.2. Advanced practice RN:
D.14.2.1. Uses advanced knowledge to provide consultation services to the organization to achieve high-quality, cost-effective outcomes for populations of patients across settings.
D.14.2.2. Promotes system-wide communication to reduce costs by avoiding unnecessary duplication of diagnostic tests.
D.14.2.3. Collects and evaluates data regarding the effectiveness of care, cost-benefit relationship of the care being provided, and patient satisfaction.
D.14.2.4. Maintains knowledge of the organization's methods of financing the delivery of care.
D.14.2.5. Implements a cost-benefit evaluation of new technology and participates in product review committees.
D.14.2.6. Considers health care access, fiscal responsibility, efficacy, and quality when providing advanced nursing care.

D.15. Standard 15: Leadership

The perioperative RN provides leadership in the profession and professional practice setting.

Measurement

D.15.1. Perioperative RN:
D.15.1.1. Supervises peers, colleagues, allied health personnel, and support staff members as assigned and appropriate.
D.15.1.2. Delegates tasks and responsibilities according to law, regulation, and accrediting agency standards.
D.15.1.3. Holds self and team members accountable to the patient, the organization, and other internal and external stakeholders.
D.15.1.4. Creates and maintains a healthy work environment.
D.15.1.5. Embraces lifelong learning for self and others.
D.15.1.6. Advocates for a culture of safety for patients and staff members in the workplace.
D.15.1.7. Actively has input into organizational operations. Activities include, but are not limited to, the following:
- influencing policy-making to improve patient care;
- advocating for issues that affect perioperative care;
- participating in quality improvement activities;
- participating on committees;
- being a role model when new policies, procedures, or processes are implemented;

- supporting change while considering short- and long-term organizational goals;
- operationalizing the mission, vision, and values of the organization; and
- encouraging peers and colleagues to be active.

D.15.1.8. Participates in ongoing quality improvement workplace activities as appropriate to the individual's position, education, and practice environment.

D.15.1.9. Enhances perioperative nursing through involvement with professional organizations. Activities include, but are not limited to, the following:
- taking an active role in the association;
- encouraging peers and colleagues to be active;
- sharing information received through associations with team members; and
- presenting pertinent information to individuals and groups of lay and professional audiences.

D.15.1.10. Participates in legislative and policy-making activities that influence perioperative care.

Additional measurement

D.15.2. **Advanced practice RN:**

D.15.2.1. Uses advanced knowledge to act at the organizational level and beyond to promote change by identifying and influencing variables affecting health care practices and outcomes.

D.15.2.2. Promotes interdisciplinary cooperation and collaboration to implement outcome-based patient care programs to meet the needs of individual patients, designated support person(s), or patient populations or local, regional, or state communities.

D.15.2.3. Uses advanced team building, negotiation, and conflict resolution skills to promote teamwork to build partnerships within and across health care systems.

D.15.2.4. Initiates legislative and policy-making activities that influence perioperative care.

D.15.2.5. Collaborates to prevent and reduce the incidence of surgical site infections, health care-associated infections, and other adverse events related to surgical patients.

D.15.2.6. Facilitates staff member access to and compliance with current local, state, and federal regulations; professional standards; and accreditation guidelines.

D.15.2.7. Advances the profession through writing, publishing, and presenting pertinent information to individuals and groups of lay and professional audiences.

E. Standards of Perioperative Administrative Practice

E.1. Standard 1: Assessment

The perioperative RN administrator collects comprehensive data necessary to support perioperative and organizational services.

Measurement

E.1.1. Uses evidence-based processes to collect pertinent data in a systematic and ongoing manner to support perioperative services.

E.1.2. Sets priorities for data collection activities based on the needs of the department, the organization, and perioperative patients.

E.1.3. Involves internal and external stakeholders, as appropriate, in systematic data collection.

E.1.4. Develops mechanisms to resolve missing or insufficient data, information, and knowledge resources.

E.1.5. Develops, maintains, and evaluates retrievable data management systems to support perioperative services.

E.2. Standard 2: Identifies Issues or Trends

The perioperative RN administrator analyzes data to develop ideas and support decisions relevant to the delivery of perioperative nursing care.

Measurement

E.2.1. Synthesizes available data to identify issues, patterns, trends, and variances involving perioperative nursing services.

E.2.2. Collaborates with internal and external stakeholders when analyzing data as appropriate.

E.2.3. Validates the issues and trends with internal and external stakeholders as appropriate.

E.2.4. Reports issues or trends to internal and external stakeholders as appropriate.

E.2.5. Documents issues and trends in a retrievable format to facilitate outcome identification and planning.

E.3. Standard 3: Outcomes Identification

The perioperative RN administrator identifies expected outcomes for perioperative services.

Measurement

E.3.1. Develops outcomes for perioperative nursing service using assessment findings and analysis.

E.3.2. Develops and maintains policies and procedures that support the outcomes.

E.3.3. Identifies evidenced-based outcomes using standardized perioperative nursing language.

E.3.4. Supports perioperative RNs and other health care personnel to achieve quality patient care outcomes.

STANDARDS OF PERIOPERATIVE NURSING

E.3.5. Promotes acquisition of appropriate technologies to provide patient and worker safety.
E.3.6. Identifies a physically, emotionally, and psychologically safe work environment as a priority.
E.3.7. Identifies a time frame in which to achieve the outcomes.
E.3.8. Modifies outcomes based on issues, trends, and research.

E.4. Standard 4: Planning

The perioperative RN administrator develops the process and strategic plan to attain expected outcomes for perioperative services.

Measurement

E.4.1. Considers organizational and departmental structure, as well as lines of authority, when planning to meet the outcomes.
E.4.2. Develops a strategic plan that is consistent with the mission, vision, and values of the organization.
E.4.3. Establishes a timeline for processes and strategies to carry out the plan.
E.4.4. Uses current laws, regulations, and standards to guide the planning process.
E.4.5. Bases the plan on current research and other evidence.
E.4.6. Assigns duties and responsibilities to carry out the plan with job descriptions, scope of practice, and regulatory and accrediting agencies.
E.4.7. Considers the physical, psychosocial, and economic effect of the plan.
E.4.8. Modifies the strategic plan based on issues and trends in the department.
E.4.9. Documents the strategic plan in a retrievable format.

E.5. Standard 5: Implementation

The perioperative RN administrator implements a strategic plan within the organizational and departmental structure.

Measurement

E.5.1. Implements the strategic plan by following the defined timeline with special consideration to the perioperative patient and workplace safety.
E.5.2. Provides those implementing the plan with sufficient time and material, as well as intellectual, human, and financial resources.
E.5.3. Uses health care organization and community resources to support implementation.
E.5.4. Coordinates and documents implementation of the plan, including modifications.
E.5.5. Communicates with internal and external stakeholders regarding implementation and modifications.
E.5.6. Encourages the development of organizational systems and processes that support implementation.

E.5.a. Standard 5a: Coordination

The perioperative RN administrator coordinates implementation of the plan, using appropriate human and capital resources.

Measurement

E.5.a.1. Organizes implementation with consideration for budgetary, health care organization, and community resources.
E.5.a.2. Promotes efficient integration of services to implement the plan.
E.5.a.3. Leads the coordination of efforts related to perioperative care and associated services when implementing the plan.

E.5.b. Standard 5b: Health Teaching and Health Promotion

The perioperative RN administrator employs strategies to promote workplace safety and health.

Measurement

E.5.b.1. Uses regulatory and evidence-based professional guidelines to implement workplace safety practices.
E.5.b.2. Promotes workplace safety by applying wellness techniques.
E.5.b.3. Commits to practicing self-care and promoting wellness with others.

E.5.c. Standard 5c: Consultation

The perioperative RN administrator provides consultation to communicate the identified plan.

Measurement

E.5.c.1. Acts as a resource to internal and external stakeholders regarding perioperative nursing care, perioperative patient outcomes, and perioperative services.
E.5.c.2. Uses assessment data, theoretical frameworks, current research, and evidence related to perioperative nursing care when providing consultation.
E.5.c.3. Provides consultation based on experience and knowledge of perioperative standards of care, recommended practices, laws, and regulations.

E.6. Standard 6: Evaluation

The perioperative RN administrator evaluates the effectiveness of the plan toward achieving desired outcomes.

Measurement

E.6.1. Measures progress toward strategic planning goals at regular intervals to determine their validity.
E.6.2. Reviews the plan for compliance with legal, regulatory, and credentialing requirements and guidelines.

E.6.3. Includes internal and external stakeholders when evaluating progress toward or achievement of outcomes.
E.6.4. Takes action based on the results of the evaluation to modify processes or structures.
E.6.5. Reports evaluation results to internal and external stakeholders.
E.6.6. Documents results of progress toward attaining outcomes.

E.7. Standard 7: Quality of Practice

The perioperative RN administrator guides improvement of care delivery using key indicators.

Measurement

E.7.1. Coordinates efforts and assigns personnel to systematically collect and record data in a retrievable format related to quality indicators.
E.7.2. Tracks data to develop performance improvement initiatives that support the delivery of high-quality patient care.
E.7.3. Develops written plans to monitor organizational or departmental outcomes at regular intervals.
E.7.4. Uses data to initiate organizational or departmental changes to provide high-quality patient care.
E.7.5. Identifies pertinent evidence to establish appropriate benchmarks.
E.7.6. Compares benchmark data to challenge current practice and organizational or departmental outcomes.
E.7.7. Incorporates research and current evidence to enhance quality and improve delivery of care.
E.7.8. Analyzes data to identify trends, variances, and patterns that affect perioperative nursing services.
E.7.9. Uses analysis to develop and enact new policies and procedures to improve perioperative nursing services.
E.7.10. Validates privileges, credentials, or certifications to schedule procedures appropriately.
E.7.11. Reports quality outcomes to internal and external stakeholders in compliance with state and federal requirements.

E.8. Standard 8: Education

The perioperative RN administrator has advanced educational preparation and management experience to direct perioperative services.

Measurement

E.8.1. Achieves advanced education in nursing or a related field.
E.8.2. Demonstrates management and leadership skills.
E.8.3. Validates experience in perioperative nursing.
E.8.4. Participates in ongoing educational activities related to leadership, management, and perioperative nursing.
E.8.5. Upholds local, state, federal, legislative, and regulatory activities affecting perioperative nursing services.
E.8.6. Recognizes professional standards, recommended practices, and guidelines pertinent to perioperative nursing services.
E.8.7. Maintains professional records to document ongoing competence.

E.9. Standard 9: Professional Practice Evaluation

The perioperative RN administrator follows regulatory, accrediting, and professional guidelines and regulations to evaluate professional practice of self and members of the department.

Measurement

E.9.1. Engages in self-evaluation of perioperative practice on a regular basis, identifying areas of strength as well as opportunities for professional development.
E.9.2. Validates competency of self and others at regular intervals.
E.9.3. Participates in a systematic peer review of self and others.
E.9.4. Provides a rationale for practice beliefs, decisions, and actions as part of the informal and formal evaluation processes.
E.9.5. Respects diversity in all interactions.
E.9.6. Ensures ongoing departmental compliance with local, state, national, and professional legislative and regulations.
E.9.7. Conducts formal performance reviews at regular intervals based on patient and departmental outcomes.
E.9.8. Solicits informal and formal feedback regarding departmental performance from appropriate internal and external stakeholders.

E.10. Standard 10: Collegiality

The perioperative RN administrator promotes the professional development of others.

Measurement

E.10.1. Serves as a professional role model and mentor to motivate, develop, recruit, and retain perioperative RNs and colleagues.
E.10.2. Establishes a learning environment that is open and respectful to others.
E.10.3. Shares expertise to advance the mission, vision, and values of the organization and promote positive perioperative outcomes.
E.10.4. Provides opportunities and support for continuing education, professional development, and formal education.
E.10.5. Promotes specialty certification.
E.10.6. Promotes active membership and participation in professional organizations.
E.10.7. Encourages staff member participation on multidisciplinary teams that improve perioperative nursing practice.

STANDARDS OF PERIOPERATIVE NURSING

E.10.8. Enhances own professional perioperative nursing practice and role performance through interactions with peers and colleagues.

E.11. Standard 11: Collaboration

The perioperative RN administrator collaborates with internal and external stakeholders to improve perioperative services.

Measurement

E.11.1. Participates on system-wide committees as a perioperative resource to influence organizational decisions, policies, and procedures.
E.11.2. Oversees departmental activities, providing expert input regarding perioperative and organizational interests.
E.11.3. Interacts with health care providers to promote positive perioperative outcomes.
E.11.4. Partners with internal and external stakeholders to influence health care policy decisions affecting perioperative services and outcomes.
E.11.5. Documents collaborative efforts toward improving perioperative services, including planning, implementation, and effectiveness.

E.12. Standard 12: Ethics

The perioperative RN administrator ensures that ethical processes are used to deliver perioperative services.

Measurement

E.12.1. Establishes an environment where perioperative team members engage in competent, ethical, and legal practices.
E.12.2. Ensures the protection of human rights for all individuals in the perioperative setting.
E.12.3. Maintains privacy and confidentiality of individuals and health information within the perioperative setting.
E.12.4. Fosters a nondiscriminatory climate within the perioperative setting.
E.12.5. Maintains sensitivity to diversity within the perioperative setting.
E.12.6. Uses resources within the organization to address ethical issues.

E.13. Standard 13: Research

The perioperative RN administrator supports and integrates current research and other available evidence into perioperative services.

Measurement

E.13.1. Evaluates and updates practice decisions based on available evidence and current research findings.
E.13.2. Creates a supportive environment with sufficient resources for nurses to investigate research findings and initiate evidence-based best practices.
E.13.3. Promotes dissemination of knowledge gained from evidence-based activities via presentations, publications, and consultation.
E.13.4. Ensures that departmental research priorities align with the mission, vision, values, and strategic plan of the organization.
E.13.5. Aligns departmental research priorities with those set by professional nursing organizations, regulatory agencies, and accrediting bodies.
E.13.6. Incorporates evidence-based practice to improve perioperative patient outcomes.
E.13.7. Incorporates evidence-based practice to improve and support a positive work environment.
E.13.8. Supports research activities that contribute to perioperative nursing knowledge.

E.14. Standard 14: Resource Utilization

The perioperative RN administrator uses human and material resources to deliver safe, high-quality, and cost-effective perioperative services.

Measurement

E.14.1. Considers safety and effectiveness when analyzing the cost-benefit ratios that affect perioperative services.
E.14.2. Allocates resources to promote quality patient outcomes.
E.14.3. Allocates fiscal resources to support the perioperative services strategic plan.
E.14.4. Advocates for human and material resources by using patient acuity and nursing workload guidelines to deliver safe patient care.
E.14.5. Advocates for human and material resources to support a safe work environment.
E.14.6. Identifies strategies for cost-effective and efficient practices without compromising perioperative patient safety or outcomes.
E.14.7. Promotes creative thinking among staff members, peers, and colleagues to develop new and innovative devices, practices, and strategies to advance and improve perioperative nursing services.
E.14.8. Advocates for environmental consciousness when using and managing resources in the perioperative setting.
E.14.9. Provides documentation for internal and external stakeholders to demonstrate costs, risks, and benefits that support decisions for perioperative practices.

E.15. Standard 15: Leadership

The perioperative RN administrator provides leadership within the organization and the profession.

Measurement

E.15.1. Maintains membership in relevant professional organizations related to leadership and perioperative nursing.
E.15.2. Strives to achieve relevant professional specialty certification(s).

E.15.3. Acts as a leader on administrative teams participating in decision making that affects perioperative services.

E.15.4. Participates in activities to influence legislative or regulatory decisions that affect perioperative services and perioperative nursing practice.

E.15.5. Leads committees, task forces, councils, and teams to make decisions that positively influence perioperative services, perioperative nursing practice, or perioperative patient outcomes.

E.15.6. Supervises perioperative personnel and supports their roles in promoting positive patient outcomes.

E.15.7. Promotes lifelong learning among personnel involved with perioperative services.

E.15.8. Inspires loyalty, teamwork, respect, and professionalism among personnel involved with perioperative services.

E.15.9. Promotes an environment that fosters independent and creative critical thinking.

E.15.10. Acts as a leader and change agent, supporting evidence-based practices in the perioperative setting.

E.15.11. Advances knowledge of perioperative services and perioperative nursing by communicating pertinent information through publishing and presenting for professional and lay audiences.

E.16. Standard 16: Advocacy

The perioperative RN administrator advocates for individuals and groups related to perioperative health and safety.

Measurement

E.16.1. Advocates for one perioperative RN circulator per patient in the intraoperative phase of care.

E.16.2. Supports perioperative patients' health care rights by involving individuals in their own care.

E.16.3. Endorses regulatory measures that provide for safe patient care and workplace safety.

E.16.4. Incorporates safe perioperative care into the design, implementation, and evaluation of policies, programs, services, and systems.

E.16.5. Allocates resources to support advocacy activities related to perioperative services and the nursing profession.

E.16.6. Supports the perioperative patient's right to access personal health data and information related to privacy, security, and confidentiality.

E.16.7. Promotes a philosophy of advocacy in the perioperative environment.

REFERENCES

1. *Nursing: Scope and Standards of Practice.* Washington, DC: American Nurses Association; 2004.
2. *Scope and Standards for Nurse Administrators.* Washington, DC: American Nurses Association; 2009.
3. Petersen C, ed. *Perioperative Nursing Data Set.* 2nd ed rev. Denver, CO: AORN, Inc; 2007.
4. *Nursing's Social Policy Statement.* 2nd ed. Washington, DC: American Nurses Association; 2003.

PUBLICATION HISTORY

Compiled from previous editions for publication in *Perioperative Standards and Recommended Practices* (Denver, CO: AORN, Inc; 2009).

Revised October 2009 for online publication in *Perioperative Standards and Recommended Practices.*

Reformatted September 2012 for publication in *Perioperative Standards and Recommended Practices*, 2013 edition.

Minor editing revisions made in November 2014 for publication in *Guidelines for Perioperative Practice*, 2015 edition.

STANDARDS OF PERIOPERATIVE NURSING

AORN gratefully acknowledges the work of the 2007–2008, 2008–2009, and 2009–2010 Nursing Practice Committees

2007–2008, 2009–2010 Chair,
2008–2009 Advisor
Antonia Hughes, MA, BSN, RN, CNOR
Perioperative Education Specialist
Baltimore Washington Medical Center
Glen Burnie, Maryland

2008–2009 Chair, 2007–2010 Member
Sharon L. Chappy, PhD, RN, CNOR
Associate Professor
University of Wisconsin Oshkosh
Oshkosh, Wisconsin

Members
Beth A. Beilein, MSM, BSN, RN, CNOR (2009–2010)
Director of Clinical Operations
Naples Day Surgery, South
Naples, Florida

James (Jay) Bowers, BSN, RN, CNOR (2007–2008)
Clinical Nurse Preceptor
West Virginia University Hospitals
Morgantown, West Virginia

Judith L. Clayton, RN, CNOR (2007–2009)
Perioperative Clinical Educator
Gwinnett Medical Center
Duluth, Georgia

Nikki A. Collier, RN, CNOR, CRNFA (2008–2010)
RN First Assistant
St Joseph Hospital
Eureka, California

Joy Crouse, MS, RN, CNOR (2007–2008)
Clinical Supervisor
St Josephs Hospital and Medical Center
Phoenix, Arizona

Jim D'Alfonso, MSN, RN, CNOR (2007–2009)
Associate Vice President
Scottsdale Healthcare Shea
Mesa, Arizona

Vicki Dreger, MSN, RN, CNOR (2007–2009)
Staff Nurse
Advocate Christ Medical Center
Oak Lawn, Illinois

Elizabeth Gasson, MSN, RN, CNOR (2009–2010)
Clinical Director
River Oaks Hospital
Jackson, Mississippi

Denise M. Jackson, MSN, RN, CNS, CRNFA (2009–2010)
RN First Assistant
Shannon Medical Center
San Angelo, Texas

Ellice M. Mellinger, MS, RN, CNOR (2008–2010)
Clinical Educator
University Medical Center
Tucson, Arizona

Barbara A. Ricker, MSN, RN, CNOR (2007–2009)
RN Clinical Development Professional
Banner Health
Phoenix, Arizona

Linda P. Voyles, BSN, RN, CNOR (2009–2010)
Perioperative Educator
Banner Estrella
Phoenix, Arizona

Dawn M. Yost, BSN, RN, RDH, CNOR (2008–2010)
Manager of Nursing Operations and Sterile Processing
West Virginia University Hospitals
Morgantown, West Virginia

2009–2010 Board Liaison
Peter Graves, BSN, RN, CNOR
Consultant
Corinth, Texas

2007–2009 Board Liaison
Jane Kusler-Jensen, MBA, BSN, RN, CNOR
Director of Perioperative Services
Ozaukee and River Woods Campuses,
Columbia-St Mary's
Milwaukee, Wisconsin

2007–2010 Staff Consultant
Bonnie G. Denholm, MS, BSN, RN, CNOR
Perioperative Nursing Specialist
AORN Center for Nursing Practice
Denver, Colorado

2007–2010 Administrative Support
Bonnie Kibbe

EXHIBIT A: HISTORICAL PERSPECTIVES ON THE AORN STANDARDS, COMPETENCY STATEMENTS, AND CERTIFICATION

AORN's first "Standards of nursing practice: OR" were developed with the American Nurses Association (ANA) Division of Medical Surgical Practice and printed in 1975. In addition to these standards, AORN began publishing recommended practices in the technical aspects of perioperative nursing in March 1975. Subsequently, AORN developed a variety of programs and activities to assist perioperative registered nurses (RNs) to become aware of and use the standards to evaluate their professional practice and the recommended practices to initiate best practices in their settings.

The standards were revised after data were collected from practicing perioperative RNs to determine the applicability and usefulness of the standards. The resulting revision, titled "Standards of perioperative nursing practice," was published in 1981. These standards were augmented by "Standards of administrative nursing practice: OR" in 1982, the "Patient outcome standards for perioperative nursing" in 1985, and the "Quality and performance improvement standards for perioperative nursing" in 2004. In 2009, the standards collection was consolidated into one document with four exhibits that included historical perspectives, perioperative patient outcomes, perioperative explications for the ANA *Code of Ethics for Nurses*, and the quality and performance improvement standards.

The Nursing Practice Committee reviewed and updated the standards collection for 2010. Advanced practice RN measurements were added and the administrative standards were revised to align with the current ANA administrative standards. The outcome statements and the quality and performance improvement standards were removed from the exhibit section of the standards collection to facilitate flexibility in updating and distributing those documents. The content changes were posted on the AORN web site for public review and comment for 30 days. The AORN Board of Directors approved the revisions in October 2009.

The standards serve as the foundation for the AORN professional competency statements, which were first published by AORN in 1986. These statements are revised periodically to provide a means for perioperative nurses to validate and measure the quality of their practice. AORN developed competency statements for the perioperative advanced practice nurse, the perioperative care coordinator, and the RN first assistant in 1994, 1999, and 2002, respectively, to define other professional roles of the perioperative nurse. All four sets of competencies were published in a collection titled *Competencies for Perioperative Practice* in 2008. Together with the *Perioperative Nursing Data Set*, recognized by ANA in 1999 and published by AORN in 2000, these resources provide a comprehensive framework for creating job descriptions, performance appraisals, competency checklists, and credentialing documents that affirm and support the contribution of the perioperative RN in providing safe, effective patient care.

Certification in perioperative nursing (CNOR®) demonstrates the perioperative RN's individual commitment to excellence in practice in the clinical setting as well as AORN's ongoing commitment to fostering excellence in the clinical setting. The first perioperative RN certification program was approved by the AORN House of Delegates in 1978 to "enhance quality patient care" and to "demonstrate accountability to the general public for nursing practice." From this vote, a Certification Council was appointed by the AORN Board of Directors to oversee the development, direction, implementation, and evaluation of the entire certification process. The Council was incorporated in January 1980. Evolution in its organizational mission and structure resulted in name changes in 1985 and 1997. In 2005, the organization became the Competency and Credentialing Institute (CCI). Today, it offers credentialing, nursing competency assessment, education, and consulting on nursing competency issues.

AORN continues to encourage the achievement and maintenance of additional certifications applicable to various arenas of perioperative practice, such as first assisting (CRNFA®), administration, nursing informatics, and other subspeciality areas. Resolutions and statements adopted by the House of Delegates consistently reiterate the primacy of the Association's concern for quality and safety in patient care. Striving for excellence in practice, perioperative nurses actively participate in shaping the practice environment and identifying clinical and organizational indicators for quality patient care, patient and workplace safety, and performance improvement.

EXHIBIT A: HISTORICAL PERSPECTIVES

Editor's note: CNOR and CRNFA are registered trademarks of the Competency and Credentialing Institute, Denver, CO.

EXHIBIT B: PERIOPERATIVE EXPLICATIONS FOR THE ANA *CODE OF ETHICS FOR NURSES*

Editor's note: The following is reprinted with permission from American Nurses Association, Code of Ethics for Nurses with Interpretive Statements, © 2001 American Nurses Publishing, American Nurses Foundation/American Nurses Association, Washington, DC.

About This Document

The ANA *Code of Ethics for Nurses with Interpretive Statements*, updated in 2001, is composed of nine provisions, with each provision further subdivided under provision headings. In the following document, the nine ANA provisions are listed with AORN's Explications. Each "Perioperative explication" is illustrated by "Perioperative examples" that pertain to a particular ANA provision heading.

The ANA *Code of Ethics for Nurses with Interpretive Statements* can be purchased online at http://nursingworld.org/MainMenuCategories/ThePracticeofProfessionalNursing/EthicsStandards/CodeofEthics.aspx.

ANA Code of Ethics for Nurses With Interpretive Statements

Preface

Ethics is an integral part of the foundation of nursing. Nursing has a distinguished history of concern for the welfare of the sick, injured, and vulnerable and for social justice. This concern is embodied in the provision of nursing care to individuals and the community. Nursing encompasses the prevention of illness, the alleviation of suffering, and the protection, promotion, and restoration of health in the care of individuals, families, groups, and communities. Nurses act to change those aspects of social structures that detract from health and well-being. Individuals who become nurses are expected not only to adhere to the ideals and moral norms of the profession but also to embrace them as a part of what it means to be a nurse. The ethical tradition of nursing is self-reflective, enduring, and distinctive. A code of ethics makes explicit the primary goals, values, and obligations of the profession.

The *Code of Ethics for Nurses* serves the following purposes:

- It is a succinct statement of the ethical obligations and duties of every individual who enters the nursing profession.
- It is the profession's nonnegotiable ethical standard.
- It is an expression of nursing's own understanding of its commitment to society.

There are numerous approaches for addressing ethics; these include adopting or subscribing to ethical theories, including humanist, feminist, and social ethics, adhering to ethical principles, and cultivating virtues. The *Code of Ethics for Nurses* reflects all of these approaches. The words "ethical" and "moral" are used throughout the *Code of Ethics*. "Ethical" is used to refer to reasons for decisions about how one ought to act, using the above mentioned approaches. In general, the word "moral" overlaps with "ethical" but is more aligned with personal belief and cultural values. Statements that describe activities and attributes of nurses in this *Code of Ethics* are to be understood as normative or prescriptive statements expressing expectations of ethical behavior.

The *Code of Ethics for Nurses* uses the term "patient" to refer to recipients of nursing care. The derivation of this word refers to "one who suffers," reflecting a universal aspect of human existence. Nonetheless, it is recognized that nurses also provide services to those seeking health as well as those responding to illness, to students and to staff, in health care facilities as well as in communities. Similarly, the term "practice" refers to the actions of the nurse in whatever role the nurse fulfills, including direct patient care provider, educator, administrator, researcher, policy developer, or other. Thus, the values and obligations expressed in this *Code of Ethics* apply to nurses in all roles and settings.

The *Code of Ethics for Nurses* is a dynamic document. As nursing and its social context change, changes to the *Code of Ethics* are also necessary. The *Code of Ethics* consists of two components: the provisions and the accompanying interpretive statements. There are nine provisions. The first three describe the most fundamental values and commitments of the nurse, the next three address boundaries of duty and loyalty, and the last three address aspects of duties beyond individual patient encounters. For each provision, there are interpretive statements that provide greater specificity for practice

EXHIBIT B: PERIOPERATIVE EXPLICATIONS

and are responsive to the contemporary context of nursing. Consequently, the interpretive statements are subject to more frequent revision than are the provisions. Additional ethical guidance and detail can be found in ANA or constituent member association position statements that address clinical, research, administrative, educational, or public policy issues.

The *Code of Ethics for Nurses with Interpretive Statements* provides a framework for nurses to use in ethical analysis and decision-making. The *Code of Ethics* establishes the ethical standard for the profession. It is not negotiable in any setting, nor is it subject to revision or amendment except by formal process of the House of Delegates of the ANA. The *Code of Ethics for Nurses* is a reflection of the proud ethical heritage of nursing, a guide for nurses now and in the future.

Preamble

The American Nurses Association (ANA) *Code of Ethics for Nurses with Interpretive Statements* expresses the moral commitment to uphold the goals, values, and distinct ethical obligations of all nurses. As nursing is practiced in a changing social context, the *Code of Ethics for Nurses* becomes a dynamic document. AORN's Ethics Task Force detailed the specific perioperative nursing explications that correspond to the nine provisions from the ANA *Code of Ethics for Nurses with Interpretive Statements* (ANA, 2001). The primary goals and values of a profession are made explicit in a code of ethics.

Together, the ANA code and the explications for perioperative nursing provide the framework within which perioperative nurses can make ethical decisions. The code establishes the profession's nonnegotiable ethical standard. This document demonstrates accountability and responsibility to the public, to other members of the health care team, and to the profession. This document helps perioperative nurses relate the ANA *Code of Ethics* to their own areas of practice and provides examples of behaviors that reflect the ethical obligations of perioperative nurses.

Introduction

Ethical decisions for the perioperative nurse are often difficult but necessary during the care of the surgical patient. Additionally, perioperative nurses need to be able to recognize ethical dilemmas and take action. Perioperative nurses are responsible for nursing decisions that are not only clinically and technically sound but also morally appropriate and suitable for the specific problems of the particular patient being treated. The technical or medical aspects of the decision answer the question, "What can be done for this patient?" The moral component involves the patient's wishes and answers the question, "What should be done for this patient?"

The strength of the ethical perspective is its resolute nature. It promotes an action guide for nurses to follow in the realm of patient care. Ethics, as a branch of philosophy, incorporates multiple approaches to take when dealing with or applying actions to real life situations. Thus, each perioperative nurse may experience a situation differently, as well as addressing the situation and identifying the ethical conflict issues, his or her feelings, behaviors, actions, analysis, and resolution of the situation differently.

Health care delivery provided via a team format, such as the surgical team, does not necessarily create ethical conflicts, but it may highlight the conflicts if the values of the team members emphasize different priorities. Additionally, new roles of health care team members may carry expectations about how members should interact with each other and how standards of care should be met.

The perioperative nurse, by virtue of the nurse-patient relationship, has an obligation to provide safe, professional, and ethical patient care. It is important that nurses know how to manage ethical decisions appropriately so that patients' beliefs can be honored without compromising the nurse's own moral conscience. Ethical practice is thus a critical aspect of nursing care, and the development of ethical competency is paramount for present and future nursing practice.

1: **The nurse, in all professional relationships, practices with compassion and respect for the inherent dignity, worth, and uniqueness of every individual, unrestricted by considerations of social or economic status, personal attributes, or the nature of health problems.**

1.1 Respect for human dignity

A fundamental principle that underlies all nursing practice is respect for the inherent worth, dignity, and human rights of every individual. Nurses take into account the needs and values of all persons in all professional relationships.

Perioperative explications
The perioperative nurse is morally obligated to respect the dignity and worth of each individual patient. Perioperative nursing care is provided to each patient undergoing a surgical or other invasive procedure in a manner that preserves and protects patient autonomy, dignity, and human rights.[1] Each nurse has an obligation to be knowledgeable about the moral and legal rights of all patients and to protect and support those rights. As health care does not occur in a vacuum, the perioperative nurse must take into account both the individual rights and the interdependence of individuals in decision-making.

Perioperative examples
- Respects patient's decision for surgery.
- Respects patient's wishes (eg, advance directives, end-of-life choices).

Code of Ethics for Nurses with Interpretive Statements reprinted with permission from American Nurses Association, © 2001 Nursesbooks.org, Silver Spring, MD.

EXHIBIT B: PERIOPERATIVE EXPLICATIONS

- Implements institutional advance directive policy in the practice setting.
- Restrains patient only when patient poses a direct or potential danger to self or others.

1.2 Relationships to patients

The need for health care is universal, transcending all individual differences. The nurse establishes relationships and delivers nursing services with respect for human needs and values, and without prejudice. An individual's lifestyle, value system, and religious beliefs should be considered in planning health care with and for each patient. Such consideration does not suggest that the nurse necessarily agrees with or condones certain individual choices, but that the nurse respects the patient as a person.

Perioperative explications

It is the responsibility of the perioperative nurse to provide care for each patient without prejudicial behavior. The care should be planned with consideration for the patient's values, religious beliefs, lifestyle choices, and age. The perioperative nurse respects the worth and dignity of the patient regardless of the diagnosis, disease process, procedure, or projected outcome. When the perioperative nurse is ethically opposed to interventions or procedures in a particular case, the nurse is justified in refusing to participate if the refusal is made known in advance and in time for other appropriate arrangements to be made for the patient's nursing care. When the patient's life is in jeopardy, the perioperative nurse is obliged to provide for the patient's safety, to avoid abandonment, and to withdraw only when assured that alternative sources of nursing care are available to the patient.

Perioperative examples

- Applies standards of nursing practice consistently to all patients with sensitivity to disability and economic, educational, cultural, religious, racial, age, and sexual differences.[2]
- Provides nursing care respecting the worth and dignity regardless of diagnosis, disease process, procedure, or projected outcome.[3]
- Respects the Patient's Bill of Rights.
- Refrains from derogatory comments about patients, families and significant others, colleagues, and other associates.
- Seeks guidance for resolving personal belief conflicts with the patient (eg, from supervisor, ethics committee, colleagues with appropriate authority).
- Uses principles of ethical analysis and moral reasoning to resolve ethical questions.[4]
- Provides spiritual comfort, arranges for appropriate substitute nursing care if personal beliefs conflict with required care, and respects the patient's decision for surgery.

1.3 The nature of health problems

The nurse respects the worth, dignity, and rights of all human beings irrespective of the nature of the health problem. The worth of the person is not affected by disease, disability, functional status, or proximity to death. This respect extends to all who require the services of the nurse for the promotion of health, the prevention of illness, the restoration of health, the alleviation of suffering, and the provision of supportive care to those who are dying.

The measures nurses take to care for the patient enable the patient to live with as much physical, emotional, social, and spiritual well-being as possible. Nursing care aims to maximize the values that the patient has treasured in life and extends supportive care to the family and significant others. Nursing care is directed toward meeting the comprehensive needs of patients and their families across the continuum of care. This is particularly vital in the care of patients and their families at the end of life to prevent and relieve the cascade of symptoms and suffering that are commonly associated with dying.

Nurses are leaders and vigilant advocates for the delivery of dignified and humane care. Nurses actively participate in assessing and assuring the responsible and appropriate use of interventions in order to minimize unwarranted or unwanted treatment and patient suffering. The acceptability and importance of carefully considered decisions regarding resuscitation status, withholding and withdrawing life-sustaining therapies, forgoing medically provided nutrition and hydration, aggressive pain and symptom management, and advance directives are increasingly evident. The nurse should provide interventions to relieve pain and other symptoms in the dying patient even when those interventions entail risks of hastening death. However, nurses may not act with the sole intent of ending a patient's life even though such action may be motivated by compassion, respect for patient autonomy, and quality of life considerations. Nurses have invaluable experience, knowledge, and insight into care at the end of life and should be actively involved in related research, education, practice, and policy development.

Perioperative explications

Perioperative nurses provide nursing care directed to meet the comprehensive needs of all patients, regardless of diagnosis, taking into consideration aspects of culture, language, perception of pain, significant others, values, and beliefs.[5] Nurses, as individuals, bring to their practice assumptions from their own culture, as well as about the cultures of others. In order to provide care that is culturally relevant to a diverse patient population, it is vital that nurses recognize the importance of each patient's values, beliefs, and health practices. In many instances, nurses provide care across cultures; thus, it becomes an ethical imperative for

Code of Ethics for Nurses with Interpretive Statements *reprinted with permission from American Nurses Association,* © 2001 Nursesbooks.org, Silver Spring, MD.

EXHIBIT B: PERIOPERATIVE EXPLICATIONS

nurses to develop the skill of culturally competent caring.

To most effectively care for patients of other cultures, the nurse must be a conscientious observer, a perceptive listener, and thorough assessor. Acquiring information about the patient's culture and gaining further personal insight provides the nurse with an increased understanding of culture and values from both perspectives (the patient's and the nurse's) as they relate to providing culturally competent care.

Perioperative examples
- Provides nursing care respecting the patient's worth and dignity regardless of diagnosis, disease process, procedure, or projected outcome.[6]
- Overcomes communication barriers to allow patients and their significant others to express preferences for care, providing interpreters when necessary.[7]

1.4 The right to self-determination

Respect for human dignity requires the recognition of specific patient rights, particularly the right of self-determination. Self-determination, also known as autonomy, is the philosophical basis for informed consent in health care. Patients have the moral and legal right to determine what will be done with their own person; to be given accurate, complete, and understandable information in a manner that facilitates an informed judgment; to be assisted with weighing the benefits, burdens, and available options in their treatment, including the choice of no treatment; to accept, refuse, or terminate treatment without deceit, undue influence, duress, coercion, or penalty; and to be given necessary support throughout the decision-making and treatment process. Such support would include the opportunity to make decisions with family and significant others and the provision of advice and support from knowledgeable nurses and other health professionals. Patients should be involved in planning their own health care to the extent they are able and choose to participate.

Each nurse has an obligation to be knowledgeable about the moral and legal rights of all patients to self-determination. The nurse preserves, protects, and supports those interests by assessing the patient's comprehension of both the information presented and the implications of decisions. In situations in which the patient lacks the capacity to make a decision, a designated surrogate decision-maker should be consulted. The role of the surrogate is to make decisions as the patient would, based upon the patient's previously expressed wishes and known values. In the absence of a designated surrogate decision-maker, decisions should be made in the best interests of the patient, considering the patient's personal values to the extent that they are known. The nurse supports patient self-determination by participating in discussions with surrogates, providing guidance and referral to other resources as necessary, and identifying and addressing problems in the decision-making process. Support of autonomy in the broadest sense also includes recognition that people of some cultures place less weight on individualism and choose to defer to family or community values in decision-making. Respect not just for the specific decision but also for the patient's method of decision-making is consistent with the principle of autonomy.

Individuals are interdependent members of the community. The nurse recognizes that there are situations in which the right to individual self-determination may be outweighed or limited by the rights, health, and welfare of others, particularly in relation to public health considerations. Nonetheless, limitation of individual rights must always be considered a serious deviation from the standard of care, justified only when there are no less restrictive means available to preserve the rights of others and the demands of justice.

Perioperative explications

Patients have the right to self-determination (ie, the ability to decide for oneself what course of action will be taken in various circumstances). The perioperative nurse provides care to each patient undergoing surgical intervention in a manner that preserves and protects patient autonomy, dignity, and human rights. The patient's autonomy in the decision-making process is acknowledged and supported by the perioperative nurse, who provides accurate, appropriate, and reasonable information to assist the patient in making an informed choice.[8] The perioperative nurse elicits the patient's response regarding perception of the surgical procedure and the implications of decisions. The perioperative nurse ensures that the patient has access to additional and accurate information.[9]

When individual rights must be temporarily overridden to preserve the life of the patient or of another person, the suspension of those rights must be considered a deviation to be tolerated as briefly as possible.

Perioperative examples
- Provides information and explains the Patient Self-Determination Act (eg, informed consent, living will, power of attorney for health care, do-not-resuscitate order, organ procurement).[10]
- Confirms that informed consent has been granted for planned procedure[11]; when possible, obtains surrogate's permission for emergency surgery.
- Explains procedures before initiating action.
- Restrains patient only when patient poses a direct danger to self or others.
- Respects advance directives and end-of-life choices.
- Implements institutional advance directive policy in practice setting.

Code of Ethics for Nurses with Interpretive Statements *reprinted with permission from American Nurses Association, © 2001 nursesbooks.org, Silver Spring, MD.*

EXHIBIT B: PERIOPERATIVE EXPLICATIONS

- Participates in perioperative teaching; answers patient's questions accurately and honestly.
- Allows choices within RN scope of practice (eg, child's preference for transport to the operating room, wagon versus cart).
- Formulates ethical decisions with assistance of available resources (eg, ethics committee, ethicists).

1.5 Relationships with colleagues and others

The principle of respect for persons extends to all individuals with whom the nurse interacts. The nurse maintains compassionate and caring relationships with colleagues and others with a commitment to the fair treatment of individuals, to integrity-preserving compromise, and to resolving conflict. Nurses function in many roles, including direct care provider, administrator, educator, researcher, and consultant. In each of these roles, the nurse treats colleagues, employees, assistants, and students with respect and compassion. This standard of conduct precludes any and all prejudicial actions, any form of harassment or threatening behavior, or disregard for the effect of one's actions on others. The nurse values the distinctive contribution of individuals or groups, and collaborates to meet the shared goal of providing quality health services.

Perioperative explications

Perioperative nurses must recognize the individuality not only of their patients, but also of their colleagues and others. As health care is not provided in a vacuum, nurses must be able to interact with a variety of other professionals and ancillary providers in the perioperative environment. In working with colleagues, perioperative nurses display the same nondiscriminatory and nonjudgmental behavior as they do with their patients. Treating others with professionalism and respect will enhance the performance of the health care team.

Perioperative nurses are compelled to treat colleagues and all people in a just and fair manner regardless of disability, economic status, level of education, culture, religion, race, age, and sexuality. Just as nurses have the right not to be abused or harassed in the workplace, so must they treat others in their workplace with respect and compassion. The nurse recognizes the contributions of each member of the health care team and works to collaborate to achieve quality patient care.

Perioperative examples
- Integrates cultural differences of coworkers.
- Recognizes and respects the value of all team members, including students and ancillary and support staff members.
- Provides education and information to coworkers, including ancillary and support staff.

- Promotes comparable levels of care in all practice settings in which invasive procedures are performed.
- Uses medical devices in a safe manner and complies with the Safe Medical Devices Act and other laws and regulations.

2: The nurse's primary commitment is to the patient, whether an individual, family, group, or community.

2.1 Primacy of the patient's interests

The nurse's primary commitment is to the recipient of nursing and health care services—the patient—whether the recipient is an individual, a family, a group, or a community. Nursing holds a fundamental commitment to the uniqueness of the individual patient; therefore, any plan of care must reflect that uniqueness. The nurse strives to provide patients with opportunities to participate in planning care, assures that patients find the plans acceptable, and supports the implementation of the plan. Addressing patient interests requires recognition of the patient's place in the family or other networks of relationship. When the patient's wishes are in conflict with others, the nurse seeks to help resolve the conflict. Where conflict persists, the nurse's commitment remains to the identified patient.

Perioperative explications

The perioperative nurse supports both the interdependence and the individual rights of the patient when making decisions. The perioperative nurse collaborates in a manner that preserves and protects the patient's autonomy, dignity, and human rights. When individual rights must be temporarily overridden to preserve the life of the patient or of another person (eg, in the case of violent patients or patients with communicable diseases), the suspension of those rights must be considered a deviation to be tolerated as briefly as possible.

Perioperative examples
- Collaborates with patient regarding health care whenever possible.
- Collects patient health data.
- Analyzes assessment data and utilizes the *Perioperative Nursing Data Set* (PNDS) to formulate a nursing diagnosis and plan nursing care.
- Identifies expected outcomes unique to the patient.[12]
- Considers assessment information, including patient preferences and unique needs, when developing an individualized plan of care to attain designated patient outcomes.[13]
- Includes family/significant others in planning care.[14]
- Provides for spiritual comfort to the patient and significant others (eg, contacts religious counselor).

Code of Ethics for Nurses with Interpretive Statements *reprinted with permission from American Nurses Association,* © 2001 Nursesbooks.org, Silver Spring, MD.

EXHIBIT B: PERIOPERATIVE EXPLICATIONS

- Acts as patient advocate.
- Provides interpreters when necessary.
- Respects patient's decision to choose or refuse care or interventions.

2.2 Conflict of interest for nurses

Nurses are frequently put in situations of conflict arising from competing loyalties in the workplace, including situations of conflicting expectations from patients, families, physicians, colleagues, and in many cases, health care organizations and health plans. Nurses must examine the conflicts arising between their own personal and professional values, the values and interests of others who are also responsible for patient care and health care decisions, as well as those of patients. Nurses strive to resolve such conflicts in ways that ensure patient safety, guard the patient's best interests, and preserve the professional integrity of the nurse.

Situations created by changes in health care financing and delivery systems, such as incentive systems to decrease spending, pose new possibilities of conflict between economic self-interest and professional integrity. The use of bonuses, sanctions, and incentives tied to financial targets are examples of features of health care systems that may present such conflict. Conflicts of interest may arise in any domain of nursing activity, including clinical practice, administration, education, or research. Advanced practice nurses who bill directly for services and nursing executives with budgetary responsibilities must be especially cognizant of the potential for conflicts of interest. Nurses should disclose to all relevant parties (eg, patients, employers, colleagues) any perceived or actual conflict of interest and in some situations should withdraw from further participation. Nurses in all roles must seek to ensure that employment arrangements are just and fair and do not create an unreasonable conflict between patient care and direct personal gain.

Perioperative explications

Conflicts may arise from financial considerations in the perioperative setting that may contribute to conflicting loyalties between the perioperative nurse and the patient. While the perioperative nurse needs to be fiscally responsible, the perioperative nurse's primary responsibility is to ensure that the patient's safety is maintained.

The perioperative nurse does not give or imply endorsement to advertising, promotion, or sale of commercial products or services in a manner that may be interpreted as reflecting the opinion or judgment of the profession as a whole.

Perioperative examples

- Identifies and resolves conflicts of interest effectively.
- Abstains from influencing purchasing decisions involving companies in which nurses have ownership to make financial gains (eg, stocks, other equity interest).
- The perioperative nurse does not solicit or accept gifts, gratuities, or other items of value that reasonably could be interpreted by others as influencing impartiality.

2.3 Collaboration

Collaboration is not just cooperation, but it is the concerted effort of individuals and groups to attain a shared goal. In health care, that goal is to address the health needs of the patient and the public. The complexity of health care delivery systems requires a multidisciplinary approach to the delivery of services that has the strong support and active participation of all the health professions. Within this context, nursing's unique contribution, scope of practice, and relationship with other health professions needs to be clearly articulated, represented, and preserved. By its very nature, collaboration requires mutual trust, recognition, and respect among the health care team, shared decision-making about patient care, and open dialogue among all parties who have an interest in and a concern for health outcomes. Nurses should work to assure that the relevant parties are involved and have a voice in decision-making about patient care issues. Nurses should see that the questions that need to be addressed are asked and that the information needed for informed decision-making is available and provided. Nurses should actively promote the collaborative multidisciplinary planning required to ensure the availability and accessibility of quality health services to all persons who have needs for health care.

Intraprofessional collaboration within nursing is fundamental to effectively addressing the health needs of patients and the public. Nurses engaged in nonclinical roles, such as administration or research, while not providing direct care, nonetheless are collaborating in the provision of care through their influence and direction of those who do. Effective nursing care is accomplished through the interdependence of nurses in differing roles—those who teach the needed skills, set standards, manage the environment of care, or expand the boundaries of knowledge used by the profession. In this sense, nurses in all roles share a responsibility for the outcomes of nursing care.

Perioperative explications

The perioperative nurse respects the interdependence of all health care providers in achieving positive outcomes for patients undergoing a surgical or other invasive procedure. As a fundamental member of the surgical team, the perioperative nurse actively participates with other health care professionals when planning and providing patient care. The perioperative nurse, nurse managers, educators, and researchers need to

Code of Ethics for Nurses with Interpretive Statements *reprinted with permission from American Nurses Association,* © 2001 nursesbooks.org, Silver Spring, MD.

EXHIBIT B: PERIOPERATIVE EXPLICATIONS

participate in direct and indirect multidisciplinary planning and decision-making regarding patient care protocols and activities.

Perioperative examples
- Collaborates with the surgeon and anesthesia care provider to plan care specific to the procedure and the patient's needs.
- Collaborates and consults with nursing colleagues in the perioperative setting and practicing in other specialty areas (eg, RN first assistant [RNFA], critical care, psychiatry, pain management, pediatrics, postanesthesia care, home health).
- Demonstrates collaborative practice among subspecialties within and outside the perioperative arena.
- Collaborates with ancillary and support staff to enhance communication and work patterns that are mutually beneficial for staff and for efficient patient care.
- Collaborates with the public, industry, and health care workers regarding environmental and cost-containment issues.
- Formulates ethical decisions with assistance of available resources (eg, ethics committee, counselors, and ethicists).

2.4 Professional boundaries

When acting within one's role as a professional, the nurse recognizes and maintains boundaries that establish appropriate limits to relationships. While the nature of nursing work has an inherently personal component, nurse-patient relationships and nurse-colleague relationships have, as their foundation, the purpose of preventing illness, alleviating suffering, and protecting, promoting, and restoring the health of patients. In this way, nurse-patient and nurse-colleague relationships differ from those that are purely personal and unstructured, such as friendship. The intimate nature of nursing care, the involvement of nurses in important and sometimes highly stressful life events, and the mutual dependence of colleagues working in close concert all present the potential for blurring of limits to professional relationships. Maintaining authenticity and expressing oneself as an individual, while remaining within the bounds established by the purpose of the relationship, can be especially difficult in prolonged or long-term relationships. In all encounters, nurses are responsible for retaining their professional boundaries. When those professional boundaries are jeopardized, the nurse should seek assistance from peers or supervisors or take appropriate steps to remove her/himself from the situation.

Perioperative explications
Perioperative nurses promote and maintain professional relationships with patients, peers, coworkers, and all members of the surgical team. Perioperative nurses are aware of the intimate nature of nursing care, the highly stressful nature of the surgical environment, and the collegial nature of the surgical team. The perioperative nurse respects professional boundaries in the nurse-patient relationship and does not convey undue influence on patient decisions. Perioperative nurses play a critical role in providing information to patients so that decisions affecting that patient will be appropriate and effective.

The nurse should seek the assistance of peers or supervisors, without hesitation, when professional boundaries are unclear or in jeopardy. Perioperative nurses deliver patient care in a nondiscriminatory and nonjudgmental manner according to published, legal, agency, professional, and regulatory standards.[15]

Perioperative examples
- Plans for appropriate substitute nursing care if personal beliefs conflict with required care.
- Avoids unprofessional behavior toward patients, coworkers, and other health care professionals.
- Demonstrates respect toward colleagues and students.
- Recognizes the professional nature of the nurse-patient relationship and its inherent boundaries.

3: The nurse promotes, advocates for, and strives to protect the health, safety, and rights of the patient.

3.1 Privacy

The nurse safeguards the patient's right to privacy. The need for health care does not justify unwanted intrusion into the patient's life. The nurse advocates for an environment that provides for sufficient physical privacy, including auditory privacy for discussions of a personal nature, and policies and practices that protect the confidentiality of information.

Perioperative explications
The perioperative nurse has an obligation to protect patients from undue exposure or unwarranted invasions of privacy. Maintaining the patient's privacy is essential to preserving the trust developed in the nurse-patient relationship. Actions demeaning the dignity of the individual could destroy this relationship and jeopardize the patient's welfare. Maintaining the patient's privacy is reflected by securing mechanisms to protect the patient's physical privacy, all forms of identifiable personal information (ie, verbal, written, electronic), personal belongings, and valuables.

Perioperative examples
- Avoids needless exposure of patient's body.
- Keeps doors to OR or procedure rooms closed except during movement of patients, personnel, supplies, or equipment.[16]

Code of Ethics for Nurses with Interpretive Statements *reprinted with permission from American Nurses Association,* © 2001 Nursesbooks.org, Silver Spring, MD.

EXHIBIT B: PERIOPERATIVE EXPLICATIONS

- Restricts access to patient care areas to designated, authorized personnel only.
- Provides cover, warmth, and comfort during transfer from unit to surgical suite as well as during transfer to postoperative unit.
- Provides and maintains respect for deceased.
- Provides protected area for viewing deceased by family/significant others.[17]
- Provides auditory privacy for patient and staff conversations.

3.2 Confidentiality

Associated with the right to privacy, the nurse has a duty to maintain confidentiality of all patient information. The patient's well-being could be jeopardized and the fundamental trust between patient and nurse destroyed by unnecessary access to data or by the inappropriate disclosure of identifiable patient information. The rights, well-being, and safety of the individual patient should be the primary factors in arriving at any professional judgment concerning the disposition of confidential information received from or about the patient, whether oral, written, or electronic. The standard of nursing practice and the nurse's responsibility to provide quality care require that relevant data be shared with those members of the health care team who have a need to know. Only information pertinent to a patient's treatment and welfare is disclosed, and only to those directly involved with the patient's care. Duties of confidentiality, however, are not absolute and may need to be modified in order to protect the patient, other innocent parties, and in circumstances of mandatory disclosure for public health reasons.

Information used for purposes of peer review, third-party payments, and other quality improvement or risk management mechanisms may be disclosed only under defined policies, mandates, or protocols. These written guidelines must assure that the rights, well-being, and safety of the patient are protected. In general, only that information directly relevant to a task or specific responsibility should be disclosed. When using electronic communications, special effort should be made to maintain data security.

Perioperative explications

In concert with privacy is the professional responsibility to maintain the confidentiality of the patient's personal information. The perioperative nurse has a duty to safeguard the confidentiality of all patient information. Measures must be taken to protect the confidentiality of patient information, including oral, written, and electronic forms. Information pertinent to the patient's treatment and welfare is shared only with members of the health care team directly concerned with the patient's care. While relevant patient information must be shared in an expeditious manner with other members of the health care team in order to provide safe patient care, the patient must have trust and confidence in the nurse that information related to his or her care will be protected. Safeguarding private information about patients is a core belief of nursing; however, new technologies such as electronic records, have added a challenge to protecting patient information.

Perioperative examples

- Maintains confidentiality of patient information within scope of practice.
- Closes patient record and logs off whenever leaving the computer unattended to protect patient information.
- Follows facility policies regarding electronic information documentation and storage.
- Is aware of and complies with local, state, and federal privacy and security regulations.
- Limits access to patient's record and information (eg, surgery schedule) to appropriate members of the health care team.
- Shares and discusses patient information only with appropriate health care providers and those directly involved in care.
- Protects all forms of confidential patient information (ie, verbal, written, electronic).
- Secures patient's records, belongings, and valuables.
- Maintains patient's record following agency policy, procedure, or protocol.
- Completes record of disposition of belongings and valuables following agency policy, procedure, or protocol.
- Completes operative records accurately and in an objective and nonjudgmental manner.
- Releases patient information only to individuals properly identified and in compliance with established policies, mandates, or protocols.
- Uses information for quality improvement purposes in a manner that protects patient confidentiality.[18]
- Follows regulations regarding disposal of printed records (eg, perioperative schedules, laboratory reports, face sheets).

3.3 Protection of participants in research

Stemming from the right to self-determination, each individual has the right to choose whether or not to participate in research. It is imperative that the patient or legally authorized surrogate receive sufficient information that is material to an informed decision, to comprehend that information, and to know how to discontinue participation in research without penalty. Necessary information to achieve an adequately informed consent includes the nature of participation, potential harms and benefits, and available alternatives to taking part in the research. Additionally, the patient should be informed of how the data will be protected. The patient has the right to refuse to participate in research or to withdraw at any time without fear of adverse consequences or reprisal.

Code of Ethics for Nurses with Interpretive Statements *reprinted with permission from American Nurses Association,* © 2001 Nursesbooks.org, Silver Spring, MD.

EXHIBIT B: PERIOPERATIVE EXPLICATIONS

Research should be conducted and directed only by qualified persons. Prior to implementation, all research should be approved by a qualified review board to ensure patient protection and the ethical integrity of the research. Nurses should be cognizant of the special concerns raised by research involving vulnerable groups, including children, prisoners, students, the elderly, and the poor. The nurse who participates in research in any capacity should be fully informed about both the subject's and the nurse's rights and obligations in the particular research study and in research in general. Nurses have the duty to question and, if necessary, to report and to refuse to participate in research they deem morally objectionable.

Perioperative explications

The nurse acts to protect the rights of patients involved in clinical research.[19] These rights include the right of adequately informed consent, the right of freedom from risk of injury, the right of privacy, and the right to the preservation of dignity. The perioperative nurse respects the patient's right to decline or discontinue participation in research. The perioperative nurse should be knowledgeable about the rights of the nurse as well as the patient regarding research studies.

Perioperative nurses have an obligation to (a) ensure that research is conducted by qualified people, (b) obtain information about the intent and nature of the research, and (c) confirm that the study is approved by appropriate review bodies. The researcher should disclose the rights and obligations of the patient and the perioperative nurse. Furthermore, the researcher has an obligation to provide information about the nature of the study to the staff members providing care to the participants. Perioperative nurses should be able to question, report, or refuse to participate in research to which they are morally opposed.

Perioperative examples

- Confirms informed consent of the patient, by physician or responsible researcher, prior to initiation of the study and before the use of patient information for research.
- Safeguards the patient's rights as a research subject.
- Submits research proposals to the institutional review board.
- Follows recommended guidelines and protocols when using investigational devices or when engaging in new procedures.
- Follows federal guidelines for treatment of human and animal subjects.
- Provides for patient confidentiality during data collection.
- Seeks guidance from supervisor to resolve issues regarding any research project that conflict with the nurse's personal beliefs.
- Plans for appropriate substitute nursing care if personal beliefs conflict with the research project.

3.4 Standards and review mechanisms

Nursing is responsible and accountable for assuring that only those individuals who have demonstrated the knowledge, skill, practice experiences, commitment, and integrity essential to professional practice are allowed to enter into and continue to practice within the profession. Nurse educators have a responsibility to ensure that basic competencies are achieved and to promote a commitment to professional practice prior to entry of an individual into practice. Nurse administrators are responsible for assuring that the knowledge and skills of each nurse in the workplace are assessed prior to the assignment of responsibilities requiring preparation beyond basic academic programs.

The nurse has a responsibility to implement and maintain standards of professional nursing practice. The nurse should participate in planning, establishing, implementing, and evaluating review mechanisms designed to safeguard patients and nurses, such as peer review processes or committees, credentialing processes, quality improvement initiatives, and ethics committees. Nurse administrators must ensure that nurses have access to and inclusion on institutional ethics committees. Nurses must bring forward difficult issues related to patient care and/or institutional constraints upon ethical practice for discussion and review. The nurse acts to promote inclusion of appropriate others in all deliberations related to patient care.

Nurses should also be active participants in the development of policies and review mechanisms designed to promote patient safety, reduce the likelihood of errors, and address both environmental system factors and human factors that present increased risk to patients. In addition, when errors do occur, nurses are expected to follow institutional guidelines in reporting errors committed or observed to the appropriate supervisory personnel and for assuring responsible disclosure of errors to patients. Under no circumstances should the nurse participate in, or condone through silence, either an attempt to hide an error or a punitive response that serves only to fix blame rather than correct the conditions that led to the error.

Perioperative explications

The perioperative nurse's primary obligation is to promote the health, welfare, and safety of the patient. The perioperative nurse is responsible for implementing and maintaining standards of perioperative nursing practice. The nurse follows policies, practice guidelines, and laws to safeguard the health and safety of the patient. The nurse participates in the establishment and evaluation of mechanisms to review practice. Competency validation is an essential component to providing safe and effective patient care. Perioperative nurses need to be aware of their own educational and clinical capabilities and seek the assistance of colleagues without hesitation when patient care needs

Code of Ethics for Nurses with Interpretive Statements reprinted with permission from American Nurses Association, © 2001 Nursesbooks.org, Silver Spring, MD.

EXHIBIT B: PERIOPERATIVE EXPLICATIONS

require additional skills. The perioperative nurse uses personal, institutional, professional, and regulatory resources to assist with the resolution of incompetent, unethical, and illegal practices in the work setting.

Perioperative examples
- Uses institutional ethics committee, practice committee, and peer review.
- Supports and participates in institutional ethics committee and institutional review boards.
- Participates in educational programs that enhance patient care (eg, morbidity/mortality conferences, ethics grand rounds, patient care conferences).
- Participates in quality and performance improvement processes.
- Participates in development and revision of professional standards of practice.
- Adheres to professional standards of practice, such as AORN's "Standards of perioperative clinical practice" and "Standards of perioperative professional performance."[20]
- Participates in multidisciplinary review of patient outcomes.
- Complies with institutional policies and procedures regarding competent performance of nursing activities.
- Complies with federal and state regulations such as Occupational Safety and Health Administration regulations, the Americans with Disabilities Act, and state boards of nursing regulations.
- Complies with accrediting agencies such as the Joint Commission and state regulatory agencies.
- Confirms clinicians' practice privileges and credentials (eg, RN first assistants, physicians, physician's assistants).

3.5 Acting on questionable practice

The nurse's primary commitment is to the health, well-being, and safety of the patient across the life span and in all settings in which health care needs are addressed. As an advocate for the patient, the nurse must be alert to and take appropriate action regarding any instances of incompetent, unethical, illegal, or impaired practice by any member of the health care team or the health care system or any action on the part of others that places the rights or best interests of the patient in jeopardy. To function effectively in this role, nurses must be knowledgeable about the *Code of Ethics*, standards of practice of the profession, relevant federal, state and local laws and regulations, and the employing organization's policies and procedures.

When the nurse is aware of inappropriate or questionable practice in the provision or denial of health care, concern should be expressed to the person carrying out the questionable practice. Attention should be called to the possible detrimental effect upon the patient's well-being or best interests as well as the integrity of nursing practice. When factors in the health care delivery system or health care organization threaten the welfare of the patient, similar action should be directed to the responsible administrator. If indicated, the problem should be reported to an appropriate higher authority within the institution or agency, or to an appropriate external authority.

There should be established processes for reporting and handling incompetent, unethical, illegal, or impaired practice within the employment setting so that such reporting can go through official channels, thereby reducing the risk of reprisal against the reporting nurse. All nurses have a responsibility to assist those who identify potentially questionable practice. State nurses associations should be prepared to provide assistance and support in the development and evaluation of such processes and reporting procedures. When incompetent, unethical, illegal, or impaired practice is not corrected within the employment setting and continues to jeopardize patient well-being and safety, the problem should be reported to other appropriate authorities such as practice committees of the pertinent professional organizations, the legally constituted bodies concerned with licensing of specific categories of health workers and professional practitioners, or the regulatory agencies concerned with evaluating standards or practice. Some situations may warrant the concern and involvement of all such groups. Accurate reporting and factual documentation, and not merely opinion, undergird all such responsible actions. When a nurse chooses to engage in the act of responsible reporting about situations that are perceived as unethical, incompetent, illegal, or impaired, the professional organization has a responsibility to provide the nurse with support and assistance and to protect the practice of those nurses who choose to voice their concerns. Reporting unethical, illegal, incompetent, or impaired practices, even when done appropriately, may present substantial risks to the nurse; nevertheless, such risks do not eliminate the obligation to address serious threats to patient safety.

Perioperative explications

Care providers in the perioperative environment provide health services within the scope of legitimate and ethical practice and safeguard the health and safety of their patients. The perioperative nurse is responsible for meeting legal, institutional, professional, and regulatory standards. It is the ethical obligation of the perioperative nurse to identify and appropriately report questionable practices by any member of the health care team. There should be an established process for reporting and handling incompetent, unethical, or illegal practice within the employment setting so that such reporting can go through official channels without causing fear of reprisal. The perioperative nurse should be knowledgeable about the process and be prepared to use it if necessary. Written

Code of Ethics for Nurses with Interpretive Statements *reprinted with permission from American Nurses Association,* © 2001 Nursesbooks.org, Silver Spring, MD.

EXHIBIT B: PERIOPERATIVE EXPLICATIONS

documentation of the observed practices or behaviors must be available to the appropriate authorities.

When incompetent, unethical, or illegal practice on the part of anyone concerned with the patient's care is not corrected within the employment setting and continues to jeopardized the patient's welfare and safety, the problem should be reported to other appropriate authorities, such as practice committees of the pertinent professional organizations or the legally constituted bodies concerned with licensing of specific categories of health workers or professional practitioners. Accurate reporting and documentation undergird all action.

Perioperative examples
- Acts as a patient advocate by protecting the patient from incompetent, unethical, or illegal practices.
- Questions care that appears inappropriate or substandard.
- Expresses concern to the person carrying out the questionable practice.
- Reports incompetent, unethical, or illegal practice to the responsible administrative person.
- Consults with colleagues and supervisors to resolve concerns.
- Documents observations and occurrences in an objective manner according to institutional policy.
- Complies with institutional policies in resolving problems.
- Reports verbal, psychological, and physical harassment or abuse.
- Intervenes appropriately to protect patient safety.

3.6 Addressing impaired practice

Nurses must be vigilant to protect the patient, the public, and the profession from potential harm when a colleague's practice, in any setting, appears to be impaired. The nurse extends compassion and caring to colleagues who are in recovery from illness or when illness interferes with job performance. In a situation where a nurse suspects another's practice may be impaired, the nurse's duty is to take action designed both to protect patients and to assure that the impaired individual receives assistance in regaining optimal function. Such action should usually begin with consulting supervisory personnel and may also include confronting the individual in a supportive manner and with the assistance of others or helping the individual to access appropriate resources. Nurses are encouraged to follow guidelines outlined by the profession and policies of the employing organization to assist colleagues whose job performance may be adversely affected by mental or physical illness or by personal circumstances. Nurses in all roles should advocate for colleagues whose job performance may be impaired to ensure that they receive appropriate assistance, treatment, and access to fair institutional and legal processes. This includes supporting the return to practice of the individual who has sought assistance and is ready to resume professional duties.

If impaired practice poses a threat or danger to self or others, regardless of whether the individual has sought help, the nurse must take action to report the individual to persons authorized to address the problem. Nurses who advocate for others whose job performance creates a risk for harm should be protected from negative consequences. Advocacy may be a difficult process, and the nurse is advised to follow workplace policies. If workplace policies do not exist or are inappropriate—that is, they deny the nurse in question access to due legal process or demand resignation—the reporting nurse may obtain guidance from the professional association, state peer assistance programs, employee assistance program, or a similar resource.

Perioperative explications
The perioperative nurse has an ethical responsibility to protect the patient, the public, and the profession from potential harm that could result from a colleague's impairment. It is both caring and compassionate to take action to protect the patient and ensure that the impaired person receives appropriate assistance. The nurse should follow guidelines outlined by the profession and the policies and procedures of the employing agency.

Perioperative examples
- Uses institutional procedural mechanisms to report substance abuse or impairment of colleagues.
- Consults with supervisory personnel.
- Confronts the individual in a supportive, caring manner.
- Uses agency resources for helping the individual to access treatment and care.
- Acts as patient advocate and takes action to ensure patient safety (eg, makes arrangements to remove the unsafe practitioner and replace him or her with an appropriate practitioner to continue patient care).

4: The nurse is responsible and accountable for individual nursing practice and determines the appropriate delegation of tasks consistent with the nurse's obligation to provide optimum patient care.

4.1 Acceptance of accountability and responsibility

Individual registered nurses bear primary responsibility for the nursing care that their patients receive and are individually accountable for their own practice. Nursing practice includes direct care activities, acts of delegation, and other responsibilities such as teaching, research, and administration. In each instance, the nurse retains accountability and responsibility for the

EXHIBIT B: PERIOPERATIVE EXPLICATIONS

quality of practice and for conformity with standards of care.

Nurses are faced with decisions in the context of the increased complexity and changing patterns in the delivery of health care. As the scope of nursing practice changes, the nurse must exercise judgment in accepting responsibilities, seeking consultation, and assigning activities to others who carry out nursing care. For example, some advanced practice nurses have the authority to issue prescription and treatment orders to be carried out by other nurses. These acts are not acts of delegation. Both the advanced practice nurse issuing the order and the nurse accepting the order are responsible for the judgments made and accountable for the actions taken.

Perioperative explications
The individual professional licensee protects the public by ensuring the basic competencies of the professional nurse. Moreover, society grants the nursing profession the right to regulate its own practice. Perioperative nurses bear primary responsibility for perioperative nursing care and are individually accountable for their own practice. The nurse is responsible for nursing decisions made regarding care and is accountable for individual actions. Perioperative nursing practice may include direct patient care, delegation, teaching, research, or administration. Nurses are responsible for judgments they make regarding care and accountable for actions taken.

Perioperative examples
- Maintains nursing licensure and certification.
- Accepts responsibility and accountability for perioperative nursing practice, staffing schedules, and on-call assignments.
- Assumes responsibility for continued education.

4.2 Accountability for nursing judgment and action
Accountability means to be answerable to oneself and others for one's own actions. In order to be accountable, nurses act under a code of ethical conduct that is grounded in the moral principles of fidelity and respect for the dignity, worth, and self-determination of patients. Nurses are accountable for judgments made and actions taken in the course of nursing practice, irrespective of health care organizations' policies or providers' directives.

Perioperative explications
Accountability refers to being answerable to oneself, patients, peers, the profession, and society for judgments made and actions taken as a perioperative nurse. Neither physicians' orders nor the employing agency's policies relieve the perioperative nurse of accountability for those actions and judgments. Professional accountability to society is reflected in the ANA *Code of Ethics for Nurses*, standards of practice, educational requirements for practice, certification, and a performance evaluation.

Perioperative examples
- Provides safe and competent patient care.
- Accounts for sponges, needles, instruments, and other potential foreign bodies.
- Practices according to the ANA *Code of Ethics for Nurses*; AORN's *Standards, Recommended Practices, and Guidelines*; and hospital and departmental policies and procedures.
- Practices within scope of practice.
- Evaluates self-performance and solicits peer review.
- Alerts surgeon and colleagues to potential risks to patients (eg, positioning, electrical hazards, blood loss, inadvertent laceration of a blood vessel).
- Questions orders that appear incorrect or inappropriate.

4.3 Responsibility for nursing judgment and action
Responsibility refers to the specific accountability or liability associated with the performance of duties of a particular role. Nurses accept or reject specific role demands based upon their education, knowledge, competence, and extent of experience. Nurses in administration, education, and research also have obligations to the recipients of nursing care. Although nurses in administration, education, and research have relationships with patients that are less direct, in assuming the responsibilities of a particular role, they share responsibility for the care provided by those whom they supervise and instruct. The nurse must not engage in practices prohibited by law or delegate activities to others that are prohibited by the practice acts of other health care providers.

Individual nurses are responsible for assessing their own competence. When the needs of the patient are beyond the qualifications and competencies of the nurse, consultation and collaboration must be sought from qualified nurses, other health professionals, or other appropriate sources. Educational resources should be sought by nurses and provided by institutions to maintain and advance the competence of nurses. Nurse educators act in collaboration with their students to assess the learning needs of the student, the effectiveness of the teaching program, the identification and utilization of appropriate resources, and the support needed for the learning process.

Perioperative explications
Responsibility refers to carrying out the duties associated with perioperative nursing. Perioperative nurse obligations are reflected in AORN's *Standards, Recommended Practices, and Guidelines*. The acceptance of responsibility for care is determined by an individual's educational preparation, professional competency, and

Code of Ethics for Nurses with Interpretive Statements reprinted with permission from American Nurses Association, © 2001 Nursesbooks.org, Silver Spring, MD.

EXHIBIT B: PERIOPERATIVE EXPLICATIONS

work experience. Nurses in administration, education, and research also are responsible for care through the people they supervise.

Each perioperative nurse is responsible for maintaining competency of professional knowledge and technical skills. It is the nurse's responsibility to assess when care required is beyond an individual's knowledge and to report it to the appropriate support person.

Perioperative examples

- Consults other health care providers for assistance when necessary.
- Identifies and develops a plan of corrective action related to deficits and limitations in knowledge.
- Assumes responsibility for continuous education through personal study; attendance at institutional inservice programs, staff orientation workshops, seminars, AORN chapter and other professional meetings; and reading the *AORN Journal* and other perioperative professional journals.
- Remains current on new procedures affecting practice.
- Uses the AORN competency statements in perioperative practice.
- Provides unit-based orientation.
- Provides competency-based orientation.
- Practices adult learning theory.
- Demonstrates competency in the use of new technologies.
- Engages in continued professional learning.

4.4 Delegation of nursing activities

Since the nurse is accountable for the quality of nursing care given to patients, nurses are accountable for the assignment of nursing responsibilities to other nurses and the delegation of nursing care activities to other health care workers. While delegation and assignment are used here in a generic moral sense, it is understood that individual states may have a particular legal definition of these terms.

The nurse must make reasonable efforts to assess individual competency when assigning selected components of nursing care to other health care workers. This assessment involves evaluating the knowledge, skills, and experience of the individual to whom the care is assigned, the complexity of the assigned tasks, and the health status of the patient. The nurse is also responsible for monitoring the activities of these individuals and evaluating the quality of the care provided. Nurses may not delegate responsibilities such as assessment and evaluation; they may delegate tasks. The nurse must not knowingly assign or delegate to any member of the nursing team a task for which that person is not prepared or qualified. Employer policies or directives do not relieve the nurse of responsibility for making judgments about the delegation and assignment of nursing care tasks.

Nurses functioning in management or administrative roles have a particular responsibility to provide an environment that supports and facilitates appropriate assignment and delegation. This includes providing appropriate orientation to staff, assisting less experienced nurses in developing necessary skills and competencies, and establishing policies and procedures that protect both the patient and nurse from the inappropriate assignment or delegation of nursing responsibilities, activities, or tasks.

Nurses functioning in educator or preceptor roles may have less direct relationship with patients. However, through assignment of nursing care activities to learners, they share responsibility and accountability for the care provided. It is imperative that the knowledge and skills of the learner be sufficient to provide the assigned nursing care and that appropriate supervision be provided to protect both the patient and the learner.

Perioperative explications

Perioperative nurses are accountable for patient outcomes resulting from nursing care rendered to patients during the perioperative experience. Perioperative nurses are accountable for the assignment of nursing responsibilities to other nurses and for the delegation of nursing care activities to other health care workers. The nurse retains accountability for patient outcomes resulting from delegated nursing tasks. Only the perioperative registered nurse plans and directs the nursing care of every patient undergoing operative and other invasive procedures. The core activities of perioperative nursing are assessment, diagnosis, outcome identification, planning, implementation, and evaluation. The perioperative nurse may delegate certain nursing care tasks, but the nursing activities that cannot be delegated are assessment diagnosis, outcome identification, planning, and evaluation.[21]

The nurse must be aware of specific state legal definitions and guidelines regarding delegation and assignment. The perioperative nurse follows facility policies or directives in delegating functions, but these do not relieve the nurse of accountability for making judgments about the competency of personnel and the appropriateness of delegated activities. Before delegation of patient care tasks, the perioperative nurse uses professional clinical judgment to decide to whom and under what circumstances to delegate appropriate patient care activities.[22] Prior to delegation, consideration also should be given to the patient's condition, the complexity of the procedure, the predictability of the outcome, the level of preparation and competence of the person accepting the delegation, and the amount of supervision needed.[23]

The perioperative work environment supports orientation to less experienced staff. It also provides policies to prevent nurses from accepting inappropriate assignments. This is to protect both the patient and the nurse.

Code of Ethics for Nurses with Interpretive Statements reprinted with permission from American Nurses Association, © 2001 Nursesbooks.org, Silver Spring, MD.

EXHIBIT B: PERIOPERATIVE EXPLICATIONS

Perioperative examples
- Knows state regulations and definitions regarding delegation and assignment.
- Knows organizational guidelines regarding assignment and delegation.
- Delegates nursing functions to nurses.
- Allows assistive personnel to assist with delegated nursing tasks only when competency has been established and when allowed by state scope of practice.
- Bases delegation and assignments on individual competency, patient acuity, complexity of the procedure, predictability of outcomes, amount of supervision required, staffing pattern, and staff availability.[24]
- Follows institutional policies for modifying patient care assignments that the nurse or other health care provider does not feel competent in performing.
- Participates in perioperative competency-based orientation.
- Perioperative nurses define and supervise the training of unlicensed assistive personnel to perform the delegated nursing care tasks.

5: The nurse owes the same duties to self as to others, including the responsibility to preserve integrity and safety, to maintain competency, and to continue personal and professional growth.

5.1 Moral self-respect

Moral respect accords moral worth and dignity to all human beings irrespective of their personal attributes or life situation. Such respect extends to oneself as well; the same duties that we owe to others we owe to ourselves. Self-regarding duties refer to a realm of duties that primarily concern oneself and include professional growth and maintenance of competence, preservation of wholeness of character, and personal integrity.

Perioperative explications

Perioperative nurses deliver care in a manner that is respectful not only to patients but also to themselves and their colleagues. Nurses identify areas for personal and professional development and assist others in their development. Nurses participate actively in community education about surgery, invasive procedures, and perioperative nursing, and they correct misinformation and misunderstanding about perioperative patient care.

Perioperative examples
- Promotes a positive image of nursing in the media and the community.
- Promotes professional autonomy and self-regulation of practice.
- Uses nursing titles according to demonstrated professional achievement (eg, CNOR®, CRNFA®).
- Corrects inaccurate portrayals of and misinformation about the profession.
- Promotes an environment that does not tolerate harassment and abuse.
- Provides an environment that optimizes the occupational health and safety of all employees.
- Promotes empowerment and team building.
- Supports the nurse's role as a patient advocate.

5.2 Professional growth and maintenance of competency

Though it has consequences for others, maintenance of competency and ongoing professional growth involves the control of one's own conduct in a way that is primarily self-regarding. Competency affects one's self-respect, self-esteem, professional status, and the meaningfulness of work. In all nursing roles, evaluation of one's own performance, coupled with peer review, is a means by which nursing practice can be held to the highest standards. Each nurse is responsible for participating in the development of criteria for evaluation of practice for using those criteria in peer and self-assessment.

Continual professional growth, particularly in knowledge and skill, requires a commitment to lifelong learning. Such learning includes, but is not limited to, continuing education, networking with professional colleagues, self-study, professional reading, certification, and seeking advanced degrees. Nurses are required to have knowledge relevant to the current scope and standards of nursing practice, changing issues, concerns, controversies, and ethics. Where the care required is outside the competencies of the individual nurse, consultation should be sought or the patient should be referred to others for appropriate care.

Perioperative explications

The perioperative nurse is accountable to society and the profession for appropriate, effective, and efficient nursing practice. Mechanisms are established to demonstrate professional accountability and responsibility for maintaining clinical competency. Knowledge and skill related to technological advances and surgical interventions should be incorporated into the perioperative nurse's practice. The perioperative nurse maintains responsibility for his or her own continuing education.

Perioperative examples
- Incorporates AORN's competency statements in perioperative nursing education.
- Remains current on new procedures related to perioperative clinical practice.
- Participates in certification processes (eg, CNOR, CRNFA, advanced cardiac life support).

Code of Ethics for Nurses with Interpretive Statements *reprinted with permission from American Nurses Association,* © 2001 Nursesbooks.org, Silver Spring, MD.

- Acquires new knowledge from continuous education through personal study; attendance at institutional inservice programs, staff orientation workshops, seminars, AORN Congress, AORN chapter and other professional meetings; and reading the *AORN Journal, Surgical Services Management*, and other perioperative and professional literature.
- Supports competency-based orientation and annual review process.
- Demonstrates competency in the use of new technologies.
- Participates in self-evaluation and peer evaluation of clinical competency, decision-making skills, and professional judgment.
- Seeks consultation as necessary to provide patient care.
- Confirms clinical privileges of all caregivers.
- Promotes individual accountability for maintaining competency.
- Promotes patient safety and other forms of patient advocacy initiatives recommended by professional organizations, legislation, and regulations.

5.3 Wholeness of character

Nurses have both personal and professional identities that are neither entirely separate, nor entirely merged, but are integrated. In the process of becoming a professional, the nurse embraces the values of the profession, integrating them with personal values. Duties to self involve an authentic expression of one's own moral point of view in practice. Sound ethical decision-making requires the respectful and open exchange of views between and among all individuals with relevant interests. In a community of moral discourse, no one person's view should automatically take precedence over that of another. Thus, the nurse has a responsibility to express moral perspectives, even when they differ from those of others, and even when they might not prevail.

This wholeness of character encompasses relationships with patients. In situations where the patient requests a personal opinion from the nurse, the nurse is generally free to express an informed personal opinion as long as this preserves the voluntariness of the patient and maintains appropriate professional and moral boundaries. It is essential to be aware of the potential for undue influence attached to the nurse's professional role. Assisting patients to clarify their own values in reaching informed decisions may be helpful in avoiding unintended persuasion. In situations where nurses' responsibilities include care for those whose personal attributes, condition, lifestyle, or situation is stigmatized by the community and are personally unacceptable, the nurse still renders respectful and skilled care.

Perioperative explications
The perioperative nurse must be genuine, open, and honest in interactions with patients and other health care providers. Nurses are aware of their powerful influence and offer their opinions based on scientific principles, evidence-based practices, and clinical experiences.

Perioperative examples
- Assists patients in formulating decisions affecting care as appropriate.
- Facilitates patient participation in perioperative plan of care.
- Integrates personal philosophy of nursing into the practice setting.
- Helps peers to be assertive and emotionally healthy.
- Respects views of others, but clarifies misinformation.
- Applies standards of nursing practice consistently to all patients regardless of disability, economic status, culture, religion, race, age, lifestyle choices, or sexuality.
- Plans for an appropriate substitute care provider if personal beliefs conflict with required care.

5.4 Preservation of integrity

Integrity is an aspect of wholeness of character and is primarily a self-concern of the individual nurse. An economically constrained health care environment presents the nurse with particularly troubling threats to integrity. Threats to integrity may include a request to deceive a patient, to withhold information, or to falsify records, as well as verbal abuse from patients or coworkers. Threats to integrity also may include an expectation that the nurse will act in a way that is inconsistent with the values or ethics of the profession, or more specifically a request that is in direct violation of the *Code of Ethics*. Nurses have a duty to remain consistent with both their personal and professional values and to accept compromise only to the degree that it remains an integrity-preserving compromise. An integrity-preserving compromise does not jeopardize the dignity or well-being of the nurse or others. Integrity-preserving compromise can be difficult to achieve, but is more likely to be accomplished in situations where there is an open forum for moral discourse and an atmosphere of mutual respect and regard.

Perioperative explications
The perioperative registered nurse does not compromise professional or personal integrity. Additionally, the perioperative nurse knows that the use of the title *Registered Nurse (RN)*, as granted by state licensure, carries with it the responsibility to act in the public interest. The title *RN* and all other symbols of academic degrees or other earned or honorary professional

Code of Ethics for Nurses with Interpretive Statements *reprinted with permission from American Nurses Association,* © 2001 Nursesbooks.org, Silver Spring, MD.

EXHIBIT B: PERIOPERATIVE EXPLICATIONS

symbols of recognition may be used in all ways that are legal and appropriate

The pressure to reduce costs, especially in surgical services, reflects the current emphasis on financial well-being. Perioperative nurses can be financially prudent and at the same time discharge their clinical, educational, and administrative duties in a manner that is consistent with ethical principles.

When the perioperative nurse is ethically and morally opposed to interventions or procedures in a particular case, the nurse is justified in refusing to participate if the refusal is made known in advance and in time for other appropriate arrangements to be made for the patient's nursing care. When the patient's life is in jeopardy, the perioperative nurse is obliged to provide for the patient's safety, to avoid abandonment, and to withdraw only when assured that alternative sources of nursing care are available to the patient.

Perioperative examples

- Facilitates a working environment conducive to learning, teaching, and education.
- Makes purchasing decisions equitably and justly to provide cost-effective, quality care.
- Uses and maintains supplies and equipment according to manufacturers' instructions.
- Resterilizes and reprocesses instruments and supplies in a manner consistent with standards and regulations.
- Accepts responsibility and accountability for perioperative nursing practices.
- Is aware of limitations and accepts assignments only when competent to function safely.
- Uses nursing titles (eg, CNOR, CRNFA) according to demonstrated professional achievement.
- Participates in risk management efforts and quality process improvement.
- Plans for an appropriate substitute care provider if personal beliefs conflict with required care.

6: The nurse participates in establishing, maintaining, and improving health care environments and conditions of employment conducive to the provision of quality health care and consistent with the values of the profession through individual and collective action.

6.1 Influence of the environment on moral virtues and values

Virtues are habits of character that predispose persons to meet their moral obligations; that is, to do what is right. Excellences are habits of character that predispose a person to do a particular job or task well. Virtues such as wisdom, honesty, and courage are habits or attributes of the morally good person. Excellences such as compassion, patience, and skill are habits of character of the morally good nurse. For the nurse, virtues and excellences are those habits that affirm and promote the values of human dignity, well-being, respect, health, independence, and other values central to nursing. Both virtue and excellence, as aspects of moral character, can be either nurtured by the environment in which the nurse practices or they can be diminished or thwarted. All nurses have a responsibility to create, maintain, and contribute to environments that support the growth of virtues and excellences and enable nurses to fulfill their ethical obligations.

Perioperative explications

The perioperative nurse is responsible for developing a caring environment that promotes the well-being of patients. This is accomplished by doing what is right and doing it well. The nurse provides a compassionate and therapeutic environment by promoting comfort and preventing unnecessary suffering. The working environment necessary to accomplish these goals supports the growth of virtues and excellences.

Perioperative examples

- Interacts with patients in a compassionate manner.
- Demonstrates empathy, sensitivity, and patience in difficult or stressful situations.
- Uses therapeutic communication.
- Assists families with challenging issues.
- Develops relationships with patients that support mutual involvement in planning care.
- Helps to answer patients' questions related to their care.
- Listens attentively and, when appropriate, refers the patient to other resources.

6.2 Influence of the environment on ethical obligations

All nurses, regardless of role, have a responsibility to create, maintain, and contribute to environments of practice that support nurses in fulfilling their ethical obligations. Environments of practice include observable features, such as working conditions, and written policies and procedures setting out expectations for nurses, as well as less tangible characteristics such as informal peer norms. Organizational structures, role descriptions, health and safety initiatives, grievance mechanisms, ethics committees, compensation systems, and disciplinary procedures all contribute to environments that can either present barriers or foster ethical practice and professional fulfillment. Environments in which employees are provided fair hearing of grievances, are supported in practicing according to standards of care, and are justly treated allow for the realization of the values of the profession and are consistent with sound nursing practice.

Perioperative explications

Perioperative nurses create, maintain, and contribute to a work environment that supports individuals in their nursing practice. This environment is safe and has policies, procedures, guidelines, and standards for

Code of Ethics for Nurses with Interpretive Statements *reprinted with permission from American Nurses Association,* © 2001 Nursesbooks.org, Silver Spring, MD.

EXHIBIT B: PERIOPERATIVE EXPLICATIONS

practice. The nurse is knowledgeable about the various processes and committees to support and promote a professional working environment.

Perioperative examples
- Follows process for addressing unsafe practice.
- Follows process for addressing ethical issues.
- Participates in developing policies, procedures, and standards.
- Maintains knowledge of policies and procedures.
- Promotes a positive work environment.
- Facilitates a working atmosphere conducive to education.

6.3 Responsibility for the health care environment

The nurse is responsible for contributing to a moral environment that encourages respectful interactions with colleagues, support of peers, and identification of issues that need to be addressed. Nurse administrators have a particular responsibility to assure that employees are treated fairly and that nurses are involved in decisions related to their practice and working conditions. Acquiescing and accepting unsafe or inappropriate practices, even if the individual does not participate in the specific practice, is equivalent to condoning unsafe practice. Nurses should not remain employed in facilities that routinely violate patient rights or require nurses to severely and repeatedly compromise standards of practice or personal morality.

Perioperative explications

The perioperative nurse treats colleagues and peers respectfully and fairly. The nurse, in all roles, participates in decisions that will affect practice and working conditions. The perioperative nurse identifies and supports conditions of employment that promote practice in accordance with AORN standards and recommended practices. This environment also meets accrediting and other regulatory standards. As a moral agent, if the work environment does not routinely support high quality patient care and safe practice, the nurse should seek employment elsewhere.

Perioperative nurses may need to address concerns about the work environment through appropriate channels. Perioperative nurses may need to participate in collective activities (eg, collective bargaining, workplace advocacy) to address concerns about patient care, work environment, or just compensation. These activities should be consistent with AORN standards and recommended practices, accrediting standards, state nurse practice acts, and the ANA *Code of Ethics for Nurses*. In this process, the interests of both nurses and patients must be kept in balance.

Perioperative examples
- Knows chain of command.
- Promotes environment that does not tolerate harassment and abuse.
- Facilitates work environment conducive to learning.
- Collaborates with all health care team members.
- Questions unfair employee practices.
- Identifies and reports unsafe patient practices.
- Participates in strategic planning and development of departmental and institutional goals.
- Promotes empowerment.
- Belongs to state nursing organization.
- Maintains membership in AORN.

7: The nurse participates in the advancement of the profession through contributions to practice, education, administration, and knowledge development.

7.1 Advancing the profession through active involvement in nursing and in health care policy

Nurses should advance their profession by contributing in some way to the leadership, activities, and the viability of their professional organizations. Nurses can also advance the profession by serving in leadership or mentorship roles or on committees within their places of employment. Nurses who are self-employed can advance the profession by serving as role models for professional integrity. Nurses can also advance the profession through participation in civic activities related to health care or through local, state, national, or international initiatives. Nurse educators have a specific responsibility to enhance students' commitment to professional and civic values. Nurse administrators have a responsibility to foster an employment environment that facilitates nurses' ethical integrity and professionalism, and nurse researchers are responsible for active contribution to the body of knowledge supporting and advancing nursing practice.

Perioperative explications

The perioperative nurse has a personal responsibility to contribute to the advancement of the profession by participating in professional organizations. There are various activities within employment agencies and local, state, and national organizations by which one can contribute to the profession. Perioperative educators and managers are additionally responsible for providing an environment conducive to advancing the profession. Nurses can contribute to the advancement of the profession and health care policy by participating in civic activities.

Perioperative examples
- Maintains membership in AORN.
- Serves as a committee member at place of employment.
- Actively participates in AORN local and national initiatives.

Code of Ethics for Nurses with Interpretive Statements *reprinted with permission from American Nurses Association,* © 2001 nursesbooks.org, Silver Spring, MD.

EXHIBIT B: PERIOPERATIVE EXPLICATIONS

- Volunteers at schools of nursing (eg, teaching, mentoring).
- Actively seeks the opportunity to be involved in activities related to patient care at place of employment (eg, patient care, product selection, safety initiatives, strategic planning, risk management, infection control, ethics committees).
- Supports perioperative preceptor programs.
- Serves as a leader or mentor on committees.
- Maintains awareness of changing health care policy at the local, state, and national levels.
- Participates in defining and revising scope of practice acts.
- Consults and collaborates with individuals who shape health care policy.

7.2 Advancing the profession by developing, maintaining, and implementing professional standards in clinical, administrative, and educational practice

Standards and guidelines reflect the practice of nursing grounded in ethical commitments and a body of knowledge. Professional standards and guidelines for nurses must be developed by nurses and reflect nursing's responsibility to society. It is the responsibility of nurses to identify their own scope of practice as permitted by professional practice standards and guidelines, by state and federal laws, by relevant societal values, and by the *Code of Ethics*.

The nurse as administrator or manager must establish, maintain, and promote conditions of employment that enable nurses within that organization or community setting to practice in accord with accepted standards of nursing practice and provide a nursing and health care work environment that meets the standards and guidelines of nursing practice. Professional autonomy and self-regulation in the control of conditions of practice are necessary for implementing nursing standards and guidelines and assuring quality care for those whom nursing serves.

The nurse educator is responsible for promoting and maintaining optimum standards of both nursing education and of nursing practice in any settings where planned learning activities occur. Nurse educators must also ensure that only those students who possess the knowledge, skills, and competencies that are essential to nursing graduate from their nursing programs.

Perioperative explications

Perioperative nurses are responsible for monitoring standards of practice pertinent to their role(s) and for fostering optimal standards of practice at the local, regional, state, and national levels of the health care system: "The perioperative nurse systematically evaluates the quality and appropriateness of nursing practice."[25] Perioperative educators and managers are equally responsible to provide an environment conducive to implementing and improving standards and recommended practices.

Perioperative examples

- Uses standards in nursing practice.
- Contributes to the work of AORN committees and projects to develop standards.
- Reviews and critiques practice standards (eg, responds to proposed AORN recommended practices).
- Participates in development and revision of standards of practice.
- Participates in quality and process improvement processes.
- Participates in multidisciplinary review of patient outcomes.
- Follows investigational device protocol and regulations.

7.3 Advancing the profession through knowledge development, dissemination, and application to practice

The nursing profession should engage in scholarly inquiry to identify, evaluate, refine, and expand the body of knowledge that forms the foundation of its discipline and practice. In addition, nursing knowledge is derived from the sciences and from the humanities. Ongoing scholarly activities are essential to fulfilling a profession's obligations to society. All nurses working alone or in collaboration with others can participate in the advancement of the profession through the development, evaluation, dissemination, and application of knowledge in practice. However, an organizational climate and infrastructure conducive to scholarly inquiry must be valued and implemented for this to occur.

Perioperative explications

The perioperative nurse has an obligation to the patient and to society to engage in activities that promote scholarly inquiry to identify, verify, and expand the body of perioperative nursing knowledge. Perioperative nursing roles include investigation to further knowledge, participation in research, and application of theoretical and empirical knowledge. Perioperative nurses can support the research process as content experts, data collectors, research subjects, or researchers.

Perioperative examples

- Uses research findings to support and improve clinical practice.
- Fosters an environment of intellectual curiosity.
- Identifies problems amenable to the research process (eg, questions outmoded practices).
- Disseminates research findings to colleagues.

Code of Ethics for Nurses with Interpretive Statements reprinted with permission from American Nurses Association, © 2001 Nursesbooks.org, Silver Spring, MD.

EXHIBIT B: PERIOPERATIVE EXPLICATIONS

8: The nurse collaborates with other health professionals and the public in promoting community, national, and international efforts to meet health needs.

8.1 Health needs and concerns

The nursing profession is committed to promoting the health, welfare, and safety of all people. The nurse has a responsibility to be aware not only of specific health needs of individual patients but also of broader health concerns such as world hunger, environmental pollution, lack of access to health care, violation of human rights, and inequitable distribution of nursing and health care resources. The availability and accessibility of high quality health services to all people require both interdisciplinary planning and collaborative partnerships among health professionals and others at the community, national, and international levels.

Perioperative explications

Availability of health care involves not only addressing specific health needs, but also factors that affect well-being. These factors include world hunger, environmental pollution, lack of access to care, violation of human rights, and rationing of health care. The perioperative nurse recognizes the interdependence and collaboration of all health care workers to provide quality health care to everyone.

Perioperative examples

- Collaborates with members of other professional organizations at international, national, and state levels (eg, joint education offerings, joint patient safety legislative efforts).
- Communicates with elected officials about health care needs.
- Educates elected officials about health care needs.
- Donates to health care-related charities.
- Participates in international nursing societies.

8.2 Responsibilities to the public

Nurses, individually and collectively, have a responsibility to be knowledgeable about the health status of the community and existing threats to health and safety. Through support of and participation in community organizations and groups, the nurse assists in efforts to educate the public, facilitates informed choice, identifies conditions and circumstances that contribute to illness, injury, and disease, fosters healthy lifestyles, and participates in institutional and legislative efforts to promote health and meet national health objectives. In addition, the nurse supports initiatives to address barriers to health, such as poverty, homelessness, unsafe living conditions, abuse and violence, and lack of access to health services.

The nurse also recognizes that health care is provided to culturally diverse populations in this country and in all parts of the world. In providing care, the nurse should avoid imposition of the nurse's own cultural values upon others. The nurse should affirm human dignity and show respect for the values and practices associated with different cultures and use approaches to care that reflect awareness and sensitivity.

Perioperative explications

The perioperative nurse is knowledgeable about the health status of the community and factors that threaten well-being and safety. The nurse participates in educating the public about the various factors influencing health care. The perioperative nurse recognizes cultural differences of various populations and does not allow his or her own beliefs and values to influence the care provided to patients of different beliefs and values. Nursing needs to adequately represent cultural diversity to promote the welfare and safety of all patients.

Perioperative examples

- Volunteers to teach wellness classes.
- Educates members of community about perioperative nursing.
- Collaborates with consumer, service, and support organizations related to health care.
- Fosters collaboration with and education of the public on local, state, and national health care issues.
- Prepares for disasters and threat to community.
- Provides explanations and answers to questions in the patient's primary language.
- Incorporates patient requests regarding religious preferences into practice as much as possible.
- Integrates cultural differences into patient care.
- Incorporates requests for alternative therapies into care, as appropriate.

9: The profession of nursing, as represented by associations and their members, is responsible for articulating nursing values, for maintaining the integrity of the profession and its practice, and for shaping social policy.

9.1 Assertion of values

It is the responsibility of a professional association to communicate and affirm the values of the profession to its members. It is essential that the professional organization encourages discourse that supports critical self-reflection and evaluation within the profession. The organization also communicates to the public the values that nursing considers central to social change that will enhance health.

Perioperative explications

AORN's mission is to support perioperative registered nurses in achieving optimal outcomes for patients undergoing operative and other invasive procedures. To further its goals, AORN is committed to excellence in support of its mission and values education, representation, and standards that

Code of Ethics for Nurses with Interpretive Statements *reprinted with permission from American Nurses Association,* © 2001 nursesbooks.org, Silver Spring, MD.

EXHIBIT B: PERIOPERATIVE EXPLICATIONS

are research based, current, timely, comprehensive, applicable, and achievable.[26]

Perioperative examples
- Participates in educational programs to promote lifelong learning.
- Reads professional journals and newsletters.
- Incorporates AORN's *Standards, Recommended Practices, and Guidelines* into practice.
- Uses the *Perioperative Nursing Data Set* (PNDS) to link perioperative nursing care to positive patient outcomes.
- Applies "Patient Safety First" principles to perioperative patient care.
- Provides consultative and other services to support perioperative nursing and patient care.
- Engages in legislative activities to support perioperative nursing and patient care.
- Promotes interaction with regulatory agencies (eg, FDA, CMS) to advance safe, quality patient care.
- Maintains membership in AORN.
- Participates in AORN chapters, state councils, specialty assemblies, and other organizational units to support AORN and perioperative nursing.

9.2 The profession carries out its collective responsibility through professional associations

The nursing profession continues to develop ways to clarify nursing's accountability to society. The contract between the profession and society is made explicit through such mechanisms as (a) the *Code of Ethics for Nurses*, (b) the standards of nursing practice, (c) the ongoing development of nursing knowledge derived from nursing theory, scholarship, and research in order to guide nursing actions, (d) educational requirements for practice, (e) certification, and (f) mechanisms for evaluating the effectiveness of professional nursing actions.

Perioperative explications
AORN's purpose is to unite perioperative registered nurses for the purpose of maintaining an association dedicated to the constant endeavor of promoting the highest professional standards of perioperative nursing practice for optimum patient care. AORN cooperates with other professional associations, health care facilities, universities, industries, technical societies, research organizations, and governmental agencies in matters affecting the goals and purposes of AORN.[27]

Perioperative examples
- Practices perioperative nursing incorporating AORN's *Standards, Recommended Practices, and Guidelines*.
- Participates in nursing research.
- Becomes knowledgeable about the ANA *Code of Ethics for Nurses* and the "AORN explications for perioperative nurses."
- Collaborates with other organizations (eg, American College of Surgeons, American Association of Nurse Anesthetists, American Society of Anesthesiologists) to foster optimal perioperative patient care.
- Collaborates with other nursing organizations (eg, Nursing Organizations Alliance, American Nurses Association) to enhance the nursing profession.
- Identifies partnering opportunities with educational, health care, governmental, payer, business, and professional organizations to promote mutually beneficial patient care initiatives.

9.3 Intraprofessional integrity

A professional association is responsible for expressing the values and ethics of the profession and also for encouraging the professional organization and its members to function in accord with those values and ethics. Thus, one of its fundamental responsibilities is to promote awareness of and adherence to the *Code of Ethics* and to critique the activities and ends of the professional association itself. Values and ethics influence the power structures of the association in guiding, correcting, and directing its activities. Legitimate concerns for the self-interest of the association and the profession are balanced by a commitment to the social goods that are sought. Through critical self-reflection and self-evaluation, associations must foster change within themselves, seeking to move the professional community toward its stated ideals.

Perioperative explications
The ANA *Code of Ethics for Nurses*, together with the "AORN explications for perioperative nursing," expresses the values and ethics of perioperative nursing. Use of the title *RN* carries with it the individual's responsibility to act in public's best interest. The title *RN* and all other academic degrees or other earned or honorary professional symbols of recognition may be used in all ways that are legal and reflect professional achievement.

Perioperative examples
- Promotes a positive image of nursing in the media and the community.
- Promotes professional autonomy and self-regulation of practice.
- Uses nursing titles (eg, CNOR, CRNFA) according to professional achievement.
- Identifies and resolves conflicts of interest effectively.
- Corrects inaccurate portrayals of and misinformation about the profession.

Code of Ethics for Nurses with Interpretive Statements reprinted with permission from American Nurses Association, © 2001 Nursesbooks.org, Silver Spring, MD.

- Incorporates the ANA *Code of Ethics for Nurses* into daily practice.

9.4 Social reform

Nurses can work individually as citizens or collectively through political action to bring about social change. It is the responsibility of a professional nursing association to speak for nurses collectively in shaping and reshaping health care within our nation, specifically in areas of health care policy and legislation that affect accessibility, quality, and the cost of health care. Here, the professional association maintains vigilance and takes action to influence legislators, reimbursement agencies, nursing organizations, and other health professions. In these activities, health is understood as being broader than delivery and reimbursement systems, but extending to health-related sociocultural issues such as violation of human rights, homelessness, hunger, violence, and the stigma of illness.

Perioperative explications

To promote the welfare and safety of all people, nurses need adequate representation to support effective health care delivery. Individual patients and society as a whole benefit from nursing participation in decisions made about health care.

Perioperative examples

- Participates in lobbying efforts affecting health care.
- Supports political candidates that advance health care issues.
- Participates in electoral process at the local, state, and national levels.
- Participates in institutional decision-making.
- Participates in the electoral process.
- Volunteers in community health services.
- Supports political candidates, governmental programs, and legislation agenda for improving patient care.
- Educates members of the community about perioperative nursing (eg, through health fairs, Perioperative Nurse Week activities, educational programs).
- Collaborates with consumer, service, and support organizations (eg, Lions Club, Reach to Recovery, AARP).
- Collaborates with the public, industry, and health care workers regarding environmental and cost-containment issues.
- Fosters collaboration with and education of the public regarding local, state, and national issues (eg, the environment, health care costs).

Conclusion

Perioperative nurses must be familiar with the ethical issues inherent to their practice. To develop familiarity with the issues, one can discuss them with peers and ethics committee members or consult other knowledgeable resources. Nurses may find it beneficial to have a file on ethics available in the department for review. Inservice programs focusing on ethical issues can be implemented for the department by utilizing members of the hospital's nursing ethics and/or medical ethics committees. Other departments and contacts, such as social services, also can be a resource, especially in the area of advance directives. Nurses can use values clarification to identify and understand their moral beliefs and attitudes.

Ethics provides guidelines of action for behavior with others. Such guidelines are both important and necessary when dealing with issues in the context of health care. To effectively deal with ethical situations in practice, nurses must be cognizant of limitations to scope of practice and never jeopardize patient care. Nurses need to realize they have a personal accountability to the care of the patient. As guidelines for practice, nurses can utilize many resources such as the ANA *Code of Ethics for Nurses* and knowledge of patient and individual rights, policies and procedures, standards of care, and community norms. Ultimately, the nurse must provide ethical care for all patients. Utilizing guidelines and recommended practices is a means to an end—safe, competent, and ethical patient care.

REFERENCES

1. S Beyea, ed, *Perioperative Nursing Data Set*, second ed (Denver: AORN, Inc, 2002) 182.
2. *Ibid*.
3. *Ibid*.
4. S Beyea, L Nicoll, "Using ethical analysis when there is no research," *AORN Journal* 69 (June 1999) 1261-1263.
5. S Beyea, ed, *Perioperative Nursing Data Set* (Denver: AORN, Inc, 2000) 150.
6. Beyea, *Perioperative Nursing Data Set*, second ed, 182.
7. *Ibid*, 184.
8. "ANA code for nurses with interpretive statements—Explications for perioperative nursing," in *Standards, Recommended Practices, and Guidelines* (Denver: AORN, Inc, 2002) 54.
9. Beyea, *Perioperative Nursing Data Set*, second ed, 178.
10. *Ibid*, 182.
11. *Ibid*, 183.
12. *Ibid*, 175-176.
13. *Ibid*, 178, 180.
14. *Ibid*, 179, 181.
15. Beyea, *Perioperative Nursing Data Set*, 125.
16. "Recommended practices for traffic patterns," in *Standards, Recommended Practices, and Guidelines* (Denver: AORN, Inc, 2002) 350.
17. Beyea, *Perioperative Nursing Data Set*, second ed, 184.

Code of Ethics for Nurses with Interpretive Statements reprinted with permission from American Nurses Association, © 2001 nursesbooks.org, Silver Spring, MD.

EXHIBIT B: PERIOPERATIVE EXPLICATIONS

18. Beyea, *Perioperative Nursing Data Set*, second ed, 183.

19. A Orb, L Eisenhauer, D Wynaden, "Ethics in qualitative research," *Journal of Nursing Scholarship* 33 (2001) 93-96.

20. *Standards, Recommended Practices, and Guidelines* (Denver: AORN, Inc, 2002) 157-162.

21. "AORN official statement on unlicensed assistive personnel," in *Standards, Recommended Practices, and Guidelines* (Denver: AORN, Inc, 2002) 141.

22. *Ibid.*

23. *Ibid.*

24. *Ibid.*

25. "Standards of perioperative professional performance," in *Standards, Recommended Practices, and Guidelines* (Denver: AORN, Inc, 2002) 160.

26. "AORN vision, mission, philosophy, and values," in *Standards, Recommended Practices, and Guidelines* (Denver: AORN, Inc, 2002) 5.

27. "AORN national bylaws," in *Standards, Recommended Practices, and Guidelines* (Denver: AORN, Inc, 2002) 7.

Publication History

Originally published in the 1994 edition of the AORN *Standards and Recommended Practices*.

Revised; approved by the AORN Board of Directors in November 2002.

This document was previously published as Exhibit C of the "Standards of perioperative nursing" in the 2009 edition of *Perioperative Standards and Recommended Practices*.

Reformatted September 2012 for publication in *Perioperative Standards and Recommended Practices*, 2013 edition.

Code of Ethics for Nurses with Interpretive Statements *reprinted with permission from American Nurses Association, © 2001 Nursesbooks.org, Silver Spring, MD.*

ADDITIONAL RESOURCES

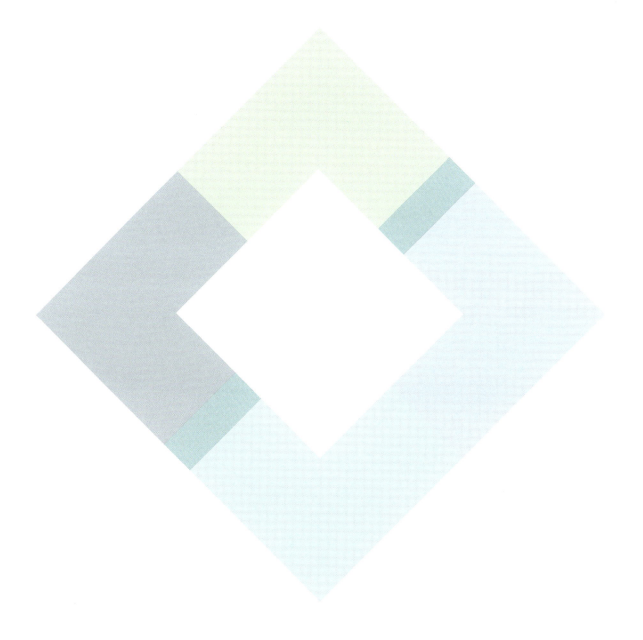

SECTION III

AORN GUIDANCE STATEMENT: SAFE PATIENT HANDLING AND MOVEMENT IN THE PERIOPERATIVE SETTING

Editor's note: Ergonomic Tool #3 and related text in this guidance statement were updated in September 2011 to reflect the revised Ergonomic Tool #3 published in the AORN Journal *(May 2011, Vol 93, No 5, page 591).*

Description of the Problem

Perioperative registered nurses and the perioperative team are routinely faced with a wide array of occupational hazards in the perioperative setting that place them at risk for work-related musculoskeletal disorders.[1-3] Musculoskeletal disorders are injuries or disorders of the muscles, nerves, tendons, joints, cartilage, or spinal discs associated with actions such as overexertion, repetitive motion, and bodily reaction.[4,5] The US Department of Labor does not include injuries caused by slips, trips, falls, motor vehicle accidents, or similar accidents in their definition of musculoskeletal disorders.[4] Musculoskeletal disorders are one of the most frequently occurring and costly types of occupational issues affecting nurses.[2,6,7] More than a third (ie, 36%) of the musculoskeletal injuries that nurses reported requiring time away from work were back injuries.[8] Among the nurses working in the private sector, nearly 9,000 had back injuries.[8,9] One study revealed that 12% of nurses planning to leave the profession indicated that back injuries were either a primary or contributing factor to their decision.[10] While back injuries are one of the most common occupational injuries in the health care industry, injuries of the shoulder and neck were more likely to prevent nurses from performing their work than low back pain.[10-13] The US Department of Health and Human Services report on nursing identified concern for personal safety in the health care environment as the reason given by 18.3% of nurses for leaving the profession.[14]

When the worker's physical ability, task, workplace environment, and workplace culture are not compatible, there is an increased risk of a musculoskeletal disorder.[1,2,15] The connection between physical risk factors and musculoskeletal disorders is greater when exposures are intense and prolonged and when several occupational risk factors are present at the same time.[16] Examples of physical stressors encountered in health care include

- forceful tasks,
- repetitive motion,
- awkward posture,
- static posture,
- moving or lifting patients and equipment,
- carrying heavy instruments and equipment, and
- overexertion.[1-3,11,12,14,17-26]

The perioperative setting poses unique challenges related to the provision of patient care and completion of procedure-related tasks. This highly technical environment is equipment intensive and necessitates the lifting and moving of heavy supplies and equipment during the perioperative team member's work period. Many of the patients having surgical or other invasive procedures are completely or partially dependent on the caregivers due to the effects of general or regional anesthesia or sedation. Patients who are unconscious cannot move, sense discomfort, or feel pain, and they must be protected from injury. This may require the perioperative team to manually lift the patient or the patient's extremities several times during a procedure. The following are among the high-risk tasks specific to perioperative nurses identified that will be addressed in the following discussion of ergonomic tools:

- transferring patients on and off OR beds,[2]
- repositioning patients in the OR bed,[2]
- lifting and holding the patient's extremities,[2]
- standing for long periods of time,[2]
- holding retractors for long periods of time,[2]
- lifting and moving equipment,[2] and
- sustaining awkward positions.

Transferring, lifting, and handling patients has been identified as the most frequent precipitating trigger of back and shoulder problems in nurses.[2,27] Certain patient handling tasks (eg, patient transfers) have been identified as high risk for musculoskeletal injuries to health care workers.[27] Lifting and moving patients is a frequent activity in the perioperative setting; for example, caregivers transfer patients to and from transport carts (eg, stretchers) and the OR bed many times during a typical work shift.

Health care providers often reposition patients once they are on the OR bed to provide appropriate exposure of the surgical site. This high-risk activity requires team members to physically lift and maneuver the patient or a patient's extremity while simultaneously placing a positioning device. The patient's weight may not be evenly distributed; the extremity's mass may be bulky and asymmetric, and it may be difficult to hold the extremity close to the health care provider's body during positioning maneuvers.[28] Additionally, concern for the patient's airway, maintaining his or her body alignment, and supporting the extremities may make it difficult for team members to position themselves in an ergonomically safe position, thus exacerbating physical demands.

SAFE PATIENT HANDLING

Several unique aspects of high-risk patient handling tasks associated with prepping a patient's limb have been identified.[29] Preparing an extremity for surgery generally requires it to be elevated to allow complete circumferential skin preparation. The limb can be suspended by a person holding the limb or by placing the limb in a holding device. In some instances, the limb may be held manually during the entire skin prep while a second person performs the skin prep. The person performing the skin prep may also hold the limb if the limb is small or if only the distal portion needs to be prepped. To maintain asepsis, the person lifting the extremity is forced to hold the limb extended away from his or her body. The size of the limb, length of prep time, posture necessary to hold the extremity, and the physical capability of the person holding the limb all contribute to the ability of the caregiver to safely suspend the limb for the required prep. The following questions should be considered when determining how to safely raise and hold a limb.

- Does the limb need to be raised for the entire surgical skin prep?
- Does the limb need to be lifted by scrubbed or unscrubbed personnel?
- Is the person holding the limb strong enough to perform the task?
- Is there an alternative practice that can be adopted?
- Is there equipment that could be used to support the task?
- Is it possible to hold a heavy limb safely without risk of injury to the nurse or the patient?[29]

Perioperative registered nurses are prone to pain and fatigue from static posture during surgical procedures. The entire perioperative team spends a significant amount of time on their feet during the course of a shift; however, sterile perioperative team members may be required to stand for much longer periods of time. The sterile team members must maintain the integrity of the sterile field, which precludes them from changing levels. They should not alternate between sitting in a chair that is lower than the sterile field and a standing position. Acute and chronic back, leg, and foot pain are frequent complaints resulting from standing in one place for long periods of time. The following factors should be considered during surgical or other invasive procedures. Are the sterile members of the team

- at the appropriate height for the level of the OR bed?
- adopting awkward positions to work effectively?
- positioned in close proximity to the patient to perform required tasks?
- stretching and relaxing muscles regularly?[29]

Perioperative nurses and other perioperative personnel are frequently required to push or pull heavy equipment (eg, OR beds, portable microscopes, video carts). This equipment is very expensive and often must be shared between several individual operating rooms. Unoccupied OR beds are very heavy and difficult to

Task Force Members

Andrea Baptiste, MA (OT), CIE
Ergonomist/Biomechanist
Patient Safety Center of Inquiry
James A. Haley Veterans' Hospital
Tampa, Fla

Edward Hernandez, RN, BSN
OR Nurse Manager
James A. Haley Veterans' Hospital
Tampa, Fla

Nancy Hughes, RN, MHA
Director, Center for Occupational and Environmental Health
American Nurses Association
Silver Spring, Md

Valerie Kelleher
Information Specialist
Patient Safety Center of Inquiry
James A. Haley Veterans' Hospital
Tampa, Fla

John D. Lloyd, PhD, MErgS, CPE
Director, Research Laboratories
Patient Safety Center of Inquiry
James A. Haley Veterans' Hospital
Tampa, Fla

Mary W. Matz, MSPH
VHA Patient Care Ergonomics Consultant and Industrial Hygienist
Patient Safety Center of Inquiry
James A. Haley Veterans' Hospital
Tampa, Fla

Karen Moser, RN, BSN, CNOR
Educator
William S. Middleton VA Hospital
Madison, Wis

Audrey Nelson, PhD, RN, FAAN
Director, Patient Safety Center of Inquiry
James A. Haley Veterans' Hospital
Tampa, Fla

Carol Petersen, RN, BSN, MAOM, CNOR
Perioperative Nursing Specialist
AORN, Inc
Denver, Colo

Lori Plante-Mallon, RN, CNOR
Perioperative RN
Strong Memorial Hospital
University of Rochester Medical Center
Rochester, NY

Kristy Robinson, RN, BSN, CNOR
Perioperative RN
Tampa General Hospital
Tampa, Fla

Manon Short, RPT, CEAS
Injury Prevention Coordinator
Tampa General Hospital
Tampa, Fla

Patrice Spera, RN, MS, CNOR, CRNFA
Director of Clinical Services
Tampa Bay Specialty Surgical Center
Pinellas Park, Fla

Deborah G. Spratt, RN, MPA, CNAA, CNOR
Clinical Specialist
University of Rochester Medical Center
Rochester, NY

Thomas R. Waters, PhD, CPE
Leader of the Human Factors Ergonomics Research Team
National Institute for Occupational Safety and Health
Cincinnati, Ohio

move. Moving an occupied OR bed is not recommended because the risk of injury increases for both the worker and the patient.

Perioperative personnel and central processing personnel are frequently required to carry sets of surgical instruments. Instrument set weights vary and may weigh as much as 40 pounds. Instrument trays are wrapped with impervious nonwoven material or contained in a ridged container system. Both packaging methods can present lifting and carrying problems. Wrapped instrument sets that are too heavy may pose an additional problem because they have no handles and are awkward to carry. Rigid container systems often have handles that make carrying easier, but the weight of the container itself adds to the total weight of a full tray. In an effort to keep costs down and conserve storage space, instrument trays may be inappropriately prepared and too heavy to lift or carry safely. Instrument sets that are flash sterilized require staff members to aseptically remove the hot trays from the sterilizer. The weight of these trays and the height of the person removing them from the sterilizer in relation to the height of the sterilizer chamber contribute to the degree of risk to that individual.

The consequences of musculoskeletal disorders are severe. Employees who experience pain and fatigue are less productive and attentive, more prone to make mistakes, more susceptible to further injury, and may be more likely to affect the health and safety of others. Nurses suffering from disabling back injuries or the fear of getting injured have contributed to the number of nurses leaving the profession, thus increasing the nursing shortage. Workplaces with high incidences of musculoskeletal disorders report increases in lost or modified workdays, higher staff member turnover, increased costs, and adverse patient outcomes.[14,29,30]

Description of the Process

The 2005–2006 Workplace Safety Task Force was charged by AORN President Sharon McNamara, RN, MS, CNOR, to prepare a guidance document for ergonomically healthy workplaces. In addition, the task force was charged with forming a collaborative arrangement with the National Institute for Occupational Safety and Health (NIOSH) and the American Nurses Association (ANA) to work together to discuss, design, and advance the agenda of healthy work sites for perioperative professionals, to include ergonomic safety. This document was developed by AORN with the assistance of a panel of experts from the Patient Safety Center of Inquiry, Tampa, Fla; the James A. Haley Veterans Administration Medical Center (VMAC); the NIOSH Division of Applied Research and Technology Human Factors and Ergonomics Research Team; and ANA.

Members of the task force examined current research, literature, and patient care practices to evaluate and make recommendations to promote patient and caregiver safety when performing activities in a perioperative setting. While there are several high-risk tasks specific to perioperative nurses, the task force identified seven key activities as the starting point for developing recommendations. Some of these recommendations are based upon current technology that can be immediately implemented. Others, such as use of ceiling lifts in operating rooms, are in development or are projected patient handling innovations. This group will continue to examine what is available and encourage manufacturers to develop new and innovative technologies to achieve the optimal safety of the patient and the care giver. Development of this equipment is critical for successful implementation of these ergonomic tools.

The ergonomic tools developed for this guidance document are based on previous work by Audrey Nelson, PhD, RN, FAAN; experts within the Veterans Administration (VA); and nationally recognized researchers.[28] The ergonomic tools for safe patient handling and movement have been designed with the goal of eradicating job-related musculoskeletal disorders in perioperative nurses. The ergonomic tools and algorithms were developed based on professional consensus and evidence from research. Plans are underway for pilot tests in several facilities.

Ergonomic Tool #1: Lateral Transfer From Stretcher To and From the OR Bed

Transferring a patient to and from the OR bed is one of the first actions of the perioperative team. The AORN "Recommended practices for positioning the patient in the perioperative practice setting" recommends that the

---

*Calculation of Design Goal

To accommodate the design goal of 75% of the US adult female working population, **maximum load for a one-handed lift** is calculated to be 11.1 lb (5.0 kg), assuming a worst-case scenario where the patient load may be handled at full arm's length. This is determined by calculating the strength capabilities for the 25th percentile US adult female maximum shoulder flexion moment (25th percentile strength = 31.2 Nm, based on mean of 40 Nm and standard deviation of 13 Nm, therefore 25th percentile = 31.2 Nm)[35] and the 75th percentile US adult female shoulder to grip length (75th percentile length = 630 mm, based on mean of 610 mm and standard deviation of 30 mm).[36] Therefore, maximum one-handed lift is calculated as 31.2 Nm divided by 0.63 m, which equals 49.5 N, or 11.1 lb.

Maximum load (for one person) for a two-handed lift (22.2 lb/10.1 kg) is calculated as twice that of a one-handed lift. According to Rohmert, muscle strength capabilities diminish as a function of time.[37] Therefore, maximum loads for two-handed holding of body parts are presented for one-, two-, and three-minute durations. After one minute, muscle endurance has decreased by 48%; by 65% after two minutes; and after three minutes of continuous holding, strength capability is only 29% of initial lifting strength.

SAFE PATIENT HANDLING

Ergonomic Tool #1. Lateral Transfer from Stretcher to and from the OR Bed

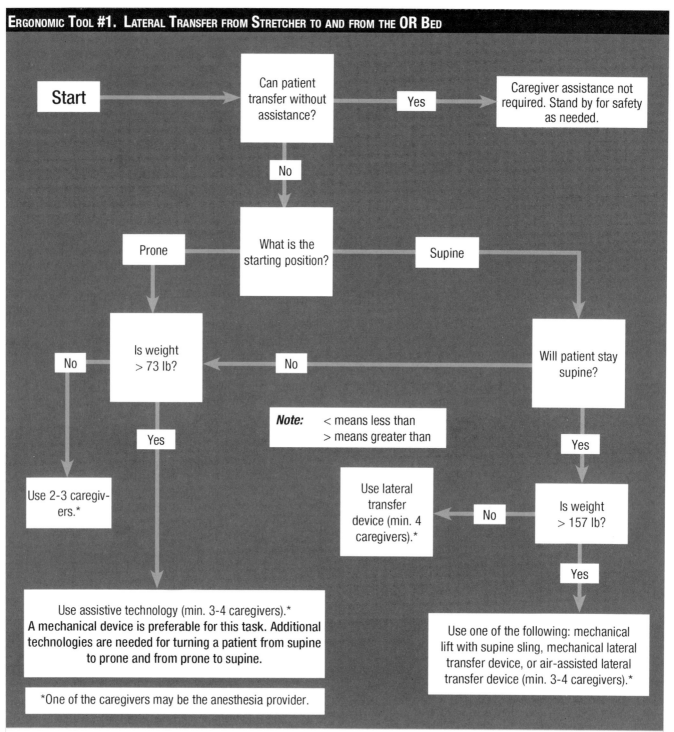

- The number of personnel to safely transfer the patient should be adequate to maintain the patient's body alignment, support extremities, and maintain patient's airway.
- For lateral transfers, it is important to use a lateral transfer device that extends the length of the patient.
- Current technologies for supine-to-prone include the Jackson frame and the spine table.
- Destination surface should be slightly lower for all lateral patient moves.
- A separate algorithm for prone-to-jackknife is not included because this is assumed to be a function of the table.
- If the patient's condition will not tolerate a lateral transfer, consider the use of a mechanical lift with a supine sling.
- During any patient transfer task, if any caregiver is required to lift more than 35 lb of a patient's weight, assistive devices should be used for the transfer.
- While some facilities may attempt to perform a lateral transfer simultaneously with positioning the patient in a lateral position (ie, side-lying), this is not recommended until new technology is available.
- The assumption is that the patient will leave the operating room in the supine position.

perioperative registered nurse perform a preoperative assessment for patient-specific positioning needs.[31] Based on that assessment and using Ergonomic Tool #1, the patient will be transferred to and from the OR bed in an ergonomically safe manner.

Supine to Prone Transfer

Assuming that one caregiver or anesthesia care provider supports the patient's head and neck during supine to prone transfers, the patient's remaining body mass equals 91.6% of his or her total body mass.[32] Using the approach for lifting and holding, a maximum two-handed load to achieve 75% US adult female design goal equals 22.2 lb (10.1 kg).* Typically one of the four caregivers moving a patient is the anesthesia care provider who maintains the airway and supports the patient's head. Two caregivers plus the anesthesia care provider can safely transfer a patient weighing up to 48.5 lb (22.0 kg) from supine to prone position. Three caregivers, plus an anesthesia care provider, can safely transfer a patient weighing up to 72.7 lb (33.0 kg). If the patient's weight is greater than 73 lb, it is necessary to use assistive technology and a minimum of three to four caregivers. Although this has been identified as a gap in technology, a mechanical device is preferable for this task and should be developed.

Supine to Supine Transfer

The desirable approach for lateral transfer of a patient involves use of a lateral transfer device (eg, friction-reducing sheets, slider board, and air-assisted transfer device). If only a draw sheet is used without a lateral transfer device, the care provider exerts a pull force up to 72.6% of the patient's weight.[33] Assuming that one caregiver or anesthesia care provider supports the patient's head and neck to maintain the airway during lateral transfers, the remaining mass of the patient's body equals 91.6% of his or her total body mass.[32] Research indicates that for a pulling distance of 6.9 ft (2.1 m) or less, where the pull point (ie, starting point for the hands) is between the caregiver's waist and nipple line, and the task is performed no more frequently than once every 30 minutes, the maximum initial force required equals 57 lb (26 kg) and the maximum sustained force needed equals 35 lb (16 kg).[34] Therefore, each caregiver can safely contribute a pull force required to transfer up to 48 lb (35 lb/0.726 as referenced above). For one caregiver, plus the anesthesia care provider, maximum patient weight equals 52.6 lb (48 lb/0.916 as referenced above). Two caregivers plus the anesthesia care provider can safely transfer a patient up to 104.8 lb ([48 x 2]/0.916 as referenced above). Three caregivers plus the anesthesia care provider can safely transfer a patient up to 157.2 lb ([48 x 3]/0.916 as referenced above). If the patient is > 157 lb, use an appropriate mechanical lifting device—ie, mechanical lift with supine sling, mechanical lateral transfer device, or air-assisted lateral transfer device—and a minimum of three to four caregivers.

Ergonomic Tool #2: Positioning and Repositioning the Patient on the OR Bed Into and From the Supine Position

The AORN "Recommended practices for positioning the patient in the perioperative practice setting" require that "the perioperative nurse should actively participate in monitoring patient body alignment and tissue integrity based on sound physiologic principles." It further states, "an inadequate number of personnel and equipment can result in patient injury."[31] Ergonomic Tool #2 provides evidence-based guidelines to assist the perioperative registered nurse and other team members to position and reposition the patient on the OR bed in a safe manner for the patient and the team.

Moving the Patient Into and Out of a Semi-Fowler Position

The mass of a patient's body from the waist up, including the head, neck, and upper extremities, equals 68.6% of the patient's total body weight.[32] Added to this is the estimated weight of the equipment (20 lb/9.1 kg). To accommodate at least 75% of the US adult female working population, the maximum load for a two-handed lift is 22.2 lb (10.1 kg). This is determined based on 25th percentile US adult female shoulder strength capabilities[35] and 75th percentile US adult female arm length.[36] Therefore, three caregivers together could lift up to 66.6 lb (10.3 kg), which equates to a 68-lb (30.1 kg) patient.‡ Mechanical devices and a minimum of three caregivers are preferable if the patient weighs more than 68 lb. An example of an appropriate mechanical device is the automatic semi-Fowler positioning feature of an electric OR bed. Further research to address gaps in technology is recommended.

Positioning the Patient Into and From the Lateral Position

Positioning or repositioning a patient into or out of a lateral position involves push/pull forces rather than lifting forces. Assuming that one caregiver or anesthesia care provider supports the patient's head and neck during lateral positioning, the patient's remaining body mass equals 91.6% of total body mass.[32] Based on the Liberty Mutual tables (see Table 3 under Ergonomic Tool #7) for a pulling distance of 6.9 ft (2.1 m) or less, with a pull point (ie, starting position of the hands) between the

---

‡Maximum patient weight = (Maximum 2-handed lift (22 lb) x 3 caregivers) − equipment weight (20 lb) = 68 lb
(68 lb)   Percentage of patient weight above the waist (0.686)

SAFE PATIENT HANDLING

ERGONOMIC TOOL #2. POSITIONING/REPOSITIONING THE PATIENT ON THE OR BED INTO AND FROM THE SUPINE POSITION

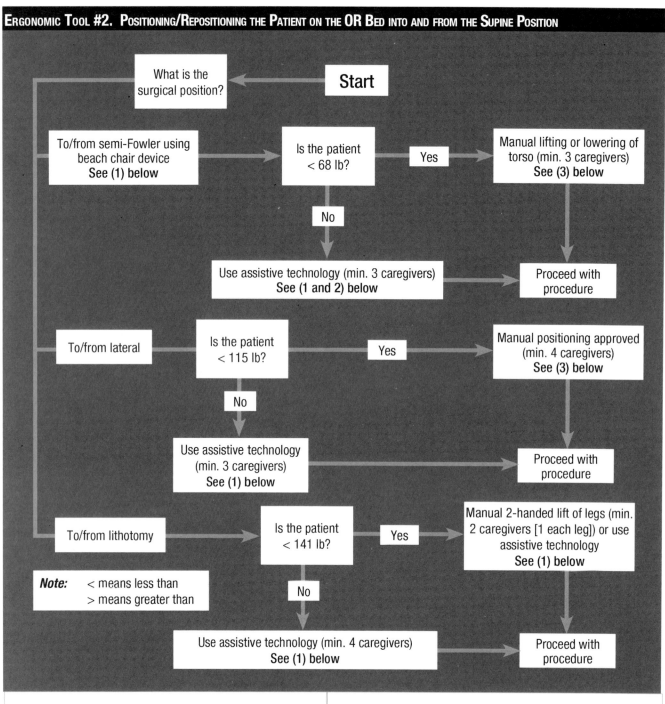

(1) *Mechanical devices are preferable for this task, but their practicality has not yet been tested. There are special slings and straps that can be used with mechanical devices. For example, turning straps can be used to turn a patient to and from lateral or supine, or limb support slings can be used to lift the legs to and from lithotomy. More research is needed.*
(2) *Use the automatic semi-Fowler positioning feature of an electric table if available.*
(3) *One of these caregivers could be the anesthesia provider to hold the head and maintain the airway.*

- During any patient handling task, if any caregiver is required to lift more than 35 lb of a patient's weight, an assistive device should be used.
- The number of personnel to safely position the patient should always be adequate to maintain the patient's body alignment.
- A separate algorithm for prone-to-jackknife is not included because this is assumed to be a function of the table.

ERGONOMIC TOOL #3. LIFTING AND HOLDING LEGS, ARMS, AND HEAD FOR PREPPING

Patient weight lb (kg)	Body part	Body part weight		Lift 1-hand	Lift 2-hand	Hold 2-hand ≤ 1 min	Hold 2-hand ≤ 2 min	Hold 2-hand ≤ 3 min
≤ 40 lb (≤ 18 kg)	Leg	< 6 lb	< 3 kg	□	□	□	□	□
	Arm	< 2 lb	< 1 kg	□	□	□	□	□
	Head	< 3 lb	< 1 kg	□	□	□	□	□
40-90 lb (18-41 kg)	Leg	< 14 lb	< 6 kg	■	□	■	■	■
	Arm	< 5 lb	< 2 kg	□	□	□	□	□
	Head	< 8 lb	< 4 kg	□	□	□	■	■
90-140 lb (41-64 kg)	Leg	< 22 lb	< 10 kg	■	□	■	□	■
	Arm	< 7 lb	< 3 kg	□	□	□	□	■
	Head	< 12 lb	< 6 kg	□	□	■	■	■
140-190 lb (64-86 kg)	Leg	< 30 lb	< 14 kg	■	■	■	■	■
	Arm	< 10 lb	< 4 kg	□	□	□	■	■
	Head	< 16 lb	< 7 kg	■	□	■	■	■
190-240 lb (86-109 kg)	Leg	< 38 lb	< 17 kg	■	■	■	■	■
	Arm	< 12 lb	< 6 kg	■	□	■	■	■
	Head	< 20 lb	< 9 kg	■	■	■	■	■
240-290 lb (109-132 kg)	Leg	< 46 lb	< 21 kg	■	■	■	■	■
	Arm	< 15 lb	< 7 kg	■	■	■	■	■
	Head	< 24 lb	< 11 kg	■	■	■	■	■
290-340 lb (132-155 kg)	Leg	< 53 lb	< 24 kg	■	■	■	■	■
	Arm	< 17 lb	< 8 kg	■	■	■	■	■
	Head	< 29 lb	< 13 kg	■	■	■	■	■
340-390 lb (155-177 kg)	Leg	< 61 lb	< 28 kg	■	■	■	■	■
	Arm	< 20 lb	< 9 kg	■	■	■	■	■
	Head	< 33 lb	< 15 kg	■	■	■	■	■
390-440 lb (177-200 kg)	Leg	< 69 lb	< 31 kg	■	■	■	■	■
	Arm	< 22 lb	< 10 kg	■	■	■	■	■
	Head	< 37 lb	< 17 kg	■	■	■	■	■
> 440 lb (> 200 kg)	Leg	> 69 lb	> 31 kg	■	■	■	■	■
	Arm	> 22 lb	> 10 kg	■	■	■	■	■
	Head	> 37 lb	> 17 kg	■	■	■	■	■

No shading: OK to lift and hold; use clinical judgment and do not hold longer than noted.
Heavy shading: Do not lift alone; use assistive device or more than one caregiver.

caregiver's waist height and nipple line, performed no more frequently than once every 30 minutes, maximum initial force equals 57 lb (26 kg), and maximum sustained force equals 35 lb (16 kg).[34] Therefore, two caregivers, plus an anesthesia care provider maintaining the patient's airway, can safely position a patient weighing up to 76 lb (34.5 kg) (35 lb x 2 care providers/0.916 as referenced above). Three caregivers plus an anesthesia care provider can safely position a patient weighing up to 115 lb (52.2 kg) (35 lb x 3 care providers/0.916 as referenced above). If the patient's weight exceeds 115 lb, lateral positioning devices are needed. Further research is needed to enhance technology to address this task.

Positioning the Patient Into and From the Lithotomy Position

When lifting and holding body parts, the maximum load for a two-handed lift is 22.2 lb (10.1 kg). Each complete lower patient extremity, including thigh, calf, and foot, weighs 15.7% of the patient's total body mass. Therefore, one caregiver can safely perform this task if the patient weighs 141 lb (64.1 kg) or less because each leg is estimated to be less than 22.2 lb.[33]

Caregivers attempting to lift the patient's legs using two hands can each safely lift one leg for patients weighing less than 141 lb. Patients weighing more than 141 lb require assistive technology or four caregivers

SAFE PATIENT HANDLING

ERGONOMIC TOOL #4. PROLONGED STANDING

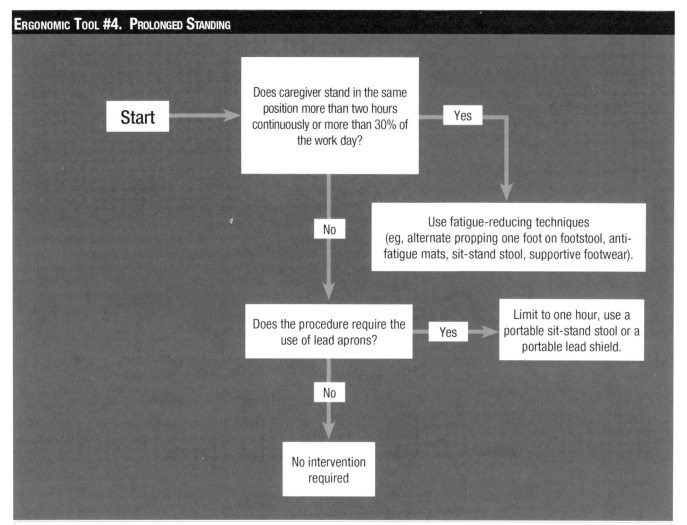

General recommendations
- Caregiver should wear supportive footwear that has the following properties:
  - does not change the shape of the foot;
  - has enough space to move toes;
  - shock-absorbing, cushioned insoles;
  - closed toe; and
  - height of heel in proportion to the shoe.
- Caregivers may benefit from wearing support stockings/socks.
- Anti-fatigue mats should be on the floors.
- Anti-fatigue mats should be placed on standing stools.
- The sit-stand chair should be set to the correct height before setting the sterile field so caregivers will not be changing levels during the procedure.*
- Be aware of infection control issues for nondisposable and anti-fatigue matting.
- Accommodations for pregnancy were considered, but the two-hour limit on prolonged standing covers this condition.
- Scrubbed staff should not work with the neck flexed more than 30 degrees or rotated for more than one minute uninterrupted.
- Two-piece, lightweight lead aprons are recommended.
- During the sit-to-stand break, staff should look straight ahead for a short while.

* "Recommended practices for maintaining a sterile field," in Standards, Recommended Practices, and Guidelines (Denver, Colo: AORN, Inc, 2007) 665-672.

SAFE PATIENT HANDLING

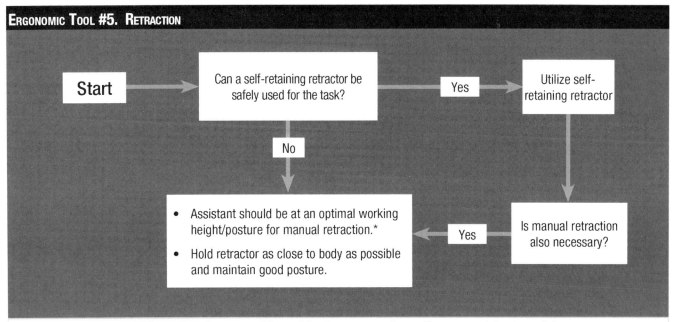

- Arm rests should be utilized as possible and be large enough to allow repositioning of the arms.
- Under optimal working height and posture, an assistive device should be used to lift or hold more than 35 lb.
- Further research is needed to determine time limits for exposure. Since this is a high-risk task, caregivers should take rest breaks or reposition when possible.
- Avoid using the hands as an approach to retraction; it is very high-risk for musculoskeletal or sharps injuries.

* *Optimal working height is defined as area between the chest and the waist height to operative field. Optimal posture is defined as perpendicular/straight-on to the operative field; asymmetrical posture may be acceptable, depending on load and duration; torso twisting should be avoided at all times.*

(ie, two to lift each leg). A mechanical device such as support slings can be used to lift the legs to and from the lithotomy position. Further research is needed to enhance availability of technology to address this task.

Ergonomic Tool #3: Lifting and Holding Legs, Arms, and Head for Prepping in a Perioperative Setting

Introduction
AORN's "Recommended practices for skin preparation of patients" states that "when indicated, the surgical site and surrounding area should be prepared with an antiseptic agent. The prepared area of skin and the drape fenestration should be large enough to accommodate extension of the incision, the need for additional incisions, and all potential drain sites."[38] To accomplish this task, a member of the perioperative team may need to hold the extremity so that the appropriate body part is prepared in the required manner.

Ergonomic Tool #3 shows the calculations for average weight for an adult patient's leg, arm, and head as a function of whole body mass, ranging from slim to morbidly obese body type. Weights are presented both in US (lb) and metric (kg) units. Maximum lift and hold loads were calculated based on 75th percentile shoulder flexion strength and endurance capabilities for US adult females, where the maximum weight for a one-handed lift is 11.1 lb and a two-handed lift, 22.2 lb.

The shaded areas of the table indicate whether it would be acceptable for one caregiver to lift the listed body parts or hold the respective body parts for 0, 1, 2, or 3 minutes with one or two hands. Respecting these limits will minimize risk of muscle fatigue and the potential for musculoskeletal disorders. Perioperative registered nurses must use clinical judgment to assess the need for additional staff member assistance or assistive devices to lift and/or hold one of these body parts for a particular period of time.

Rationale and Calculations for Ergonomic Tool #3
Note: These are guidelines for the average weight of the leg, arm, and head based upon the patient's weight. Nurses should use their clinical judgment to assess the need for additional staff member assistance or assistive devices to lift and/or hold one of these body parts for a particular period of time. The maximum weight for a one-handed lift is 11.1 lb and for a two-handed lift, 22.2 lb.

SAFE PATIENT HANDLING

Ergonomic Tool #6. NIOSH Lifting Index Value for Typical Manual Lifting of Objects

Lifting task	Lifting index	Level of risk
3,000 mL irrigation fluid	< 0.2	
Sand bags	0.3	
Linen bags	0.4	
Lead aprons	0.4	
Custom sterile packs (eg, heart or spine)	0.5	
Garbage bags (full)	0.7	
Positioning devices off shelf or rack (eg, stirrups)	0.7	
Positioning devices off shelf or rack (eg, gel pads)	0.9	
Hand table (49" x 28"); largest hand table, used infrequently	1.2	Light
Fluoroscopy board (49" x 21")	1.2	Light
Stirrups (two—one in each hand)	1.4	Light
Wilson frame	1.4	Light
Irrigation containers for lithotripsy (12,000 mL)	1.5	Light
Instrument pans	2.0	Heavy

No shading — Minimal risk—Safe to lift
Light shading — Potential risk—Use assistive technology as available
Heavy shading — Considerable risk—One person should not perform alone or weight should be reduced

Patient weight is divided into 10 categories, ranging from very light (≤ 40 lb) to very heavy (> 440 lb). Normalized weight for each leg, each arm, and the patient's head is calculated as a percentage of total body weight, where each complete lower extremity represents 15.7% of total body mass, each upper extremity (ie, upper arm, forearm, hand) represents 5.1% of total body mass, and the combination of head and neck represents 8.4% of total body mass.[32] All weights are presented in both pounds and kilograms, rounded to the nearest whole unit.

To accommodate 75% of the US adult female working population, maximum load for a one-handed lift is calculated to be 11.1 lb (5.0 kg). This is determined by calculating the strength capabilities for 25th percentile US adult female maximum shoulder flexion moment (the mean equals 40 Newton meters; standard deviation equals 13 Nm)[35] and 75th percentile US adult female shoulder to grip length (the mean equals 610 mm, the standard deviation equals 30 mm).[36] Maximum loads for one person for a two-handed lift (ie, 22.2 lb/10.1 kg) are calculated as twice that of a one-handed lift. Muscle strength capabilities diminish as a function of time; therefore, maximum loads for two-handed holding of body parts are presented for 1, 2, and 3 minute durations.[37] After 1 minute, muscle endurance has decreased by 48%, decreasing by 65% after 2 minutes, and after 3 minutes of continuous holding, strength capability is only 29% of initial lifting strength. If the limits in Ergonomic Tool #3 are exceeded, additional staff members or assistive limb holders should be used.

Ergonomic Tool #4: Prolonged Standing

Perioperative team members who are scrubbed or first assisting for long periods of time may be susceptible to injuries caused by static load.[39-44] Prolonged standing, trunk flexion, and neck flexion are all components of static load.[45,46] Ergonomic Tool #4 assists perioperative team members to take protective action to decrease the stress caused by prolonged standing.

Ergonomic Tool #5: Retraction

Sterile perioperative team members or those performing in the role of first assistant may be required to hold retractors or body parts for long periods of time, in addition to standing for long periods of time. Manual retraction used to provide exposure of the operative site for the surgeon often requires first assistants to stand in an awkward posture for long periods of time to grip and pull a retractor or to use their hands to retract or steady organs (eg, heart). The height of the surgical field in relation to the person providing retraction influences the risk for musculoskeletal injury.[47] Prolonged standing, trunk flexion, neck flexion, and arms held higher than the optimal working height place perioperative team members at risk for a musculoskeletal injury.

SAFE PATIENT HANDLING

TABLE 1. DATA USED TO CALCULATE THE NIOSH LIFTING INDEX VALUES FOR TYPICAL ITEMS LIFTED IN THE OR

Lifting task	Weight	Horizontal distance (inches)	Vertical location-origin (inches)	Vertical location-destination (inches)	Distance carried (feet)	Lifting index
3000 cc IV bags irrigation fluids	2.5 lb	6 in	42 in	30 in	49–118 ft	< 0.2
Sand bags	10.5 lb	12 in	30 in	32 in	20 ft	0.3
Linen bags	15 lb	6 in Set = 10 in	Floor Set = 0 in	42 in	140–251 ft	0.4
Lead aprons	16 lb	13 in	36 in	36 in	N/A on cart	0.4
Custom sterile packs (heart or spine)	12.4 lb	18 in	23 in	32 in		0.5
Garbage bags (full)	23.6 lb	6 in Set = 10 in	Floor Set = 0 in	42 in	140–251 ft	0.7
Positioning devices off shelf or rack (stirrups)	17 lb each (2 stirrups would be 34 lb)	18 in	36 in	36 in		0.7
Positioning devices off shelf or rack (gel pads)	8–25 Set to 25 lb	18 in	36 in	36 in	5–10 ft	0.9
Hand table (49" x 28"); largest hand table, used infrequently	15–27 lb Set to 27 lb	20 in	43 in	32 in	49–118 ft	1.2
Fluoroscopy board (49" x 21")	26 lb	20 in	43 in	32 in	49–118 ft	1.2
Stirrups (2, one in each hand)	34 lb	18 in	36 in	36 in		1.4
Wilson frame	27 lb	32 in	31.5 in	32 in	49–118 ft	1.4
Irrigation containers for lithotripsy (12,000 mL)	0–50 lb Set to 50 lb	6 in Set = 10	63 in (top shelf)	N/A Housekeeping places in bags Set to 33 in	49–118 ft	1.5
Instrument pans	3–38 lb Set to 38 lb	19 in	6–50 in Set to 6 in	Varies Set to 34 in	5–10 ft	2.0

Ergonomic Tool #6: Lifting and Carrying Supplies and Equipment

Members of the perioperative team may need to lift and carry many different types of unsterile and sterile supplies, instrument trays, and equipment. This tool is intended to assist caregivers in evaluating these tasks and taking measures to protect themselves. Information from Association for the Advancement of Medical Instrumentation, the organization that sets standards for safety and efficacy of medical instrumentation, recommends that instrument trays weigh a maximum of 25 lb.[48]

Manual lifting and carrying of objects is physically demanding and may place the worker at substantial risk of low back pain. The NIOSH has developed an equation for calculating the recommended weight limit and lifting index for assessing the physical demands of manual lifting tasks.[49,50] A description of the NIOSH lifting equation is presented in the section entitled "Other background materials."

Typical lifting tasks performed by perioperative nurses were identified and evaluated for potential risk of low back pain due to manual lifting using the Revised NIOSH Lifting Equation (RNLE). Ergonomic Tool #6 lists the lifting index values for these tasks. According to NIOSH, tasks with a lifting index value greater than 1.0 place some workers at risk of low back pain and a lifting index value greater than 3.0 places many workers at risk of low back pain. In a subsequent

SAFE PATIENT HANDLING

Ergonomic Tool #7. Recommendations for Pushing, Pulling, and Moving Equipment on Wheels

OR equipment	Pushing		Max push distance ft/(m)		Ergonomic recommendation
Electrosurgery unit	8.4 lbF	(3.8 kgF)	> 200 ft	(60 m)	
Ultrasound	12.4 lbF	(5.6 kgF)	> 200 ft	(60 m)	
X-ray equipment portable	12.9 lbF	(5.9 kgF)	> 200 ft	(60 m)	
Video towers	14.1 lbF	(6.4 kgF)	> 200 ft	(60 m)	
Linen cart	16.3 lbF	(7.4 kgF)	> 200 ft	(60 m)	
X-ray equipment, C-arm	19.6 lbF	(8.9 kgF)	> 200 ft	(60 m)	
Case carts, empty	24.2 lbF	(11.0 kgF)	> 200 ft	(60 m)	
OR stretcher, unoccupied	25.1 lbF	(11.4 kgF)	> 200 ft	(60 m)	
Case carts, full	26.6 lbF	(12.1 kgF)	> 200 ft	(60 m)	
Microscopes	27.5 lbF	(12.5 kgF)	> 200 ft	(60 m)	
Hospital bed, unoccupied	29.8 lbF	(13.5 kgF)	> 200 ft	(60 m)	
Specialty equipment carts	39.3 lbF	(17.9 kgF)	> 200 ft	(60 m)	
OR stretcher, occupied, 300 lb	43.8 lbF	(19.9 kgF)	> 200 ft	(60 m)	
Bed, occupied, 300 lb	50.0 lbF	(22.7 kgF)	< 200 ft	(30 m)	Min two caregivers required
Specialty OR beds, unoccupied	69.7 lbF	(31.7 kgF)	< 100 ft	(30 m)	
OR bed, unoccupied	61.3 lbF	(27.9 kgF)	< 25 ft	(7.5 m)	Recommend powered transport device
OR bed, occupied, 300 lb	112.4 lbF	(51.1 kgF)	< 25 ft	(7.5 m)	
Specialty OR beds, occupied, 300 lb	124.2 lbF	(56.5 kgF)	< 25 ft	(7.5 m)	

No shading   Minimal risk—Safe to lift
Light shading   Potential risk—Use assistive technology as available
Heavy shading   Considerable risk—One person should not perform alone or weight should be reduced

study that examined the effects of the NIOSH lifting index as a predictor, the risk of back pain increases when the lifting index exceeds 2.0.[51] As can be seen in the table, tasks with a lifting index value less than 1.0 can easily be performed manually. For those tasks with a lifting index value greater than 1.0, however, caution should be used. Alternate handling procedures may help reduce risk of low back pain due to lifting these objects. The list is not all inclusive; the NIOSH equation can be used to calculate a lifting index value for other two-handed manual lifting tasks not on the list.[50]

Note: *Assistive devices include adjustable-height lift tables, rolling carts, two-wheeled carts, dollies, or mechanical transport devices.*

Rationale and Calculations for Ergonomic Tool #6

A series of typical operating room lifting tasks were identified and evaluated with the NIOSH Lifting Equation (NLE) for potential risk of low back pain due to manual lifting of objects in support of patient care (see Table 1). The NLE is a tool for assessing manual lifting of objects that allows the user to calculate the recommended weight limit for a specified two-handed manual lifting task. In addition, the lifting index for the task can be calculated by dividing the actual weight of the load lifted by the recommended weight limit (for details, see "Other background material").

Ergonomic Tool #7: Pushing, Pulling, and Moving Equipment on Wheels

Introduction

Case preparation is a combination of many activities. The movement of patients, supplies, and equipment in and out of the OR contributes to physical stress and should be performed based on scientific evidence. The recommendations in Ergonomic Tool #7 are a result of research done by task force members and include some, but not all, of the necessary activities undertaken to prepare for a case.

Pushing forces were measured for equipment listed in the following table. Maximum pushing distances were determined based on Liberty Mutual's psychophysical limits. All results are presented in both US and metric units.

Based on these results, it is clear that pushing an occupied standard hospital bed or standard or specialty OR beds, whether occupied or not, presents a moderate to high risk of injury to the caregiver. For these situations it is strongly recommended that a minimum of two

SAFE PATIENT HANDLING

TABLE 2. Measured Push Forces for Operating Room Equipment

Equipment	Type of force	Trial 1 (N)	Trial 2 (N)	Trial 3 (N)	Trial 4 (N)	Trial 5 (N)	Mean (N)	Mean (lbF)	Max push distance (ft)
Electrosurgical unit	initial force	30	35	35	30	30	32.0	7.2	> 200
	sustained force	10	10	10	10	10	10.0	2.2	> 200
	initial-wheels turned	40	35				37.5	8.4	> 200
OR stretcher, unoccupied	initial force	62	70	65	75		68.0	15.3	> 200
	sustained force	20	20	25	25	25	23.0	5.2	> 200
	initial-wheels turned	113	110				111.5	25.1	> 200
OR stretcher, occupied, 300 lb	initial force	120	120	120	115	120	119.0	26.8	> 200
	sustained force	30	35	30	40	40	35.0	7.9	> 200
	initial-wheels turned	210	180				195.0	43.8	< 50
Bed, unoccupied	initial force	115	120	125	110	105	115.0	25.9	> 200
	sustained force	30	25	30	25		27.5	6.2	> 200
	initial-wheels turned	130	135				132.5	29.8	> 200
Bed, occupied, 300 lb	initial force	170	160	167	135	155	157.4	35.4	> 200
	sustained force	40	50	50	40	60	48.0	10.8	> 200
	initial-wheels turned	230	215				222.5	50.0	< 25
OR bed, unoccupied	initial force	218	275	245	280	270	257.6	57.9	< 25
	sustained force	120	125	120	100	120	117.0	26.3	< 25
	initial-wheels turned	270	275				272.5	61.3	< 25
OR bed, occupied, 300 lb	initial force	425	432	445	405	325	406.4	91.4	< 25
	sustained force	180	180	180			180.0	40.5	< 25
	initial-wheels turned	485	515				500.0	112.4	< 25
Specialty OR beds, unoccupied	initial force	175	182	190	260	200	201.4	45.3	< 25
	sustained force	100	100	100			100.0	22.5	< 100
	initial-wheels turned	305	315				310.0	69.7	< 25

continued on next page

caregivers participate in the transport task, or ideally, that a powered transport device is used.

Recommendations

The recommendations in Ergonomic Tool #7 are based on Liberty Mutual's psychophysical limits for push forces, where hands are positioned at a middle push point of 3 ft (0.92 m) from the floor or above and task is performed no more frequently than once every 30 minutes.[34]

- Pushing tasks are ergonomically preferred over pulling tasks.[34]
- Ensure that handles are at a correct push height of approximately 3 ft (0.92 m) from the floor.[34]
- For tasks where the push point is lower than 3 ft (0.92 m), maximum and sustained push forces will be decreased by approximately 15%.[34]
- For tasks performed more frequently than once every 30 minutes, maximum and sustained push forces will be decreased by approximately 6%.[34]
- If push force limits are exceeded it will be necessary to reduce the weight of the load, use two or more caregivers to complete the task together, or use a powered transport device.
- Equipment casters need to be properly maintained to assist in moving equipment more easily.
- For OR equipment not listed above, compare physical effort to that required to push an unoccupied standard hospital bed. If greater effort is required, then additional caregivers and/or use of powered transport device is recommended.

Rationale/Calculations Used for Ergonomic Tool #7

Push forces were measured in Newtons (N) for each item of equipment listed in Table 2. Initial forces

SAFE PATIENT HANDLING

Table 2 continued. Measured Push Forces for Operating Room Equipment

Equipment	Type of force	Trial 1 (N)	Trial 2 (N)	Trial 3 (N)	Trial 4 (N)	Trial 5 (N)	Mean (N)	Mean (lbF)	Max push distance (ft)
Specialty OR beds, 300-lb patient	initial force	365	290	320	305	305	317.0	71.3	< 25
	sustained force	140	160	140	115	115	134.0	30.1	< 25
	initial-wheels turned	560	545				552.5	124.2	< 25
Microscopes	initial force	62	75	80	75	75	73.4	16.5	> 200
	sustained force	20	25	20	25	25	23.0	5.2	> 200
	initial-wheels turned	125	120				122.5	27.5	< 50
Case cart, full	initial force	62	108	75	108		88.3	19.8	> 200
	sustained force	30	40	40	40		37.5	8.4	> 200
	initial-wheels turned	122	115				118.5	26.6	> 200
Case cart, empty	initial force	60	65	65	62	65	63.4	14.3	> 200
	sustained force	40	30	35	40	35	36.0	8.1	> 200
	initial-wheels turned	120	95				107.5	24.2	> 200
X-ray equipment, C-arm	initial force	100	75	100	75	85	87.0	19.6	> 200
	sustained force	20	25	25	25	25	24.0	5.4	> 200
	initial-wheels turned	N/A	N/A				N/A	N/A	N/A
X-ray equipment, portable	initial force	60	55	55	60	58	57.6	12.9	> 200
	sustained force	25	30	30	30	30	29.0	6.5	> 200
	initial-wheels turned	N/A	N/A				N/A	N/A	N/A
Video towers	initial force	35	40	40	35	35	37.0	8.3	> 200
	sustained force	15	20	20	15	20	18.0	4.0	> 200
	initial-wheels turned	60	65				62.5	14.1	> 200
Ultrasound	initial force	35	40	45	45	40	41.0	9.2	> 200
	sustained force	20	20	25	20	20	21.0	4.7	> 200
	initial-wheels turned	55	55				55.0	12.4	> 200
Specialty equipment carts	initial force	105	90	120	125	145	117.0	26.3	> 200
	sustained force	25	30	30	25	25	27.0	6.1	> 200
	initial-wheels turned	165	185				175.0	39.3	< 200
Linen cart	initial force	50	70	55	55	65	59.0	13.3	> 200
	sustained force	20	25	20	25	20	22.0	4.9	> 200
	initial-wheels turned	75	70				72.5	16.3	> 200

were measured as the peak force to initially propel the item. Sustained force was measured as the minimum force required to maintain equipment propulsion. Initial-wheels turned were measured as the peak initial force where the wheels on the equipment were turned perpendicular to the desired direction of travel. The average force measured across five repeated trials for each condition and equipment item was computed and converted into US units.

Maximum pushing distances were determined and reported in Table 2, based on Liberty Mutual's push force limits.[34] The shortest acceptable push distance, considering both initial and sustained forces, was accepted (see Table 3). These values are based on the operator with his or her hands positioned at a middle push point of 3 ft (0.92 m) from the floor or above and performing a task no more frequently than once every 30 minutes.

Measuring Pushing/Pulling Forces

To measure OR equipment not listed in Table 2, a measuring device can be applied to measure applicable pushing/pulling forces. Commercially available measuring instruments can be used to measure push/pull forces (eg, strain gage, force meters, precision springs). A simple low-cost method for measuring the required forces for pushing or pulling objects, such as beds, carts, and transfer equipment, is shown in Figure 1. As illustrated, a broom handle or other lightweight cylindrical object can be taped to a bathroom scale and used to measure push forces. Required pull forces would be identical to the required pushing force. The scale is placed against the object to be pushed and a force is then slowly applied to the handle until the object moves. The maximum required pushing force is read off the weight scale. The scale should provide a continuous readout of applied force to obtain the maximum value. To obtain the best estimate of the actual maximum force, the measurement should be repeated several times and the average value should be used for assessment. This force can then be compared to the maximum recommended push force values shown in Table 3. For example, assume that the force required to push a cart was measured to be 60 lb. According to Table 3, this task would not be acceptable for one caregiver for any distance, but would be acceptable for two caregivers (assuming each pushed 26 lb) for a distance of up to 25 feet. A powered transport device would be recommended if one caregiver is performing the task.

Other Background Materials

The Revised NIOSH Lifting Equation

The Revised NIOSH Lifting Equation (RNLE) provides a mathematical equation for determining the recommended weight limit (RWL) and lifting index (LI) for selected two-handed manual lifting tasks. The RWL is the principal product of the RNLE and is defined for a specific set of task conditions and represents the weight of the load that nearly all healthy workers could perform over a substantial period of time (eg, up to 8 hours) without an increased risk of developing lifting-related low back pain. By "healthy workers," NIOSH means workers who are free of adverse health conditions that would increase their risk of musculoskeletal injury.

The concept behind the RNLE is to start with a recommended weight that is considered safe for an "ideal" lift (ie, load constant equal to 51 lb or 23 kg) and then reduce the weight as the task becomes more stressful (ie, as the task-related factors become less favorable). The RWL equation consists of a fixed load constant of 51 lb that is reduced by six factors related to task geometry (ie, location of the load relative to the worker at the initial liftoff and setdown points), task frequency and duration, and type of handhold on the object. Assessment of patient handling tasks was specifically excluded as a restriction for use of the RNLE due to limitations in the data used to derive the equation. For some patient handling tasks, however, where the person being lifted is noncombative or where there is little or no movement of the patient during the lifting task, the RNLE may be applicable, and it should be possible to determine whether the lift exceeds the RWL for those tasks. For example, the RNLE was used to derive the 35-lb weight limit for patient lifting in the VA and AORN ergonomic tools.[52] The precise formulation of the revised lifting equation for calculating the recommended weight limit is based on a multiplicative model that provides a weighting (ie, multiplier) for each of six task variables, which include the

- horizontal distance of the load from the worker (H),
- vertical height of the lift (V),
- vertical displacement during the lift (D),
- angle of asymmetry (A),
- frequency (F) and duration of lifting, and
- quality of the hand-to-object coupling (C).

The weightings are expressed as coefficients that serve to decrease the load constant, which represents the maximum RWL to be lifted under ideal conditions. For example, as the horizontal distance between the load and the worker increases, the recommended weight limit for that task would be reduced from the ideal starting weight (see Table 4).

The term *task variables* refers to the measurable task-related measurements that are used as input data for the

Table 3. Push Force Limits

Push/pull forces based on 75% acceptable for women design goal					
Distance (ft)	25	50	100	150	200
Initial (lb)	51	44	42	42	37
Sustained (lb)	30	25	22	22	15

Adapted from Manual Materials Handling Guidelines, *http://libertymmhtables.libertymutual.com/CM_LMTablesWeb/pdf/LibertyMutualTables.pdf. Reprinted with permission from the Liberty Mutual Research Institute for Safety.*

Figure 1. Simple Device for Measuring Required Push Force

Photo by Tom Waters, PhD, CPE. Used with permission.

SAFE PATIENT HANDLING

Table 4. Recommended Weight Limit

	Variable		Metric	US Customary
The recommended weight limit is defined as follows: RWL = LC x HM x VM x DM x AM x FM x CM Where:	LC =	Load Constant =	23 kg	51 lb
	HM =	Horizontal Multiplier =	(25/H)	(10/H)
	VM =	Vertical Multiplier =	1−(.003|V−75|)	1−(.0075|V−30|)
	DM =	Distance Multiplier =	.82 + (4.5/D)	.82 + (1.8/D)
	AM =	Asymmetric Multiplier =	1−(.0032A)	1−(.0032A)
	FM =	Frequency Multiplier =	From Table 5	From Table 5
	CM =	Coupling Multiplier =	From Table 6	From Table 6

formula (ie, H, V, D, A, F, C), whereas the term *multipliers* refers to the reduction coefficients in the equation (ie, HM, VM, DM, AM, FM, CM).

The following list briefly describes the measurements required to use the RNLE. Details for each of the variables are presented later in this chapter (see section entitled "Obtaining and using the data").

H = Horizontal location of hands from midpoint between the inner ankle bones. This is measured in centimeters or inches at the origin and the destination of the lift.

V = Vertical location of the hands from the floor. This is measured in centimeters or inches at the origin and destination of the lift.

D = Vertical travel distance in centimeters or inches between the origin and the destination of the lift.

A = Angle of asymmetry; angular displacement of the load from the worker's sagittal plane. This is measured in degrees at the origin and destination of the lift.

F = Average frequency rate of lifting measured in lifts/min. Duration is defined as follows: short-duration (< 1 hour); moderate-duration (> 1 but < 2 hours); or long-duration (> 2 but < 8 hours), assuming appropriate recovery allowances (see Table 5).

C = Quality of hand-to-object coupling (quality of interface between the worker and the load being lifted). The quality of the coupling is categorized as good, fair, or poor, depending upon the type and location of the coupling, the physical characteristics of load, and the vertical height of the lift (see Table 6).

The LI is a term that provides a relative estimate of the level of physical stress associated with a particular manual lifting task. The estimate of the level of physical stress is defined by the relationship of the weight of the load lifted and the RWL.

The LI is defined by the following equation:

$$LI = \frac{\text{Load weight}}{\text{Recommended Weight Limit}} = \frac{L}{RWL}$$

Where Load weight (L) = Weight of the object lifted (lb or kg).

According to NIOSH, the lifting index may be used to identify potentially hazardous lifting jobs or to compare the relative severity of two jobs for the purpose of evaluating and redesigning them. From the perspective of NIOSH, it is likely that lifting tasks with a lifting index > 1.0 pose an increased risk for lifting-related low back pain for some fraction of the work force.[49] Lifting jobs should be designed to achieve a lifting index of 1.0 or less whenever possible. Some experts believe that worker selection criteria may be used to identify workers who can perform potentially stressful lifting tasks (ie, lifting tasks that would exceed a lifting index of 1.0) without significantly increasing their risk of work-related injury above the baseline level.[49,50] Those who endorse the use of selection criteria believe that the criteria must be based on research studies, empirical observations, or theoretical considerations that include job-related strength testing and/or aerobic capacity testing.

Even these experts agree, however, that many workers will be at a significant risk of a work-related injury when performing highly stressful lifting tasks (ie, lifting tasks that would exceed a lifting index of 3.0). "Informal" or "natural" selection of workers may occur in many jobs that require repetitive lifting tasks. According to some experts, this may result in a unique workforce that may be able to work above a lifting index of 1.0, at least in theory, without substantially increasing their risk of low back injuries above the baseline rate of injury.

To gain a better understanding of the rationale for the development of the recommended weight limits and lifting index, the *Revised NIOSH Equation for the Design and Evaluation of Manual Lifting Tasks* provides a discussion of the criteria underlying the lifting equation and of the individual multipliers.[49] This article also identifies both the assumptions and uncertainties in the scientific studies that associate manual lifting and low back injuries. For more detailed information about how to use the RNLE, the reader should consult the *Applications Manual for the Revised NIOSH Lifting Equation*.[50]

Glossary

Air-assisted lateral transfer device: A mattress that is inflated with air by a portable air supply, thus facilitating a smoother lateral transfer.

SAFE PATIENT HANDLING

Anti-fatigue mats: A special mat designed with friction-reduction properties, used for workers who stand for long periods of time.

Anti-fatigue technique: Any technique that will reduce fatigue experienced by the worker.

Assistive devices/technology: Equipment that can be used to take all or a portion of a load, such as the weight of a body part, off of the person performing a high-risk task.

Clinical tools: A standardized process or set of rules by which a provider makes decisions about a complex process (eg, which equipment and techniques to use when performing high-risk patient handling and movement tasks).

Compressive force: Mechanical force directed along the Y (ie, vertical) axis, brought about by the combined effect of internal and external load bearing.

Ergonomics: Applied science of designing and arranging things for people to use efficiently and safely; matching job tasks to workers' capabilities.

Ergonomist: A practitioner in the field of ergonomics.

Friction-reducing devices: Low-friction (slippery) material assistive aids for lateral transfer of patients.

Lateral position: Side-lying.

Lateral transfer: Movement of a patient in a supine position on a horizontal plane, such as transferring a patient from a bed to a stretcher.

Lateral transfer device: A device that is used to move a patient from one surface to another while in a supine position.

lbF: A unit of force equal to the mass of 1 lb with an acceleration equal to 1 gravitational constant (32 ft/s^2). Acceleration due to gravity (g) equals 9.8 meters per second squared (9.8 m/s^2) or 32 feet per second squared (32 ft/s^2).

Lifting index: Relative estimate of physical stress associated with one specific task. It is equal to the load of the object/recommended weight limit.

TABLE 5. FREQUENCY MULTIPLIERS

Frequency lifts/min (F)	< 1 hour		> 1 but < 2 hours		> 2 but < 8 hours	
	V < 30	V > 30	V < 30	V > 30	V < 30	V > 30
0.2	1.00	1.00	.95	.95	.85	.85
0.5	.97	.97	.92	.92	.81	.81
1	.94	.94	.88	.88	.75	.75
2	.91	.91	.84	.84	.65	.65
3	.88	.88	.79	.79	.55	.55
4	.84	.84	.72	.72	.45	.45
5	.80	.80	.60	.60	.35	.35
6	.75	.75	.50	.50	.27	.27
7	.70	.70	.42	.42	.22	.22
8	.60	.60	.35	.35	.18	.18
9	.52	.52	.30	.30	.00	.15
10	.45	.45	.26	.26	.00	.13
11	.41	.41	.00	.23	.00	.00
12	.37	.37	.00	.21	.00	.00
13	.00	.34	.00	.00	.00	.00
14	.00	.31	.00	.00	.00	.00
15	.00	.28	.00	.00	.00	.00
> 15	.00	.00	.00	.00	.00	.00

TABLE 6. COUPLING MULTIPLIER

	Coupling multiplier	
	V < 30 inches (75 cm)	V > 30 inches (75 cm)
Good	1.00	1.00
Fair	0.95	1.00
Poor	0.90	0.90

Lithotomy position: Supine position with the hips and knees flexed and the thighs abducted and rotated externally.

Manual retraction: When a member of the perioperative sterile team (ie, scrubbed team) provides exposure of underlying anatomical parts during surgery with his or her hand or by physically holding and/or pulling with a sterile device designed to hold back the edges of tissue and organs.

Maximum sustained force: Force needed to pull or lift for a period of time.

Mechanical lateral transfer device: A powered device that moves a patient horizontally from one surface to another while in a supine position.

Mechanical lift device: Patient transfer device that uses a sling and mechanical lift to transfer patients and/or lift body parts (includes ceiling-mounted and floor-based lifts as well as sit-to-stand lifts).

Musculoskeletal: Relating to or involving the muscles and the skeleton.

Newton (N): A metric unit of measure for forces. (1 Newton = 0.2248 lb)

Newton meter (Nm): A metric unit of measure for moments (ie, force × length). One Newton meter = .738 ft·lb.

Optimal posture: Perpendicular/straight on to the operative field.

Optimal working height: Area between the chest and waist height to the operative field.

Prone: With the front (or ventral) surface of the body positioned face downward.

Recommended weight limit: Recommended weight limit is the principal product of the revised NIOSH lifting equation defined for a specific set of task conditions as the weight of the load that 75% of the population could perform safely.

Revised NIOSH Lifting Equation: Mathematical equation for determining the recommended weight limit and lifting index for selected two-handed manual lifting tasks.

Self-retaining retractor: A sterile device designed to mechanically hold back the edges of tissue and organs to provide exposure to underlying anatomical structures during a surgical procedure.

Semi-Fowler position: The upper half of the body raised to an incline of 30 to 45 degrees; also called the beach-chair position.

Sit-stand stool: A stool that allows the worker to sit or stand while working without changing levels.

Spinal compression: Forces acting along the length of the spine.

Spine loading: Overall mechanical force acting on the spine calculated as root-mean-square value of compressive, lateral, and anterior-posterior components.

Static posture: Postures requiring a sustained position for a long period of time (eg, standing in one position during surgery).

Supine: With the back or dorsal surface of the body positioned downward (ie, lying face up).

References

1. B D Owen, A Garg, "Reducing risk for back pain in nursing personnel," *AAOHN Journal* 39 (January 1991) 24-33.

2. B D Owen, "Preventing injuries using an ergonomic approach," *AORN Journal* 72 (December 2000) 1031-1036.

3. J R Garb, C A Dockery, "Reducing employee back injuries in the perioperative setting," *AORN Journal* 61 (June 1995) 1046-1052.

4. "NIOSH facts: Work-related musculoskeletal disorders," National Institute for Occupational Health and Safety, http://www.cdc.gov/niosh/muskdsfs.html (accessed 1 Oct 06).

5. A B Hoskins, "Occupational injuries, illnesses, and fatalities among nursing, psychiatric, and home health aides, 1995–2004," Bureau of Labor Statistics, http://www.bls.gov/opub/cwc/content/sh20060628ar01pl.stm (accessed 28 Sept 2006).

6. A Converso, C Murphy, "Winning the battle against back injuries," *RN* 67 (February 2004) 52-58.

7. A Nelson, G Fragala, N Menzel, "Myths and facts about back injuries in nursing," *AJN* 103 (February 2003) 32-41.

8. US Department of Labor, "Table R10, Number of nonfatal occupational injuries and illnesses involving-days away from work by occupation and selected parts of body affected by injury or illness, 2001," Bureau of Labor Statistics, http://www.bls.gov/iif/oshwc/osh/case/ostb1165.pdf (accessed 1 Oct 2006).

9. "Lost-worktime injuries and illnesses: characteristics and resulting time away from work, 2004," US Department of Labor, Bureau of Labor Statistics, http://www.bls.gov/news.release/archives/osh2_12132005.pdf (accessed 28 Nov 2006).

10. D A Stubbs et al, "Backing out: Nurse wastage associated with back pain," *International Journal of Nursing Studies* 23 no 4 (1986) 325-336.

11. B D Owen, "The magnitude of low-back problems in nursing," *Western Journal of Nursing Research* 11 (April 1989) 234-242.

12. A Vasiliadou et al, "Occupational low-back pain in nursing staff in a Greek hospital," *Journal of Advanced Nursing* 21(January 1995) 125-130.

13. M J Lusted et al, "Self-reported symptoms in the neck and upper limbs in nurses," *Applied Ergonomics* 27 no 6 (1996) 381-387.

14. E B Moses, *The Registered Nurse Population: Findings From the National Sample Survey of Registered Nurses, 1992*, (Rockville, Md: US Department of Human Services, 1992) 65; also available at Health Resources and Services Administration, ftp://ftp.hrsa.gov/bhpr/nursing/samplesurveys/1992sampsur.pdf (accessed 11 Dec 2006).

15. ECRI, "Workplace hazard reduction through ergonomic evaluation," *Operating Room Risk Management* (September 2005) 1-5.

16. B P Bernard, ed, "Musculoskeletal disorders (MSDs) and workplace factors: A critical review of epidemiological evidence for work-related musculoskeletal disorders of the neck, upper extremity, and low back," US Department of Human Services, National Institute for Occupational Safety and Health, http://www.cdc.gov/niosh/ergosci1.html (accessed 16 Feb 2006).

17. C B Stetler et al, "Evidence for prevention of work-related musculoskeletal injuries," *Orthopedic Nursing* 22 (January/February 2003) 32-41.

18. National Occupational Research Agenda for Musculoskeletal Disorders: Research Topics for the Next Decade—A Report by the NORA Musculoskeletal Disorders Team (Washington, DC: US Department of Health and Human Services, 2001) 1-33.

19. P M McGovern, "Toward prevention and control of occupational back injuries," *Occupational Health Nursing* (April 1985) 180-183.

20. G Cust, J C G Pearson, A Mair, "The prevalence of low back pain in nurses," *International Nursing Review* 19 no 2 (1972) 169-179.

21. P Harber et al, "Occupational low-back pain in hospital nurses," *Journal of Occupational Medicine* 27 (July 1985) 518-524.

22. T Videman et al, "Low-back pain in nurses and some loading factors of work," *Spine* 9 no 4 (1984) 400-404.

23. K Williamson et al, "Occupational health hazards for nurses, part 2," Image: *Journal of Nursing Scholarship* 20 (Fall 1988) 162-168.

24. D Stubbs et al, "Back pain research," *Nursing Times* 77 (May 14, 1981) 857-858.

25. F Bell et al, "Hospital ward patient-lifting tasks," *Ergonomics* 22 no 11 (1979) 1257.

26. J Greenwood, "Back injuries can be reduced with worker training, reinforcement," *Occupational Health Safety* (May 1986) 26-29.

27. A L Nelson, G Fragala, "Equipment for safe patient handling and movement," in *Back Injury Among Healthcare Workers*, W Charney, A Hudson, eds (Washington, DC: Lewis Publishers, 2004) 121-135.

28. Patient Safety Center of Inquiry, *Patient Care Ergonomic Resource Guide: Safe Patient Handling and Movement*, A L Nelson, ed (Tampa, Fla: Department of Veterans Affairs, April 2005) 1-71.

29. P Wicker, "Manual handling in the perioperative environment," *British Journal of Perioperative Nursing* 10 (May 2000) 255-259.

30. K Tuohy-Main, "Why manual handling should be eliminated for resident and career safety and how," *Geriaction* 15 no 4 (1997) 10-14.

31. "Recommended practices for positioning the patient in the perioperative practice setting," in *Standards, Recommended Practices, and Guidelines* (Denver: AORN Inc, 2006) 587-592.

32. D B Chaffin, G B J Anderson, B J Martin, *Occupational Biomechanics*, third ed (New York: J Wiley & Sons, 1999) 73.

33. J D Lloyd, A Baptiste, "Friction-reducing devices for lateral patient transfers: A biomechanical evaluation," *American Association of Occupational Health Nurses* 54 (March 2006) 113-119.

34. S H Snook, V M Ciriello, "The design of manual handling tasks: Revised tables of maximum acceptable weights and forces," *Ergonomics* 34 no 9 (1991) 1197-1213.

35. D B Chaffin, G B J Anderson, B J Martin, *Occupational Biomechanics*, third ed (New York: J Wiley & Sons, 1999) 114.

36. S Pheasant, *Bodyspace* (London: Taylor & Francis, Ltd, 1992) 111.

37. D B Chaffin, G B J Anderson, B J Martin, *Occupational Biomechanics*, third ed (New York: J Wiley & Sons, 1999) 49.

38. "Recommended practices for skin preparation of patients," in *Standards, Recommended Practices, and Guidelines* (Denver: AORN, Inc, 2006) 603-606.

39. "Standing problem," *Hazards Magazine*, http://www.hazards.org/standing (accessed 8 May 2006).

40. E Ha et al, "Does standing at work during pregnancy result in reduced infant birth weight?" *Journal of Occupational and Environmental Medicine* 44 (September 2002) 815-821.

41. T B Hendriksen et al, "Standing and walking for > 5 hours per work day increased the risk for preterm delivery," *American College of Physicians* 1 (November/December 1995) 28-30.

42. A P Keomeester, J P J Broesen, P E Treffers, "Physical work load and gestational age at delivery," *Occupational & Environmental Medicine* 52 (May 1995) 313-315.

43. M J Saurel-Cubizolles et al, "Employment working conditions, and preterm birth: Results from the Europop case-control survey," *Journal of Epidemiology and Community Health* 58 (May 2004) 395-401.

44. B Luke et al, "Obstetrics. The association between occupational factors and preterm birth: A United States nurses' study," *American Journal of Obstetrics and Gynecology* 173 (September 1995) 849-862.

45. J Mathias, "New research looks at ergonomic stresses on operating room staff," *OR Manager* 21 (July 2005) 1, 6-7.

46. R Berguer et al, "A comparison of surgeon's posture during laparoscopic and open surgical procedures," *Surgical Endoscopy* 11 (1997) 139-142.

47. R Berquer, W D Smith, D Davis, "An ergonomic study of the optimum operating table height for laparoscopic surgery," *Surgical Endoscopy* 16 (2002) 416-421.

48. Association for the Advancement of Medical Instrumentation, *Comprehensive Guide to Steam Sterilization and Sterility Assurance in Health Care Facilities, ANSI/AAMI ST79:2006* (Arlington, Va: Association for the Advancement of Medical Instrumentation, 2006) 62.

49. T Waters et al, "Revised NIOSH equation for the design and evaluation of manual lifting tasks," *Ergonomics* 36 no 7 (1993) 749-776.

50. T Waters, A Garg, V Putz-Anderson, *Applications Manual for the Revised NIOSH Lifting Equation*, NIOSH publication no 94-110 (Cincinnati, Ohio: Department of Health and Human Services, National Institute for Occupational Safety and Health, Division of Biomedical and Behavioral Science, January 1994) 1-119.

51. T R Waters et al, "Evaluation of the revised NIOSH lifting equation: A cross-sectional epidemiologic study," *Spine* 24 (February 1999) 386-394.

52. T R Waters, "Using the NIOSH Lifting Equation to Determine Maximum Recommended Weight Limits for Manual Patient Lifting Tasks," presentation at the 6th Annual Safe Patient Handling and Movement Conference, Clearwater Beach, Fla, 1 March 2006.

PUBLICATION HISTORY

Approved by the AORN Board of Directors, November 2006.

This document was formerly published as part of *AORN Guidance Statement: Safe Patient Handling and Movement in the Perioperative Setting*. Denver, CO: AORN, Inc; 2007.

Reformatted September 2012 for publication in *Perioperative Standards and Recommended Practices*, 2013 edition.

SAFE PATIENT HANDLING

AORN gratefully acknowledges the following individuals for reviewing the content of this guidance document:

Darlene Ace, MS
Industrial Hygienist; Environmental Health and Safety Specialist
University of Rochester
Environmental Health & Safety
Industrial Hygiene Unit
Rochester, NY

Kay Ball, RN, BSN, MSA, CNOR, FAAN
Nurse Consultant/Educator
K & D Medical Inc.
Lewis Center, Ohio

Joan Blanchard, RN, MSS, CNOR, CIC
Perioperative Nursing Specialist
AORN Center for Nursing Practice
Denver, Colo

Jay Bowers, RN, BSN, CNOR
Charge Nurse
West Virginia University Hospitals
Morgantown, WVa

Byron Burlingame, RN, MS, CNOR
Perioperative Nursing Specialist
AORN Center for Nursing Practice
Denver, Colo

Camille Collette, RN, MS, CNOR
Patient Safety Coordinator
Risk Management, Health Care Quality
Beth Israel Deaconess Medical Center East
Boston, Mass

Alice Comish, RN, BSN, CNOR
Director, Surgical Technology Program
Our Lady of the Lake College
Baton Rouge, La

Ramona Conner, RN, MSN, CNOR
Perioperative Nursing Specialist
AORN Center for Nursing Practice
Denver, Colo

Bonnie Denholm, RN, MS, CNOR
Perioperative Nursing Specialist
AORN Center for Nursing Practice
Denver, Colo

Guy Fragala, PhD, PE, CSP
Director of Compliance Programs
Environmental Health and Engineering
Newton, Mass

Sharon Giarrizzo-Wilson, RN, MS, CNOR
Perioperative Nursing Specialist
AORN Center for Nursing Practice
Denver, Colo

Judi Goldberg, RN, BSN, CNOR
Clinical Educator
The William W. Backus Hospital
Norwich, Conn

Linda Groah, RN, MSN, CNOR, CNAA, FAAN
Chief Operating Officer
San Francisco Medical Center
Kaiser Foundation Hospital
San Francisco, Calif

Pamela C. Hagan, MSN, RN
Chief Programs Officer
American Nurses Association
Silver Spring, Md

Katherine Halverson-Carpenter, RN, MBA, CNOR
Director, Perioperative Services
University of Colorado Hospital
Denver, Colo

Stephen D. Hudock, PhD
Ergonomics, Certified Safety Professional
Team Leader, Human Factors and Ergonomics Research
National Institute for Occupational Safety and Health
Robert A. Taft Laboratories
Cincinnati, Ohio

Stephanie Lackey, RN
Clinical Nurse Manager
Fannin Surgicare
Houston, Tex

Nancy Menzel, PhD, RN, COHN-S
Associate Professor
School of Nursing
University of Nevada Las Vegas
Las Vegas, Nev

Donna Pritchard, RN, BSN, MA, CNOR, CAN
Director Perioperative Service
Kingsbrook Jewish Medical Center
Brooklyn, NY

Patricia Seifert, RN, MSN, CNOR, CRNFA, FAAN
Education Coordinator, CVOR
Inova Fairfax Hospital
Falls Church, Va

Victoria Steelman, PhD, RN, CNOR
Advanced Practice Nurse
Perioperative Nursing
University of Iowa Healthcare
Iowa City, Iowa

Dawn L. Tenney, RN, MSN
Associate Chief Nurse
Perioperative Services
Massachusetts General Hospital
Boston, Mass

Dawn M. Yost, RDH, RN, BSN, CNOR
Perioperative Nurse Clinician/Preceptor
West Virginia University Hospitals
Morgantown, WV

LISTING OF AORN POSITION STATEMENTS

The following is a listing of AORN's official position statements on a variety of topics. These position statements represent the Association's official position on current health care issues affecting perioperative nursing practice and the profession.

AORN position statements are approved by the AORN Board of Directors. All current AORN position statements are available online at http://www.aorn.org/Clinical_Practice/Position_Statements/Position_Statements.aspx.

AORN Position Statements as of November 2014:

Allied Health Care Providers and Support Personnel in the Perioperative Practice Setting
APRNs in the Perioperative Environment
Care of the Older Adult in Perioperative Settings
Creating a Practice Environment of Safety
Criminalization of Human Errors in the Perioperative Setting
Distractions and Noise in the Perioperative Practice Setting
Entry into Practice
Environmental Responsibility
Healthy Perioperative Work Environment
One Perioperative Registered Nurse Circulator Dedicated to Every Patient Undergoing a Surgical or Other Invasive Procedure
Orientation of the Registered Nurse and Certified Surgical Technologist to the Perioperative Setting
Patient Safety
Perioperative Care of Patients with Do-Not-Resuscitate (DNR) Orders
Preventing Wrong-Patient, Wrong-Site, Wrong-Procedure Events
Responsibility for Mentoring
RN First Assistants
Role of the Health Care Industry Representative in the Perioperative Setting
Safe Staffing and On-Call Practices
Value of Clinical Learning Activities in the Perioperative Setting in Undergraduate Nursing Curricula

LISTING OF AORN POSITION STATEMENTS

AACD GLOSSARY OF TIMES USED FOR SCHEDULING AND MONITORING OF DIAGNOSTIC AND THERAPEUTIC PROCEDURES

The following glossary was developed by the Association of Anesthesia Clinical Directors (AACD) and was approved by their board of directors in October 1995. It has been endorsed by AORN, Inc, and the Society for Technology in Anesthesia and has been accepted without revision by the American Society of Anesthesiologists Committee on Quality Improvement and Practice Management. It is reprinted here with permission of the AACD.

Background

Elevated concerns regarding the economics of health care are dramatically intensifying the pressure for health care providers to establish critical pathways and/or total quality management programs. In addition, negotiating fiscally sound managed care contracts with health maintenance organizations and health insurance carriers, as well as meeting state and federal government documentation requirements, requires justification for each aspect of patient care as well as improved techniques in cost factor analysis and accounting. Few hospital administrators would deny that operating rooms/procedure rooms (OR/PR) are expensive to run, and all would concur that economic analyses of running OR/PRs are not readily available.

During the planning for multicenter studies of OR/PR scheduling, utilization, and efficiency, members of the Association of Anesthesia Clinical Directors (AACD) felt semantics were introducing a major impediment to data comparison and economic analysis. To provide a universal lexicon for the acquisition of data, the AACD has developed a glossary which inclusively, yet restrictively, defines the procedural times that permit comprehensive analyses of OR/PR scheduling, utilization, and efficiency. The AACD proposes adopting this lexicon as a standardized "Glossary of Times Used for Scheduling and Monitoring of Diagnostic and Therapeutic Procedures."

The glossary is divided into four sections: 1) Procedural Times, 2) Procedural and Scheduling Definitions and Time Periods, 3) Utilization and Efficiency Indices, and 4) Patient Categories. The terms defined under Procedural Times are listed in what is the usual chronological order, while terms defined in the other sections are presented in alphabetical order.

1. Procedural Times

(For purposes of analyzing efficiency, each of the times defined below may be further classified by the subscripts S and A, for "Scheduled" and "Actual," respectively.)

1.1 Patient in Facility (PIF) = Time patient arrives at health care facility (applicable to outpatient or same day admission patients).

1.2 Patient Ready for Transport (PRT) = Time when all preparations required prior to transport (eg, labs, consent, gowning) have been completed.

1.3 Patient Sent-for (PS) = Time when transporting service is notified to deliver patient to the OR/PR.

1.4 Patient Available (PA) = Time the patient arrives in the OR/PR preprocedure area.

1.5 Room Set-up Start (RSS) = Time when personnel begin setting up, in the OR/PR, the supplies and equipment for the next case.

1.6 Anesthesia Start (AS) = Time when a member of the anesthesia team begins preparing the patient for an anesthetic.

1.7 Room Ready (RR) = Time when room is cleaned and supplies and equipment necessary for beginning of next case are present (see Discussion).

1.8 Patient In Room (PIR) = Time when patient enters the OR/PR.

1.9 Anesthesiologist, First Available (AFA) = Time of arrival in OR/PR of first anesthesiologist who is qualified to induce anesthesia in patient (see Discussion).

1.10 Procedure Physician, First Available (PPFA) = Time of arrival in OR/PR of first physician/surgeon qualified to position and prep the patient (see Discussion).

1.11 Anesthesiologist of Record In (ARI) = Time of arrival in OR/PR of anesthesiologist of record (see Discussion).

1.12 Anesthesia Induction (AI) = Time when the anesthesiologist begins the administration of agents intended to provide the level of anesthesia required for the scheduled procedure.

1.13 Anesthesia Ready (AR) = Time at which the patient has a sufficient level of anesthesia established to begin surgical preparation of the patient, and remaining anesthetic chores do not preclude positioning and prepping the patient (see Discussion).

1.14 Position/Prep Start (PS) = Time at which the nursing or surgical team begins positioning or prepping the patient for the procedure.

AACD PROCEDURAL TIMES GLOSSARY

1.15 Prep-Completed (PC) = Time at which prepping and draping have been completed and patient is ready for the procedure or surgery to start.

1.16 Procedure Physician of Record In (PPRI) = Arrival time of physician/surgeon of record (see Discussion).

1.17 Procedure/Surgery Start Time (PST) = Time the procedure is begun (eg, incision for a surgical procedure, insertion of scope for a diagnostic procedure, beginning of exam under anesthesia [EUA], shooting of x-ray for radiological procedure).

1.18 Procedure/Surgery Conclusion Begun (PCB) = Time when diagnostic or therapeutic maneuvers are completed and attempts are made by the physician or surgical team to end any noxious stimuli (eg, beginning of wound closure, removal of bronchoscope).

1.19 Procedure Physician of Record Out (PPRO) = Time when physician/surgeon of record leaves the OR/PR (see Discussion).

1.20 Procedure/Surgery Finish (PF) = Time when all instrument and sponge counts are completed and verified as correct; all postoperative radiological studies to be done in the OR/PR are completed; all dressings and drains are secured; and the physician/surgeons have completed all procedure-related activities on the patient.

1.21 Patient Out of Room (POR) = Time at which patient leaves OR/PR.

1.22 Room Clean-up Start (RCS) = Time housekeeping or room personnel begin clean-up of OR/PR.

1.23 Arrival in PACU/ICU (APACU) = Time of patient arrival in PACU or ICU.

1.24 Anesthesia Finish (AF) = Time at which anesthesiologist turns over care of the patient to a postanesthesia care team (either PACU or ICU).

1.25 Room Clean-up Finish (RCF) = Time OR/PR is clean and ready for set-up of supplies and equipment for the next case.

1.26 Ready-for-Discharge from Postanesthesia Care Unit (RDPACU) = Time that patient is assessed to be ready for discharge from the PACU.

1.27 Discharge from Postanesthesia Care Unit (DPACU) = Time patient is transported out of PACU.

1.28 Arrival in Same Day Surgery Recovery Unit = Time of patient arrival in same day surgery recovery unit.

1.29 Ready-for-Discharge from Same Day Surgery Recovery Unit (RDSDSR) = Time that patient is assessed to be ready for discharge from the same day surgery recovery unit.

1.30 Discharge from Same Day Surgery Recovery Unit (DSDSR) = Time patient leaves SDSR unit (either to home or other facility).

2. Procedural and Scheduling Definitions and Time Periods

(For purposes of analyzing efficiency, each of the time periods defined below may be further classified by the subscripts E and A for "Estimated" and "Actual," respectively.)

2.1 Anesthesia Preparation Time (APT) = Time from Anesthesia Start to Anesthesia Ready Time.

2.2 Average Case Length (ACL) = Total hours divided by total number of cases performed within those hours.

2.3 Block Time (BT) = Hours of OR/PR time reserved for a given service or physician/surgeon. Within a defined cutoff period (eg, 72 hours prior to day of surgery), this is time into which only the given service may schedule. (NB: In some institutions, this is known as available or allocated time.)

2.4 Case Time (CT) = Time from Room Set-up Start to Room Clean-up Finished (see Discussion).

2.5 Early Start Hours (ESH) = Hours of Case Time performed prior to the normal day's start time when it is not expected that the Patient Out of Room Time will be before the normal start time for that day.

2.6 Evening/Weekend/Holiday Hours (EWHH) = Hours of Case Time performed outside of Resource Hours.

2.7 In-own Block Hours (IBH) = Hours of Case Time performed during a service's own Block Time. (NB: For a case to be counted in IBH, it must begin during that given service's Block Time.)

2.8 Open Time (OT) = Hours of OR/PR time not reserved for any particular service, into which any service or physician/surgeon may schedule according to the rules established by the given institution. (NB: In some institutions, this is known as discretionary time).

2.9 Outside-own Block Hours (OBH) = Hours of Case Time performed during Resource Hours but outside of the service's Block Time.

2.10 Overrun Hours (OVRH) = Hours of Case Time completed after the scheduled closure time of the OR/PR (ie, after the end of that day's Resource Hours).

2.11 Released Time (RT) = Hours of OR/PR time that are released from a service's Block Time and converted to Open Time (typically done when a service anticipates that it will be unable to use the Block Time due to meetings or vacation).

2.12 Resource Hours (RH) = Total number of hours scheduled to be available for performance of procedures (ie, the sum of all available Block Time and Open Time). This is typically provided for on a weekly recurring basis, but may be analyzed on a daily, weekly, monthly, or annual basis (see Discussion).

2.13 Room Clean-up Time (RCT) = Time from Patient Out of Room to Room Clean-up Finished.

2.14 Room Close (RC) = Time at which the room should be empty and the assigned personnel free to be discharged.

2.15 Room Open (RO) = Time when appropriate staff are scheduled to be present and are expected to have the OR/PR available for patient occupancy.

2.16 Room Set-up Time (RST) = Time from Room Set-up Start to Room Ready.

2.17 Service = A group of physicians or surgeons that together perform a circumscribed set of operative or diagnostic procedures (eg, cardiothoracic surgery, interventional radiology). Generally, any member of a service may schedule into that service's block time. Similarly, OR/PR time used by a given physician or surgeon is credited to his/her service's Total Hours.

2.18 Surgical Preparation Time (SPT) = Time from Position/Prep Start to Procedure/Surgery Start Time.

2.19 Start Time (ST) = Patient In Room Time (see Discussion).

2.20 Total Cases (TC) = Cumulative total of all cases done in a given time period. May be subdivided by service or physician/surgeon.

2.21 Total Hours (TH) = Sum of all Case Times for a given period of time. TH = IBH + OBH + EWHH. May be subdivided by service or individual physician/surgeon.

2.22 Turnover Time (TOT) = Time from prior Patient Out of Room to succeeding Patient In Room Time for sequentially scheduled cases (see Discussion).

3. Utilization and Efficiency Indices

3.1 Adjusted-Percent Service Utilization (ASU) = (IBH + OBH) x 100 ÷ BT. This measures the percentage of time a service utilizes their Block Time during Resource Hours. It is adjusted, compared to Raw Utilization, in that it gives a service "credit" for the time necessary to set up and clean up a room, during which time a patient cannot be in the room. It may exceed 100% because of the inclusion of cases performed during Resource Hours that are Outside-own Block Hours (see Discussion).

3.2 Adjusted-Percent Utilized Resource Hours (AURH) = (Total Hours-Evening/Weekend/Holiday Hours) ÷ Resource Hours x 100. This calculation provides the percentage of time that the OR/PRs are being prepared for a patient, are occupied by a patient, or are being cleaned after taking care of a patient during Resource Hours. It is adjusted, compared to Raw Utilization, in that it includes the time necessary to set up and clean up a room, during which time a patient cannot be in the room (see Discussion).

3.3 Delays may be due to:
    3.3.1   Patient issues
              Insurance problems
              Patient arrived late
              Patient ate/drank
              Abnormal lab values
              Surgery issues
              Complications arose
    3.3.2   System issues
              Test results unavailable
              Blood unavailable
              Patient not ready on floor
              Transport delay
              Elevator delay
              Previous case ran late
              Case bumped for emergency case
              Equipment unavailable
              Equipment malfunction
              X-rays unavailable
              X-ray technician unavailable
              Delay in receiving floor bed
              Insufficient post procedure care beds
              ICU delay
              Instrument problem
    3.3.3   Practitioner issues
              Needs more workup (eg, labs, consults)
              No consent
              Physician/surgeon arrived late
              Anesthesiologist arrived late
              Physician/surgeon unavailable
              Anesthesiologist unavailable
              Inaccurate posting
              Prolonged set-up time

3.4 Early Start = When Patient In Room, Actual, is prior to Patient In Room, Scheduled.
    3.4.1   With overlap—When a case starts early but prior to the Room Clean-up Finished, Actual, of the case originally scheduled to precede it (this occurs when either the preceding or following case is moved to a different OR/PR than originally scheduled).
    3.4.2   Without overlap—When a case starts early but after the Room Clean-up Finished, Actual, of the case originally scheduled to precede it (this may occur because there is no preceding case or because the preceding case finishes earlier than scheduled).

3.5 Late Start = When Patient In Room, Actual, is after Patient In Room, Scheduled.
    3.5.1   With no interference—when the Room Clean-up Finished, Actual, of the preceding case occurs before the Room Set-up Start, Scheduled, of the following case (ie, the OR/PR is available prior to or at the time that preparation for the next case is supposed to begin).
    3.5.2   With interference—When Room Clean-up Finished, Actual, of the preceding case occurs after the Room Set-up Start, Scheduled, of the following case (ie, the OR/PR is not available at the time that preparation for the next case is supposed to begin, either because it is still occupied or because it has not been cleaned).

3.6 Overrun = When Room Clean-up Finished, Actual, for the last scheduled case of the day is later than Room Close. This may be caused by a late start; a Case Time, Actual, greater than Case Time, Scheduled; or a combination of late start and longer than scheduled Case Time.

3.7 Productivity Index (PI) = Percent of time per hour that a patient is in the OR/PR during the prime shift time (eg, first 8 hours).

AACD PROCEDURAL TIMES GLOSSARY

3.8 Raw Utilization (RU) = For the system as a whole, this is the percent of time that patients are in the room during Resource Hours (see Adjusted-Percent Utilized Resource Hours). For an individual service, this is the percent of its Block Time during which a service has a patient in the OR/PR (see Adjusted-Percent Service Utilization).

3.9 Room Gap = Time OR/PRs are vacant during Resource Hours.

- 3.9.1 Empty Room (or Late Start) Gap (LSG) Planned—When Patient In Room, Scheduled, is later than Room Open Unplanned—When Patient In Room, Actual, is later than Room Open.
- 3.9.2 Between Case Gaps (BCG) Planned—When Patient In Room, Scheduled, is later than the Room Clean-up Finished, Actual, of the preceding case. Unplanned—When Patient In Room, Actual, is later than the Room Clean-up Finished, Actual, of the preceding case.
- 3.9.3 End of Schedule Gaps (ESG) Planned—When Room Clean-up Finished, Scheduled, occurs before Room Close. Unplanned—When Room Clean-up Finished, Actual, occurs before Room Close.
- 3.9.4 Total Gap Hours (TGH) = LSG + BCG + ESG.

4. Patient Categories

4.1 In-house (IH) = Patient admitted to and residing in the hospital prior to scheduled surgery/procedure.

4.2 Outpatient (OP) = Patient who is coming in on the day of surgery/procedure and is expected to return home following the procedure.

4.3 Same Day Admit (SDA) = Patient who is coming in on the day of surgery/procedure and will be admitted to the hospital following the procedure.

4.4 Overnight-Recovery (ONR) = Patient who comes in on the day of surgery/procedure but requires overnight recovery prior to returning home. These patients are never admitted to the hospital as inpatients, but may remain in the recovery facility for 12 to 23 hours post surgery/procedure.

Discussion

The foregoing list of the procedural times was intentionally made exhaustive in order to be all inclusive. This by no means suggests that all of the data points defined need to be collected by all institutions. Where problems with OR/PR efficiency exist, whether they are real or perceptual, collecting the appropriate times listed above, and calculating the pertinent time periods, will permit objective evaluation of where the real problems lie. Use of common definitions across the country will also permit inter-institutional comparisons that have been previously impossible.

Several terms listed in the "Procedural Times Glossary" have not had heretofore universally accepted definitions. For several of these, the authors, the board of directors of the Association of Anesthesia Clinical Directors, and the Society for Technology in Anesthesia National Database Committee felt that there existed significant controversy over which definition should be chosen. Although for each of these a consensus was generated which led to the definition chosen, general acceptance of these choices may be improved if the logic behind the decision is known. For those terms which created serious debate, the following discussion of terms is provided.

Adjusted-Percent Service Utilization (ASU) = (IBH + OBH) x 100 ÷ BT. This measures the percentage of time a service utilizes its Block Time during Resource Hours. It is adjusted, compared to raw utilization, in that it gives a service "credit" for the time necessary to set up and clean up a room, during which time a patient cannot be in the room. It may exceed 100% because of the inclusion of cases performed during Resource Hours that are Outside-own Block Hours.

Adjusted-Percent Utilized Resource Hours (AURH) = (Total Hours-Evening/Weekend/Holiday Hours) ÷ Resource Hours x 100. This calculation provides the percentage of time that the OR/PRs are being prepared for a patient, are occupied by a patient, or are being cleaned after taking care of a patient during Resource Hours. It is adjusted, compared to raw utilization, in that it includes the time necessary to set up and clean up a room, during which time a patient cannot be in the room.

Raw Utilization (RU) = For the system as a whole, this is the percent of time that patients are in the room during Resource Hours (see Adjusted Percent Utilization Resource Hours). For an individual service, this is the percent of its Block Time during which a service has a patient in the OR/PR (see Adjusted-Percent Utilization).

Frequently, institutions attempt to assess the extent to which a service uses its allotted Block Time by calculating a utilization percentage. Such a calculation should be performed for the system as a whole to measure the extent to which the "normal" hours of operation are actually used for patient care. If one considers only the time that a patient is in the OR/PR (raw utilization), then the percent of time that a service uses its Block Time is artificially lowered because the time necessary to set up and clean up a room, during which time a patient cannot be in the room, is not accounted for. Similarly, the calculation of percentage utilization of Resource Hours is artificially reduced if only Patient In Room time is used. The larger the number of procedures done in a given room during Resource Hours, the greater the error.

Cost-effective utilization requires highly effective scheduling and optimum utilization of the Resource Hours, with minimal overtime and/or uses of more highly paid on-call personnel. For proper assessment of the extent to which a service or system utilizes its

Block or Resource Hours, respectively, the utilization calculations should be adjusted as defined above. For the individual service, this provides a fairer determination of how much of its Block Time is truly used. For the system as a whole, it provides the actual percentage of time that the OR/PRs are being used for patient care. Perhaps as important, it provides an accurate percentage of time that is not used and therefore available for efficiency improvements.

Anesthesiologist, First Available (AFA) = Time of arrival in OR/PR of first anesthesiologist who is qualified to induce anesthesia in patient.

Procedure Physician, First Available (PPFA) = Time of arrival in OR/PR of first physician/surgeon qualified to position and prep the patient.

If delays in starting cases are thought to be due to the late arrival of either a qualified anesthesiologist or surgeon, recording of these times will allow documentation of the extent of that cause of delay.

Anesthesia Ready (AR) = Time at which the patient has a sufficient level of anesthesia established to begin surgical preparation of the patient, and remaining anesthetic chores do not preclude positioning and prepping the patient.

To maximize efficiency, surgical preparation of the patient should begin as soon as an adequate level of anesthesia has been obtained. In some instances however, the anesthesiologist may need to continue anesthetic preparation of the patient (eg, insertion of Swan-Ganz catheter) that precludes moving or prepping the patient. Anesthesia Ready is thus defined as that time when the anesthesiologist may allow surgical preparation to begin.

Anesthesiologist of Record In (ARI) = Time of arrival in OR/PR of anesthesiologist of record.

Procedure Physician of Record In (PPRI) = Arrival time of physician/surgeon of record.

In academic settings, delays may be due to the late arrival of either the attending anesthesiologist or surgeon. Recording of these times will allow one to determine if tardiness of either attending contributes to delays. Further, in the future, accrediting bodies and insurance carriers may require documentation of the time of presence of the physicians of record.

Case Time (CT) = Time from Room Set-up Start to Room Clean-up Finished.

This definition includes all of the time for which a given procedure requires an OR/PR. It allows for the different duration of Room Set-up and Room Clean-up Times that occur because of the varying supply and equipment needs for a particular procedure. For purposes of scheduling and efficiency analysis, this definition is ideal because it includes all of the time that an OR/PR must be reserved for a given procedure.

Procedure Physician of Record Out (PPRO) = Time when physician/surgeon of record leaves the OR/PR.

Because perceptual differences of turnover times abound, it is important to note when the physician of record leaves the OR/PR, as this may be significantly earlier than when the patient leaves the OR/PR. In those situations when an anesthesiologist is supervising another anesthesia care provider (resident or CRNA), the anesthesiologist of record may be in and out of the OR/PR multiple times, and thus no analogous definition has been provided for.

Resource Hours = Total number of hours scheduled to be available for performance of procedures (ie, the sum of all available Block Time and Open Time). This is typically provided for on a weekly recurring basis, but may be analyzed on a daily, weekly, monthly, or annual basis.

For a given institution, this is the time during which an optimum number of appropriate personnel are available to do cases. This may include more than one shift of personnel, or personnel working extended shifts (ie, greater than 8 hours), in order to gain vertical expansion of OR/PR hours. It may also include electively scheduled time on weekends to gain horizontal expansion of OR/PR hours. Resource hours do not include time gained through overtime or use of on-call personnel, even though this time may be routinely accrued at a given institution.

Room Ready (RR) = Time when room is cleaned and supplies and equipment necessary for beginning of next case are present. To maximize efficiency, the patient should be brought into the OR/PR as early as possible. Although some wish to have all the supplies and equipment necessary for the entire case present and open before the patient is brought in, institutions that have minimized turnover times move patients into the OR/PR as soon as it is clean and only the minimum supplies and equipment (ie, those needed to start the case) are present, but not necessarily open. In those institutions, room preparation continues as anesthesia in induced, allowing an overlap of processes (anesthesia induction and room preparation) that saves time.

Start Time (ST) = Patient in Room Time. Significant debate, indeed, even argument, exists over the proper definition of Start Time. Operating and procedural room nurses generally feel that they have properly accomplished their preparatory tasks if the room is ready at the scheduled start time (Room Ready = Start Time, Estimated), regardless of where the patient is at that time. Anesthesiologists often feel that they are "on time" if anesthesia induction has been completed by the scheduled start time (Anesthesia Ready = Start Time, Estimated). Surgeons generally believe start time should be the time at which the procedure is begun (Procedure/Surgery Start Time = Start Time, Estimated). Since Room Set-up Time is procedure specific and therefore generally known at the time of scheduling, one can reasonably predict Room Ready Time. Anesthesia Preparation Time, however, depends on both the procedure and patient needs. It is thus more variable and not known at the time a procedure is scheduled, making accurate prediction of Anesthesia Ready Time impossible.

This variability in Anesthesia Preparation Time also makes prediction of Procedure/Surgery Start Time inaccurate. Variability in Case Times, due to varying length of surgery, makes prediction of Start Times after the first scheduled case of the day even more inaccurate.

Much of the concern over Start Time is for the first case of the day, particularly when a service or surgeon follows herself/himself in the same OR/PR throughout the day. Prediction, then, of accurate Start Times for the first case of the day appears to be most critical. Once the procedure is known, it is almost always possible to have the Room Ready at any time that is desired for the start of the day. It should also be possible, and desirable for maximizing efficiency, to have the patient in the room for the first case of the day as soon as the room is ready. For maximizing scheduling accuracy and attempting to encourage the most efficient patient flow, the authors have elected to define Start Time as Patient In Room Time.

Turnover Time (TOT) = Time from prior Patient Out of Room to succeeding Patient In Room Time. Strong perceptual differences exist over the definition of Turnover Time. Anesthesiologists and OR/PR nurses usually consider turnover time to be the time between cases when the room is not occupied by a patient. Surgeons consider any time when they are unable to operate as "down time," and thus more often consider turnover time to be the time between the end of surgery on one case and the beginning of surgery on the next case. The latter may appear to be particularly long to an academic surgeon who leaves an OR before the wound is closed (allowing the residents to close and dress the incision) and does not re-enter the OR until the next patient is ready for incision.

As with Start Time, the variability of Anesthesia Preparation Time (APT) makes prediction of turnover times inaccurate if APT were to be included. Thus, to maximize scheduling accuracy and to encourage distinction of time spent preparing the OR/PR from time spent preparing the patient, the authors have elected to define Turnover Time as time from prior Patient Out of Room to succeeding Patient In Room Time for sequentially scheduled cases. As this definition attempts to include the time spent cleaning and preparing the OR/PR for the next case, it should only be calculated if a subsequent case is scheduled to immediately follow. With nonsequential cases, idle time between Room Clean-up Finished for the prior case to Room Set-up Start for the subsequent case should be identified and recorded under the appropriate room-gap category.

Copyright © Association of Anesthesia Clinical Directors, 1997. Reprinted with permission.

Editor's note: *The Association of Anesthesia Clinical Directors changed its name to the American Association of Clinical Directors in 2004. The purpose of the society is to provide a forum for anesthesiologists whose primary responsibility is operating room management. ("About us," American Association of Clinical Directors, http://aacdhq.org [accessed 28 Dec 2006].)*

QUALITY AND PERFORMANCE IMPROVEMENT STANDARDS FOR PERIOPERATIVE NURSING

The 2002 AORN Nursing Practices Committee (NPC) was charged with the review and revision of the "Quality improvement standards for perioperative nursing" developed by the 1990 NPC.

Over time, health care has used many different terms to denote the processes used to improve patient care, such as quality assurance (QA), continuous improvement (CI), and continuous quality improvement (CQI). Quality cannot be assured, but it can be measured, assessed, and improved. Perioperative nurses should strive continuously to improve the care provided to patients in the perioperative setting.

Quality improvement (QI) and performance improvement (PI) are the newest terms used in the quest for excellence. They are two different methodologies that are linked together and continuously developing. "QI examines processes in order to improve them. PI addresses human performance within organizations at the individual, process, and organizational levels."[1] The origin of QI is based in industry and has more of a management and process focus; PI focuses more on the people, their motivation, and the tools (eg, work design, technical support, supervision, safety) they use to achieve the goals of the organization.

Government-funded peer review organizations (PROs), Medicare/Medicaid reimbursement regulations, laws generated at the federal and state levels, and private health insurers' standards have refocused the efforts required to assess patient care systematically. The recent focus of regulatory bodies and the Joint Commission on Accreditation of Healthcare Organizations (JCAHO) has placed greater emphasis on patient safety and reducing the errors that have resulted, at times, in patient deaths. The Institute of Medicine's 1999 report, *To Err Is Human: Building a Safer Health System,"* states, "Although there are many kinds of standards in health care, especially those promulgated by licensing agencies and accrediting organizations, few standards focus explicitly on issues of patient safety."[2]

The Joint Commission states, "The goal of the improving organization performance function is to ensure that the organization designs processes well and systematically monitors, analyzes, and improves its performance to improve patient outcomes. Value in health care is the appropriate balance between good outcomes, excellent care and services, and costs. To add value to the care and services provided, organizations need to understand the relationship between perception of care, outcomes, and costs, and how the three issues are affected by processes carried out by the organization. An organization's performance of important functions significantly affects the quality and value of its services."[3] JCAHO bases its evaluation of an institution's QI/PI activities on
- designing processes,
- monitoring performance through data collection,
- analyzing current performance, and
- improving and sustaining improved performance.

An effective quality/performance improvement plan should be consistent with the philosophy, mission, and strategic goals of the organization. Departmental initiatives should be systematic, written, and communicated to leaders, practitioners, and staff. The plan should provide reliable data that is integrated into an organization-wide plan. Implementation of QI/PI standards may provide the basis for selecting mechanisms that measure outcomes and maintain systems to analyze and trend data and corrective actions that result in improved, safer patient care.

Staff participation and a multidisciplinary approach to the program enhance the awareness of personnel providing direct and indirect care and enable challenges to be funneled into opportunities for improvement. Documentation should show that all aspects of care in the department conform to contemporary standards of clinical practice and that data are used to study and improve the quality of care.

AORN's *Guidelines for Perioperative Practice* should be used as a resource when establishing a QI/PI program. Organizations, depending on their size, resources, and commitment to QI/PI, may have a central department, task force, or steering committee to oversee, expedite, and guide departments in achieving the goals of their QI/PI plan.

Standard I

Assign responsibility for monitoring and evaluation activities.

Interpretive statement 1:
The director and/or the designee (eg, manager or other individual[s] responsible for the department) assume overall responsibility for the monitoring and evaluation processes within the department and in the department's participation in the organization-wide performance improvement plan.

Criteria:
1. The director actively participates in and supports the program.

QUALITY IMPROVEMENT

2. The director may select an individual (ie, designee) to be responsible for the department's overall participation in the QI/PI plan.
3. The director/designee selects the individual/team responsible for each QI/PI project. The team may include, but is not limited to,
   - staff nurses,
   - ancillary staff members,
   - educators,
   - medical director/chief of services,
   - members of the medical staff,
   - OR director/supervisor,
   - QI/PI coordinator, and
   - representatives from any departments involved in the process.
4. The director collaborates with other disciplines and departments that share responsibility for QI/PI activities.

Interpretive statement 2:
The director/designee or other responsible individual(s) develops a mechanism for ensuring that departmental initiatives are congruent with the organization-wide QI/PI plan. The departmental initiatives are integrated and communicated throughout the organization.

Criteria:
1. The plan reflects a departmental and organization-wide commitment to patient care excellence.
2. The plan is communicated through organization-wide and unit-based staff development programs.
3. The plan is evaluated and revised at least annually to determine program appropriateness and effectiveness.
4. The plan describes the roles and responsibilities of those involved in quality improvement/performance improvement. This plan may be in the form of a narrative statement, outline, flow chart, or team charter.
5. The plan describes the monitoring and evaluation activities. These may include, but are not limited to,
   - delineating scope of care,
   - identifying important functions and processes,
   - prioritizing areas for improvement,
   - collecting and analyzing data,
   - evaluating patient care,
   - resolving problem areas and/or improving processes that affect patient care,
   - documenting results,
   - communicating findings, and
   - maintaining improvements.
6. The plan identifies collaborating disciplines/departments that share responsibilities and are interdependent in QI/PI. These activities may include, but are not limited to,
   - contracted services,
   - engineering,
   - environmental services,
   - infection control,
   - laboratory,
   - materials management,
   - medical staff,
   - nursing units,
   - pharmacy,
   - radiology,
   - risk management/safety, and
   - special care units.
7. The plan describes the schedule of the quality QI/PI plan. This may include, but is not limited to, schedule of meetings, schedule of times, and locations of monitoring and evaluation activities.
8. The plan reflects the uniqueness of nursing activities performed in the perioperative setting and the outcomes of perioperative patient care.

Standard II

Delineate the scope of patient care activities or services.

Interpretive statement:
The scope of patient care activities or services describes who is served, what services are provided, who provides the services, physical sites, and times that services are provided.

Criteria:
1. The patient population assessment/description may include, but is not limited to,
   - patient acuity,
   - patient socioeconomic status,
   - demographics,
   - support systems, and
   - clinical conditions/diagnoses.
2. Customers are identified, and they are relevant to the type of service provided. Customers may include, but are not limited to,
   - employees,
   - patients,
   - families,
   - practitioners,
   - purchasers, and
   - suppliers.
3. Clinical care activities and nursing services are determined. These may include, but are not limited to,
   - circulating;
   - scrubbing;
   - first assisting;
   - patient education;
   - resource nurses/advanced practitioners (eg, clinical nurse specialists, nurse practitioners); and
   - others identified in AORN's *Guidelines for Perioperative Practice.*
4. Services provided in the department are inventoried. Services may include, but are not limited to,
   - cardiovascular/thoracic,
   - endoscopy,
   - general surgery,
   - ophthalmology,
   - orthopedics,

QUALITY IMPROVEMENT

- otolaryngology,
- obstetrics and gynecology,
- neurosurgery,
- pediatrics, and
- pain management.

5. Departmental practitioners are listed by job title and level of expertise. Individuals who contribute to departmental care and activities may include, but are not limited to,
   - advanced practice nurses,
   - registered nurses,
   - licensed practical/vocational nurses, and
   - unlicensed assistive personnel.
6. Other practitioners/personnel who share patient care responsibilities are listed. These may include, but are not limited to,
   - ancillary departments,
   - contracting agencies,
   - employed caregivers, and
   - physicians.
7. The physical site is described. The description may include, but is not limited to,
   - number and type of suites/rooms,
   - their proximity to each other, and
   - support areas.
8. Dates, days, and hours of operation are described.
9. Suites/rooms are identified by type of service provided.
10. Staffing plans/patterns that support services are identified.[4] A rationale is given for the chosen staffing, and a mechanism is in place to evaluate the effectiveness.

Standard III

Identify processes impacting the quality and safety of patient care.

Interpretive statement:
High-volume, high-risk, and/or problem-prone processes are identified.

Criteria:
1. High-volume types of patient care activities are those performed on a frequent or daily basis to a large volume of patients. High-volume types include, but are not limited to,
   - procedures that occur frequently (eg, cholecystectomy, laparoscopy, cataract extraction);
   - nursing activities frequently performed for patients (eg, placement of electrosurgical dispersive pad, administration of medication, aseptic technique); and
   - nursing care that affects a large number of patients (eg, patient assessments, patient education, discharge planning, intravenous therapy, pain management).
2. High-risk processes are those that carry a greater potential for liability and/or patient injury. High-risk areas may include, but are not limited to,
   - patients at risk of serious consequences (eg, patients with a history of difficult airway management or a high risk assessment for DVT/PE, physiologically compromised patients, elderly patients, children, neonatal patients);
   - complex or high-risk procedures that are performed infrequently;
   - care delivered that was inconsistent with nursing standards or guidelines (eg, incorrect counts, wrong site/side surgery or failure to verify procedure[s] or patient identity, medication errors, improper positioning, breaks in aseptic technique, lack of appropriate patient education);
   - acts of omission/commission;
   - patients receiving moderate or deep sedation (refer to JCAHO Standards [TX2]); and
   - patients undergoing multiple procedures or recurrent surgeries.
3. Problem-prone processes identify departmental problem areas. Problem-prone areas may include, but are not limited to,
   - procedures and/or care that cause patient and/or staff anxiety;
   - activities known to generate a number of incident reports;
   - activities needing increased efficiency (eg, surgery schedule management, instrument processing); and
   - equipment known to have a high risk or incidence of user error (eg, new equipment, infrequently used equipment, equipment that has been modified).

Standard IV

Systematic performance measures (ie, indicators) and/or priority areas are identified as opportunities for improvement based on the functions and processes of the perioperative episode.

Interpretive statement:
Performance measures (ie, indicators) should relate to the structure, process, or outcome of care and/or service.

Criteria:
1. Structure measures based on the AORN "Standards of perioperative administrative practice" relate to physical, fiscal, and organizational elements that require
   - establishing, controlling, and monitoring a safe perioperative environment (eg, technical and aseptic practice, electrical safety, physical facilities, occupational safety);
   - assessing, managing, and monitoring fiscal resources (eg, equipment, supplies, personnel, time); and
   - communicating and implementing organizational elements (eg, standards of nursing practice, such as care and professional performance, policies and procedures, staffing

763

patterns, orientation, staff development activities, quality assessment plans).
2. Process measures based on the AORN "Standards of perioperative clinical practice" and "Standards of perioperative professional practice" focus on activities of the nurse or process of nursing that require
   - implementation of the nursing process;
   - management of complications; and
   - adherence to policies and procedures (eg, correct site/side and identity verification, safe medication administration, specimen labeling, counting, positioning).
3. Outcome measures based on the AORN "Perioperative patient outcomes" relate to patient status following delivery of care that requires
   - emphasis on adverse events and complications; and
   - evaluation of measurable changes in patient health status (eg, free from injury, infection, nerve damage, altered skin integrity).
4. When selecting performance measures (ie, indicators), consideration should be given to the following issues:
   - departmental and organizational quality and safety goals;
   - accreditation standards and regulatory requirements;
   - perioperative clinical and service topics of national or local interest;
   - topics of greatest concern to patients and the community; and
   - trends of near misses for the purposes of improving processes.

Standard V

Establish performance expectations.

Interpretive statement 1:
The baselines for each of the measures are determined based on the measurement of the current process.

Criteria:
1. Baseline data should be gathered to establish the current level of performance.
2. Baseline data is used as a starting point for measurement.

Interpretive statement 2:
The baseline is evaluated and a determination is made whether there is an opportunity for improvement.

Criteria:
1. Evaluation of the baseline may be accomplished through analysis of collected data, peer review, literature review, etc.
2. A plan for improvement is thoughtfully designed. Tools such as flowcharts and process diagrams may be used to assist in identifying areas of the process with potential for failure.

Standard VI

Collect and organize data for evaluation.

Interpretive statement 1:
Data sources and methods of data collection/organization for each indicator are identified to establish a baseline of performance.

Criteria:
1. Existing sources of data are used. These may include, but are not limited to,
   - surgery schedule log,
   - staffing schedule,
   - incident reports,
   - perioperative documentation,
   - occurrence screens,
   - patient questionnaires,
   - patient records,
   - personnel credentialing/inservice records, and
   - postoperative visit/call log.
2. Other sources for data collection are used. These may include, but are not limited to,
   - direct observation of and inquiries regarding staff and patient care activities, and
   - physical site inspections.
3. Individuals collecting data have appropriate skill levels for the task being monitored and have the information system—or access to an individual who does—for inputting data and formulating meaningful reports.
4. Methods of data collection are concurrent and retrospective. These methods may include, but are not limited to,
   - chart review,
   - departmental reporting forms,
   - focused review,
   - occurrence screening,
   - peer review,
   - interviews, and
   - questionnaires/surveys.
5. Personnel are provided adequate time to participate in data collection and entry.
6. Personnel are encouraged to report incidents, adverse events, and hazardous conditions without fear of punitive action or retribution.

Interpretive statement 2:
The frequency of data collection and the sample size are sufficient to accumulate the necessary data.

Criteria:
1. The frequency of data collection is determined by the type of care or activity being monitored. This may include, but is not limited to,
   - the number of patients affected,
   - the degree of risk involved,

- the frequency of the event,
- the significance of the event or activity being monitored, and
- the extent to which the important aspect of care has been demonstrated to be problem free.
2. Data collection includes all sentinel events (eg, deaths, serious perioperative complications, near misses).
3. Data collection for performance measures is ongoing. A calendar of events is established to determine frequency of data collection for each indicator.
4. Sampling can be used to gather measurement data. Criteria such as volume, risk, and new procedure or provider can be used to determine an adequate sample size.[5]

Interpretive statement 3:
Data are organized, synthesized, and reported to allow for an accurate analysis of performance.

Criteria:
1. The quality of the data is evaluated to determine accuracy. This may be evaluated by answering questions such as the following.
   - Have all cases that were to be included in the study population been identified and reviewed?
   - Have all required data fields on the data collection instrument been completed?
   - Did the data gatherer(s) follow their explicit data collection instructions?
   - If the data were entered into a computerized database, did the edit/validation checks confirm the accuracy of the data?
   - If the data were obtained through electronic data transfer, did the edit/validation checks confirm the accuracy of the data?
2. Data collected over a period of time for each measure are aggregated for analysis purposes.
3. Aggregated measurement data are used to identify trends or patterns of performance that might not otherwise be evident in case-by-case review.
4. Statistical analysis techniques and comparative measurement data from outside sources are used to evaluate aggregated measurement data to identify significant undesirable variation from expected performance.

Standard VII
Evaluate care based on data collected.

Interpretive statement 1:
Analysis and evaluation of ongoing, collected data determines the need for action to improve the process(es).

Criteria:
1. Action is taken on adverse trends and patterns. The goal is for the care given to be congruent with perioperative nursing standards.
2. Analysis and evaluation of data collection is timely and provides efficacious opportunities for modifying actions/processes.

Interpretive statement 2:
Measurement data are compared with performance expectations.

Criteria:
1. Performance expectations are compared with actual performance to evaluate compliance with perioperative nursing standards of care and other important aspects of patient care and service.
2. Analysis of measurement data determines the need for more in-depth evaluation and/or initiation of an improvement project.
3. When performance consistently meets or exceeds expectations, the need for continued monitoring of that aspect of care/service is evaluated.
4. Evaluation of performance measurement data is timely.

Interpretive statement 3:
Initiate evaluation of important single events.

Criteria:
1. When an important single event occurs, a root cause analysis will be initiated in accordance with the organization's patient safety policies.
2. People knowledgeable about the systems and processes that affected the occurrence of the event are involved in the evaluation.
3. Evaluation of important single events are coordinated with other involved disciplines or departments.

Standard VIII
Take actions to improve care and services.

Interpretive statement 1:
Action plans/solutions are developed, supported, and approved at the appropriate levels and enacted to solve problems or improve care.

Criteria:
1. Identify the cause(s) of undesirable performance.
2. Corrective action plans are developed based on a thorough understanding of the process problems that are contributing to undesirable performance.
3. Actions are taken to correct defects in systems and/or processes. Actions may include revision of policies and procedures, staffing modifications, judicious use of equipment and supplies, and/or

QUALITY IMPROVEMENT

correction of communication or teamwork problems.

4. Relevant knowledge-based information is considered when developing action plans.
5. The plan of corrective action includes who or what is expected to change, individual(s) responsible for implementing the change, what action is needed to bring about the change, and when the change is expected to occur.
6. The action plan/solutions are forwarded to the body that has the authority to act, if the needed action exceeds the authority of the department. This may include, but is not limited to, the
   - administration,
   - board of trustees,
   - chief of service,
   - nursing/medical staff peer review committees,
   - ethics committee, and
   - OR committee.

Interpretive statement 2:
Actions for improvement are appropriate to the cause, scope, and severity of the problem.

Criteria:
1. Active reporting of errors and breaches in patient safety should be embraced without punitive action.
2. Whenever possible, corrective actions should be of a nonpunitive nature. They should be viewed as an opportunity for education and process improvement of the individual(s) involved, the department, and even the institution.
3. Punitive measures can be counterproductive to the goals of QI/PI and should only be used when appropriate (eg, blatant failure to follow policy resulting in injury and/or liability).
4. Actions are taken to correct knowledge deficits. Actions related to insufficient knowledge may require staff development, referral to other resources, and/or recommendations for continuing education.
5. Actions are taken to correct defects in the system. Actions related to systems may require revision of policies and procedures, staffing modifications, judicious use of equipment and supplies, a change in process, and/or correction of communication problems.
6. Actions are taken to correct deficient behavioral performances. Actions related to behavior or performance may require, but are not limited to,
   - education and training;
   - mentoring;
   - counseling;
   - increased supervision;
   - peer review; and
   - transfer, suspension, termination, or other disciplinary action.

Standard IX

Assess the effectiveness of action(s) and document outcomes.

Interpretive statement 1:
Actions are evaluated based on outcomes.

Criteria:
1. Actions delegated to individuals or disciplines for problem solving are monitored.
2. Effectiveness of actions is assessed through continuous monitoring of care. If an opportunity to improve care is identified and improvement does not occur, the action needs to be reevaluated.
3. A time line is established for reevaluation.
4. Further investigation of the cause of the problem and evaluation to identify the less obvious elements that contributed to the failure of the action plan must take place.

Interpretive statement 2:
Document the action plan and the method of communication.

Criteria:
1. A system is established to document the problem-solving process and the effectiveness in improving care or resolving the problem.
2. A system is established to document the results of the action plan, including trends and patterns that affect action.

Standard X

Communicate relevant information to the appropriate individuals, organization-wide, while maintaining confidentiality.

Interpretive statement 1:
The written organization-wide QI/PI plan identifies appropriate channels of communication.

Criteria:
1. Intradepartmental communication channels include, but are not limited to,
   - minutes of departmental meetings,
   - staff meetings, and
   - summary reports.
2. Conclusions, recommendations, actions, and findings are communicated to
   - departmental staff,
   - appropriate medical staff committees,
   - administration,
   - interdisciplinary committees,
   - organization-wide QI/PI committee,
   - governing body, and
   - accreditation and/or regulatory agencies as appropriate.

3. Confidentiality of QI/PI data is maintained. Maintenance of QI/PI data and all related communications shall comply with
   - federal Health Insurance Portability and Accountability Act (HIPAA) privacy and confidentiality regulations,
   - pertinent state regulations governing privacy and confidentiality of peer review and quality/performance data, and
   - organizational privacy and confidentiality policies and procedures.

Interpretive statement 2:
Personnel are informed of the conclusions, recommendations, actions, and findings.

Criteria:
1. Regularly scheduled staff and/or departmental meetings include quality improvement/performance improvement reports and activities.
2. Identified opportunities to improve care are addressed through staff development offerings, deploying changes in process and practice to staff.

Interpretive statement 3:
Results of the organization-wide quality improvement/performance improvement monitoring activities provide the opportunity to improve care and may have applicability in other areas in the organization.

Criteria:
1. Medical staff, administration, and the governing body use outcomes to determine clinical privileges and credentialing decisions.
2. Departmental managers use outcomes to objectively monitor staff performance, develop short- and long-range plans, measure performance, and contain costs.
3. Clinical practitioners use the outcomes of the QI/PI activities for self-assessment and peer review activities.

Models and Improvement Processes

The models and processes for performing QI/PI are numerous. More than one model can be used in an effective QI/PI program. No matter which method or model is used, the goal is to "Do the right thing, and do the right thing well."[3] AORN and the NPC are not endorsing any one model or any accrediting body. **Note:** More information is available in the *Notes* and *Resources* listed, or by using the Internet and searching under the terms *quality improvement* and *performance improvement*.

Glossary

Assessment: For purposes of performance improvement, the systematic collection and review of patient-specific data.

"For purposes of patient assessment, the process established by an organization for obtaining appropriate and necessary information about each individual seeking entry into a health care setting or service. The information is used to match an individual's need with the appropriate setting, care level, and intervention."[6]

Baseline: "A set of critical observations or data used for comparison or a control."[7]

Clinical practice guidelines: Systematically developed statements to assist practitioner and patient decisions about appropriate health care for specific clinical circumstances.

Concurrent: An activity that takes place in real time; care in progress.

Failure Mode and Effects Analysis (FMEA): A proactive approach to prevent or lessen the chances of a sentinel event from occurring, or reducing the risk/liability when an event occurs. This differs from root cause analysis, which is done after a sentinel event occurs and is a retrospective review of a process or processes. As with other QI/PI models, FMEA is an analysis technique drawn from non-medical industry. FMEA is an exercise that allows identification of the probabilities for "failure" at any point in the implementation of a process. In utilizing this technique, three questions must be answered:
- What are the steps of the process?
- Where is the process most likely to fail?
- How can we minimize the effects of these failures?

FMEA incorporates many of the same tools that are used in other QI/PI models. In determining the possible effects of potential failures, it is possible to quantify the likelihood, severity, and probability of detecting and preventing each failure. This allows providers to determine how critical each failure will be and give it a priority ranking. It allows one to avoid errors or failures before putting new processes in place.

JCAHO, in its leadership standards, addresses the requirements for the use of FMEA and root cause analysis by organizations seeking accreditation. These requirements are specific to the level of care provided by the organization.

Focused review: A formal review of one particular indicator, procedure, or practitioner over a specified time frame. It can be retrospective or concurrent.

Goal: The result that a department, service, or organization aims to accomplish. Also, a statement of attainment/achievement that is proposed to be accomplished or attained.[8]

Hazard analysis: The process of collecting and evaluating information on the circumstances leading to a higher risk for adverse outcomes. These circumstances or conditions are not related to the disease process or the condition for which the patient is being treated.

High risk: Patients at risk if the aspect of care is not provided correctly and in a timely manner. It may be that the patients themselves are at risk due to physical status, or it may be that the complexity and/or risk of complications related to the procedure puts the patients at risk.

High volume: The procedures or treatments that occur frequently, on a regular basis, or affect a large patient population.

Important aspects of care: Clinical or service-related activities that involve a high volume of patients, entail a high degree of risk for patients, or tend to produce problems for staff or patients. Such activities are deemed most important for purposes of monitoring and evaluation.[8]

Indicator: Well-defined, measurable, objective statement related to the structure, process, or outcomes of care; direct attention to problems or opportunities to improve care.[8]

Methodology: The strategies, models, or steps for gathering and analyzing the data in the quality improvement/performance improvement process.

Near miss: "Any process variation that did not affect the outcome, but for which a recurrence carries a significant chance of a serious adverse outcome. Such a near miss falls within the scope of the definition of a sentinel event, but outside the scope of those sentinel events that are subject to review by the Joint Commission under its Sentinel Event Policy."[6]

Nursing process: A systematic approach to nursing practice utilizing problem-solving techniques, including the components of assessment, planning, implementation, and evaluation.

Occurrence screens: Data that are used to identify individual variations in care, which are reviewed and confirmed by peer review and entered into a database to identify trends and/or patterns.[8]

Outcome identification: The intended, or realistically expected, correction of the patient's problem by a certain point in time.

Peer review: The examination and evaluation by associates of a practitioner's clinical practice. Individuals are evaluated by recognized, established standards. Physicians review physicians, registered nurses review registered nurse, etc.

Performance expectation: The desired condition or target level for each performance measure.

Performance measure: A quantitative tool (eg, rate, ratio, index, percentage) that provides an indication of an organization's performance in relation to a specified process or outcome. (See also *process measure* and *outcome measure.*)[6]

Population: The entire set of individuals sharing some common characteristics (eg, all patients with a particular disease, undergoing the same procedure, or of the same demographics).

Problem-prone: Those processes or steps that commonly generate incidents or barriers for patients and/or staff.

Process: A goal-directed, interrelated series of actions, events, mechanisms, or steps. An interrelated series of events, activities, actions, mechanisms, or steps that transform inputs into outputs.[6]

Retrospective: A review that begins with a current manifestation and links this effect to some occurrence in the past; post-discharge or post-procedure; not concurrent.

Root cause analysis: "A process for identifying the basic or causal factors that underlie variation in performance, including the occurrence or possible occurrence of a sentinel event. A root cause analysis focuses primarily on systems and processes, not individual performance. It progresses from special causes in clinical processes to common causes in organizational processes and identifies potential improvements in processes or systems that would tend to decrease the likelihood of such events in the future, or determines, after analysis that no such improvement opportunities exist."[9]

Sentinel event: "An unexpected occurrence involving death or serious physical or psychological injury, or the risk thereof. Serious injury specifically includes loss of limb or function. The phrase 'or the risk thereof' includes any process variation for which a recurrence would carry a significant chance of a serious adverse outcome. Such events are called 'sentinel' because they signal the need for immediate investigation and response."[9]

Standard: "A statement that defines the performance expectations, structures, or processes that must be substantially in place in an organization to enhance the quality of care."[6]

Structure: Organizational characteristics, fiscal resources, and management qualifications of health professionals; physical facilities and equipment; environment where care takes place.[10]

REFERENCES

1. T Bornstein, "Quality improvement and performance improvement: Different means to the same end?" *QA Brief* 9 (Spring 2001) http://www.qaproject.org/pdf/engv9n1.pdf (accessed 5 March 2003).

2. Institute of Medicine, *To Err is Human: Building a Safer Health System* (Washington, DC: National Academy Press, 2000) 114.

3. Joint Commission on Accreditation of Healthcare Organizations, "Improving organization performance," in *Hospital Accreditation Standards* (Oakbrook Terrace, Ill: Joint Commission on Accreditation of Healthcare Organizations, 2002) 161, 163.

4. Joint Commission on Accreditation of Healthcare Organizations, "Management of human resources," in *Hospital Accreditation Standards* (Oakbrook Terrace, Ill: Joint Commission on Accreditation of Healthcare Organizations, 2002) 234.

5. Joint Commission on Accreditation of Healthcare Organizations, "Management of information," in *Hospital Accreditation Standards* (Oakbrook Terrace, Ill: Joint Commission on Accreditation of Healthcare Organizations, 2002) 254.

6. Joint Commission on Accreditation of Healthcare Organizations, "Glossary," in *Hospital Accreditation Standards* (Oakbrook Terrace, Ill: Joint Commission on Accreditation of Healthcare Organizations, 2002) 331, 346, 351, 354, 360.

7. *Merriam-Webster's Collegiate Dictionary,* 10th ed (Springfield, Mass: Merriam-Webster, Inc., 1993) 95.

8. L A Kepler, E A Stuart, J Kiefel, "Ten-step template," *QRC Advisor* 6 (April 1990) 1-3.

9. Joint Commission on Accreditation of Healthcare Organizations, "Sentinel events," in *Hospital Accreditation Standards* (Oakbrook Terrace, Ill: Joint Commission on Accreditation of Healthcare Organizations, 2002) 51, 52.

10. Joint Commission on Accreditation of Healthcare Organizations, "Official accreditation policies and procedures," in *Hospital Accreditation Standards* (Oakbrook Terrace, Ill: Joint Commission on Accreditation of Healthcare Organizations, 2002) 48-49.

Resources

AORN, Inc. *Standards, Recommended Practices, and Guidelines.* Denver: AORN, Inc. Annual edition.

Joint Commission Resources. *Failure Mode and Effects Analysis in Health Care: Proactive Risk Reduction.* Oakbrook Terrace, Ill: Joint Commission on Accreditation of Healthcare Organizations, 2002.

Joint Commission Resources. *A Guide to Performance Measurement for Hospitals.* Oakbrook Terrace, Ill: Joint Commission on Accreditation of Healthcare Organization, 2000.

Joint Commission Resources. *A Pocket Guide to Using Performance Improvement Tools.* Oakbrook Terrace, Ill: Joint Commission on Accreditation of Healthcare Organization, 1996.

Joint Commission Resources. *Tools for Performance Measurement in Health Care: A Quick Reference Guide.* Oakbrook Terrace, Ill: Joint Commission on Accreditation of Healthcare Organization, 2002.

Organizational Dynamics. *Quality Action Teams: Team Members' Workbook.* Burlington, Mass: Organizational Dynamics, 1987.

Schroeder, P, ed. *Journal of Nursing Care Quality* Published quarterly by Lippincott Williams & Wilkins, Philadelphia.

Shewhart, W A; Deming, W E. *Statistical Method from the Viewpoint of Quality Control.* New York: Dover Publications, 1986.

Spath, P L. *Fundamentals of Health Care Quality Management.* Forest Grove, Ore: Brown-Spath & Associates, 2000.

Publication History

Originally published as "Quality improvement standards for perioperative nursing" in the 1992 *Standards and Recommended Practices for Perioperative Nursing.*

Revised; approved by the AORN Board of Directors in June 2003.

This document was previously published as part of the "Standards of perioperative nursing" as Exhibit D in the 2009 edition of *Perioperative Standards and Recommended Practices.*

Reformatted September 2012 for publication in *Perioperative Standards and Recommended Practices*, 2013 edition.

Minor editing revisions made in November 2014 for publication in *Guidelines for Perioperative Practice*, 2015 edition.

QUALITY IMPROVEMENT

INDEX

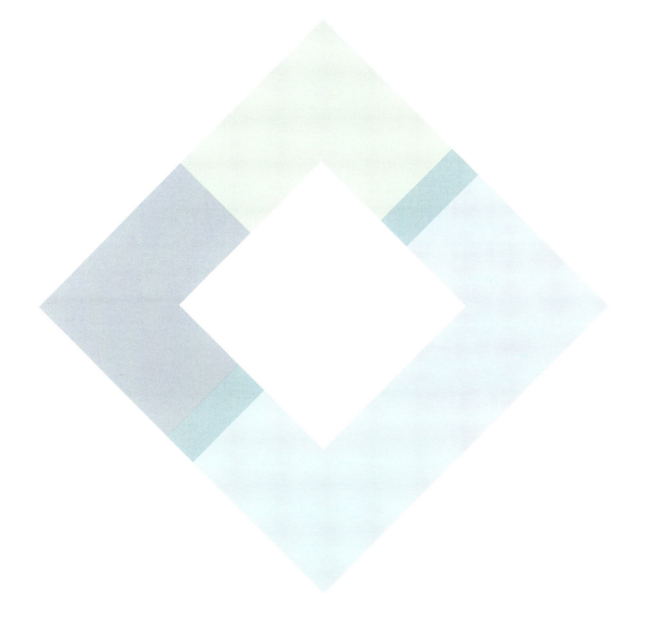

INDEX TO THE 2015 EDITION

A

absorbed dose, 341–342
accessories for electrosurgery, 121, 134, 599
accountability, 721–724
accreditation requirements, 499–500
accuracy of health care record, 499–500
active electrode. *See also* electrode
    bipolar, 129
    capacitive coupling, shielding for, 133, 546
    defined, 133, 546
    direct coupling from, 128
    for electrosurgery, 123–125
    gas emboli with, 128–129
    indicator shaft, 121, 133, 546
    injury minimization using, 123–125
    insulation failure of, 128
    insulation testing device for, 121, 133, 546
    monitoring, 95, 133, 546
    shielding of, 128
active skin warming, 484, 486
acupressure, 461
acupuncture, 461
addendum, 499–501, 503
additional complementary care interventions, 464–465
adjunct technologies, 356–357
administration, 301–308, 553
adsorption, 638–639, 644
adverse effects/reactions, 226–231
    of local anesthesia, 516–521
    to medication, 308
advocacy, 707
aeration/aerator, 674–675, 689
aerosol, 637, 644
aftercare instructions for medication, 308–310
agreement state, 399, 414
air
    dynamic removal of, 684, 686, 690
    laminar delivery system, 271, 285
    laser-generated contaminants from, 143, 150
    lateral transfer device using, 737, 748
    medical-grade compressed, 632, 644
    overhead delivery system for, 285
    ultra low particulate filter, 134, 150
airborne precautions, 424–426, 444, 452
airborne transmission
    contamination through, 13
    defined, 444
    infection isolation and, 425–426, 444
    in room, 425
air filter, high-efficiency particulate, 130, 143, 150
airflow displacement system, 284
alcohol
    antiseptic surgical hand rub based with, 34–35
    hand rub based with, 34, 40
    isopropyl, 593
    rinsing with, 593

alert alarm, 247, 258
alignment of body, 575–576
allograft, 215–216, 221, 231
alternate site injury, 127, 133, 533, 547
ambient temperature, 481, 486
Ambulatory Supplement: Guidelines, 5
    for medication safety, 330–334
    for radiological exposure, 345
    for retained surgical items, 364
    for safe environment of care, 264
    for transmissible infection, 452–454
amendments, 499–500, 503
American Association of Tissue Banks (AATB), 187, 231
American National Standards Institute, 121, 150
American Nursing Association (ANA)
    Code of Ethics for Nurses, 711–732
American Recovery and Reinvestment Act (ARRA), 493, 503
analgesia. *See* sedation
analytical phase, 405, 414
anesthesia. *See also* local anesthesia
    general, 555–556, 559
    intravenous regional, 153, 158–160, 165–166
    neuraxial, 486
Anesthesia Clinical Directors (AACD) glossary, 755–760
anesthetists, 568–575
anhydrous items, 689
anodized coating, 142, 150
anti-fatigue mats, 749
anti-fatigue technique, 749
antimicrobial surgical scrub agent, 34–35
antisepsis. *See* skin antisepsis
antiseptic agents. *See also* skin antisepsis
    alcohol-based surgical hand rub as, 34–35
    application of, 55–60
    in bath, 45–47
    defined, 61
    disposing, 60–61
    flammable, 60–61
    handling, 60–61
    manufacturer's instructions for, 60–61
    for perioperative skin, 49–55
    safety data sheets for, 60–61
    selecting, 49–55
    in shower, 45–47
    storing, 60–61
    surgical, 40
antiseptics. *See* antiseptic agents
anxiolytic, 559
apoptosis, 206, 231
apron, leaded, 340, 342
argon-enhanced coagulation (AEC), 133, 535, 547
aromatherapy, 461–462
artificial nails, 40, 46
aseptic technique/practices, 90. *See also* cleaning
    for high-level disinfection, 607

for packaging systems for sterilization, 654–655
assay, 394, 414
assessment, 695, 703, 767. *See also* specific types of
    in health care record, 491–492
assistant for laser, 141, 150
assisted gloving, 90
assistive devices/technology, 741, 745, 749
Association of periOperative Registered Nurses (AORN)
    Guidance Statement of, 733–751
    position statements of, 753
    Standards of, 709–710
attenuation, 338, 342
authentication, 498–503
authorized laser operator, 150
authorized operator for laser, 150
authorized user, 340–342
autograft, 221–222, 231. *See also* autologous tissue
    autotransplantation of, 211–217
    contaminated, 211–217, 223–226
    damaging, 223–226
    discarding, 211–217
    protecting, 220–226
    replantation of, 211–217
    securing, 220–226
autologous tissue. *See also* autograft; autologous tissue management
    autotransplantation of, 217–226
    bloodborne pathogen exposure and, 218–223
    defined, 231
    integrity of, 220
    labeling of, 218–220
    packaging of, 218–220
    replantation of, 217–226
    sterile technique for handling, 223–226
    storage of, 218–223
    tracking, 218–220
    transferring of, 217–218
    transporting of, 220
autologous tissue management, 187–232. *See also* autologous tissue
    competency assessment on, 227
    continuing education on, 227
    for cranial bone flap preservation/replantation, 194–203
    cross-contamination and, 218–220
    documentation during, 227–228
    evidence review on, 187–189
    during labeling, 218–220
    mix-ups during, 218–220
    multidisciplinary team for, 211–217
    during packaging, 218–220
    for parathyroid tissue cryopreservation/autotransplantation, 203–207
    patient confidentiality and, 220
    performance improvement during, 228–231
    for periodontal ligament cell validity, 189–194
    policies and procedures for, 226–227

principles of, 228–231
process of, 228–231
purpose of, 187
quality management program for, 228–231
risk assessment and, 211–217
safety during, 218–220
for skin preservation/autotransplantation, 207–209
sterile technique for, 223–226
during storing process, 220–223
for tracking purposes, 218–220
during transfers, 217–218
during transports, 220
for vein preservation/autotransplantation, 210–211
vs. other treatment options, 211–217
autolysis, 408, 414
automated endoscope reprocessor, 592, 598, 605, 610, 619
automated fluid management system, 542, 547
autotransplantation, 231
of autograft, 211–217
of autologous tissue, 217–226
of parathyroid tissue, 203–207
vein, 210–211
avulsion/avulsed tooth, 189–194, 231

B

baby, 479, 484, 486
background radiation, 398, 414
barrier material, 70, 77, 90
baseline, 352–353, 359, 764, 767
bath/bathing, 45–47
beam, 336–338, 342
bed for procedure, 575, 579
benzodiazepine, 555, 559
bioburden, 595, 598, 610, 627, 689
bioengineering services personnel, 123, 133
biofilms, 590, 598, 603, 610
biological indicator, 684–689
biomarker, 393, 414
biopsy forceps, 595
bipolar active electrode, 129
bipolar resection devices, 535, 547
blades, saw, 371–374
blood, transmissible infection through, 426–427
bloodborne pathogens, 382
from autologous tissue, 218–223
from sharps, 367–369
transmissible infection through, 426–427
Bloodborne Pathogen Standard (OSHA), 426–427
body alignment, 575–576
body mass index (BMI), 566, 578
body mechanics, 566–567
body temperature, core
defined, 486
hypothermia and, 481–482
during minimally invasive surgery, 543
monitoring of, 481–482
bone
cancellous, 225, 231
cranial, 194–203
cutters for, 371–374
fragments of, 371–374
borescope, 629, 644

borrowed laser, 139–140
Bowie-Dick test (Class 2 chemical indicator), 686, 689
Braden scale, 565, 578
brushes
for cleaning, 595
cytology, 595
building regulations, 525–529
burrs, 371–374

C

cancellous bone, 225, 231
cap, 595
capacitance, 128, 134, 534, 547
capacitive coupling, 121, 128, 134, 533, 547
active electrode shielding for, 133, 546
defined, 134, 547
electrosurgical unit, injury from, 123–124, 130
during minimally invasive procedures, 121, 128, 533
pad for, 127
risk of, 128, 533–534
capacitively coupled return electrode, 134
capacitor, 547
capillary interface pressure, 563, 575, 578
cavitation, 610, 627–628, 644
chain of custody, 397, 414
channels of flexible endoscope, 592
characteristic wastes, 256, 258
chemical disinfectants, 599, 604–607, 610
disposal of, 607
federal regulations on, 607
local regulations on, 607
safe environment of care, 607
state regulations on, 607
chemicals
disinfection using, 599, 604–607, 610
high-level disinfection using, 604–607
indicators for, 655–656, 661, 689–690
liquid, 678–679
in perioperative setting, 253–255
procurement of, 294–298, 330
safe environment of care using, 253–255
storage of, 294–298
chondrocyte, 215, 231
circulating-fluid garment, 486
Class 4 laser, 139, 150
Class 3 laser, 139, 150
cleaner, enzymatic, 596, 599. *See also* cleaning
cleaning. *See also* disinfection; environmental cleaning; surgical instrument cleaning and care
brushes for, 595
competency assessment on, 23–24
during construction, 20–23
continuing education on, 23–24
defined, 26, 599, 644
enhanced, 26, 445
evidence review on, 9–10
of flexible endoscope, 589–594
frequencies of, 10–12
high-level disinfection and, 601–604
manual, 592
multidisciplinary team for, 10–12
in perioperative practice setting, 10–12, 16–18
pneumatic tourniquet, 168
policies and procedures for, 20–24

precautionary measures during, 19–20
procedures for, 10–12
purpose of, 9
quality management program for, 24–26
of rigid sterilization container system, 657–658
for safe environment, 12–14
schedule for, 18–19
special procedures for, 20–23
sterilization guidelines and, 668–669
terminal, 16–18, 26
clinical practice
guidelines for, 767
information systems for, 493, 497, 503
support technologies for, 503
tools for, 749
closed assisted gloving, 90
closed gloving, 90
closing count, 355–356, 364
Clostridium difficile, 20–23
coagulation, argon-enhanced, 133, 535, 547
code key, 499, 503
Code of Ethics for Nurses with Interpretive Statements, 711–732
accountability, 721–724
collaboration with health professionals, 729
commitment to patient, 715–717
compassion, 712–715
conclusion, 731–732
health care environment, 726–727
introduction, 712
patients rights, 717–721
preamble, 712
preface, 711–712
professional advancements, 727–728
purpose of, 711
relationships, 712–715
respect, 712–715
self-care, 724–726
values, 729–731
cold ischemic time, 393–394, 414
collaboration, 700–701, 706
collegiality, 700, 705–706
colony forming unit, 70, 86, 90
combustible substance, 243, 255, 258
commissioning process, 266, 284
commitment to patient, 715–717
compartment syndrome, 168, 171, 572, 578
compassion, 712–715
competency assessment
autologous tissue management, 227
computer-assisted technologies, 543–544
deep vein thrombosis, 474–475
electrosurgery, 131–132
environmental cleaning, 23–24
flexible endoscope, 596–597
hand hygiene, 36
health care information management, 501
high-level disinfection, 607–608
hypothermia, 485
laser safety, 147
local anesthesia, 516–521
medication safety, 312–314
minimally invasive surgery, 543–544
packaging systems for sterilization, 658–659
patient information transfer, 585–586
pneumatic tourniquet, 168–169
product selection, 183

retained surgical items, 357
safe environment of care, 256–257
sedation/analgesia, 557–558
sterile technique, 89–90
sterilization guidelines, 682
transmissible infection, 436–438, 452
complementary patient care interventions
acupressure as, 461
acupuncture as, 461
additional, 464–465
aromatherapy as, 461–462
evidence review on, 455–456
hypnosis as, 462–463
massage therapy as, 460–461
music as, 456–460
purpose of, 455
Reiki therapy as, 463–464
compliance requirements, 494–498
compounding, 300–301, 323
compressed air, medical-grade, 632, 644
compressed medical gas cylinders, 249–250, 258, 264
compressive force, 749
computed tomography (CT), 200, 231
computer-assisted technologies/procedures, 544, 547
competency assessment on, 543–544
complications associated with, 536–539
continuing education on, 543–544
documentation during, 544–545
electrosurgical units used during, 533–536
injuries associated with, 536–543
minimally invasive surgery and, 533–539
multidisciplinary team approach to, 525–529
policies and procedures for, 545
risks of, 540–543
concurrent, 764, 767
Conference of Radiation Control Program Directors (CRCPD), 342
confidentiality
health care information management and, 498–499
of health care record, 498–499
for patient, 220
construction, 20–23
consultation, 697–698, 704
contact
direct, 421–423, 445
indirect, 422–423, 445
precautions during, 421–423, 444
return-electrode quality monitoring during, 134
transmissible infection through, 421–423
containers for specimens, 403–408
contamination/contaminants
through airborne transmission, 13
of autograft, 211–217, 223–226
of autologous tissue, 218–220
defined, 599
devices for, 653, 661
environmental, 20–23
of flexible endoscope, 590–591, 594–595
high-level disinfection and, 607
laser-generated airborne, 143, 150
microbial, 594–595
safe environment of care and preventing, 271–272

of sharps, 377–378
of specimens, 402–403, 414
sterile technique for preventing, 85–87
surgical instrument, 620–621, 623–624
continuing education
autologous tissue management, 227
cleaning, 23–24
computer-assisted technologies, 543–544
deep vein thrombosis, 474–475
electrosurgery, 131–132
electrosurgical units, 131–132
environmental cleaning, 23–24
hand hygiene, 36
health care information management, 501
high-level disinfection, 607–608
hypothermia, 485
laser safety, 147
local anesthesia, 516–521
medication safety, 312–314
minimally invasive surgery, 543–544
packaging systems for sterilization, 658–659
patient information transfer, 585–586
pneumatic tourniquet, 168–169
positioning of patient, 576–577
radiological exposure, 341
retained surgical items, 357
safe environment of care, 256–257
sharps safety, 378–379
sterile technique, 87–88
sterilization guidelines, 682
surgical instrument cleaning and care, 641
transmissible infection, 436–438, 452
contoured tourniquet cuffs, 159, 171
controlled access area, 150
controlled environment, 666–668
controlled terminology, 503
controls, engineering, 369–370, 382
cooling fluid, 530–531
coordination of care, 697, 705
cords, electrical, 123
core body temperature
defined, 486
equipment for, 481–482
hypothermia and, 481–482
during minimally invasive surgery, 543
monitoring of, 481–482
physiologic response to, 543
reliability of, 481–482
corneal eye shield, 143, 150
corrections, 503
to health care record, 499–500
counting discrepancies, 355–356, 364
coupling capacitor, 134, 547
active electrode shielding for, 133, 546
defined, 134, 547
electrosurgical unit, injury from, 123–124, 130
during minimally invasive procedures, 121, 128, 533
pad for, 127
risk of, 128, 533–534
cove base, 271, 284
cranial bone flap preservation/replantation, 194–203
craniectomy, 224, 231
cranioplasty, 225, 231
Creutzfeldt-Jakob disease, 603, 644
critical item, 599, 601, 610

cross-contamination, 218–220
cryopreservation, 203–207, 218, 231
cryoprotectant, 218, 231
cuff
contoured tourniquet, 159, 171
for pneumatic tourniquet, 162–165
cumulative effect, 34–36, 40
current, 132, 134
current orders for medication, 301–302
customization, 503
cytology brushes, 595
cytotoxicity, 214, 231

D

data
assessment of, 516
mining of, 502–503
quality of, 502–503
repository for, 500–501, 503
decontamination. See also cleaning; decontamination area; high-level disinfection (HLD)
defined, 599, 610, 644
of flexible endoscope, 595
prior to high-level disinfection, 601–604
of surgical instruments, 617–619, 624–626
decontamination area, 690. See also decontamination
for flexible endoscope, 590–591, 595–596
for surgical instrument, 617–624
for surgical instrument cleaning and care, 620–624
decontaminator, 644
deemed status, 495, 503
deep dose equivalent, 338, 342
deep sedation, 559
deep vein thrombosis (DVT)
competency assessment on, 474–475
continuing education on, 474–475
documentation on, 475
mechanical prophylaxis for, 471–472
perioperative assessment for, 471
pharmacologic prophylaxis for, 473–474
plan of care for, 469–470
policies and procedures for, 475
preventing, 469–470, 473–474
prophylactic measures for, 473–474
protocol for, 469–470
purpose of, 469
quality improvement program for, 475
risk factors for, 471
defective surgical instrument, 629–630
deflation of pneumatic tourniquet, 165–168
delivery/delivering
of items following high-level disinfection, 607
medication, 294–298, 330
devices. See equipment; positioning equipment/devices
diagnosis. See nursing diagnosis
diagnostic radionuclides, 339–340, 345
digital OR, 527, 547
digital signature, 499, 503
digitized inked signatures, 499, 503
dilutional hyponatremia, 542–543, 547
direct contact, 421–423, 445

2015 INDEX

direct coupling, 128, 134, 547
direct radiological exposure, 340–341
discharge, 308–310, 557
disinfectants. *See also* disinfection
    chemical, 599, 604–607, 610
    hospital, 602, 610
    low-level, 115
disinfection. *See also* disinfectants; high-level disinfection (HLD)
    aseptic technique for, 607
    chemical, 604–607
    cleaning prior to, 601–604
    competency assessment on, 607–608
    continuing education on, 607–608
    of critical item, 601
    decontamination prior to, 601–604
    defined, 22–24, 26, 599, 610
    documentation during, 608–609
    high-level, 599, 610
    intermediate-level, 610
    low-level, 26, 611
    of noncritical item, 601
    pasteurization and, 604
    policies and procedures for, 20–23
    policies and procedures on, 609
    procedures for, 10–12
    purpose of, 601
    quality management program for, 609–610
    safe environment for, 607
    of semicritical item, 601
    thermal, 604
    using chemicals, 599, 604–607, 610
dispensing medication, 300–301, 330–332
dispersive electrode, 132, 134
displacement airflow system, 284
displacement of gravity, 603, 639, 690
disposing/disposal
    of antiseptic agents, 60–61
    of chemical disinfectants, 607
    of medication, 311–312, 332–333
    of sharps, 377–378
    of surgical attire, 109–113
distance, 339, 342
distention media, 530–531
distilled water, 631–633, 644
distraction, 284–285
documentation. *See also* nursing documentation
    autologous tissue management, 227–228
    computer-assisted technologies, 544–545
    deep vein thrombosis, 475
    electrosurgery, 132
    flexible endoscope, 597
    health care information management, 492–498
    high-level disinfection, 608–609
    hypothermia, 485–486
    laser safety, 148–149
    local anesthesia, 516
    medication safety, 314–316
    minimally invasive surgery, 544–545
    patient information transfer, 586
    pneumatic tourniquet, 169–170
    positioning of patient, 577–578
    product selection, 184
    radiological exposure, 340–341
    retained surgical items, 357–358
    safe environment of care, 257
    sedation/analgesia, 558–559

sharps safety, 379–380
specimen management, 413–414
sterile technique, 88–89
sterilization guidelines, 682
surgical instrument cleaning and care, 640–641
synchronized, 492–493
transmissible infection, 439–440, 452
donning, 71–76
donning gloves, 34–35
dosage/dosing
    absorbed, 341–342
    deep, equivalent, 338, 342
    external, 342
    internal, 342
    occupational, 338, 342
    shallow, 342
    total effective, 342–343
dosimeter, 340, 342
downtime, 499, 503, 688, 690
drapes, 69–71, 76–78
drill bits, 371–374
droplet precautions, 423–424, 445, 452
dry-heat sterilization guidelines, 677–678
dual foil electrode, 134
Dulbecco's modified Eagle's medium, 205, 231
duration of limiting-exposure, 150
dust cover, 651, 661
dwell time, 11, 26
dynamic air removal, 684, 686, 690

E

Eagle's minimum essential medium, 222, 231
ears, 113–114
ebonized finish, 142, 150
education, 699, 705. *See also* patient education
electrical cords, 123
electrical equipment injury, 246–247
electrical hazard, 145
electrode. *See also* active electrode
    capacitively coupled return, 134
    dispersive, 132, 134
    dual foil, 134
    return, 134
electronic health record (EHR), 493, 503
electronic information systems, 702
electronic medical record (EMR), 493, 503
electronic signature, 503
electroplating, 627, 644
electrosurgery. *See also* electrosurgical units (ESUs)
    accessories for, 121
    active electrodes for, 123–125
    argon enhanced coagulation for, 129–130
    bipolar, 133–134
    bipolar active electrodes for, 129
    competency assessment on, 131–132
    continuing education on, 131–132
    defined, 134
    dispersive electrode for, 125–128
    documentation during, 132
    improvement process for, 133
    injuries during, 122–123
    during minimally invasive surgery, 128–129
    monopolar, 125–128, 134

    policies and procedures for, 132–133
    purpose of, 121
    quality management program for, 133
    risks of, 121
    safety during, 121
    surgical smoke during, hazards of, 130–131
    vessel occluding devices for, 129
electrosurgical accessories, 121, 134, 599
electrosurgical tips, 371–374
electrosurgical units (ESUs)
    capacitive coupling, injury from, 123–124, 130
    computer-assisted technologies and, 533–536
    continuing education on, 131–132
    defined, 134
    electrical cords for, 123
    ground-referenced, 127–128, 134
    injury from, minimization when using, 121–123
    isolated, 134
    minimally invasive surgery and, 533–536
    new, 121
    plugs on, 123
    purchasing, 121
    refurbished, 121
    safety features of, 121
    selecting, 121
    ultrasonic, 129
emergency spill plan, 675, 690
endoscope. *See also* flexible endoscope
    accessories for (*See* flexible endoscope)
    automated reprocessor for, 592, 598, 605, 610, 619
    minimally invasive procedure using, 134
    surgery using, 547
energy transfer pads, 483, 486
engineering controls, 369–371, 382
engrafting, 195, 231
enhanced cleaning, 26, 445
environment. *See also* safe environment of care
    contamination in, 20–23
    controlled, 666–668
    in health care, 726–727
    oxygen-enriched, 125, 134, 146, 150
    reestablishment of clean, 14–16
environmental care. *See* safe environment of care
environmental cleaning. *See also* safe environment of care
    competency assessment on, 23–24
    during construction, 20–23
    continuing education on, 23–24
    enhanced, 26, 445
    evidence review on, 9–10
    following transfers, 14–16
    frequencies of, 10–12
    microorganism transmission and, 19–20
    multidisciplinary team for, 10–12
    for patient, 12–14
    performance improvement program for, 24–26
    in perioperative practice setting, 10–12, 16–18
    policies and procedures for, 20–24
    precautionary measures during, 19–20
    procedures for, 10–12
    purpose of, 9

quality management program for, 24–26
reestablishment of clean environment, 14–16
for safe environment, 12–14
schedule for, 18–19
special procedures for, 20–23
terminal, 16–18
enzymatic cleaner, 596, 599
equipment, 18–19, 342. *See also* instruments; personal protective equipment (PPE); positioning equipment; surgical instruments
for core body temperature, 481–482
Guidance Statement of AORN, 743–748
operator for, 342
radiographic, 341
ergonomics, 567, 578, 735, 749
ergonomist, 749
errors in medication, 292–294, 298–300, 330
eschar, 124, 134
ethics, 701, 706
ethyl, 593
ethylene oxide, 673–675
evaluation, 698, 704–705
of health care record, 491–492
of packaging systems for sterilization, 652–653
of perioperative administrative practice standards, 704–705
of perioperative nursing standards, 698
of products, 184
of professional practice, 699–700, 705
of surgical instrument cleaning and care, 629–630
event-related sterility, 90
evidence, forensic, 396, 414
evidence-based design, 266, 285
examination, gross, 412–414
exposure, 342. *See also* radiological exposure
bloodborne pathogens, 367–369
incidents of, 445
laser beam, 141–142
limiting, 150
maximum permissible, 141, 150
short-term, 690
exsanguination, 162, 171
external dose, 342
extravasation, 543, 547
eye shield, corneal, 143, 150
eyewear, 142–143

F

facial hair, 113–114
Failure Mode and Effects Analysis (FMEA), 767
family members, 585
federal regulations, 499–500
on chemical disinfectants, 607
on medication, 311–312
on operating rooms, 525–529
fibroblasts, 192–193, 231
filter
high-efficiency particulate air, 130, 143, 150
hydrophobic insufflation, 547
ultra low particulate air, 134, 150
filtration masks, high, 131, 144, 150
fingernails, 31–33

fire retardant material, 150
fire safety, 242–246
flame retardant material, 150
flammable antiseptic agents, 60–61
flammable hazard, 145–146
flammable substance, 256, 258
flash point, 243, 258
flexible endoscope
alcohol rinse for, 593
automatic endoscope reprocessor for, 592, 598, 605, 610, 619
channels of, 592
cleaning of, 589–594
competency assessment on, 596–597
contamination of, 590–591, 594–595
damaging, 594–595
decontamination area for, 590–591, 595–596
decontamination of, 595
documentation for, 597
flushing, 593
function of, 593–594
high-level disinfection of, 592–593
inspection of, 593–595
integrity of, 593–594
leak testing capabilities of, 591–592
manual cleaning of, 592
manufacturer's written instructions for, 589–590, 593
microbial contamination of, 594–595
organic material on, 590–592, 595–596
personal protective equipment for handling, 596
policies and procedures for, 597–598
precleaning of, 590–591
pressure tests on, 591–592
purpose of, 589
quality management program for, 598
rinsing, 593
sterilization of, 592–593
storage of, 589–590, 594–595
fluid
automated management system for, 542, 547
circulating garment, 486
complications associated with, 540–543
cooling, 530–531
deficit in, 547
injuries from, 540–543
irrigation, 530–531, 540–543
management of, 531–533
for minimally invasive surgery, 530–533, 540–543
retention of, 543
temperature of, 530–531
warming, 530–531
fluoroscopy, 338, 342
flush/flushing, 593
focused review, 767
fomite, 12, 26, 114
force, 749
maximum sustained, 737, 739, 749
forced-air warming, 483–484, 486
forceps for biopsy, 595
forensic evidence, 396, 414
free-rinsing, 610
friction, 575–576, 578
devices for reducing, 749

G

gamma radiation, 335, 342
garment for circulating fluid, 486
gas
cylinders for, 249–250, 258, 264
hydrogen peroxide, 653, 661
industrial, 249, 258
gas distention media, 539–543
gas embolism, 128–129
general anesthesia, 555–556, 559
generator, 129, 134
germicide. *See* disinfectant
gloves/gloving
assisted, 90
closed, 90
closed assisted, 90
donning, 34–35
open, 76, 90
open assisted, 73, 90
sterile technique, 69–76
for surgical procedures, 34–35
goal, 767
gonad, 342
gonad shield, 342
gossypiboma, 349, 359
gowns, 69–76
gravity displacement, 603, 639, 690
gross examination of specimen, 412–414
gross soil, 626–627, 644
ground-referenced electrosurgical units, 127–128, 134
Guidance Statement of AORN, 733–751
equipment, 743–748
lifting of patient, 741–742
positioning of patient, 737–741
prolonged standing, 742
retraction, 742–743
safe handling patient, 734–752
transferring of patient, 735–737

H

hair, 47–49, 113–114
hand hygiene
competency assessment on, 36
continuing education on, 36
defined, 40
fingernails and, 31–33
improvement programs for, 37–40
jewelry and, 31–33
in perioperative setting, 31–33
policies and procedures for, 36–37
purpose of, 31
quality management program for, 37–40
skin cleansing and, 31–33
standardized procedure for, 33–34
surgical hygiene product for, 34–36
US Food and Drug Administration requirements for, 34–35
hand rub, alcohol-based, 34, 40
hands-free technique, 372, 382
Hank's Balanced Salt Solution, 189–191, 231
hazards
analysis of, 767
electrical, 145
flammable, 145–146
of lasers, 142–143
of medication, 310–311
nominal zone, 142–143, 150
with positioning of patient, 567

surgical smoke, 130–131, 143–144
head, 113–114
health-care acquired transmissible infection, 430–433
health care information management. *See also* health care record; nursing documentation
    accreditation requirements and, 499–500
    competency assessment on, 501
    compliance requirements for, 494–498
    confidentiality and, 498–499
    continuing education on, 501
    documentation for, 492–498
    federal regulations on, 499–500
    national practice guidelines for, 499–500
    nursing diagnosis and, 491–492
    outcome identification and, 491–492
    patient assessment and, 491–492
    plan of care and, 491–492
    policies and procedures for, 501–502
    progress evaluation and, 491–492
    purpose of, 491
    quality management program for, 502–503
    security and, 498–499
    state regulations on, 499–500
    unauthorized disclosure and, 498–499
health care laser system, 140, 150
health care organization policies, 311–312
health care personnel activity restrictions, 435–436
health care record. *See also* medical care record
    accuracy of, 499–500
    addendums in, 499–500
    amendments to, 499–500
    assessment in, 491–492
    confidentiality of, 498–499
    corrections to, 499–500
    diagnosis in, 491–492
    electronic, 493, 503
    evaluation in, 491–492
    interoperable, 493, 504
    modification of, 499–500
    outcome identification in, 491–492
    patient care continuum in, 493–494
    plan of care in, 491–492
    security of, 498–499
    unauthorized disclosure of, 498–499
health care system. *See also* health care information management; medical care; patient care
    environment in, 726–727 (*See also* safe environment of care)
    important aspects of, 768
    laser in, 139–140, 150
    laundry facilities accredited in, 99, 102, 114
Health Information Technology for Economic and Clinical Health (HITECH), 503–504
health professionals, collaboration with, 729
health promotion, 697, 704
health teaching, 697, 704
heat-stable items, 669–671, 673–679
helmet system, surgical, 74–75, 90
hemacytometer, 205, 231
high-efficiency particulate air filter (HEPA), 130, 143, 150

high filtration masks, 131, 144, 150
high-level disinfection (HLD)
    aseptic technique for, 607
    chemical, 604–607
    cleaning prior to, 601–604
    competency assessment on, 607–608
    contamination and, 607
    continuing education on, 607–608
    of critical item, 601
    decontamination prior to, 601–604
    delivery of items following, 607
    documentation during, 608–609
    of flexible endoscope, 592–593
    of noncritical item, 601
    pasteurization and, 604
    policies and procedures on, 609
    purpose of, 601
    quality management program for, 609–610
    reprocessing of items using, 601
    safe environment for, 607
    of semicritical item, 601
    surgical instrument, 617–619
    thermal, 604
    US Food and Drug Administration-cleared agents for, 604–607
high radiation area, 342
high risk, 767–768
high touch, 21, 25–26
high volume, 763, 768
homogenate tissue, 638, 644
hospital disinfectant, 602, 610
HVAC system, 272–278
hybrid OR, 529, 544, 547
hydrogen peroxide gas plasma sterilization, 653, 661
hydrogen peroxide vapor sterilization, 653, 661, 676
hydrophobic, 540, 638, 644
hydrophobic insufflation filter, 547
hygiene for hands
    competency assessment on, 36
    continuing education on, 36
    defined, 40
    fingernails and, 31–33
    improvement programs for, 37–40
    jewelry and, 31–33
    in perioperative setting, 31–33
    policies and procedures for, 36–37
    purpose of, 31
    quality management program for, 37–40
    skin cleansing and, 31–33
    standardized procedure for, 33–34
    surgical hygiene product for, 34–36
    US Food and Drug Administration requirements for, 34–35
hypervolemia, 539–540, 547
hypnosis, 462–463
hypodermic needles, 371–374
hyponatremia, 542–543, 547
hypothermia
    competency assessment on, 485
    continuing education on, 485
    core temperature monitoring for, 481–482
    defined, 547
    documentation and, 485–486
    improvement program for, 486
    injuries caused by, 485
    interventions for preventing, 483–486
    mild, 486
    patient assessment for, 485–486

    performance improvement process for, 486
    plan of care for, 481, 485–486
    policies and procedures for, 486
    purpose of, 479
    quality management program for, 486
    redistribution, 487
    risk assessment for, 479–481
    unplanned perioperative, 479–481, 483–485
    warming devices for minimizing, 485
hysteroscopy, 534–535, 547

I

iatrogenic transmission, 604, 610
identification
    issues, 703
    outcome, 491–492, 703–704, 768
    radio-frequency, 360, 406, 414
    site, 392, 414
    specimen, 392–393, 414
    trend, 703
immediately available, 558, 560
immediate surgical instruments cleaning and care, 619–620
immediate use steam sterilization (IUSS), 671–673, 690
immunizations, 433–435
implementation, 696–697, 704
improvement program
    electrosurgery, 133
    hand hygiene, 37–40
    hypothermia, 486
    medication safety, 320–323, 333–334
indicator, 768
    for chemicals, 655–656, 661, 689–690
indicator shaft for active electrode, 121, 133, 546
indirect contact, 421–423, 445
indirect radiological exposure, 340–341
industrial gases, 249, 258
infant, 479, 484, 486
infection. *See also* transmissible infection
    airborne transmission and isolation of, 425–426, 444
infection preventionist, 179, 211–217, 424, 445
inflation of pneumatic tourniquet, 162–165
information management in health care. *See also* health care record; nursing documentation
    accreditation requirements and, 499–500
    competency assessment on, 501
    compliance requirements for, 494–498
    confidentiality and, 498–499
    continuing education on, 501
    documentation for, 492–498
    federal regulations on, 499–500
    national practice guidelines for, 499–500
    nursing diagnosis and, 491–492
    outcome identification and, 491–492
    patient assessment and, 491–492
    plan of care and, 491–492
    policies and procedures for, 501–502
    progress evaluation and, 491–492
    purpose of, 491
    quality management program for, 502–503

security and, 498–499
state regulations on, 499–500
unauthorized disclosure and, 498–499
information systems. *See also* information management in health care; information transfer for patient care
clinical, 493, 497
clinical practice, 503
electronic, 702
perioperative, 501–503
information transfer for patient care
competency assessment on, 585–586
continuing education on, 585–586
development of process for, 583–585
documentation during, 586
evidence for, 583–585
family members involvement in, 585
patients involvement in, 585
policies and procedures for, 586
purpose of, 583
quality management program for, 586–587
significant others involvement in, 585
standardization process for, 583–585
injuries
from active electrode, 123–125
alternate site, 127, 133, 533, 547
from computer-assisted technologies, 536–543
from electrical equipment, 246–247
from electrosurgery, 122–123
from electrosurgical units, 121–123
from fluid, 540–543
from gas distention media, 539–543
from hypothermia, 485
from minimally invasive surgery, 536–539
musculoskeletal, 742, 749
occupational, 240–241
from positioning of patient, 563–564, 576
from sharps, 378, 382
thermal, 247–248
inspection
of flexible endoscope, 593–595
of packaging systems for sterilization, 656
of positioning equipment, 565
of rigid sterilization container system, 657–658
sterilization guidelines and, 668–669
of surgical instrument, 629–630
during surgical instrument cleaning and care, 629–630
instructions for use (IFU)
for packaging/package, 654–658
surgical instruments cleaning and care, 616–619, 624–629
instruments, 359. *See also* equipment; surgical instruments
case/cassette for, 661
loaned, 679–680
retained, 353–354
insufflate/insufflation, 539, 547
insulation
failure of, 128, 134
passive, 487
testing devices for, 121, 133, 546
insulator, 134
integrated OR, 527, 544, 547
integrity, 504
of autologous tissue, 220

of flexible endoscope, 593–594
of package, 661
of skin, 575–576
of specimen, 393–402
interdisciplinary collaboration, 553–554
internal dose, 342
interoperable health records, 493, 504
interruption in work, 282, 285
interventional radiology, 525–529
interventions, 483–486. *See also* complementary patient care interventions
intracorporeal mobile devices, 525, 547
intraocular ophthalmic surgical instrument, 630–633
intraoperative positioning of patient, 576
intraoperative monitoring, 482
intravasation, 541–542, 547
intravenous regional anesthesia, 153, 158–160, 165–166
invasive procedure, 83, 86, 90
positioning equipment/devices for, 564–565
retained surgical items for, 348–349
sterile technique during, 68–69, 78–81
in vitro, 520, 610
iodism, 54–55, 61
ionizing radiation, 335, 342
irrigation fluid, 530–533, 540–543
isolated electrosurgical units, 134
isolation
precautions during, 443, 445
techniques for, 79, 90
isopropyl alcohol rinse/flush, 593
isotonic solution, 225, 231
issues identification, 703

J

jewelry, 31–33

K

Krebs-Ringer solution, 210, 231
K-wires, 371–374

L

labeling
of autologous tissue, 218–220
autologous tissue management during, 218–220
of packaging systems for sterilization, 658
of specimen, 414
sterilization guidelines and, 680–681
Lactobacillus reuteri, 190–191, 231
laminar air delivery system, 271, 285
laparoscopy, single-port access, 547
laryngoscope blades/handles, 633–635
laser assistant, 141, 150
laser beam exposure, 141–142
lasers. *See also* laser safety
airborne contaminants generated by, 143, 150
authorized operator for, 139, 150
borrowed, 139–140
Class 4, 139, 150
Class 3, 139, 150
controlled access to area for, 141
defined, 150
hazard zone for, 142–143

in health care system, 139–140, 150
leased, 139–140
treatment area for, 141, 145, 150
unintentional beam exposure from, 141–142
users of, 141–142, 150
laser safety
competency assessment on, 147
continuing education on, 147
documentation and, 148–149
electrical hazard and, 145
eyewear for, 142–143
flammable hazard and, 145–146
laser area, controlled access to, 141
laser beam exposure and, 141–142
Laser Safety Officer's role in, 142–143
performance program for, 149–150
policies and procedures for, 148
program for, 139–140
purpose of, 139
quality management program for, 149–150
surgical smoke hazard and, 143–144
unintentional beam exposure and, 141–142
Laser Safety Officer (LSO), 142–143, 145, 147, 150
laser safety specialist, 139, 140, 150
lateral position, 737–739, 749
lateral transfer, 749
air-assisted device for, 737, 748
mechanical device for, 570, 749
laundering of surgical attire, 109–113
laundry facility, health care-accredited, 99, 102, 114
leaded apron, 340, 342
leadership, 702–703, 707
leak testing capabilities, 591–592
leased laser, 139–140
licensed independent practitioner, 553, 555, 560
lift device, mechanical, 749
lifting index, 747–749
lifting of patient, 565–567, 741–742
light cable, 537–538, 547
limb occlusion pressure (LOP), 159, 163, 171
limiting-exposure duration, 150
liquid chemicals, 678–679
liquid oxygen containers, 249–250, 264
lithotomy position, 739–741, 749
loaned instruments, 617–619, 679–680
loaned items, 617, 644
local anesthesia
adverse effects of, 516–521
competency assessment on, 516–521
continuing education on, 516–521
contraindications for, 516–521
data assessment and, 516
documentation during, 516
evidence review on, 513–514
monitoring during, 516
nursing diagnosis and, 516
patient education on, 521–522
pharmacology for, 516–521
physiological response to, 516
plan of care and, 516
policies and procedures for, 522
preoperative nursing assessment for, 514–516
psychological response to, 516
purpose of, 513

2015 INDEX

resuscitation and, 516–521
systemic toxicity of, 518–519, 522
local regulations, 607
  on medication, 311–312
  on operating rooms, 525–529
log reduction, 50, 61
long-term expansion services, 525–529
low-temperature hydrogen peroxide gas plasma sterilization, 675–676
low-temperature hydrogen peroxide vapor sterilization, 676–677
lumen, 632–633, 644

M

malware, 498, 504
manual cleaning, 592
manual count procedures, 356–357
manual retraction, 742, 749
manufacturer instructions/guidelines
  antiseptic agents, 60–61
  flexible endoscope, 589–590, 593
  medication, 311–312
  packaging/package, 654–655
  pneumatic tourniquet, 168
  positioning equipment, 567–568
  rigid sterilization container system, 657–658
  skin antisepsis, 60–61
  sterilization, 666–668
  surgical instrument cleaning and care, 616–617
masks
  for high filtration, 131, 144, 150
  for procedure, 430, 445
  surgical, 106–107, 115, 420, 445
massage therapy, 460–461
materials
  barrier, 70, 77, 90
  fire retardant, 150
  flame retardant, 150
  labeling of, 680–681
  nonwoven, 653, 661
  organic, 590–592, 595–596
  for packaging/package, 652–654
  potentially infectious, 379–380, 382
  viscoelastic, 564, 644
  wastes, 19–20
mats, anti-fatigue, 749
maximum permissible exposure, 141, 150
maximum sustained force, 737, 739, 749
McCoy's 5A medium, 209, 231
mechanical lateral transfer device, 570, 749
mechanical lift device, 749
mechanical prophylaxis, 471–472
medical care record
  accuracy of, 499–500
  addendums in, 499–500
  amendments to, 499–500
  assessment in, 491–492
  confidentiality of, 498–499
  corrections to, 499–500
  diagnosis in, 491–492
  electronic, 493, 503
  evaluation in, 491–492
  interoperable, 493, 504
  modification of, 499–500
  outcome identification in, 491–492
  patient care continuum in, 493–494
  plan of care in, 491–492
  security of, 498–499

unauthorized disclosure of, 498–499
medical gas cylinders, compressed, 249–250, 258, 264
medical-grade compressed air, 632, 644
medical waste, regulated, 20, 26
medication
  administration of, 301–308
  adverse reactions to, 308
  aftercare instructions for, 308–310
  competency assessment on, 312–314
  continuing education on, 312–314
  current orders for, 301–302
  delivering, 294–298, 330
  discharge and, 308–310
  dispensing of, 300–301, 330–332
  disposal of, 311–312, 332–333
  documentation of, 314–316
  errors in, 292–294, 298–300, 330
  federal regulations on, 311–312
  handling, 307–308
  hazardous, 310–311
  health care organization policies on, 311–312
  history of, 301–302
  irrigation fluid and, 531–533
  local regulations on, 311–312
  management of, 292–294
  manufacturer's instructions on, 311–312
  monitoring of, 308
  nursing medication plan for, 302–303
  patient assessment for, 301–302
  patient education plans on, 308–310
  perioperative, 300–301
  plan of care and, 302–303, 332
  preparing, 303–307
  procurement of, 294–298, 330
  safety while handling, 307–308
  sedation, 555–556
  special care when handling, 310–311
  state regulations on, 311–312
  storage of, 294–298, 330
  therapeutic effect of, 308
  transcribing of, 300
  transfers of, 307–308
  verifying, 303–307
medication safety. See also medication
  aftercare instructions for, 308–310
  Ambulatory Supplement, 330–334
  competency assessment on, 312–314
  continuing education on, 312–314
  documentation for, 314–316
  during handling, 307–308
  following discharge, 308–310
  improvement programs for, 320–323, 333–334
  medication plan for, 302–303
  multidisciplinary team approach to, 292–294, 330
  patient education plan for, 308–310
  performance improvement process for, 320–323
  perioperative assessment and, 301–302
  by pharmacists, 300–301, 330–332
  policies and procedures for, 316–320, 333
  purpose of, 291–292
  quality management programs for, 320–323, 333–334
  in sterile field, 307–308
medicine. See medication
meshed skin, 208, 231
methodology, 768

metric weight, 301–302
microbial contamination, 594–595
microorganism transmission, 19–20
mild hypothermia, 486
minimally invasive surgery (MIS)
  capacitive coupling during, 121, 128, 533
  competency assessment on, 543–544
  complications associated with, 536–539
  computer-assisted devices for, 533–539
  continuing education on, 543–544
  contraindications during, 531–533
  core body temperature during, 543
  defined, 359, 547
  documentation during, 544–545
  electrosurgery during, 128–129
  electrosurgical units used during, 533–536
  endoscope, 134
  fluids for, 530–533, 540–543
  gas distention media from, 539–543
  injuries associated with, 536–539
  multidisciplinary team approach to, 525–529
  in operating rooms, 525–529
  patient assessment for, 531–533
  performance improvement during, 545–546
  physiologic response to, 543
  policies and procedures for, 545
  precautions during, 531–533
  purpose of, 525
  quality management program for, 545–546
  risks of, 536–539
minimum effective concentration, 590, 599, 605, 611
miscellaneous items, 351–353, 359
missing items, 355–356, 364
mitochondria, 206, 231
mobile devices, intracorporeal, 525, 547
moderate sedation, 560
moisture-stable items, 669–671, 673–679
monitor/monitoring
  active electrode, 95, 133, 546
  core body temperature, 481–482
  intraoperative, 482
  local anesthesia, 516
  medication, 308
  physical, 685, 690
  pneumatic tourniquet, 164–165
  postoperative, 482
  preoperative, 482
  radiological exposure, 340
  return-electrode contact quality, 134
  sedation, 555–557
  sterile technique, 83–85, 690
  sterilization process device, 690
monolithic surface, 271, 285
monopolar electrosurgery, 125–128, 134
morbid obesity, 574, 578
Morus rubra, 191, 231
moving patient, 565–567
multidisciplinary team/committee
  autologous tissue management, 211–217
  cleaning, 10–12
  computer-assisted technologies, 525–529
  environmental cleaning, 10–12
  medication safety, 292–294, 330
  minimally invasive surgery, 525–529

product selection, 179–183
retained surgical items, 348–349
safe environment of care, 265–266
skin antisepsis, 49–55
multidose vial, 312, 323
multidrug-resistant organisms, 20–23
musculoskeletal injury, 742, 749
music, 456–460
Mylar, 656–657

N

nails, artificial, 40, 46
nanotechnologies, 525, 547
national practice guidelines, 499–500
natural orifice transluminal endoscopic surgery (NOTES), 538, 547
natural rubber latex protocol, 251–253
near miss incidents, 360, 644, 765, 768
needles, 371–374
neonate, 484, 486
neuraxial anesthesia, 486
neutral zone, 372–373, 382
newborn, 479, 484, 486
new electrosurgical units, 121
new surgical instrument, 617–619
Newton (N), 742, 745, 749
Newton meter (Nm), 742, 749
nidus, 611
noise, 283–285
nominal hazard zone, 142–143, 150
noncritical item
  defined, 26
  high-level disinfection of, 601
non-functioning clinical alarm, 247
noninfectious waste, 20, 26
nonwoven material, 653, 661
normothermia, 485–487
no-touch technique, 373, 382
nursing diagnosis, 695–696
  health care information management, 491–492
  local anesthesia, 516
  nursing documentation, 491–492
nursing documentation. *See also* documentation
  of diagnosis, 491–492
  electronic perioperative, 493–494
  of radiation exposure, 340–341
  regulatory compliance requirements for, 494–498
nursing process, 492–494, 764, 768
nursing work flow, 492–494

O

obesity, 574, 578
occupational dose, 338, 342
occupational injury, 240–241
occupational radiological exposure, 336–338
occurrence screens, 764, 768
open assisted gloving, 73, 90
open gloving, 76, 90
operating rooms (ORs)
  design of, 525–529
  digital, 527, 547
  federal regulations on, 525–529
  hybrid, 529, 544, 547
  integrated, 527, 544, 547
  local regulations on, 525–529
  long-term expansion services for, 525–529
  minimally invasive surgery, 525–529
  positioning equipment/devices for, 564–565
  safety of, 525–529
  state regulations on, 525–529
operator for equipment, 342
opioid, 555, 560
optical density, 142, 150
optimal posture, 749
optimal working height, 742, 750
oral rehydration solution, 191, 231
organic material on flexible endoscope, 590–592, 595–596
organizing tray, 657, 661
OSHA Bloodborne Pathogen Standard, 426–427
osmolality, 191–192, 231
osmosis, reverse, 622, 644
osseointegration, 195, 231
osteoblasts, 214–215, 231
osteoclasts, 214–215, 231
osteoconduction, 195, 231
osteocytes, 197, 215, 231
osteoinduction, 195, 231
outcome identification, 703–704, 768
  health care information management, 491–492
overhead air delivery system, 285
oxygen-enriched environment, 125, 134, 146, 150
ozone, 677

P

packaging/package. *See also* packaging systems for sterilization
  autologous tissue management during, 218–220
  chemical indicators for, 655–656
  instructions for use for, 654–655
  integrity of, 661
  labeling of, 658
  manufacturer's instructions, 654–655
  materials for, 652–654
  sterilization guidelines, 669
packaging systems for sterilization
  aseptic technique for, 654–655
  chemical indicators specific to, 655–656
  compatibility of, 653–654
  competency assessment on, 658–659
  continuing education on, 658–659
  evaluation of, 652–653
  evidence review on, 651–652
  inspection of, 656
  instructions for use (IFU) on, 654–658
  labeling of, 658
  peel pouches for, 656–657
  performance improvement process for, 659–661
  policies and procedures on, 659
  processing of, 654
  purpose of, 651
  quality management program for, 659–661
  quality of, 654
  reusable woven, 656
  rigid sterilization container for, 657–58
  selection of, 658–659
  storage of, 654
pads
  for capacitive coupling, 127
  energy transfer, 483, 486
paper-plastic pouch, 653, 656–657, 661
parathyroid tissue, 203–207
par level, 318, 323
passive insulation, 487
pasteurization, 604, 611
pathogens, bloodborne, 382
  from autologous tissue, 218–223
  from sharps, 367–369
  transmissible infection through, 426–427
patient. *See also* specific topics on
  confidentiality for, 220
  environmental cleaning for, 12–14
  health care record of, 493–494 (*See also* patient care record)
  hypnosis of, 462–463
  lifting of, 565–566, 741–742
  metric weight of, 301–302
  moving, 565–566
  patient care information transfer and, 585
  rights of, 717–721
  transporting, 565–566
patient assessment
  health care information management, 491–492
  hypothermia, 485–486
  medication, 301–302
  sedation, 554–556
patient care complementary interventions
  acupressure as, 461
  acupuncture as, 461
  additional, 464–465
  aromatherapy as, 461–462
  evidence review on, 455–456
  hypnosis as, 462–463
  massage therapy as, 460–461
  music as, 456–460
  purpose of, 455
  Reiki therapy as, 463–464
patient care information transfer
  competency assessment on, 585–586
  continuing education on, 585–586
  development of process for, 583–585
  documentation during, 586
  evidence for, 583–585
  family members involvement in, 585
  patients involvement in, 585
  policies and procedures for, 586
  purpose of, 583
  quality management program for, 586–587
  significant others involvement in, 585
  standardization process for, 583–585
patient care record
  accuracy of, 499–500
  addendums in, 499–500
  amendments to, 499–500
  assessment in, 491–492
  confidentiality of, 498–499
  corrections to, 499–500
  diagnosis in, 491–492
  electronic, 493, 503
  evaluation in, 491–492
  interoperable, 493, 504
  modification of, 499–500
  outcome identification in, 491–492
  patient care continuum in, 493–494
  plan of care in, 491–492

security of, 498–499
unauthorized disclosure of, 498–499
patient education
  on local anesthesia, 521–522
  on medication safety, 308–310
peel pouch, 653, 656–657, 661
peer review, 768
perforation indicator system, 74, 90, 375, 382
performance. *See also* performance improvement program
  expectation of, 765, 768
  measurement of, 765, 768
performance improvement program/standards
  autologous tissue management, 228–231
  environmental cleaning, 24–26
  hypothermia, 486
  laser safety, 149–150
  medication safety, 320–323
  minimally invasive surgery, 545–546
  packaging systems for sterilization, 659–661
  pneumatic tourniquet, 170–171
  positioning of patient, 578
  product selection, 184
  quality and, 761–769
  retained surgical items, 358
  sharps safety, 381–382
  sterilization guidelines, 683–689
  transmissible infection, 442–444, 453
perfusion of tissue, 575–576
periodontal ligament (PDL), 189–194, 231
Perioperative Administrative Practice Standards, 703–707
  advocacy, 707
  assessment, 703
  collaboration, 706
  collegiality, 705–706
  consultation, 704
  coordination, 705
  education, 705
  ethics, 706
  evaluation, 704–705
  health promotion, 704
  health teaching, 704
  implementation, 704
  issues/trend identification, 703
  leadership, 707
  outcomes identification, 703–704
  planning, 704
  professional practice evaluation, 705
  quality of practice, 705
  research, 706
  resource utilization, 706–707
perioperative assessment
  deep vein thrombosis, 471
  medication safety, 301–302
  positioning of patient, 564–565
perioperative information systems, 501–503
perioperative medication, 300–301
Perioperative Nursing Practice
  defined, 694–695
  goals for, 694
  role functions in, 695
  scope of, 694–695
  settings of, 695
  span of, 695
Perioperative Nursing Standards, 695–698
  assessment, 695
  consultation, 697–698

coordination of care, 697
diagnosis, 695–696
evaluation, 698
health promotion, 697
health teaching, 697
implementation, 696–697
planning, 696
prescriptive authority, 698
Perioperative Patient Focused Model, 693–694
  conceptual framework of, 693
  domains of, 694
  outcome focused, 694
  patient centered, 694
Perioperative Practice Setting
  chemicals in, 253–255
  cleaning in, 10–12, 16–18
  environmental cleaning in, 10–12, 16–18
  hand hygiene in, 31–33
Perioperative Professional Practice Standards, 698–703
  collaboration, 700–701
  collegiality, 700
  education, 699
  ethics, 701
  leadership, 702–703
  professional practice evaluation, 699–700
  quality of practice, 698–699
  research, 701–702
  resource utilization, 702
perioperative RN, defined, 694
perioperative skin, 49–55
persistence, 34, 40
personal protective equipment (PPE), 382, 445, 599, 611
  defined, 26
  for flexible endoscope, 596
  sharps safety, 374–377
  surgical instruments cleaning and care, 623–624
  transmissible infection, 427–430
pharmacists, 300–301, 330–332
pharmacologic prophylaxis, 473–474
pharmacology, 516–521
physical monitor, 685, 690
physiological response
  to core body temperature, 543
  to local anesthesia, 516
  to minimally invasive surgery, 543
  to pneumatic tourniquet, 170–171
plan of care/planning, 696, 704
  deep vein thrombosis, 469–470
  health care information management, 491–492
  hypothermia, 481, 485–486
  local anesthesia, 516
  medication, 302–303, 332
  pneumatic tourniquet, 158–160
  positioning equipment/devices, 564–565
  specimens management, 391–392
Plasma-Lyte, 211, 232
plasma sterilization, 653, 661
plugs on electrosurgical units, 123
pneumatic tourniquet
  cleansing of components of, 168
  competency assessment on, 168–169
  continuing education on, 168–169
  contraindications related to, 154–158
  cuff for, 162–165

deflation of, 165–168
documentation during, 169–170
evidence review on, 153–154
inflation of, 162–165
manufacturer's written instructions for, 168
monitoring during, 164–165
outcome of, 166–168
performance improvement program for, 170–171
physiologic response to, 170–171
plan of care related to, 158–160
policies and procedures on, 170
postoperative assessment following, 166–168
preoperative assessment for, 154–158
purpose of, 153
quality management program for, 170–171
risks of, 154–158
safety during, 160–162, 170–171
pneumoperitoneum, 540, 547
point-of-care testing, 407, 414
policies and procedures
  autologous tissue management, 226–227
  cleaning, 20–24
  computer-assisted technologies, 545
  deep vein thrombosis, 475
  electrosurgery, 132–133
  environmental cleaning, 20–24
  flexible endoscope, 597–598
  hand hygiene, 36–37
  health care information management, 501–502
  high-level disinfection, 609
  hypothermia, 486
  laser safety, 148
  local anesthesia, 522
  medication safety, 316–320, 333
  minimally invasive surgery, 545
  packaging systems for sterilization, 659
  patient care information transfer, 586
  pneumatic tourniquet, 170
  positioning of patient, 578
  product selection, 184
  for radiological exposure, 341
  retained surgical items, 358–359, 364
  safe environment of care, 257, 264
  sedation, 559
  sharps safety, 380–381
  specimens management, 412
  sterile technique, 88–89
  sterilization guidelines, 682–683
  surgical instruments cleaning and care, 641–642
  transmissible infection, 440–442, 452–453
population, 563–564, 765, 768
porosity detector, 630, 644
portable water, 599
positioning equipment/devices, 579
  design of, 563–564
  inspection of, 565
  for invasive procedures, 564–565
  maintenance of, 565
  manufacturer's instructions for using, 567–568
  for operative procedures, 564–565
  patient care plan for, 564–565
  population and, 563–564
  purchasing, 563–564

research on, 563–564
risks of, 563–564
safety when using, 563–564, 567–568
semi-Fowler, 737, 750
supine, 737–741, 750
transporting, 565
positioning of patient. *See also* positioning equipment
    anesthetist's role in, 568–575
    body alignment following, 575–576
    body mechanics for, 566–567
    competency assessment on, 576–577
    continuing education on, 576–577
    documentation during, 577–578
    Guidance Statement of AORN, 737–741
    hazards with, 567
    injury resulting from, 563–564, 576
    intraoperative, 576
    lateral, 737–739, 749
    lifting and, 566–567
    lithotomy, 739–741, 749
    moving and, 566–567
    performance improvement program for, 578
    perioperative assessment for, 564–565
    policies and procedures on, 578
    precautions when, 565–566
    procedure-specific, 565–566
    prone, 737, 750
    purpose of, 563
    quality management program for, 578
    safety during, 567
    skin integrity following, 575–576
    surgeon's role in, 568–575
    tissue perfusion following, 575–576
    transferring and, 567
    transporting and, 566–567
Position Statements of AORN, 753
postanalytical phase, 389–390, 414
postoperative assessment, 166–168
postoperative monitoring, 482
postoperative patient caregiver, 576
potentially infectious material, 379–380, 382
pounds per force (lbF), 745, 749
powered air-purifying respirator, 429, 445
power failures, 278–279
preadmission, 493–494
preanalytical phase, 414
precautions
    airborne, 424–425, 444
    cleaning, 19–20
    contact, 423, 444
    droplet, 423–424, 445, 452
    environmental cleaning, 19–20
    isolation, 443, 445
    positioning of patient, 565–566
    standard, 26, 382, 445
precleaning of flexible endoscope, 590–591
preconditioning, 171
preoperative assessment, 154–158, 514–516
    for minimally invasive surgery, 531–533
    specimens management, 392–393
preoperative monitoring, 482
prescriptive authority, 698
preservation
    of cranial bone flap, 194–203
    of specimens, 393–401, 408–411, 414
    vein, 210–211
pressure
    capillary interface, 563, 575, 578
    flexible endoscope tests on, 591–592

limb occlusion, 159, 163, 171
static, 750
prevacuuming, 669, 690
prion disease, 20–23, 635–640
problem-prone process, 763, 768
procedures. *See also* specific types of
    bed for, 575, 579
    for cleaning, 10–12
    mask for, 430, 445
    positioning of patient for specific, 565–566
    room for, 275–276, 285
process
    commissioning, 266, 284
    defined, 184, 768
    problem-prone, 763, 768
process challenge device (PCD), 684–686, 690
procurement, 294–298, 330
products. *See also* product selection
    evaluation of, 184
    life of, 656
    quality assurance testing of, 644
    reposable, 181–182, 184
    reusable, 184–185
product selection
    competency assessment on, 183
    development of mechanism for, 179
    documentation during, 184
    multidisciplinary committee for, 179–183
    performance improvement program, 184
    policies and procedures for, 184
    purpose of, 179
    quality management program for, 184
professional advancements, 727–728
professional practice evaluation, 699–700, 705
prolonged standing, 742
prone position, 737, 750
prophylaxis, 472–474
protective eyewear, 142–143
psychological response to local anesthesia, 516
pulsatile lavage, 224–225, 232

Q

qualification testing, 687–688, 690
quality
    data, 502–503
    of packaging systems for sterilization, 654
    performance improvement standards and, 761–769
    of practice, 698–699, 705
    sterile/sterilization, 654
quality assurance testing, 618, 644
quality improvement program
    autologous tissue management, 228–231
    cleaning, 24–26
    deep vein thrombosis, 475
    electrosurgery, 133
    environmental cleaning, 24–26
    flexible endoscope, 598
    hand hygiene, 37–40
    health care information management, 502–503
    high-level disinfection, 609–610

hypothermia, 486
laser safety, 149–150
medication safety, 320–323, 333–334
minimally invasive surgery, 545–546
packaging systems for sterilization, 659–661
patient care information transfer, 586–587
pneumatic tourniquet, 170–171
positioning of patient, 578
product selection, 184
retained surgical items, 358
safe environment of care, 257–258
sedation, 559
sharps safety, 381–382
sterile technique, 89–90
sterilization guidelines, 683–689
surgical instruments cleaning and care, 642–644
transmissible infection, 442–444, 453

R

rad, 342
radiation. *See also* radiological exposure
    background, 398, 414
    gamma, 335, 342
    high area, 342
    ionizing, 335, 342
    scatter, 335–336, 342
    therapeutic, 340
radiation safety officer, 340
radioactivity, 342
radio-frequency identification (RFID), 360, 406, 414
radiographic equipment, 341
radiological exposure
    Ambulatory Supplement, 345
    competency assessment on, 341
    continuing education on, 341
    from diagnostic radionuclides, 339–340, 345
    direct, 340–341
    documentation of, 340–341
    dosimeter for, 340
    indirect, 340–341
    minimization of, 336
    monitor for, 340
    occupational, 336–338
    policies and procedures for, 341
    purpose of, 335–336
    radiological training on, 341
    shielding devices for, 338–339
    from therapeutic radiation, 339–340, 345
    unnecessary, 336
radiological training, 341
radiology, interventional, 525–529
radionuclide, 339–340, 342, 345
radiopaque surgical soft goods, 349–351
razors, 371–374
reagents, 294–298, 330
recommended weight limit, 747, 750
record of health care
    accuracy of, 499–500
    addendums in, 499–500
    amendments to, 499–500
    assessment in, 491–492
    confidentiality of, 498–499
    corrections to, 499–500
    diagnosis in, 491–492

2015 INDEX

evaluation in, 491–492
modification of, 499–500
outcome identification in, 491–492
patient care continuum in, 493–494
plan of care in, 491–492
security of, 498–499
unauthorized disclosure of, 498–499
redistribution, 487
reestablishment of clean environment, 14–16
refurbished electrosurgical units, 121
refurbished surgical instrument, 617–619
regulated medical waste, 20, 26
regulations on building, 525–529
Reiki therapy, 463–464
relationships, 712–715
rem, 338, 342
repaired surgical instrument, 617–619, 629–630
replantation
    of autologous tissue, 217–226
    of cranial bone flap, 194–203
    defined, 232
reposable product, 181–182, 184
reprocessing, 184, 601
research, 701–702, 706
    on positioning equipment/devices, 563–564
resection devices, 535, 547
resource utilization, 702, 706–707
respect, 712–715
respirator, 429, 445
restricted areas, 99–109
resuscitation, 516–521
retained surgical items (RSIs)
    adjunct technologies for, 356–357
    Ambulatory Supplement, 364
    competency assessment on, 357
    continuing education on, 357
    counting discrepancies and, 355–356, 364
    documentation for preventing, 357–358
    instruments as, 353–354
    during invasive procedures, 348–349
    manual count procedures and, 356–357
    miscellaneous items as, 351–353
    multidisciplinary approach for preventing, 348–349
    performance improvement process for, 358
    policies and procedures on, 358–359, 364
    purpose of, 347
    quality management program for, 358
    radiopaque surgical soft goods as, 349–351
    sharps as, 351–353
    standardized methods for, 355–356, 364
    during surgical procedures, 348–349
    unretrieved device fragments as, 354
retention of fluid, 543
retraction, 742–743, 749
retractors, 371–374, 750
retrospective review, 768
return electrode, 134
reusable items, 666
reusable products, 184–185
reusable woven packaging, 656
reusing medical devices, 185
reverse osmosis, 622, 644
revised NIOSH Lifting Equation, 750
rigid sterilization container system, 661
cleaning of, 657–658
inspection of, 657–658
maintenance of, 657–658
manufactures written instructions on, 657–658
packaging systems for sterilization, 657–58
repairing, 657–658
rinse/rinsing
    alcohol, 593
    flexible endoscope, 593
    free-, 610
    isopropyl alcohol, 593
risk assessment
    autologous tissue management, 211–217
    capacitive coupling, 128, 533–534
    computer-assisted technologies, 540–543
    deep vein thrombosis, 471
    electrosurgery, 121
    hypothermia, 479–481
    minimally invasive surgery, 536–539
    pneumatic tourniquet, 154–158
    positioning equipment/devices, 563–564
room
    airborne transmission in, 425
    temperature of, 530–531
root cause analysis, 360, 414, 768
Roswell Park Memorial Institute 1640
    culture medium, 206, 232
rub for hands, 34, 40

S

safe environment of care
    alert alarm failure and, 247
    Ambulatory Supplement, 264
    chemical disinfectants, 607
    chemical usage in perioperative setting, 253–255
    cleaning for, 12–14
    competency assessment on, 256–257
    compressed medical gas cylinders and, 249–250, 264
    contamination prevention and, 271–272
    continuing education on, 256–257
    distraction minimization and, 284–284
    documentation for, 257
    electrical equipment injury and, 246–247
    environmental cleaning for, 12–14
    evidence review on, 239–240, 265
    fire safety and, 242–246
    for high-level disinfection, 607
    for HVAC system, 272–278
    liquid oxygen containers and, 249–250, 264
    multidisciplinary team for, 265–266
    natural rubber latex protocol and, 251–253
    noise minimization and, 283–284
    non-functioning clinical alarm, 247
    occupational injury and, 240–241
    performance improvement process for, 257–258
    policies and procedures for, 257, 264
    for power failures, 278–279
    purpose of, 239, 265
    quality management program for, 257–258
    for structural surfaces, 278
    in surgical suite, 266–271, 279–281
    thermal injury and, 247–248
    waste anesthesia gas and, 250–251
    waste handling and, 255–256
safety. *See also* laser safety; medication safety; safe environment of care; sharps safety
    autologous tissue management, 218–220
    electrosurgery, 121
    electrosurgical units, 121
    fire, 242–246
    operating rooms, 525–529
    pneumatic tourniquet, 160–162, 170–171
    positioning equipment/devices, 563–564, 567–568
    skin antisepsis, 55–60
safety data sheets (SDSs), 60–61
safety-engineered sharps, 369–371
Salvia officinalis, 191, 232
saturated steam under pressure, 669–671
saw blades, 371–374
scalpels, 371–374
scatter radiation, 335–336, 342
schedule for cleaning, 18–19
scissors, 371–374
scope of nursing practice, 553
scrub attire, 112–115. *See also* surgical attire
sealed and unsealed sources, 342
security
    autograft, 220–226
    health care information management and, 498–499
    of health care record, 498–499
sedation
    administration of, 553
    competency assessment on, 557–558
    deep, 559
    discharge criteria following, 557
    documentation during, 558–559
    interdisciplinary collaboration for, 553–554
    medications used during, 555–556
    moderate, 560
    monitoring during, 555–557
    patient assessment prior to, 554–556
    policies and procedures on, 559
    purpose of, 553
    quality assessment program for, 559
    scope of nursing practice for, 553
sedative, 560. *See also* sedation
self-care, 404, 724–726
self-retaining retractor, 750
semicritical item, 599, 601
semi-Fowler position, 737, 750
semi-restricted areas, 99–109
sentinel event, 359–360, 414, 768
sequential wrapping, 655, 661
shallow dose equivalent, 342
sharps. *See also* sharps safety
    containment of, 377–378
    defined, 360, 382
    disposal of, 377–378
    with engineered sharps injury protection, 382
    retained surgical items and, 351–353
    safety-engineered, 369–371

sharps safety. *See also* sharps
   bloodborne pathogens exposure and, 367–369
   continuing education on, 378–379
   documentation for, 379–380
   engineer controls for, 369–371
   evidence review on, 366–367
   injury prevention and, 378
   performance improvement process for, 381–382
   perioperative RN's responsibility for, 378
   personal protective equipment and, 374–377
   policies and procedures for, 380–381
   purpose of, 365–366
   quality assessment program for, 381–382
   work place controls for, 371–374
shearing, 159, 171, 568, 579
shelf life, 654, 661
shielding, 342
   active electrode, 128
   for radiological exposure, 338–339
short-term exposure limits, 690
shower/showering, 45–47
signature
   digital, 499, 503
   digitized inked, 499, 503
   electronic, 503
signature legend, 499, 504
significant others, 585
single-port access laparoscopy, 547
single-use devices, 666
site identification, 392, 414
sit-stand stool, 750
skin. *See also* skin antisepsis
   autotransplantation of, 207–209
   cleansing of, 31–33
   hooks for, 371–374
   integrity of, 575–576
   meshed, 208, 231
   perioperative, 49–55
   preservation of, 207–209
   warming of, 484, 486
skin antisepsis. *See also* antiseptic agent
   antiseptics for, 45–47, 49–60
   bathing and, 45–47
   evidence review on, 43–45
   hair removal and, 47–49
   manufacturer's instructions for, 60–61
   multidisciplinary team for, 49–55
   purpose of, 43
   safety data sheets for, 60–61
   safety during, 55–60
   showering and, 45–47
   soap for, 45–47
smoke, surgical, 130–131, 143–144
soap, 45–47. *See also* antiseptic agents
soft goods, radiopaque surgical, 349–351
soiled surgical instrument, 629–630
solutions
   isotonic, 225, 231
   Krebs-Ringer, 210, 231
   oral rehydration, 191, 231
specimens. *See also* specimens management
   collecting, 392–393, 414
   containers for, 403–408
   containment of, 402–403, 414
   defined, 414
   disposition of, 414
   gross examination of, 412–414
   handling of, 414
   identification of, 392–393, 414
   integrity of, 393–402
   labeling of, 414
   preservation of, 393–401, 408–411, 414
   protecting, 393–401
   transferring, 401–402, 414
   transporting, 411–412, 414
specimens management. *See also* specimen
   containers for, 403–408
   containment for, 402–403
   documentation for, 413–414
   evidence review on, 390–391
   plan of care for, 391–392
   policies and procedures for, 412
   preoperative assessment for, 392–393
   for preservation, 393–401, 408–411
   purpose of, 389–390
   during transfers, 401–402
   during transporting, 411–412
spinal compression, 750
spine loading, 750
sponges, 349–351, 360
squames, 103, 115
standard, 768. *See also* standardized procedures/process
standardized procedures/process
   hand hygiene, 33–34
   patient care information transfer, 583–585
   retained surgical items, 355–356, 364
standard precautions, 26, 382, 420–421, 445
Standards of AORN, 709–710
standing, prolonged, 742
state agreement, 399, 414
state regulations
   chemical disinfectants, 607
   health care information management, 499–500
   medication, 311–312
   operating rooms, 525–529
State-Trait Anxiety Inventory (STAI), 457, 465
static pressure, 750
sterile/sterilization, 90, 307–308, 599. *See also* packaging systems for sterilization; rigid sterilization container system; sterile technique; sterilization guidelines
   chemical indicators for, 655–656
   defined, 599, 611, 690
   event-related, 90
   of flexible endoscope, 592–593
   hydrogen peroxide gas plasma, 653, 661
   hydrogen peroxide vapor, 653, 661, 676
   immediate use steam, 671–673, 690
   monitoring device for process of, 690
   qualities required for, 654
   terminal, 690
   validation studies on, 661
sterile technique. *See also* sterile/sterilization; sterilization guidelines
   for autologous tissue management, 223–226
   competency assessment on, 89–90
   for contamination, 85–87
   continuing education on, 87–88
   defined, 90
   documentation during, 88–89
   donning and, 71–76
   drapes for, 69–71, 76–78
   evidence review on, 67–68
   gloves for, 69–76
   gowns for, 69–76
   during invasive procedures, 68–69, 78–81
   monitoring, 83–85
   policies and procedures for, 88–89
   purpose of, 67
   quality assessment during, 89–90
   during surgical procedures, 78–81
   for transferring items, 81–83
   transmissible infection and, 68–69
sterility maintenance cover, 651, 661
sterilization guidelines. *See also* sterile/sterilization; sterile technique
   cleaning and, 668–669
   competency assessment on, 682
   continuing education on, 682
   in controlled environment, 666–668
   documentation and, 682
   dry-heat, 677–678
   ethylene oxide, 673–675
   evidence review on, 665–666
   formalized program for, 679–680
   for heat-stable items, 669–671, 673–679
   immediate use steam, 671–673
   inspections and, 668–669
   labeling of materials and, 680–681
   liquid chemical, 678–679
   for loaned instruments, 679–680
   low-temperature hydrogen peroxide gas plasma, 675–676
   low-temperature hydrogen peroxide vapor, 676–677
   manufacturer's, 666–668
   for moisture-stable items, 669–671, 673–679
   ozone, 677
   packaging and, 669
   performance improvement process and, 683–689
   policies and procedures for, 682–683
   purpose of, 665
   quality assessment program for, 683–689
   for reusable items, 666
   for saturated steam under pressure, 669–671
   for single-use devices, 666
   transportation and, 681–682
   of US Food and Drug Administration, 666
sterilizer manufacturers, 654–655
storage
   antiseptic agents, 60–61
   autologous tissue, 218–223, 220–223
   chemicals, 294–298
   flexible endoscope, 589–590, 594–595
   medication, 294–298, 330
   packaging systems for sterilization, 654
storage medium, 226, 232
structure, 768
subgaleal space, 201, 232
subungual area, 35, 40
superheating, 654, 661
supine position, 737–741, 750
supplies. *See also* equipment
   procurement of, 294–298, 330
   storage of, 294–298
support technologies, 503
surgeons, 568–575
surgical antiseptic agents, 34–35, 40
surgical attire

defined, 115
disposable, 109–113
for ears, 113–114
evidence review on, 97–99
for facial hair, 113–114
for hair, 113–114
for head, 113–114
laundering of, 109–113
purpose of, 87
in restricted areas, 99–109
in semi-restricted areas, 99–109
surgical hand antisepsis, 34–35
surgical hand hygiene products, 35–36
analysis of, 35–36
effectiveness of, 35–36
requirements for applying, 35–36
user acceptance for, 35–36
surgical hand scrub, 34–35, 90
surgical helmet system, 74–75, 90
surgical instruments. *See also* surgical instrument cleaning and care
contaminated, 620–621, 623–624
decontamination area for, 620–624
decontamination of, 617–619, 624–626
defective, 629–630
evaluation of, 629–630
high-level disinfection of, 617–619
inspection of, 629–630
intraocular ophthalmic, 630–633
loaned, 617–619
new, 617–619
prion disease from, 635–640
refurbished, 617–619
repaired, 617–619, 629–630
soiled, 629–630
transporting, 620–621
surgical instruments cleaning and care. *See also* surgical instrument
containment during, 620–621
continuing education on, 641
in decontamination area, 620–624
documentation of, 640–641
evaluation following, 629–630
evidence review on, 615–616
immediate, 619–620
inspection following, 629–630
instructions for use on, 616–619, 624–629
of laryngoscope blades/handles, 633–635
manufacturer's instructions on, 616–617
personal protective equipment for, 623–624
policies and procedures for, 641–642
purpose of, 615
quality management program for, 642–644
special precautions during, 630–633
US Food and Drug Administration (FDA) approval for, 616–617
water used for, 624
surgical mask, 106–107, 115, 420, 445
surgical procedures
gloves/gloving for, 34–35
retained surgical items for, 348–349
sterile technique, 78–81
surgical scrub agent, antimicrobial, 34–35
surgical smoke, 130–131, 143–144
surgical suite, 266–271, 279–281
suture needles, 371–374

T

tailored health care information, 497, 504
tap water, 593, 599
telepresence, 527, 547
temperature. *See also* core body temperature
ambient, 481, 486
of fluid, 530–531
room, 530–531
terminal cleaning, 16–18, 26
terminal sterile/sterilization, 690
tests/testing
leak, 591–592
point-of-care, 407, 414
qualification, 687–688, 690
quality assurance, 618, 644
textiles, 349–351
therapeutic effect, 308
therapeutic radiation, 340
therapeutic radionuclides, 339–340, 345
thermal high-level disinfection, 604
thermal injury, 247–248
thermistor, 481, 487
thermocouple, 481, 487
thermometer, 481, 487
thermostat, 487
time
cold ischemic, 393–394, 414
dwell, 11, 26
factor of, 343
warm ischemic, 415
TiProtec, 210, 232
tissue. *See also* autologous tissue
bank for, 232
homogenate, 638, 644
parathyroid, 203–207
perfusion of, 575–576
tooth avulsion, 189–194, 231
tooth pulp, 192, 232
total dosage, 516–521
total effective dose equivalent, 342–343
tourniquet cuffs, contoured, 159, 171
towel clips, 371–374
towels, 349–351
toxic anterior segment syndrome (TASS), 630, 644
toxicity, local anesthetic systemic, 518–519, 522
tracking, 218–220
transcribing, 300
transfer of patient care information
competency assessment on, 585–586
continuing education on, 585–586
development of process for, 583–585
documentation during, 586
evidence for, 583–585
family members involvement in, 585
patients involvement in, 585
policies and procedures for, 586
purpose of, 583
quality management program for, 586–587
significant others involvement in, 585
standardization process for, 583–585
transfers/transferring. *See also* transfer of patient care information
autologous tissue management during, 217–218
environmental cleaning following, 14–16
Guidance Statement of AORN, 735–737
lateral, 737, 748–749
of medication, 307–308
positioning of patient for, 567
specimens, 401–402, 414
sterile technique, 81–83
transmissible infections
airborne precaution for, 424–426, 452
Ambulatory Supplement, 452–454
through blood, 426–427
competency assessment on, 436–438, 452
contact precautions for, 421–423
continuing education on, 436–438, 452
through direct contact, 421–423
documentation of, 439–440, 452
droplet precaution for, 423–424, 452
evidence review for, 419–420
health-care acquired, 430–433
health care personnel activity restrictions and, 435–436
immunizations against, 433–435
through indirect contact, 421–423
OSHA Bloodborne Pathogen Standard for, 426–427
performance improvement process for, 442–444, 453
personal protective equipment for reducing, 427–430
policies and procedures for, 440–442, 452–453
purpose of, 419
quality management program for, 442–444, 453
standard precautions for, 420–421
sterile technique and, 68–69
vaccinations against, 433–435
transmissible spongiform encephalopathy (TSEs), 232, 604, 644
transmission. *See also* airborne transmission
iatrogenic, 604, 610
microorganism, 19–20
precautions based on, 445
transporting/transportation
autologous tissue management during, 220
of patient, 565–566
positioning equipment/devices, 565
positioning of patient, 566–567
specimens, 411–412, 414
sterilization guidelines, 681–682
surgical instrument, 620–621
transurethral resection (TUR) syndrome, 541, 547
treated water, 622, 644
treatment area/options
autologous tissue management vs. other, 211–217
laser, 141, 145, 150
for laser, 141
trend identification, 703
trocars, 371–374
tulle gras, 208, 232
Tyvek, 656–657

U

ultra low particulate air (ULPA) filter, 134, 150
ultrasonic cleaner, 644
ultrasonic electrosurgical units, 129

ultrasonic scalpel, 134
unauthorized disclosure, 498–499
unintentional beam exposure, 141–142
US Food and Drug Administration (FDA)
    hand hygiene, 34–35
    high-level disinfection, 604–607
    sterilization guidelines, 666
    surgical antiseptic agents, 34–35
    surgical instruments cleaning and care, 616–617
US Nuclear Regulatory Commission (NRC), 338, 343
unnecessary radiological exposure, 336
unplanned perioperative hypothermia, 479–481, 483–485
unretrieved device fragments, 354
useful life, 185, 661
user
    acceptance of, 35–36
    authorized, 340–342
    laser, 141–142, 150

V

vaccinations, 433–435
validation studies, 644, 661
values, 729–731
vapor sterilization, 653, 661, 676
variant Creutzfeldt-Jakob disease (vCJD), 603, 644
vein autotransplantation, 210–211
vein preservation, 210–211
versioning, 500, 504
vessel occluding devices, 129
vessel sealing device, 134
viscoelastic material, 564, 644
visual analog scale (VAS), 457, 465

W

waived count, 360
warming
    devices for, 485
    fluid, 530–531
    forced-air, 483–484, 486
warm ischemic time, 415
washer, 644
washing hands, 33–34. See also hand hygiene
waste
    characteristic, 256, 258
    medical, regulated, 20, 26
    microorganism transmission and handling, 19–20
    noninfectious, 20, 26
    safe environment of care and handling, 255–256
waste anesthesia gas, 250–251
water
    bottle for, 590, 595
    distilled, 631–633, 644
    intoxication of, 543, 547
    portable, 599
    for surgical instruments cleaning and care, 624
    tap, 593, 599
    treated, 622, 644
    tubing, 595
weight
    metric, 301–302
    recommended limit for, 747, 750
wet packs, 655, 661
white balancing, 538, 547
work
    interruption in, 282, 285
    practice controls at, 371–374, 382
woven textile, 656, 661

X

x-ray, 338–339, 343
X-Vivo 10, 210–211, 232

Stay Current. Network with Peers. Influence Perioperative Practice.

AORN connects perioperative professionals who share a passion for nursing. Together, we have the power to advance perioperative nursing and the dedication to influence optimal outcomes and patient safety every day. Become a member today.

AORN Journal
Award-winning, peer-reviewed

ORNurseLink
Hot topic discussions, networking, peer advice

Nurse Consultation
Answers to your clinical questions

Over 40 Free CEs
Meet your CE requirements

Patient Safety Tool Kits
Implement evidence-based practices

Periop Insider e-newsletter
Stay current with industry news & trends

Free ANA Affiliate membership
Access to ANA online resources

PLUS, exclusive member discounts on CNOR© certification, AORN Surgical Conference & Expo, education programs, AORN publications, and practice tools to help implement AORN Guidelines.

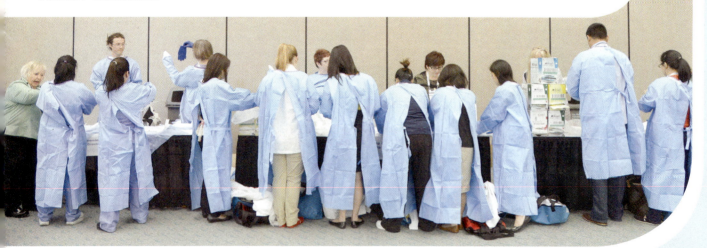

www.aorn.org/membership

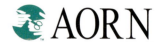

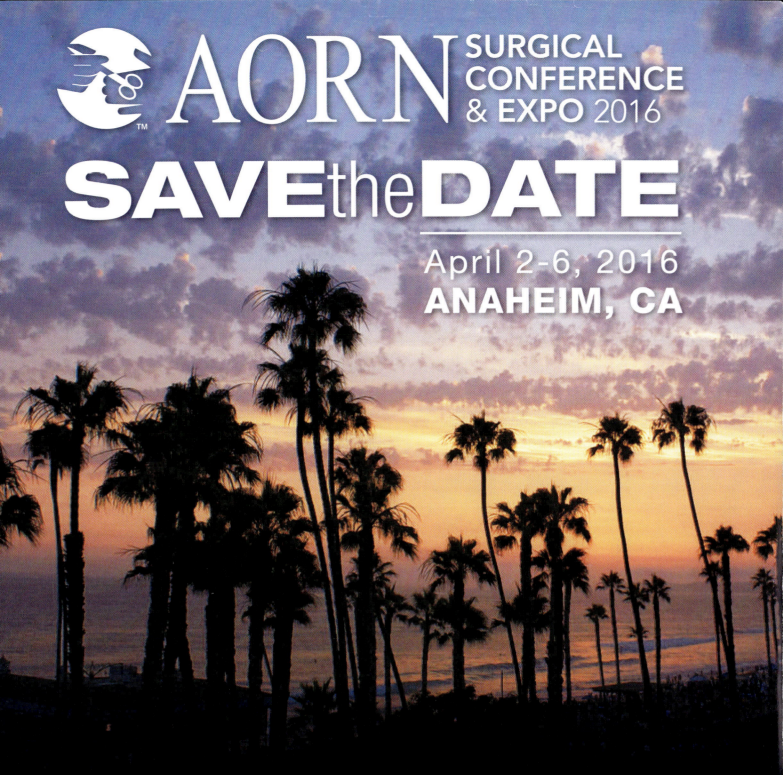

AORN SURGICAL CONFERENCE & EXPO 2016

SAVE the DATE

April 2-6, 2016
ANAHEIM, CA

It's not too early to get ready for next year.

- Reserve your room to get the best hotel
- Submit your paid time off
- Check out Anaheim

www.aorn.org/surgicalexpo

PERIOP 101:
A CORE CORRICULUM™

Experience Periop 101 through a free preview and see first-hand the benefits of this online learning resource

Reduce patient risk through standardized, evidence-based education. Periop 101 is the essential perioperative education program that:

- builds confidence in OR nurses to practice safely
- enables cost savings related to reduced turnover and increases retention
- accessible online, on demand

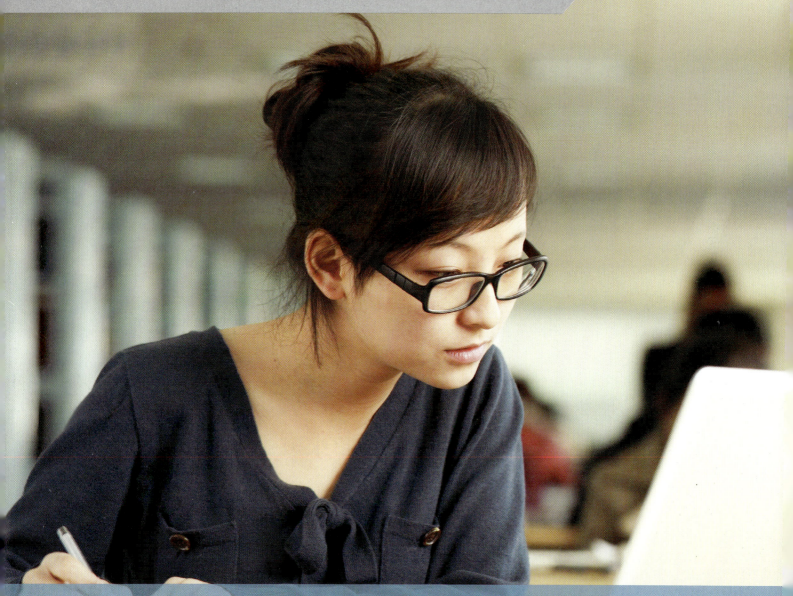

Request the Periop 101 free preview at
aorn.org/Periop101

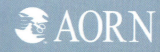